PREMIER EDITION

Nonprescription Drug Reference for Health Professionals

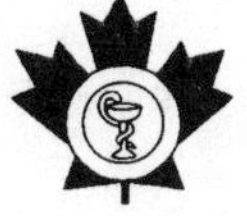

Canadian Pharmaceutical Association

Nonprescription Drug Reference for Health Professionals

PUBLISHED BY
Canadian Pharmaceutical Association
Ottawa, Ontario, Canada

President	Bev Allen, BSP
Executive Director	Leroy Fevang, BScPharm, MBA
Publisher	Leesa D. Bruce

Editor	Patricia Carruthers-Czyzewski, BScPhm, MSc(Pharmacology)
Project Manager	Louise Travill, BSP
Managing Editor	M. Claire Gillis, BSc(Pharm)
Associate Editor	Dianne Letwin

The editors gratefully acknowledge the assistance of Saj Butt, Jane Dewar, Frances Hachborn, Robin McIntosh and Carol Repchinsky.

Published by Canadian Pharmaceutical Association
1785 Alta Vista Drive
Ottawa, Ontario, Canada
K1G 3Y6

Tel. (613) 523-7877, (800) 917-9489
Fax (613) 523-0445

Cover Illustration
Joanne Purich, Purich Design Studio

Interior Format and Design
Brian Berube

Cover Design and Production
Marilyn Birtwistle, Manager, Special Projects, CPhA

Typesetter/Desktop Publisher
Lucienne Prévost, CPhA

Illustrations by *Lianne Friesen*

Index by Editor's Ink

Third printing April 2001

Printed in Canada by Webcom Limited

Canadian Cataloguing in Publication Data
Main entry under title: Nonprescription drug reference for health professionals

Previously publ. under title: Self-medication reference for health professionals.
Includes index. ISBN 0-919115-47-0
1. Self medication. 2. Drugs, Nonprescription.
I. Carruthers-Czyzewski, Patricia A., 1952- II. Gillis,
M. Claire, 1961- III. Canadian Pharmaceutical Association.

RM671.5.C3C35 1996 616.02'4 C96-900712-4

TABLE OF CONTENTS

AUTHORS ____ vii

REVIEWERS ____ ix

FOREWORD ____ xiii

INTRODUCTION ____ xv

Chapters

1 NONPRESCRIPTION DRUGS IN HEALTH CARE ____ 1
John Bachynsky

2 CONSUMER COUNSELLING ____ 13
Brenda J. McBean Cochran

3 SPECIAL PATIENT GROUPS ____ 39
Eileen Yoshida

4 ACNE ____ 57
Debra J. Sibbald

5 ALLERGY AND COLD PRODUCTS ____ 79
Keith J. Simons

6 ANTIPARASITIC AND ANTHELMINTIC PRODUCTS ____ 101
Susan Mansour

7 DERMATITIS, SEBORRHEA, DANDRUFF AND DRY SKIN PRODUCTS ____ 121
Dale E. Wright

8 EAR CARE PRODUCTS ____ 149
Lynn Torsher

9 EYE CARE PRODUCTS ____ 163
Lynn R. Trottier/David S. Wing

10 FIRST AID PRODUCTS ____ 223
Kimberley Rowat White

11 FOOT CARE PRODUCTS ____ 261
Betsy Miller

12 GASTROINTESTINAL PRODUCTS ____ 275
Patrick S. Farmer

13 HEMORRHOIDAL PRODUCTS — 325
Patricia Carruthers-Czyzewski

14 HERBAL PRODUCTS — 335
R. Frank Chandler

15 HOMEOPATHIC PRODUCTS — 361
Heather Boon/Michael Smith/Linda Muzzin

16 MEDICAL DEVICES — 375
Marie Berry

17 MEN'S HEALTH CARE PRODUCTS — 411
Denis Bélanger

18 NUTRITION PRODUCTS — 425
Nadeem Bhanji/Shirley Heschuk

19 ORAL HEALTH CARE PRODUCTS — 489
Linda G. Suveges

20 PAIN AND FEVER PRODUCTS — 531
Yvonne M. Shevchuk/Alfred J. Rémillard

21 PERSONAL HYGIENE PRODUCTS — 567
Deanne P. Wong/Stephanie Edwards

22 SLEEP AIDS AND STIMULANTS — 585
Sandra Naidoo

23 SMOKING CESSATION PRODUCTS — 597
Melanie Rantucci

24 SPORTS MEDICINE PRODUCTS — 613
Lily Lum

25 SUNSCREEN AND TANNING PRODUCTS — 623
Sanna G. Pellatt

26 TRAVEL HEALTH PRODUCTS — 643
Helen Ng

27 WOMEN'S HEALTH CARE PRODUCTS — 655
Laura-Lynn Pollock

REFERENCES — 693

GENERAL INDEX — 755

AUTHORS

John Bachynsky, Ph.D.
Professor of Pharmacy Administration
Faculty of Pharmacy and Pharmaceutical Sciences
University of Alberta
Edmonton, Alberta

Denis Bélanger, B.Sc.Phm.
Drug Information Specialist
Ottawa Valley Regional Drug Information Service
Ottawa General Hospital
Ottawa, Ontario

Marie Berry, B.Sc.(Pharm.), B.A., LL.B.
Vimy Park Pharmacy
Winnipeg, Manitoba

Nadeem Bhanji, B.Sc.(Pharm.)
Pharmacist, University of Alberta Hospital
Heritage Park Pharmacy
Clinical Instructor, Faculty of Pharmacy
University of Alberta
M.D. Student, Faculty of Medicine, University of Alberta
Edmonton, Alberta

Heather Boon, B.Sc.Phm.
Doctoral Candidate
Faculty of Pharmacy
University of Toronto
Toronto, Ontario

Patricia Carruthers-Czyzewski, B.Sc.Phm., M.Sc.(Pharmacology)
Scientific Advisor, Patented Medicine Prices Review Board
Ottawa, Ontario

R. Frank Chandler, B.Sc.Pharm., M.Sc., Ph.D.
Director and Professor
College of Pharmacy
Dalhousie University
Halifax, Nova Scotia

Stephanie Edwards, B.Sc.Pharm.
Drug Information Pharmacist
Ontario College of Pharmacists
Drug Information Service
Toronto, Ontario

Patrick S. Farmer, B.S.P., M.Sc., Ph.D.
Associate Professor
College of Pharmacy
Dalhousie University
Halifax, Nova Scotia

Shirley Heschuk, B.Sc.(Pharm.), M.Sc.(Pharmacology)
Clinical Assistant Professor
Faculty of Pharmacy and Pharmaceutical Sciences
University of Alberta
Edmonton, Alberta

Lily Lum, B.Sc.Pharm.
Drug Information Pharmacist
Ontario College of Pharmacists
Drug Information Service
Toronto, Ontario

Susan Mansour, B.Sc.Pharm., M.B.A.
Assistant Professor
College of Pharmacy
Dalhousie University
Halifax, Nova Scotia

Brenda J. McBean Cochran, B.Sc.Pharm., M.Sc.Pharm.
Consumer Health Education Consultant
President
BMC Health Associates Limited/Practical Touch Publications Incorporated
Halifax, Nova Scotia

Betsy Miller, B.Sc.Pharm.
Janssen-Ortho Inc.
Faculty of Pharmacy
University of Toronto
Toronto, Ontario

Linda Muzzin, Ph.D.
Associate Professor
Faculty of Pharmacy
University of Toronto
Toronto, Ontario

Sandra Naidoo, B.Sc.Phm.
Faculty of Pharmacy
University of Port Elizabeth
Port Elizabeth, Republic of South Africa

Helen Ng, B.Sc.Phm.
Drug Information Pharmacist
Ontario College of Pharmacists
Drug Information Service
Toronto, Ontario

Sanna G. Pellatt, B.Sc.(Pharm.)
British Columbia Cancer Agency
Vancouver Island Cancer Centre
Victoria, British Columbia

Laura-Lynn Pollock, B.Sc.(Pharm.)
Clinical Pharmacist Consultant
Victoria, British Columbia

Melanie Rantucci, M.Sc.Phm., Ph.D.
Pharmacist/Consultant
MJR Pharmacy Communications
Mississauga, Ontario

Alfred J. Rémillard, B.Sc., B.Sc.(Pharm.), Pharm.D.
Professor of Pharmacy
College of Pharmacy and Nutrition
University of Saskatchewan
Saskatoon, Saskatchewan

Kimberley Rowat White, B.Sc.(Pharm.)
Clinical Pharmacist
Victoria General Hospital
Victoria, British Columbia

Yvonne M. Shevchuk, B.S.P., Pharm.D.
Associate Professor of Pharmacy
College of Pharmacy and Nutrition
University of Saskatchewan
Saskatoon, Saskatchewan

Debra J. Sibbald, B.Sc.Phm.
Coordinator, Pharmaceutical Care I
Faculty of Pharmacy, University of Toronto
President, Debary Dermatologicals
Staff Pharmacist, Mississauga Hospital
Mississauga, Ontario

Keith J. Simons, B.Sc.(Pharm.), M.Sc., Ph.D.
Professor and Head
Division of Pharmaceutical Sciences
Faculty of Pharmacy
University of Manitoba
Winnipeg, Manitoba

Michael Smith, B.Pharm., Hons., N.D.
Pharmacist/Licensed Naturopath
Director of Clinical Services
Hooper's Pharmacy
Toronto, Ontario

Linda G. Suveges, B.S.P., M.Sc., Ph.D.
Professor of Pharmacy
College of Pharmacy and Nutrition
University of Saskatchewan
Saskatoon, Saskatchewan

Lynn Torsher, B.Sc.Pharm.
Staff Pharmacist
Mayo Medical Center
Rochester, Minnesota

Lynn R. Trottier, B.Sc.(Pharm.)
Clinical Pharmacist, Vancouver Hospital and Health Sciences Centre, UBC Site
Clinical Instructor, Faculty of Pharmaceutical Sciences
University of British Columbia
Adjunct Professor, Gerontology Program
Simon Fraser University
Vancouver, British Columbia

David S. Wing, B.S.P., M.S.
Consultant Pharmacist
Calgary, Alberta

Deanne P. Wong, B.Sc.Phm.
Drug Information Pharmacist
Ontario College of Pharmacists
Drug Information Service
Toronto, Ontario

Dale E. Wright, B.S.P., M.Sc.(Pharmacol.)
Consultant Pharmacist
Calgary, Alberta

Eileen Yoshida, B.Sc.Phm.
University of Chicago Hospitals
Chicago, Illinois

REVIEWERS

Susan Ablen
North York, Ont.

Peter Alberti
Toronto, Ont.

Dean Ast
Regina, Sask.

Sylvia Baran
Red Deer, Alta.

William Bartle
North York, Ont.

Ken Bayerlin
Markham, Ont.

David Beaudin
Saint John, N.B.

Françoise Becquey
Markham, Ont.

Marty Belitz
Toronto, Ont.

Colline Blanchard
Ottawa, Ont.

Teresa Bosse
Edmonton, Alta.

Ann Boucher
Nepean, Ont.

Pierre Boucher
Pierrefonds, P.Q.

Ken Boughton
Don Mills, Ont.

Janet Bradshaw
Dysart, Sask.

Colin J. Briggs
Winnipeg, Man.

Debra Buffum
Red Deer, Alta.

Mary Carman
Ottawa, Ont.

Siu C. Chan
Calgary, Alta.

Suzanne Chatterjee
Weston, Ont.

Praveen Chawla
North York, Ont.

John Collins
Mississauga, Ont.

Morna Cook
Winnipeg, Man.

Garry Cruickshank
London, Ont.

Peter Cummins
Guelph, Ont.

Doug Danforth
Coquitlam, B.C.

Lisa Dare
Calgary, Alta.

Diana deRond
Nepean, Ont.

John Derry
Mississauga, Ont.

Michael Doughtey
Glasgow, Scotland

Mervin Dusyk
Red Deer, Alta.

Pauline Dusyk
Red Deer, Alta.

Paul Duval
Mississauga, Ont.

Ron Elliott
St. Thomas, Ont.

Hugh Ellis
Moncton, N.B.

Susanne Essensa
Summerside, P.E.I.

Greg Etue
Ottawa, Ont.

Leo Fleming
Ottawa, Ont.

Desmond Fonn
Waterloo, Ont.

Walter Forgiel
Mississauga, Ont.

Dawn M. Frail
Halifax, N.S.

Marilyn Gaw
Mississauga, Ont.

Rick Gazzola
Fort Erie, Ont.

Alan Gervais
Ottawa, Ont.

Jane Gloor
London, Ont.

Ruby Grymonpre
Winnipeg, Man.

Lyn Guenther
London, Ont.

Dan Haas
Toronto, Ont.

Geoff Hadrill
Mississauga, Ont.

Leanne Harris
Smiths Falls, Ont.

F.P. Haugen
Duncan, B.C.

Linda Hensman
St. John's, Nfld.

Maryann Hopkins
Nepean, Ont.

Lawrence Hough
Don Mills, Ont.

James R. Hull
North York, Ont.

Danica Irwin
Ottawa, Ont.

Michelle Jacob
Mississauga, Ont.

Reta Johnson
Prince George, B.C.

Doris Kalamut
Toronto, Ont.

Sarah Kemp
Montreal, P.Q.

Peter Kertes
Ottawa, Ont.

David Knoppert
London, Ont.

Marian Kremers
Winnipeg, Man.

Brenda Kuzyk
Edmonton, Alta.

Lise Lafoley
Ottawa, Ont.

Diane Lamarre
Longueuil, P.Q.

Claudette Landry
Moncton, N.B.

Rebecca M. Law
St. John's, Nfld.

Daniel Lebouef
Disraeli, P.Q.

Ruth N.F. Lee
Toronto, Ont.

Helen Leeds
Winnipeg, Man.

Joel Lexchin
Toronto, Ont.

Susan Lovell
London, Ont.

Barb Marriage
Edmonton, Alta.

Louise Matte
Cap-Rouge, P.Q.

Christiane Mayer
St. Leonard, P.Q.

Susan McFaul
Ottawa, Ont.

Claudia McKeen
Ottawa, Ont.

Grace Meehan
Manotick, Ont.

John Meehan
Mississauga, Ont.

Brian Meloche
Ottawa, Ont.

Ivy Michel
Ottawa, Ont.

Penny Miller
Vancouver, B.C.

Stephen Molnar
London, Ont.

Alexander H. Murray
Halifax, N.S.

Bob Nakagawa
Coquitlam, B.C.

Linda Nemerofsky
Kirkland, P.Q.

John O'Mullane
Weston, Ont.

K. Orr
Mississauga, Ont.

Julie Palmer-Redl
Yorkton, Sask.

Gillian Panini
Montreal, P.Q.

David Pao
Agincourt, Ont.

William Parker
Timberlea, N.S.

Jennifer Peddlesden
Chestermere, Alta.

Anita Pedvis Leftick
Vanier, Ont.

Peter Peko
Toronto, Ont.

David Pellow
Walkerton, Ont.

Stephen Pennisi
White Plains, N. Y.

Susan Pierce
Halifax, N.S.

T. Pierscianowski
Ottawa, Ont.

Edward Pollock
Mississauga, Ont.

Virginia Pora
Ottawa, Ont.

Jeff Poston
Ottawa, Ont.

Grazia Prochazka
Winnipeg, Man.

Ken Redl
Yorkton, Sask.

David Reichert
Markham, Ont.

Gordon Riddle
Orleans, Ont.

Michael Roberts
Nepean, Ont.

Huguette Roy
Pickering, Ont.

Glenwood H. Schoepp
Victoria, B.C.

Neil Shear
North York, Ont.

Debra J. Sibbald
Mississauga, Ont.

Solange Simard
Montreal, P.Q.

Brenda Simec
Mississauga, Ont.

Don Skeffington
Mississauga, Ont.

David Skinner
Ottawa, Ont.

Joanne Smith
Toronto, Ont.

Simon Soucy
Ville St. Laurent, P.Q.

Carolyn Stang
Edmonton, Alta.

Roy Steeves
Rothsay, N.B.

Ernest Stefanson
Gimli, Man.

Alison Stephen
Saskatoon, Sask.

Philloza Suleman
Scarborough, Ont.

Jim Swann
Guelph, Ont.

Jack E. Taunton
Vancouver, B.C.

Caryll Tawse
Halifax, N.S.

Patti Taylor
Kensington, P.E.I.

Michael G. Tierney
Ottawa, Ont.

T.A. Toriglia
Parksville, B.C.

Nghia Truong
Ottawa, Ont.

Leanne Wagner
Weston, Ont.

Linda Wein
Toronto, Ont.

Barbara Wells
Toronto, Ont.

Anne Marie Whelan
Halifax, N.S.

Bill Whiteside
Mississauga, Ont.

Norma Wildeman
Regina, Sask.

Joanne Willoughby
Guelph, Ont.

Mark Wise
Thornhill, Ont.

Irene Worthington
North York, Ont.

Barbara Young
Mississauga, Ont.

Joanne Zevenhuizen
Halifax, N.S.

Foreword

Given all of the changes taking place in health care, it is fitting that this volume has been completely revamped. Originally known as *Self-Medication Reference for Health Professionals*, this reference work first became available in 1980. At that time, few of its readers would have understood the importance of the subject matter to Canada's health care system the way we do today.

Professor John Bachynsky's introductory chapter on the role of nonprescription drugs in health care sums up well all the factors that have contributed to the increasing importance of self-medication: the more health conscious and self-driven consumer, the economic need for reducing health care costs, the increasing number of Rx to OTC switches and the greater availability of pharmacist counselling. It is the critical importance of this last factor that makes this volume so important.

As a result of patients becoming more autonomous and taking on the role of "consumers" of health services, the fundamental relationship between patients and health professionals is changing rapidly from one that is prescriptive to one that is consultative. Opportunities abound for the health professionals who are willing to share their knowledge with these information-hungry consumers and help them to make the health care choice that is right for them.

Patient education comes from many sources: the pharmacist who counsels on prescription and nonprescription drug use; the physician or nurse who gives self-care advice to patients presenting with minor or self-manageable illnesses; and public information materials that help patients make responsible self-care choices. The true value of this volume is its ability to bring consistency to these various sources. Whether in the hands of pharmacists, physicians, nurses or consumers themselves (in the case of the patient information summaries contained in another CPhA publication, *Compendium of Nonprescription Products*), the information in the reference text is equally valuable toward ensuring responsible self-medication. The Nonprescription Drug Manufacturers Association of Canada is committed to using the information in this reference text as the "gold standard" upon which all of the Association's patient education efforts will be based.

We congratulate the Canadian Pharmaceutical Association for this important contribution to cost-effective health care.

David S. Skinner
President
Nonprescription Drug Manufacturers Association of Canada

Introduction

Since 1980, the Canadian Pharmaceutical Association (CPhA) has published *Self-Medication* as the main reference textbook on nonprescription drugs for pharmacy students and pharmacists in practice. Since then, the contents of the book have evolved over four subsequent editions and have seen important enhancements to the scope and depth of its information. When it was time to research the next edition, focus groups were conducted. It was identified that, although pharmacists are the main source of information for other health care professionals and consumers on nonprescription drugs, there is an emerging need for these professionals to have access to reliable and authoritative information on nonprescription drugs. This is a result of increased demand from consumers seeking this information from a variety of sources. On the basis of this research, it was recognized that the traditional format of *Self-Medication* could no longer meet this need. This provided an opportunity to review the scope of the publication and to redesign it to meet the information needs of a broader group of users. The one element that has not changed is that the authors of all the chapters are pharmacists, as was the case for *Self-Medication.* To ensure that the needs of this broader group of users were met, an exhaustive review process was elaborated and included practitioners from a variety of settings including other pharmacists, nurses, physicians, and scientists and representatives from the pharmaceutical industry. It has truly been a team effort.

This team effort required a vision and a willingness on the part of the Canadian Pharmaceutical Association to change its approach to meet the needs of pharmacy students and pharmacist members at the practice level while reaching out to other health care professionals seeking this information. Carmen Krogh provided the seed for this vision, and the CPhA Board of Directors provided the support to move in this new direction. To translate this vision into a deliverable required the expertise of a skilled project manager to work with a team of 32 authors and over 100 reviewers in defining a unified focus for the book. I personally wish to thank Louise Travill of Travill Consulting for undertaking this huge task, for bringing her creative ideas to the enhancement of this publication and for persevering through the ups and downs of the project. I believe that she, as a practising pharmacist, brought a unique focus to the book and a greater understanding of the information needs of colleagues and other health care professionals.

The resulting book is a reflection of the pharmacist's unique knowledge of nonprescription drugs and provides a mechanism for sharing this expertise with other health care professionals. To obtain information on specific nonprescription products, the reader is referred to the *Compendium of Nonprescription Products*, also a publication of the Canadian Pharmaceutical Association.

Patricia Carruthers-Czyzewski
Editor

1

NONPRESCRIPTION DRUGS IN HEALTH CARE

JOHN BACHYNSKY

CONTENTS

Introduction 1

Nonprescription Drug Therapy 2
- Terminology
- Self-treatment
- Appropriate Use
- Economics

Regulations 5
- Regulatory Process
- Drug Schedules—Conditions of Sale

Changes Influencing Nonprescription Drugs 7
- Consumers
- Patient Education—Knowledge
- Professional Issues
- Industry Issues
- Switch from Prescription to Nonprescription Status

Conclusion 10

Recommended Reading 11

INTRODUCTION

A nonprescription drug has been defined as a product the average consumer can use to treat minor, self-limiting illnesses without the intervention of a health professional.

Though nonprescription drugs are used by 90% of the population, they rarely come to mind when health care and costs are discussed. Their wide distribution seems to blur their role as an important component of the system.

The variety of products available makes the limits of the category difficult to establish. They blend into other common groups that are not clearly health care related. For example, the category includes dandruff shampoo but not ordinary shampoo, medicated soap but not ordinary soap, dressings with anti-infectives but not ordinary wound dressings.

The size of the market is equally difficult to estimate. The Health Information Division of Health Canada has estimated the 1993 nonprescription drug market at $2.5 billion, less than half the estimated $5.9 billion spent on prescription drugs.

Our current definition of health emphasizes the maintenance or restoration of the ability to function. Health maintenance behavior is a complex area of human response that is not well understood and changes over time. A wide range of health problems and an equally wide range of responses are based on an individual's life experiences and beliefs. This includes many ordinary actions not thought of as specific health activities, such as washing our hands or hair. The range extends through to professional health care procedures. In the same way, many nonprescription drugs, such as vitamins, skin creams and anticaries products, are routinely used to preserve or maintain health when there is no apparent problem or symptom.

As health care has grown and become more effective, scientific and complex, so has the nonprescription drug component. A recent revision of procedures at the Health Protection Branch of Health Canada allows it to deal more effectively with nonprescription drug issues. There has also been a coordinated attempt by the profession of pharmacy to achieve a more uniform system of control in Canada.

The goal is to make safe and effective products widely available. There are now many new, effective products coming on the nonprescription drug market. Some of them are in new therapeutic categories and require patient education to ensure safe use. This poses a challenge to the regulatory agencies.

NONPRESCRIPTION DRUG THERAPY

TERMINOLOGY

Over the years, the terms used in the sale of nonprescription drugs have changed. Historically, the products promoted to the public were known as **proprietary** or **patent medicines**. They were extensively advertised to the public and were a major force in the growth of advertising at the turn of the century. The composition of the products was secret, and they were sold through a variety of retail outlets. In Canada, manufacturers selling them were represented by an organization known as the Proprietary Association of Canada.

The products and promotion methods have also changed. Manufacturers now are more likely to be divisions of major prescription manufacturers and have a more scientific orientation. They are now represented by the Nonprescription Drug Manufacturers Association of Canada (NDMAC).

Another group, known as **ethical OTC products**, was promoted to pharmacists and physicians for recommendation to their patients: ethical, because they were promoted to the health professions and OTC because they could be sold "over the counter," without a prescription.

The two groups have been integrated as the companies adapted to new regulatory requirements. In Canada, they are increasingly referred to as nonprescription drugs. In the United States, the term OTC continues to dominate, although the U.S. organization representing the manufacturers has also taken the name of Nonprescription Drug Manufacturers to replace Proprietary Association.

SELF-TREATMENT

A comprehensive survey of consumer use and attitudes to nonprescription drugs was sponsored by the NDMAC and conducted by Canadian Facts in 1991. This survey showed the most common ailments among Canadians and their response (Tables 1 and 2).

In Table 2, the use of nonprescription medication is the most common method of responding to ailments. The high rate of consultation with physicians and pharmacists, the frequent use of other forms of therapy and the number of instances where no action is taken emphasize the overlap between various patient responses.

In another community survey, 40% of the sample reported that laypersons understand their state of health better than most doctors. A similar percentage stated that some home remedies are still better than prescribed drugs.

APPROPRIATE USE

Safety Issues

The public is aware of the risk from nonprescription drugs. With increasing media reporting of adverse reactions and the perception that "chemical drugs" are more dangerous than natural products there may be more sensitivity by consumers to the potential threat of nonprescription drugs. It should be noted that public perception of safety and intrinsic safety do not always equate.

The elderly, who are likely to be taking prescription drugs that may interact with nonprescription drugs, are, for physiological reasons, more prone than younger people to side effects. In addition, the drugs they are inclined to use (e.g., analgesics and hypnotics) are those most likely to result in harm.

The high rate of nonprescription drug use by children has caused concern. In one recent study it was reported that during the 30 days preceding the study, 53.7% of all 3-year-old children had been given a nonprescription drug. In 70% of recent child illnesses, some nonprescription drug had been used.

Drug Interactions

The use of nonprescription drugs by people being treated with prescription drugs poses a serious and growing problem. More work needs to be done on the significance of the interactions between nonprescription and prescription drugs, as well as with alcohol. Patients must be made aware that their nonprescription drugs should also be recorded on their medication profile. Both industry and the profession of pharmacy should vigorously promote this.

In the marketing of a product, health professionals are concerned with the context of drug use. Is it to be used in conjunction with prescription drugs and what is the potential outcome? Is it likely to be used with alcohol and are there problems associated with this use? Will elderly or debilitated patients with reduced organ function be able to use this drug safely at the recommended dosage levels? Will the product be safe when used by nursing mothers? Can the directions for use be adequately conveyed to people who are visually impaired? Do the users of the product have enough knowledge of the disease state and forms of therapy available to make an informed choice? Looking at these questions, one is faced with the kind of scientific evidence required for deciding to give a drug nonprescription status. The submissions to a regulatory agency do not contain unequivocal answers on the safety and effectiveness of the product. The benefits to individuals and the population at large are balanced against the potential for harm and misuse.

There is widespread knowledge that nonprescription drugs and alcohol do interact, but there is little information available to patients when they purchase the nonprescription drug unless they are prepared to take the time to discuss it with the pharmacist. This is not being done in most cases.

ECONOMICS

The current economic environment has changed the emphasis from hospital and medical care to self-treatment, community services and prevention of disease. In response, the number of services, both conventional (nonprescription drugs) and alternative (health foods, herbal remedies) has increased.

As the use of these services substitutes for insured health care, there is a potential saving for the health care system. In the Canadian Facts survey, 60% of the respondents agreed and only 17% disagreed with the statement, "Using nonprescription medications whenever possible reduces costs to our health care system." Similarly, 71% agreed with the statement, "The availability of nonprescription drugs helps avoid the cost of a doctor or hospital visit."

TABLE 1: Ailments From Which Canadians Suffer

	Percent of Canadian Adults (n = 1860)		
Ailments/Conditions	**Past Year**	**Past 6 Months**	**Frequently**
Colds	60	41	8
Headache/migraine	40	34	15
Muscle aches and pains	40	34	19
Upset stomach	29	22	9
Allergies	22	19	11
Eye irritation/redness	16	14	6
Skin irritation/rashes	15	11	6
Irregularity	11	9	4
Hemorrhoids	9	6	3
Foot odor	8	6	3
Fungal foot infections	5	4	1
None	12	20	45

Reprinted with permission from: Consumer usage and attitude study vol. 1—report. Ottawa: Nonprescription Drug Manufacturers Association of Canada, 1991.

TABLE 2: Usual Practice to Deal with Ailments/Conditions

Ailments/Conditions	Number of Adults	Percent of Canadian Adults				
		Consult with Doctor	Consult with Pharmacist	Use Nonprescription Drugs	Use Other Form of Treatment	Take No Action
Colds	(1119)	21	17	72	14	16
Headache/migraine	(749)	22	10	81	10	10
Muscle aches and pains	(737)	39	8	43	20	30
Upset stomach	(543)	28	9	55	12	27
Allergies	(417)	45	22	55	17	17
Eye irritation/redness	(300)	36	13	37	16	30
Skin irritation/rashes	(277)	57	15	32	34	20
Irregularity	(206)	37	15	46	26	28
Hemorrhoids	(160)	36	11	53	15	29
Foot odor	(143)	3	5	46	10	46
Fungal foot infections	(85)*	35	17	52	22	19

*Figures percentaged on a base of less than 100 should be interpreted with caution.

Reprinted with permission from: Consumer usage and attitude study vol. 1—report. Ottawa: Nonprescription Drug Manufacturers Association of Canada, 1991.

REGULATIONS

REGULATORY PROCESS

The Food and Drugs Act and Regulations is the legislation that deals with nonprescription drugs. Within the Health Protection Branch of Health Canada, the Bureau of Pharmaceutical Assessment administers these regulations. The products may be assigned a Drug Identification Number (DIN) or a General Public (GP) number.

The regulatory process for both prescription and nonprescription products has been undergoing significant change that will likely continue. Gradually, it has become more open to the public and more reliant on advisory groups. The Health Protection Branch, which is overburdened with drug submissions, is committed to a major regulatory reorganization based on the Gagnon report, *Working in Partnerships...Drug Review for the Future.*

Manufacturers planning to switch a prescription drug to nonprescription status are sensitive to the regulatory delays in getting the product to market. A combination of factors serve as a disincentive: the high cost of initial promotion, the slowness of regulatory clearance, and the provincial regulations that require the products to be placed in a non-public access area in pharmacies, which often results in lower sales.

Internally, the Health Protection Branch is organizing itself to handle nonprescription drugs more effectively. There is an increasing emphasis on postmarketing surveillance and it is likely that some form of postmarketing surveillance for nonprescription products will be established in the near future. Overall, the concern with safety remains strong, and though the agency bases its decisions on scientific proof of toxicity, it is also sensitive to perceptions of toxicity, which may influence decisions in the future.

Policies at the Food and Drug Administration in the United States will increasingly influence the direction taken by the Health Protection Branch. Free trade and a movement to make regulations more uniform between the two countries is beginning to have a greater effect on drug control policies.

DRUG SCHEDULES—CONDITIONS OF SALE

Federal legislation regulates conditions of sale for nonprescription drugs. Provincial Pharmacy Acts may further specify the conditions of sale. Not all provinces provide this additional level of control, thus creating disharmony in drug scheduling.

The Canadian Drug Advisory Committee, a group of drug experts mandated to make recommendations to provincial regulators about drug scheduling, published a final report in May 1995 *(Final Recommendations for National Drug Schedules)* that advocates a harmonized four-part drug schedule structure across Canada. This report and its recommendations, a central expert advisory committee, and corresponding principles of practice for pharmacists in the distribution of schedule drugs have been approved by provincial regulators for implementation in each province.

The harmonized drug schedule model for implementation across Canada consists of four schedules:

- I Prescription;
- II Pharmacist monitored, no public access;
- III Pharmacy-only sale; and
- IV Sale in any retail outlet.

The central advisory committee was formed in August 1995 and is called the National Drug Scheduling Advisory Committee. This committee will advise the federal government and provincial regulators as to which schedule a nonprescription drug should be assigned.

Currently, schedules to pharmacy legislation have the same categories of control, but they are not used in all of the provinces and they are not applied consistently from province to province.

Nonprescription, Pharmacist Monitored

These products are sold by a pharmacist and are not directly accessible to the public.

There appears to be general agreement by governments, pharmacists and industry that this is an acceptable and reasonable approach. However, it applies to only a small number of products that are complex to use or are potentially risky.

How do customers know the products are available? Will they be advertised to the public? Will the public ask pharmacists for the products? These key questions will force the pharmaceutical system to adapt to the needs of the public for the products while maintaining some level of control. Optimal use would be based on patients asking pharmacists about symptoms they were not certain about treating. This approach restricts the availability and sales of products but balances access with public safety.

Pharmacy-Only Products

Currently, this classification is used because of the relative risk posed by drugs in this schedule. It is accepted and will continue to be an important channel of distribution in Canada. Drugs in this category are deemed to be sufficiently safe to be distributed without direct involvement by the physician or pharmacist, and available through public self-selection, but there still exists sufficient risk to warrant a pharmacist's availability for advice.

Sale in Any Retail Outlet

There are many drugs outside this schedule that are now available through grocery stores and other retail outlets, and this will continue even with drug schedule harmonization.

These products have demonstrated their safety, and the public is familiar with their use.

Two major criticisms are that there is no more counselling in pharmacies than in any other outlet and that prices will be higher in the pharmacies if sales are restricted only to pharmacies. In reply, pharmacists point to the trend to more counselling on nonprescription drug use and a growing awareness by patients that counselling is available. There is vigorous competition among pharmacies, and the price levels are unlikely to be significantly different if other outlets distributed the products.

It cannot be assumed that products will be more readily available to the public if they are not restricted to pharmacies. This is because grocers and other retailers only stock very high-turnover drug products. Pharmacies are accessible to most of the population by virtue of their locations and extended hours.

Some opposition may flow from the United States where there is no such category, although the pharmacy organizations there have been pressing for a "third class" of drugs for some time. To have products readily available while ensuring that information is available for their safe use, the system should meet future needs rather than review what has been done in the past. In this regard, the experience in the United States is not particularly useful.

CHANGES INFLUENCING NONPRESCRIPTION DRUGS

Publicly funded health care in Canada is undergoing rapid, major change, driven by financial constraint. The changes being made reflect a shift from institutional to ambulatory care, which gives more emphasis to self-care and the use of pharmaceuticals, both prescribed and nonprescribed. With a perception of difficult access to traditional care along with the promotion of other forms of care, the public now seems to be more open to alternative approaches.

The boutique health care system (shops that sell weight loss diets, specialized foot care, specialized eye products and nutritional health products, and individuals who sell health-related services, such as psychological counselling, transcendental meditation, naturopathy and massage) has developed into the major competition for nonprescription drugs.

Current health care planning emphasizes public expenditures but excludes some prescription drugs and most nonprescription drugs from public-funded drug plans. Representation of the role of nonprescription drugs at professional and institutional health care meetings would bring a greater recognition that the use of these drugs is an important component of health care.

CONSUMERS

The general population has shown an enormous interest in health subjects and health maintenance, and a number of publications have emerged to meet the demand for information. While there is a great deal more knowledge, it is likely the amount of misinformation is also growing, posing the question of the public's understanding of self-treatment.

The public has demonstrated a willingness to spend money on health care and on maintaining physical well-being, particularly to improve physical performance and reduce fat.

That there will be a decrease in prescription drug benefits and more copayment in the future, is now clear. The amount paid in copayments will likely be similar to the amount patients pay for nonprescription drugs. When equal payment levels for prescription and nonprescription medication is added to other factors, such as difficulty in seeing physicians and the need to control costs, there may be an increase in the use of some nonprescription drug products.

It is difficult to know if there is widespread concern in the population with the safety of nonprescription drugs. A survey of the public by Decima Research, sponsored by the Department of National Health and Welfare in 1990, showed that people generally regarded both prescription and nonprescription drugs with caution.

PATIENT EDUCATION—KNOWLEDGE

There is a need for public instruction on the use of nonprescription drugs. This is different from product information, which is now available but gives only instructions for use rather than details on the use of the products in treating a symptom or problem. To date, much of the information on a product comes from advertising and product labels. This is seen to be inadequate.

Sixty-four percent of pharmacists questioned on the adequacy of label information disagreed with the statement, "Package labels help people make responsible choices when buying nonprescription drugs," according to a survey of community pharmacists in 1992 by ABM Research Ltd. The majority did agree with the statement, "Cautions and warnings on nonprescription drugs are often ignored."

Some information on nonprescription drug use has been in pamphlet form with uneven distribution and uncertain acceptance. Audiotapes, videotapes, community and school presentations, public health clinic programs, television public service programs and presentations by the health professions could all be used. Some companies have been actively involved in innovative approaches.

Consumers request information on nonprescription products as shown in Table 3 (listed by frequency of response by pharmacists).

Some issues that might be included in an educational campaign, in addition to the specific aspects of various products, are comprehension of the label and the meaning of various words, auxiliary information that is available when products are used, the dose to be used for infants, sources of information for the visually impaired and interactions with substances such as alcohol.

TABLE 3: Nonprescription Drug Information Requests by Category

Category	%	Category	%
Cold remedy	77%	Laxative	14%
Cough remedy	64.2%	Sunscreen product	10.5%
Antihistamine	26.1%	Head lice	7.8%
Multivitamin	17.9%	Blood glucose monitor	6.2%
Headache remedy	15.6%	Contact lens soaking solution	6.2%
Antacid	15.6%	Pregnancy test	1.6%
Diarrhea remedy	15.6%		

Reprinted with permission from: A survey of drugstore trends. Toronto: Drug Merchandising and Le Pharmacien, 1992.

PROFESSIONAL ISSUES

Nonprescription drugs account for about 25% of pharmacy sales. More than 75% of all nonprescription drug sales in Canada are through pharmacies, compared to about 50% in the United States. In the 1988 Upjohn Canadian Pharmacy Services Study, the purpose given by 23% of respondents for their last visit to a pharmacy was to buy nonprescription drugs. For economic reasons pharmacists have a strong vested interest in maintaining nonprescription drug sales in pharmacies. They also have a professional interest in the control of these products. There has been some standardization (harmonization) of regulatory controls in the provinces, which will likely continue and lead to a more uniform national system.

Pharmacy graduates are now more patient oriented, and the amount of counselling available to patients on both prescription and nonprescription drugs has increased in the past decade. In the future there is potential for even more patient counselling, health information and surveillance of nonprescription drugs. Interactions between prescription and nonprescription drugs will be important.

In the Canadian Facts Survey about one-third of respondents sought the advice of a pharmacist or physician. When consultation was sought from a pharmacist, the customer approached the pharmacist in 96% of the cases. When pharmacists were asked about the initiation of discussion of nonprescription drugs, they reported that the customer initiated about 55% of the discussions while pharmacists initiated about 40%. Pharmacists are reporting more counselling and this is beginning to deal with the continuing problem of pharmacy being an underutilized resource in health care and patient monitoring.

Physicians have traditionally been an important resource for the patient in recommending nonprescription drugs. This will likely continue and manufacturers continue to keep physicians informed of their products. Physicians often resist the shift of products from prescription to nonprescription status, partly due to concern with the risk of improper use, but also because they lose valuable products to prescribe. Patients are often less satisfied because nonprescription drugs are not covered by drug benefit programs.

In Saskatchewan, a research project has been funded to assess methods of collecting information from pharmacists on adverse reactions of nonprescription drugs.

INDUSTRY ISSUES

In the past 20 years, the nonprescription pharmaceutical industry has become more health oriented with closer ties to health professionals and government. As some of the prescription manufacturers move into the nonprescription field, they have established consumer products divisions that have specialized skills for advertising and promotion to the public.

Regulatory standards demand clear evidence of the efficacy and safety of the products sold. In Canada there are few problems with quality of products, misleading claims or toxic ingredients. Many of the problems that do occur are likely to originate outside the country. For example, advertisements for nonprescription products from the United States are often shown on Canadian television through a cable service and the standards for them may be significantly different.

Following extensive consumer advertising, some products have achieved very high volume sales through a large number of outlets. This trend has developed rapidly in Canada. The potential for this kind of promotion and distribution has increased with the movement of grocery stores into the pharmacy business.

Selected groups of products, at this time a small and fragmented market, will continue to rely on professional recommendation rather than media promotion. Normally counselling by a professional is required to ensure proper use and their relatively low sales volume does not warrant the cost of mass promotion.

SWITCH FROM PRESCRIPTION TO NONPRESCRIPTION STATUS

The movement of some prescription drugs to the nonprescription drug category, once unthinkable, is now acceptable to consumers, governments and pharmaceutical manufacturers. Health professionals are less enthusiastic.

The process has proceeded more slowly in Canada than in the United States for several reasons. First, many of the drugs moved to nonprescription status in the United States were already nonprescription drugs in Canada. Second, there was no thought that this might occur in Canada until it began in the United States. The Health Protection Branch now has guidelines for this process and has organized itself to deal expeditiously with nonprescription drugs.

Prescription drugs that became available as nonprescription products in the United States had strong consumer acceptance and their sales increased several fold (one estimate is that a prescription drug would increase its sales four fold as a nonprescription item). For a number of older products with decreasing sales, and at risk of being replaced by newer improved prescription drugs, it was a strong incentive for manufacturers to promote them actively in the nonprescription market.

Historically in Canada the movement of products to nonprescription status has been similar, but product growth was limited by the no-public-access requirement. Also, the impact of the switching in the United States was reinforced in Canada by pressure from the provincial drug benefit programs to reduce the number of benefit products in their formularies.

Drug benefit programs have attempted to control costs by removing nonprescription drugs as benefits. As products are switched from prescription to nonprescription status and are no longer available as a benefit, the assumption is made that there is a saving. To the extent that the products are not substituted by other prescription drugs, this may be a saving to the programs.

In one study the extent of possible savings to the health care system in having nonsedating antihistamines as nonprescription products rather than as prescription drugs was calculated as $11.6 million in Ontario (1994). This included the costs of physician visits, pharmacists' professional fees and the cost of the medication.

Candidates for Switch

The manufacturer initiates the process to switch. Considerations for change include the length of time the product has been established and its safety record. There is a relatively small pool of suitable prescription products with the required characteristics that can be moved into the nonprescription drug market.

One of the major problems in the movement of drugs to nonprescription status is the ability of the patient to diagnose the condition the medication will be used to treat. This will slow the switch of products. There is, however, substantial potential for products to be used in self-limiting or recurring conditions where the initial diagnosis has been established by a physician. The patient would use the nonprescribed medication following the directions carefully to control the condition (e.g., miconazole and clotrimazole for vaginal yeast infections). This treatment is acceptable to health professionals, patients and third-party payers. The emphasis is on education, and the companies must show physicians and pharmacists how to obtain the best possible results from the product.

Historically, drugs moved from prescription to nonprescription status would first be placed in the no-public-access (pharmacist-monitored) category. The process now followed is that when the Health Protection Branch makes a decision to recommend a switch to nonprescription status (e.g., removal from Schedule F) for a drug, it will advise the National Drug Scheduling Advisory Committee (NDSAC). NDSAC then makes a recommendation as to which nonprescription drug category the drug should be assigned, based on consideration of a cascading system of factors for inclusion. This recommendation will be published in the Canada Gazette.

CONCLUSION

In Canada there is widespread use of nonprescription drugs in the prevention and treatment of health problems. The low cost and high effectiveness of these products provides significant scope for growth in the market and potential for a large number of new products. Greater use poses potential problems of harm to the patient and the need for education and monitoring.

The marketplace has evolved a system of graduated controls for drugs, from prescription to pharmacist only, to pharmacy only, to open distribution based on their potential for harm.

A surveillance program for nonprescription drugs that will provide information for the evaluation and control of these products is needed. Health professionals will have a greater input into the control processes as newer forms of regulation occur.

The documentation of the sale of drugs in the pharmacist-monitored and pharmacy-only schedules, when appropriate or requested by the patient, has been recommended as a standard of practice for pharmacists by the Canadian Drug Advisory Committee. This principle of practice was endorsed by the provincial regulatory bodies. It is a subject that needs more publicity to create consumer knowledge, acceptance and demand.

Patient education is needed from a variety of sources and in new and innovative ways for the public to obtain maximum benefits from nonprescription drugs.

Canadian regulatory control of nonprescription drugs is good and there are few problems of product quality, misleading advertising or inappropriate regulatory action.

RECOMMENDED READING

ABM Research Ltd. Community pharmacists and self-medication, A report prepared for the Canadian Pharmaceutical Association, the Conference of Pharmacy Registrars of Canada, the Health Protection Branch of Health and Welfare Canada, and the Nonprescription Drug Manufacturers Association of Canada, 1992.

Anon. The 1994 pharmacy business trends report. Toronto: Pharmacy Post/Eli Lilly, 1994.

Anon. To the year 2000: the changing roles of nonprescription medicines and the practice of pharmacy. Ottawa: Nonprescription Drug Manufacturers Association of Canada,1992.

Canadian Facts. Consumer usage and attitude study vol. 1. Ottawa: Nonprescription Drug Manufacturers Association of Canada, 1991.

Decima Research. Attitudes, perceptions and behaviour relating to ethical medicines. Ottawa: Ministry of Supply and Services, 1990.

Manley R. 1994 Survey on OTC counselling and recommendations. Pharm Post 1994;2:1,15-16.

Newton GD, Pray WS, Popovich NG. New OTCs: a selected review. Am Pharm 1993;NS33:28-36.

Skinner D. Consumer use of nonprescription drugs. Can Pharm J 1985;118(5):206-14.

A survey of drug store trends. Toronto: Drug Merch andising and Le Pharmacien, 1992.

2

CONSUMER COUNSELLING

BRENDA J. MCBEAN COCHRAN

CONTENTS

Introduction 13

The Health Professional and Self-Care 14

Information-Gathering Communication Skills 16
- Questioning Techniques
- Facilitation

Systematic Approach to Self-Care Counselling 19
- Step I: Define the Problem
- Step II: Identify Factors That May Affect Product Choice
- Step III: Select Suitable Product
- Step IV: Counsel Consumer About Product
- Step V: Nonpharmacological Approaches
- Step VI: Follow-up and Monitoring

Nonverbal Communication 28
- Body Language
- Paralinguistics
- Proxemics
- Personal Style
- Nonverbal Communication from Consumers

Special Counselling Situations 31
- Potentially Embarassing Subjects
- Talkative Consumers
- Older Consumers

Summary 36

Recommended Reading 37

INTRODUCTION

A step-by-step counselling guide describes the art of questioning, assessing an individual's symptoms and medical history, recommending a suitable course of action, counselling on nonprescription products and nonpharmacological measures, and encouraging appropriate follow-up of self-treated symptoms. Discussions of nonverbal communication and special counselling situations—such as dealing with potentially embarrassing subjects, talkative consumers or the hearing-impaired—complete the chapter.

Advising on self-treatment can be a complex process because of the amount of information that needs to be exchanged between a health professional and consumer. In most cases, a thorough description of the problem is required before advice can be given. When self-medication is indicated, consumers need information about the safe and effective use of nonprescription products. And the workload of most health professionals requires that these activities be completed in a reasonable amount of time.

During the past several decades, scientists studying communication and learning behavior have contributed much knowledge that applies to self-care counselling. An understanding of information-gathering skills, adult education principles and the influence of nonverbal behavior can help the health professional make the most productive use of counselling time. Some situations, such as potentially embarrassing discussions, require special communication awareness and skills so both the health professional and consumer are comfortable discussing a health problem.

THE HEALTH PROFESSIONAL AND SELF-CARE

Self-care may be broadly defined as all the things that people do to protect, maintain or improve their own health. Within this context, self-treatment refers to the process of selecting suitable drug and nondrug measures for the prevention and treatment of diseases or symptoms. About 85% of symptoms are self-treated, and of all ill people, about 30% are known to use nonprescription drugs. Although valid reasons exist for self-medication, uninformed reliance on this form of treatment may result in inaccurate or delayed diagnosis of significant disease, adverse drug-drug or drug-disease interactions, unnecessary adverse reactions and risks, and/or delayed treatment with more effective measures.

All health professionals are in a position to help ensure safe and effective self-treatment by consumers. After discussing an individual's specific situation, recommendations may include: referral to a different health professional; self-treatment with nonprescription drugs, nondrug measures, or both; or reassurance that no intervention is necessary at this time. A critical element in this process is the ability to exclude certain diagnoses before recommending self-treatment measures.

There are guidelines to help health professionals meet this responsibility. Following the initial work of an ad hoc committee of the Canadian Pharmaceutical Association (CPhA), a task force was formed in 1983 to help pharmacists respond to questions from consumers and establish criteria for referring consumers for medical attention. A number of broad guidelines were developed by this committee, many based on a comprehensive report by the Pharmaceutical Society of Great Britain. Figure 1 summarizes the task force recommendations. These guidelines, along with the right communication and interviewing skills, should help all health professionals meet the self-medication needs of consumers in an effective, efficient and comfortable manner.

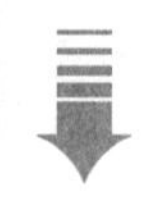

FIGURE 1

Pharmacists' Responses to the Self-Medicating Consumer

I GENERAL PRINCIPLES

A. The standard of care

When responding to the self-medicating consumer, a pharmacist is able to assess those presenting symptoms to determine the most appropriate action:

- refer for medical opinion
- recommend nonprescription drug and/or nonpharmacologic treatment
- reassure the consumer that no treatment is necessary at that time.

B. Regarding a medical diagnosis

A pharmacist does not have the knowledge, skills nor training to make a medical diagnosis. However, he or she should be able to differentiate between those symptoms indicative of a serious condition and those treatable by obtaining symptomatic relief.

C. Consumer/Pharmacist communications

To achieve effective communication with consumers, a pharmacist must consider:

- developing a systematic approach when responding to a request for advice
- establishing an appropriate degree of privacy
- eliminating physical barriers
- phrasing the technical information in nontechnical terms
- establishing good eye contact and understanding the meaning of body language.

II SCREENING

A pharmacist is able to review a variety of factors and symptoms to judge when to refer consumers to a practitioner or when to suggest self-treatment.

General factors

The following are to be considered whenever a pharmacist is determining how to respond to a request for advice:

- age
- sex
- allergies
- general health of the individual and the clustering of several symptoms
- other medication being taken
- pregnancy
- lactation
- previous medical diagnosis for these symptoms
- duration of symptoms

Referral for medical advice

Consumers with the following symptoms or conditions should be immediately referred for medical advice as these symptoms are strongly associated with a serious health condition.

CAUTION: This list is not exhaustive. Other symptoms should be evaluated especially when associated with a General Factor.

- anorexia
- loss of blood from any orifice
- yellowing of the skin
- increasing breathlessness
- any discharge from the penis or vagina
- increased urinary frequency
- pain upon urination
- swelling and/or lumps of any size, including those around the joints
- persistent or recurrent fever, cough and/or hoarseness
- skin or mouth conditions that fail to heal or change in size
- loss of weight
- spontaneous bruising
- ankle swelling
- unusual changes in the sputum, particularly if it is yellow or green
- discoloration of urine
- menstrual abnormalities
- difficulty in swallowing
- severe pain in the chest, abdomen, head or ears
- diarrhea, particularly with infants
- reduced ability to see, hear or taste

Responding to symptoms

The following symptoms are often associated with minor or self-limiting conditions and frequently respond to a specific regimen of self-treatment by the consumer. When recommending self-medication, a pharmacist is able to give advice on the dosage, storage, administration, adverse effects and precautions associated with the particular medications recommended.

CAUTION: These symptoms may be part of a more serious condition, and pharmacists must vigilantly assess them in light of "General Factors".

- insomnia
- fever
- common cold
- diarrhea
- foot problems, warts, corns
- symptoms of the eye, ear or mouth
- burns
- headache
- sinus congestion
- constipation
- pain
- rash, itching of skin
- allergic symptoms
- fatigue

III EVALUATING RESULTS

When medications are recommended, a pharmacist is able to suggest a time period within which the suggested treatment should be effective along with a reassessment or referral at that time.

Special considerations: A pharmacist is to emphasize the following points:

- Symptomatic treatment should never be continued for more than a few days.
- Repeated use of symptomatic medications may mask serious conditions.
- Any adverse change in the original symptoms could indicate a more serious underlying condition that should be reported to the physician.

Adapted from: Pharmacists' responses to the self-medicating patient (Draft). Ottawa: Canadian Pharmaceutical Association, 1985.

INFORMATION-GATHERING COMMUNICATION SKILLS

Most, if not all, self-care counselling requires assessment of an individual's problem. The importance of effective information-gathering skills cannot be overemphasized because consumers' self-reports are often the sole basis for recommending a course of action.

Professional inquiries can range from simple questions, such as determining someone's age, to more involved problems, such as defining what is meant by stomach upset. Although this process may seem straightforward, experience and research show the quality of information received from consumers is not always the best. The way a health professional asks a question influences the accuracy, breadth and depth of this information. For example, to the question "Do you use any other drugs?" people may respond with an emphatic "No!" if they think the professional is referring to street drugs, or if they do not consider nonprescription items to be drugs.

The effective use of information-gathering skills can improve the questioning process. Often called probes, information-gathering skills may be defined as virtually any behavior that elicits a response from the other person. In this discussion, these skills are addressed under the general headings of questioning techniques and facilitation.

QUESTIONING TECHNIQUES

Closed Questions

Also referred to as direct or specific questions, closed questions are those that ask for specific information and limit the answer options of the patient. Although it may not be the questioner's intention, closed questions often restrict answers to "Yes." or "No." For example, "Have you had the pain long?" and "Are you nauseated?" are two closed questions that might be used to assess the need for referral to a doctor.

Although there are times when closed questions are helpful, their routine use is discouraged for several reasons.

First, because closed questions seek specific information, a series of them may be needed to get the necessary information, adding to the time it takes to assess an individual's symptoms.

Second, the health professional is more likely to miss potentially significant information about the complaint. The restrictive or rapid-fire nature of these questions can create an air of interrogation, which causes many people to become passive or closed in their communication. If the health professional neglects to ask about a particular aspect of a condition, the subsequent decision may be based on incomplete data.

Third, many closed questions leave the health professional unsure of what the response means. For example, a "Yes." to the question "Do you know how to use this product?" does not tell the health professional what the consumer actually knows. The health professional must then rephrase or ask additional questions to ensure the individual has appropriate information.

Fourth, people can respond to some closed questions without really knowing the answer. For example, an individual may answer "No." to the question "Do you have any allergies?" simply to avoid having to say "I don't know." Similarly, closed questions allow people to give an answer they think the health professional wants to hear, or to avoid discussing a potentially uncomfortable topic. "Do you drink much alcohol?" elicits a "No." from many people, a response that may or may not be accurate.

Open Questions

The best information is usually obtained with open questions. In contrast to the closed format, these questions cannot be answered "Yes." or "No." and usually require a response of more than a few words. Open questions are often built around the words "what" or "how" and the topic is normally specified in broad terms. "What symptoms are you experiencing?" and "How do you normally use this product?" are examples of two open questions used in self-care counselling.

Initially, open questions may be more difficult to formulate, and a certain skill is required to minimize repetitive, confused or less relevant responses. With practice, however, these questions can provide a significant amount of information with minimal effort. Their use is encouraged for several reasons.

First, because open questions are nonrestrictive, consumers may spontaneously provide all the information the health professional needs to make an appropriate recommendation.

Second, the open format increases the possibility of obtaining unsolicited information about a condition. For example, an individual may reveal details that the health professional would not have addressed with the closed format, or a response may provide clues to other questions that should be asked.

Third, open questions encourage people to talk with minimum guidance and input from the health professional, allowing the practitioner more time to listen and observe. This is especially important in self-care counselling where observation may reveal important details about an individual's condition.

Fourth, because the open format allows people to express symptoms in their own words, the health professional will be able to use similar terminology and avoid words that might alarm or antagonize. The health professional can also assess the consumer's current level of knowledge and focus counselling efforts on misconceptions or gaps in understanding.

Finally, open questions are easier to answer because respondents can do so from their own point of reference. This is particularly helpful with nontalkative people, although some studies suggest that for all people, the more an individual is allowed to speak, the more successful the interview. Similarly, the open format conveys a willingness to listen, a factor likely to promote a positive and ongoing relationship.

Despite these advantages, open questions should not be used exclusively. As described later, most successful interviews use a combination of open and closed questions.

Follow-up Questions

An initial question may not provide the specific information being sought. Follow-up or secondary questions are needed. These questions seek more detail in a specific area and indicate a larger perspective is required. For example, "In what way do you feel worse?" or "Can you tell me more about how the medication affected you?" are helpful when the response to an initial question—whether open or closed—is incomplete, vague or suggests a problem area. Follow-up questions are usually asked in relatively general terms. Even though some can be answered "Yes." or "No." they imply the need for more than a one-word answer.

Multiple Questions

A common pitfall in assessment is the multiple question. These are questions with more than one point of inquiry ("How long have you been taking this, and has it helped?") or that ask for more than one item of information ("Do you have any vision changes, stomach upset or dizziness?"). Multiple questions should always be avoided. They are confusing; people may not know how, or to which portion, they should respond. Similarly, if answered "Yes." or "No." the health professional may not be sure which part the respondent is referring to, and the efficiency of the interview decreases. In addition, people often answer only one part of the question, and important information may be lost as other parts are forgotten.

Leading Questions

Another pitfall is leading the consumer. Leading questions, a form of closed question, strongly imply a desired answer. Questions such as "You take your blood pressure pills all the time, don't you?" and "The pain isn't worse after meals, is it?" can be threatening, and leave little room for disagreement by the respondent. Leading questions, or any nonverbal behavior that suggests a desired response, should always be avoided.

Why Questions

Questions beginning with why should also be avoided. Although the intention is to obtain information, "Why didn't you tell your doctor about this?" and "Why didn't you follow the directions?" can put respondents on the defensive, implying they must justify their behavior. Why questions are almost impossible to answer completely and can result in a response that becomes complicated even for a highly trained psychologist. Because the health professional has little control over a person's answer, the efficiency of the discussion is reduced. Alternatives to why questions are those using "what", "how" or "was there a special reason."

FACILITATION

Other approaches to obtaining information fall under the broad heading of facilitation. Defined as the purposeful encouragement to continue talking, facilitation techniques are nondirective and can include any manner, gesture or word that encourages people to say more about a particular topic. Reflection and attentive silence are particularly helpful for guiding a discussion without biasing an individual's response.

Reflection

As the name implies, reflection is the technique of mirroring or repeating back the last few words of a person's sentence. The words usually take on the inflection of a question, and may simply repeat the area in which a questioner wishes more information. For example, a person may say "I've had this stomach ache for the last few days." Reflection with "Stomach ache?" encourages description of that symptom in greater detail.

Reflection is especially useful for nontalkative people, although everyone responds favorably to hearing their own words. As with all facilitation techniques, reflection should not be overused. As a general rule, no more than one or two reflective statements about the same topic are appropriate.

Attentive Silence

Silence is one of the most powerful tools for obtaining information. Although practitioners—particularly those new to counselling—may be uncomfortable with periods of silence, people often need time to organize their thoughts. Interrupting this silence may destroy the opportunity to get valuable information.

During periods of silence, it is important to attend to the other person, as nothing will end a discussion faster than the health professional appearing not to listen. Continued listening is usually conveyed nonverbally, with gestures like a nod of the head or leaning forward with an interested, expectant facial expression. Equally effective is the use of encouraging comments such as "Hmmm-mmm." or the interjection of "Yes." or "I see." These comments are useful alternatives to head-nodding, which tends to be overused. If a person stops talking about a subject on which more information is needed, a simple "Tell me more about that." will encourage further description.

As with reflection, silence must not be used excessively. Too much silence, especially when someone expresses feelings of anxiety or depression, may be interpreted as cold or distant. Similarly, pauses may occur when the listener does not understand a question or comment; the health professional must be aware of faulty communication as a cause of silence.

Other communication skills, such as empathy and assertiveness, can help the health professional obtain information from a consumer. A description of these skills is beyond the scope of this chapter; the reader is referred to the recommended reading section for a discussion of these subjects.

SYSTEMATIC APPROACH TO SELF-CARE COUNSELLING

According to Dr. Lawrence Weed, father of the problem-oriented medical record, a basic criterion for problem-solving is "how well a clinician can identify patients' problems and organize them for solution." An important interviewing principle related to this goal is that counselling will be more successful if the health professional uses a preplanned, structured approach during discussions with consumers. In other words, counselling will be more effective and efficient if the health professional has a logical sequence for questioning and educating patients, and a mental image of the order in which this information ideally is exchanged.

Figure 2 illustrates one such approach for self-care counselling. Both the broad and specific steps in the Systematic Approach are based on principles of medical interviewing, therapeutic drug monitoring and adult education. At least four reasons can be identified for why this type of approach increases productivity of health professionals' self-care counselling.

First, although the health professional may be aware in principle of the questions needed to define a problem, without a predetermined course of action it is easy to become sidetracked and miss potentially significant information. A mental image of the order of information exchange increases the likelihood that all factors are considered before a recommendation is made.

Second, the health professional has better control over the flow of information. People seldom articulate their history in a concise, logical manner. Health professionals who have a clear idea of the information they need at each step are better able to guide an orderly discussion.

Third, and equally important, asking questions in a logical order can prevent unnecessary questions. For instance, if near the beginning the health professional determines that back pain has persisted more than a few days, or is accompanied by pain on urination, additional assessment is not needed, and the consumer can be immediately referred to a physician.

Finally, because information required by consumers is organized into stages in the health professional's mind, he or she will be better able to transmit these ideas one at a time. In turn, the educational process will be more effective.

The following sections describe the Systematic Approach in detail. Examples of questions for assessing symptoms are provided along with suggestions for wording with which consumers are more familiar. As with any counselling tool, health professionals must use their own judgment when applying this approach in practice. Although the broad headings are a helpful memory aid, all steps will not apply to each consumer. Based on information in Step I, for example, the health professional may choose simply to reassure a consumer and, skipping Steps II through V, provide advice about appropriate follow-up if the symptoms change in any way (Step VI). Or if a consumer is referred to a physician, the health professional can also recommend appropriate nondrug measures for

FIGURE 2

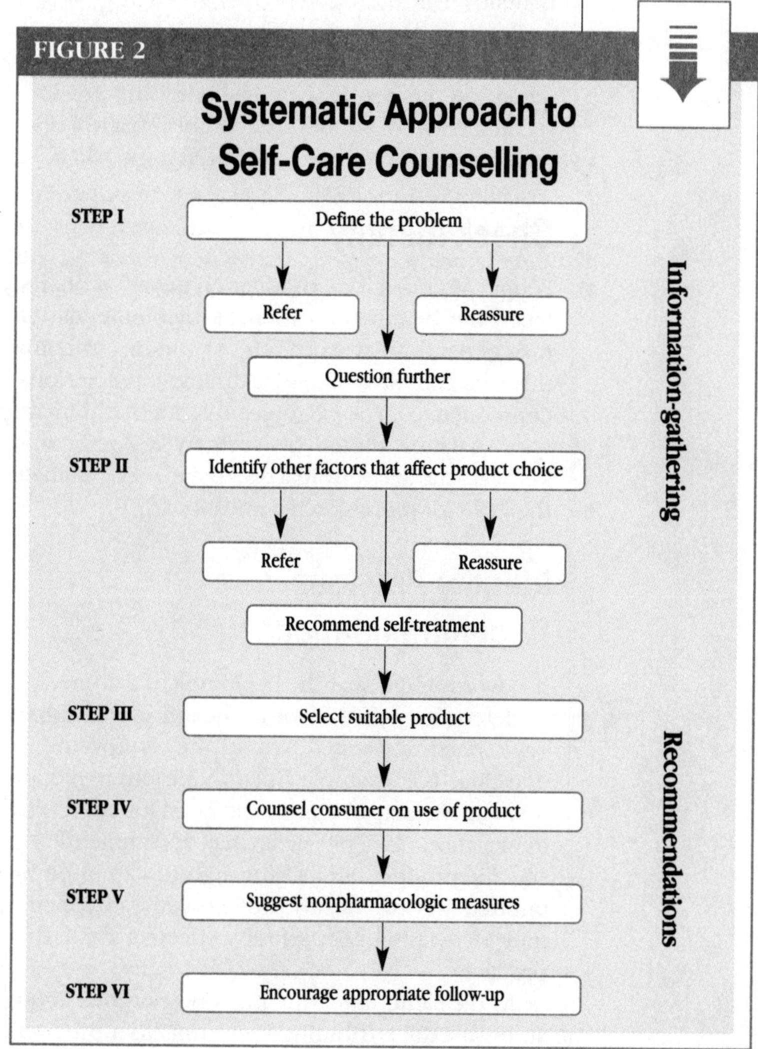

reducing, alleviating or preventing symptoms (Step V). Note also that nondrug suggestions (Step V) may be made before a specific product (Step III) is recommended.

STEP I: DEFINE THE PROBLEM

The first logical step with any request about self-treatment is to find out more about the person's problem. Step I has two objectives. First and foremost is the need to rule out more serious health conditions; if the health professional cannot be reasonably certain symptoms are self-treatable, individuals should be encouraged to see the appropriate health care professional (e.g., physician, dentist). Second, when self-medication seems appropriate, details in Step I will provide initial information about nonprescription products or ingredients from which the consumer might benefit.

Before symptom-specific questions are asked, three introductory steps need to be considered: identity of the person with the complaint; previous recommendations about that complaint; and a brief explanation of why questions need to be asked.

Check Identity

People often ask for a product on behalf of others. Since the health professional's recommendation may depend on who has the symptoms, missing this step can have time-consuming, if not serious, consequences. For example, a 9-month-old infant with diarrhea should be seen by a doctor and knowing the age early in a discussion may eliminate the need for more specific questions.

Identify Previous Recommendations

It is worthwhile near the beginning of a discussion to determine whether other health professionals have been consulted about the symptoms in question. For example, identifying other recommendations may eliminate the need for additional information. If a physician has recommended a specific product, Steps I through III can often be omitted and the health professional can concentrate on details for the safe and effective use of that product.

At the same time, one must be cautious about automatically attributing symptoms to a previous diagnosis, since other pathological factors might have developed. Additionally, the health professional must establish whether other instructions were given at the time of the original diagnosis. For example, some people may have been advised to return to their doctor if symptoms recur or worsen. Closely related, people often self-diagnose their ailments and request specific medications based on these self-assessments. The health professional must be careful about accepting these assessments at face value and encourage referral if there is any question about the advisability of self-treatment.

Explain Purpose of Further Questions

People respond best when they understand why questions are being asked. Especially when detailed or personal questions are needed, it is helpful to preface those questions with an explanation of their purpose.

The explanation should include the amount of time or number of questions to be asked, subjects to be covered, and benefits to the consumer. For example, the statement "To help you find the best treatment for your symptoms, I'll need to ask you a few questions about. . . ." is a succinct way of indicating that questions are asked not out of superficial curiosity, but out of a genuine desire to help.

Clarify Symptoms

Although identifying a problem in general terms is straightforward (a cold or stomach upset), obtaining a thorough description of that problem may be more complex. For example, Table 1 illustrates eight categories of questions used in medical history-taking, and Part II of the Canadian Pharmaceutical Association guidelines shows other factors that need to be considered when assessing the advisability of self-treatment with nonprescription drugs (Figure 1).

The best approach to obtaining this information is to gradually restrict the openness of a series of questions. This key principle for any information-gathering situation is especially important when the health professional attempts to identify the nature of a medical problem. In practice, this approach can be broken into three distinct stages to help the health professional achieve a smooth and efficient flow of information: ask the

TABLE 1: Dimensions of Present Illness

Chronology	How long has the consumer had the symptom? Has the consumer had this symptom before?
Related symptoms	What other symptoms does the individual have? Is there any clustering of symptoms? What is their chronological relationship to each other?
Bodily location	Where does the symptom occur? Specific questions related to depth, radiation and area(s) may be needed to localize the symptom.
Quality	How is the symptom described? If pain, is it sharp, dull, constant, throbbing, etc.? Descriptions will range from mild to severe and need to be evaluated in light of temperament.
Quantity	Specific questions about frequency (how often?), size (how big?) and volume (how much?) may be necessary.
Setting	Under what circumstances does the symptom occur? Is it worse (or better) at a particular time of day? Can it be related to factors in environment or lifestyle?
Aggravation or alleviation	Is there anything that makes the symptom worse or that relieves the symptom? What medication has been tried? What were the results?
Possible health-related causes	Does the individual have other health conditions that might explain the current symptoms? Is it a side effect of other medication being taken?

Note: Some diseases do not manifest in all dimensions and others have symptoms not fully covered by these categories. By and large, however, their use in history-taking is reliable and can serve as a guide to the clinician in organizing a description of the illness.

broadest possible question first; identify all general symptoms; and ask specific questions to fill in gaps.

Ask the broadest question first: For example, when someone asks for a cold remedy, an appropriate first question might be "What symptoms do you have?" This approach allows people to respond in their own words. In some cases, the health professional may be able to make an immediate recommendation on the basis of this information.

Identify all general symptoms: The efficiency of many information-gathering situations can be improved if the next set of questions identifies all general symptoms. For the person with a cold, the presence or absence of nasal involvement, cough, sore throat, fever, aches or pains should be determined before detailed questions are asked about each symptom. A nonspecific question, such as "Do you have any other symptoms?" is appropriate. Alternatively, the health professional may ask directly about the presence of symptoms commonly associated with the presenting complaint, or that might suggest the person has something other than a minor, self-limiting condition.

There are four reasons why identifying all symptoms at this stage can decrease counselling time. First, finding out about certain symptoms early in the discussion may eliminate the need for more detail. For example, symptoms listed in Part IIB of the CPhA guidelines strongly suggest more serious health problems, and people describing any of these should be referred for medical advice.

Equally important is clustering of symptoms. As a general rule, the presence of related symptoms is a criterion for referral to a physician; again, the health professional may save time by obtaining this information near the beginning of a discussion.

Identifying symptoms in a general way also helps the health professional focus next on those more likely to need medical attention. For example, a sore throat is potentially more serious than a stuffy nose and investigating that symptom first may eliminate the need for details about the nasal symptoms.

Finally, identifying all general symptoms allows the health professional to begin narrowing the range of nonprescription products that might be helpful. For instance, if a cold is confined to the head, products containing expectorants and antitussives can mentally be eliminated from the list of possibilities.

Ask specific questions to fill in gaps: The health professional should now have a fairly clear picture of an individual's problem. Some symptoms may, however, require further elaboration. This stage of assessment is perhaps the most difficult, particularly when complaints are vague or when a substantial amount of information is still needed. Since a goal at this stage is to rule out the need for referral, the most productive questions will be those that help the health professional differentiate between serious conditions and those that are minor or self-limiting.

Of the eight dimensions in Table 1, chronology is the most important. The time required to make a decision about referral can be substantially reduced if the health professional asks about the duration of symptoms early in the line of questioning. For example, a headache that has lasted 3 days may indicate serious disease; one that has lasted 2 hours is less likely to require immediate medical assessment. Information about recurring symptoms may be equally important. Symptoms that return frequently may indicate a major pathologic condition and should be referred, particularly since the repeated use of symptomatic medications can mask the condition and delay appropriate diagnosis.

The relative importance of the remaining categories in Table 1 varies with individual symptoms. As with all assessment questions, the ability to elicit this information efficiently requires an understanding of disease states and their presentation. Each chapter in this text provides a list of formulated questions to ask about specific conditions. The reader is referred to these as well as basic therapeutic textbooks to develop priorities for the order of questions at this stage.

Referring a Consumer

Although there are no hard and fast rules, the above discussion identifies three guidelines for referring consumers to a physician: the presence of symptoms strongly suggesting serious disease; clustering of symptoms; and long-lasting or recurring symptoms. Another consideration is general appearance. If the person with a 2-hour history of headache looks ill, the possibility of a potentially serious condition cannot be excluded, and medical assessment should be advised.

These guidelines are not meant to be exhaustive. During discussions with consumers, other considerations of a more general nature may emerge. Some people simply may be seeking encouragement to see a physician; an individual's perception of symptoms must always be taken into account. In other cases, referral may be in order when symptoms might respond better to prescribed medication. Finally, a cardinal rule of assessment is to discourage self-treatment if any uncertainty exists about the cause of the symptom. If the health professional cannot reasonably exclude the possibility of a more serious underlying condition, the person must be referred for medical opinion.

A proper referral reflects three factors: whom the person should see; when that person should be seen; and why referral is recommended. The health professional should use both tact and firmness so the person understands the importance of follow-up without becoming unduly alarmed. Wording similar to the following can be effective in most situations: "From what you have told me, I think it is a good idea (or important) to see your doctor. It may be a simple case of . . . , but it is better to be safe, and I'm sure your doctor would want to see you about this."

People are more likely to follow this advice if they understand why they have been referred. If a consumer appears reluctant to bother a doctor for seemingly minor complaints, the importance of having symptoms medically evaluated may need to be stressed. Questions such as "Do you have a regular doctor?" or "Can you reach your doctor today (or within an appropriate time frame)?" and "Do you want me to call and explain your symptoms?" may provide needed encouragement.

STEP II: IDENTIFY FACTORS THAT MAY AFFECT PRODUCT CHOICE

When self-medication seems advisable, the next step is to evaluate other factors in the consumer's history that may affect the choice of product. Depending on the situation, it may be necessary to find out about some or all of the following areas.

Health of the consumer: Are there any other illnesses or health conditions that affect the choice of product? For example, when considering a sympathomimetic, the health professional must know if there is a history of diseases like high blood pressure or diabetes. Since conditions such as pregnancy and lactation may affect the choice of product, questions about health should not be restricted to illness or disease.

Other drugs: Is the person taking any other drugs, including nonprescription drugs, natural or home remedies, that may interact with the ingredients being considered? Classic examples include tetracycline for people requesting an antacid and warfarin when ASA is considered.

Allergies and previous adverse effects: Does the person have an allergy to specific ingredients? Has the person had adverse reactions to the product or product category under consideration? For example, people react differently to different antihistamines. Past drowsiness from one may make another choice more appropriate.

Some of this information may have been obtained in Step I. If not, direct or closed questions are usually the most efficient at this stage. These questions may follow an initial broad question, and a technique known as bridging may be useful. For example, when considering an analgesic, the statement "You mentioned you take . . .. Are you taking any other prescription or nonprescription medicines?" can be followed with questions about blood thinners, medicines for gout and other classes of drugs that interact with the product the health professional has in mind.

STEP III: SELECT SUITABLE PRODUCT

In the absence of drug or disease interactions, the next step in the Systematic Approach is to select a suitable product. This process is guided primarily by information obtained in Steps I and II. Another important consideration is the safety and efficacy of products. Many health professionals evaluate products within a category and have two or three in mind for each type of symptom.

Other drug variables, such as dosage form and side effects, should be matched with consumer variables, such as lifestyle or work conditions. A topical decongestant may be more appropriate than an oral antihistamine combination for someone who needs to be alert. Or, children's dosage forms may be better for certain age groups. Because elderly people sometimes have difficulty swallowing, liquid preparations or coated tablets might be more suitable.

A person's past experience with a product is also important. By finding out which products have been used, the health professional can avoid recommending those found unsuitable in the past. Conversely, if a product gave excellent results, the health professional can accept and encourage that choice, as long as other criteria for selection have been met.

Finally, although not a sole criterion, the health professional should consider the relative cost of products. Different dosage forms may represent a cost saving, and people will appreciate receiving a less expensive remedy.

STEP IV: COUNSEL CONSUMER ABOUT PRODUCT

Although consumers today are relatively well informed, a number of studies suggest errors occur with nonprescription drugs. Often these errors are due to lack of knowledge. Once a product is chosen, the health professional must ensure the consumer has sufficient information to use that product in the most beneficial and least toxic manner. Although the type and amount of information varies with each person, five general categories need to be considered: intended benefits; administration instructions; potential side effects; potential interactions; and storage instructions.

For each category the health professional's goal is to provide accurate, understandable and practical information. One principle of adult education states that people are more likely to remember and follow advice if they understand the reason for doing so. Therefore the health professional should explain the rationale for advice and instructions whenever possible. This explanation not only helps ensure proper use of nonprescription products, but reinforces that these items are drugs and must be used carefully. The time spent educating consumers can be more productive if the health professional begins by finding out what the consumer knows about a product. This allows them to identify and correct any misconceptions, and in many cases avoid unnecessary duplication of information. In accord with another principle of adult education, new information will have more meaning, because it can be related to what an individual already knows. As well, the health professional will be able to use more appropriate terminology, taking cues from words the individual uses.

Intended Benefits

An integral part of nonprescription drug counselling is an explanation of the intended benefits of a product. This usually is as simple as explaining why that product was chosen and, in the case of multiple-ingredient preparations, describing the purpose of each ingredient.

Explanations should be brief, specific to the consumer's problem and in understandable terms.

Systematic Approach to Self-Care Counselling

A health professional might recommend a combination product for nasal congestion and nonproductive cough, but a person told it contains a sympathomimetic and antitussive seldom learns the benefits of the product. A more meaningful explanation might be: "This ingredient (referring to the package) will help relieve nasal stuffiness, and this one (the antitussive) helps stop coughing so there is less irritation to the throat."

When explaining the choice of product, the health professional should also bear in mind the power of the placebo effect. Statements such as "This medicine is often helpful for conditions such as yours." or "This is an excellent product for. . ." go a long way toward relieving symptoms. This approach is particularly important with products that have become so common the public tends to underestimate their efficacy, and with conditions such as pain that have a large psychological component. For similar reasons, the health professional should avoid appearing hesitant about a product. Statements like "Well, I guess this might help." do little to inspire confidence in the value of the product.

Consumers should also be told when benefits are likely to appear. Symptom relief may be almost immediate, but products such as bulk-forming laxatives, acne remedies or dandruff treatments do take longer to work. People who expect immediate relief may become discouraged unless they know what to expect. Also, certain people may need to be cautioned about benefits. For example, masking muscular pain with an analgesic may lead to overactivity of the injured muscle.

Administration Instructions

Nonprescription drugs may be ineffective simply because they are administered improperly. Although most labels give complete instructions, studies show that some people do not read, let alone correctly interpret, this information. In some cases, the print may be too small for visually impaired people, and several studies show that some information is written at a level higher than the average consumer can comprehend. An estimated 18% of Canadian adults, and up to 67% of those over age 55, do not have the reading skills to deal with most written material encountered in everyday life. Numeracy skills, or the ability to read and interpret numbers, can be equally poor. About 38% of the population are believed to have difficulty in this area, and an estimated 14% have skills so limited they are unable to reliably read medication instructions.

For these reasons, it is important for the health professional to verbally review or supplement package information in some or all of the following areas: the amount per single dose; the number of doses per day; the times of administration; the specific method of administration; and the suggested length of treatment.

The amount per single dose: A review of manufacturers' single-dose recommendations is important. Since consumers may view nonprescription drugs as safe and may believe that if one is good, two are better, it is especially important to outline the consequences of exceeding these recommendations. On the other hand, individuals who are sensitive to drugs may want to reduce initial doses when trying new preparations.

Number of doses per day: For similar reasons, the maximum amount of medication that may be taken in a 24-hour period, as well as the suggested interval between doses, needs to be pointed out. Undercompliance, on the other hand, is seldom a problem, as most people are motivated by symptoms to use a nonprescription product. However, the health professional may encounter people who take a nonprescription drug for a chronic problem on the advice of their physician. In these cases, the importance of using the medication regularly needs to be stressed. It is best to be extremely specific in this explanation. The following example, which can be adapted for most medical conditions, illustrates a succinct way of conveying information to a person with arthritis: "Some people take ASA only when required for the relief of pain. However, in your case, it is important to take it 4 times a day, even when you feel well, to help prevent the pain and swelling that comes from arthritis."

Times of administration: Depending on the drug, information about specific times of administration may include: when to take the drug in relation to food (e.g., ASA); when to take the drug in relation to other medication (e.g., antacids); or when during a 24-hour period the effects of the medication are least disruptive (e.g., certain laxatives).

Specific method of administration: Many self-care products require special administration. People receiving suppositories, vaginal products, or otic, ophthalmic or nasal preparations should receive detailed explanations of how those products should be used. When products feature diagrams on the package, it may be sufficient to point these out, encouraging consumers to call if they have questions. A less obvious consideration is drugs with a special coating. Elderly people often have difficulty swallowing products like enteric-coated ASA, and it is not unusual for these people to crush or chew their drugs.

Length of therapy: The appropriate length of therapy usually is discussed in relation to a person's symptoms (Step VI: Follow-up and Monitoring). However, there may be instances—as with the number of consecutive days for nose drops—when this information is more drug-specific.

As a general rule, symptomatic treatment should not be continued for more than a few days without medical supervision. Little harm can be done in advising self-medication if the health professional follows this guideline, although longer or shorter recommendations are appropriate in some cases. For instance, using an acne or dandruff product beyond a few days is reasonable, but may not be for an antinauseant.

Side Effects

Common concerns about discussing side effects are that people will experience those effects through the power of suggestion, or become too frightened to take the drug. Numerous studies indicate that few people react this way. Most people want to know what side effects drugs might cause. Perhaps more importantly, these concerns must be weighed against the potential consequences of an inadequately informed consumer.

A discussion about every adverse drug reaction associated with nonprescription products is seldom necessary. As a rough guideline, people should be advised about those effects they can recognize and for which appropriate precautionary measures can be taken. About 70 to 80% of side effects can be predicted as an extension of pharmacologic action. Within this category, consumers should be informed about the following:

- annoying side effects that can be minimized or eliminated by consumer initiated measures. For example, a dry mouth can be resolved by chewing sugarless gum or taking small, frequent sips of ice water.
- side effects that might otherwise cause undue alarm. For example, drug-induced urine or stool color changes should be discussed before these changes occur.
- bothersome side effects that are transient. For example, some acne treatments cause initial peeling or reddening of the affected area, and people are more likely to tolerate this side effect, and continue with treatment, if they understand the effect's short-term nature.
- side effects that impair ability to perform. Any person receiving a product that causes drowsiness, dizziness, blurred vision or other impairment of physical or mental capacity needs to be forewarned of these effects. Of all side effects, this is perhaps the most important, as failure to inform may result in serious harm to the user.

The remaining 20 to 30% of side effects includes more serious, usually unpredictable, toxicities, such as allergic or idiosyncratic reactions. The former may be prevented by questioning the consumer's medical history. The latter as a rule do not require detailed discussion, since people usually do not administer nonprescription products for prolonged periods. On the other hand, advising against long-term use without a physician's advice becomes doubly important for drugs associated with more serious adverse effects over time.

The potential for alarming consumers or for psychologically inducing side effects can be reduced considerably by following a few general principles.

Avoid definitive statements about the drug's side effects. Comments like "This drug causes stomach problems." or "You'll probably feel drowsy after you take this." not only are more likely to produce a side effect, but the health professional does not know whether the user will experience the reaction in question. A less alarming, and more accurate approach, is to avoid the word you in favor of general descriptions like: "Some people find this upsets their stomach." and "A few people find they are drowsy after taking this product."

Set the stage, if necessary. If several side effects are to be discussed, it may help to preface information with a general phrase putting these in perspective. For example, "Some people experience unwanted effects with this product. You may not necessarily get these, as the drug affects different people in different ways. However, it is important to be aware of these effects and what to do if they occur."

Gauge the consumer's initial reaction. The health professional should be particularly observant at the beginning of a side effects discussion. If a person appears concerned, additional reassurance about the nature and likelihood of a side effect may be needed.

Provide practical advice. Consumers need to be told more than "This drug may cause dizziness, drowsiness, stomach upset. . . ." They also need to know when a side effect is likely to appear and, more important, what to do to minimize its occurrence. For example, if a product causes gastric irritation, the user should be advised to take the drug with food, or crackers and water. It is also helpful to encourage people to call back if a side effect occurs, as an alternate product or self-treatment measure can often be recommended.

Interactions

Any person taking a product that interacts with alcohol needs to be forewarned. The phrasing of this information is important, so not to leave the impression that alcohol-drug combinations are similar to increased alcohol consumption. Some people see this as a beneficial outcome. To help prevent this interpretation you might say: "You may experience an unpleasant feeling, such as extreme drowsiness or disorientation, if you drink alcoholic beverages around the time you take. . . ."

Counselling about alcohol consumption also requires tact. All health professionals have heard people react to statements about alcohol with an indignant, "I don't drink!" Often these reactions occur before the health professional has a chance to provide relevant information. The following response might be helpful in these situations: "I like to mention this point because a number of people have wine with their meals or the odd beer, and this product should be avoided within . . . hours of having a drink." Alternatively, to prevent this reaction, phrases like social drink or wine with meals are preferable to alcohol or drink(ing). Another effective approach is to preface any statement about alcohol with "This may not apply to you, but. . . ."

Depending on the product, other drug interaction advice may be needed. Reviewing all future possibilities at the time of sale, however, is usually an inefficient use of time, as people are unlikely to remember this much detail. The most efficient way to address potential drug interactions is to provide general information, along with encouragement to contact a health professional as situations arise. For example: "This product can affect the way other medicines work (avoiding the word interact), so if you start any new medicines while using this product, be sure to call your doctor or me first so we can tell you whether there is any problem."

Storage

Information about storing nonprescription products may be relevant in some cases, e.g., diabetic testing supplies. Health professionals should emphasize that the bathroom may not be the best place to store medication since higher temperatures and moisture can cause certain medicines to break down. As well, the statement "Keep out of the reach of children." can be emphasized by suggesting storage in a locked cupboard to prevent accidental poisoning.

STEP V: NONPHARMACOLOGICAL APPROACHES

Apart from product-specific information, a major component of self-care counselling is advice about nonpharmacological approaches. Information may be given in conjunction with a product, e.g., water with expectorants, or on its own. Nonpharmacological advice is particularly helpful when contraindications to drug therapy exist and a physician cannot be seen immediately, e.g., in the evening or on weekends.

The health professional needs to be aware of nonpharmacological measures for both prevention and treatment. Such advice may include eating and other lifestyle habits to relieve constipation, the use of a humidifier for cold symptoms and the application of warm or cold compresses for headache. Many excellent pamphlets are available through health agencies, provincial and federal health departments, and pharmaceutical companies. Supplying this information not only adds to consumers' appreciation of the health professional, but is an efficient way to educate people about their symptoms.

STEP VI: FOLLOW-UP AND MONITORING

Consumer counselling should be concluded with encouragement for appropriate follow-up. Since most nonprescription drugs should be used only for minor or self-limiting conditions, the health professional needs to ensure the consumer has a clear understanding of what action to take if relief is not obtained.

The foremost consideration for follow-up is an allowable duration of symptoms. Self-treatment, with or without drugs, should be continued only for the time normally required for a particular symptom to resolve on its own. The actual number of days varies with each condition—simple indigestion usually clears within 24 hours, but the common cold typically lasts a week. When recommending appropriate follow-up periods, the health professional must consider the duration of symptoms before advice was sought.

Follow-up is also recommended if a nonprescription drug fails to relieve symptoms within an expected period of time. As well, information about symptoms that may indicate a more serious disease is needed in some instances. The appearance of new symptoms, such as fever with a cold, or a change in original symptoms, such as green sputum, may suggest an underlying pathology that should be assessed by a physician. Similarly, the repeated use of nonprescription drugs may mask serious problems, and people should be encouraged to see their physicians if symptoms recur frequently.

Encouraging appropriate follow-up requires the same tact and firmness as referral for initial medical advice. In addition, the following phrase may be helpful: "If your symptoms are not relieved by this product or if you are not better in (the time period appropriate for that condition), contact your doctor. Be sure to explain you have been using this product." This latter statement reinforces that nonprescription items are drugs and of interest to the physician.

As a concluding statement, many health professionals find it helpful to encourage feedback. A comment such as "Please call and let me know how you manage." or "I will call you in a day or so to see how you are doing." indicates an interest consumers appreciate. Equally important, it gives health professionals an opportunity to evaluate the appropriateness of their advice.

NONVERBAL COMMUNICATION

Effective communication depends not only on words, but the nonverbal behavior of the people involved. Consumers are as likely to respond to the way the health professional looks, the manner in which words are delivered and accompanying facial expressions, as they are to spoken words.

The importance of nonverbal communication, which encompasses all behavior outside the spoken word, is underlined by findings that up to 90% of meaning in face-to-face discussions can be attributed to nonverbal sources. Unlike verbal communication, nonverbal communication is a continuous process. It begins before the first word is spoken and continues until a particular encounter ends, regardless of how much, or how little, is said.

Nonverbal communication is more spontaneous than verbal communication and often reflects the true feelings of a speaker. When verbal and nonverbal messages contradict each other, the nonverbal are more believable. For example, if someone stalks out of the room, slams the door and shouts "I'm not the least bit angry!" the nonverbal behavior obviously is the most credible.

Nonverbal signs are highly subject to misinterpretation and can be misleading. Without verbal information, a listener can only infer the meaning of a particular behavior and does so in a totally personal manner. A quick look at a wristwatch during a conversation may mean: it is a boring conversation, it is time for coffee, or simply that the listener has a new wristwatch. Similarly, the person who appears to be loitering may be preparing to shoplift or may simply be embarrassed about purchasing a particular product.

The health professional's ability to send and receive nonverbal messages influences the quality of relationships with consumers. Though nonverbal behavior is an unconscious process in everyday life, it can be controlled if one is aware of the elements involved. Elements particularly relevant to counselling include: kinesics or body language; proxemics or the study of space, position and objects in relation to communication; paralanguage or nonword vocalizations; and the personal style of people engaged in communication. The application of these elements in counselling is described briefly below. Several excellent references are available for more complete information on nonverbal communication.

BODY LANGUAGE

One of the richest categories of nonverbal communication is body language or kinesics. Often mistakenly equated with the entire process of nonverbal communication, this category refers to the wide range of body movements and facial expressions that accompany the spoken word. Of all nonverbal elements, the use or misuse of body language can have the most dramatic impact on a message.

Within this category, the presence or absence of eye contact is critical. Many health professionals, without realizing it, do not look at consumers when talking to them. Lack of eye contact is one of the largest barriers to communication. People may interpret it as lack of interest or lack of confidence on the part of the health professional. Particularly in self-care counselling, not looking at an individual also limits the health professional's ability to watch for clues about the severity of a condition, or for people's reactions to information. At the same time, good eye contact does not mean continually staring at another person. Prolonged eye contact may be interpreted as a sign of arrogance or disrespect. Generally speaking, the best approach is brief eye contact that continues throughout the conversation.

Closely related, the health professional's overall facial expression is important. For instance, mannerisms such as biting the lips, puckering the mouth, knitting or lowering the eyebrows in response to a question, could be interpreted as suspicion, disapproval or a lack of knowledge. Health professionals need to be aware of how they unintentionally send messages, especially ones that do not communicate **competence** as a health professional and **respect** for the consumer.

The health professional's willingness to talk to consumers can be detected on the basis of body stance, e.g., closed posture: arms are folded across the chest, legs are crossed at the knees and the head faces downward. Individually these body positions can be appropriate, but the combination of such nonverbal actions (called cue clusters) can signal a desire to be doing something other than talking to the consumer.

The best approach for counselling is an open cue cluster. Communicating openness generally includes: brief, consistent eye contact throughout the discussion; a relaxed facial expression that conveys interest and willingness to listen; a relaxed posture with legs uncrossed and arms by the side; a frontal appearance with shoulders square or rotated toward the other person; an erect body position, with head up and shoulders back; a slight lean toward the other person, if sitting; appropriate comfortable gestures, for example, with the hands; and absence of distracting motions.

The open posture contributes to the perception that the health professional is willing to devote time to individual consumers. Several studies show a positive relationship between consumer satisfaction and the degree of interest communicated nonverbally by a health professional. In addition, the open posture may influence people's ability to understand and recall information. One study of physicians' nonverbal behavior found that a greater degree of openness, expressed through a forward lean and body orientation, resulted in higher levels of understanding. The authors postulated that the positive interest shown by the practitioner motivated people to listen more closely and, therefore, to retain more information.

PARALINGUISTICS

A second major element of nonverbal communication is the manner in which words are delivered—the tone, rate, pitch and volume of voice and the presence of nonword vocalizations, such as uh, throat clearings or nervous giggles. As much as one-third of nonverbal communication takes place through such vocal cues or paralanguage.

A varied and interesting voice is ideal, but as long as one's speech is not too extreme, there should be little interference with communication. On the other hand, people can become remarkably upset because an inappropriate tone of voice has been used, often creating an entirely different meaning than the speaker intended. Similarly, a monotone or flat voice is difficult to listen to; adding even modest inflection can help keep the listener's attention. Listening to the inflection, rate and volume of one's voice on tape is a helpful exercise; many people find they sound far different than expected.

Vocal cues can also be used to give and request permission to speak. Four identifiable vocal cues that indicate turn-taking have been postulated: turn-yielding cues in the form of silence, or a higher or lower pitch at the end of a comment; turn-requesting cues such as an audible inspiration of breath during pauses; turn-maintaining cues, which include increasing one's volume and rate when the listener indicates a desire to speak; and turn-denying cues, which include silence and slower than normal reinforcement of the other person's comment. Missing any of these cues from a consumer may appear rude or inconsiderate. On the other hand, these cues may be helpful during telephone conversations where nonverbal signals such as facial expression are absent. They can also be effective during discussions with talkative people.

PROXEMICS

The most familiar example of proxemics (the structure and use of space in communication) is the typical dispensary design. Many prescription counters act as a physical and psychological barrier, and communication is often improved when the pharmacist steps out from behind the counter to talk to a consumer. This gesture is especially important when the dispensary platform is elevated. High-low physical relationships can suggest a superior-inferior relationship, and consumers who perceive themselves to be in the inferior position are less likely to participate in a discussion.

A less familiar component of proxemics is the closeness of body position between the health professional and the consumer. There are four identifiable distances in North American culture that reflect the purpose of an interaction as well as the acquaintance level of the participants. Anything less than 45 cm is reserved for those with whom one has an intimate relationship. When a stranger or nonintimate associate enters this space, anxiety or anger at the invasion of privacy may result. The next level is 45 to 120 cm (casual-personal distance), which represents the most comfortable distance for conversation between friends and acquaintances. The most accepted distance between two people involved in professional transactions lies between 1 and 4 m (social-consultative distance). Distances over 4 metres are generally reserved for occasions when one speaks to an audience (public distance) and imply that little or no interruption will occur.

Obviously, the health professional who counsels from a public distance—a pharmacist shouting advice or directions from a dispensary platform—does little to encourage active participation by the consumer. The distance the health professional chooses to counsel a person depends on the relationship with that person as well as the context and topic of discussion. Many health professional-consumer exchanges occur at the social-consultative level, but for explanations about products such as vaginal or rectal medication, the health professional may choose the outer limits of the casual-personal distance—close enough for privacy, but with enough room for each person to feel comfortable.

In pharmacy settings, the ideal situation is to have a private area near the dispensary. In the absence of this service, there are ways to provide psychological privacy. A particularly helpful arrangement is to form a triangle using the consumer, pharmacist and wall shelf or gondola as the three sides. This positioning signals to others that the conversation is private and not to be interrupted. Even in the most crowded pharmacy, a sense of privacy can also be achieved by stepping into a quieter aisle.

The environment in which counselling takes place also projects a nonverbal image and can convey a positive, or negative, message about the health professional. Colors, lighting, background noise, and the general use of space have all been documented as important communication channels. Dirt, clutter and general untidiness in any environment have a negative impact that is even stronger in a health care setting.

PERSONAL STYLE

Just as an untidy or unclean environment can project a negative image, so too can the appearance of the health professional and his or her associates. Style and cleanliness affect how consumers will respond to the health professional. People are quick to make assumptions about intelligence, credibility, reliability, breadth of experience and a host of personality characteristics on the basis of physical appearance. If there is any question about the power of personal style, consider how one reacts to people with dirty clothes, dirty hands and fingernails, and unwashed hair.

NONVERBAL COMMUNICATION FROM CONSUMERS

Effective communication requires the detection of nonverbal behavior in others. The elements described above apply equally to consumers, and the health professional needs to observe consumers' nonverbal behavior when counselling them about the selection and use of nonprescription drugs.

Awareness of consumers' nonverbal behavior often provides valuable feedback on the effectiveness of counselling efforts. Body language and paralinguistics are particularly relevant. For example, a quizzical look in response to questions or product information should alert the health professional to the need for further explanation. Similarly, hesitations in speech or a concerned look may suggest that more discussion about a particular topic is needed.

The health professional should also be familiar with nonverbal signs indicating anxiety, anger and embarrassment, as these emotions may mean a different style of interaction is needed. Swinging a leg, tapping a foot or drumming fingers may all suggest a state of nervousness. Repeatedly clenching and unclenching one's fist might indicate a certain level of anxiety, or even hostility. People often demonstrate a unique set of body movements for expressing reactions to illness, including self-manipulating movements, such as wringing the hands, licking the lips or scratching the nose and face during stressful situations. Since a person's emotional state influences how much is gained from counselling, the health professional is well advised to address these emotions before providing advice and information about drug therapy.

Finally, nonverbal behavior is influenced by cultural background. For example, although lack of eye contact in American culture is tantamount to denying another person's existence, Oriental people are taught to communicate respect by decreasing eye contact. In the Bulgarian culture, shaking the head from side to side is a sign of agreement. Middle Eastern people may not have the same need for intimate space discussed under proxemics. Health professionals who provide services to populations of particular racial or cultural origin can find out more about nonverbal behaviors of these groups by reading appropriate texts. However, one must be cautious, as the nonverbal behavior of individuals raised in North America is likely to reflect that background.

SPECIAL COUNSELLING SITUATIONS

Some situations in self-care counselling require additional attention to communication skills. Although it is difficult to generalize, the following sections outline approaches to help the health professional in three areas: discussing potentially embarrassing subjects; counselling overtalkative people; and counselling hearing-impaired older consumers.

POTENTIALLY EMBARRASSING SUBJECTS

In self-care counselling, the health professional often encounters subjects that embarrass the consumer. It is easy to forget that some people are acutely distressed by any discussion relating to sex, intimate body parts or bodily functions. Purchasers of laxatives, suppositories, enemas, hemorrhoid preparations or vaginal creams may be reluctant to discuss problems with the health professional. The social implications of certain products may also cause embarrassment, as when teenagers buy their first package of condoms or parents purchase a pediculicide for their children.

Most embarrassing situations can be predicted and handled in a smooth, professional manner. With attention to specific communication skills, health professionals can reduce the likelihood of embarrassing an individual and can take appropriate steps to set obviously embarrassed people at ease.

As a first step, the health professional should anticipate topics that might be embarrassing. In these cases, the discussion should be general at first with questions structured from less personal to more personal areas. This gives people time to observe the health professional's approach and see that sensitive issues will be addressed in a professional manner.

When personal questions must be asked, it is best to avoid open ones. People usually find it easier to answer closed questions in embarrassing situations. For example, someone requesting a pediculicide may be uncomfortable responding to the question "Where do you have the problem?" If the health professional explains that the area to be treated affects the choice of product, it becomes relatively easy to answer "Yes." or "No." to "Is it in the groin area?" Another approach is to provide relevant information and let the consumer choose the proper formulation. For instance, with the information "The lotion or shampoo is used for the groin area, the shampoo for the scalp, and cream or lotion for the skin," most consumers can choose the best product for their symptoms.

In any potentially sensitive situation, the health professional should provide as much privacy as possible for the discussion. (See the section on nonverbal communication.) Voice level is also important: when other people are near, the health professional should use a low tone so consumers understand their privacy is respected. At the same time, a hushed voice may suggest there is something to be embarrassed about and should be avoided.

Health professionals also need to project a degree of comfort with subjects of a personal nature. Apart from avoiding a subject altogether, one of the worst things a health professional can do is discuss a delicate problem vaguely or euphemistically. For example, if the health professional says, "Does it hurt down there where, uh, you know." may make consumers feel they must also avoid using words like vagina or groin.

At the other extreme, some health professionals may attempt to compensate for discomfort by using street language or making light of a situation. Or they may feel they are creating an open and relaxed atmosphere by speaking bluntly. Although important advice may be given, consumers may be so embarrassed by the brash approach, they tune out anything useful the health professional says.

The best terminology for potentially sensitive topics is straightforward, matter-of-fact words. Technical terminology is especially awkward in sensitive situations; if people do not know the meaning of a word, they may be too embarrassed to ask. In these instances, extra effort should be made to use understandable terms, and to rephrase a question or response if the other person seems confused.

Closely related, certain terms may have emotional overtones. Saying symptoms rather than naming a particular problem (e.g., lice) and choosing words like fluid instead of pus, and pain reliever rather than narcotic, reduce the chances of upsetting an individual. An open approach at the beginning of the interview helps identify words with which the consumer is comfortable. By using a common vocabulary, the health professional can help people feel more comfortable discussing sensitive issues.

Despite the health professional's best intentions, people may still be embarrassed in sensitive situations. Sometimes the response is obvious—a blush or stammer is relatively easy to read—but often the message is more subtle, and the health professional must pay close attention to the consumer's nonverbal behavior. Signals such as indirect or seemingly pointless questions, general evasiveness, or hesitations may point to a consumer who is embarrassed or concerned that the discussion will not be kept in confidence.

A natural tendency in these situations is to tell the person not to be embarrassed. Although some form of reassurance may be in order, judgments about a person's reaction should be avoided. Health professionals who say "There's no reason to be embarrassed." have not solved the problem—people are embarrassed whether they should be or not. Similarly, one should avoid any tendency to laugh or tease. If someone thinks a health professional is intentionally poking fun at a delicate situation, an automatic barrier to effective communication is created. Even lighthearted teasing, such as sometimes accompanies the need for a laxative or antidiarrheal, should be avoided.

If embarrassment interferes with the transfer of information, two techniques may be appropriate. A comment like "You seem to be having difficulty talking about this." is intended to encourage discussion about the source of embarrassment. Closely related, a statement that recognizes the feelings of the other person (empathy) may be helpful. An empathic statement might be something like "I know it can be difficult to talk about this subject." followed by attentive silence. Again, once people are given an opportunity to verbalize their embarrassment, they may be better able to continue the discussion.

No more than one or two such statements are appropriate in any given discussion. It is important not to push too far with pointed and detailed questions. Despite the health professional's attempts to respect a person's privacy, to use appropriate language and to provide opportunities to discuss a problem, some people do not want to open up. The best route in these situations is to provide as much information as possible and leave an opening, such as "If you have any questions about these products, I'll be happy to answer them." As well, written material is one alternative for informing consumers in these situations.

TALKATIVE CONSUMERS

A difficult problem for experienced and beginning practitioners alike is the talkative consumer. These people are often seen as barriers to efficiency and may be a major source of irritation. Although complete control is usually impossible, a number of techniques can increase the productivity of discussions with these people.

One type of talkative person is the obsessive individual, who insists on giving an overdetailed account of symptoms. When interviewing such people, health professionals should be particularly aware of their own nonverbal behavior, avoiding overfacilitation with encouraging nods, gestures or phrases. Instead, health professionals should limit their show of interest in trivial data, and show greater interest when relevant information is provided. Closed questions can be introduced earlier in the questioning. A courteous interruption when enough information has been obtained about a given point, followed by another specific question, keeps the interview focused and makes it possible to obtain information in a reasonable period of time. A mental image of the order in which questioning is to proceed is particularly helpful in these situations, because it increases the health professional's ability to refocus the discussion into areas where information is required.

Another type of talkative person is one who rambles or shows similar evidence of confusion and poor organization. A polite interruption is appropriate when these people wander away from the topic at hand. Bridging, or transition, is a particularly useful technique. The following example illustrates how bridging and the use of specific questions might work with a talkative person:

Consumer (with stomach upset): And my husband—he's a teacher you know—he's going to take March break off—he usually doesn't but I insisted this time—and we're going skiing. I think we'll probably go to Lake Louise—maybe not, maybe we'll go to that new place (slight pause). . . .

Health professional: It sounds like a wonderful time and I can see you are excited about getting away. Since you'll be travelling, it might be best if I gave you a tablet form of antacid. Are you having any gas with the stomach upset?

Written material also is helpful with these people. Pointing out directions or instructions on a product container or written sheet attracts consumers' attention. Since they are concentrating on the written word, they are less likely to interrupt with unrelated thoughts.

A third type of talkative person is the one who makes every attempt to prolong a discussion. Many of these people simply cannot be hurried. The health professional may choose to continue chatting (depending on the time available), or several techniques for closing an interview can help one exit these situations gracefully. The first is a summation of important points covered during the interview. Not only does this technique reinforce information, but it subtly indicates that the discussion is coming to a close. Following summation, the health professional can use sentences that have concluding words, such as "Well, I think that about covers it. Do you have any questions?" or "If you have any questions, please feel free to call." Certain nonverbal behavior can also be a powerful form of communication; adopting a closed stance is an effective but discreet way to signal that the discussion is finished. Last but not least, health professionals may indicate they need to terminate the discussion. Most people respect a clinician whose manner suggests strength and self-assurance. They are not offended by an assertive but polite statement, such as "I'd really like to hear more about . . . sometime, but I do need to get back to these prescriptions."

OLDER CONSUMERS

Counselling older consumers can present a challenge for the health professional. In addition to increased pharmacological and therapeutic considerations, some seniors have a degree of sensory loss that makes the exchange of information difficult and frustrating for both parties.

The most common sensory deficit accompanying aging is hearing-impairment, a general term used to describe all hearing problems from minute loss to profound deafness. Compared to a rate of about 10% in the total population, an estimated 60% of individuals over age 65 have some degree of impairment. At least 35% of these individuals experience enough hearing loss to interfere with normal conversation.

The older adult is extremely susceptible to drug-use problems and often benefits most from a discussion with the health professional. Declining physical function usually requires multiple medications, and although seniors represent one-tenth of the population, they consume one-quarter of all prescribed medication. In addition, several surveys have identified this group as major consumers of certain nonprescription products. This use of drug products, coupled with the fact that several physicians are likely to be involved in an older person's care, makes screening for drug interactions particularly important. Physiological changes associated with aging may also alter the presentation of certain illnesses (e.g., older people may not mount fevers to the same degree as younger people), which complicates the assessment of certain conditions. Similarly, altered response to drugs places seniors at greater risk for adverse reactions, a factor that must be taken into account when assessing complaints and recommending products.

The growing number of older people makes it increasingly important to understand and respond to their needs. Currently about 10% of the Canadian population, this age group is projected to increase to about 17.6% of the population in the next 50 years.

Counselling the Hearing-Impaired

The most common form of hearing loss in older people is presbycusis, a communication disorder characterized by progressive degenerative breakdown in auditory function. It causes a loss in level as well as clarity of hearing, which makes speech difficult to hear and understand. Specific techniques for communicating with these people are divided into nonverbal, or attending, communication skills and verbal communication skills.

Attending communication skills refer to all nonverbal considerations in communication. Although important in any counselling situation, these are crucial for the hearing-impaired, who are as dependent on nonverbal communication as they are on the spoken word.

The first consideration is to select a quiet environment for the discussion. A common misconception about hearing-impairment is that the level at which a person can hear simply declines. However, a major characteristic of hearing-impairment (called auditory discrimination difficulty) is a disproportionate and increased sensitivity to sounds. This sensitivity, coupled with distortion of sound within the auditory system, makes it extremely difficult to differentiate between background noise and a speaker's voice.

Hearing aids generally do not correct auditory discrimination difficulties, so the need for a quiet environment applies equally to these people.

Second, ensure there is good lighting. Many hearing-impaired people rely on lipreading. The counselling area should provide good lighting for the health professional's face and upper body so people can take advantage of important visual cues. Similarly, individuals should be positioned so they do not have to look into bright or concentrated sources of light (such as lamps or sunshine) to see the health professional. Looking into light makes it extremely difficult to see a speaker's face, and attempts at lipreading will be quickly frustrated. Other distractions that make lipreading difficult include pencil-chewing, placing hands near or on the lips, and moustaches that cover the mouth.

Third, the health professional should face the consumer. It is important to look directly at the individual, as even a slight turn of the head can obscure the lips. If the consumer is sitting, it will help to sit or bend down so the conversation takes place face-to-face. Good eye contact helps convey a feeling of direct communication.

Finally, the health professional should indicate when he or she is ready to speak. A common cue when someone is about to speak is an audible intake of breath immediately before the first word. The hearing-impaired often miss this cue. To ensure the first parts of a sentence are not missed, health professionals should use another cue to indicate when they are ready to speak. Attention can be attracted with an upraised hand, a tap on the shoulder or arm, or simply by making eye contact before speaking.

Pathophysiological changes within the auditory system make attention to verbal communication skills equally important.

First, the health professional should consider voice level. A natural tendency with the hard-of-hearing is to shout. However, since increased sensitivity and distortion of loud sounds is characteristic of hearing-impairment, a shouted message is less likely to be understood. The best results are achieved when one speaks slowly and distinctly, using a well-modulated and firm tone of voice. At the same time, exaggerating or overemphasizing words makes lipreading difficult. The best rule is to speak clearly and naturally.

Second, the health professional should pay attention to voice pitch. Most older people have difficulty hearing high-frequency sounds. Lowering the pitch may help. Female health professionals, in particular, may need to adjust the pitch of their voices when speaking with seniors.

Third, pacing needs to be considered. Older adults, particularly the hearing-impaired, may have difficulty understanding speech as a result of delayed central processing and reaction time. Because these people take longer to process a message, a slow and relaxed pace should be consciously maintained. Particularly during the assessment phase, ample time must be given for responses to the health professional's questions. Consumers also should be encouraged to ask for repetition when a message is not understood.

Periods of silence are common when talking with the hearing-impaired older adult. Silence should not be regarded as a breakdown in communication unless it persists for an extended period of time, for example, more than 20 or 30 seconds. These pauses may simply reflect an attempt to interpret an instruction or recall a fact. As noted earlier, the health professional should wait attentively during these silences.

Finally, the health professional should pay close attention to vocabulary. Consonant discrimination is often more difficult for the hearing-impaired. Short, simple sentences and a familiar vocabulary consisting of words of as few syllables as possible (e.g., drug or pills instead of medication or prescription) are usually easier to comprehend. Re-emphasizing the same point in various ways is also preferable to repeating the same phrase several times. The health professional should be careful not to overload the individual with information. Elderly people in particular may be confused by large amounts of information and, confronted with an abundance of facts, may decide to ignore part or all of what is said. As well, sudden changes in subject matter are hard to follow with diminished hearing acuity; explaining when a new subject is about to be discussed helps avoid confusion.

An attitude of respect and consideration is vital to effective communication with the hearing-impaired person. The health professional must keep in mind that hearing-impairment is not a problem of intelligence, but rather of physical disability. If individuals interpret altered and simplified patterns of speech as condescending, they are likely to dismiss the health professional's advice.

Counselling the Deaf Person

Many of the above techniques are equally applicable to deaf people. In addition, some people communicate with paper and pencil, in which case the health professional should do the same. Others use interpreters who are familiar with their sign language. If an interpreter is present, the health professional should speak directly to the deaf person, maintaining eye contact throughout the discussion to convey a feeling of direct communication. Addressing the interpreter with questions such as, "Does he always take it in pill form?" or "Will she remember to mix it with water?" should be avoided. This approach to a deaf person can be both degrading and impersonal.

Recognizing the Hearing-Impaired

Many people are reluctant to disclose a hearing problem. They may accept hearing loss as an inevitable part of aging and not feel the need to mention it. Conversely, they may ignore the disability because they are uncomfortable with the idea of getting older. Others are so fed up with having to say "Pardon?" they eventually give up all attempt to communicate. With any of these people, the health professional needs to be alert to characteristic behaviors of hearing loss so appropriate communication techniques can be implemented.

A common clue to partial hearing-impairment is when a person tilts his or her head so the good ear is directed toward the speaker. Other important nonverbal behaviors include a blank facial expression during conversation, restless limb movements or irregular posture shifts, and noticeable attempts to read lips. Verbal clues include frequent requests for repetition, special difficulty with rapid speech, a loud voice, abnormal spacing or pauses while speaking, and the omission of word endings, especially those with high-frequency sounds such as t, s, sh, f and v.

Although not always receptive to this advice, individuals identified as hearing-impaired should be encouraged to seek audiology assessment and therapy. Most, if not all, communities have a Canadian Hearing Society office or contact person who can help. Along with a number of excellent programs and services for the hearing-impaired, this group offers a variety of materials for the health professional who deals with the hearing-impaired.

SUMMARY

Self-care counselling has undergone renewed interest in the past several years. Increasing numbers of people are moving toward self-care as a treatment alternative, and studies show that health professionals are seen as a valuable source of information. To help meet the growing demand for this service, the health professional needs to be able to make the best use of time available for counselling consumers about self-treatment.

Health professionals must be able to elicit and define an individual's problem so the best advice can be given. Interviewing is the principle tool used; other communication skills described in this chapter will help improve the effectiveness, efficiency and ease with which self-care counselling is conducted. As with other skills, the ability to counsel individual consumers takes practice and continued awareness of ways in which this process can be improved.

RECOMMENDED READING

Ley P. Communicating with Patients. Improving Communication, Satisfaction and Compliance. New York: Croom Helm, 1988.

Smith CE, ed. Patient Education: Nurses in Partnership with Other Health Professionals. Orlando: Grune & Stratton, 1987.

Rantucci MJ. Talking with Patients: a Pharmacist's Guide to Patient Counselling. Kingston, Ontario: Weathervane Books, 1990.

Tindall WN, Beardsley RS, Kimberlin CL. Communication in Pharmacy Practice: A Practical Guide for Students and Practitioners. Philadelphia: Lea & Febiger, 1994.

3

SPECIAL PATIENT GROUPS

EILEEN YOSHIDA

CONTENTS

Older Individuals 39
- Physiological Changes
- Other Considerations

Infants and Children 44
- Pharmacokinetic Principles
- Reye's Syndrome
- General Administration Instructions

Pregnancy and Lactation 46
- Pregnancy
- Lactation

Individuals with Chronic Diseases 51
- Hypertension
- Cardiovascular Disease
- Hyperthyroidism
- Glaucoma
- Benign Prostatic Hypertrophy and Bladder Neck Obstruction
- Diabetes

Recommended Reading 56

OLDER INDIVIDUALS

In 1950 there were about one million Canadians 65 years of age or older, less than 8% of the population; in 1979 there were two million, 9% of the population. By the year 2025, people 65 years of age or older will number almost six million, 17% of the Canadian population.

The elderly are the greatest consumers of health care resources, including pharmaceuticals. The Canada Health Survey showed that in 1981, about 75% of those 65 years of age or older (compared to less than half of the general population) were taking at least one prescription or nonprescription drug, and that 1 in 5 were taking multiple drugs. Still another report claimed that in 1986, 25% of all prescription drugs were taken by those 65 years of age or older.

Because the elderly may have more than one chronic illness, multiple drug use is common and can present a number of problems. Individuals may see more than one physician, each (perhaps unknowingly) prescribing independently, potentially leading to duplication of therapy, drug-drug interactions or the prescribing of agents that may aggravate another condition. Patients may not volunteer information about nonprescription drug use as they may be unaware these medications are harmful in some situations and can modify the desired effects of prescription drugs. The incidence of serious reportable adverse effects increases with age and the number of drugs taken. In North America, 10 to 25% of all hospital admissions for the elderly are the result of untoward drug effects, including falls associated with drugs that may be sedating, have hypotensive effects, or impair balance or reaction time.

Cultural influences, undesirable side effects of some medications and complicated regimens—especially those that require significant changes in an individual's lifestyle, are inconvenient or costly—may all be contributing factors. Physical limitations, such as difficulty opening childproof vials or swallowing problems, may also result in noncompliance. Memory deficits, inability to read written directions due to poor eyesight or hear verbal instructions due to hearing loss, may prevent a patient from taking their medications as directed.

Certain nonprescription drugs that should be used with caution in the elderly are presented in Table 1.

PHYSIOLOGICAL CHANGES

A number of physiological changes occur in older individuals as a normal consequence of aging. Because there is great variation, physiological age is much more important than chronological age. This is only a brief review; expanded information should be sought elsewhere.

Senses: Visual and auditory acuity are diminished and the visual field somewhat reduced. These changes require special consideration when counselling the elderly. For example, it may be impossible for an older patient to identify each tablet by color, size or shape due to impaired vision. There is a reduction in the number of taste buds with a diminished ability to taste sweet, sour and bitter, but not salty foods. Liquid medications, although palatable to most people, may not taste good to older individuals.

Central Nervous System (CNS): With age there is a decline in some intellectual functions involving speed of response, unfamiliar material and complexity of task. There are also changes in memory, particularly recall of information in short-term memory. Complicated drug regimens should be simplified as much as possible and instructions to patients made clear to decrease the risk of noncompliance. Older individuals can be particularly sensitive to the adverse CNS effects of nonprescription narcotic analgesics, first generation antihistamines and skeletal muscle relaxants.

Gastrointestinal Tract: Gastrointestinal transit time is increased in older individuals, and the ingestion of nonprescription products containing iron, calcium carbonate, or first-generation antihistamines may cause constipation, especially in those less mobile.

The elderly may suffer from dry mouth as a normal consequence of aging, which can be further exacerbated by the anticholinergic effects of some drugs, including first-generation antihistamines. Because of xerostomia they may have difficulty tasting, masticating and even swallowing food. Decreased secretion of salivary enzymes that initiate carbohydrate digestion impairs digestion. These changes may ultimately contribute to malnutrition. Individuals with dry mouth are also more susceptible to secondary bacterial and fungal infections including candidiasis.

Musculoskeletal System: Age-related changes in skeletal profile, a change in the centre of gravity, decreased muscle strength as well as sensory input and nerve conduction impairment make balance more precarious for older individuals and cause them to fall. The use of drugs that are sedating (e.g., first-generation antihistamines), hypotensive or that further impair balance or reaction time increases the likelihood of a fall. Osteoporosis and osteopenia increase the risk of fractures following even relatively minor trauma.

Skin: With age there is an increase in epidermal permeability to water and certain chemicals (e.g., nonprescription steroid preparations).

Endocrine System: Impaired glucose tolerance and thyroid dysfunction are common problems in older patients, and drugs affecting glucose metabolism and thyroid function should be used with caution. Decreased estrogen production predisposes elderly women to osteoporosis.

There is no change in temperature perception in older individuals, although the thermoregulatory response to cold may be impaired. This complex response involves the integration of numerous systems, any one of which may be deficient. The elderly may have an increased pain threshold, and falls and fractures can occur without much apparent distress.

OTHER CONSIDERATIONS

Pharmacokinetics

Pharmacokinetics refers to all aspects of drug disposition in the body including absorption, distribution, metabolism and elimination. The aging process is associated with several physiological changes that can modify the pharmacokinetics of many drugs, resulting in an altered pharmacological response.

Absorption: Various changes that could theoretically modify the absorption of many drugs occur in the elderly (Table 2). Decreased gastric acidity could affect the absorption of weakly acidic drugs, resulting in a delayed onset of action. Absorption may be decreased for drugs that require an acid pH in the stomach (e.g., iron salts). Slower gastric emptying times may result in potentially ulcerogenic drugs, such as NSAIDs, having more contact with the stomach; drugs predominantly absorbed in the upper intestine may have a delayed onset of action. A reduction in the number of absorbing

TABLE 1: Nonprescription Drugs That Should be Used with Caution in Older Individuals

Drug	Effect	Explanation/Examples
Antacids	Drug interaction	Aluminum- and/or magnesium-, calcium-containing antacids form insoluble, poorly absorbed compounds with tetracycline, quinolone antibiotics, iron, digoxin
		Ketoconazole requires acidic medium for dissolution and absorption; antacids increase gastric pH, therefore, may inhibit ketoconazole absorption
	Toxicity	Chronic and/or excessive use of sodium bicarbonate, calcium-, aluminum- and/or magnesium-containing antacids may result in ion accumulation and subsequent toxicity in older individuals with poor renal function
Nonprescription narcotic analgesics, first-generation antihistamines	Toxicity	Chronic and/or excessive use may result in CNS toxicity (sedation, dizziness, confusion, disturbed coordination) especially in older individuals taking other drugs with CNS side effects
Saline laxatives	Toxicity	Chronic and/or excessive use may result in accumulation of component ions (magnesium, sulfate, phosphate), especially in older individuals with poor renal function; dehydration may also occur
Mineral oil laxatives	Toxicity	Lipid pneumonia may result from aspiration, especially when ingested orally at bedtime by the elderly, debilitated or dysphagic
NSAIDs	Drug interaction	Chronic and/or high doses of NSAIDs may decrease antihypertensive and/or antidiuretic effects of beta-blockers, ACE inhibitors, diuretics secondary to inhibition of prostaglandin synthesis
		Concurrent administration of chronic NSAID therapy and oral anticoagulants may result in increased risk of bleeding episodes
First-generation antihistamines, scopolamine	Toxicity	Anticholinergic (side) effects may be particularly troublesome to older individuals who have chronic conditions which may be exacerbated or are receiving other drugs with significant anticholinergic side effects
Calcium	Drug interaction	Calcium ingestion from calcium-containing antacids may inhibit activity of calcium channel blockers by increasing the extracellular calcium concentration
		Co-administration of large doses of calcium with thiazide diuretics can result in the development of milk-alkali syndrome
Iron	Drug interaction	Iron salts inhibit quinolone antibiotic absorption by binding to it in the gastrointestinal tract

cells minimizes the surface area available for drug absorption. Impaired active transport mechanisms can limit the absorption of calcium, thiamine and iron.

However, despite these physiological changes, impaired absorption does not appear to be a major clinical problem in older individuals. The most common cause of altered drug absorption in the elderly is drug-drug interactions. For example, many older individuals use and misuse antacids, which can decrease the absorption of certain drugs (e.g., tetracycline, quinolone antibiotics, ketoconazole, digoxin) if administered concurrently, resulting in therapeutic failures.

Distribution: The volume of distribution of many drugs is likely altered in older individuals in comparison with younger adults. Although body weight

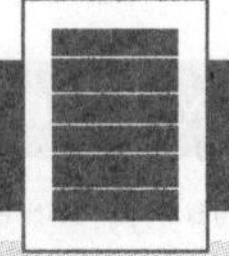

TABLE 2: Physiologic Changes in the Elderly That May Affect Drug Absorption

Increased gastric pH

Delayed gastric emptying

Decreased GI motility

Decreased number of absorbing cells

Decreased splanchnic blood flow

Impaired active transport

remains constant, there are changes in the relative proportions of body composition that affect both water-soluble and fat-soluble drugs. There is a 25 to 30% loss in lean body mass and a doubling of adipose tissue weight. Total body water decreases by 17%, decreasing the volume of distribution of water-soluble drugs with a resultant increase in drug serum concentration levels and greater risk of toxicity. This decrease in total body water may also render older individuals more sensitive to fluid and electrolyte disturbances caused by aggressive laxative use. In addition, adipose tissue can serve as a drug reservoir for lipophilic drugs, increasing drug accumulation, prolonging duration of action and delaying onset of action.

Drug distribution can also be affected by serum protein binding. The elderly have a decrease in plasma proteins, such as albumin, and an increase in α_1-acid glycoprotein (AAG), which accounts for the majority of serum protein binding. For example, albumin is the major protein to which acidic drugs are bound. The serum concentration of albumin may decline between 10 and 20% in old age (although the decline may be minimal in healthy older individuals). Since unbound (e.g., free) drug is the active form of the drug, the effect of highly protein bound drugs, such as phenytoin or warfarin, may be intensified. However, unbound drug is also more susceptible to clearance from the body; thus, the clinical consequences of altered protein binding in the elderly will depend on the degree of protein binding, the specific protein(s) to which the drug is predominantly bound and the clearance characteristics of the drug in question. The relationship between age and AAG concentration is not as well defined.

Metabolism: Metabolism is the sum of all chemical reactions involved in the biotransformation of foreign compounds to more polar, water-soluble, ionized structures that can be eliminated more easily. Various age-related physiological changes occur in the liver that could affect drug metabolism.

Specific liver changes in older individuals include a decline in liver weight, decreased hepatic blood flow, increased liver dysfunction and decreased intrinsic enzyme activity affecting drugs metabolized by the mixed-function oxidase system. In general, phase I oxidation reactions decrease with age while phase II reactions are usually unaffected. A decrease in hepatic blood flow is important for drugs that are highly extracted by the liver as their clearance is dependent on their rate of delivery to the liver by the hepatic circulation. The bioavailability of flow-dependent drugs may be increased due to a reduction in the presystemic metabolism secondary to a decrease in the liver blood flow. Finally, the aging liver may be influenced by some inducing agents to a lesser degree than that observed in younger individuals.

Elimination: Renal elimination is often considered the most important route of drug elimination from the body. Changes that occur in older individuals include a decrease in the number of functioning nephrons and decreased renal perfusion secondary to arteriosclerosis and decreased cardiac output. These changes can significantly alter the elimination of drugs and metabolites that are predominantly renally excreted. Judicious use of aluminum- and/or magnesium-, calcium- or sodium bicarbonate-containing antacids, and magnesium-, sulfate-, or phosphate-containing laxatives is cautioned in patients with poor renal function, or accumulation and resultant toxicity of the component ion occur. Reduced doses and/or prolonged dosing intervals for many drugs are often necessary in the elderly.

Pharmacodynamics

Older individuals may have an altered tissue responsiveness that renders them more or less sensitive to the pharmacologic actions of some drugs. Baroreceptor sensitivity declines with age, which increases the risk of postural hypotension. Drugs that affect blood pressure or produce postural hypotension as a side effect should be used with caution in the elderly as it has been well documented that these medications have been associated with falls, and subsequent fractures, in the elderly.

Compliance

Noncompliance, either intentional or unintentional, is another problem in older individuals that may have serious consequences. Various authors disagree on whether age, per se, is a risk factor for problems with compliance. However, most agree that patients who have insight into their illness and perceive benefits from taking their medications are more likely to comply with medication instructions than those who do not. By identifying these issues, drug-taking behavior in the elderly can be optimized.

In summary, the aging process is associated with a number of physiological changes that affect the pharmacokinetics and pharmacodynamics of many drugs or require special attention by health care professionals and other caregivers. Some general recommendations can be made when considering drug therapy in older individuals. Nonpharmacological management should be tried first. If drugs are needed, lower doses and/or prolonged dosing intervals, with slow upward titration as needed, are prudent. Drug regimens should be kept as simple as possible to minimize the risk of adverse drug reactions, drug-drug interactions and to enhance compliance. Older individuals (or their caregivers) should be encouraged to have only one primary care physician and to frequent one pharmacy. The importance of sharing information as much as possible with all health care professionals (e.g., specialists) so that they can make informed decisions should be stressed. All patients should have a clear understanding of what drugs they are taking and why. Any modification to drug therapy (e.g., drug addition and deletion, changes in dose or frequency) should be explained to the individual. Taking someone else's medication should be discouraged. Alternative dosage formulations may benefit those who have difficulty swallowing tablets or capsules; many medications are available as oral liquids or suppositories. Additionally, some tablets may be crushed (e.g., acetaminophen, dimenhydrinate) and some capsules may be opened and their contents suspended in food or water for increased ease of administration. Patients who have difficulty opening childproof vials should make special arrangements to have their medications dispensed in easy-to-open vials or dosettes. Finally, when counselling older individuals, possible deficits in hearing, eyesight or memory should be considered. Written instructions that are clearly visible to the patient may help reinforce clear verbal communication.

INFANTS AND CHILDREN

The effects of many drugs in infants and children can vary significantly from those seen in adults. Dosage regimens extrapolated from adult data and merely adjusted for body weight or surface area of pediatric patients are not always appropriate. Intensified or even toxic effects of drugs administered to children may reflect variations in drug disposition. The absorption, distribution, metabolism and elimination of many drugs may also differ among pediatric patients because of differences in age, organ function and disease states.

The first step when using drugs in the pediatric population is understanding the age-related alterations in drug disposition.

PHARMACOKINETIC PRINCIPLES

Absorption: The absorption of many drugs from the gastrointestinal tract is dependent on a number of factors, all of which may vary according to age.

Many drugs are absorbed by passive diffusion that is pH-dependent in the gastrointestinal tract. In a full-term infant, gastric pH ranges from 6 to 8 at birth but declines to 1 to 3 within 24 hours. The gastric pH in premature infants may remain elevated initially because of immature acid secretion. It is not until 3 to 7 years of age that adult levels of gastric acidity are attained. A higher gastric pH means that drugs that are weak acids (e.g., phenobarbital, phenytoin) may be more slowly absorbed in pediatric patients while weak bases (e.g., penicillin) are preferentially absorbed.

Gastric emptying time is prolonged up to 6 to 8 hours in the immediate newborn period (0 to 24 hours) for both full-term and preterm neonates and does not approach adult values until 6 to 8 months of age. Thus, drugs that may not be well absorbed in adults may be better absorbed in infants because of prolonged contact time with the gastrointestinal mucosa.

Another factor influencing drug absorption is the changing biochemistry of the developing gastrointestinal tract. Differences in the activity of various enzymes and the continued development of the intestinal bacterial flora must be considered.

Percutaneous absorption may be substantially increased in newborns because of an underdeveloped epidermal barrier and increased skin hydration. Skin vascularization and glandular development are also important. Pediatric drug absorption from intramuscular sites may be highly erratic compared to older children and adults because of differences in relative muscle mass, blood flow to various muscles, peripheral vasomotor instability and insufficient muscle contraction.

Distribution: Drug distribution is determined by the physicochemical properties of a drug and the physiological factors specific to the patient. While the physicochemical properties of a drug are constant, patient physiology varies among different age groups.

Body composition differs markedly with age. The infant body is composed of a much higher proportion of water and lower proportion of fat compared to adults. As the infant ages, water content progressively decreases and fat content increases. Since drugs are distributed between the extracellular fluid and fat according to the lipid-water partition coefficient, the relative proportions of these two body constituents influence drug distribution.

Age-related changes in drug-protein binding can substantially alter the pharmacokinetics of a drug. Plasma protein binding is decreased in newborns because of decreased plasma protein concentration, lower binding capacity of protein, decreased affinity of proteins for drug binding, and competition for certain binding sites by endogenous compounds, such as bilirubin. The free (unbound) fraction of drug is the active form but is also subject to immediate body clearance.

Metabolism: The capacity to metabolize drugs varies throughout development. In general, metabolism is slower in infants compared with older children and adults although the various pathways of metabolism mature at different rates. For example, the sulfation pathway is well developed, but the glucuronidation pathway is not matured in infants. Oxidation is impaired in newborns.

Elimination: Drugs and their metabolites are often eliminated by the kidney. The processes of glomerular filtration, tubular secretion and reabsorption determine the efficiency of renal excretion, and each of these processes matures at a different rate. Neonates may have prolonged elimination half-lives of some drugs because of their inefficiency in eliminating drugs.

REYE'S SYNDROME

Reye's syndrome is an infrequent but serious disease, primarily affecting children 5 to 15 years of age and, rarely, young adults. Reye's syndrome typically occurs in a child recovering from a viral illness (e.g., influenza, chickenpox) and is characterized by vomiting, lethargy, confusion, irritability or aggressiveness. Mortality is high, between 22 and 42%. Autopsy reveals fatty infiltration of the liver, cerebral edema and encephalopathy. Although the evidence is not conclusive, several large epidemiological studies have supported an association between salicylate ingestion and the development of Reye's syndrome. Currently, ASA is not recommended as first-line therapy in the pediatric population, especially in influenza-like illnesses or chickenpox. Acetaminophen is the current drug of choice in children.

GENERAL ADMINISTRATION INSTRUCTIONS

Administration of medications to the pediatric population can be a challenge from a number of perspectives. Not all drugs are approved for use in children; therefore, official dosing recommendations may be difficult to obtain and the prescriber may have to rely on case reports in lieu of rigorous scientific data. Secondly, suitable dosage forms may not be available, and dilution of highly concentrated drugs intended for adult administration may be necessary, although it is preferable to use an accurate measuring device, such as an oral syringe, rather than dilute an appropriately flavored and stabilized product.

In general, children less than 5 years of age often cannot take solid oral dosage forms and may require reformulation of an existing product to an oral liquid preparation. Any modification of the original drug product must be supported by stability data. Whenever possible, it is preferable to crush tablets or open capsules immediately prior to use, and administer the dose suspended in a small amount of applesauce, ice cream or some other pleasant-tasting food or liquid. Note this may destroy the enteric-coating or slow-release formulation of a product.

If a liquid oral dosage formulation is prepared, the solid oral dosage form is reduced to a powder and an appropriate vehicle incorporated in geometric proportions to make a smooth uniform mixture. If an injectable product is used as the basis for the formulation, an appropriate volume is mixed with the vehicle to give a uniform solution. Suspending agents that are inert, nonreactive and pH-neutral are highly desirable. Common suspending vehicles include Simple Syrup B.P., methylcellulose 1 to 2%, Aromatic Elixir DTC, distilled water and sorbitol 70%; many children's hospitals have formulated their own vehicles. Preservatives and flavorings may be added if necessary. The number of ingredients included in extemporaneous formulations for neonates, especially premature infants, are kept to a minimum. The pH of a product is also a consideration if the drug exhibits pH-dependent degradation. If pH adjustment is necessary, it is usually to the acidic range by adding citric acid and using a pH indicator paper to determine the endpoint. Many formulations for oral liquid dosage preparations are documented in the literature or may be obtained by contacting the local children's hospital. If used, the formulations should be followed exactly when preparing the dosage form.

Drug therapy in the pediatric population can present a number of problems, unique to this age group. Table 3 lists certain nonprescription drugs that should be used with caution in children.

TABLE 3: Nonprescription Drugs That Should be Used with Caution in Children

Drug	Effect
First-generation antihistamines e.g., dimenhydrinate, promethazine, chlorpheniramine	Usually cause sedation in adults but children sometimes develop paradoxical excitation, manifested as restlessness, nervousness, palpitations, seizures
Laxatives	Excess use can lead to diarrhea and problems with dehydration

PREGNANCY AND LACTATION

The risks versus the benefits must always be weighed when treating patients with drugs. Nowhere is this problem better illustrated than in the treatment of pregnant and lactating women.

PREGNANCY

It is important to realize that even if a woman does not take any medication during pregnancy, there is always a baseline risk of 1 to 3% for major malformations. This risk is based on chance or factors not yet identified, so there is no way to reduce or eliminate it. On top of this uncertainty, most medications have an unknown risk of teratogenicity, and only a few are specifically indicated for use during pregnancy. The paucity of information available does not represent drug manufacturers' indifference to pursuing this information, but the difficulties in obtaining it. Ethically, studies cannot be performed in this population to ascertain outcome and, unfortunately, animal studies do not always correlate with human fetal risk. Additionally, conclusions drawn from one particular observation made in isolation may not be appropriate for prediction in another situation because of high genetic heterogeneity and exposure to different environments; drug-drug, drug-disease and drug-lifestyle interactions may all render innocuous agents, teratogenic.

Placental transport of maternal substrates to the fetus and vice versa is established by approximately the fifth week of fetal life; low molecular weight substances diffuse freely across the placenta, driven primarily by the concentration gradient. Almost every substance can and does pass from mother to fetus, but what is important is whether the rate and extent of transfer are sufficient to result in significant concentrations within the fetus. The first three months of gestation may be the most critical in terms of physical malformation; however, functional and behavioral defects are associated with later exposure when the brain is still developing. In addition to teratogenesis, health care professionals must be cognizant that the fetus is susceptible to the pharmacological actions of drugs administered in the latter half of pregnancy.

Despite our lack of knowledge, pharmacotherapy is sometimes necessary and vital for the pregnant patient and her unborn child. A recent survey revealed that pregnant women are important consumers of drugs, with an average of 3.1 prescription drugs plus prenatal vitamins during gestation. Of concern to some is the fact that not all drugs are necessary; some people feel that many individuals are overly concerned with their own comfort. Pregnant women may also seek to self-medicate with nonprescription drugs assuming that because of their ease of availability, nonprescription drugs do not produce toxic effects. Health care professionals have a responsibility to ensure that pregnant women understand the potential benefits and risks when taking any medication. Table 4 summarizes important factors to consider when recommending drug therapy for pregnant women. Accurate information should be provided in a calm nonalarming manner. There are many excellent resource centres that can be consulted by health care professionals or patients. Table 5 lists a number of common ailments for which pregnant women may seek nonprescription drugs and the preferred nondrug and drug methods of treatment.

LACTATION

In recent years we have come to appreciate the benefits of breast-feeding our children. The American Academy of Pediatrics' (AAP) position paper emphasizes breast-feeding as the best nutritional mode for infants for the first six months of life. Breast milk also remains a valuable source of immunity and nutrition for infants beyond their first year. Mother's milk contains nutritional and immunologic properties superior to those found in infant formula.

Sometimes, breast-feeding women may require medication, including nonprescription drugs, or may seek them, thinking that because they are available without a prescription, they cannot be too strong and, therefore, could not harm their child.

Nearly all drugs will be present in breast milk following maternal ingestion. Water-soluble nonionized molecules with molecular weights less than 200 pass into breast milk by simple diffusion via the aqueous-filled pores in the capillaries of the breast. The passage of larger molecules depends on their lipid solubility, state of ionization and degree of binding to milk or plasma proteins. Drugs can affect the breast-fed child in two ways: indirectly by suppressing lactation and also directly through excretion in breast milk.

TABLE 4: Drug Therapy for Pregnant and Lactating Women
The use of any drug should be avoided unless absolutely necessary.
Is the drug necessary?
The benefits of drug therapy must outweigh the risks.
Nondrug interventions should be tried first, if appropriate.
The most beneficial agent with the least amount of risk in the lowest possible dose for the shortest possible duration should be chosen; consider local application of drugs to maternal site to minimize systemic drug absorption e.g., nasal decongestants would be preferred over oral products.
A physician should approve prolonged and continuous use and must be contacted if drugs fail to provide relief.
In breast-feeding women, choose drugs that pass poorly into breast milk and that have no active metabolites; consider age of infant as it affects their ability to metabolize and eliminate drugs and plays role in quantity of breast milk received (e.g., younger infants are usually almost entirely breast-fed while infants greater than 6 months require supplemental nutrition); if drug therapy is required, schedule doses so that least amount gets into milk (e.g., have mother take medication just after she has breast-fed her infant or just before infant is due to have lengthy sleep); consider possibility of short abstinence period from breast-feeding if anticipated length of drug therapy is short; remember that drugs which can be given directly to infant, can probably be given to mother during lactation.
Along with any discussion of the risks to the infant of drug ingestion via breast milk one must weigh the risks of not breast-feeding and the risks of use of artificial milk on the infant.

Although they may be present in breast milk, many drugs will have negligible effects on the suckling infant as, in most cases, only very low concentrations of drugs are available (e.g., decreased bioavailability in infants for drugs degraded by acid). Generally, the occasional ingestion of therapeutic doses of most drugs by breast-feeding mothers will have no ill effects on their children. Noncompliance with prescription drugs may be a concern when the breast-feeding mother is overly concerned with the effects of the drug on her infant. They should be counselled that taking drugs during breast-feeding has much less risk to the infant than drug therapy during pregnancy. According to the AAP, with only a few exceptions, most drugs are safe to use during lactation. Of greater concern, is the chronic ingestion of large doses of drugs as drug accumulation is more likely. Neonates may not be able to metabolize and excrete drugs as efficiently as their mothers.

A number of lists of drugs that are acceptable to ingest during lactation have been developed. Unfortunately, many have drawn different conclusions, depending on the authors' interpretation of the data. In fact, the effects of maternal ingestion of most drugs on the suckling infant have not been well studied. Most of the published data come from single case reports that do not provide adequate information; reports of drug concentration in breast milk are often based on single dose measurements and do not account for drug accumulation with repeated doses. Therefore it is difficult to interpret the clinical significance of this information. Table 6 is a compilation of a few of these lists for nonprescription medications.

Each case of maternal ingestion of drugs and its effect on the suckling infant should be evaluated individually. Table 4 lists some important general principles to remember when considering drug therapy. Breast-feeding women should be counselled to consult a health care professional before taking any nonprescription medication. Accurate information should be provided in a calm nonalarming manner. A list of reference texts and articles appears in the Recommended Reading section. All mothers should be aware of the potential risks of drug therapy.

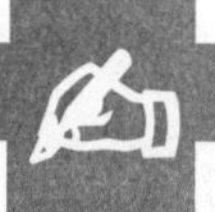

Resource List

Motherisk
Toronto, ON
(416) 813-6780
Ottawa, ON
(613) 737-1100

Safe Start
Hamilton, ON
(905) 525-9140
(ext 2278); or
(905) 521-2100
(ext 2780)

FRAME Program
London, ON
(519) 439-3271
(ext 4378)

B.C. Medical Genetics Program
Vancouver, BC
(604) 875- 2157

TABLE 5: Treatment of Common Medical Problems in Pregnancy

Complaint	Nonpharmacological Intervention	Agent	Contraindications/Comments
Nausea and vomiting	Get plenty of rest Eat small meals at frequent intervals; for early morning symptoms, eat a few dry crackers before getting out of bed Avoid noxious food or odors e.g., spicy or greasy food Increase carbohydrate intake Take vitamin and iron supplementation after meals	*Diclectin* (prescription-requiring); contains doxylamine (antihistamine) and pyridoxine (vitamin B_6)	Nonprescription drugs may be used under direct supervision of physician only; dimenhydrinate has been used
Allergic rhinitis	Avoid allergens Stay indoors	Nonprescription drugs may be used under direct supervision of physician Chlorpheniramine, brompheniramine, diphenhydramine and promethazine have been used Classic antihistamines may be safer than newer agents	Prescription topical corticosteroids may provide relief with minimal risk to patient
Heartburn	Avoid large meals Eat slowly Avoid foods that give you heartburn e.g., greasy or spicy foods; some women avoid coffee and cigarette smoke Drink warm milk Avoid eating just before going to bed Elevate the head of the bed using blocks or use extra pillows to raise the head Avoid stooping, bending or assuming other positions that tend to worsen reflux	Aluminum-and/or magnesium-containing antacids as well as products containing magaldrate Calcium products may provide additional benefits in pregnancy and lactation Alginic acid	Sodium bicarbonate; ASA-containing antacids should be avoided especially in 3rd trimester as it alters normal blood clotting processes and could increase risk of bleeding in mother and/or baby immediately after birth; other potential problems: prolonged gestation and labor, premature closure of ductus arteriosus, neonatal jaundice ASA is a particular risk in 3rd trimester but probably should be avoided throughout pregnancy except under direction of physician
Constipation	Eat foods high in fiber Increase fluid intake Exercise	Bulk laxatives are safest; emollient agents have also been used Osmotic agents may be acceptable for short-term use	Repeat administration of osmotic and stimulant laxatives, including castor oil, should be avoided due to excess fluid and electrolyte loss; mineral oil and castor oil may interfere with absorption of nutrients and fat-soluble vitamins, respectively

TABLE 5: Treatment of Common Medical Problems in Pregnancy *(cont'd)*

Complaint	Nonpharmacological Intervention	Agent	Contraindications/Comments
Hemorrhoids	Avoid constipation and straining An ice pack may help relieve itching Keep anal area clean to avoid irritation Warm sitz baths for 15 minutes, 2–3 times daily may also provide some relief	Nonprescription drugs may be used under direct supervision of physician External products are preferred Products containing astringents, protectants or local anesthetics have been used	
Backache, headache	Relaxation exercises Massage Good posture and lifting techniques; rest in recumbent position; moderate exercise; pelvis tilts; one leg elevation while standing Cool wet cloth to forehead for headaches	Acetaminophen with codeine if necessary; codeine should only be used in smallest dose for shortest treatment period possible	ASA (see notes on heartburn) Other NSAIDs should only be taken under supervision of physician
Common cold	Bed rest Maintain fluids Humidify air	Should only be used under direct supervision of physician; many products contain more than one ingredient including analgesic, decongestant, cough suppressant or expectorant and/or antihistamine Use of topical decongestants is preferred over systemic products Cough and throat lozenges are unlikely to have systemic effects If drugs are needed, they should be used sparingly and for the shortest treatment period possible	
Vitamin and mineral supplementation	Eat a well-balanced diet	Folic acid supplementation (400 µg daily) is recommended for all women planning to become pregnant, starting before conception to the 12th week of gestation. Folic acid decreases the risk of neural tube defects Should be supplemented under supervision of physician	Megadoses of any vitamin or mineral, especially A, C, D and iron

TABLE 6: Maternal Nonprescription Medication Usually Compatible with Breast-feeding

Drug Category	Comment
Analgesics	Analgesics such as acetaminophen, ASA, ibuprofen and codeine are compatible with breast-feeding when taken occasionally at therapeutic doses; chronically administered ASA, especially at high antirheumatic doses has been associated with bleeding and metabolic acidosis (one case)
Vitamins	When used in normal doses
Laxatives	The safest are bulk-forming agents (at recommended doses) as they do not contain absorbable compounds; other laxatives including anthraquinones have been used with little or no adverse effect to suckling infant; mineral oil, magnesium salts are generally safe
Antidiarrheals	May be safest to prescribe least absorbable compounds such as salicylates or clays, bismuth salts, pectin or charcoal; loperamide has been used safely
Nasal decongestants	Pseudoephedrine has been used Nasal sprays or drops preferred
Antihistamines	Generally thought to pose no hazard to nursing infant; may be associated with symptoms of irritability and lethargy
Antacids	Problems related to acid-base balance are minimal with nonsystemic antacids since they are relatively nonabsorbable; however, cations such as magnesium and aluminum are absorbed from gastrointestinal tract and in theory, may pass into breast milk in significant amounts

INDIVIDUALS WITH CHRONIC DISEASES

HYPERTENSION

Sympathomimetics: Sympathomimetics are found in many cough and cold preparations as nasal decongestants and in ophthalmic decongestants as eye whiteners (vasoconstrictors). These drugs can raise blood pressure, although a compensatory reflex decrease in heart rate may prevent measurable effects. Concomitant ingestion of drugs that increase heart rate may antagonize the reflex buffering effect, resulting in hypertension. Sympathomimetics are available in both oral and topical (nasal and ophthalmic) formulations. Usually, at recommended doses, significant increases in blood pressure do not occur; however, with overuse or overdose, enough drug can be absorbed systemically for hypertension to occur.

The phenylamine group of sympathomimetics include ephedrine, pseudoephedrine, phenylpropanolamine and phenylephrine. These drugs can provoke the release of neuronal norepinephrine with varying degrees of affinity for alpha- and beta-receptors and directly stimulate the receptor site. Few studies have examined the cardiovascular effects of the phenylamines and those that have include small samples of normotensive patients. The effects of these agents on hypertensive patients are not clear.

Significant increases in blood pressure do not usually occur with ephedrine unless single doses greater than 5 to 15 mg are ingested. Single doses of 60 mg have increased blood pressure while 90 mg doses have affected heart rate. Pseudoephedrine, a stereoisomer of ephedrine, has less vasopressor activity than ephedrine, and its decongestant activity occurs at doses lower than that required to cause significant increases in blood pressure. Two studies involving a small number of subjects found that single doses of at least 120 mg of pseudoephedrine (one of the studies indicated 210 mg) were needed to increase the pulse rate and blood pressure in healthy volunteers. Pseudoephedrine is considered to have a very high therapeutic index. Phenylpropanolamine has been studied by a number of investigators with varying results; however, significant increases in blood pressure have been reported with doses of 50 to 85 mg. Although there are concerns regarding the drug's potentially narrow therapeutic index, the Expert Advisory Committee of Health Canada has concluded that doses found in Canadian products pose no significant risk of cardiovascular side effects. Finally, ingestion of 2 to 3 times the recommended single dose quantity of phenylephrine has caused significant elevations in blood pressure in normotensive individuals. Doses of 40 to 60 mg of phenylephrine are required for clinically significant cardiovascular effects; at doses of 25 mg, blood pressure may increase by 7 mmHg. Adverse reactions have also been reported with topical phenylephrine application.

The imidazoline group of sympathomimetic agents includes naphazoline, oxymetazoline, tetrahydrozoline and xylometazoline. These agents possess alpha-agonist activity with no beta-stimulation and are used topically as nasal decongestants. However, they have the potential to cause systemic effects, and occasionally enough drug may be absorbed to produce hypertension.

The health care professional can help patients with hypertension alleviate their cough and cold symptoms. Nonpharmacological treatment is recommended as first-line therapy; however, if drug therapy is required, the use of single entity products is encouraged over multi-ingredient preparations. Cough suppressants and expectorants, as well as antihistamines usually have little or no effect on the cardiovascular system. Patients specifically seeking relief from nasal congestion may benefit from the short-term use of a topical decongestant. Oral decongestants should be reserved for patients whose symptoms do not respond to topical treatment. Of the phenylamines, pseudoephedrine may be the agent least likely to cause a significant rise in blood pressure. Phenylpropanolamine should probably be avoided in patients with hypertension. Recommended doses should not be exceeded and short treatment periods encouraged.

Similar principles guide the use of ocular decongestants in this patient population. Systemic side effects can occur if enough drug is absorbed via the conjunctival vessels or absorption following drainage through the nasolacrimal system. Antihistamines, either systemic or topical, may be a safer choice if an allergic reaction is the cause of irritation.

Nonsteroidal Anti-inflammatory Drugs (NSAIDs): NSAIDs including ASA and ibuprofen, should be used with caution in patients with hypertension.

A meta-analysis has estimated that NSAIDs elevate mean blood pressure by approximately 5 mmHg, over a period of several weeks. However, the magnitude of the effect can vary substantially among patients. In addition, some drugs, including thiazide and loop diuretics, beta-blockers, alpha-blockers and ACE inhibitors, exert their antihypertensive effects through prostaglandins, and will, therefore, have their effects reduced by NSAIDs because they inhibit prostaglandin synthesis. The exact mechanism of NSAIDs' effects on blood pressure is unknown.

Health care professionals should be aware of the possible deterioration in blood pressure control when patients are started on NSAID therapy. Because of the large interpatient variability in response, close monitoring of blood pressure should be encouraged in all patients, especially during the initial period. Older individuals may be at increased risk of adverse effects as they have the highest prevalence of chronic illnesses, including musculoskeletal disorders and hypertension. Acetaminophen should be used if analgesic or antipyretic activity is desired.

CARDIOVASCULAR DISEASE

The use of nonprescription drugs in cardiovascular diseases other than hypertension also requires special consideration.

The development of adverse cardiac effects (e.g., torsades de pointes, ventricular tachycardia or ventricular fibrillation, heart block or cardiac arrest) has been reported in patients ingesting therapeutic doses of terfenadine and astemizole. Reports have been rare and usually develop in patients with a recognizable condition that predisposes them to toxicity.

Any condition or drug that inhibits the body's ability to metabolize terfenadine may result in potentially toxic terfenadine blood concentrations. Concurrent administration of erythromycin (all salts) or ketoconazole and terfenadine has been implicated. Significant interactions have also been reported in patients with liver disease or dysfunction (e.g., hepatitis, alcoholic liver cirrhosis). Although less well established, concurrent ingestion of drugs that increase the QT interval of the ECG (e.g., antiarrhythmics, phenothiazines, tricyclic/tetracyclic antidepressants) or drugs that influence electrolyte balance (e.g., diuretics, corticosteroids, amphotericin B, cisplatin, β_2-agonists) may also predispose patients to develop cardiotoxicity from terfenadine as does pre-existing cardiac or metabolic disease that may cause disturbances in electrolyte balance.

No reports of an interaction between astemizole and ketoconazole or erythromycin have been reported although it is important to note that astemizole is metabolized by the liver and the potential for an interaction with any drug that inhibits hepatic metabolism exists. Patients with severe liver dysfunction may also be unsuitable candidates to receive astemizole. In addition, patients with pre-existing cardiac or metabolic disease that may cause disturbances in electrolyte balance or drugs that increase the QT interval of the ECG or influence electrolyte balance, also predispose patients to develop astemizole-associated cardiotoxicity.

Patients without any predisposing risk factors can safely use terfenadine or astemizole at the recommended dosing regimens. Clinical manifestations of these adverse cardiac events include hypotension, palpitations, tachycardia, fainting/dizziness, chest pain and shortness of breath. Loratadine, chlorpheniramine or cetirizine (not hepatically metabolized but has occasionally caused elevated liver enzymes) are acceptable alternatives for patients in whom either drug is contraindicated.

Patients with congestive heart failure are usually on sodium-restricted diets and should avoid the use of any medications with high sodium content. A number of nonprescription drugs contain a significant amount of sodium (e.g., sodium bicarbonate antacids). These agents should be avoided and the safer calcium carbonate, magnesium and/or aluminum hydroxide, magaldrate or bismuth subsalicylate preparations employed, especially in this patient population. Additionally, NSAIDs, including ASA, which have occasionally been associated with edema and water retention, presumably secondary to the inhibition of prostaglandin synthesis, should be used judiciously in patients with congestive heart failure.

Patients with severely compromised cardiac status, including postmyocardial infarction patients, should avoid straining during defecation. The regular use of a bulk-forming or emollient laxative is recommended for chronic constipation. Mineral oil is another alternative but should be reserved for short treatment periods only.

HYPERTHYROIDISM

Sympathomimetics are found in many cough and cold preparations as nasal decongestants and in ophthalmic decongestants as eye whiteners (vasoconstrictors). These agents should be used with caution in patients with hyperthyroidism because their cardiac-stimulating properties (as discussed in detail under Hypertension) can aggravate the cardiac symptoms of hyperthyroidism.

GLAUCOMA

A number of medications have been associated with the propensity to increase intraocular pressure (IOP) or carry label information cautioning use in glaucoma. The potential for a medication to produce or worsen glaucoma depends on the type of glaucoma, and whether or not the patient is adequately treated.

The most common mechanism by which systemic drugs elevate IOP is pupillary dilation, causing further obstruction of an already narrow angle. In patients with normal open angles, there is less danger that IOP will increase than in patients with narrow angle glaucoma. Topical use of drugs with anticholinergic or sympathomimetic activity is most likely to result in angle closure. Systemic agents should also be used with caution in such patients. Sympathomimetics can be found in many cold preparations because of their decongestant activity and in ophthalmic products as eye whiteners. The first-generation antihistamines, used in the treatment of allergic rhinitis and insomnia, have dose-dependent anticholinergic activity and should be used judiciously.

BENIGN PROSTATIC HYPERTROPHY AND BLADDER NECK OBSTRUCTION

Benign prostatic hypertrophy (BPH) is the benign enlargement of the prostate gland that develops in the aging male population. Hypertrophy of the bladder neck can also occur and cause problems in voiding.

The bladder and prostate receive both adrenergic and cholinergic innervation. Sympathomimetic drugs found in many cough and cold preparations worsen the symptoms of BPH and bladder neck obstruction because their α_1-adrenergic stimulating properties cause smooth muscle contraction of the urethra and subsequent urinary retention. Additionally, the first-generation antihistamines (e.g., dimenhydrinate, diphenhydramine) and drugs such as scopolamine exacerbate these diseases because their anticholinergic effects cause bladder smooth muscle relaxation and urinary retention.

DIABETES

The Caloric Content of Medications

Diabetic individuals often monitor their caloric intake as part of their disease management. Insulin-dependent diabetics are susceptible to dramatic swings in their blood glucose levels and the unknowing ingestion of medications with high caloric content may be problematic. Individuals with non-insulin-dependent diabetes may experience less dramatic swings in their blood glucose levels but may be on caloric restriction diets to lose weight.

Diabetics may be unaware that many nonprescription preparations contain sugar, alcohol and other calorigenic substances. In addition, the labels sugarless or dietetic may be misleading as the former may contain significant amounts of carbohydrates or calories while the latter may contain up to half the amount of glucose of the regular product. In general, the caloric content of solid oral dosage forms is usually small while that of liquid oral dosage forms may be more significant. Oral liquid preparations may be sweetened with sorbitol or mannitol to increase palatability. Although these substances are not sugars, they are calorigenic.

Health care professionals, as well as diabetic individuals themselves should be aware of the potential caloric contribution of all medications. The *Compendium of Pharmaceuticals and Specialties* contains a list of alcohol-free and low alcohol (less than or equal to 1%) products and some individual monographs also contain calorie information.

Diabetics should limit alcohol consumption for a number of reasons. In addition to being a high source of energy, alcohol can depress the capacity of the liver for gluconeogenesis, impairing the body's ability to recover from hypoglycemia. Alcohol may also interact with certain oral hypoglycemic agents. Finally, the signs and symptoms of hypoglycemia may be mistaken for alcohol intoxication.

Diabetic individuals may seek nonprescription drug relief for many common ailments including the common cold, nasal congestion, sore throat, constipation, pain and heartburn. In general, the ingestion of high calorigenic medications should be avoided if possible. In many cases, preparations containing fewer calories are available. If alternative agents are unavailable, the occasional or short-term use of highly calorigenic products should not be problematic for most well-controlled patients; however, long-term use in patients with poorly controlled disease should be evaluated carefully.

Medications That May Affect Blood Glucose Levels

In addition to the caloric content of medications, diabetic individuals and health care professionals should be aware of the potential impact of certain classes of nonprescription medications on glycemic control.

Sympathomimetic agents are available in many nonprescription cold products as decongestants. Many sympathomimetics contain warning labels cautioning against their use in diabetic individuals although there is little evidence that supports this claim. Parenterally administered epinephrine can increase blood glucose concentration secondary to increased gluconeogenesis, glycogenolysis and other catecholamine-induced mechanisms; however, nonprescription decongestants seldom have as potent an effect on blood glucose as epinephrine. Diabetic patients seeking relief from nasal congestion may benefit from the use of a topical, or if necessary, an oral decongestant. The short-term or occasional use of sympathomimetics is not contraindicated in individuals with diabetes; however, it may be prudent to use these agents under the advice or supervision of a physician as their use may require closer blood glucose level monitoring.

Diabetics will occasionally require the use of an oral analgesic or antipyretic agent. Occasional use of low dose ASA, acetaminophen or ibuprofen will have no effect on blood glucose concentrations. However, the high doses of salicylates (e.g., 4 to 6 g of ASA daily) that are required for anti-inflammatory effects may decrease blood glucose concentrations because they can heighten insulin response to glucose and the peripheral utilization of glucose. Furthermore, non-insulin-dependent diabetic patients receiving oral sulfonylureas may be at an even greater risk of hypoglycemia because salicylates may displace sulfonylureas from protein binding sites, resulting in an increased free fraction of the hypoglycemic agent.

Diabetic individuals who require high doses of salicylates, especially those on oral hypoglycemic agents, should monitor their glycemic control with their physician when initiating or modifying the dose. In addition, diabetics and health care professionals caring for these patients should be aware that many products contain ASA as one of their active ingredients (e.g., cold preparations).

Nonprescription Medications That Interfere With Blood Glucose Testing

One study has evaluated the in vitro effects of ASA, acetaminophen and ascorbic acid on the accuracy of blood glucose testing by three home blood

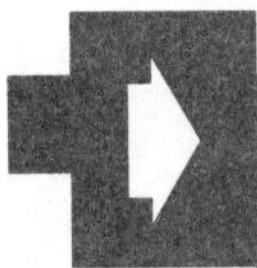

ADVICE FOR THE PATIENT

Diabetic Foot Care

- Inspect feet daily for breaks in skin, especially between toes. Use a mirror to observe the underside. Have someone help you if you have poor eyesight.
- Wash feet daily in tepid water with mild nonmedicated soap. Pat dry thoroughly, especially between the toes. Apply moisturizer to feet.
- Cut toenails straight across.
- Keep feet dry and warm.
- Cover any breaks in skin with a mild antiseptic and sterile nonocclusive bandage.
- Have your doctor, podiatrist or nurse inspect your feet on visits.
- Have shoes fitted professionally; never wear ill-fitting shoes. Wear new shoes for a few hours at a time to break them in.
- Never walk barefoot or in open-toed shoes or sandals.
- Avoid constricting hosiery, stockings and socks.
- Do not cut calluses or corns. Do not apply strong chemicals or corn removers to your feet.
- Do not use a hot water bottle or heating pad on your feet.
- Do not self-medicate warts on the feet. See your doctor or podiatrist.

glucose monitoring systems. Strong reducing substances can prevent the oxidation of the indicator dyes used in the glucose oxidase test strips, thereby modifying or impairing color development. The three drugs were capable of depressing the test results obtained by the *Visidex II*, *Accu-chek bG* and *Dextrostix* systems significantly (i.e., to the extent that insulin dose would most likely be modified). The extent of interference depended on the drug and its concentration and the system used as each system used a different dye. The authors concluded that switching between systems should be avoided and that diabetic patients taking ASA, acetaminophen or ascorbic acid should not use home blood glucose monitoring systems. Results from this study should be, in general, interpreted with caution until further clinical studies evaluate the effect of drug interference in diabetics.

Diabetic Foot Care

Diabetic individuals are more prone to develop foot complications for numerous reasons. Peripheral neuropathy impairs the sensations felt in their feet. Therefore, they are at risk of developing soft tissue infections as well as bone and joint injuries as minor cuts and scratches can go unnoticed. Pressure sores can also develop from poorly fitted shoes. Diabetics also suffer from autonomic neuropathy, and they have decreased sweating in their feet. The skin becomes dry and cracked and may allow bacteria to enter more easily.

Vascular disease, both micro- and macrovascular, decreases blood supply to the feet, while trauma and infection increase the demand. Thickening of the capillary basement membrane leads to increased permeability of fluid and protein that may inhibit migration of leukocytes into interstitial tissue, decreasing the individual's ability to fight infection. Other factors that may contribute to impaired host defences in diabetic patients include reduced leukocyte chemotaxis and adherence, and decreased intracellular killing.

It is important that individuals with diabetes practice preventive foot care to minimize their chance of developing complications. Health care professionals should be aware of the potential problems that can develop in this patient population and know how to counsel them.

RECOMMENDED READING

Infants and Children

Benitz WA, Tatro DS. The Pediatric Drug Handbook. 2nd ed. Chicago: Mosby-Year Book, 1988.

Dupuis LL, Smith JL, Secker D, eds. HSC Formulary of Drugs and Nutritional Products. Toronto: Hospital for Sick Children, published annually.

Extemporaneous Oral Liquid Dosage Preparations. Ottawa: Canadian Society of Hospital Pharmacy, 1988.

Gellis SS, Kagan BM, eds. Current Pediatric Therapy. Philadelphia: WB Saunders, 1994.

Greene MG, ed. Harriet Lane Handbook. 13th ed. St. Louis: Mosby-Year Book, 1993.

Nahata MC, Hipple TF. Pediatric Drug Formulation. Cincinnati: Harvey Whitney Books, 1990.

1991 Red Book (Report of the Committee on Infectious Diseases) American Academy of Pediatrics, 1991.

Pediatric Drug Dosage Handbook. 6th ed. Winnipeg: Health Sciences Centre, 1988.

Pregnancy and Lactation

American Academy of Pediatrics Committee on Drugs. The transfer of drugs and other chemicals into human milk. Pediatrics 1994;93:137–50.

Anderson PO. Drug use during breast-feeding. Clin Pharm 1991;10:594–624.

Atkinson SA. Drugs in breast milk. In: Raddle IC, MacLeod SM, eds. Pediatric Pharmacology and Therapeutics. 2nd ed. St. Louis: Mosby 1993:443–56.

Briggs GG, Freeman RK, Yaffe SJ, ed. Drugs in Pregnancy and Lactation: A Reference Guide to Fetal and Neonatal Risk. 4th ed. Baltimore: Williams & Wilkins, 1994.

Koren G, ed. Maternal-Fetal Toxicology: A Clinician's Guide. 2nd ed. Toronto: Marcel Dekker, 1994.

4

ACNE

Debra J. Sibbald

CONTENTS

Acne 57
- Pathophysiology
- Pathogenesis
- Predisposing Factors
- Signs and Symptoms
- Differential Diagnosis
- Treatment

Pharmaceutical Agents 73
- Exfoliants
- Antibacterials
- Other Agents

Summary 76

Recommended Reading 77

ACNE

Acne vulgaris is a common, self-limiting skin disorder, present in about 80% of people between the ages of 12 and 25 years. It is not limited to teenagers, can begin as early as the neonatal period, and in 20 to 30% of individuals, in their late twenties, thirties, and sometimes forties. The intensity and duration varies for each individual; in most cases, it becomes less active as adolescence ends. It is often more severe in males, but more persistent in females, who may have periodic premenstrual flares until menopause.

Although perceived as benign, its associated physical and psychological problems are well known: onset is generally during adolescence when any stigma interferes with the establishment of social identity. Early treatment is advisable because the disease slowly progresses, resulting in permanent scarring and psychological problems.

PATHOPHYSIOLOGY

At puberty, androgenic hormonal stimulation leads to increased development of pilosebaceous units, a combination of hair follicles and sebaceous glands. These are large and numerous in the midline of the back and external auditory meatus, on the forehead, face and anogenital surface, and acne is common in these sites. Sebaceous glands connect via short ducts to a deep, wide hair canal containing a fine, vellus hair that seldom extends out of the follicle.

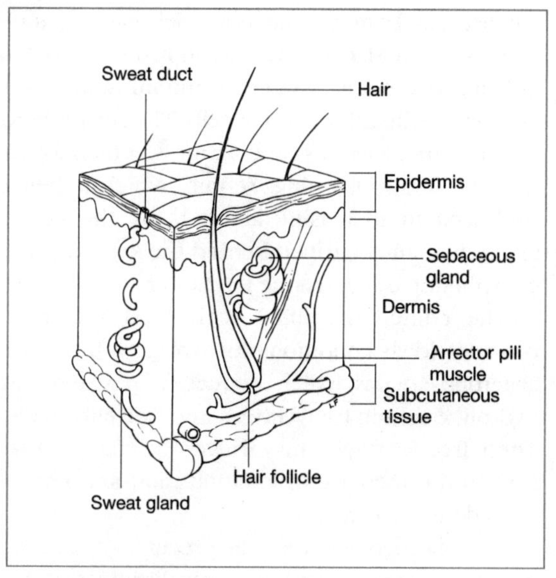

FIGURE 1: The Skin

The hair follicle, sebaceous gland and overlying epidermis represent different types of epithelium. The upper portion of the hair follicle, the acroinfundibulum, is a continuation of surface epithelium and shedding of cells proceeds normally. The lower portion, the infrainfundibulum, is larger and keratinizes a thin noncoherent layer of cells that slough quickly into the canal. Sebaceous glands form sebum, a yellow lipid mixture of triglycerides and wax esters, which empties into the hair follicle canal (Figure 1).

Acne

Besides sebum and shed cells, the canal contains a mixed microbial population, primarily the anaerobe *Propionibacterium acnes*, in its depths. The yeasts *Pityrosporum ovale* and *Pityrosporum orbiculare* are found in the upper canal while aerobic cocci, mostly *Staphylococcus epidermidis*, colonize the skin surface.

As sebum moves up the canal, a lipase produced by *P. acnes* hydrolyzes the triglycerides to irritating free fatty acids and glycerol.

PATHOGENESIS

The pathogenesis of acne progresses through four major stages:

1) increased follicular keratinization;
2) increased sebum production;
3) bacterial lipolysis of sebum triglycerides to free fatty acids; and
4) inflammation.

Acne begins with the development of a plugged follicle, called a microcomedone. Sebaceous glands increase their size and activity in response to circulating androgens while the infrainfundibulum increases its keratinization of cells. The cells adhere to each other in an expanding mass, which forms a dense keratinous plug. Sebum, which is being produced in increasing amounts by the active gland, becomes trapped behind the keratin plug, contributing to comedone formation.

The comedone, filled with lipid substrate, provides ideal conditions for overgrowth of the anaerobe *P. acnes*, which produces a lipase that can hydrolyze sebum triglycerides into free fatty acids. These free fatty acids may trigger the changes that lead to the increase in keratinization and microcomedone formation.

This microcomedone is the precursor of all acne lesions and may not be noticeably distended at this stage. Widening of the follicular infundibulum with horny material produces a flask-shaped, closed comedone, or whitehead. This is the first clinically visible lesion of acne and takes approximately 5 months to develop. The closed comedone is almost completely obstructed to drainage and has a tendency to rupture (Figure 2).

As the plug extends to the upper canal and dilates its opening, an open comedone, or blackhead, is formed. Its dark color is not due to dirt but to either oxidized lipid and melanin or to the impacted mass of horny cells. The cylindrically shaped, open comedone is very stable and may persist for a long time as soluble substances and liquid sebum escape more easily (Figure 3). Acne that is characterized by open and closed comedones is called noninflammatory acne.

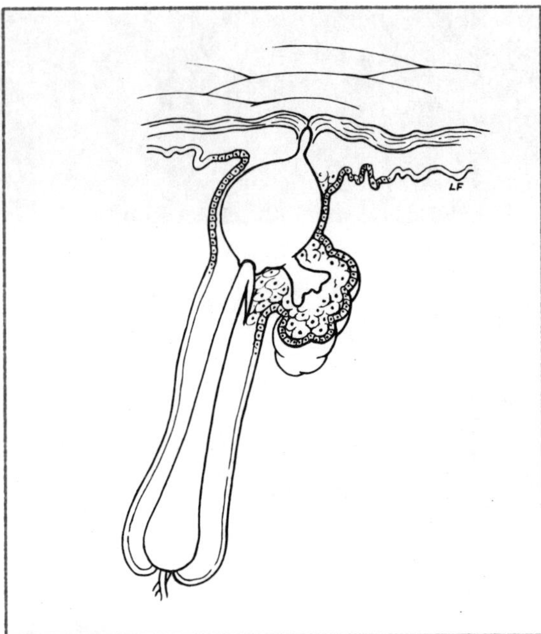

FIGURE 2: Closed comedone

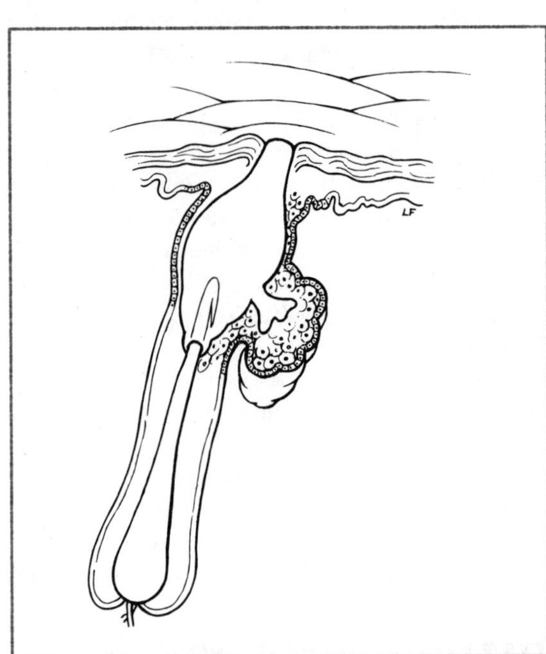

FIGURE 3: Open comedone

Rupture of the follicular wall of a comedone releases follicular contents into the dermis and can produce various inflammatory lesions. The critical trigger for this rupture is *P. acnes*, which produces extracellular phosphatases, hyaluronidases, proteases and neuraminidases. These enzymes are thought to increase the permeability of the follicular epithelium. *P. acnes* also releases low molecular weight chemotactic factors that diffuse through the thinned follicular epithelium and attract neutrophils into the lumen of the comedone. While these factors phagocytize the bacterium, hydrolases are liberated that damage the follicle wall and cause it to rupture.

Other processes contribute to the inflammation. The keratin, hair and lipids in the extruded sebum initiate inflammation directly by a foreign body reaction. The free fatty acids are cytotoxic. The bacteria activate complement pathways to produce additional chemotactic factors that exacerbate the inflammation.

When the contents of the follicle are spilled into the dermis, several different types of inflammatory lesions may form. A superficial aggregation of neutrophils forms a **pustule**, a raised white lesion filled with pus, usually less than 5 mm in diameter. Superficial pustules usually resolve within a few days without scarring. A deeper, dermal, inflammatory reaction will produce a **papule**, which is an erythematous (red), raised, solid lesion, similar in size to pustules. They take a longer time to heal and may result in scarring. Extensive inflammatory infiltration will produce a **nodule**, the most severe variant of acne. They are warm, tender, firm lesions, with a diameter of 5 mm or greater. They may be suppurative or hemorrhagic within the dermis, may involve adjacent follicles and sometimes extend down to fat. Suppurative nodules can be called **cysts** because they resemble inflamed epidermal cysts.

The inflammation may extend to involve nearby follicles and produce significant scarring. Scars are the dreaded aftermath of acne.

Atrophic scars can be shallow and broad-based or a deep, ice-pick shape, while hypertrophic scars are elevated and often seen on the chest and back. For some patients with mild scarring, nonprescription alpha-hydroxy acids may be used, while severe scarring may be corrected with other treatment modalities that require a dermatologist consultation. Dermabrasion, local excision, collagen implants and chemical peels have all been used as techniques to improve scarring. Usually the scar is not completely removed but a more cosmetically acceptable result is achieved. It is important to note that scarring can be prevented with the conscientious use of modern treatments.

PREDISPOSING FACTORS

Drugs: Certain drugs may cause acneiform eruptions (drug-induced acne). Systemic corticosteroids can cause a pustular inflammatory form of acne, especially on the trunk. Onset is abrupt, 2 to 6 weeks after initiation of therapy. Small uniform, erythematous papules and pustules are the classical lesions while comedones are usually absent initially. Acne has also been associated with most of the potent topical steroids, but not with hydrocortisone, which lacks the ability to inhibit protein synthesis. Discontinuation of the steroid results in an initial worsening of the appearance due to removal of the anti-inflammatory action of the steroid itself. Patients should be cautioned about this reaction, which can be subdued through judicious use of topical hydrocortisone.

Halogens, especially an excess of iodide in seafood, salt and health foods, can worsen acne. Other drugs that may induce acne include heavy metals (lithium and cobalt in vitamin B_{12}), antiepileptics and tuberculostatics. A more detailed list is found in Table 1.

Maternal androgens: Newborns or infants between 2 and 3 months may develop closed comedones, and sometimes open comedones, papules and pustules due to placental transfer of maternal androgens (neonatal acne). The stimulated sebaceous glands involute within a few months and the acne subsides. Boys are affected more often than girls because of a transient increase in testosterone secretion during the third and fourth month of intrauterine life. Parents should be reassured that resolution will usually occur without therapy. Baby oil should be avoided as it may aggravate follicular occlusion.

Topical agents: The application of some topical agents may promote the formation of acne (contact acne). This can be due to the use of cosmetics or topical medications or to occupational hazards.

Comedone formation through mechanically occluded follicles (pomade acne) may occur with the use of oil-based scalp preparations on the forehead and temples, oily lubricants in infants and children, and the application of topical tar products. Tar folliculitis can be minimized by applying the tar in the direction the hair grows out at the skin surface, leaving the angle beneath the hair free of tar to allow secretion of duct contents.

In some postadolescent women, acne can be caused or made worse by the liberal use of oily

TABLE 1: Drugs That May Produce Acne-like Eruptions

Hormones:	**Antiepileptic drugs:**	**Miscellaneous:**
androgenic hormones in women	hydantoin derivatives	cyclosporine
corticosteroids	phenobarbital	cyanocobalamin
corticotrophin (ACTH)	trimethadione	dantrolene
oral contraceptives		gold salts
	Tuberculostatic drugs:	lithium salts
Halogens:	ethambutol	maprotiline
bromides	ethionamide	psoralens
chlorides	isoniazid	quinidine
halothane		quinine
iodides		
Drugs That May Produce Papular Pustular Eruptions or Folliculitis		
carbamazepine	dactinomycin	norfloxacin
cephalexin	diltiazem	piperazine
cefazolin	furosemide	pyrimethamine
chloramphenicol	isoniazid	streptomycin
cotrimoxazole	naproxen	tetracyclines

Source: Bruisma W. A Guide to Drug Eruptions. 5th ed. Oosthuizen, The Netherlands: European Book Service, 1990:6.

cosmetics (cosmetic acne). This commonly occurs in a perioral distribution with a clear zone around the lips; acne due to application of hair spray may develop around the hair margins.

Patients should be advised to stop using their oil-containing cosmetics and avoid cosmetic programs that advocate applying multiple layers of cream-based cleansers and coverups. Various creams and cosmetics used during a beauty salon facial may precipitate acne in such patients. Instead, the patient should wash twice daily with a mild soap, and restrict cosmetic use to products labeled oil-free rather than water-based, including makeup, moisturizers or sunscreens.

Water-based cosmetics may contain significant amounts of oil-phase in the form of undiluted vegetable oils, lanolin, fatty acid esters (butyl stearate, isopropyl myristate), fatty acids (stearic acid), fatty acid alcohols, cocoa butter, coconut oil, red veterinary petrolatum, and sunscreens containing benzophenones. Flesh-tone tinted acne formulations may be recommended.

Occupational hazards: Closed comedones, papules, pustules and nodules may be induced by contact with acnegenic industrial agents such as coal, tar, pitch, mineral oil and petroleum oil (occupational acne). Ingestion, inhalation or transcutaneous penetration of halogenated aromatic hydrocarbons, including the polychlorobiphenyls in paint, varnishes, lacquers, fungicides, insecticides, herbicides, wood preservatives and various oils will produce a distinct form of occupational acne (chloracne). Within a few months of sufficient exposure, open and closed comedones appear on the chest, temples and behind the ears. Inflammatory lesions may follow. Exposure should be minimized and the patient referred to a physician.

Physical pressure: Pressure from headbands, violins, chin straps, sports helmets, guitar straps and orthopedic braces have induced localized acne (acne mechanica). Mechanical friction should be eliminated or reduced.

Manual manipulation: Acne patients will manipulate their comedones and pustules with finger pressure in an attempt to drain lesions, often subconsciously or during sleep (acne excoriée). Crusting, erosions, scarring and hyperpigmentation may result from the ensuing rupture and inflammation.

Diet: Acne is uninfluenced by diet, and a healthy balanced diet should be advised. Some patients wish to restrict certain foods they perceive exacerbate acne (chocolate, cola drinks, milk and milk products, and iodides).

Environmental factors: Heat and humidity may induce comedones while pressure, friction and excessive scrubbing or washing can exacerbate existing acne by causing microcomedones to rupture. Hair styles low on the forehead or neck may cause excess sweating and occlusion and make acne worse.

Stress: Emotional stress and intense anger can exacerbate acne. Patients may develop social problems, such as a low self-esteem, phobias or depression. Acne should never be trivialized, for the psychosocial scars and trauma are often deeper and more disastrous than the blemishes. By being empathetic and informative during counselling, the health professional may motivate the patient to continue long-term therapy.

SIGNS AND SYMPTOMS

Acne vulgaris may be noninflammatory or inflammatory. Noninflammatory acne vulgaris is characterized by open and closed comedones. Inflammatory acne vulgaris traditionally is characterized as papulo-pustular and/or nodular. The severity grading is based on a lesion count approximation, as shown in Table 2. Mild inflammatory acne has a few to several papules and/or pustules and no nodules. Moderate inflammatory acne has several to many papules and/or pustules and few to several nodules. Severe inflammatory acne has numerous and/or extensive papules and/or pustules and many nodules. Lesions are usually located on the face, back, neck and chest, but may extend to buttocks or extremities. Often resolution of these lesions leaves erythematous or pigmented macules that can persist for months or longer. The cascade of the pathogenesis of acne is shown in Figure 4.

DIFFERENTIAL DIAGNOSIS

Acne vulgaris is rarely misdiagnosed. The most commonly mistaken condition is acne rosacea. It is a chronic relapsing condition, occurring after age 30, commonly in people of Celtic complexion. The first sign is easy flushing (redness or erythema), followed by development of inflammatory lesions with edema, papules, pustules, and telangiectasia appearing on the nose, cheeks and forehead. Chronic deep inflammation of the nose leads to sebaceous hypertrophy called rhinophyma (enlargement of the nose). The etiology is unknown, but aggravating factors include alcohol, sun or wind exposure, spicy foods and hot drinks such as coffee, which can lead to flushing. Patients should be referred to a physician for treatment.

Acne that is asymmetric usually indicates an external factor. Whiteheads may be confused with milia, which are whiter and usually infraorbital. Acneiform drug eruptions can be misdiagnosed. Gram-negative organisms may complicate acne, and folliculitis may occur due to staphylococci. Warts may cause confusion. Zinc deficiency produces a severe papulo-pustular eruption. Acne cysts may be confused with dental or epidermoid cysts. Acne may be the presenting sign in adrenal and ovarian tumors, Cushing's disease, and polycystic ovarian disease. Women who present with moderate to severe acne and signs of androgen excess, such as hirsutism (usually hair appearing on the upper lip or chin) or irregular menses, and children with persistent or severe acne should be referred to their physician. A summary is provided in Table 3.

TREATMENT

The goals of treatment for acne vulgaris focus on prevention of both psychological and physical scarring. It is impossible to standardize a formula, as individual regimens must consider such variables as

TABLE 2: Severity Grading of Inflammatory Acne Lesions

Severity	Papules/Pustules	Nodules
Mild	Few to several	None
Moderate	Several to many	Few to several
Severe	Numerous and/or extensive	Many

Source: Pochi PE, Shalita AR, Straus JC, et al. Report of the consensus conference on acne classification. J Am Acad Dermatol 1991;24(3):495–500.

FIGURE 4

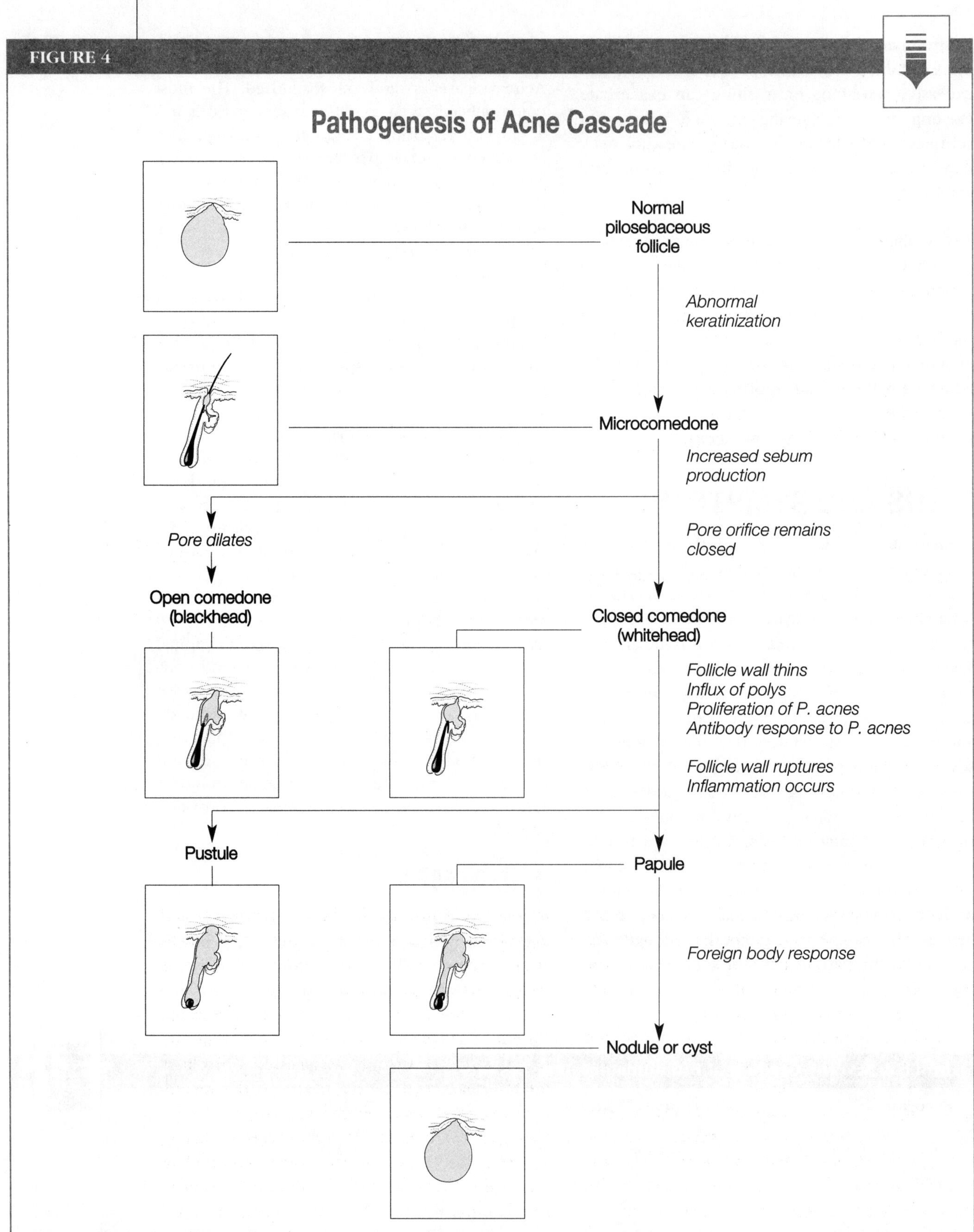

Adapted with permission from: Habif TP. Acne, rosacea, and related disorders. In: Klein EA, Menczer BS, eds. Clinical Dermatology. Toronto: CV Mosby, 1990:114.

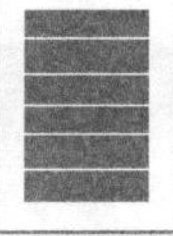

TABLE 3: Differential Diagnosis

OTHER KINDS OF ACNE

Acne Variant	Comedones Open	Comedones Closed	Pustules	Papules	Nodules	Other
Vulgaris	X	X	X	X	X	
Drug-induced		+/−	X	X		
Neonatal		X	X	+/−		
Conglobata			X	XX	XX	cysts, abscesses, sinus tracts
Fulminans			X	XX	XX	ulcerating cysts
Contact:						
— pomade		XX	X			
— cosmetic	X	XX	XX	X		
— occupational (oil)		XX	X	X		
— chloracne	XX	XX	X	X		
Endocrine			XX	X	X	
Excoriated			X	X		crusts, scars, erosions, hyperpigmentation
Mechanica		XX	XX	X		
Rosacea			X	X	+/−	erythema, edema, telangiectasia

OTHER CONDITIONS

Milia
Folliculitis—gram-negative, staphylococcal, candida
Warts
Dental sinuses or epidermoid cysts

severity, predominating type of lesion, sex of the patient, lesion distribution, allergies or sensitivities, previous treatments, other medications, cosmetic acceptance, cost and compliance. Key points include patient education, cleansing the skin and treatment of noninflammatory (comedonal) and inflammatory lesions. In certain cases a physician referral is warranted (Table 4).

A rational approach must begin with a counselling session with the patient or parent. Emphasize to the individual that improvement usually takes 4 to 6 weeks to be noticeable and 3 to 5 months to achieve control. The natural self-limiting course of the disorder should be a reassuring point, but the dangers of permanent damage due to scarring should be stressed. Anxiety, aggravating factors and a balanced diet should be reviewed, and diary keeping suggested: lesion count in relation to stress, menses, and cosmetics can be recorded as well as manual manipulation.

A good history, following the guidelines in the Patient Assessment Questions section, must be taken before any therapy is suggested. Guidelines for information gathering, based on the recommendations of the American Academy of Dermatology, are found in Table 5. An algorithm detailing a systematic approach to patient counselling for acne vulgaris may be found in Figure 5. Both nonpharmacological and pharmacological measures are needed for most patients, and their expectations should be discussed to encourage long-term treatment.

TABLE 4: When to Refer an Acne Patient to a Physician

Some patients may require further investigation, prescription therapy or other modalities
If the etiology of the acne is drug-induced or an endocrinopathy
If acne is moderate to severe
Patients who are non-responsive to nonprescription therapy
Patients who experience scarring, especially if moderate to severe

TABLE 5: Guidelines for Information Gathering

The following variables should be considered in determining individual therapy:

Duration and severity of the condition		
Seasonal variation		
Aggravation by stress		
For women:	premenstrual flare-up pregnancy status oral contraceptives: use and effect on acne cosmetics and moisturizers—types and frequency	
Current treatments: topical and systemic:	— for acne — for other diseases	
Family history of acne		
Allergies:	drug topical preparations atopy	
General health and medical conditions		
Lesion types:	noninflammatory	— open comedones — closed comedones
	inflammatory	— papules — pustules — nodules and/or cysts
Location:	face/neck back anterior chest extremities	
Gradation:	mild moderate severe for each lesion type	
Complications:	scarring pigmentation excoriations	

The dangers of picking their own lesions should be carefully explained to the patient and behavior modified by keeping a daily diary of the number of times they touch their lesions. Fingernails should be kept short and comedone expression suggested to certain patients.

Nonpharmacological Treatment

Basic nonpharmacological measures include discontinuing aggravating factors, using oil-free make-up, maintaining a balanced diet and controlling stress factors. Patients should wash twice daily with a mild nonalkaline soap.

Acne patients tend to wash too frequently in an attempt to remove surface oils; however, there is no evidence that this is helpful. Surface lipids removed by soap and water are not involved in the pathogenesis of acne: lipids deep in the pilosebaceous unit are contributory factors, and these are not eliminated through washing. Similarly, while antiseptic cleansers will effectively remove dirt and oil from the skin surface, leaving a clean refreshed feeling, antibacterial soaps and washes may destroy surface aerobic bacteria without any significant effect on *P. acnes* in the anaerobic depths of the follicle.

Patients should understand that cleansing will improve an oily appearance and promote comfort, but will not rinse away their acne. There is no evidence to indicate that one washing regimen is better than another. They should be instructed to wash with a mild, gentle soap or soapless cleanser no more than twice a day. Scrubbing should be minimized or avoided as this type of trauma may rupture follicles, producing inflammation leading to more papules and pustules. It is not necessary to use a medicated cleanser, but such agents require increased skin contact time. With the use of any soap, the patient should be told to expect a drying effect on the skin due to detergent action. This

FIGURE 5

Suggested Approach for Treating Acne with Nonprescription Medication

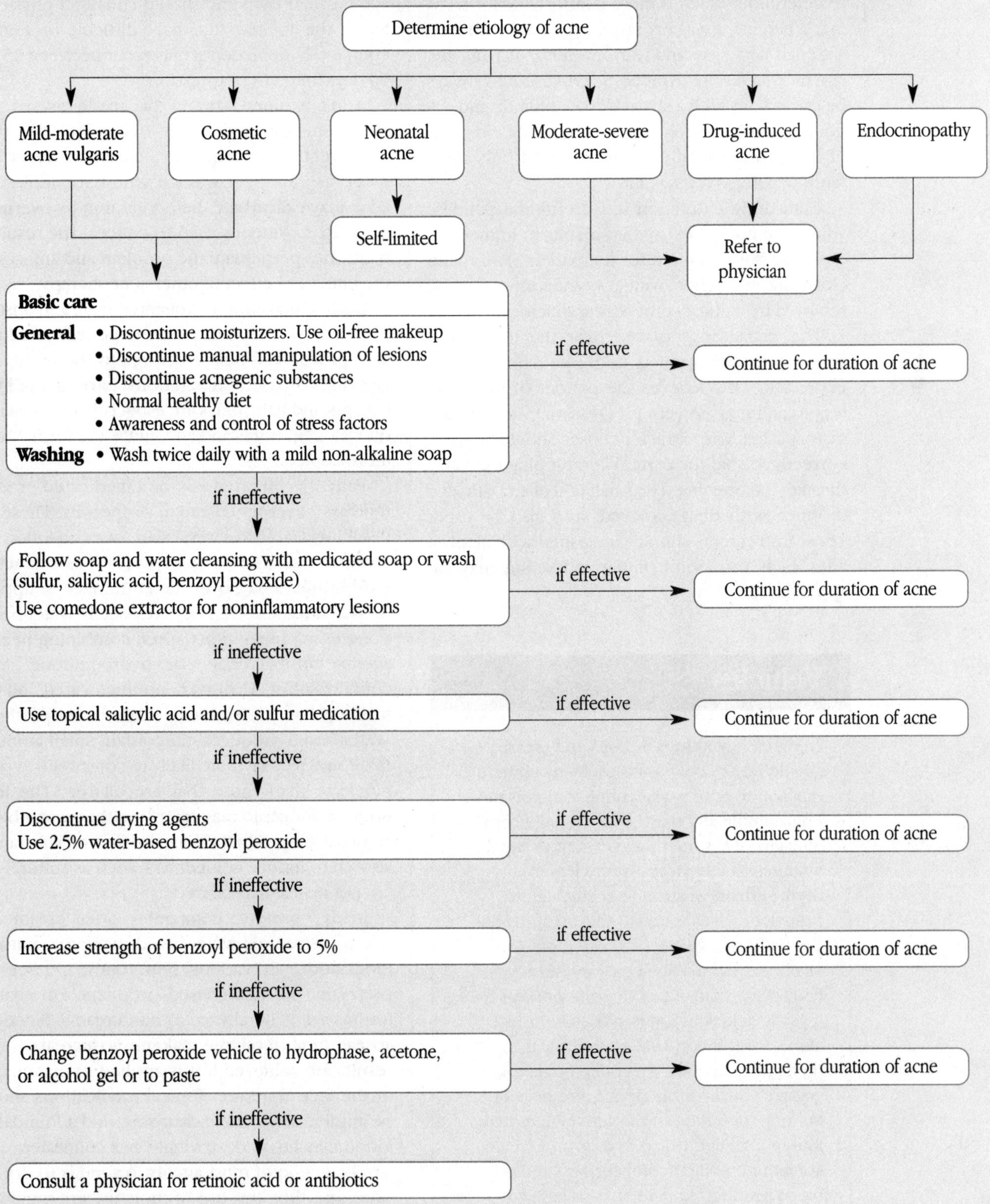

Determine etiology of acne

- Mild-moderate acne vulgaris → Basic care
- Cosmetic acne → Basic care
- Neonatal acne → Self-limited
- Moderate-severe acne → Refer to physician
- Drug-induced acne → Refer to physician
- Endocrinopathy → Refer to physician

Basic care

General
- Discontinue moisturizers. Use oil-free makeup
- Discontinue manual manipulation of lesions
- Discontinue acnegenic substances
- Normal healthy diet
- Awareness and control of stress factors

Washing
- Wash twice daily with a mild non-alkaline soap

if effective → Continue for duration of acne

if ineffective ↓

Follow soap and water cleansing with medicated soap or wash (sulfur, salicylic acid, benzoyl peroxide)
Use comedone extractor for noninflammatory lesions

if effective → Continue for duration of acne

if ineffective ↓

Use topical salicylic acid and/or sulfur medication

if effective → Continue for duration of acne

if ineffective ↓

Discontinue drying agents
Use 2.5% water-based benzoyl peroxide

if effective → Continue for duration of acne

If ineffective ↓

Increase strength of benzoyl peroxide to 5%

if effective → Continue for duration of acne

if ineffective ↓

Change benzoyl peroxide vehicle to hydrophase, acetone, or alcohol gel or to paste

if effective → Continue for duration of acne

if ineffective ↓

Consult a physician for retinoic acid or antibiotics

is more pronounced with products that contain peeling agents. Cream-based cleansers should be avoided.

Males should try both electric and safety razors to determine which is more comfortable for shaving. When using a safety razor, the beard should be softened with soap and warm water or shaving gel, and nicking lesions avoided. Shaving should always be carried out with a sharp blade, as lightly and seldom as possible. Strokes should be in the direction of hair growth, and each area shaved only once without going over it again.

Comedone extraction is a useful and painless adjunct to acne therapy that results in immediate cosmetic improvement for the patient. Following cleansing with hot water, comedones can be removed by using a comedone extractor.

The extractor is placed over the lesion and gentle pressure applied until the contents are expressed. This relieves the patient of unsightly lesions and may prevent progression to the inflammatory stage. The extractor chosen should be sized correctly so that the central keratin plug extrudes through the opening. The small end of a plastic eye dropper, with bulb removed, may also be used. These instruments should be cleaned with alcohol after each use. Some initial reddening may be apparent.

Vehicles

Nongreasy solutions, lotions and creams should be selected as bases. Many contain ethanol or isopropyl alcohol, which is more lipid soluble and may be preferred. Propylene glycol is sometimes present in small amounts to add viscosity and lessen the drying effects of strong peeling agents. Propylene glycol gels are easy to apply and dry without a visible or sticky film. Nonalcoholic gels may be equal in efficacy and less drying than alcoholic solutions. An 8% glycolic acid solution is available for use alone or for incorporation in topical antibiotic preparations. Alcoholic or acetone gels are usually more drying and provide better penetration of the active ingredient; lotions are slightly less drying, and creams are more emollient. Moisturizers and oil-based products should be discouraged.

If the contents are not expressed with modest pressure, patients should not continue since improper extraction may irritate the skin further. Some may find this technique too difficult to manage on their own and should consult a physician. Since the follicle sheath is difficult to remove completely, comedones may recur between 25 and 50 days following expression.

Adult women should be made aware that persistent low-grade acne, occurring after their mid-twenties, is frequently caused by heavy cosmetic use. Younger women who have adolescent acne may exacerbate their condition by overusing makeup. Cosmetics used to conceal the resultant blemishes perpetuate the problem and antagonize the beneficial effect of other acne therapy.

Oil-free makeups are tolerated well, and lipstick, eye shadow, eyeliner, eyebrow pencils and loose face powders appear to be relatively innocuous. Heavier, oil-based preparations, particularly moisturizers and hair sprays are especially troublesome: they clog up pores and encourage the formation of more comedones.

Patients will often ask for a medicated product that has cover-up cosmetic properties. These are usually available in several skin tones, in lotion and cream forms. They may be applied as cosmetics, 2 or 3 times a day, over the entire face or applied to individual lesions. They are usually water-based, nongreasy preparations, often combining peeling agents, antibacterials, or hydroquinone. Most contain sulfur. However, nonmedicated, oil-free makeups are preferable to water-based products. Water-based products still contain small amounts of oil, and may be more likely to contribute to pore-blockage than those that are oil-free. The term noncomedogenic may refer to either water-based vehicles or products that are free of substances known to induce comedones, such as sulfur. They are not necessarily oil-free.

Many cosmetic companies offer cream and liquid oil-free, or water-based makeups, without medication, in various skin tones. Oil-free are preferable to water-based products. Foundation lotions are generally safer than creams. Since the spread time of oil-free makeup is decreased, best results are achieved if it is applied to one-quarter of the face at a time. Topical medications should be applied after gentle cleansing, and a foundation lotion may be used, sparingly, as a concealer.

The action of most agents in acne is to dry the skin, and thus the use of moisturizers would be counterproductive. The use of moisturizers should be restricted to oil-free products unless absolutely necessary because of treatment with strong drying agents or isotretinoin.

In the past, ultraviolet light was recommended for desquamation. This peeling technique is no longer advised since the carcinogenesis and photoaging effects of ultraviolet exposure are now well established. Moreover, inflamed skin is more susceptible to the damaging effects of ultraviolet light. Acne patients should apply sunscreens in alcohol or oil-free bases and avoid using the acnegenic benzophenones. The sunscreen should be applied as the first product.

Pharmacological Treatment

While nonpharmacological measures should always be the first step, most cases of acne also need them combined with pharmacological

Medicated Soaps and Washes

- Medicated soaps and washes may contain topical antiseptics, or peeling agents such as salicylic acid, sulfur or benzoyl peroxide, alone or in combination. Most washes require thorough rinsing from 15 seconds to 5 minutes after application. This limits the amount of time the active ingredient is in contact with the skin. Other cleansers are applied after washing and left on the skin without rinsing. Quaternary ammonium compounds are cationic detergents that are inactivated quickly in the presence of organic material, such as sebum. The duration of action of these products is short.
- Bacteriostatic soaps, such as hexachlorophene, carbanilides and salicylanilides (halogenated hydroxyphenols), have been found to be acnegenic. It should be emphasized that few ordinary soaps induce acne. However, acne patients are particularly susceptible to comedogenic contactants, and if these soaps are applied several times daily for long periods, they may become troublesome. Soaps containing coal tar, which can induce folliculitis, are not indicated for acne.
- Chlorhexidine inhibits the in vitro growth of *P. acnes.* A 4% chlorhexidine gluconate preparation in a detergent base has been shown to be as effective as benzoyl peroxide washes in patients with mild acne, and both preparations reduced the number of inflammatory and noninflammatory lesions after 8 and 12 weeks, compared to vehicle alone.
- Polyester cleansing sponges (e.g., *Buf-Puf*) are synthetics that abrade the skin surface, removing superficial debris. They are unlikely to unseat comedones, considering the structure of these lesions. The sponges are available in soft or coarse textures, with or without soap. Patients should be cautioned against using a circular or rubbing motion that will increase irritation, but instructed to use single, gentle, continuous strokes on each side of the face, from the midline out towards the ears.
- Alcohol-detergent medicated pads, impregnated with salicylic acid 0.5 % have reduced inflammatory lesions and open comedones in mild to moderate acne. This type of medication is less abrasive, is not rinsed off and is convenient to use.
- Abrasives consist of finely-divided particles of fused aluminum or plastic together with cleansing and wetting agents. Abrasives peel and remove skin surface debris and may assist resorption of papules and pustules. Despite vigorous rubbing, removal of comedones is not accomplished. Particles, such as sodium tetraborate decahydrate, dissolve on use and their abrasiveness is limited.
- The effectiveness of an abrasive cleanser containing polyethylene granules and the same cleansing agent without the abrasive granules has been compared in patients with mild to moderate acne. No significant difference was noted. These products are not indicated in most cases but may be used in a patient who responds empirically.

Acne

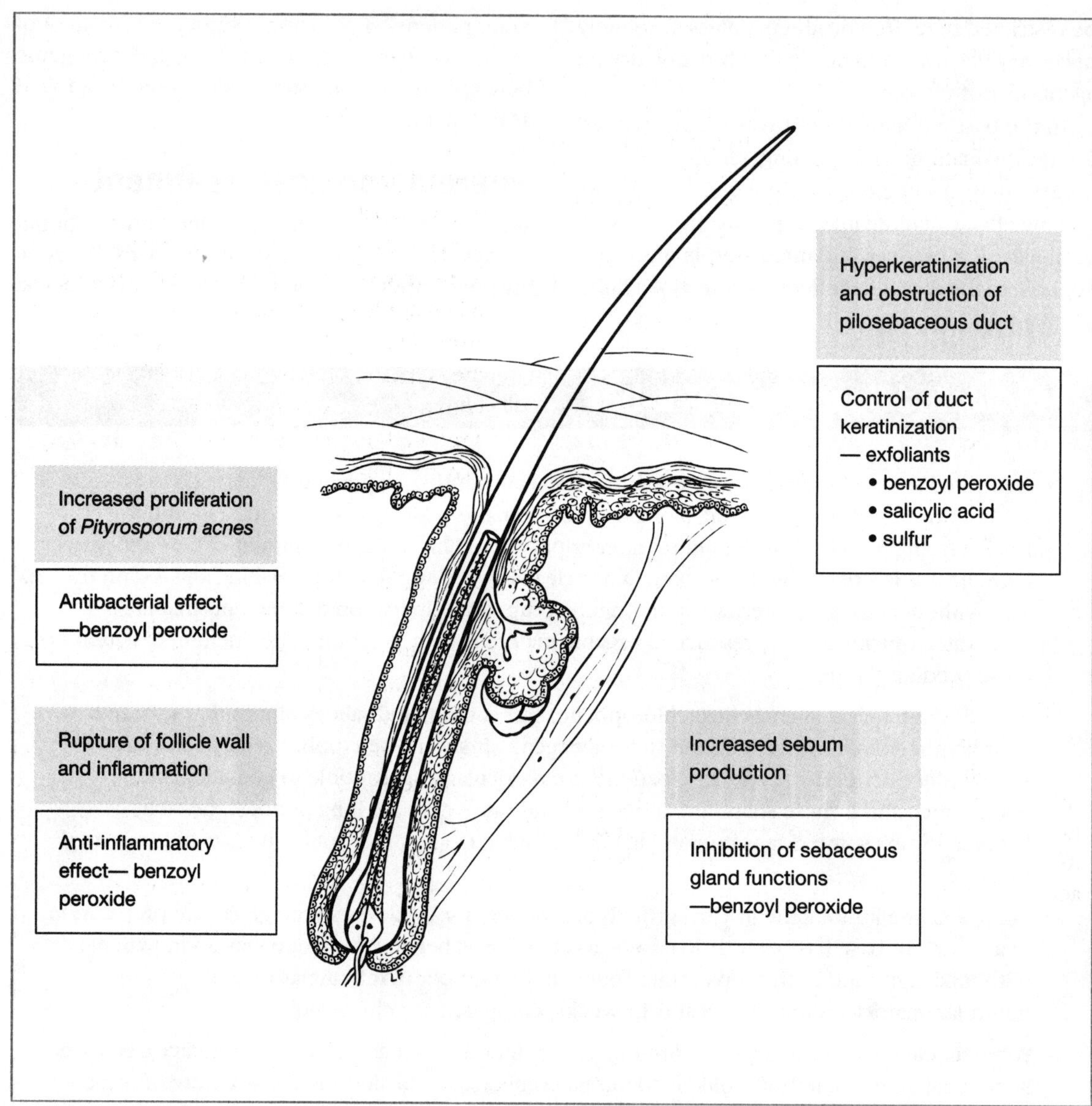

FIGURE 6: Mechanism of Action of Nonprescription Acne Medication

treatment. First, determine the severity and cause of acne. Mild to moderate acne vulgaris and cosmetic acne can be treated with nonprescription medication; moderate to severe acne, drug-induced acne, acne rosacea or endocrinopathies should be referred to a physician. Excellent treatment is available for severe acne provided it is started early.

Although acne cannot be cured, it can be controlled. Improvement may be noted after 8 to 12 weeks although the condition may worsen after initial application of peeling agents. The therapeutic outcome should be to maintain chronic control of lesions, adjusting therapy to the lowest dosing schedules that suppress symptoms until natural resolution, in men when they reach their early twenties and in women somewhat later. A patient who is nonresponsive to nonprescription therapy should be referred to a physician.

If nonprescription therapy is appropriate, the first determinant is the type of acne: noninflammatory or inflammatory. Feasible treatment alternatives for either type will depend on the mechanism of action of the topical agent. Pharmacological treatments counteract 1 or more of 4 major factors that cause noninflammatory or inflammatory acne: abnormalities in follicular keratinization, increased sebum production, bacterial lipolysis of sebum triglycerides to free fatty acids, and conversion of a noninflamed lesion into an inflammatory one. Topical agents act at various stages in the evolution of an acne lesion and may be used either alone or in combination to enhance efficacy (Figure 6). Combination therapy is more effective when drugs exerting different mechanisms are used together.

Keratinization of the duct of the pilosebaceous unit is controlled with exfoliants or peeling agents that prevent or eliminate comedones. Peeling is the best treatment for most forms of acne, especially milder cases, and even severe forms will benefit noticeably. The most powerful peeling agents, however, are prescription medications. Increased sebum production, formation of free fatty acids through bacterial lipases, and conversion to inflammatory lesions may all be counteracted by benzoyl peroxide. Other agents that affect these mechanisms are prescription drugs. Resolution of inflammatory lesions is accomplished by any drugs that enhance local blood flow and accelerate tissue clearance of toxic products, such as counterirritants.

Mild to moderate comedonal, noninflammatory acne can generally be controlled with self-treatment and can be treated exclusively with a topical peeling agent or exfoliant. Extraction of comedones, especially blackheads, is therapeutically and cosmetically worthwhile. Mild inflammatory acne of the papulo-pustular type may be controlled by benzoyl peroxide, and this should be the first step. After considering type of acne and mechanisms of action, selection of the most appropriate nonprescription therapy should also involve the patient's preference with respect to side effects, vehicles, and cost.

How to Use Topical Preparations

Topical preparations should not be applied to individual lesions but to the whole area affected by acne to prevent new lesions from developing. Care should be taken when applying peeling agents to areas around the eyelid, mouth and neck since they chafe easily. Lotions should be applied with a cotton swab once or twice a day after washing. Those leaving visible residue may be applied at bedtime.

Inflammatory lesions often heal with altered pigmentation, even though residual scarring may not develop. This may take 6 months to 1 year to resolve. In patients with fair skin, residual erythema or a violaceous hue is often present for months after the active lesions have cleared. Hydroquinone reversibly damages melanocytes and is used as a nonprescription hypopigmenting agent in concentrations of 2 to 4%.

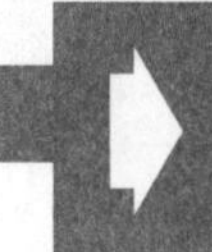

ADVICE FOR THE PATIENT

Acne

- ➤ Treat acne as soon as it appears to avoid complications such as scarring.
- ➤ Allow 6 to 8 weeks of treatment before assessing improvement. Some medications cause initial reddening or worsening that subsides with treatment. These may need to be introduced gradually. If acne does not improve with an adequate course of nonprescription medication, consult a physician.
- ➤ Discontinue use of greasy cosmetics, coversticks, moisturizers, hair pomades, scalp oils, eye creams and hair spray. Even one application of a greasy cosmetic can perpetuate acne for months.
- ➤ Do not use makeup regularly. If necessary, use an oil-free preparation and remove carefully at bedtime.
- ➤ Discuss any current medications for acne, other conditions, or any materials you may contact at work with the health professional who is advising you about treatment. Some substances may cause acne.
- ➤ Wash your skin gently twice daily with a mild, nonalkaline soap or soapless cleanser. Do not rub or scrub your skin. Water alone is fine.
- ➤ Shampoo hair regularly: if it is oily, wash it more frequently. Keep your hair off your face as much as possible and tie it back during sleep.
- ➤ Do not manipulate acne lesions: avoid picking, scratching, popping or squeezing. Keeping a daily diary of the number of times you touch your skin may help to decrease this habit. If necessary, a comedone extractor may be used.
- ➤ Eliminate mechanical friction: e.g., from headbands, violins, chin straps, sports helmets, guitar straps and orthopedic braces.
- ➤ Males with acne who shave should try both an electric and a safety razor to determine comfort. If using a safety razor, soften your beard thoroughly with soap and warm water. Shave as lightly and as seldom as possible and always use a sharp blade. Stroke in the direction of hair growth over each area only once.
- ➤ Eat a healthy balanced diet. Foods are usually not aggravating factors.
- ➤ Be aware that stress may aggravate acne. Try to minimize its effect through relaxation or exercise.
- ➤ Apply acne medication to the entire affected area. In most cases, it is best not to spot-treat lesions. Use a clean swab for each application and discard.
- ➤ Use an oil-free sunscreen, usually in an alcohol lotion or gel form. Apply the sunscreen after cleansing and before acne medication. If using benzoyl peroxide, apply the sunscreen during the day and the benzoyl peroxide at night.
- ➤ Continue proper skin care until the tendency to have acne has passed.

?

PATIENT ASSESSMENT QUESTIONS

Q At what age did your acne begin and how long have you had it?

Acne is predominantly a disease of puberty and adolescence that usually resolves spontaneously by the early twenties. A small percentage of teenagers develop severe nodular acne that may not resolve for 10 to 15 years. Some patients, particularly women, develop acne in their twenties that may last longer than a decade. Acne appearing at an unusual age is frequently due to a drug or an internal disease. Neonates may develop an acne that is self-limiting.

Q What makes your acne worse? Is it aggravated by stress or emotional upsets?

Acne has long been considered the special curse of anxious adolescents who may magnify the smallest lesion or the mildest case of acne into a severe disease. This is a result of psychological pressure emphasizing the importance of physical appearance at this age. Acutely stressful situations may cause sudden flares, but anxiety does not cause this disease. There may also be an increase in mechanical manipulation as a response to the stress. Drawing the patient's attention to the sequence of events is often helpful.

Q Does your acne change with the seasons? Is sunlight beneficial?

Summer sun may diminish acne activity in dry conditions, whereas humidity and heavy sweating may lead to duct obstruction and exacerbate inflammatory acne. A distinct type of acne (acne aestivale) may occur up to 2 to 3 months after exposure to strong ultraviolet light, which can induce duct obstruction. These patients may benefit from an application of sunscreen 1 hour prior to sun exposure.

Q Do you have any habits that may aggravate acne?

Cradling the chin in the hands or greasy hair worn low over the forehead may exacerbate acne lesions. Patients should be cautioned against picking, excoriating, pinching, pressing, or otherwise traumatizing the skin. Wool or other rough textured fabrics, occlusive clothing and sports equipment (helmets) may also be irritants.

Q Are you exposed to heavy oils, greases or tars at work?

People who work with grease, coal tar, pitch, insecticides, chlorinated hydrocarbons and tar distillates may develop an acneiform eruption.

Q Do you notice any differences with changes in diet?

In the past, severe restrictions of chocolate, cola, fried foods, cheese, nuts and milk were advised. Essentially, acne is uninfluenced by diet, and a healthy balanced diet is all that is required. If the patient believes certain foods exacerbate acne, these may be restricted if the diet remains nutritionally sound.

Q Is there a premenstrual flareup?

Approximately 70% of females may complain of this phenomenon. The pilosebaceous duct opening is significantly smaller between days 15 to 20 of the menstrual cycle, leading to increased duct obstruction and resistance to sebum flow. There may be additional changes in keratin hydration.

Q Are you pregnant? Are you taking oral contraceptives? If so, which one?

There may be a change in the appearance of acne with hormonal change in pregnancy. Oral contraceptives that contain the androgenic and antiestrogenic progestogens may provoke an acneiform eruption.

Q Are you taking any medications other than those for acne?

Acne occurring in postadolescent years may be precipitated by medication.

Q Are you using any greasy cosmetics?

Acne can be produced by greasy hair care products (pomade acne) or cosmetics (cosmetic acne).

Q Where are the lesions located?

Acne vulgaris lesions are seen primarily on the face, but the neck, chest, shoulders, back, thighs and upper arms may be involved.

PATIENT ASSESSMENT QUESTIONS (*cont'd*)

Q ***Are you under a physician's care? What treatments have you taken or are you still taking for your acne?***

Treatment failures may be due to improper dosage, such as tetracycline taken with meals or antacids, or discontinuing therapy before an adequate period of assessment has elapsed. Clearing takes approximately 3 months, and drug effects should not be judged sooner than 8 weeks. Other drying agents should be discontinued when initiating therapy with benzoyl peroxide or prescription exfoliants. Retinoic acid and benzoyl peroxide should not be applied at the same time.

Q ***Do you have any allergies to topically applied or oral medications? Do you have atopic dermatitis?***

Patients may confuse acne with an allergic eruption. Patients with allergies should avoid any acne medications that may cross-react with allergens. Atopics may be more sensitive to irritant acne therapy.

Q ***What types of lesions do you have? What percentage of the skin is involved?***

Acne lesions are classified as whiteheads, blackheads, papules, pustules, nodules and scars. The types of lesions, the area of involvement and the number of lesions will determine the appropriate therapy.

Q ***Are the lesions mild, moderate or severe? Are they itchy or painful?***

The severity of the lesions will also determine if self-treatment with nonprescription medications is appropriate. Inflammatory lesions may itch as they erupt and may be very painful on pressure.

Q ***Do you have any residual damage from acne lesions?***

Patients with scarring, pigmentation and excoriations can be referred to a physician for cosmetic improvements. Patients should be reminded of the dangers of manipulating their lesions.

PHARMACEUTICAL AGENTS

EXFOLIANTS

Peeling Agents

Exfoliants induce continuous mild drying and peeling by primary irritation, damaging the superficial layers of the skin and inciting inflammation. This stimulates mitosis, leading to a thickening epidermis, an increase in horny cell production, scaling, and often erythema. Exfoliants may decrease sweating, creating the appearance of a dry, less oily surface, and may provide superficial resolution of pustular lesions.

The ability of several topical exfoliants to retard the formation of comedones or to accelerate their loss (comedolytic activity) has been assessed by using the external ear canal in an experimental rabbit model. Retinoic acid (also known as tretinoin) (available by prescription) was the most active and benzoyl peroxide and salicylic acid were active, while most other traditional exfoliants contained in nonprescription products were weak or ineffective. These included phenol, resorcinol, betanapthol, sulfur, Vleminckx's solutions and sodium thiosulfate. Because these peeling agents affect only the epidermis and not the middle of the hair canal, they are not comedolytic. As nonprescription treatments, their marginal benefits are now largely supplanted by the superior effects of retinoic acid, benzoyl peroxide and salicylic acid. Patients requiring an exfoliant but who may be allergic to benzoyl peroxide, or who find its peeling action too strong, can be effectively treated with salicylic acid alone, or in combination with other peeling agents such as sulfur or resorcinol. Because the primary action of benzoyl peroxide is its suppressant effect on *P. acnes*, it will be discussed under antibacterials.

Resorcinol, a phenol derivative, is less keratolytic than salicylic acid. It is an irritant and sensitizer and is said to be both bactericidal and fungicidal. Products containing resorcinol 1 to 2% have been used for acne, often in combination with other peeling agents, such as sulfur or salicylic acid. While the U.S. Food and Drug Administration (FDA) considers resorcinol 2% and resorcinol monoacetate 3%, in combination with sulfur 3 to 8%, to be safe and effective, it is not convinced that resorcinol and resorcinol acetate are safe and effective when used as single ingredients, and has placed such products in Category II (not generally recognized as safe and effective, or misbranded). However, there are several products containing these single ingredients currently on the Canadian market.

Salicylic acid has comedolytic activity, although the concentrations in commercial preparations, less than 2 to 3%, are generally low. While concentrations less than 2% may actually increase keratinization, concentrations between 3 and 6%, are keratolytic, softening the horny layer and shedding scales. This occurs by solubilizing the intercellular cement and by decreasing cell to cell cohesion. However, lower concentrations are sometimes combined with sulfur to produce an additive keratolytic effect. Concentrations of up to 5 to 10% can be used for acne, beginning with a low concentration and increasing as tolerance to the irritation develops. It is an effective agent, although as a peeling agent, slightly less potent than equal strength benzoyl peroxide. Its keratolytic effect may enhance the absorption of other agents. The FDA monograph on OTC topical acne drug products recognizes salicylic acid as safe and effective.

Sulfur is used in the precipitated or colloidal form in concentrations of 2 to 10%. Sulfur compounds (e.g., sulfides, thioglycolates, sulfites, thiols, cysteines and thioacetates) are also available and somewhat weaker. Sulfur helps resolve comedones by its exfoliant action. It has been shown that elemental sulfur, but not sulfur compounds, induces comedone formation. Its popularity is due to its ability to quickly resolve pustules and papules, mask and conceal lesions (similar to a thick foundation lotion), and mild antibacterial action. It is often combined with salicylic acid or resorcinol to increase its effect. However, its use is limited by its offensive odor and the availability of more effective agents.

It has met the criteria of the FDA Advisory Review Panel for OTC topical acne products, although the claim for antibacterial effects was disallowed. Sodium thiosulfate, zinc sulfate, and zinc sulfide were not recognized in the monograph as safe and effective.

ANTIBACTERIALS

Benzoyl peroxide preparations are the single most useful group of topical agents and the agents of first choice for most patients with acne vulgaris.

Pharmaceutical Agents

Benzoyl peroxide has three principle actions that make it useful in both noninflammatory and inflammatory acne. It has powerful anaerobic antibacterial activity by a slow release of oxygen, comedolysis and depression of sebum production.

Benzoyl peroxide has a rapid (within 2 hours) bactericidal effect that lasts at least 48 hours. As a result, it may decrease the number of inflamed lesions within 5 days. Its anti-acne effect is augmented because it increases blood flow, producing erythema, is a dermal irritant, has local anesthetic properties and may promote healing.

Since the primary effect of benzoyl peroxide is antibacterial, it is most effective for inflammatory acne. Many patients with noninflammatory comedonal acne will respond due to its peeling action.

Cleansers containing benzoyl peroxide are available as nonprescription liquid washes and solid bars of various strengths. The desquamative and antibacterial effectiveness in a soap or wash is minimized due to the limited contact time on the skin and its removal with proper rinsing.

When applied topically, benzoyl peroxide penetrates unchanged through the stratum corneum and into the follicle, diffusing into the epidermis and the dermis where it is converted by follicular bacteria to benzoic acid. This metabolite is transported to the kidneys and excreted unchanged in urine.

Stable lotions are available in 2.5, 5 and 10%. Alcohol and acetone gels facilitate bioavailability and may be more effective, while water-based vehicles are less irritating and better tolerated. A 4% hydrophase gel (*Solugel*) is available that suspends crystals of benzoyl peroxide in a dimethylisosorbide solvent as the water in the base evaporates. The resulting solution is absorbed by the skin, leaving no film. The manufacturer claims the resulting efficacy is equal to 10% benzoyl peroxide with the minimal irritation of a 2.5% aqueous base gel. This may be an alternative for the patient who requires additional potency but whose skin is easily irritated. Paste vehicles are stiffer and more drying than ointments or creams, facilitate absorption and allow the active ingredients to stay localized.

Concentrations of 2.5, 5 and 10% in a water-based gel have been compared with the vehicle alone. The 2.5% formulation was more effective than its vehicle and equivalent to the 5 and 10% formulation in reducing the number of inflammatory lesions. Irritant side effects with the 2.5% gel were less frequent than with the 10% gel but equivalent to the 5% gel. The lowest concentration of benzoyl peroxide should be useful for treating patients with easily irritated skin and might lessen the expected degree of irritation when used in combination topical therapy with comedolytic agents.

Benzoyl peroxide may bleach hair and clothing, and may produce a mild primary irritant dermatitis that settles over continued use. This is more likely to occur with fair complexions, those who have a tendency to skin irritancy or who sunburn easily. There are rare reports of contact allergic dermatitis. Cross-reactions with other sensitizers, notably Peruvian balsam and cinnamon, are well-established. It may cross-sensitize to other benzoic acid derivatives such as topical anesthetics. Concomitant use of an abrasive cleanser may initiate or enhance sensitization. Another side effect includes a body odor that remains on clothing and bed sheets.

As a producer of free radicals, benzoyl peroxide can act as a promoter of skin cancer in mice or hamsters pretreated with the potent cancer-inducer, DMBA (7,12-dimethylbenz(a)anthracene), although this has not been shown in humans. There is no indication that the normal use of benzoyl peroxide in the treatment of acne is associated with an increased risk of facial skin cancer. The overall cutaneous use of benzoyl peroxide is relatively safe. The FDA determined that additional studies are needed to address concerns about benzoyl peroxide's possible tumor-initiating and promotion potential but acknowledges that this process may take several years. In the meantime, in August 1991, the FDA downgraded it from Category I (safe and effective) to Category III (data insufficient to permit classification).

Benzoyl peroxide has been used in combination with other anti-acne medications, such as sulfur and chlorhydroxyquinoline, or in formulations with urea to facilitate drug delivery. No significant improvement has been demonstrated. Since benzoyl peroxide has a different mechanism of action from retinoic acid, combination treatment has produced additive effects. By making the skin more permeable, retinoic acid may increase the tissue concentration of benzoyl peroxide. To avoid chemical incompatibility these two products should not be applied at the same time of day.

Preparations of benzoyl peroxide are available without prescription in concentrations up to 5%. The weakest concentration, 2.5%, in a water-based formulation should be recommended for anyone with a history of skin irritancy, or who must use combination therapy. There are many suggested routines to initiate therapy. One is to gently cleanse the skin and apply the preparation for 15 minutes the first evening, avoiding the eyes and mucous membranes. A mild stinging and reddening will appear. Each evening the time should be doubled until it is left on for 4 hours and subsequently all night. Dryness and peeling will appear after a few days. Once the patient can tolerate the medication, the strength may be increased to 5% or the base changed to the hydrophase, acetone or alcohol gels, or paste. Alternatively, benzoyl peroxide can be applied for 2 hours for 4 nights, 4 hours for 4 nights, and then left on all night. It is important to wash the product off in the morning. Other drying agents should be discontinued.

A sunscreen is recommended if benzoyl peroxide is used. To avoid interactions, apply the sunscreen during the day and the benzoyl peroxide at night.

OTHER AGENTS

Azaleic acid, a dicarboxylic acid, is a recently released nonprescription medication for mild to moderate acne. A 20% cream has been effective in clinical trials. Its mechanism of action is unclear, but it has antibacterial properties, reduces 5-alpha-reductase activity and modifies keratinization. It also inhibits melanocytes, improving postinflammatory hyperpigmentation.

Hydroquinone reversibly damages melanocytes and is used as a nonprescription hypopigmenting agent in concentrations of 2 to 4%. Preparations are available as clear or tinted gels, which are more drying, and vanishing or opaque, flesh-tinted creams, and may contain alpha-hydroxy acids or sunscreen. Epidermal but not dermal pigmentation will fade. Onset of response is usually 3 to 4 weeks, and the depigmentation lasts for 2 to 6 months but is reversible.

SUMMARY

Appearance and social acceptance have become important concepts today. The patient with acne needs encouragement and support as even the most inconspicious lesion may cause acute embarrassment. Once an appropriate ongoing treatment plan has been decided on with the patient, continuous monitoring and follow-up of his or her progress should be the responsibility of the health care professional. Teenagers should be reassured about the eventual self-limiting nature of the disease.

RECOMMENDED READING

Arndt KA. Acne. In: Arndt KA, editor. Manual of Dermatologic Therapeutics. Toronto: Little, Brown and Co, 1989:3-13.

Habif TP. Acne, rosacea, and related disorders. In: Klein EA, Menczer BS, eds. Clinical Dermatology. Toronto: CV Mosby & Co, 1990:756.

Lever L, Marks R. Current views on the aetiology, pathogenesis and treatment of acne vulgaris. Drugs 1990;39(5): 681-92.

Leyden J, Shalita AR. Rational therapy for acne vulgaris: an update on topical treatment. J Am Acad Dermatol 1986;15:907-14.

Puissegur-Lupo M. Acne vulgaris, treatments and their rationale. Postgrad Med 1985;78(7):76-88.

Taylor MB. Treatment of acne vulgaris. Postgrad Med 1991;89(8):40-47.

Winston MH, Shalita AR. Acne vulgaris. Pediatr Clin North Am 1991;38(4):889-903.

5

ALLERGY AND COLD PRODUCTS

KEITH J. SIMONS

CONTENTS

Rhinitis 79
- Introduction
- Symptoms
- Treatment

The Common Cold 86
- Introduction
- Symptoms
- Differential Diagnosis
- Treatment

Pharmaceutical Agents 93
- Analgesics/Antipyretics
- Antihistamines
- Antitussives
- Decongestants
- Expectorants
- Lozenges
- Vitamin C

Recommended Reading 100

RHINITIS

INTRODUCTION

Rhinitis may be defined as a noninfectious nasal disorder characterized by inflammation and hyperreactivity of the nasal mucosa to environmental stimuli. Symptoms include nasal discharge, congestion, itching and recurrent sneezing. The three most prevalent types of rhinitis are allergic, eosinophilic and vasomotor.

In allergic rhinitis, acute or perennial, symptoms may have a seasonal pattern and often include itching, erythema, and tearing of the eyes; itching of the nose; nasal discharge; congestion; and sneezing. Specific antigens such as pollens or animal danders that provoke symptoms can be identified by the patient history and positive skin tests or in vitro quantitation of specific immunoglobulin E to the allergen(s) implicated. Eosinophilic rhinitis and vasomotor rhinitis are nonallergic in nature. Eosinophilic rhinitis is characterized by paroxysmal sneezing and watery rhinorrhea, with numerous eosinophils in the nasal discharge, but negative allergy tests to inhaled antigens. Vasomotor rhinitis is characterized by chronic, watery nasal discharge and intermittent nasal congestion. Nasal secretions do not contain eosinophils and patients have no evidence of sensitization to inhaled antigens. Seasonal allergic rhinitis occurs yearly at specific times, for example, with ragweed pollination, from July to October. The term chronic rhinitis is applied when the duration is more than 8 weeks (Table 1).

Epidemiology

Discussion here will focus on allergic rhinitis, a commonly occurring disease that affects from 5 to 20% of the world's population. About 15% of Canadians, most under the age of 20, are afflicted.

Etiology

Allergic rhinitis is an antibody-mediated inflammatory disease of the nasal mucous membranes. When a genetically predisposed individual is exposed to an antigenic substance, antibodies or

Rhinitis

TABLE 1: Differential Diagnosis of Rhinitis

Sign/ Symptom	Common Cold	Acute Allergic Rhinitis	Perennial Allergic Rhinitis	Nonallergic Rhinitis
General symptom grade	Acute; symptoms present throughout the entire day; symptoms change somewhat over episode	Acute; symptoms wax and wane daily; usually worse in the morning	Chronic, low-grade; vary in severity, often unpredictably, throughout the year	Persistent symptoms; resembles perennial allergic rhinitis
Symptom time frame	Most episodes subside within a week	Weeks to months; symptoms correlate to seasons and to pollen count	No distinct seasonal pattern; intermittent or continuous throughout year	Remissions and exacerbations
Nasal discharge	Initially clear and watery, then changes consistency to mucopurulent; occurs mainly during days 1 through 3 of a cold	Copious, watery; clear	Rhinorrhea mild but chronic	Rhinorrhea mild but chronic
Congestion	Nasal and sinus congestion is common	Common	Chronic nasal obstruction is often prominent and may extend to eustachian tube obstruction, especially in children	Nasal congestion alternating with watery rhinorrhea
Conjunctivitis	Not common, except initially	Common; prominent ocular lacrimation and itch	Uncommon, but lacrimation can occur; lesser grade than acute allergic rhinitis	Uncommon, but lacrimation can occur
Sneezing	Uncommon, except at initial stages; occurs if congestion irritates nasal mucosal linings	Common, hallmark feature; sneezing often precedes appearance of rhinorrhea	Less common than with acute allergic rhinitis	Less common than with acute allergic rhinitis
Fever	Rare; more frequent in children	Absent	Absent	Absent
Pruritus	Nose and eyes can be somewhat affected	Common; nose, roof of mouth and eyes	Less common than with acute allergic rhinitis	Less common than with acute allergic rhinitis
Cough	Common, especially in later stages of cold	Coughing and asthmatic wheezing may develop as the season progresses; may be associated with postnasal drip	Rare; as for acute allergic rhinitis	Rare unless irritant-related, where inhalation of irritant induces cough reflex
Sore throat	Generally appears in early stages of cold; mild; may persist with accompanying postnasal drip or irritation via cough	Uncommon; may appear with postnasal drip	Uncommon; may appear with postnasal drip	Uncommon
Other	Mild constitutional symptoms; sinus headaches	Allergic shiners (dark circles under eyes); crease in nose from habitual rubbing; sinus headaches; recurring otitis media	As for acute allergic rhinitis	
Causative factor	Viral	Allergic; usually airborne pollens	Allergic; allergens present throughout the year, e.g., house dust	Etiology is uncertain; lacks evidence of any allergic basis; can be aggravated by dry air or inhaled irritants

Adapted from: Taylor JG. Allergic rhinitis. In: Carruthers-Czyzewski P, ed. Self-medication. Reference for Health Professionals. 4th ed. Ottawa: Canadian Pharmaceutical Association, 1992.

immunoglobulins of the IgE class specific to that antigen (allergen) are generated by the body's defence mechanisms. Common antigens include the protein components of pollens from trees, grasses and weeds, mold components and spores, animal dander (including saliva proteins), house dust components including mites, plant derived proteins such as enzymes (e.g., papain, kapok, food and saw dusts) and small molecular weight chemicals (e.g., penicillin, ethylenediamine, phthalic anhydride, etc.). Mast cells, generally located near small blood vessels and nerves as well as in connective tissue, lymphoid tissue and respiratory epithelium, and basophils that circulate in the blood stream, are target cells for IgE.

Following subsequent challenge with the same antigen, IgE production is stimulated. When the antigenic proteins cross-link two or more IgE molecules affixed to the membranes of mast cells and basophils, a complex chain of events requiring the presence of calcium and involving cyclic AMP occurs. This culminates in the degranulation of the mast cells and subsequent release of preformed and generated mediators of immediate and late phase hypersensitivity. The action of the chemical mediators, histamine, prostaglandins, kinins, leukotrienes, platelet activating factor (PAF) and others, on the blood vessels, goblet cells and mucosal glands produces the symptoms of allergic rhinitis.

The activity of histamine, mediated primarily through H_1-receptors with the possible minor involvement of H_2-receptors, produces capillary dilation that in turn causes the surrounding tissue to swell. With increased capillary permeability plasma proteins and fluid leak and various nerve endings are stimulated leading to the sensation of itching. Other mediators, such as prostaglandin D_2, the leukotrienes, thromboxane and PAF, are mildly vasoactive but also contribute to the inflammation through their chemotactic activity, attracting the inflammatory cells, eosinophils, basophils and neutrophils to the area.

SYMPTOMS

The most prevalent symptoms of allergic rhinitis are profuse and clear rhinorrhea; nasal congestion; lacrimation, with reddened and swollen conjunctiva; periorbital swelling; palatal, nasal and ocular pruritus; sneezing, often in intense bouts; eustachian tube obstruction, with or without ear ache; and frontal headaches. The nose, palate, pharynx and eyes usually begin to itch soon after exposure to an allergen followed by lacrimation, sneezing and rhinorrhea. Periods of nasal congestion, intermittent sneezing and rhinorrhea may last for 0.5 to 1 hour after exposure to a specific antigen, are frequently worse in the morning and improve towards the end of the day. Secondary sinusitis from persistent inflammatory obstruction of the sinus cavity openings, and coughing and asthmatic wheezing may be present. These physical discomforts can produce irritability, anorexia and insomnia in allergic patients. In children, chronic serous otitis media secondary to eustachian tube blockage; "allergic shiners," dark circles under the eyes due to periorbital edema; and the nose crease from the "allergic salute" (persistent upward rubbing of the tip of the nose with the palm of the hand) may be present in one-third to one-half of patients. The severity of symptoms of allergic rhinitis correlates to the degree of allergen exposure or pollen count. Primary exposure to one allergen can affect subsequent exposures (the "priming" effect), not only to the primary allergen, but also to other allergens. For example, during pollen season more severe reactions to house dust may occur.

Symptoms persisting for more than 8 weeks are considered chronic and, although similar to seasonal effects, are usually of lower severity. Chronic nasal congestion may lead to hearing problems in children when it affects the function of the eustachian tube, and may promote mouth breathing that results in dry mouth and throat, and cough.

The diagnosis of allergic rhinitis depends on the documentation of a careful history to correlate symptoms to the inciting agent, circumstances, duration, type and severity of symptoms as well as history of other family members who may be atopic or asthmatic. Positive identification of the offending allergen depends on skin prick testing, or RAST testing, a radioimmunoassay for measuring specific IgE serum concentrations. It is important to differentiate between the nasal congestion, rhinorrhea and pruritus of allergic rhinitis and similar symptoms of the common cold.

Symptoms of rhinitis vary in intensity throughout the day; cold symptoms are more persistent. The rhinorrhea from allergies remains clear and watery and does not progress to mucopurulent as with a cold. Sneezing and itching of the eyes, throat and nose are more evident in allergic rhinitis. Rhinitis medicamentosa from the overuse of topical decongestants as well as the adverse effects of other medications, such as antihypertensives, antipsychotics, ASA and oral contraceptives, must also be considered. The dry throat, a symptom of mouth breathing, should be distinguished from the infected sore throat.

TREATMENT

The goals of therapy for the treatment of allergic rhinitis are to assist the patient to reduce and possibly eliminate the symptoms through information that helps the patient learn how to avoid or reduce their exposure to allergens, preventing the allergic reaction. Complete avoidance of allergens is usually impossible, so recommendation of optimal pharmacological therapy to suppress and control symptoms should also be included.

Nonpharmacological Treatment

Once the causative allergen(s) have been positively identified, optimal treatment is allergen avoidance, either by elimination of that allergen from the environment or reduction or avoidance of exposure to the allergen. Control of house dust, mold and animal dander requires rigorous and possibly expensive measures. Careful housecleaning routines include the use of mattress covers and rigorous vacuuming of carpets. The areas should be assessed to determine whether the expense of replacing carpets with vinyl or wooden floors is necessary. There are commercial cleaners containing benzyl benzoate that can be brushed onto carpets, left to dry, and then vacuumed away. They will kill dust mites and their larvae. Meticulous laundry methods, including hot water in the rinse cycle, will kill mites on bedding. Extensive filtration, including electrostatic filters for forced air heating systems and reduction of humidity will reduce dust, mites and mold. Elimination of active smoking and passive exposure to tobacco smoke should be encouraged.

Animal dander may also be reduced by careful cleaning and vacuuming, but severe hypersensitivity may require removal of the pet from the environment. Persistence of animal allergens requires up to several months of intensive cleaning and filtration of air before complete elimination of the offending allergens can be guaranteed. This should be considered when removal of the pet for a trial period is being evaluated.

Pollen counts can be reduced to zero in a closed, well-filtered, air-conditioned room; in rooms with open windows they approach one-third of that found outdoors. Avoiding rural areas or driving with closed car windows, discouraging atopic children from playing in open fields, bathing and changing clothes after playing outside, and careful weed control in the high-use areas are recommended. If symptoms are severe, leaving the area of exposure during peak pollen periods or even permanently, may have to be considered.

Pharmacological Treatment

Total elimination or avoidance of the offending allergen may not be possible and immunotherapy may not be available or warranted. Self-medication treatment of the symptoms of allergic rhinitis involves the use of nonprescription antihistamines and/or decongestants.

H_1-receptor antagonists are effective in the management of seasonal and perennial allergic rhinitis symptoms such as rhinorrhea, nasal itching and sneezing. They also control ocular itching, tearing and erythema. Topical formulations are also now available. None of the H_1-receptor antagonists prevent nasal blockage in allergen challenge tests and none relieve nasal blockage as well as they prevent rhinorrhea, itching or sneezing (Table 2). Individuals should start taking medications before the allergen exposure and continue taking them regularly until the end of the season or exposure for maximum effectiveness.

The addition of a sympathomimetic agent such as pseudoephedrine or phenylpropanolamine to an H_1-antagonist significantly improves relief of nasal congestion compared to the H_1-antagonist alone. Topical application of lubricant formulations containing polyethylene glycol/propylene glycol may provide some relief from nasal congestion. A management algorithm for allergic rhinitis is provided at Figure 1.

Prescription agents include mast cell stabilizing agents, cromolyn and nedocromil, topically applied corticosteroids such as beclomethasone, flunisolide, budesonide, and triamcinolone and the anticholinergic, ipratropium bromide. Immunotherapy is long-term, controversial and depends on the availability of appropriate antigenic material. It may become of increasing importance as purified, specific allergen extracts become available.

TABLE 2: Antihistamines: Classification, Characteristics, Doses

Class	General Comments	Representative Agents	Dosage (24-hour maximum)
First-Generation Antihistamines			
Alkylamines	Drowsiness most common reaction, but overall incidence is low. Cause less CNS depression than members of other groups. Some CNS stimulation is possible, especially in young children. Low incidence of side effects	brompheniramine	*Adults:* 4 mg every 4–6 hr (24 mg) *6 to 11 yrs:* 2 mg every 4–6 hr (12 mg) *2 to 5 yrs:* 1 mg every 4–6 hr (6 mg) Alternate children's dose: 0.5 mg/kg/day in 3 or 4 divided doses
		chlorpheniramine	*Adults:* 4 mg every 4–6 hr (24 mg) *6 to 11 yrs:* 2 mg every 4–6 hr (12 mg) *2 to 5 yrs:* 1 mg every 4–6 hr (6 mg) Alternate children's dose: 0.35 mg/kg/day in 4 divided doses
		dexbrompheniramine	*Adults:* 2 mg every 4–6 hr (12 mg) *6 to 11 yrs:* 1 mg every 4–6 hr (6 mg) *2 to 5 yrs:* 0.5 mg every 4–6 hr (3 mg)
		triprolidine	*Adults:* 2.5 mg every 4–6 hr (10 mg) *6 to 11 yrs:* 1.25 mg every 4–6 hr (5 mg) *4 to 5 yrs:* 1 mg every 4–6 hr (3.75 mg) *2 to 3 yrs:* 0.625 mg every 4–6 hr (2.5 mg) *4 mo to under 2 yrs:* 0.313 mg every 4–6 hr (1.25 mg)
Ethanolamines	Diphenhydramine and doxylamine can cause marked drowsiness Drowsiness is the most frequent side effect reported with clemastine but sedative effect is considered low Carbinoxamine has lowest incidence of drowsiness of this group Significant anticholinergic activity Relatively low incidence of gastrointestinal side effects	carbinoxamine	*Adults:* 4–8 mg 3 to 4 times daily *6 to 11 yrs:* 4 mg 3 to 4 times daily *3 to 5 yrs:* 2–4 mg 3 to 4 times daily *1 to 2 yrs:* 2 mg 3 to 4 times daily Alternate children's dose: 0.2–0.4 mg/kg/day in 3 or 4 doses
		clemastine	*Adults:* 1 mg twice daily (6 mg) *Children up to 12 yrs:* 0.5–1 mg twice daily
		diphenhydramine	*Adults:* 25–50 mg every 4–6 hr (300 mg) *6 to 11 yrs:* 12.5–25 mg every 4–6 hr (150 mg) *2 to 5 yrs:* 6.25 mg every 4–6 hr (37.5 mg) Alternate children's dose: 5 mg/kg/day in 4 divided doses
		diphenylpyraline	*Adults:* 2 mg every 4 hr (10 mg) *6 to 11 yrs:* 2 mg every 6 hr (6 mg) *2 to 5 yrs:* 1–2 mg every 8 hr (4 mg)
		doxylamine	*Adults:* 7.5–12.5 mg every 4–6 hr (75 mg) *6 to 11 yrs:* 3.75–6.25 mg every 4–6 hr (37.5 mg) *2 to 5 yrs:* 2–3.125 mg every 4–6 hr (18.75 mg)
Ethylenediamines	Incidence of side effects 20–35% Relatively weak CNS effects, but drowsiness may occur in some people Gastrointestinal side effects common Incidence of sedation with tripelennamine lower than with diphenhydramine, but dizziness is common	pyrilamine	*Adults:* 25–50 mg every 6–8 hr (200 mg) *6 to 11 yrs:* 12.5–25 mg every 6–8 hr (100 mg) *2 to 5 yrs:* 6.25–12.5 mg every 6–8 hr (50 mg)
		tripelennamine	*Adults:* 25–50 mg every 4–6 hr (600 mg) *Children:* 5 mg/kg/day in 4 to 6 divided doses (300 mg)

TABLE 2: Antihistamines: Classification, Characteristics, Doses (*cont'd*)

Class	General Comments	Representative Agents	Dosage (24-hour maximum)
Phenothiazines	All precautions applicable to phenothiazines may apply Sedative effects prominent Significant anticholinergic activity Promethazine also used as an antiemetic	promethazine	*Adults:* 25 mg at bedtime; if necessary, 12.5 mg 4 times daily. Alternatively, 20–100 mg/day, in divided doses at meals, with the highest dose given at bedtime. *Children:* 0.5 mg/kg at bedtime or 0.125 mg/kg as needed (*Note: promethazine should not be administered to children less than 2 years of age due to a possible association with sleep apnea.**)
Piperadines	Drowsiness is the most common side effect; sedative potential is comparable to that of the ethylenediamine class Moderate anticholinergic effects Although cyproheptadine stimulates appetite in children, weight gain is inconsistent, transient and quickly reversible after withdrawal of the drug	azatadine	*Adults:* 1–2 mg twice daily *6 to 12 yrs:* 0.5–1 mg twice daily
		cyproheptadine	*Adults:* 4 mg 3 times daily. Most adults require 12–16 mg daily *6–14 yrs:* 4 mg 2 to 3 times daily *2 to 5 yrs:* 2 mg 2 to 3 times daily (8 mg) Not recommended in children less than 2 yrs
		phenindamine	*Adults:* 25 mg every 4–6 hr *6 to 12 yrs:* 12.5 mg every 4–6 hr (75 mg) *Less than 6 yrs:* as directed by physician
Second-Generation Antihistamines			
	Although sedation is the most commonly reported side effect, it occurs at a rate similar to placebo groups The CNS effects of alcohol are not enhanced by these agents Negligible anticholinergic effects Astemizole may have a slower onset of action in relation to other agents	astemizole	*Adults:* 10 mg daily (*Note: use of astemizole in children less than 12 years of age should be under the guidance of a physician.*) *6 to 12 yrs:* 5 mg daily *Less than 6 yrs:* 2 mg/10 kg/day
		cetirizine	*Adults:* 5–10 mg daily (20 mg)
		loratadine	*Adults:* 10 mg daily Use should be limited to no longer than 6 months unless recommended by a physician Safety and efficacy in children less than 12 yrs have not been established
		terfenadine	*Adults:* 60 mg twice daily or 120 mg daily *7 to 12 yrs:* 30 mg twice daily *3 to 6 yrs:* 15 mg twice daily *Less than 3 yrs:* as directed by physician Use in children should be limited to periods of 1 week unless otherwise directed by a physician

*Kahn A, Hasaerts D, Blum D. Phenothiazine-induced sleep apneas in normal infants. Pediatrics 1985;75:844–47.
Adapted from: Taylor JG. Allergic rhinitis. In: Carruthers-Czyzewski P, ed. Self-medication. Reference for Health Professionals. 4th ed. Ottawa: Canadian Pharmaceutical Association, 1992.

FIGURE 1

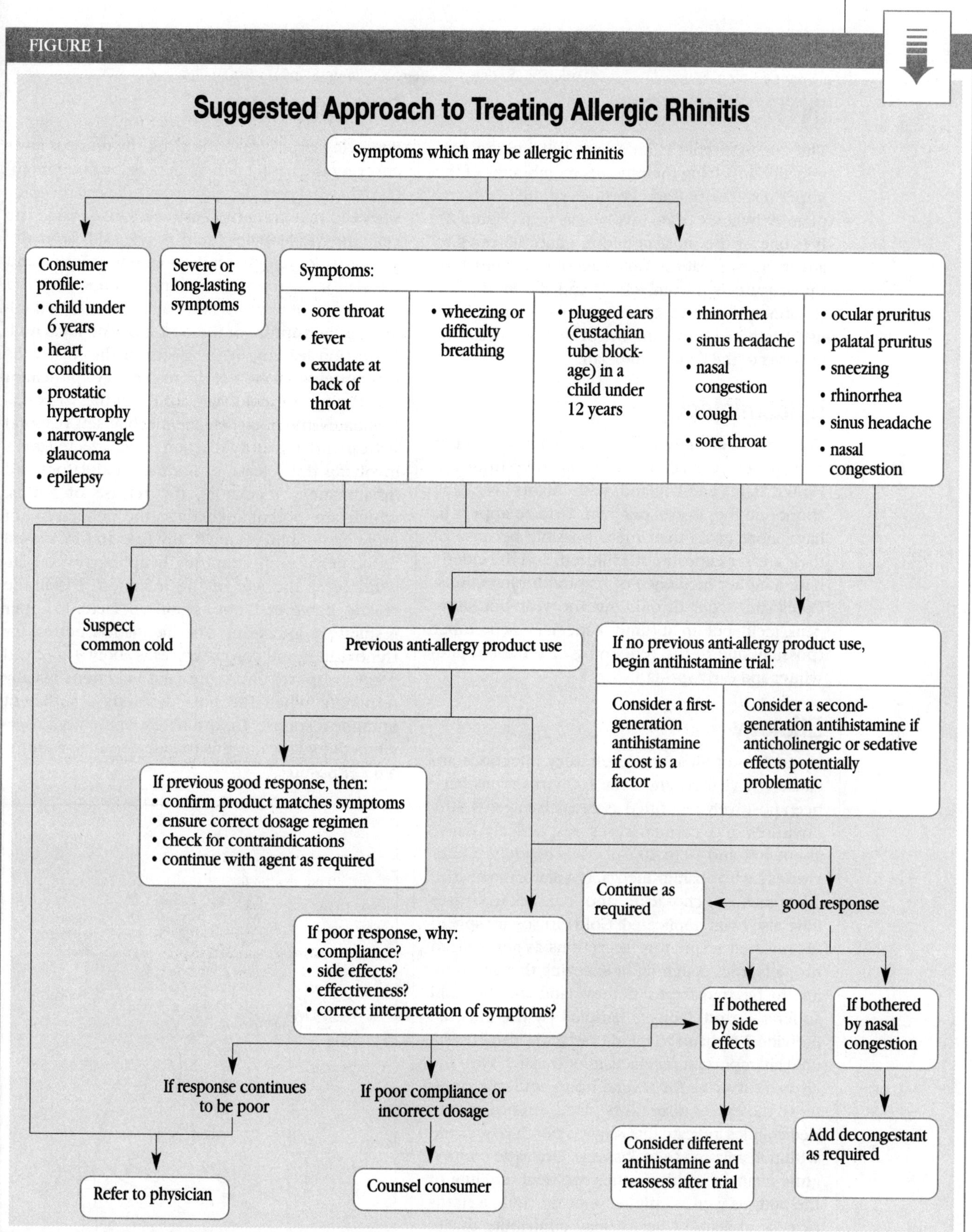

Adapted from: Taylor JG. Allergic rhinitis. In: Carruthers-Czyzewski P, ed. Self-medication. Reference for Health Professionals. 4th ed. Ottawa: Canadian Pharmaceutical Association, 1992.

THE COMMON COLD

INTRODUCTION

The common cold is an acute, self-limiting viral infection involving the mucous membranes of the upper respiratory tract. Portions of the lower respiratory tract are often involved as well (Figure 2). It is one of the most common acute illnesses to affect the population. Colds account for much of the absenteeism from school and the workplace (in about 50% of cases, at least 1 day away from usual activities), and are one of the major reasons for visits to the family physician.

Epidemiology

Colds occur at a rate of about 1 to 3 episodes per person per year according to surveys from the United States and England, with infants averaging about 6 to 8 episodes per year. Women appear to have more colds than men, possibly because of their greater exposure to children, and the elderly have a higher incidence of respiratory infections. Colds can occur throughout the year but show peak incidence in autumn, especially September (possibly due to the reopening of schools), midwinter and early spring.

Etiology

Up to 90% of all acute respiratory infections are caused by viruses, and over 100 virus types have been positively identified as causative agents. Rhinoviruses and coronaviruses respectively cause about 40% and 10 to 20% of colds in adults. Other viruses such as parainfluenza, respiratory syncytial, adenosackie, echosackie and coxsackie viruses have also been implicated. Cold viruses are spread via infected respiratory secretions as aerosolized droplets from coughing or sneezing that are more apt to be transferred if they land on the cold sufferer's hand. Objects handled by the infected individual or hand to hand contact is also considered an important mechanism of transfer, with the viruses surviving for several hours until the transfer to the eye or nose takes place. Studies of married couples indicate that saliva is poorly associated with transmission (e.g., kissing). Dramatic temperature changes, cold weather, wet feet, chilling of the body as well as fatigue, poor nutritional status or general state of health may contribute to the severity of the cold, but exposure to the causative virus must occur first.

Pathophysiology

Following exposure to the virus, the mucous layer covering the nasal epithelium must be penetrated, then the viral particles bind to specific cell receptor sites and penetrate the host cell. Once inside the cell, the viral nucleic acid is released from the protective envelope, replication, transcription and translation of the viral genome occurs with the production of new viruses, which are released following the rupture of the host cell. The local multiplication leading to the death of the host cells causes desquamation of the respiratory epithelium and the typical cold symptoms. As the virus disseminates, the body defence mechanisms respond with an inflammatory reaction in the affected areas involving the release of immunomodulators and inflammatory mediators, the release of kinins, which are potent autocoids, the generation of immunoglobulins, specifically IgA, and increased tissue perfusion, permitting lymphocytes to concentrate at the site of the infection. Histamine release, however, is not a significant factor in upper respiratory infections. The incubation period for rhinoviruses and coronaviruses is about 1 to 2 and 3 days respectively. Acute viral infections usually terminate when the host develops a sufficient immune response. Unfortunately, immunity to specific cold viruses begins to fade about 18 months after exposure.

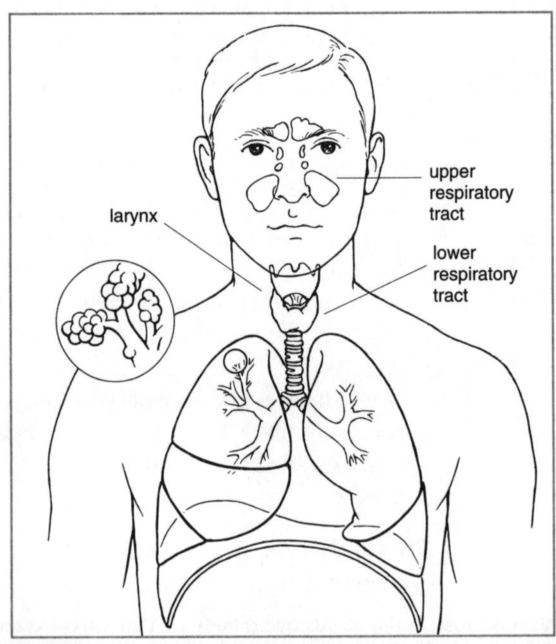

FIGURE 2

SYMPTOMS

The most common symptoms of the common cold are nasal discharge and congestion (80 to 100%), sneezing (50 to 70%), sore throat (50%) and cough (40%). In most cases, symptoms persist for about 7 days with peak effects occurring on days 2 and 3, while in about 25% of cases symptoms may last for 2 weeks. The extent and sequence of appearance of these symptoms generally follows a pattern.

The initial symptom is usually the discomfort of a sore throat, often described as dryness, scratchiness or soreness rather than pain. This is usually followed by varying degrees of nasal congestion and rhinorrhea. The initial nasal discharge is clear, then becomes thicker and opaque as the infection progresses due to the large number of epithelial and white blood cells being shed, and may become purulent if secondary bacterial infection occurs. The congestion may lead to sinusitis, headache, nasal irritation resulting in sneezing, and, especially in children, otic symptoms such as pain or a plugged sensation. Postnasal drip can cause coughing or laryngitis, and conjunctivitis and watering eyes are initially present.

The cough accompanying a cold usually starts as dry and nonproductive, but becomes productive as the increased bronchial secretions and cellular debris from phagocytic activity accumulate. The cough is most frequently caused by the common cold, and is the symptom of an underlying condition accounting for a large percentage of visits to the physician, especially during the winter months. In association with the cold, coughs last for no longer than 1 to 2 weeks. Coughs can also be induced by sinusitis, postnasal discharge that irritates receptors in the pharynx, or by stimulation of receptors in the sinus, or even just the result of mouth breathing, which allows poorly conditioned air to dry the upper airways.

Dry, nonproductive coughs that persist for some weeks after the other symptoms of a cold have disappeared may indicate any of the following: an exaggerated response to virus-induced respiratory damage or bronchitis; asthma in a child, especially if the cough is worse at night; gastroesophageal reflux if associated with heartburn and sour taste in the mouth; chronic obstructive lung disease; lung cancer; or even the symptom of left ventricular heart failure. Environmental irritants such as cigarette smoke or volatile chemicals can also cause cough by irritating receptors in the larynx, trachea and bronchi. Dry, nonproductive coughs can also be present as an adverse effect of certain medications, such as angiotensin converting enzyme (ACE) inhibitors.

Fever of any significant degree is seldom present, but chill sensations are common, while children are more prone to develop fever, 38 to 39°C. These symptoms, although discomforting, seldom cause serious complications or residual pathologic damage to the respiratory tract. Sinusitis, otitis media, exacerbation of asthma and infectious exacerbations in cases of chronic obstructive pulmonary disease have occurred, while increased chest involvement with purulent sputum suggests secondary bacterial infection.

DIFFERENTIAL DIAGNOSIS

Since individual symptoms of the common cold are similar to those of other conditions such as pharyngitis, influenza, sinusitis, bronchitis, allergic rhinitis, it is important to differentiate between them (Table 3), assess for self-treatment or, if deemed necessary, refer the patient to a physician.

Bronchitis

Bronchitis is an inflammation of the tracheobronchial tree due to infection with common organisms as *S. pneumoniae*, *H. influenzae*, *M. pneumoniae*, and common cold viruses. It may often follow an episode of a cold. The main symptom is cough, initially dry and nonproductive but becoming productive over time as sputum becomes more abundant and mucopurulent. The cough is essential to the removal of bronchial secretions, and wheezing after coughing may be present. In severe bronchitis, fever and chest pain may be present, and if persistent, indicate complicating pneumonia. In young children, it is best treated empirically with antibiotics, while cultures should be taken in adults prior to such treatment. Initially, a cough suppressant may be used if the dry, nonproductive cough interferes with sleep, while an expectorant may be required as the cough becomes productive.

Pharyngitis

Streptococcal pharyngitis (strep throat) in which *Streptococcus pyogenes*, group A ß-hemolytic streptococcus is the main causative agent, is characterized by sore throat, fever often greater than 38.3°C, a beefy-red pharynx and exudate over the tonsils. The onset of pain is more rapid and severe than in viral infections and is aggravated by swallowing.

Although it accounts for the minority of all sore throats, a sore throat alone or with other symptoms not consistent with the common cold, especially in children, should be referred to a physician. A throat culture is usually required to confirm diagnosis, and treatment with antibiotics is based on the risk of the individual developing serious sequelae, such as acute rheumatic fever and acute glomerulonephritis.

Sinusitis

Sinusitis, the inflammation of the mucosal lining of the nasal sinuses, is commonly caused by *Staphylococcus*, *Streptococcus* and *Haemophilus influenzae* bacteria. The congestion created by a cold blocks natural drainage of the sinus creating an environment conducive to bacterial infection. The distinguishing symptoms include purulent discharge from the sinus cavities, headache and facial tenderness if the pain can be localized to the sinus area, and possibly fever. In addition, chronic sinusitis may yield a postnasal discharge with a musty odor or a nonproductive cough. In children, persistent cough and purulent rhinorrhea associated with irritability and tiredness are likely symptoms. Systemic antibiotics and oral and topical decongestants are first-line therapies, so referral to a physician is mandatory.

Influenza

Although the terms common cold and flu are often used interchangeably, influenza is a much more serious acute respiratory infection caused by *myxovirus A, B* or *C*. Type A-influenza is the most virulent and causes annual outbreaks of infection that may reach epidemic proportions every 2 or 3 years, usually in winter. True influenza is a serious disease and an estimated 5,000 Canadians, principally those over 65 years of age, die every year from influenza-aggravated illness. Annual immunization can prevent influenza and is recommended for patients at high risk of complications, and the elderly.

Similar to the common cold, influenza is contracted from exposure to the respiratory secretions of those infected with the virus. Systemic symptoms, including fever, chills, headache, myalgias predominately in the back and legs, and malaise occur rapidly following exposure. The face is flushed, the skin hot and moist with a marked and rapidly rising fever of 38 to 40°C within 12 hours of onset. Symptoms such as sore throat, nonproductive cough and rhinorrhea increase in severity during the illness. As the fever subsides, systemic symptoms diminish. Accompanying coughs, usually nonproductive, develop in more than 75% of cases and may persist for more than 2 weeks. A major complication of influenza is pneumonia due to the overgrowth of the influenza virus, or more commonly bacterial, which results in fever, chills, chest pain and a cough that produces purulent or rust-colored sputum.

TREATMENT

Nonpharmacological Treatment

Generally a cold is self-limiting and usually disappears in 7 to 10 days regardless of treatment. Warmth and bed rest are certainly preferable to cool temperatures and the workplace or school. Bed rest for 1 or 2 days when the initial symptoms are severe is often recommended and will definitely protect colleagues from the virus. Performance at work or school may be less than efficient during this time.

Good nutrition will help patients to maintain their strength, and extra fluids will be beneficial if fever is present and help reduce the tenacity of mucus. Hot fluids may be superior to cold fluids and the addition of alcohol (hot toddy) tops the list of home cold remedies for adults, but not young children. Since these are usually administered prior to sleep, the interaction of alcohol with other medications, such as H_1-antagonists, will not be a problem, and may ensure an undisturbed night's sleep. Chicken soup will probably work as well as any other hot nourishing liquid. Salt water gargles, one-quarter of a teaspoonful of salt to 250 mL of warm water, for about 15 seconds, repeated frequently during the day are said to help clean the back of the throat and provide local relief of pain, but the duration is short, usually less than 1 hour. Humidification of room air, either by steam or cool mist, may relieve the symptoms of the sore throat, the dry cough, and the nasal and chest congestion by reducing mucus viscosity, making it easier to blow the nose and expectorate respiratory secretions. Vaporizers (either steam, cool mist or ultrasonic) can be used. Cool mist vaporizers are safer for areas with children as there is no chance of scalding; however, the reservoir must be kept scrupulously clean to prevent contamination with bacteria or molds. Reservoirs of steam vaporizers require little cleaning; however, if the water is hard, mineral build-up on the electrodes or in the container may occur. Aromatic compounds, either home remedies or commercial formulations, may be placed in the medication cup and be vaporized and dispersed by the stream of vapor. In addition to the medicine-like odor, decongestant and antitussive activity may result, mainly due to the increased humidity.

Nasal congestion in infants, especially when breast- or bottle-fed, may be alleviated by 1 or 2 drops of saline into each nostril followed by gentle nasal suction. This procedure should only be performed on the advice of a physician. Propping up the infant's head or having the child sleep in a car seat may assist nasal drainage.

Pharmacological Treatment

Treatment of the common cold is primarily symptomatic. Initially, it is important to try to identify the condition, allergic rhinitis, common cold, strep throat, sinusitis, bronchitis or influenza, or a more serious underlying condition, and establish whether nonprescription therapy is appropriate or referral to a physician is indicated.

The treatment algorithm (Figure 3) provides guidelines for selecting therapy. Nonpharmacologic measures should always be recommended along with product recommendations.

Nasal Congestion and Discharge

The sympathomimetic effects of decongestants are useful in treating nasal mucosal congestion in the common cold. Topical and oral preparations are available.

Because there is no evidence of histamine release associated with the nasal symptoms of the common cold, the use of antihistamines is questionable. Recent studies have had conflicting results. Older first generation, sedating H_1-receptor antagonists with anticholinergic activity may be preferable to second generation, nonsedating agents, since the drying effect on the upper respiratory tract secretions is the most noticeable relief of symptoms observed by patients. Intranasal lubricant formulations containing polyethylene glycol/ propylene glycol may provide some relief from nasal congestion if used routinely.

Cough

If a dry, nonproductive cough is accompanying a cold and is uncomplicated but annoying, especially at night, treatment with an antitussive (cough suppressant) is indicated. If the cough is productive, e.g., during the later stages of a cold or with bronchitis, recommendation of an expectorant to help loosen phlegm and bronchial secretions and rid the bronchial passageway of mucus is desirable. Expectorants may also relieve irritated membranes in the respiratory tract by preventing dryness through increased mucus flow.

Sore Throat

Sucking a sour hard candy to stimulate saliva flow or the use of a warm, saline gargle to soothe inflamed tissue should be tried first. If not effective, lozenges containing antimicrobial agents, local anesthetics, aromatic compounds or demulcents can be recommended.

Fever and Headache

Fever, common in children, should not be treated with ASA due to its association with the development of Reye's syndrome. Acetaminophen may be used safely, provided there is strict adherence to the recommended dosage regimens.

Product Selection

The availability of hundreds of nonprescription products containing almost every combination and permutation of the major classes of pharmaceutical agents for the treatment of the symptoms of the common cold presents a challenge to the health professional.

Once it has been established that self-treatment is appropriate, individual component formulations should be recommended to treat specific symptoms; an H_1-antagonist for rhinorrhea, a decongestant for nasal blockage, an antipyretic for fever, an antitussive for a dry, nonproductive cough, or an expectorant for a productive cough. By using these products, the patient can individualize the therapy as the cold progresses and the symptoms change. While there is a loss of flexibility when multiple ingredient formulations are used, H_1-antagonist and decongestant or decongestant and analgesic or decongestant and antitussive products may be recommended since patients often present with multiple symptoms. Reduced costs may be considered, as well as improved patient compliance from the reduced number of doses. A focus on the most annoying symptoms rather than a blanket approach is preferable. Diabetics, while very knowledgeable about their condition, may require assistance to distinguish between *dietetic* (calorie reduced) and *diabetic* (calorie-free) products, or alternative therapy such as antitussives in calorie-free tablet formulations instead of cough syrups.

The Common Cold

PATIENT ASSESSMENT QUESTIONS

Q Do you think you have a cold or allergic rhinitis?

The following will assist to differentiate between allergic rhinitis and the upper respiratory symptoms of the common cold.

Rhinorrhea, congestion and ocular or palatal itchiness, acute bouts of sneezing, and the persistence of these symptoms longer than the typical 10 to 14 days of a common cold, suggest rhinitis. Identification of trigger factors may suggest allergic rather than nonallergic rhinitis.

Symptoms of the common cold include mild to moderate sore throat, changing to rhinorrhea followed by nasal congestion, watery eyes and a cough. Terms such as "head" cold and "chest" cold will assist in differentiating upper or lower respiratory symptoms that need to be treated. Persistence of cough with greenish-colored sputum exudate may indicate a more serious lower respiratory tract infection.

If rhinitis is indicated by the symptoms:

Q Have you used or are you currently using any medications?

It is important to know if medications such as topical steroids are being used, and if antihistamines, alone or in conjunction with decongestants have been recommended or prescribed.

Q Are you using antihistamine and/or decongestant products?

Antihistamines are the nonprescription drugs of choice and the addition of a decongestant, either as an additional dosage form or in a combination form will provide relief of the rhinorrhea, congestion and ocular tearing and itching. Administration before the onset of symptoms usually provides better relief rather than after symptoms appear. This is especially important if exposure to known allergens is anticipated. Regular dosing is the most efficient way to control symptoms rather than intermittent use when symptoms occur.

Q Are you experiencing any adverse effects?

The central nervous system and anticholinergic adverse effects of the first-generation antihistamines may be reduced or eliminated by recommending a switch to the relatively nonsedating second-generation compounds. Conditions such as narrow-angle glaucoma, heart disease, epilepsy or prostate enlargement may be complicated by the side effects of the first-generation antihistamines.

Q Are you benefitting from your antihistamine therapy?

A number of anecdotal reports and some prospective studies have demonstrated development of subsensitivity to chronic users of antihistamines. Patients in well-designed studies have not demonstrated subsensitivity for up to 3 to 4 months. Reduced patient compliance, due to irritating side effects, or the development of tolerance to the CNS effects may persuade patients that the medications are no longer relieving symptoms. Even if this is only a perception by the patient, changing to another antihistamine may produce beneficial effects.

If the common cold is indicated by the symptoms:

Q Are the symptoms runny nose and congestion?

The rhinitis, congestion and ocular symptoms may be treated with antihistamines and/or decongestants, oral or topical, alone or in combination. Some of the first-generation antihistamines may be more beneficial because of the sedative effects and the anticholinergic effects, especially at nighttime. Dosing once daily at bedtime might reduce the sedative symptoms for the following day. The addition of a decongestant may not only relieve the nasal congestion but also reduce the sedative effects of the antihistamine. The second-generation antihistamines are less sedating and have no anticholinergic effects so may not seem to be as effective. In combination with decongestants, wakefulness may occur at nighttime due to the lack of sedative effects of the antihistamine.

Q Is the cough productive or nonproductive and/or distracting due to frequency?

A cough that produces sputum exudate should not be suppressed. Increased fluid intake and possibly expectorants should be recommended. Under certain circumstances, suppressants might be recommended if the exudate is minimal and sleep disturbance is a problem. The dry, nonproductive cough should be treated with cough suppressants.

TABLE 3: Differential Diagnosis of the Common Cold

Symptom	Common Cold	Acute Sinusitis	Strep Throat	Influenza
Nasal discharge	Common; clear, copious rhinorrhea initially, followed by a more mucopurulent appearance; nasal congestion is common	Purulent, often colored	Rare	Present, but overshadowed by systemic symptoms; clear discharge initially, becoming more purulent; nasal obstruction is uncommon
Fever	Rare; low grade if any	Over 38°C; variable with severity of the infection; present in less than one-half of sufferers; mainly children	Over 38°C in 90% of children; spiking	39 to 40°C; sudden onset, lasting 3 to 4 days
Sore throat	Common but mild; should be gone within 3 days	None, unless associated with postnasal drip	Pain onset is severe and sudden; inflamed; exudate at back of throat and on tonsils; voice could be hoarse	Sometimes
Cough	Mild to moderate, dry, hacking cough; may change presentation during course of cold	None, unless associated with postnasal drip	Rare	Common; can be severe
Headache	Rare; more frequent with sinus congestion	Occurs via sinus congestion; pain over involved areas; typically is worse during the day and subsides in evening; varies with a change in body position	Occurs in 70% of children	Prominent; throbbing, frontal headache; severity is related to the level of the fever
General aches and pain/ fatigue and weakness	Mild	Rare	Malaise possible	Common; often severe; fatigue and weakness can last up to 2 to 3 weeks
Other		Acute maxillary sinusitis may cause a feeling of pain in the area of the teeth; chronic sinus infection may produce minimal symptoms	Breath odor; cervical lymphadenopathy; abdominal pain in 20% of children	Chills: GI symptoms, e.g., diarrhea, vomiting; the main symptoms are sudden and severe in onset
Duration of illness	5 to 7 days	Days; months if not treated	Commonly 3 days; up to a week	Approximately 10 days
Cause	Viral	Bacterial (*Staphylococcus*, *Streptococcus*, *Haemophilus influenzae*); usually follows an acute upper respiratory infection or nasal allergies, or less frequently, swimming and dental abscess	*S. pyogenes*; note that other bacteria can cause sore throat	Influenza virus

Adapted from: Taylor JG. Allergic rhinitis. In: Carruthers-Czyzewski P, ed. Self-medication. Reference for Health Professionals. 4th ed. Ottawa: Canadian Pharmaceutical Association, 1992.

FIGURE 3

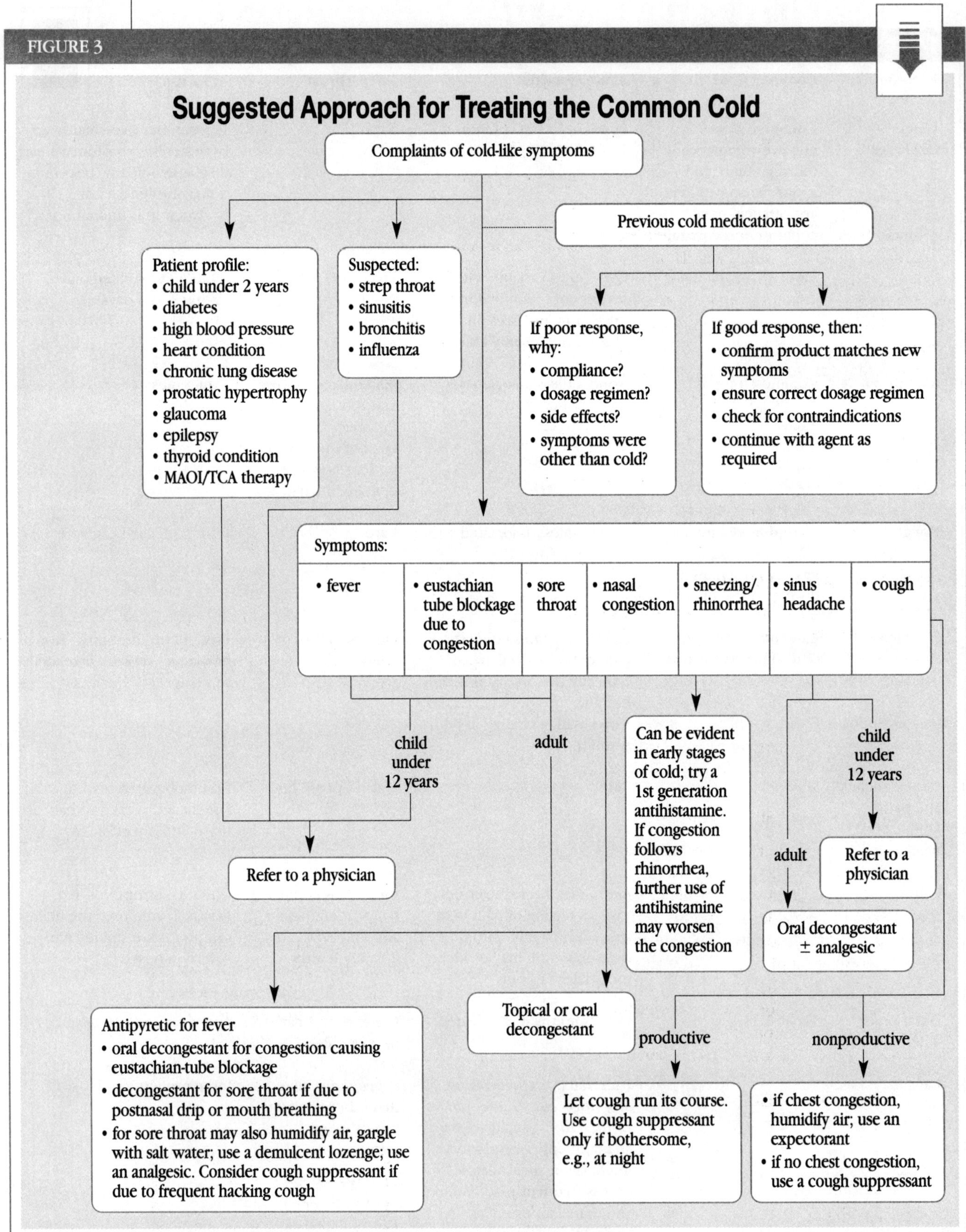

Adapted from: Taylor JG. Allergic rhinitis. In: Carruthers-Czyzewski P, ed. Self-medication. Reference for Health Professionals. 4th ed. Ottawa: Canadian Pharmaceutical Association, 1992.

PHARMACEUTICAL AGENTS

ANALGESICS/ANTIPYRETICS

(See the Pain and Fever Products chapter)

ANTIHISTAMINES

Antihistamines are H_1-receptor antagonists. They block histamine from binding with H_1-receptors on target cells such as pruritus receptors, the mucous glands in the nasal mucosa and nasal blood vessels, thereby preventing itching, mucous secretion and vasodilation. Some H_1-receptor antagonists also prevent release of inflammatory mediators from sensitized mast cells and basophils; while others have anticholinergic and antiserotonin and local anesthetic properties. The H_1-receptor antagonists are generally divided into two distinct classes, the first-generation sedating H_1-antagonists and the second-generation, nonsedating H_1-antagonists. For a listing of agents see Table 2.

First-Generation Antihistamines

Most of the first-generation H_1-antagonists contain the core antihistamine structure and are divided into subclasses on the basis of chemical structure. Structural modification was intended to achieve more specific H_1-receptor activity and reduce the cross-reactivity to anticholinergic, antiserotonin, and α-adrenergic blocking activity to prevent the primary adverse effects of sedation and dry mouth.

Second-Generation Antihistamines

The second-generation H_1-antagonists, although containing structures such as piperadine rings, are not generally classified by chemical structure. These include astemizole, loratadine, terfenadine and cetirizine; those not yet available in Canada such as acrivastine and azelastine; and those on prescription such as the topically applied levocabastine. These compounds are relatively lipophobic and are extensively bound to plasma proteins so they do not cross the blood brain barrier, thus resulting in no more central nervous system sedative effects than placebo, which can range from 15 to 25%.

Efficacy

Allergic Rhinitis

In manufacturers' recommended doses, most of the new relatively nonsedating H_1-antagonists are equal in efficacy. They are superior in efficacy to placebo and comparable in efficacy to chlorpheniramine or other first-generation H_1-antagonists in relieving nasal discharge, itching and sneezing. In many studies astemizole has a demonstrated longer lag time to peak onset of action than other H_1-antagonists and is perhaps not suited for sporadic use. Astemizole should be discontinued for at least 4 to 6 weeks prior to allergy testing, while for other agents a 1 week washout is satisfactory. In well-designed prospective studies, where compliance has been vigorously monitored, no evidence of subsensitivity has been demonstrated for up to 4 months of continuous therapy.

Common Cold

Studies to evaluate the benefit of the H_1-antagonists in the treatment of the symptoms of the common cold have yielded conflicting results. This may be due to poor study design: the effect of an H_1-antagonist in combination with a decongestant does not allow for individual evaluation of separate entities, the lack of a placebo control, subjective evaluation techniques, the use of large multicenters, the difficulty in selecting homogeneous populations, and the lack of a good simulation model of the symptoms of the common cold that can be experimentally-induced. In multicenter studies it is more difficult to obtain uniform results due to location and range of study staff.

Dosage

Most of the first-generation H_1-antagonists are administered 3 to 4 times daily because of the short serum elimination half-life. Chlorpheniramine and brompheniramine have an average half-life of about 20 hours in adults, and once daily dosing should be possible. The short-acting formulations are still recommended for 3 to 4 times daily dosing with 2 to 3 times daily dosing of sustained-release formulations. Triprolidine, and its nonsedating analogue, acrivastine, have short half-lives and require 3 to 4 times daily dosing. Once daily dosing is suitable for astemizole, cetirizine and loratadine due to the relatively long elimination half-lives, although when the latter is combined with pseudoephedrine, the dose is reduced by half and dosing is every 12 hours. In this product, the pseudoephedrine is formulated for sustained release. Terfenadine is available as 60 mg every 12 hours or 120 mg once daily, with the twice daily dosing regimen considered superior, providing more uniform serum concentrations, and possibly effect, although improved patient compliance may be possible with the once-daily dosing.

Adverse Effects

The major central nervous system (CNS) adverse effects of the first-generation agents, which cross the blood brain barrier, can range from drowsiness to deep sleep as well as altered co-ordination, dizziness, lassitude and inability to concentrate. These effects have been attributed to central histamine receptor antagonism as well as serotonin antagonism, anticholinergic activity and blockade of the central α-adrenoreceptors.

This appears to be less of a problem with the alkylamines over the ethanolamine and phenothiazine-type agents. However, some objective impairment of CNS function may occur in about 50% of subjects after diphenhydramine or chlorpheniramine. CNS effects caused by first-generation H_1-antagonists are potentiated by alcohol or diazepam. Sedating effects may be beneficial in some circumstances, but are hazardous in day-time activities requiring alertness. Tolerance to sedation is reported to occur after a few days, but there is minimal scientific data to support this.

Administration of a single dose at bedtime for these compounds may be an alternative, but there is now evidence that even with this approach, alertness is still diminished in the morning. Six hours after a 50 mg diphenhydramine dose, the sedative effect was comparable to that experienced with alcohol and triazolam. The mild central stimulatory properties of the sympathomimetic agents (decongestants) when used in combination with first-generation, sedating H_1-antagonists, may decrease the antihistamine drowsiness. Some first-generation H_1-antagonists may also cause paradoxical restlessness, palpitations, tremors and difficulty in sleeping, especially in children.

In objective, single-dose studies, the incidence of somnolence and impairment of CNS function associated with manufacturers' recommended doses of the second-generation H_1-antagonists is similar to that produced by placebo, and is significantly lower than that produced by the first-generation agents. In most studies, the second-generation H_1-antagonists have not potentiated the adverse CNS effects of alcohol or diazepam.

A combination of terfenadine and pseudoephedrine produced insomnia in 25% of patients, headache in 15% and CNS excitation, including restlessness, nervousness, jitter, anxiety, irritability, increased energy, stimulation, disorientation, tension, trembling and agitation in 12% of patients. These results were no different from those obtained when pseudoephedrine was administered alone, namely, 27%, 15% and 7% respectively.

Gastrointestinal adverse effects rarely occur. Anticholinergic adverse effects such as blurred vision, urinary retention, constipation and tachycardia may occur, especially with diphenhydramine and promethazine, requiring caution in persons with enlarged prostate, narrow-angle glaucoma and cardiac disease. Drying of the mouth and mucous membranes may also occur, which may be of concern to asthmatics, but they are not contraindicated.

The second-generation H_1-antagonists terfenadine and astemizole have been reported to prolong the QT interval and cause polymorphic ventricular tachycardia, torsades de pointes and other potentially fatal cardiac dysrhythmias. Deaths have occurred, consequently products containing these agents require the consultation of a pharmacist when sold. Risk factors, which must be assessed for these rare events, include large doses or an overdose, pre-existing hepatic, cardiac or metabolic disorders or in the case of terfenadine, concurrent administration of some macrolide antibiotics such as erythromycin, imidazole antifungals such as ketoconazole and itraconazole, or other hepatic cytochrome P450 inhibitors. Terfenadine was not affected by the concurrent administration of cimetidine. Loratadine and cetirizine have not been implicated to date.

Information for Special Populations

There are very few well-designed, prospective studies published in the literature evaluating the efficacy and safety of the pharmacological agents used in the treatment of allergic rhinitis and colds in pregnancy, during lactation, or in children or the elderly.

The first-generation H_1-antagonists have been used in pregnancy but when the medications were ingested close to term, withdrawal symptoms have been observed in the neonates shortly after birth. The second-generation H_1-antagonists are classified for use in pregnancy where the benefits would outweigh the risks. In well-designed studies, loratadine and the active metabolite of terfenadine have been measured in breast milk from mothers ingesting these compounds during lactation. No terfenadine was detected. The potential doses received by the nursing infants have been calculated to be of the order of 0.5% of that ingested by the mother, and are not considered to put the infants at risk.

There are a few pharmacokinetic and pharmacodynamic studies in children of the first-generation H_1-antagonists, chlorpheniramine, diphenhydramine and hydroxyzine, and of the second-generation H_1-blockers, terfenadine, astemizole, loratadine and cetirizine. In most cases, the elimination of these compounds is much more rapid than found in young adults. However, apart from the recommended, empirically-defined doses, which are smaller than those recommended for adults, no modification of the frequency of dosing has been established.

There are no published studies of the pharmacokinetics and pharmacodynamics of the decongestants pseudoephedrine and phenylpropanolamine in children to date. However, in recently published abstracts it has been reported that the elimination of these compounds occurs more rapidly in children than in young adults. Although relatively high doses were administered, no clinically significant increases in pulse rate or blood pressure were reported.

In the elderly, it has been demonstrated that some of these compounds are eliminated more slowly than in healthy young adults, but there are few recommendations regarding reduction of amount or frequency of dosing for these compounds.

In view of the paucity of information about the safety and efficacy of medications used in the treatment of allergic rhinitis and common colds in pregnancy, during lactation, in children and the elderly, recommendations for their use in these patients should be tempered with caution based on the above information.

TABLE 4: Recommended Doses of Centrally-acting Antitussives

Agent/Age	Dosage (daily maximum)
Codeine	
<2 yrs	Not recommended
2 to 5 yrs*	On advice of a physician; 1 mg/kg/day in 4 divided doses
6 to 11 yrs	5–10 mg every 4–6 hr (60 mg)
12 yrs and over	10–20 mg every 4 to 6 hr (120 mg)
Dextromethorphan	
<2 yrs	On advice of a physician
2 to 5 yrs†	2.5 to 5 mg every 4 hr or 7.5 mg every 6 to 8 hr (30 mg)
6 to 11 yrs†	5 to 10 mg every 4 hr or 15 mg every 6 to 8 hr (60 mg)
12 yrs and over	10 to 20 mg every 4 hr or 30 mg every 6 to 8 hr (120 mg)
Diphenhydramine	
2 to 5 yrs	On advice of a physician
6 to 11 yrs	12.5 mg every 4 hr (75 mg)
12 yrs and over	25 mg every 4 hr (150 mg)

*Measure with calibrated measuring device.
†Alternatively, children can be given 1 mg/kg per day in 3 or 4 divided doses.
Source: Marchessault J, Boyd J, Crocker J, et al. Second report of the Expert Advisory Committee on nonprescription cough and cold remedies to the Health Protection Branch. Antitussives, expectorants and bronchodilators. Ottawa: Health and Welfare Canada, 1989.

ANTITUSSIVES

Recommended for the dry, nonproductive, irritating cough that may disturb sleep, the centrally acting antitussives inhibit coughing through a direct effect on the cough centre in the medulla by raising the threshold for cough stimulus (Table 4).

Codeine, a narcotic agent, has been thoroughly evaluated and produces effective cough suppression, the peak effect occurring within 1 to 2 hours and persisting for up to 4 hours.

The most common adverse effects are nausea, dizziness, sedation and pruritus while repeated doses may cause constipation. The abuse potential is low. Codeine is not recommended for use in children under 2 years of age and only after a physician's advice for 2 to 5 year olds. Because codeine can cause the release of histamine and appears to dry the respiratory tract mucosa and increase the viscosity of bronchial secretions, it is not recommended for asthmatics. The maximum codeine content in nonprescription liquid cough formulations is 3.3 mg/5 mL, so that doses of 5 to 10 mL for adults do not achieve the recommended antitussive dose of 15 mg. Codeine-containing tablets contain 8 mg, so two tablets may provide an alternative means of easily achieving an antitussive dose, an additional benefit to diabetic patients who want to avoid the ingestion of cough syrups.

Dextromethorphan, a modified narcotic agent devoid of analgesic or addictive properties, has a similar mechanism of action and is considered to have equal or near-equal antitussive potency to that of codeine. Its effect is observed within 15 to 30 minutes after ingestion and may persist for 3 to 6 hours. It is especially useful for children. Sustained-release formulations may provide relief for up to 12 hours in adults, but are not usually recommended for use in children.

Dextromethorphan has a low degree of sedative, gastric-irritating, constipating and addictive properties, but drowsiness, nausea and dizziness may occur infrequently, and it has the potential to release histamine. It requires doses greater than 5 times the antitussive dose to cause excitation, bizarre behavior, mental confusion or depression, ataxia or opiate-like respiratory depression, and no fatalities have occurred, even at 100 times the recommended dose. Dextromethorphan is the antitussive choice for children.

Diphenhydramine, an H_1-antagonist with antitussive activity that appears to be independent of any sedative effect, is reported equivalent to codeine when doses of 25 to 50 mg are used. Minimal sedation appears at the lower dose, but can occur at the higher. The added sedative effect may be beneficial in cases of nighttime cough.

Noscapine, an opiate derivative with no narcotic activity, is reported to have questionable effectiveness compared to codeine's antitussive effects. Agents such as camphor, menthol and eucalyptus oil in appropriate doses, administered in lozenges, applied as topical ointment formulations or inhaled via steam vaporizers have antitussive properties.

DECONGESTANTS

Stimulation of the α_1- and α_2-receptors in the human nasal mucosa causes constriction of the subepithelial precapillary sphincters, arterioles and venous sinuses. Medications that stimulate either of these receptors cause nasal decongestion and consequently decrease edema and blanching of the nasal mucosa, but do not prevent the nasal response to inhaled antigen.

Classes

The two main classes of sympathomimetic agents used as nasal decongestants are the phenylamines (including ephedrine, pseudoephedrine, phenylephrine and phenylpropanolamine), usually administered orally (Table 5), and the imidazolines (xylometazoline and its hydroxy derivative, oxymetazoline, and naphazoline), usually administered topically (Table 6).

Ephedrine, phenylephrine and the imidazolines when applied topically have a faster onset of action than the oral agents. Oral agents may provide a more prolonged effect due to the removal of topically applied medication by respiratory tract fluids. However, xylometazoline and oxymetazoline are purported to relieve nasal congestion for up to 10 and 12 hours respectively, longer than oral products, except in sustained-release formulations. Absorption of topically applied agents from application sites tends to be minimal; however, excess product may flow over the nasal mucosa into the pharynx to be swallowed and absorbed orally. Spray formulations are recommended for adults since a more uniform application is possible over a larger area. For the symptomatic treatment of sinusitis, drops applied when the head is upside down will provide better coverage to the sinus cavities than sprays. For children, especially under the age of 6, drops are preferred, since the nasal surface area is smaller. Drops or sprays can be used in children 6 to 12 years of age, but application by an adult is desirable.

Adverse Effects

Overuse, or prolonged use of topical agents may result in rebound congestion called rhinitis medicamentosa in as little as 3 to 7 days. The nasal mucosal membranes become more congested and swollen than before treatment. This condition is more likely to occur with the shorter-acting agents, ephedrine and phenylephrine, rather than the longer-acting imidazoline compounds. Rebound congestion does not occur in the first 3 days of oxymetazoline use, and xylometazoline, 1 mg/mL applied 3 times daily for 6 weeks does not produce adverse effects, diminished mucociliary function or morphological changes. Topical application of an α-adrenergic agonist may cause local burning or stinging, sneezing or dryness of the mucous membranes.

Nasal congestion as a result of rhinitis medicamentosa can usually be identified by detailed questioning of the patient. There is no specific treatment apart from the withdrawal of the offending agent. If a short-acting topical decongestant is the cause, substitution of a longer-acting agent with a reduced dosage regimen may help, although the patient should be encouraged to discontinue the use of the medication entirely over time. If a long-acting agent has caused the problem, the frequency

TABLE 5: Recommended Dosages of Oral Decongestants

Agent	Adults	6–11 yrs	2–5 yrs	<2 yrs
Ephedrine	8 mg every 6–8 hr	Under review	Under review	Under review
Pseudoephedrine	60 mg every 4–6 hr (240 mg daily max)	30 mg every 4–6 hr* (120 mg daily max)	15 mg every 4–6 hr* (60 mg daily max)	On advice of physician
Phenylpropanolamine	25 mg every 4 hr or 37.5 mg every 6 hr (150 mg daily max)	12.5 mg every 4 hr (75 mg daily max)	6.25 mg every 4 hr (37.5 mg daily max)	On advice of physician
Phenylephrine	10 mg every 4 hr (60 mg daily max)	5 mg every 4 hr (30 mg daily max)	2.5 mg every 4 hr (15 mg daily max)	On advice of physician

*Alternatively, children may receive 1 mg/kg 4 times daily.
Do not give sustained-release formulations to children less than 12 years of age.
Source: Marchessault J, Boyd J, Crocker J, et al. First report of the Expert Advisory Committee on nonprescription cough and cold remedies to the Health Protection Branch. Antihistamines, nasal decongestants and anticholinergics. Ottawa: Health and Welfare Canada, 1988; and McEvoy GK, ed. AHFS Drug Information. Bethesda: American Society of Hospital Pharmacists, 1992:703–4.

TABLE 6: Recommended Dosages of Topical Decongestants

Agent	Dose and Frequency	Concentration of solution: Adults	6–11 yrs	2–5 yrs*	<2 yrs
Phenylephrine	2–3 drops or sprays not more than every 4 hr	0.25–1.0%	0.25%	0.125%	On advice of physician
Naphazoline	1–2 drops or sprays not more than every 6 hr	0.05%	———On advice of physician———		
Oxymetazoline	2–3 drops or sprays not more than every 10–12 hr (max 2 applications/24 hr)	0.05%	0.025–0.05%	0.025%	On advice of physician
Xylometazoline	2–3 drops or sprays not more than every 8–10 hr	0.1%	0.05%	0.05%	On advice of physician

*Drops are recommended for children under 6 years of age.
Single-drop and spray dosage formulations are available with some preparations.
Source: Marchessault J, Boyd J, Crocker J, et al. First report of the Expert Advisory Committee on nonprescription cough and cold remedies to the Health Protection Branch. Antihistamines, nasal decongestants and anticholinergics. Ottawa: Health and Welfare Canada, 1988.

of use should be reduced gradually over time with the ultimate goal of eliminating it altogether. Treatment of nasal congestion with oral agents should be recommended for future use, although the patient should be advised that the rapid relief given by topically applied agents might not be repeated.

The oral agents pseudoephedrine and phenylpropanolamine can be administered alone or in combination with an H_1-antagonist. Dosing every 12 hours can only be achieved by sustained-release formulations. Therefore if a once daily dosed H_1-antagonist is used in the combination, it will require dosing every 12 hours as well as dose reduction. Oral agents are less beneficial on a mg/mg basis than when applied directly to the nasal mucosa, but they are more effective than placebo in relieving nasal congestion. Oral agents potentially provide a more complete decongestant action by reaching parts of the nasopharyngeal and sinus mucosa via the systemic circulation. In predisposed patients phenylpropanolamine administration may cause cardiovascular problems, such as hypertension, postural hypotension, cardiac arrhythmias, myocardial injury, and CNS amphetamine-like adverse effects, such as seizures, hallucinations and memory loss. However, doses higher than recommended for relief of nasal congestion were used in these studies, and there may be some bias against this drug in the literature as conflicting data have been published. A high dose of ephedrine, 60 mg instead of the usual 10 to 20 mg, may increase systolic and diastolic blood pressure and increase heart rate in normal subjects, and other effects, such as insomnia and palpitations, may occur. Pseudoephedrine is reported to have fewer cardiac and CNS stimulating effects in the usual nasal decongestant doses; however, hallucinations have occurred in children and urinary retention in adults. Individuals with heart disease, high blood pressure, thyroid disease, diabetes, glaucoma, prostatic enlargement, and those who are pregnant or breastfeeding should use these products with caution unless directed by a physician. These agents should be used with caution in patients on MAO inhibitor (MAOI) therapy because coadministration of indirect-acting sympathomimetics and MAOIs has resulted in serious hypertension. Orally administered decongestants do not cause rebound congestion.

EXPECTORANTS

During the course of viral infections, there is an increase in the volume and consistency of phlegm, so coughs may change from dry, irritating and nonproductive to congested. Increased fluid intake is the simplest, nonpharmacological treatment for reducing the viscosity of bronchial fluids to aid expectoration. Agents that make bronchial secretions more mobile should improve expectoration but may initially increase the frequency of coughing. The use of such agents has been controversial due to the difficulty of understanding what changes to the properties of respiratory secretions correlate best with ease of expectoration. Also, most research has been conducted on chronic coughing associated with chronic obstructive pulmonary disease, rather than cough due to the common cold.

Guaifenesin (glyceryl guaiacolate) a derivative of guaiacol, is considered safe and effective and used almost exclusively in cough formulations. It appears to cause an indirect increase in the output of respiratory tract fluid, enhancing the flow of less viscid secretions, promoting ciliary action and facilitating the removal of mucus, or it may be absorbed and taken up by the bronchial glands and directly stimulate secretions by these glands. In spite of the controversial results, guaifenesin is considered safe and effective, with doses every 6 hours of 200 to 400 mg in adults, 100 mg in children 6 to 11 years, 50 mg in children 2 to 5 years, and to children under 2 years only following the advice of a physician.

LOZENGES

The initial sore throat is often treated with lozenges containing antimicrobials, local anesthetics, aromatic compounds and demulcents. Lozenges dissolved in the mouth increase salivation and exert a demulcent effect on the throat by coating irritated or inflamed mucous membranes, even relieving the dryness associated with mouth breathing. The duration of action is relatively short, and usually disappears as soon as the locally acting agents are washed away by the saliva.

The quaternary ammonium compounds, cetylpyridinium chloride, domiphen bromide and benzalkonium chloride, have bactericidal activity against gram-positive organisms but are relatively ineffective against viruses. Phenol and hexylresorcinol may have some activity against both gram-positive and gram-negative organisms and certain viruses, as well as a slight local anesthetic effect. Local anesthetics, primarily benzocaine, can temporarily relieve soreness in the throat but may numb the tongue as well. Benzocaine can sensitize the oral mucosa, but this seldom occurs with the use of a topical anesthetic in lozenge form. Patients should be warned against eating too soon after use so that injuries from hot liquids or biting the cheek or tongue do not occur. Volatile aromatics such as menthol and eucalyptus oil produce a cooling sensation to mask minor throat discomfort and may also relieve nasal congestion or act as antitussives if therapeutic doses are used. To provide relief, nonmedicated lozenges may be used frequently, but those containing medicinal agents, including antihistamines and decongestants, must be taken only as directed.

VITAMIN C

Experiments have failed to produce any strong evidence that doses of vitamin C greater than

1 g/day and as high as 4 to 10 g/day protect against or ameliorate the symptoms of the common cold. Some studies have shown a reduction of no more than one-half day in the duration of cold symptoms in the vitamin C ingesting group compared to the control placebo group. Abdominal distress and diarrhea, interference with diabetic urine tests, and the effect of acidification of the urine on drug excretion following doses of 1 g/day, and lack of positive results support the recommendation that the prophylactic or therapeutic use of large doses of vitamin C for common colds is unwarranted.

RECOMMENDED READING

Fireman P. Pathophysiology and pharmacotherapy of common upper respiratory diseases. Pharmacotherapy 1993;13(Pt 2):101S–09S.

Simons FER, Simons KJ. Optimum pharmacological management of chronic rhinitis. Drugs 1989; 38:313–31.

Smith MBH, Feldman W. Over-the-counter cold medications. A critical review of clinical trials between 1950 and 1991. JAMA 1993;269: 2258–63.

Simons FER, Simons KJ. The pharmacology and use of H_1-receptor-antagonist drugs. N Engl J Med 1994;330:1663–70.

Hilding DA. Literature review: The common cold. Ear Nose Throat J 1994;73:639–47.

Horak F. Seasonal allergic rhinitis. Newer treatment approaches. Drugs 1993;45:518–27.

6

ANTIPARASITIC AND ANTHELMINTIC PRODUCTS

SUSAN MANSOUR

CONTENTS

Pediculosis	101
Types of Lice	
Symptoms	
Treatment	
Scabies	108
Introduction	
Symptoms	
Treatment	
Enterobiasis	113
Symptoms	
Treatment	
Pharmaceutical Agents	117
Recommended Reading	120

PEDICULOSIS

Lice are small insects that are ectoparasites of mammals. The head louse, *Pediculus humanus capitis*, the pubic louse, *Phthirus pubis,* and the body louse, *Pediculus humanus corporis* are obligate parasites of humans. Of the three, head and pubic lice are the most common. Head, pubic and body lice vary somewhat in size, shape, and area of the body they infest. They are similar in that the adults have 3 pairs of legs and range from a tan to a grey color. They do not have wings, are unable to fly, nor do they jump. Adult females may lay up to 10 eggs per day and live for about 25 days. Lice, at any stage of their life cycle, are unlikely to survive longer than 30 days away from a host.

TYPES OF LICE

Head Lice

As the name implies, head lice live on the scalp. The adults are about the size of a sesame seed, 1 to 4 mm in length. The adult female glues her eggs, also known as nits, on to hair shafts close to the scalp. The eggs are oval, a grey, yellow or tan color, about the size of a pinhead, 0.3 mm wide and 0.8 mm long, and often found at the nape of the neck or behind the ears.

After 5 to 10 days the eggs will hatch leaving behind the empty egg cases. This time period corresponds to about 0.64 cm of hair growth. The egg cases may remain attached to the hair shaft for a prolonged period of time and are removed by the natural growth and subsequent cutting of the hair. They may also be removed manually with a fine-toothed comb. If the egg cases are seen about 1.25 cm away from the scalp, they are likely empty. Once the eggs hatch, the louse will mature in 7 or more days. Unfed adult lice may survive up to 10 days away from a host.

Head lice are transmitted by direct hair to hair or head to head contact. Although there is little data supporting other types of transmission, it is possible they are transmitted by sharing contaminated objects such as clothing, brushes, and head gear. Lice are believed to prefer clean scalps to dirty or dandruffed scalps. There is usually no relationship to length of hair.

Between 6 and 10 million cases of head lice are reported annually in the United States. Children are the most commonly infested, perhaps from head to head contact while playing or napping. An estimated 1 to 10% of Canadian elementary school children are infested at any one time, although it is believed that only 10% of infestations are acquired through school. Head lice infest women more, whites more often than blacks, and are more common in larger families. Although there appears to be little research into the seasonality of infestations, peaks have been reported in the winter months. Those infested, or having children infested with head lice, often have a sense of shame.

Pubic Lice

Infestation with pubic lice is also known as phthiriasis. Pubic lice are about 1 to 2 mm long and rounded in shape, resembling a crab. They attach themselves to coarser body hair, such as pubic hair, hair in the perianal area, on the thighs and trunk, axillary or facial hair, eyebrows and eyelashes. Like the eggs of head lice, the eggs of pubic lice are glued to hair shafts. The nits tend to be smaller than those of head or body lice. Unfed adults usually cannot survive more than 24 hours away from a host.

Transmission of pubic lice is through direct person to person contact, most commonly sexual contact. Rarely, toilet seats, beds or other shared objects, including clothing or towels have been implicated.

The incidence of pubic lice is highest in single people between the ages of 15 to 40 years of age. About one-third of patients also have another sexually transmitted disease.

Body Lice

The body louse looks the same as the head louse but is slightly larger. Body lice most often infest the homeless, individuals living in crowded, unhygienic conditions who are unable to wash and change clothing. They do not live on the skin of the host but feed on the host and live in the seams of clothing worn close to the body. They attach their eggs to the fibres or seams of clothing and are transmitted through clothes and bedding. Unfed adult lice may survive for up to 10 days away from the host. Body lice can transmit certain diseases such as *Rickettsia quintana* (Trench fever), as seen in the First and Second World Wars and *Rickettsia prowazekii* (typhus) and *Borrelia recurrentis* (relapsing fever), seen primarily in parts of Africa and exacerbated by famine and war.

SYMPTOMS

Symptoms are often nonexistent or mild. The original bite may manifest as a slight stinging sensation. Allergic sensitization may occur from 5 to 30 days after a louse bite. The allergic reaction may develop to the puncture wound, fecal material from the louse, or digestive juices. At the onset of the allergic reaction, the primary symptom will be local pruritus, sometimes extreme, accompanied by scratching, redness, irritation and inflammation. Crusts and excoriations may be present and bacterial or fungal infection may result if scratching is excessive. Differential diagnosis may include eczema, impetigo, seborrheic dermatitis, psoriasis and pyoderma.

Occasionally, an individual with many bites in a short period of time will have a mild fever and malaise. If sensitized, an individual may also have generalized pruritus and urticaria.

Head Lice

Specifically, symptoms of head lice include an itchy scalp and red, pruritic papules around the ears, face, neck or shoulders. Since there are generally few adult lice on the scalp (often less than 10), and they avoid light, they are difficult to detect. They may appear when combing the hair with a fine-toothed comb over a white paper or cloth.

Observation of the nits firmly attached to the hair shaft is also helpful in identifying the problem. Sometimes confused with dandruff or cosmetics, the nits may be differentiated in that they are difficult to remove. Once hatched, the empty nit cases appear translucent. If nit cases are observed but are 1.25 cm or more away from the scalp, they likely will be empty. If adult lice are not detected, this indicates an old infestation rather than new. Examination of a nit under a microscope is recommended to confirm diagnosis.

Pubic Lice

Anogenital pruritus is one of the symptoms of infestation by pubic lice. There may be few, or many, difficult to find adult pubic lice of a yellow to grey color. Nits may be found with a magnifying glass at the base of the hair shaft. The presence of small brownish specks of lice excreta on undergarments or skin aids identification. Bites may result in small blue-grey spots on the skin known as maculae cerulea, believed due to local hemorrhage or signifying the presence of lice excreta. Verification by microscopic examination is often necessary.

Infestation of the eyelids with pubic lice may result in symptoms such as itching, scaling, crusting and discharge in the area of the eye. When present in children, there is sometimes concern that this may be an indicator of child abuse.

Body Lice

Persistent, pruritic red lesions about 1 mm in diameter, most noticeable on the back, accompany infestation with body lice. These may cause both sleep and mood changes. The insect will more likely be found in the seams of clothing than on the body.

TREATMENT

Nonpharmacological Treatment

Head Lice

When treating head lice, combs and brushes should be soaked in a combination of pediculicidal shampoo and water, alcohol or a 2% *Lysol* solution for 1 hour. Alternatively, they may be immersed in 65°C (149°F) water for 5 to 10 minutes. Bed linens, towels and clothing must be washed in hot 50°C (125°F) water and dried in a dryer for 20 minutes. Other articles may be drycleaned or stored in a sealed plastic bag for 2 weeks. Vacuuming carpets and stuffed furniture is considered as useful as pediculicidal sprays in eliminating any environmental lice. As noted, inanimate objects are considered a minor route of transmission. This, in addition to cost and potential hazards, should lead to the discouragement of the use of pediculicidal sprays.

Nit removal following treatment is controversial since it is time consuming and the effect may be primarily cosmetic. However, some schools have a no nit policy: children may not re-enter school until they have been found nit free.

To remove nits, hold the hair at its distal end and comb in towards the scalp with a fine-toothed comb. Since they may be difficult to dislodge, treatment with an 8% formic acid cream rinse (*Step 2*) has been shown effective by dissolving the glue that binds them to the hair shaft. Alternatively, rubbing alcohol, full or half strength, or vinegar mixed half and half with water, may be used to loosen nits. These should be applied for several minutes, the hair shampooed, dried and then brushed. If vinegar is used, it must be applied only to the scalp to avoid facial burns. Daily combing may help remove any nits that have survived.

Good hygiene habits and routine scalp inspections in institutions are considered useful as prevention strategies. Schools should be notified of cases of head lice.

Body Lice

The treatment of body lice requires adequate cleaning of clothing. This includes laundering in hot water, at least 50°C (125°F), hot tumble drying or drycleaning to kill the lice and their eggs. Alternatively, boiling clothing followed by ironing of seams or storing of clothing in a sealed plastic bag for at least 2 weeks may be useful in the eradication of body lice.

Pharmacological Treatment

All available pediculicides kill lice, but they have varying degrees of ovicidal activity. It is usually recommended that both head and pubic lice be treated with 2 applications of pediculicide, about 1 week apart because the egg incubation period is 6 to 10 days. However, the second application should occur only if, after 1 week following initial treatment, the patient is examined and viable lice, or nits at the base of the hair shaft are found.

Head Lice

Agents used in Canada to treat head lice include: lindane 1%, permethrin 1%, pyrethrins, allethrins, or bioallethrin combined with piperonyl butoxide

Instructions for Use

Pyrethrins with Piperonyl Butoxide Shampoo or Foam for Head Lice

- Saturate dry hair with the product.
- Leave on for 10 to 20 minutes.
- Add small amounts of water, massaging in to create a lather.
- Rinse thoroughly.
- Maximum use is 2 applications in a 24-hour period.
- Avoid the eyes and mucous membranes.

For products containing an additional cream rinse:

- apply cream rinse after shampoo has been rinsed out, massage in and leave on for 1 minute;
- remove nits with a nit comb.

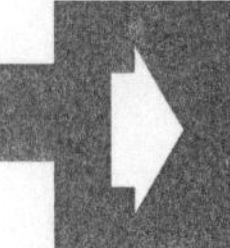

ADVICE FOR THE PATIENT

Head Lice

- Head lice is a common condition among children that is usually associated with CLEAN hair.
- There are several effective medications available to treat head lice—permethrin is most often recommended.
- Certain types of medication may be better for certain age groups, so it is best to check with your pharmacist.
- Each type of medication is used slightly differently, and it is important to use it only as directed.
- Medication should not be left on any longer than directed, nor should it be used more often than directed. For some medications, one treatment may be enough, although most require two treatments, separated by about 7 days.
- All medication should be kept out of the eyes, away from the mouth, nose and other sensitive areas, and out of the reach of children.
- When applying lindane, it may be a good idea to use rubber gloves, especially if it is being applied to more than one person.
- Combs and brushes should be cleaned by soaking in alcohol, *Lysol*, or medication for 1 hour or in 65°C water for 5 to 10 minutes.
- Bedding, towels and clothing should be washed in hot water and dried in a dryer for 20 minutes.
- Other items may be drycleaned or stored in a plastic bag for 2 weeks.
- Vacuuming of carpets and furniture is also a good idea.
- To remove nits, hold the hair at its end and comb towards the scalp with a fine-toothed comb. Dispose of nits in a sealed plastic bag.
- Itching may remain after treatment and need to be treated with other types of medications.
- It is important to notify schools of any problems with lice so they can be easily controlled.
- Close contacts should be examined and treated if lice are present.

and a combination product containing acetic acid, camphor, lemon oil and sodium lauryl ether sulfate. Permethrin is considered the treatment of choice, followed by pyrethrins with piperonyl butoxide and lindane.

There are no adequate or well controlled studies available regarding the use of permethrin, pyrethrins or lindane in pregnant women. Percutaneous absorption of permethrin is low, but it should be used in pregnancy only if clearly needed. Since the topical absorption of pyrethrins with piperonyl butoxide is also poor, this agent should be less toxic than lindane, more of which is absorbed through the skin.

It is not known if permethrin is present in human breast milk after topical application. Since animal studies have identified some tumorigenic potential, it may be advisable to discontinue breast-feeding while using permethrin or to avoid permethrin use in women who are breast-feeding. It is also unknown if pyrethrins are present in breast milk after topical application.

Low concentrations of lindane are excreted in breast milk. Although it is unlikely that levels in breast milk would be sufficient to cause serious adverse reactions in the infant, an alternate method of feeding may be used for 2 days following lindane application.

Instructions for Use

Lindane Shampoo for Head Lice

- Saturate dry hair with the product.
- Work the shampoo through the area for 4 minutes.
- Add water in small amounts to form a lather and continue shampooing for 4 minutes.
- Rinse thoroughly, towel dry briskly.
- Avoid the eyes and mucous membranes.
- Flush eyes with water if contact occurs.
- Do not use on open cuts or extensive excoriations.
- Avoid unnecessary skin contact and wear rubber gloves when applying lindane, especially if applying it to more than one person.

Permethrin 1% cream rinse may be used on children over 2 years of age. Lindane should not be used in premature infants, and the risk of toxicity is greater in young children. The manufacturer recommends that it be used on children under the age of 6 only on the advice of a physician, nurse or pharmacist.

Permethrin and pyrethrins are contraindicated in those with hypersensitivities to any pyrethrins, ragweed and chrysanthemum. Lindane should not be used in anyone with seizure disorders or hypersensitivity to lindane.

Permethrin use is reported to result in easier to comb hair, but it is not necessary to remove nits from the hair. Permethrin exhibits 70 to 80% ovicidal activity but persists on the hair shaft for at least 10 days: if viable nits remain after the initial treatment, the larvae will be killed as they hatch. It is not necessary to repeat the treatment with permethrin unless there is evidence of the problem 7 to 10 days after the original treatment. One 10-minute treatment is believed effective in over 95% of cases. Lice are killed quickly, within 30 minutes.

Pyrethrins with piperonyl butoxide may be less effective than permethrin, although 2 applications of the pyrethrin combination have been shown to be equal in efficacy to one application of permethrin. They are reportedly at least equal in effect to lindane. They do not have complete ovicidal activity; therefore, treatment should be repeated in 7 to 10 days. Ovicidal activity is estimated at about 70 to 75%, similar to that of lindane. However, the insect dies in 10 to 23 minutes compared to 3 hours with lindane.

Lindane is also an effective treatment for head lice but has been shown less effective with two treatments than permethrin with one treatment.

Since lindane and the pyrethrins with piperonyl butoxide may not be completely ovicidal, nits should be removed or the product reapplied within 2 weeks, usually 7 to 10 days after the initial application.

An additional product (*SH-206 Shampoo*) marketed in Canada for the treatment of head lice contains a combination of acetic acid, camphor, lemon oil, and sodium lauryl ether sulfate. The mechanism of action and effectiveness are unclear, although the manufacturer cites highly positive results. It should not be used on those sensitive to the product or its ingredients, or on children less than 30 months of age. Adverse effects include slight pruritus.

Household contacts should be examined, and family and close friends may also need to be treated.

Instructions for Use

SH-206 Shampoo for Head Lice

- Wet hair and apply enough shampoo to cover the hair (about 2 teaspoons) and then lather.
- Ensure that the shampoo does not come in contact with any mucous membranes, especially the eyes, nose and mouth.
- Scrub vigorously for 2 minutes, paying particular attention to the area around the base of the skull and around the ears.
- Allow the shampoo to remain on the hair for 10 minutes, then rinse well with lukewarm water.
- Remove dead lice and nits with a fine-toothed comb.
- Repeat the treatment 48 hours later.

Pubic Lice

The treatment of choice for pubic lice is identical to that of head lice. Permethrin is reported 95% effective compared to 75 to 85% effectiveness for lindane, although the product indication for permethrin does not include pubic lice.

Lindane 1% shampoo is used in the same way for pubic lice as in treating head lice. Alternatively, the cream or lotion may be applied to the affected and surrounding area and left on for 8 to 12 hours. Clean clothing should be worn. The cream or lotion is then removed by thorough washing. The manufacturer suggests that treatment may need to be repeated once in 4 to 7 days.

The method of application for the pyrethrins with piperonyl butoxide combination is also the same as with head lice.

Other body areas should be checked for infestation, and treatment should include the trunk, thighs and axillae, since these areas are often involved, especially in hairy individuals. General treatment recommendations include repeating treatment in at least 7 to 10 days. Some recommend

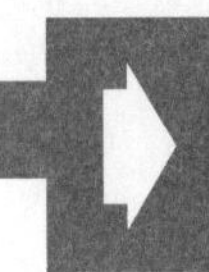

ADVICE FOR THE PATIENT

Pubic Lice

- There are several effective medications available to treat pubic lice.
- Certain types of medication may be better for certain age groups, so it is best to check with your pharmacist.
- Each type of medication is used slightly differently, and it is important to use it only as directed.
- Medication should not be left on any longer than directed, then washed off well.
- Medication should not be used more often than directed.
- All medication should be kept out of the eyes, away from the mouth, nose and other sensitive areas, and out of the reach of children.
- When applying lindane, it may be a good idea to use rubber gloves, especially if it is being applied to more than one person.
- Bedding, towels and clothing should be washed in hot water and dried in a dryer for 20 minutes.
- Other items may be drycleaned or stored in a plastic bag for 2 weeks.
- To remove nits, hold the hair at its end and comb towards the scalp with a fine-toothed comb. Dispose of nits in a sealed plastic bag.
- Close contacts should be examined and treated if lice are present.

removing all nits with a fine-toothed comb, washing and hot drying of bed linen and clothes and treatment of sexual contacts to effectively eradicate the infestation.

Pubic lice found in the eyelashes should be mechanically removed, and thick applications of petrolatum may be applied twice daily for 8 days. Other regimens include applying the petrolatum 3 to 5 times daily. This is believed to asphyxiate the lice and eggs.

Symptomatic Treatment

Pruritus may persist for weeks after adequate treatment with pediculicides. Antipruritic or anti-inflammatory agents used topically may aid in symptom control. It may also be necessary to use oral antihistamines.

Instructions for Use

Permethrin Cream Rinse for Head Lice

- Wash hair with a regular shampoo.
- Rinse the hair and towel it dry.
- Shake well.
- Apply the permethrin cream rinse so that the hair and scalp are wetted thoroughly and leave it on for 10 minutes.
- Rinse off well and dry with a clean towel.
- Avoid contact with mucous membranes and eyes.
- Flush eyes with water if contact occurs.

?

PATIENT ASSESSMENT QUESTIONS

Q ***What are the symptoms? Have you seen any live lice or nits?***

The presence of live lice indicates infestation. Nits seen about 1.25 cm (½ inch) away from the scalp or skin are likely to be empty. Itching may indicate a need for antipruritics in addition to a pediculicide.

Q ***Is the individual pregnant or breast-feeding?***

None of the available agents have been adequately assessed in pregnancy. Lindane absorption is the greatest, with the highest potential for adverse fetal effects. Alternate methods of feeding should be recommended for breast-feeding women using any available products.

Q ***What are the ages of the people affected?***

This will help determine an appropriate treatment. Lindane is not recommended for use in infants and children.

Q ***Do they have any allergies, especially to ragweed, chrysanthemum or pyrethrins?***

If so, pyrethrins and permethrin should be avoided.

Q ***Do they have any medical conditions, in particular epilepsy?***

Lindane should be avoided in those with neurological disorders.

SCABIES

INTRODUCTION

Etiology

Scabies is caused by an obligate human parasite known as *Sarcoptes scabiei,* an arachnid of the genus *Acarus*. The female mite is about twice the size of the male and at about 0.3 by 0.4 mm is just visible to the naked eye. The mite is whitish with brownish legs and mouthparts. The female may be fertilized by the male once she is present on the human host. Once impregnated, she burrows into the stratum corneum and lays her eggs. It is possible that she burrows to layers beyond the stratum corneum, but she does not invade the dermis. In 3 to 5 days, the eggs hatch and become larvae, which mature through a nymph stage to an adult stage in 1 to 3 weeks. In a typical scabies infestation there are about 10 to 12 mites present on an adult human. Adult mites are believed able to survive off the host for at least 34 to 96 hours at normal room temperatures and conditions.

Sites

Typical sites of infestation on the adult human include the interdigital web spaces, flexor surfaces of the wrists, flexor surfaces of the elbows, axillae, the back, lower abdomen, navel, between the buttocks, inframammary folds and nipples in women, and the penis in men. These sites are also most often affected in older children. Infestation above the neck is rare but may occur in younger children, infants and the bedridden. Infestation of the palms and soles is also rare. The condition is generally more widespread in smaller children and infants with the entire body being affected, particularly areas such as the head, neck, palms, soles, intergluteal cleft, umbilicus, axillae, postauricular folds, and the genitals.

Transmission

Close person-to-person contact is the most common means of transmission of the mite. Prolonged intimate contact appears to be necessary, and among single adults the most common means of transmission is sexual contact. However, since infested sites often include the web spaces between the fingers, it has been suggested that hand to hand contact may be a route of transmission. Contact with contaminated bedding, towels or clothing may result in transmission of the disease since the mite may live off the host for a period of time. However, this is considered a minor route.

Incidence

Scabies seems to appear in epidemics due to unknown factors with no regular cycle, and immunity does not develop. An estimated 300 million people worldwide suffer from scabies. In North America, blacks are more commonly affected than whites. Scabies is not limited to any population but is seen more commonly in those living in crowded conditions, children and mothers, presumably due to increased chances of direct contact with an affected individual.

Other scabies mites may cause mange in the specific species of animal that they infest. They may feed on humans but cannot reproduce or form burrows. This may, however, result in a papulovesicular eruption in humans that is usually less severe than infestation caused by the human mite. Since the infestation is self-limiting, removal or treatment of the animal will result in resolution of any symptoms in the humans. Animals should be treated by a veterinarian.

SYMPTOMS

Although the disease may present in different forms, the primary symptom is typically intense pruritus magnified by warmth and especially prevalent during the night when the female is more active. This will develop within 2 to 6 weeks after an initial infestation, the result of an inflammatory and immune response to the mites, their eggs, saliva, feces, other body secretions, and possibly other antigens from the mite's body. The pruritus is initially present in the area of the burrows but may become generalized later in the infestation. Prior to the development of the pruritus, individuals may be asymptomatic carriers and, occasionally, may remain asymptomatic. Those previously infested may develop symptoms as rapidly as 24 hours after reinfestation.

Other symptoms include burrows that appear as either inflamed linear or S-shaped markings or a linear grey-white papule about 1 mm in diameter and 2 to 20 mm in length. Difficult to detect with the naked eye (visible in less than 25% of patients), burrows may be identified by a physician using topical ink or topical tetracycline. Microscopic examination of skin scrapings may permit the mite, ova or excrement (also known as scybala) to be seen, thus confirming the diagnosis.

Emergence of larvae from the burrows may result in the formation of papules. Vesicles, pustules, excoriation, thickening of the skin, and hyperpigmentation may result from prolonged scratching and inflammation. Pustules and vesicles occur primarily on the palms and soles of infants and children, and bullae and urticaria may also be present. Secondary bacterial infections from scratching the area are a risk, especially in areas of poor hygiene.

Variations

In general, scabies must be differentiated from other types of skin disorders including contact dermatitis, atopic dermatitis, seborrheic dermatitis, other insect bites or infestations, papular urticaria, lichen planus, syphilis, folliculitis, psoriasis and others. In children or infants with vesicles, pustules, or nodules, differential diagnosis includes heat rash, palmoplantar pustuloses of infancy, histiocytosis and possibly, syphilis. Scabies should be considered in any individual complaining of pruritus and a rash of vesicles and papules.

Nodular scabies consists of a small number of nodules about 1 cm in size, commonly in the inguinal and axillary areas. These nodules may persist for some time after successful treatment of the infestation.

Scabies incognita refers to an infestation where the lesions are only slightly inflamed due to the use of corticosteroids or other immunosuppressants.

Neonatal or pediatric scabies may be found in infants and often presents with red crusted or eczematous lesions. Irritability and poor feeding may result. Children are usually infected by close, nonsexual contact.

Norwegian or crusted scabies occurs most commonly in senile, debilitated, and immunodeficient individuals, including those with HIV infection. Large areas of the body are often affected, and the skin is often thick, crusted and scaly. The typical erythematous papules and burrows of scabies are not obvious. The pruritus accompanying this infestation is variable in intensity. There are often hundreds of thousands of mites infesting the patient in this state as compared to about a dozen in the more typical presentation. This infestation is difficult to differentiate from other skin conditions such as eczema, seborrheic dermatitis, or contact dermatitis and is a particular problem in nursing homes or institutions where it is most often found. It is highly contagious and may be difficult to manage.

TREATMENT

Pharmacological Treatment

The method of application of scabicides is important to the success of treatment. Treatment must be applied to all body areas from the head downward. Since scabies may affect the scalp of infants, scabicide should be applied to this area as well. Some suggest the use of a 5 cm paint brush to aid in the application of the scabicide. To avoid treatment failures, areas such as the interdigital webs, wrists, elbows, breasts, buttocks, genitalia, head, under

Instructions for Use

Esdepallethrin with Piperonyl Butoxide for Scabies

- If a bath has been taken, allow the skin to dry and cool.
- Use the spray in a well ventilated area, and avoid contact with the eyes.
- If using on children under 5 years of age, protect their mouth and nose with a clean handkerchief.
- Do not spray the face and scalp. If that area is affected, apply the spray to cotton, and rub the cotton on the area.
- Spray the rest of the body surface area paying special attention to any folds of skin and areas between the fingers and toes.
- When spraying, hold the can about 20 to 30 cm (8 to 12 inches) away from the skin.
- After 12 hours remove the product from the skin with soap and water.
- A second treatment is not usually needed unless itching persists beyond 2 weeks after treatment.

the nails, axillae, skin folds or soles must be adequately treated. It may also be useful to trim the nails to decrease damage to the skin during scratching and to ensure that any mites under the nails are adequately treated. Fomites may play a minor role in treatment failures. Fresh clothing and linen should be used after the last applications. Laundering of clothing and bed linens in hot water and hot drying are recommended. It is likely that good hygiene plays a role in treatment and personal prevention but serves as little protection against general outbreaks. Drycleaning and storage of objects for 5 to 10 days are also effective ways to eliminate the scabies mite from inanimate objects. Insecticide sprays are effective in killing mites on inanimate objects such as furniture. Vacuuming and sweeping are recommended. Multiple applications of scabicide may be required in the treatment of Norwegian scabies. Following the use of the scabicide, a gentle bath using a mild soap followed by the application of a moisturizer may minimize irritation from the products.

Permethrin 5% cream is considered the treatment of choice for scabies. Lower strength permethrin products are not effective.

Lindane is equally effective in the treatment of scabies, although resistance may be developing. It has been replaced by permethrin as drug of choice due to its potential for toxicities.

It is not known how much time is required to eradicate the mite, but 4 to 6 hours is likely enough. Some believe that patients are no longer contagious 24 hours after treatment.

Approximately 10% of patients or less will not respond to a single treatment of either permethrin or lindane. This may be from incorrect application technique, reinfestation, or the presence of environmental reservoirs. Two or three retreatments over a 1-month period are unlikely to be a problem.

There are no adequate or well controlled studies available regarding the use of permethrin or lindane in pregnant women. Percutaneous absorption of permethrin is low, but it should be used in pregnancy only if clearly needed. Lindane is absorbed through the skin.

It is unknown if permethrin is present in human breast milk after topical application. Since animal studies have identified some tumorigenic potential, it may be advisable to discontinue breast-feeding while using permethrin or to avoid permethrin use in women who are breast-feeding. Low concentrations of lindane are excreted in breast milk. Although it is unlikely that levels in breast milk would be sufficient to cause serious adverse reactions in the infant, an alternate method of feeding may be used for 2 days following lindane application.

Permethrin 5% cream may be used on children between 2 and 23 months, with medical supervision. Lindane should not be used in premature infants, and the risk of toxicity is greater in young children. The manufacturer recommends that it be used on children under the age of 6 years only on the advice of a physician, nurse or pharmacist.

Permethrin is contraindicated in those with hypersensitivities to any pyrethrins and chrysanthemum. Lindane should not be used in anyone with a seizure disorder or hypersensitivity to lindane.

Instructions for Use

Lindane for Scabies

- If there are crusts, use a warm bath, then let skin cool and dry.
- Apply to dry, cool skin to avoid absorption through the skin and possible side effects such as seizures.
- Apply the cream or lotion in a thin layer to the entire body from the neck down, paying particular attention to areas under the arms and breasts, in the umbilicus, and up to the openings of the genitalia.
- One 30 to 120 mL application of lotion or 30 to 60 g of cream should be sufficient to cover the entire body of an adult.
- After 8 to 12 hours, remove the lindane by washing.
- Put on clean clothing.
- One application is curative in about 96% of cases, although a reapplication 1 week later is often recommended to allow for inadequate coverage of all body areas during the initial treatment.
- A reapplication is necessary if evidence of active infestation remains or if the patient has been re-exposed.
- Avoid eyes, mucous membranes, open cuts or extensive excoriations.
- Mild burning and stinging may occur with lindane use.

Another synthetic pyrethroid, esdepallethrin, combined with piperonyl butoxide, is available in Canada in an aerosol form for the treatment of scabies. Data comparing this agent to lindane and permethrin are not available. It should not be used by those with sensitivities to synthetic pyrethroids. The manufacturer indicates that it may be used for the treatment of scabies in infants, children and adults, but that it should be used in pregnancy only when potential benefits outweigh risks. Possible adverse effects include transient cutaneous tingling, slight ocular tingling and respiratory tract irritation.

Sulfur and crotamiton may be the preferred treatments for pregnant and lactating women, although there is a lack of evidence regarding their toxicity. Some recommend avoiding crotamiton in these groups.

Crotamiton 10% cream is used as both an antipruritic and scabicide although it is not as effective as other therapies. It is applied 2 to 5 times consecutively, 24 hours apart, followed by bathing 24 hours after the final application. There are other regimens including twice daily application for 5 days, which is believed to have a 70% success rate.

Sulfur in a 5 to 10% concentration in petrolatum or an oil-in-water emulsion is applied at bedtime for

Instructions for Use

Permethrin for Scabies

- Soften any crusted lesions with a warm bath prior to application of permethrin.
- Apply the cream from the head to the soles of the feet, and massage into clean, dry skin (if using in infants, include the scalp).
- Pay particular attention to the fingernails, waist and genitalia when applying the cream (a tube of 30 g is often sufficient for an adult).
- Leave the cream on for 12 to 14 hours, then wash off.
- One treatment is considered adequate, although some authorities recommend a repeat application after 1 week. Others recommend retreatment only if there is clear evidence of treatment failure.

ADVICE FOR THE PATIENT

Scabies

- There are several effective medications available for the treatment of scabies.
- Certain types of medication may be better for certain age groups, so it is best to check with your pharmacist.
- Each type of medication is used slightly differently, and it is important to use it only as directed.
- Medication should not be left on any longer than directed, then should be washed off well.
- Medication should be applied to cool, dry skin.
- Certain medications should not be used if the skin is damaged.
- Medication should not be used more often than directed.
- One treatment may be effective.
- All medication should be kept out of the eyes, away from the mouth, nose and other sensitive areas, and out of the reach of children.
- When applying lindane, it may be a good idea to use rubber gloves, especially if it is being applied to more than one person.
- If using lindane in children, long-sleeved shirts, pants and mittens should be used to be sure they do not swallow any of the medication.
- When applying medication, special attention must be given to the fingernails, the waist, the umbilicus and the genital area.
- Bedding, towels and clothing should be washed in hot water and dried in a dryer for 20 minutes.
- Other items may be drycleaned or stored in a plastic bag for 2 weeks.
- Close contacts should be examined and treated if scabies is present.

2 to 5 nights. A 2.5% concentration has been recommended for infants, followed by bathing 24 hours after the final treatment, or the sulfur product can be applied for 8 hours before washing off, with another application 48 hours later. The toxicity is unknown but considered less than the other pediculicides. It is messy and odorous.

Benzyl benzoate may also be used in the treatment of scabies although it is not considered as effective as other remedies. The most common concentration recommended is 25%. Various regimens have been recommended: 2 to 3 applications either on successive days, separated by a week, or within a 24-hour period. It is also possible that a single application for a period of 24 hours may be effective. A bath should follow, 24 hours after the last treatment. Benzyl benzoate should be used half-strength in children and one-third strength in infants, to lessen the irritating effect.

Although pruritus usually subsides within a few days of effective scabicide treatment, it may continue for up to 4 weeks to 2 months due to irritation from the dead mites and their feces, irritation from the scabicide, or hypersensitivity reactions. This should not be interpreted as treatment failure, but lesions should be re-examined for the presence of mites. The pruritus may require additional treatment with agents such as oral or intralesional corticosteroids, topical steroids, antihistamines, topical calamine lotion, emollients or lotions containing menthol and phenol. Oral antibiotics may be necessary to treat secondary bacterial infections that have developed and prevent complications such as septicemia, glomerulonephritis, or rheumatic fever.

Other household members, close friends, those sharing quarters with the infested individual, and sexual contacts should be either evaluated or treated at the same time. In some situations, it may be advisable for day-care or nursing home workers to be treated simultaneously. Treatment of asymptomatic contacts may only be necessary for the caregiver of an infested child or those sharing a bed. Since scabies may be sexually transmitted, it may be advisable that patients be evaluated for other types of sexually transmitted diseases.

?

PATIENT ASSESSMENT QUESTIONS

Q ***What are your symptoms?***

Typical symptoms include itching that is most intense at night and may be accompanied by various types of rashes. Itching may require antipruritic medication in addition to the scabicide.

Q ***Have you had the condition diagnosed?***

There are many conditions with symptoms similar to scabies and an accurate diagnosis should be obtained.

Q ***Have you been in contact with someone diagnosed with scabies?***

This may help determine the need for treatment.

Q ***Are there any allergies, especially to ragweed or chrysanthemum?***

If so, permethrin should be avoided.

Q ***Are there any medical conditions, in particular epilepsy?***

Lindane should be avoided in those with neurological disorders.

Q ***Is the individual pregnant or breast-feeding?***

None of the available agents have been adequately assessed in pregnancy. Lindane absorption is the greatest, with the highest potential for adverse effects on the fetus. Alternate methods of feeding should be recommended for breast-feeding women using any available products.

ENTEROBIASIS

Enterobiasis refers to human infestation by *Enterobius vermicularis*, the pinworm. This is probably the most common helminth (parasitic worm) infestation, estimated to affect 500 million people worldwide. As many as 15 to 20% of the population of the United States may be affected. *Enterobius vermicularis* is thought to be the only helminth more common in temperate than tropical climates. It is the most common helminth infestation in Canada. Many other parasitic worms are soil borne, and the Canadian climate is too cold for their survival. About half of the world's population harbors one or more helminths. This is a particular problem in developing countries, and international travel and refugees may increase the risk of other types of helminth infestations in the wider population.

Enterobiasis is more common in children, affecting 11 to 43% of those living at home and 65% of those in institutions. There may be a higher incidence with the increased use of day-care facilities. An estimated one-third of Canadian children will be infested during their childhood. Pinworms are found most commonly in children 5 to 10 years of age living in crowded conditions. Transmission within families is common.

The infestation is also more common in homosexual men. Other high risk populations include institutionalized patients, residents of native reserves, and travellers to areas of high incidence, such as India and Iran.

Enterobiasis is not a sign of unclean living conditions. It is the only helminth spread from person to person. The eggs of *Enterobius vermicularis* enter the human through several possible routes: ingestion from contaminated hands or food, through the air from contaminated bed linen, from dust into the mouth or nose and, less often, from contaminated water. The eggs may be viable for several weeks away from the human. Occasionally larvae migrate from the anal area into the colon and can spread through sexual activity.

Once ingested, the eggs hatch in the upper small intestine. The larvae then migrate to the ileum and attach to the mucosal surface of the lower ileum, cecum or ascending colon, where they mature and copulate. When the female ovary is full of eggs, she migrates to the anus and deposits eggs on the perianal surface and perineum. The eggs become infective within 6 hours. This full cycle takes about 15 days. The adult pinworm is light yellowish white and shaped like a spindle with a long thin pointed tail. The adult female measures 8 to 13 mm, the male 2 to 5 mm. A few to several hundred adults may be present in an infected person.

There is a high likelihood of autoinfection due to scratching of the infested area followed by inadequate hand washing. This may lead to subsequent reingestion of the eggs, starting the cycle all over again. Reinfection may also occur from exposure to soiled objects and contaminated dust. The high rate of reinfection makes the problem difficult to combat. Theoretically the infestation would be self-limiting in several weeks if no reinfection occurred.

SYMPTOMS

Enterobiasis is generally considered a nuisance problem, but the pinworm has been known to migrate to other areas including the liver, spleen, kidney, lung and appendix. Eosinophilic granulomas of the colon and rectal area, local hemorrhages, secondary infections, perianal eczema, and appendicitis may be complications. In females, endometritis, salpingitis, pelvic peritonitis, and urinary tract infections have occurred.

Common symptoms include an intense pruritus known as pruritus ani, described as severe itching or sometimes even pain. The itching is worse at night when the females lay eggs, which are attached to the perianal area by a sticky substance that causes this pruritus. In heavy infestation, anorexia, weight loss, restlessness, and irritability due to disrupted sleep may occur.

If the worm migrates to the genital area in females, vulvovaginitis, vaginal discharge and irritation, nocturnal enuresis and diurnal urinary incontinence may be seen. If the pinworm carries colonic bacteria to the urinary tract, urinary tract infections may result. Asymptomatic granulomas of the female genitalia may also be seen.

Diagnosis is made by a swab obtained by placing scotch tape with the sticky side out on the end of a glass slide or tongue depressor. On awakening and before bathing or defecating, the device is pressed against the perianal area and then examined microscopically. This method is quite accurate in that one swab will identify 50% of cases and three will identify 90% of cases. The pinworm is rarely seen in the feces. Sometimes it is possible to see the white thread-like worm in the perianal area at night with a flashlight.

TREATMENT

Nonpharmacological Treatment

In addition to treatment with an anthelmintic, there are a number of measures that must be taken to ensure the treatment is successful. Proper hygiene is very important and includes handwashing and nailcleaning after defecation, scratching of the perianal area, and before eating. Keeping the fingernails short, and wearing tightfitting light pyjamas and cotton gloves may decrease nocturnal scratching and reinfestation. The use of antipruritic ointments may also be helpful. Bathing each morning is recommended. Regular cleaning of bedclothes, sleeping garments, undergarments and hand towels is considered useful. It is important to fold bedclothes or clothes before laundering rather than shaking them to prevent the spread of eggs. Boiling sheets and cleaning rooms daily is probably not necessary although keeping the bedroom floor clean should be helpful. Household disinfectants have little effect on pinworm eggs, and the use of damp cloths in cleaning may spread any eggs present, so this is not considered essential.

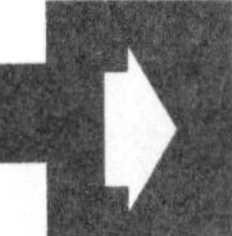

ADVICE FOR THE PATIENT

Pinworms

- Pinworms are a common infection in children aged 5 to 10 years.
- The condition should be diagnosed before using medication.
- The infection is easily transmitted in families, so all family members should be treated at once.
- There are a number of effective medications available to treat pinworms, pyrantel pamoate is most commonly recommended.
- Pregnant women and people with children under 2 years of age should check with their pharmacist or physician when choosing a medication.
- It is important to take the medication in the correct dose and exactly as prescribed.
- Medication usually needs to be repeated about 2 weeks after the first dose to be sure the infection is gone.
- Proper hygiene is important when treating pinworm infections.
- Wash hands and clean nails after defecation, scratching the anal area and before eating.
- Keep fingernails short and wear tight fitting pyjamas or cotton gloves to prevent scratching.
- Bathe and clean bedclothes, sleeping garments and undergarments daily, folding them instead of shaking to avoid spreading eggs.
- Ensure that sleeping areas are kept clean.

Pharmacological Treatment

It is recommended that pinworm infestations be treated only after diagnosis as anthelmintics are not prophylactic. All family members should be treated, however, since the probability of becoming infested is high. The treatment of uncomplicated cases is relatively straightforward, while family groups and institutions may be more difficult due to inadequate cures or reinfections. Treatment may need to be repeated in about 2 weeks since the available drugs are not ovicidal, and reinfection from various sources can occur. This time period corresponds to the pinworm life cycle.

The nonprescription drug of choice is pyrantel pamoate, and the prescription drug of choice is mebendazole. Other nonprescription agents available include pyrvinium pamoate and piperazine adipate. Evidence of effectiveness consists of a negative swab on 7 consecutive days. Gentian violet has been used in the past but is believed to have low efficacy, requires a 10-day course of therapy and may be a carcinogen and a mutagen.

If prescribed, mebendazole is given as a single 100 mg dose to adults and children over the age of 2. The dose is repeated after 2 weeks. It is available in chewable tablets that may be mixed with food. It should not be used in pregnancy.

In the treatment of pinworm in children over 1 year of age and adults, pyrantel pamoate is given in a dose of 11 mg/kg to a maximum of a 1 g single dose (Table 1). This should be repeated in 2 weeks to kill any newly ingested eggs. It can be given on either an empty or full stomach. The liquid form should be shaken well before use. Safety in pregnancy has not been definitively established, and it should not be used in the first trimester. It is not recommended in patients with liver dysfunction and should not be given in conjunction with

TABLE 1: Dosage Information for Nonprescription Drugs for Pinworm Infection

Drugs	Drug Dose	Body Weight	Product Dose
Piperazine adipate	75 mg/kg* for 7 days	<13.5 kg	5 mL/day for 7 days
		13.5–27.5 kg	10–15 mL/day for 7 days
		27.5–41 kg	15–25 mL/day for 7 days
		>41 kg	max. 25 mL/day for 7 days
Pyrantel pamoate	11 mg/kg	12–23 kg	2.5–5 mL
		23–45 kg	5–10 mL or 2–4 tablets
		45–68 kg	10–15 mL or 4–6 tablets
		>68 kg	max. 8 tablets
Pyrvinium pamoate	5 mg/kg	10–20 kg	5–10 mL
		20–40 kg	10–20 mL
		40–50 kg	20–25 mL
		50–70 kg	25–35 mL
		>70 kg	max. 35 mL

* 75 mg piperazine adipate is equivalent to 65 mg piperazine hexahydrate.
Adapted from: Farmer PS. Anthelmintics. In: Carruthers-Czyzewski P, ed. Self-Medication: Reference for Health Professionals. 4th ed. Ottawa: Canadian Pharmaceutical Association, 1992:281.

piperazine adipate as the mechanisms of action of the two drugs are antagonistic.

Pyrvinium pamoate for the treatment of pinworm is given as a 5 mg/kg single dose to a maximum of 350 mg, repeated in 2 weeks. Since the drug is a promutagen, it is not recommended for use in pregnancy. Pyrvinium pamoate is well tolerated and not well absorbed. The drug stains feces, vomitus, and clothing. Tablets should be swallowed whole to avoid staining the teeth.

Piperazine adipate is also used in the treatment of pinworm at 50 to 65 mg/kg per day (maximum 2.5 g/day) for 7 days, repeated in 1 to 4 weeks. Safety in pregnancy has not been established, and it should definitely not be used during the first trimester. If used during breast-feeding, the infant should be fed first, the mother should then take the dose of piperazine adipate and not breast-feed the baby for 8 hours. Milk produced in between should be discarded. The drug should not be used with phenothiazines, chlorpromazine and pyrantel pamoate. Piperazine adipate should not be used in epileptics or in patients with impaired renal or hepatic function. Use in impaired renal function may result in an increased neurotoxicity known as "worm wobble." This presents as gait instability, incoordination, vertigo, dysphasia, confusion, and myoclonic contractions.

The use of laxatives to facilitate removal of pinworms is not necessary after anthelmintic therapy.

It is recommended that an asymptomatic pregnant woman be treated after delivery since there are no harmful effects to mother or child from the infection. Treatment during the first trimester is to be avoided.

PATIENT ASSESSMENT QUESTIONS

Q *What are your symptoms?*
Nighttime itching in the perianal area is the most common symptom of pinworms. Intense itching may require an antipruritic in addition to an anthelmintic.

Q *How long have the symptoms been present?*
This may determine whether this is a new infection or a recurrence of one incorrectly treated.

Q *Have you been in contact with others who have pinworms?*
Transmission is common among children and families, and close contacts usually need to be treated.

Q *Have you had this problem before and how did you treat it?*
This will help to identify any problems with usage.

Q *How many people are in the household and what are their ages?*
This information will help in choosing a product and calculating the dosages.

Q *Is anyone pregnant, have health conditions or take medications?*
This information will also help in choosing a product or deciding whether or not treatment is appropriate.

PHARMACEUTICAL AGENTS

Benzyl Benzoate

Benzyl benzoate has been used in the treatment of scabies. It occurs naturally in balsam of Peru but is generally manufactured synthetically. This chemical is known to be irritating when applied topically, producing stinging and contact dermatitis, especially when applied to excoriated skin. It has a strong odor. Ingestion can produce convulsions, and its efficacy and toxicity have not been well established.

Crotamiton

Crotamiton 10% has been used as a treatment for scabies, sometimes as an alternative to lindane. However, it has exhibited effectiveness of less than 50% in children. It should not be used in pregnant or lactating women since there is a lack of evidence regarding its toxicity.

Lindane

Lindane 1% (gamma benzene hexachloride) is a chlorinated hydrocarbon with insecticidal activity used in the treatment of lice and scabies. About 10% of a topical dose may be absorbed, and absorption is very high in the scrotal area. Lindane has been known to result in neurotoxicity, including seizures and death in infants and children, and has been associated with aplastic anemia. Toxicity has usually occurred when the drug was used as a pesticide for agricultural purposes, and often with chronic exposure, in older individuals, and in situations of misuse, such as overuse due to long application times, frequent reapplications, use on infants with skin disease, or by ingestion. It is possible that certain conditions such as inflammation or other skin disorders may result in increased absorption. The risk of absorption and adverse effects is also greater in young children due to their higher surface area to body mass ratio. Additionally, malnourished patients and premature infants may be at increased risk. Applying lindane to wet skin could also increase the risk of absorption. Lindane used to treat head lice should have a lower risk of toxicities than when used for the treatment of scabies due to the shorter contact time and smaller body surface area to which it is applied.

Alternate therapy should be recommended for infants, children, pregnant and nursing women, patients with neurologic disorders, or those who may overuse products containing lindane. Measures to decrease the risk of toxicity when using lindane include: using the drug with caution, if at all, when skin is excoriated or the epidermal barrier function is otherwise compromised; applying the agent to cool, dry skin and avoiding a hot, soapy bath immediately prior to application; when treating head lice, applying the agent to the affected areas only; using the agent for the shortest recommended time possible; washing the drug off well, especially in the scrotal area; repeating usage only if active infestation can be demonstrated, not sooner than 7 to 8 days between treatments and not more frequently than twice monthly; using long-sleeved shirts, pants and mittens to minimize the possibility of young children ingesting the drug by licking.

Irritant contact dermatitis occurs fairly regularly with the use of lindane. Burning and stinging, pruritus, erythema, tingling and rash have been reported. Resistance to lindane has been reported in Central and South America as well as some areas of the United States and Australia; however, it is still believed to be low in North America.

Piperazine Adipate

As an anthelmintic, this drug causes flaccid paralysis of the worm resulting in removal by the host through normal peristaltic action.

The drug is well absorbed and mostly excreted in the urine within 24 hours. More common adverse effects include nausea, vomiting, cramps and diarrhea. Rarely, CNS effects such as transient dizziness, paresthesia, some incoordination and difficulty in focusing may be experienced. Hypersensitivity reactions such as fever and joint pain are signals to withdraw the drug. Safety in pregnancy has not been established, and it should definitely not be used during the first trimester. If used in breast-feeding, the infant should be fed first, the mother should then take the dose of piperazine adipate and not breast-feed the baby until 8 hours later. Milk produced in between should be discarded.

The drug produces increased extrapyramidal effects when given with phenothiazines. It should not be used with chlorpromazine as there may be a potentiated risk of seizures. It should not be given with pyrantel pamoate due to an antagonistic mechanism of action.

Piperazine adipate may exacerbate seizures and should not be used in epileptics. It is contraindicated in impaired renal or hepatic function; it may result in an increased neurotoxicity known as "worm wobble." This presents as gait instability, incoordination, vertigo, dysphasia, confusion, and myoclonic contractions.

Pyrantel Pamoate

Pyrantel pamoate is an anthelmintic that causes paralysis of the worm by producing neuromuscular blockade. Since the worm depends on its muscular activity to remain attached to the host, this blockade permits expulsion by the host's normal intestinal peristalsis.

The neuromuscular junction in helminths is much more sensitive than that of humans, thus there is little toxicity to the host. Adverse effects that may occur include nausea, vomiting, abdominal cramps and diarrhea, which may be decreased by giving the drug with food or milk. Pyrantel pamoate is not well absorbed. Most of the drug is excreted unchanged in the feces, although some drug is metabolized in the liver. It is not recommended in patients with liver dysfunction. Alternatively, it may be possible to use lower doses. Pyrantel pamoate may cause some dizziness, drowsiness and insomnia. It should not be given in conjunction with piperazine adipate as the mechanisms of action of the two drugs are antagonistic.

Safety in pregnancy has not been definitively established, and it should not be used in the first trimester.

Pyrethrins, Synthetic

Development of synthetic agents similar to the natural pyrethrins for the treatment of lice and scabies has been based on efforts to increase effectiveness, lower toxicity and produce products that are more photostable and biodegradable. The synthetic agents available in Canada include allethrin, bioallethrin, esdepallethrin and permethrin. Allethrin is similar to the natural pyrethrins in both insecticidal activity and lack of stability to light.

Permethrin: Permethrin is a synthetic pyrethroid that acts by delaying repolarization on the neural cell membrane resulting in paralysis of the insect. It is effective in treating lindane resistant cases of scabies. It is photostable, thermostable and an active residue persists for as long as 10 days so that any nymphs that hatch will be killed. It is considered more effective than lindane, crotamiton and pyrethrins in a single dose due to this residual activity. It also has about 70 to 80% ovicidal activity. The incidence of adverse effects is reported to be low although it has been reported to cause increased pruritus following treatment. Burning and stinging, erythema, and other skin reactions have also been reported. It is less toxic than lindane and has been found safe in children over 2 years of age. The 5% cream may be used on children between the ages of 2 and 23 months with medical supervision. Less than 2% is absorbed through the skin, and it is almost entirely excreted in the urine in 72 hours as inactive metabolites. Rarely, reports of respiratory difficulty and musculoskeletal shaking have been reported. Individuals with a sensitivity to chrysanthemums and ragweed may exhibit allergic contact dermatitis to permethrin, although it is unlikely due to the chemical purity of the substance. It is odorless and will not stain clothing.

Pyrethrins with Piperonyl Butoxide

Pyrethrins combined with piperonyl butoxide are used in the treatment of lice infestations. Pyrethrins are insecticidal chemicals found in pyrethrum, which is the dried flower from the *Chrysanthemum* genus of plants. These agents cause paralysis and death of the louse by interfering with neural transmission. They are combined with piperonyl butoxide which serves as a synergist by inhibiting enzymes in the louse that metabolize pyrethrins. This results in a 2- to 12-fold increase in activity of pyrethrins. Concentrations found in commercial products range from 0.17 to 0.33% for pyrethrins and from 2 to 4% for piperonyl butoxide. Absorption of these compounds is not extensive, and they are rapidly metabolized when absorption does take place. Adverse effects are uncommon but may include contact dermatitis and other allergic manifestations including anaphylactoid reactions. Cross-sensitivity may occur in individuals allergic to ragweed and chrysanthemums. Thus, patients with sensitivities to ragweed, chrysanthemums or other pyrethrins should avoid the use of products containing pyrethrins. There are reports of corneal damage associated with these agents. Ingestion of products with a petroleum distillate solvent may be fatal.

Pyrvinium Pamoate

The mechanism of action of pyrvinium pamoate as an anthelmintic may be through flaccid paralysis of the worm or the depletion of the worm's energy sources.

The drug is well tolerated and is not well absorbed. Adverse effects include nausea, vomiting, abdominal cramps and diarrhea. It is a photosensitizer and stains feces, vomitus, and clothing. Tablets should be swallowed whole to avoid staining the teeth.

Since the drug is a promutagen, it is not recommended for use in pregnancy.

Sulfur

Sulfur preparations are considered by some to be the treatment of choice for scabies infestations in pregnant or lactating females due to the lack of reported toxicities. However, there is also a lack of controlled trials regarding the efficacy and toxicity of sulfur. Sulfur preparations stain clothing and bedclothes and are odorous.

RECOMMENDED READING

Pediculosis and Scabies

Burns DA. The treatment of human ectoparasite infection. Br J Dermatol 1991;125:89-93.

Chunge RN, Scott FE, Underwood JE, et al. A review of the epidemiology, public health importance, treatment and control of head lice. Can J Public Health 1991;82:196-200.

Chunge RN, Scott FE, Underwood JE, et al. A pilot study to investigate transmission of headlice. Can J Public Health 1991;82:207-08.

DeSimone EM, McCracken G. September lice alert. US Pharm 1994;19(9):32-40.

Drugs for parasitic infections. Med Lett Drugs Ther 1995;37(961):99-108.

Gossel TA. Head lice: coping with the yearly infestation. US Pharm 1990;15(9):39-46.

Hogan DJ, Schachner L, Tanglertsampan C. Diagnosis and treatment of childhood scabies and pediculosis. Pediatr Clin North Am 1991;38: 941-57.

Lane AT. Scabies and head lice. Pediatr Ann 1987;16:51-54.

Rasmussen JE. The problem of lindane. J Am Acad Dermatol 1981;5:507-16.

Taplin D, Meinking TL. Scabies, lice and fungal infections. Prim Care 1989;16:551-68.

Taplin D, Meinking TL. Pyrethrins and pyrethroids in dermatology. Arch Dermatol 1990;126: 213-20.

Enterobiasis

Cook GC. Enterobius vermicularis infections. GUT 1994;35:1159-62.

Cook GC. Threadworm infection and its treatment. Pharm J 1990;244(June 23):765-67.

Drugs for parasitic infections. Med Lett Drugs Ther 1995;37(961):99-108.

Katz M. Anthelmintics: current concepts in the treatment of helminthic infections. Drugs 1986; 32: 358-71.

Keusch GT. Anthelmintic therapy: the worm has turned. Drug Ther 1982;12(Aug):213-17, 220-22.

Pray WS. Pinworms: a common family nuisance. US Pharm 1993;18(4):30-35.

Rosenblatt JE. Antiparasitic agents. Mayo Clin Proc 1992;67(3):276-87.

van Riper G. Pyrantel pamoate for pinworm infestation. Am Pharm 1993;NS33(2):43-45.

7

DERMATITIS, SEBORRHEA, DANDRUFF AND DRY SKIN PRODUCTS

DALE E. WRIGHT

CONTENTS

Introduction 121
- Anatomy and Physiology of the Skin

Atopic Dermatitis 123
- Symptoms
- Treatment

Contact Dermatitis 128
- Irritant Contact Dermatitis
- Allergic Contact Dermatitis
- Treatment
- Diaper Dermatitis

Seborrhea and Dandruff 134
- Symptoms
- Treatment
- Cradle Cap

Dry Skin 137
- Symptoms
- Treatment

Pharmaceutical Agents 141
- Antipruritics
- Astringents
- Bath Products
- Bufexamac
- Cleansing Products
- Coal Tar
- Corticosteroids
- Cytostatic Shampoos
- Emollients
- Keratolytics
- Soaks

Recommended Reading 147

INTRODUCTION

Dermatitis is a nonspecific term describing acute and chronic inflammatory lesions of the skin. Nonprescription drug treatment is suitable for some eczematous dermatoses, including atopic dermatitis, irritant and allergic contact dermatitis, seborrheic dermatitis and an associated condition, dandruff. Dry skin is an underlying feature of some of these conditions or may, on its own, pose a problem for the patient.

ANATOMY AND PHYSIOLOGY OF THE SKIN

The skin consists of the epidermis and dermis overlying a subcutaneous fatty layer that acts as a cushion between the outer layers and the underlying bone (Figure 1). The most important function of the skin is as a barrier preventing penetration of the body by chemicals and radiation and loss of body water and electrolytes. It also protects against mechanical injury, regulates heat loss, mediates sensation, initiates immunological response to antigens, is involved in the synthesis of vitamin D and allows some ingested toxins to be excreted. By appearance, feel and smell, it is integral to sociosexual communication.

The barrier function of the skin lies in the epidermis, which is composed mainly of keratinocytes with a smaller number of Langerhans cells and melanocytes. Keratinocytes produce an insoluble fibrous protein, keratin, which is ultimately responsible for the barrier properties. They also contain melanin, a protein that protects the skin from ultraviolet radiation. Melanin is produced in melanocytes and transferred to keratinocytes in

Introduction

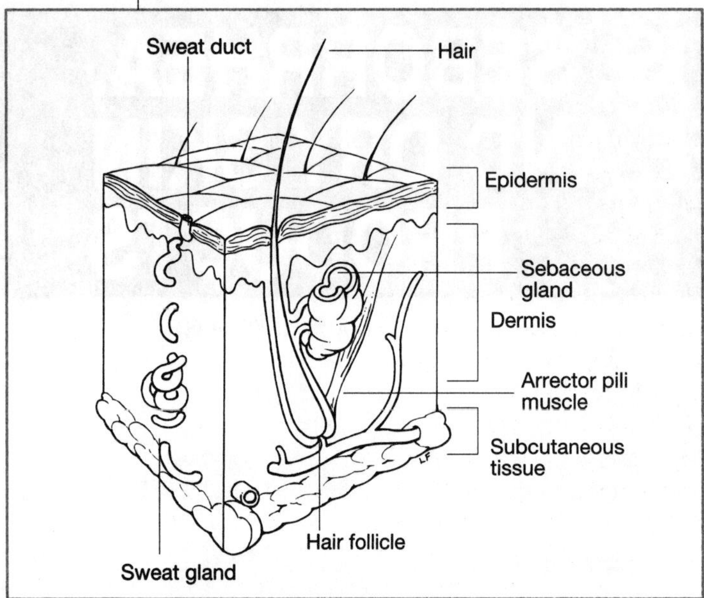

FIGURE 1: The Skin

pigment granules called melanosomes. Keratinocytes also produce a number of immune system factors important in the pathogenesis of inflammatory skin conditions. Langerhans cells, the other component of the immune system in the epidermis, process antigens in contact with the skin. Constant renewal of the epidermis is achieved by migration of keratinocytes from the basal layer to the surface about every 28 days. As the keratinocytes migrate outward, they gradually flatten, lose their nuclei and die. In the outermost layer of the epidermis, the stratum corneum, keratin-filled corneocytes arranged in orderly stacks are responsible for the resilience and water-holding capacity of the epidermis. The intercellular matrix is composed mainly of lipids such as ceramides, cholesterol and free fatty acids that aid in corneocyte cohesion and provide the barrier to water loss. The stratum corneum is constantly renewed as the keratin-filled scales gradually loosen and fall away.

The dermis underlies and supports the epidermis. Its major function is to protect the body from mechanical injury, but it is also a source of nutrients to the avascular epidermis. The dermis is composed of collagen and elastin fibres in an aqueous matrix of glycosaminoglycans. Collagen, a protein with high tensile strength, makes up 70% of the weight of the dermis and is responsible for its mechanical properties. Elastin is a resilient protein that helps the skin maintain its tonus and returns deformed skin to the resting state. Other elements of the dermis include capillary blood vessels arising from arteries in the subcutaneous fat, sensory and autonomic nerves, and cells important to the inflammatory response: mast cells, lymphocytes, macrophages, eosinophils and basophils.

ATOPIC DERMATITIS

Atopic dermatitis, commonly referred to as eczema, is a chronic inflammatory pruritic dermatosis usually associated with a personal or family history of allergic disease. Seventy-five to 80% of patients with atopic dermatitis have a family or personal history of allergic disease and nearly 80% will demonstrate positive reactions to allergens in immediate hypersensitivity skin testing.

It affects 0.5 to 1% of the general population, but is particularly common in young people: 10 to 20% of persons born after 1970 have been affected at some point. It is most prevalent in young children: 80% of cases develop before 1 year of age and 95% before age 5. Onset before 3 months or after age 30 is unusual. Infants younger than 3 months of age with dermatitis probably have seborrheic dermatitis, as the itch-scratch reflex is not yet developed. Some infants appear to have a combined form of atopic dermatitis–seborrheic dermatitis with atopy greater than that of normal controls but less than that of individuals with atopic dermatitis. Up to 50% of children with atopic dermatitis will develop asthma or allergic rhinitis as they age, often as the dermatitis improves. The dermatitis will resolve in many infants by the age of 2, and over 65% of children will have outgrown it between the ages of 5 and 25.

Atopic dermatitis is an immune system disorder. Patients have defective cell-mediated immunity with abnormal biochemical responsiveness and mediator release by immune system cells in the epidermis and dermis. All patients with atopic dermatitis appear to have dry skin, with increased transepidermal water loss, reduced water-binding capacity and low water content.

Exposure to a flare factor such as psychic stress, irritants (e.g., soaps, chemicals), environmental factors (e.g., heat, humidity), trauma or food allergens initiates an intensely pruritic erythematous flush in areas subject to dermatitis.

Patients with atopic dermatitis are often colonized with *Staphylococcus aureus* and/or the yeast *Pityrosporum ovale* in active areas. They are prone to developing viral, bacterial and fungal skin infections.

SYMPTOMS

Pruritus is the most common and least tolerated symptom of atopic dermatitis.

Characteristic lesions of atopic dermatitis result from scratching and may include weeping erosions, vesicles, and excoriated reddened, scaling papules or plaques. Chronically, the skin may become thickened secondary to rubbing and scratching (lichenification), and there may be postinflammatory pigmentation changes that gradually resolve over 6 to 12 months. In infants and young children the scalp, face and extensor surfaces of the extremities are primarily involved. Hair may be lost, but returns after the dermatitis remits. In children over 2 years of age and adults, lesions are most commonly found on the neck, inner surfaces of the elbows and knees, wrists, ankles, hands and feet. Important conditions in the differential diagnosis include seborrheic dermatitis, contact dermatitis, and icthyosis vulgaris (Table 1).

TREATMENT

The main priorities in managing atopic dermatitis are to decrease the dryness of the skin and control the often debilitating itching that perpetuates the skin lesions. Dry skin creates a defective barrier that permits penetration of irritants, allergens and infectious agents that exacerbate the condition. Refer to Figure 2 for the suggested treatment approach.

Nonpharmacological Treatment

In counselling the patient or parent of a child with atopic dermatitis, it is important to stress that it is a condition of dry, sensitive, easily irritated skin. Patients should minimize their use of soaps and solvents, including bubble baths. Cleansing agents should have minimal defatting activity and a neutral pH. A mild synthetic detergent cleanser can be suggested for patients sensitive to soaps. Their use should be confined to intertriginous areas such as the axillary or groin regions. Laundry soap residue can be reduced by adding a second rinse cycle to ensure removal of soap from clothing and bedding. Avoid bleach and fabric softener. Cold air humidifiers can help reduce room dryness (especially bedrooms), thereby helping to relieve itching.

To reduce itching caused by sweating, ideally the work and home environment should be kept at a constant cool temperature and humidity. Open-weave loose-fitting garments made of cotton or cotton blends will help. Avoid wool, nylon or rough fabrics.

Atopic Dermatitis

TABLE 1: Differential Diagnosis of Atopic Dermatitis, Contact Dermatitis, Dry Skin, Seborrheic Dermatitis, Dandruff

Condition	Symptoms	Distribution	Appearance	Trigger Factors
Atopic dermatitis	Cycles of itching and scratching. Dry sensitive skin.	*3 months–2 yr:* cheeks, scalp, extensor surface of arms/legs. *2–12 yr:* flexural areas, neck, wrists, ankles. *12 yr–adult:* flexural areas, face, hands, feet.	*Acute:* pruritic papules and vesicles on erythematous area; may be erosions with exudate from scratching. *Subacute:* scaling papules/plaques, erythema. *Chronic:* thickened, dry skin with pigmentation changes.	Psychic stress, irritants, environmental factors (no humidity), trauma, food allergens, molds/pollens, infections.
Irritant contact dermatitis	*Acute:* burning or stinging at contact site. *Chronic:* itching, irritated skin.	*Acute/chronic:* restricted to contact area in pattern consistent with irritant (e.g., hand dermatitis, diaper dermatitis).	*Acute:* blisters, erosions or erythematous plaques at contact site; oozing. *Chronic:* reddened, chapped skin initially, then dry, thickened inflamed plaques.	*Strong irritants* (e.g., acids, alkalies) cause immediate damage. *Mild irritants* (e.g., water, soap, detergents, solvents) cause chronic injury.
Allergic contact dermatitis	Delayed itching at contact site: initial contact—1 to 3 weeks; repeat contact—24 to 48 hours.	Exposed or contact area. Allergen inadvertently spread by touch. Often in patterns with straight margins, unusual shapes corresponding to contact area.	Reddened areas with weeping, crusted papules and vesicles. May progress to thickened, scaling chronic lesions.	Numerous contact allergens exist (e.g., poison ivy, cosmetic creams, nail lacquers, glues, rubber, metal—see Table 2).
Dry skin	Usually none. Occasional itching.	Front of lower legs, back of hands, forearms. Face, trunk less commonly.	Roughness, flaking, scaling, chapping of skin. Redness may occur. Fissuring in severe cases.	Low humidity, dry cold wind, mechanical abrasion, exposure to soaps/solvents/detergents.
Seborrheic dermatitis		*Infants (cradle cap):* scalp, central face, forehead, ears. *Adults:* scalp, eyebrows, eyelids, cheek, nasal and beard area, chest, back, ears. Less common—intertriginous areas.	Patchy areas with dry or oily yellowish scales and slight redness of underlying skin.	Stress, low humidity, low temperatures. Worse in winter.
Dandruff	Usually none. Flakes are cosmetically unappealing.	Scalp.	Thin white or greyish flakes spread evenly on scalp.	Relatively stable. May be exacerbated by inadequate washing, dry climate.

Adapted from Ricciatti-Sibbald DJ. Dermatitis. In: Carruthers-Czyzewski P, ed. *Self-medication. Reference for Health Professionals.* 4th ed. Ottawa: Canadian Pharmaceutical Association, 1992:65.

Although ultraviolet (UV) light may be beneficial in atopic dermatitis, patients should avoid sunburn and hot or humid conditions that can increase pruritus. Use sunscreens to avoid sunburn.

Allergen avoidance is a controversial aspect of management but may benefit a subset of patients with identified allergic triggers. The major food antigens appear to be eggs, cows' milk, soy products, wheat, peanuts and fish. Aeroallergens such as house mite dust and pollens and microbial allergens such as *Pityrosporum* yeasts and *S. aureus* can be a problem for some patients.

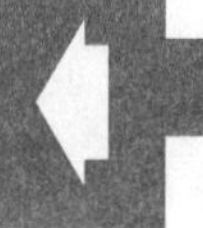

ADVICE FOR THE PATIENT

Atopic Dermatitis

This is a condition of dry, sensitive, easily irritated skin. Itchy rashes will come and go in unpredictable cycles.

Some of the possible causes of an atopic dermatitis rash are:

- stress;
- skin irritants, such as soaps or chemicals;
- environmental factors, such as high heat or humidity;
- foods, molds or pollens to which you may be allergic.

Things you can do to protect your skin include:

- Minimize your use of soaps and solvents, including bubble baths. Use only a mild skin cleanser for groin, underarms and feet.
- Water can dry the skin too much so restrict bathing to once or twice a week with sponge baths other days.
- Wear cotton or cotton-blend clothing; avoid wool, nylon or rough fabrics.
- Remove laundry soap residue from clothing and bedding by adding a second rinse cycle. Soap flakes may be less irritating than laundry detergents. Do not use fabric softener or bleach.
- Keep the work and home environment at a constant cool temperature and humidity if possible.
- Use sunscreens to avoid sunburn.
- Avoid foods to which you know you are allergic.

When you have a rash, some of the things you can do to relieve the itching include:

- Soak the area in cool water, or bathe in warm water for 15 to 20 minutes.
- Add an oatmeal product or baking soda to the water for a soothing effect. If bath oil is used, add it only in the last 5 minutes of the bath.
- Pat the area dry then rub in an ointment.
- Oral antihistamines may relieve itching. If they cause too much drowsiness, use them at bedtime or try a nonsedating antihistamine.
- Rub a moisturizing cream into the skin 3 or 4 times a day to prevent skin dryness.
- Try a nonprescription hydrocortisone ointment if the above suggestions don't work.
- Avoid ointments or creams that contain antihistamines or local anesthetics (especially benzocaine) because these can be irritating. Ask your pharmacist if you are unsure which creams to avoid.

If the rash covers a large area, is blistered or oozing or does not respond to these measures, see your doctor.

Pharmacological Treatment

The first step in the treatment of atopic dermatitis is to alleviate the dry skin. Hydrate the skin by soaking the affected area(s) or bathing in tepid water for 15 to 20 minutes. Bath oils can be added in the last 5 minutes of the bath. After bathing, remove excess water by patting with a soft towel and apply an emollient. A water-in-oil emollient should be applied within 3 to 5 minutes to help the skin retain the water. Petrolatum may also be applied to improve the barrier function. Note that in some patients using an emollient that is too greasy can irritate eczematous as well as uninvolved skin.

In the maintenance phase, water-in-oil moisturizers should be applied at least 3 to 4 times a day.

Atopic Dermatitis

Moisturizers will help keep the skin supple and reduce drying and cracking that can perpetuate the inflammatory cycle. Products containing urea or lactic acid may be beneficial in more resistant dry skin. They should be introduced cautiously because they can be irritating. Applying these products to dampened skin will minimize stinging and burning.

For severely affected or persistent areas of dermatitis, wet wraps may help promote hydration, uptake of medications and cooling of the skin.

For localized, weeping lesions, Burow's solution compresses will provide astringent and antibacterial effects. They should be used for 2 to 3 days only, however, as Burow's solution is very drying and may lead to increased itching and cracking.

To alleviate the itch associated with atopic dermatitis, the mainstay of treatment is topical corticosteroids. They should be applied immediately after hydration for better penetration, but no more than 3 to 4 times a day. Low-potency nonprescription hydrocortisone products are unlikely to be effective for an acute flare-up but may be used to combat the itch of resolving lesions and for maintenance therapy. Bufexamac 5% ointment is a nonprescription topical nonsteroidal anti-inflammatory drug that may be used as an alternative to low-potency hydrocortisone preparations. In an acute flare-up, mild- to high-potency corticosteroids are prescribed for several days, with the choice determined by location and extent of lesions. The choice of vehicle depends on the patient's needs. Creams and lotions are preferable for acute weeping lesions. Ointments are preferred for chronic dry lesions. Therapy should be discontinued when the lesions are gone. Chronic use for prolonged periods can cause thinning of the skin.

Colloidal oatmeal products or sodium bicarbonate can be added to bath water to reduce itching.

Although antihistamines are widely used, they are considered to have only minor benefit because the pruritus of atopic dermatitis is only partially related to histamine release. Traditional antihistamines (e.g., hydroxyzine, diphenhydramine, chlorpheniramine) are preferred. Their sedative effect is thought to provide relief by reducing itching. The newer nonsedating antihistamines may provide an alternative when sedative and anticholinergic side effects (e.g., dry mouth) of the traditional agents are troublesome. Loratadine 5 to 10 mg daily and terfenadine 30 mg twice daily have both been shown to provide relief of itching in some children with atopic dermatitis. Cetirizine may provide some benefit because in addition to its antihistamine effects it also blocks mast cell mediator release and some IgE-mediated immunologic effects. Avoid the use of topical antihistamines and benzocaine-containing topical anesthetics because of potential sensitization. Crotamiton 10% cream has been used as an antipruritic, but its antipruritic action is not well established.

Coal tar products are helpful adjuncts in treating eczema. They can be used in subacute and chronic eczema, but may cause folliculitis on hairy areas of the skin. Coal tar products have anti- inflammatory and antipruritic properties that may help reduce the need for topical corticosteroids in chronic atopic dermatitis. Tar products are best applied under an emollient because of their drying properties. Compliance is increased if they are only used at bedtime and washed off in the morning.

Patients with skin infection should be referred to a physician because systemic antibiotics may be needed. Antibacterial cleansers and topical antibiotics are generally not recommended, since they may irritate the skin or cause hypersensitivity reactions.

With basic therapy, significant improvement of the eczema is usually achieved in 10 to 14 days. Patients with unresponsive, infected or extensive lesions should be referred to a physician.

FIGURE 2

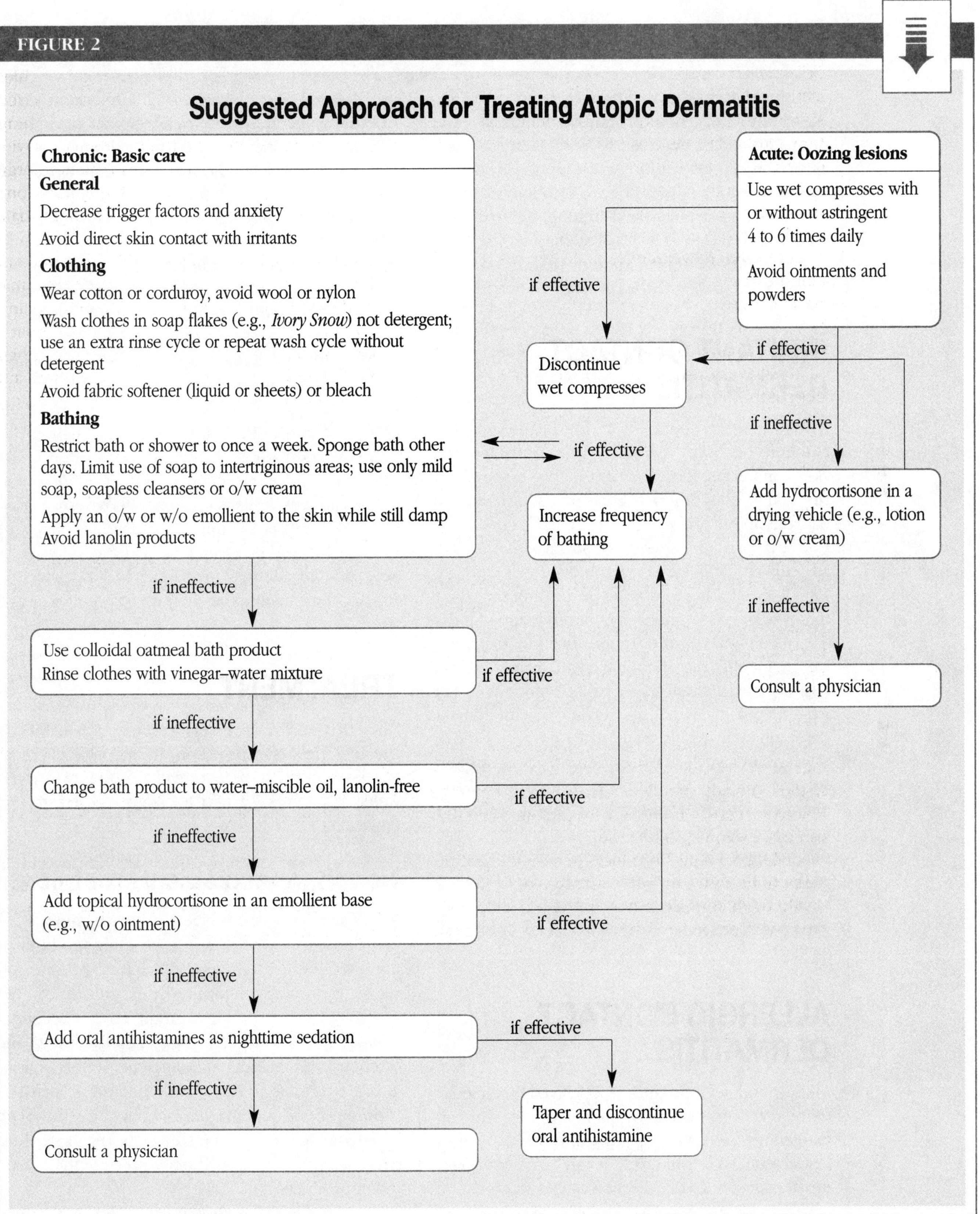

Adapted from Ricciatti-Sibbald DJ. Dermatitis. In: Carruthers-Czyzewski P, ed. *Self-medication. Reference for Health Professionals.* 4th ed. Ottawa: Canadian Pharmaceutical Association, 1992:67.

CONTACT DERMATITIS

Contact dermatitis is caused by exposure of the skin to exogenous irritants, such as in hand dermatitis and diaper dermatitis, or allergens, such as poison ivy dermatitis or cosmetic dermatitis. Patients commonly seek nonprescription treatment for chapping, redness and itching. Contact dermatitis accounts for 4 to 7% of all dermatology consults and may be severe enough to interfere with the patient's daily activities at work and home.

IRRITANT CONTACT DERMATITIS

Irritant contact dermatitis (a nonallergic skin reaction) accounts for 80% of all contact-related skin conditions. It is an inflammatory response of the skin to nonimmunologic physical or chemical damage, and may occur in anyone if the concentration of the irritant is sufficient. Strong irritants such as acids or alkalies cause immediate cell damage, initially producing a stinging or burning sensation followed by blisters or erythematous plaques at the site of contact. Onset of lesions is rapid, making it easy to identify the offending agent. Hand dermatitis and diaper dermatitis are two common forms of irritant contact dermatitis. Chronic irritant contact dermatitis can result from repeated exposure to mild irritants such as water, detergents, soaps and solvents. Initially the skin becomes reddened and chapped, which enhances penetration of the irritant and perpetuates the injury cycle. Over time, the skin becomes thickened and inflamed. Location of the rash often provides a clue to the offending agent. Patients with atopic dermatitis are more susceptible because of their impaired epidermal barrier.

ALLERGIC CONTACT DERMATITIS

Allergic contact dermatitis is a delayed hypersensitivity reaction caused by skin contact with an exogenous allergen. It is less common (20%) than irritant contact dermatitis, but can be more severe. Initial exposure to the allergen causes sensitization of the immune system that can delay appearance of symptoms 7 to 10 days and, rarely, up to 25 days. With subsequent exposure to the allergen, symptoms develop in 12 to 48 hours. Because symptoms are delayed, it is often difficult to identify the offending agent. Symptoms are similar to those of contact dermatitis: reddened, itchy skin with weeping, crusted papules and vesicles that may become infected or progress to thickened, scaling chronic lesions. Often only patch testing can confirm the allergic nature of the eruption. The most common allergens are listed in Table 2. Note that medications such as topical antihistamines or topical anesthetics that may be used to treat the reaction can also be sensitizing.

The differential diagnosis of allergic and irritant contact dermatitis includes seborrheic and atopic dermatitis (Table 1). The pattern of lesions and their distribution may be helpful in distinguishing the cause, particularly with allergic contact dermatitis (Table 2). For example, poison ivy dermatitis typically produces vesicles in streaks in exposed areas. Hand dermatitis is commonly occupational and contact in origin. Dermatitis of the ears or neck suggests an allergy to nickel in jewelry. Eye involvement suggests an allergy to cosmetics or eye drops.

TREATMENT

The first priority is symptomatic control of the acute lesions. Some nonpharmacological measures can be taken to prevent future reactions. Refer to Figures 3 and 4 for suggested treatment approaches.

Nonpharmacological Treatment

After the acute episode, the best treatment for contact dermatitis is prevention. Avoiding the offending agent, substituting an alternative product or wearing protective clothing (e.g., gloves) can be recommended depending on the type of reaction (Table 3). Barrier creams (e.g., silicone creams) are often recommended, but their clinical effectiveness is controversial. In occupational hand dermatitis, they may be of benefit by facilitating the removal of sticky oils, greases and resins from the skin, thus decreasing the need to wash with potentially irritating products.

Persons with occupational hand dermatitis should be advised to avoid the use of solvents and harsh soaps if possible. Abrasive soaps should be restricted to use on the palms where skin is thicker and more resistant to irritation from friction. If using waterless hand cleansers, patients should wash off the residue with a mild soap or synthetic detergent cleanser and routinely apply an emollient after washing. Creams or ointments containing sensitizing ingredients should be avoided. If water contact is to be avoided, the patient should wear a pair of thin cotton gloves inside rubber or vinyl gloves.

Pharmacological Treatment

Cool tap water compresses applied to the rash for 30 minutes, 4 to 6 times per day may provide some symptomatic relief and will help rehydrate dry skin in irritant contact dermatitis. Application of hydrophobic emollients will help maintain hydration of dry skin areas. Patients with hand dermatitis should frequently apply a plain cream or ointment to their hands throughout the day to keep the skin supple.

For oozing vesicles and to soothe the area, Burow's solution 1:40 or 1:20 should be applied as a damp compress. Avoid applications longer than 20 minutes as Burow's solution can be irritating.

For extensive dermatitis, colloidal oatmeal baths in tepid water may be helpful. After bathing, patients should pat dry the irritated areas of the skin and apply a thin layer of moisturizing cream.

Topical calamine, zinc oxide or aluminum hydroxide lotions may be soothing, but they are not recommended for weeping lesions as they may cake and adhere to inflamed areas.

Oral antihistamines such as hydroxyzine, promethazine and diphenhydramine may help relieve pruritus by their sedating effect. Avoid topical antihistamines in contact dermatitis. Although they may be effective, they can be sensitizing and may cause contact dermatitis.

Nonprescription topical hydrocortisone products are safe and effective in relieving symptoms of contact dermatitis. Topical hydrocortisone should be applied in a thin layer to the affected area 3 to 4 times a day immediately after hydration. Occlusion will increase drug absorption and is not recommended unless advised by a physician. If the rash does not clear after 7 days of therapy, a doctor should be consulted. A short course of oral or potent topical corticosteroids may be warranted in some cases. Nonprescription topical hydrocortisone should not be recommended for children under 2 years of age because they are more susceptible to absorption of topical steroids. Bufexamac cream is an alternative to nonprescription hydrocortisone products. It appears to be as effective as corticosteroids in relieving symptoms of contact dermatitis.

TABLE 2: Contact Allergens by Site

Area	Suspect
Eyelids	Perfume, nailpolish, handcream, cosmetics, eye medication, eyelash curlers
Ears	Earrings, glasses, perfume, hair products
Mouth	Lipstick, gum, food dyes, mouthwashes, toothpaste, pens or pencils
Face	Cosmetics, hair products, soaps, aerosol sprays
Hands	Jewelry, foods, soaps, cosmetics, occupational contacts
Feet	Leather, glue, nickel, chromium, rubber, dyes

Adapted with permission, from Walzer RA. Dermatitis and eczema: a few rash statements. In: Skintelligence: How to be Smart About Your Skin. New York: Appleton-Century-Crofts, 1981:71–87.

DIAPER DERMATITIS

Diaper dermatitis is a form of irritant contact dermatitis that can be a problem in infant and elder care. It was originally thought that urinary ammonia was the contact irritant. It is now thought that bacteria in the area contribute to an increased pH that promotes the activity of fecal enzymes that act as irritants. Occlusion maceration, abrasion, frequent bowel movements and diarrhea are contributing factors. A secondary infection with *Candida albicans* frequently occurs after 2 or 3 days.

Diaper dermatitis is found on the skin in contact with the diaper: buttocks, upper thighs, lower abdomen and genitalia. Initially it appears as shiny reddened patches with papules or vesicles. Fissures and erosions can develop in skin folds due to maceration. Pustules can develop in areas infected with *C. albicans.*

To prevent diaper dermatitis, keep the skin as dry as possible, limiting the mixing of feces and urine. Disposable diapers with absorbent gelling have been shown to reduce the prevalence of rashes, even in atopic babies.

Treatment

When a rash develops, frequent diaper changes will help keep the area clean and dry. Cleanse the area gently with warm water and pat dry. Avoid the use of wipes containing irritants or soaps. Petrolatum or zinc oxide ointment are effective protectants. Silicone barrier creams can also be used. Powders can be used sparingly to dry the area if vesicles or maceration are present. Avoid the use of cornstarch as a drying powder as it can promote fungal growth. Care should be taken when using powders such as talc because inhaling it can cause respiratory distress in infants. Rather than sprinkling the powder directly on the infant, parents should apply it to their own hand then gently pat it on the infant. If a secondary *Candida* infection develops, topical antifungal agents may be required. Topical clotrimazole or miconazole twice daily or nystatin 4 times daily are effective and resolve most candidal infections in 2 weeks.

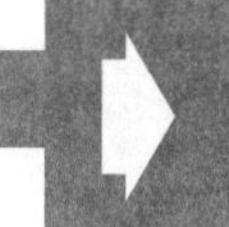

ADVICE FOR THE PATIENT

Contact Dermatitis

Contact dermatitis may result from skin contact with something that is irritating or to which you are allergic. The resulting rash is red and itchy and sometimes forms blisters that may ooze and crust. The rash usually occurs at the site of contact and is not contagious. Allergic rashes may not appear for 2 to 4 days or even up to 3 weeks. Common types of contact dermatitis include:

Irritant Contact Dermatitis
- strong chemicals that injure the skin where they touch;
- soaps, detergents or mild chemicals that cause a rash after repeated contact;
- diaper rash.

Allergic Contact Dermatitis
- nickel in costume jewelry, metal snaps or rivets;
- hair and leather dyes, including those in shoes;
- rubber, including gloves, shoes, elastic;
- medicines applied to the skin including some local anesthetics, antihistamines or antibiotics;
- preservatives in many cosmetics or personal products;
- fabrics treated to be wrinkle resistant or waterproof.

The easiest way to prevent contact dermatitis is to avoid things that you know cause sensitivity. Sometimes you can use a different product that will not give you a rash. Check with your doctor or pharmacist for advice on other products.

If you have hand dermatitis from contact with chemicals or soaps and detergents, some of the things you can do to protect your hands include:
- wear gloves to handle chemicals;
- wear plastic gloves with cotton liners for wet work and remove them often to dry your hands;
- wash hands briefly in tepid water with a mild nonsoap cleaner and rub in an ointment while your hands are still damp;
- apply moisturizers often during the day.

If you have a skin rash, you can try the following:
- apply damp, cool compresses to the rash for 20 minutes 4 to 6 times daily;
- if the rash is oozing, prepare the compress containing an astringent such as Burow's solution;
- apply refrigerated calamine lotion unless the rash is oozing;
- use an oral antihistamine every 4 to 6 hours;
- if the rash does not improve, try hydrocortisone ointment 0.5%.

If the rash does not improve over 7 to 10 days, or becomes worse despite treatment, see your doctor.

FIGURE 3

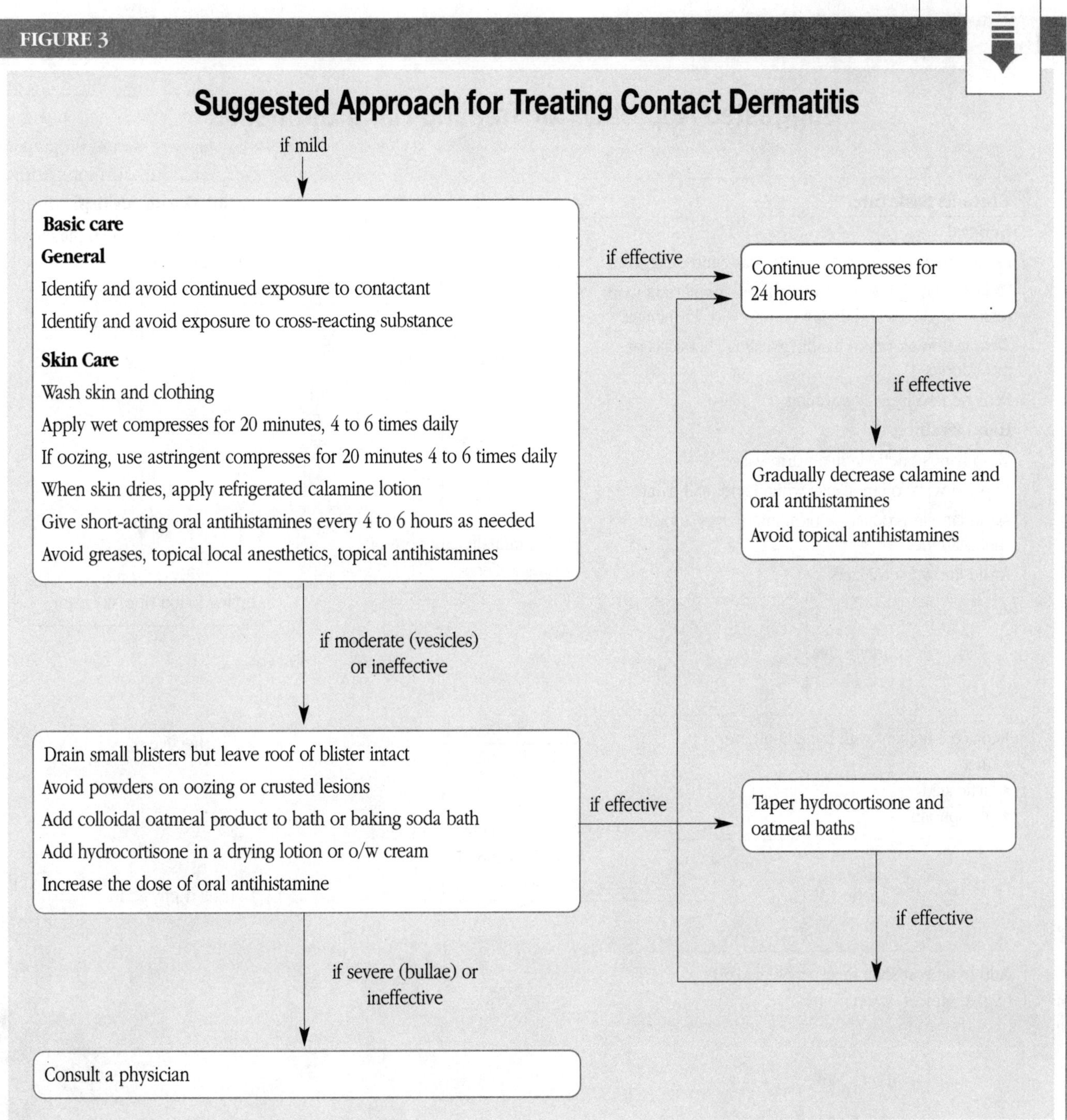

Adapted from Ricciatti-Sibbald DJ. Dermatitis. In: Carruthers-Czyzewski P, ed. *Self-medication. Reference for Health Professionals*. 4th ed. Ottawa: Canadian Pharmaceutical Association, 1992:70.

FIGURE 4

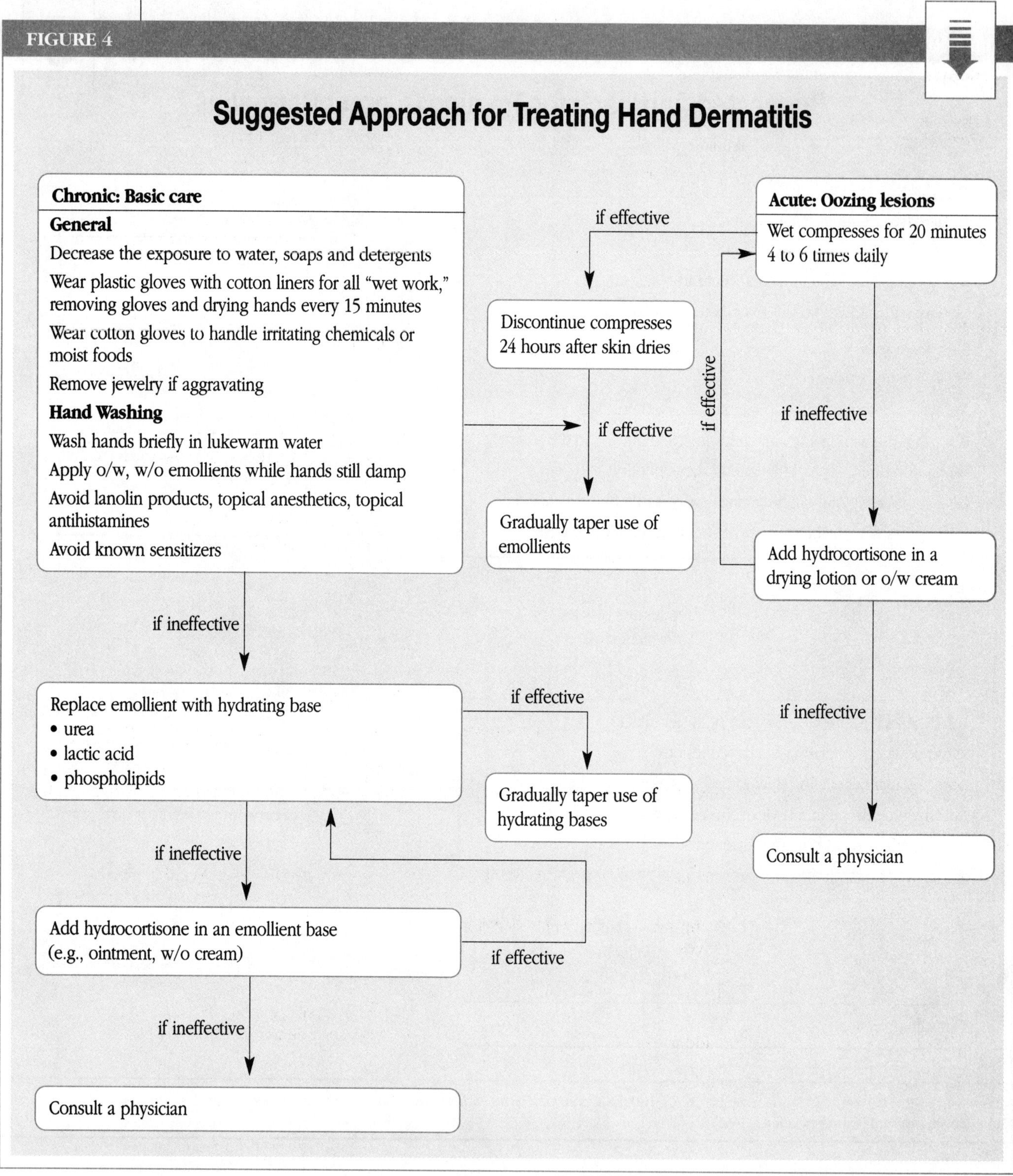

Adapted from Ricciatti-Sibbald DJ. Dermatitis. In: Carruthers-Czyzewski P, ed. *Self-medication. Reference for Health Professionals.* 4th ed. Ottawa: Canadian Pharmaceutical Association, 1992:71.

TABLE 3: Common Causes of Allergic Contact Dermatitis

Allergen	Source	Comments
Poison oak/ivy/sumac (*Toxicodendron* species)	Poison oak—west coast, B.C. to California Poison sumac—eastern Canada and U.S Poison ivy—ubiquitous in Canada and U.S	Wash exposed areas within 15 minutes. Wash clothes/equipment/pets in contact with plant. Blister fluid will not spread the rash. The rash is not contagious.
Paraphenylenediamine	"Permanent" hair dyes Fur dyes Leather products	Cross-reaction possible with PABA esters, benzocaine, topical sulfonamides. May try disperse dyes (e.g., Clairol Loving Care) or vegetable dye (e.g., henna).
Nickel	Costume jewelry, earrings, rings Metal snaps, rivets on blue jeans Car keys	Use gold/silver/stainless steel jewelry. Protect skin from metal objects (e.g., snaps, rivets).
Rubber	Rubber gloves, condoms Athletic shoes Elastic, adhesives	Controlling hyperhidrosis can prevent shoe dermatitis. Use vinyl gloves, spandex/lycra elastics. Use natural skin condoms with or without a latex condom.
Ethylenediamine	Aminophylline Stabilizer in some creams	Avoid Kenacomb preparations, topical antihistamines, tripelennamine, hydroxyzine, aminophylline.
Benzocaine	Topical anesthetics	Cross-sensitivity with local anesthetics (e.g., cocaine, procaine, ester-type, chloroprocaine, tetracaine). May use amide-type local anesthetics (e.g., bupivacaine, lidocaine, dibucaine, mepivacaine).
Neomycin	Topical ointments—antibiotic skin or eye	Some alternative OTC antibiotics (e.g., bacitracin) may also be sensitizers.
Thimerosal	Preservative (e.g., contact lens solutions) Eyedrops	Alternatives include chlorobutanol, benzalkonium chloride. Parabens do not cross-react but may also be sensitizers.
Formaldehyde	Textiles treated to be wrinkle resistant, waterproof Some shampoos: formaldehyde-releasing preservatives *Dr. Scholl's* preparations	May try untreated fabrics. Avoid cosmetics containing Dowicil 200, Germal 115, Germal II, Bronopol 200.
Epoxy resin	Adhesives Cement additives	Alternative products may be available for occupational dermatitis.
Dichromate	Cement additive Leather goods	May try synthetic leather products.
PABA, PABA esters	Sunscreens	Cross-sensitivity with paraphenylenediamine, benzocaine possible. May try sunscreens with salicylates, cinnamates, Parsol or benzophenones.
Parabens	Preservatives in topical creams, ointments, lotions, cosmetics and eye drops	Alternatives include chlorobutanol, benzalkonium chloride.

SEBORRHEA AND DANDRUFF

Seborrheic dermatitis is a scaly inflammatory dermatosis occurring most commonly in infants less than 3 months of age (cradle cap) and adults from 30 to 60 years of age. Two to 5% of the population is affected to some degree, men more frequently than women. There appears to be a higher incidence in mental retardation, idiopathic and neuroleptic-induced parkinsonism, and endocrine states associated with obesity, zinc deficiency and severe acne. Forty to 80% of patients with AIDS have a skin condition resembling seborrheic dermatitis that is resistant to treatment.

The etiology of seborrheic dermatitis is subject to debate. Although seborrhea means hypersecretion of sebum (sebaceous gland secretions), increased oil production is not always present. Seborrheic dermatitis may be due to irritation caused by an alteration in the lipid composition of sebum, a breakdown product of sebum caused by microorganisms, or infection with a yeast, *Pityrosporum ovale*. Alternatively, a secondary bacterial or yeast infection may perpetuate an underlying inflammatory process. Skin in affected areas shows increased epidermal cell turnover with scaling and inflammation.

SYMPTOMS

Lesions consist of patchy areas with dry or oily yellowish scales and slight to moderate redness of the underlying skin. They are usually found in areas with high sebaceous gland concentration, such as the centre of the chest and midback area, face (nose, lips, eyebrows, eyelids), ears, axillae and groin. Pruritus is common when the scalp or ear canal is involved. Exacerbations of seborrheic dermatitis are associated with stress, low humidity and temperature. It seems to be more severe in the winter.

Dandruff, like seborrheic dermatitis, is associated with increased cell turnover and visible excessive scaling, which may be accompanied by itching. Unlike seborrhea, dandruff is not inflammatory, is diffuse rather than patchy, and is confined to the scalp. It tends to fade in the summer, wane with age and is not influenced by emotional state. It may be exacerbated by inadequate washing and a dry climate. Dandruff scales appear as dried cell fragments that are thin, white or greyish, and are spread uniformly on the scalp. Although a few dandruff scales can be found in all adults, only 25% of adults have a troublesome amount.

TREATMENT

Seborrhea and dandruff are treated in the same manner. The objective is to remove scales and crust and alleviate associated itching or inflammation. Shampoos are the foundation of treatment. In general, nonprescription treatment adequately controls dandruff and many cases of seborrheic dermatitis. Individuals with seborrheic dermatitis that does not improve, or that worsens within 2 weeks after starting appropriate nonprescription therapy, should consult a physician. Refer to Figure 5 for the suggested treatment approach.

Pharmacological Treatment

A nonmedicated shampoo should be tried first. It may be enough to eliminate dirt and scaliness. Shampoo the scalp at least 3 times a week, massaging firmly. It is important to rinse well. After the scaling is under control, shampooing can be reduced to twice weekly.

When a nonmedicated shampoo is inadequate, the next step is to try a medicated shampoo. Both selenium sulfide 0.5 to 2%, zinc pyrithione 1 to 2.5%, and ketoconazole 2%, reduce scale equally well. The health professional should instruct the user to shampoo at least twice. The first shampooing, which may be with a nonmedicated shampoo, removes oil and dirt and wets the scalp. The second allows the medicated shampoo to work on the scalp. The shampoo should be left on for at least 5 minutes. Zinc pyrithione can be used daily to maintain control of the condition. Selenium sulfide or ketoconazole should be used only once or twice a week. Selenium sulfide may be added to a zinc pyrithione regimen in resistant cases. Zinc pyrithione can be applied to all involved areas except the eyelid to avoid contact with the eye.

When cytostatic/antiyeast shampoos are ineffective, keratolytic agents (e.g., precipitated sulfur, salicylic acid) may be tried to soften and detach flakes of keratin. Generally, keratolytics are less effective than selenium sulfide or zinc pyrithione.

For people who experience itching, tar shampoos may be tried. They are unlikely to be as effective as other agents in removing scale unless they are allowed to remain in contact with the scalp for prolonged periods. For example, resistant cases may respond to LCD (liquor carbonis detergens) in *Nivea* oil, or a tar shampoo applied to the scalp at bedtime and covered with a showercap

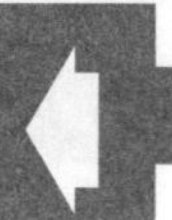

overnight. The patient then rinses and shampoos in the morning as usual and may follow with a topical steroid. Many people find tar products cosmetically unacceptable because of color and odor. However, they are safe and provide longer-lasting relief than steroids.

To lower the population of bacteria or yeast on the scalp, antiseptic shampoos containing cetrimide, povidone–iodine, triclosan or quaternary ammonium compounds have been recommended. Their efficacy in seborrhea and dandruff has never been proven and they are not recommended as first-line treatment. Combination products containing coal tar plus an antiseptic are available.

For seborrheic dermatitis of the eyelids, the patient should apply warm compresses followed by gentle débridement with a cotton-tipped applicator. Baby shampoo can be worked into the area, but medicated shampoos should not be used around the eyes.

Seborrheic dermatitis on areas other than the scalp may respond to nonprescription hydrocortisone or bufexamac creams. Prescription corticosteroids are rarely needed.

CRADLE CAP

Seborrheic dermatitis in infants usually presents as cradle cap, a dry patch of scaling skin that has become thickened to form a cap on the scalp. The etiology of cradle cap is unknown and it may not even be the same disease as the seborrheic dermatitis seen in adults. It usually appears around 3 to 4 weeks of age and disappears by 1 year of age. The scales are usually white, off-white or yellowish, overlying mildly erythematous skin. It may be accompanied by a fine diffuse scaling on the central face, forehead and ears. It is not itchy, and there is no oozing or weeping.

In mild cases, an emollient such as petrolatum is applied to soften the scales, which are then removed by gentle brushing. This can be followed by a mild, nonmedicated baby shampoo. For more resistant cases, apply warmed vegetable oil at bedtime and shampoo in the morning. Tar shampoos applied with a cotton swab and gentle scrubbing may be tried when there is no response to nonmedicated shampoos. Avoid topical steroids and shampoos with salicylic acid due to the potential for increased percutaneous absorption in infants.

ADVICE FOR THE PATIENT

Seborrhea and Dandruff

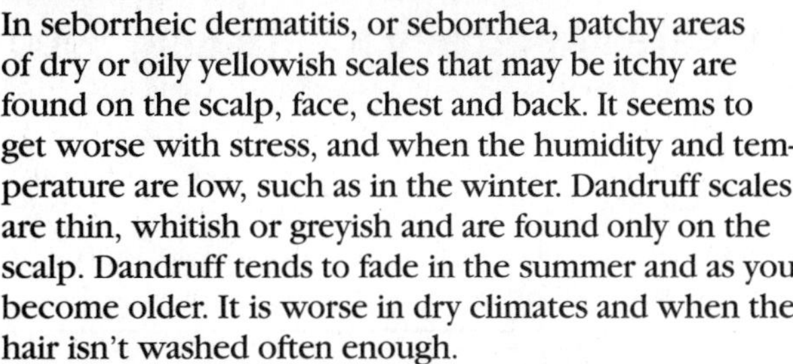

In seborrheic dermatitis, or seborrhea, patchy areas of dry or oily yellowish scales that may be itchy are found on the scalp, face, chest and back. It seems to get worse with stress, and when the humidity and temperature are low, such as in the winter. Dandruff scales are thin, whitish or greyish and are found only on the scalp. Dandruff tends to fade in the summer and as you become older. It is worse in dry climates and when the hair isn't washed often enough.

Some of the things you can do to reduce the scaling include:

- shampoo with a nonmedicated shampoo at least 3 times a week, massaging firmly; rinse well;
- if a regular shampoo does not work, try a medicated shampoo containing zinc pyrithione, selenium sulfide or ketoconazole; shampoo twice; use a regular shampoo first to clean your scalp, then follow with a medicated shampoo; the medicated shampoo has to be in contact with your scalp for at least 5 minutes for the best effect; remember, you are treating your scalp, not your hair;
- after the scaling is under control, use the medicated shampoo less often; use a regular shampoo for routine cleaning.

Some precautions to take when using selenium sulfide include:

- do not use shampoos with selenium sulfide more than 3 times a week because oily hair and hair loss can occur;
- remove all jewelry before using the shampoo and wash hands well after;
- do not use within 2 days of applying hair tints or perm solutions;
- blond or grey hair can be stained, so rinse well after use;
- do not use on inflamed or damaged skin;
- keep out of reach of children.

If you have seborrheic dermatitis, you can also try:

- cleaning bars or shampoos with salicylic acid, which may help remove flakes;
- cleansers and shampoos with tar, which may help relieve itching; combination shampoos with tar and salicylic acid or tar and zinc pyrithione are available;
- if the eyelids are affected apply warm compresses followed by gentle scrubbing with a cotton-tipped applicator; baby shampoo can be worked into the area; do not use medicated shampoos around the eyes.

If your skin condition does not improve in 2 weeks with these treatments, or worsens, see your physician.

FIGURE 5

Suggested Approach for Treating Seborrheic Dermatitis and Dandruff

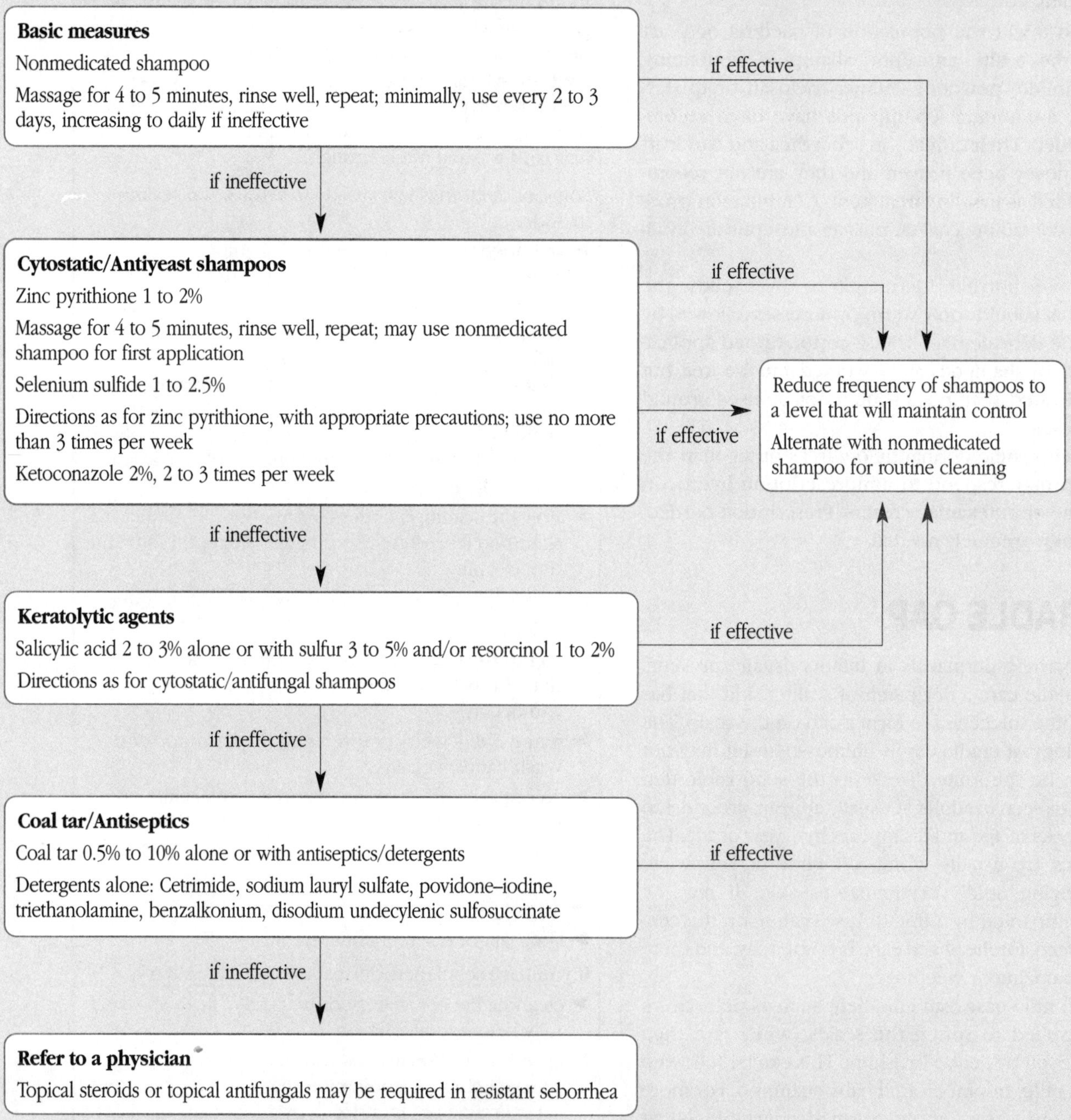

Basic measures

Nonmedicated shampoo

Massage for 4 to 5 minutes, rinse well, repeat; minimally, use every 2 to 3 days, increasing to daily if ineffective

if effective → Reduce frequency of shampoos

if ineffective ↓

Cytostatic/Antiyeast shampoos

Zinc pyrithione 1 to 2%

Massage for 4 to 5 minutes, rinse well, repeat; may use nonmedicated shampoo for first application

Selenium sulfide 1 to 2.5%

Directions as for zinc pyrithione, with appropriate precautions; use no more than 3 times per week

Ketoconazole 2%, 2 to 3 times per week

if effective → Reduce frequency of shampoos

if ineffective ↓

Keratolytic agents

Salicylic acid 2 to 3% alone or with sulfur 3 to 5% and/or resorcinol 1 to 2%

Directions as for cytostatic/antifungal shampoos

if effective → Reduce frequency of shampoos

if ineffective ↓

Coal tar/Antiseptics

Coal tar 0.5% to 10% alone or with antiseptics/detergents

Detergents alone: Cetrimide, sodium lauryl sulfate, povidone–iodine, triethanolamine, benzalkonium, disodium undecylenic sulfosuccinate

if effective → Reduce frequency of shampoos

if ineffective ↓

Refer to a physician

Topical steroids or topical antifungals may be required in resistant seborrhea

Reduce frequency of shampoos to a level that will maintain control

Alternate with nonmedicated shampoo for routine cleaning

DRY SKIN

Dehydration of the stratum corneum results in dry skin or xerosis. Water in the stratum corneum originates in the deeper epidermal layers. It moves upward to hydrate cells in the stratum corneum and is eventually lost through evaporation. There is no single substance in the skin that controls the hydration state of the stratum corneum. Skin lipids and the natural moisturizing factor that is composed of substances such as amino acids, lactate, urea and electrolytes help the stratum corneum retain water. Dry skin is noted when the moisture content is less than 10% and there is a loss of continuity of the stratum corneum. Dry skin may be a feature of other dermatoses such as atopic dermatitis, or may occur in persons with normal skin as a result of aging, illness or environmental factors.

Epidermal water loss can be accelerated by low humidity caused by air conditioning in summer and forced-air heating systems in winter; low humidity (less than 30%) and exposure to dry, cold winds in the winter; mechanical abrasion; or repeated exposure to solvents, soaps and disinfectants that remove lipid from the skin. Dry skin is more prevalent with increasing age because reduced sebum production allows increased water loss from the stratum corneum.

SYMPTOMS

Symptoms of dry skin include roughness, flaking, scaling and chapping, usually on the front of the lower legs, backs of hands and forearms. The face and trunk may be affected. If it is accompanied by inflammation and pruritus, it is called asteatotic eczema. In dry climates it is called winter itch because symptoms worsen with the onset of winter. Redness may occur in or around the involved areas, and in severe cases, fissuring can occur. Rubbing and scratching can perpetuate the irritation.

TREATMENT

The goal of treating dry skin is to maintain hydration of the skin by minimizing bathing frequency and using hydrating substances.

Hydration and emollients form the basis of treatment for dry skin. After bathing in warm water, which may contain a bath additive such as sodium bicarbonate, oatmeal or bath oil, pat the skin dry and apply an occlusive emollient (see Atopic Dermatitis). If these are not acceptable to the patient because of their greasy nature, recommend a water-in-oil moisturizer.

To keep the skin moist and supple, patients with dry skin should apply a moisturizer frequently during the day and at bedtime. Creams and ointments are generally more effective than lotions and gels, which can be drying. Creams are less occlusive and should be applied every 4 hours. Ointments can be applied less frequently because of their greater occlusive effect. Special dry skin creams formulated with urea or lactic acid are promoted to aid in hydration of the skin. They are suitable for moderate xerosis not responding to a regular emollient. Products containing urea or lactic acid should be applied to damp skin to minimize stinging or burning.

Oral antihistamines may be helpful in reducing itching that may accompany dry skin. Avoid topical antihistamines and anesthetics because of their sensitizing potential.

Topical corticosteroids will not improve dry skin but can reduce inflammation and itching in severe cases. If symptoms do not respond to topical hydrocortisone in 7 to 10 days, the patient should be referred to a physician. Long-term use of higher potency topical corticosteroids in the elderly is discouraged because they can potentially enhance atrophy of skin that is already thinned with age.

Refer to Figure 6 for the suggested treatment approach.

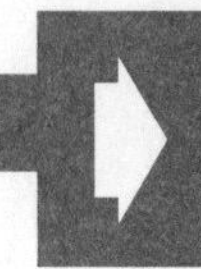

ADVICE FOR THE PATIENT

Dry Skin

Dry skin may occur with other skin conditions such as atopic dermatitis or in normal skin as a result of aging, illness, weather changes or environmental conditions (overheated homes with low humidity). It is common in the winter in dry climates. The skin may appear rough, flaky, scaly or reddened, especially on the lower legs, hands, arms and face. Rubbing and scratching will make it worse.

Some of the things you can do to prevent dry skin include:

- use a humidifier on forced-air heating systems;
- keep the room temperature at the lowest comfortable level in the winter and use a humidifier;
- avoid air conditioning when possible;
- water dries out the skin so bathe in warm water every 1 to 2 days; avoid hot water and frequent bathing;
- use a mild or superfatted soap; if dry skin continues, avoid soaps except on the groin, underarms and feet;
- avoid wool and rough clothing that will irritate the skin.

To treat dry skin, try some of the following:

- add a bath oil to the water in the last 5 minutes of your bath; adding it earlier will not allow water to be absorbed into your skin; caution: bath oil will make the tub very slippery;
- add baking soda or oatmeal to your bath if your skin is itchy;
- rub in an ointment after your bath to help the skin hold in the moisture;
- rub a moisturizer into your skin often during the day and at bedtime; special dry skin creams can be tried if regular moisturizers do not help;
- oral antihistamines can help relieve itching, especially at bedtime;
- hydrocortisone cream 0.5% can help itching and redness that may occur with some cases of dry skin; it will not cure dry skin, however; hydrocortisone should not be used for long-term control of dry skin; if the itching and redness do not improve after 7 to 10 days' treatment, see your physician.

FIGURE 6

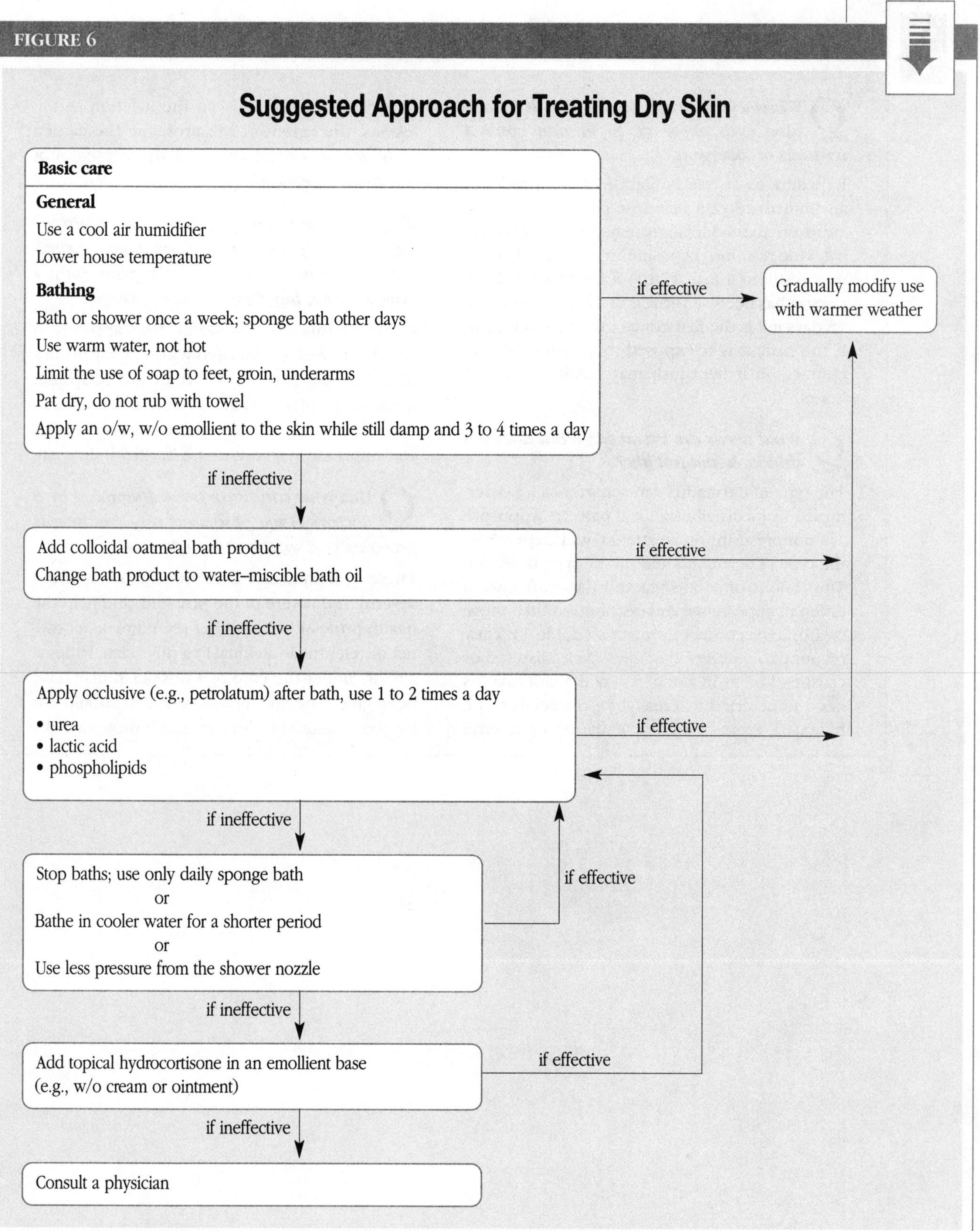

Adapted from Ricciatti-Sibbald DJ. Dermatitis. In: Carruthers-Czyzewski P, ed. *Self-medication. Reference for Health Professionals.* 4th ed. Ottawa: Canadian Pharmaceutical Association, 1992:73.

Dry Skin

? PATIENT ASSESSMENT QUESTIONS

Q When did the rash begin? Was it associated with exposure to known contact irritants or allergens?

Exposure to strong contact irritants produces an immediate skin response, whereas chronic exposure to mild irritants may produce a slowly evolving reaction. Exposure to contact allergens may result in a rash 12 to 48 hours later if the person has been sensitized in the past, or up to 25 days if it is the first contact with the allergen. If the patient is re-exposed to a strong allergic contact, an irritant rash may result in 6 to 12 hours.

Q What areas are involved? What does the skin look and feel like?

The type of dermatitis can sometimes be determined by its distribution and pattern. Appropriate nonprescription treatment will depend on the type of dermatitis and on the type of lesion. The lesions of seborrhea and dandruff have a different appearance and distribution than those of atopic or contact dermatitis (Table 1). They respond to different therapies. Wet, blistered or crusting lesions in atopic and contact dermatitis need to be dried whereas dry skin needs to be hydrated. Product recommendation or referral to a physician depends on the location of the lesions, the extent of the problem, the degree of hydration of the skin and the presence of secondary infection.

Q How long have you had this condition? Does anyone in your family have a similar condition? Does anyone in your family have asthma, hay fever or other allergies?

Atopic dermatitis commonly first appears in childhood, and is associated with a family history of allergic disorders. It is chronic and relapsing. Hand dermatitis is frequently occupational and chronic. Allergic contact dermatitis is usually an acute episode in an otherwise healthy individual.

Q Has your condition been diagnosed by a doctor? Have you used any treatments previously? If so, were they effective?

These questions can generate discussion of the severity and nature of the problem, and help the health professional to either recommend a product or refer the individual to a physician. Patients already under the care of a physician may have been given specific instructions that should not be contradicted by another health professional.

PHARMACEUTICAL AGENTS

ANTIPRURITICS

Itching is a symptom of many dermatoses that may cause considerable distress to the patient. Scratching is the patient's first choice for relief of pruritus, but it exacerbates and perpetuates inflammatory dermatoses. Relief of itching is often a higher priority for the patient than resolution of the skin condition. Topical antipruritics may contain rubefacients such as camphor or menthol, anesthetics such as phenol or benzocaine, or astringents and protectants such as calamine or zinc oxide. Oral antihistamines are often used to treat pruritus.

In low concentrations (1 to 3%), camphor and menthol induce a feeling of cold that competitively inhibits itching. While the mechanism of action of counterirritants is poorly understood, it is thought that they may depress cutaneous sensory receptors for itch while stimulating sensory receptors for cold, thus substituting one sensation for the other. Camphor is also mildly anesthetic and weakly antiseptic. Camphor and menthol may be used separately or combined with other topical antipruritics. They are irritating when used on broken or acutely inflamed skin.

Phenol in a concentration of 0.5 to 2% is antipruritic by virtue of its local anesthetic properties. It is caustic in higher concentrations. Phenol can be absorbed percutaneously, and its use is not recommended in pregnant women, children less than 6 months old or individuals with renal disease. Avoid use in intertriginous areas where the skin is more sensitive to its irritating effects and absorption can be increased.

Local anesthetics such as benzocaine, lidocaine, dibucaine and pramoxine are available in topical creams and ointments to relieve pruritus. Local anesthetics act by stabilizing the neuronal membrane of cutaneous nerve endings, preventing the generation and conduction of nerve impulses, and thus blocking the sensation of itch. Unfortunately, topically applied anesthetics may not have the desired effect since most are poorly absorbed through intact skin and many nonprescription products contain subtherapeutic amounts. Benzocaine in concentrations of 20% and lidocaine 3 to 4% are effective within 5 to 10 minutes and will relieve pruritus or pain for up to 45 minutes. Because of their short duration of action, they are most useful for short-term symptom relief (e.g., at bedtime). Benzocaine is a well recognized sensitizing agent and its topical use should be discouraged. Anesthetics of the "amide" type such as lidocaine or dibucaine, or structurally unique anesthetics such as pramoxine are rarely sensitizing and are suitable alternatives for patients sensitive to benzocaine. Lidocaine is available alone or in combination with polymyxin. Pramoxine is available alone or in combination with camphor and/or menthol. Dibucaine is available alone.

Antihistamines competitively block the action of histamine, one of the mediators of itch, at the H_1-receptor. They are most effective in pruritus related to histamine release. Antihistamines are less effective when pruritus is induced by other mediators, such as that in atopic dermatitis. First-generation antihistamines such as hydroxyzine (prescription only) and diphenhydramine are useful in this type of pruritus by virtue of their sedating effects. Diphenhydramine and promethazine are available in topical preparations; however, while topical antihistamines may have transient antipruritic effects, sensitization is common, particularly with diphenhydramine. Generally, topical antihistamines should be avoided.

ASTRINGENTS

Astringents, such as calamine, zinc oxide or aluminum salts, are protein precipitants that harden the damaged capillary lining to inhibit transcapillary movement of plasma protein. Exudation, local edema and inflammation are thereby reduced. Astringents can be added to baths or soaks or applied to the skin in a lotion.

A lotion is a suspension or solution of powder in a water vehicle. In addition to the astringent effect from the added medication, lotions provide a cooling effect by evaporation of water from the skin after application. Alcohol is frequently added to enhance the cooling effect. This makes the lotion more drying, which can actually increase itch. Lotions are most useful on lesions accompanied by pruritus where the cooling effect is soothing. The drying effect of added astringents can be useful on slightly oozing lesions. Lotions are not recommended for markedly oozing or weeping lesions. They may cake in the exudate and adhere to the inflamed area forming a crust under which infections may occur. Also, lotions should not be applied to hairy areas because they tend to crumble. Generally astringent lotions are not recommended for dry skin conditions because of their drying effect.

BATH PRODUCTS

Bath additives may contain oils such as mineral oil or lanolin, salts such as sodium bicarbonate, or colloidal solids such as oatmeal. While they may not enhance hydration, they may be soothing to itchy, irritated skin.

Bath oils consist of a mineral or vegetable oil that floats on top of the water, or may contain a surfactant to disperse the oil throughout the water. Patients may make their own bath oil by adding 60 mL olive oil or *Nivea* oil to a cup of milk. Bath oils coat the skin upon emerging to make it feel smooth and less dry. No one type of bath oil is superior to another. For optimum effect, bath oils should be added in the last 5 minutes of the bath. If they are added too soon they may prevent access of water to the skin and actually inhibit hydration. Their ability to help the skin retain moisture is limited since most of the oil is wiped from the skin when towelling dry after the bath. Patients should be cautioned that all bath oils make the bathtub slippery. If the patient wants a bath oil effect without adding oil to the bath, 5 mL (1 teaspoon) of mineral oil in 125 mL (½ cup) of warm water can be recommended as a rubdown after bathing.

Bath salts soften the water and may be soothing. Sodium bicarbonate (baking soda) 125 to 250 mg (¼-½ cup) in a tubful of water will have the same effect. If bath salts make the water too alkaline, skin itching and redness can result. In addition, bath salts may contain fragrances that can be irritating to sensitive skin.

Oatmeal releases protein and carbohydrate when dissolved in the bath and has a soothing effect on pruritic skin. A similar effect can be achieved by mixing 500 mL (2 cups) of cornstarch with 1 L (4 cups) of water and adding it to the bath. When using oatmeal products, the measured amount of powder is dispersed onto the water surface close to a jet of hot water from the faucet. Avoid direct contact with the jet of water to prevent clumping. Add cold water until the temperature of the bath is suitable then stir in any powder that may have settled.

BUFEXAMAC

Bufexamac is a topical nonsteroidal anti-inflammatory agent. Its anti-inflammatory effect may be related to its ability to inhibit prostaglandin synthesis. It has also been shown to stabilize lysosomal membranes in vitro. The best response is seen in patients with seborrheic and contact dermatitis. Resolution or improvement is usually seen in 1 to 2 weeks. Chronic dermatoses and those with moderate to severe symptoms do not respond as well. While some studies have found bufexamac cream to compare favorably to topical corticosteroids in various types of dermatitis, other studies have found it to be no more effective than placebo. It is usually well tolerated. Some patients complain of local reactions such as redness, irritation, swelling and itching.

CLEANSING PRODUCTS

There are two types of cleansing products available: soaps made by saponification of animal and/or vegetable fats and soap-like synthetic detergent cleansers. Both emulsify fats with water to remove oils and dirt from the skin. Both are available in liquid and bar form and are effective cleansers despite their differing composition. Any type of skin cleanser can aggravate skin dryness and dermatologic conditions depending on its pH, cleansing ability, composition and additives.

Normal skin has a pH of 5 to 6. In general, cleansing with a high pH product stresses the skin's buffering capacity whereas cleansing with a neutral product minimizes skin pH changes. Most soaps are alkaline with a pH of 9 to 10.5. Synthetic detergents have a broad pH range from near neutral to 9. Laboratory tests of soap irritancy have shown that pH is not a major determinant of irritancy.

Products with a high cleansing ability may be irritating by removing skin lipids that help maintain hydration of the stratum corneum. In an attempt to reduce the irritancy of some cleansers, substances such as glycerin, cocoa butter, mineral oil or lanolin are added. However, these substances also reduce the cleansing potential of the product, which alone may account for the reduced irritancy. "Superfatted" cleansers have fatty acids such as stearic acid added on the assumption that they will leave a protective coat of oil on the skin. It is more likely that irritancy is reduced by lowering the amount of cleanser that contacts the skin. It is unlikely that a product intended to remove oil and dirt from the skin would have the opposite effect of coating the skin with oil. Transparent or glycerin soaps have a higher fat content than opaque soaps as well as additives such as fatty alcohols, glycerin and sugar.

They are claimed to be more neutral and less drying than opaque soaps, although objective evaluations are lacking.

Additives such as perfumes, antibacterials in deodorant bars, colorants or preservatives all can add to the irritancy of a cleanser. Note that even unscented products may contain a masking fragrance to cover the base odor.

In general, mild synthetic detergent cleaners are usually less irritating than soaps and can be recommended in milder cases of dermatitis and dry skin. In acute eczematous states and more severe dry skin conditions, cleansers should be avoided or restricted to uninvolved areas or those areas most in need of cleaning (e.g., underarms, groin and feet). Avoid vigorous rubbing or massaging with soaps, and rinse thoroughly after use.

COAL TAR

Coal tar is a heterogeneous mixture of compounds produced from the distillation of coal at high temperatures. It is claimed to have antiseptic, antipruritic, antiparasitic, antifungal, antibacterial, keratoplastic and vasoconstrictive activities, most of which are unsubstantiated. Coal tar is available in ointments, lotions, gels, shampoos and bath preparations. Lotions and creams are suitable for application to lesions on the trunk and extremities. Gels are used on hairy areas. Although tar gel products are cosmetically acceptable, they contain alcohol and may cause burning and irritation of acutely inflamed skin. In addition, prolonged use of gel vehicles leads to drying and irritation at the site of application. Their use in dry skin conditions is discouraged. Coal tar shampoos are sometimes used for seborrhea of the scalp or cradle cap.

Side effects of tar products include folliculitis, particularly of hairy regions, tar acne, contact dermatitis and photosensitivity. To prevent folliculitis, instruct the user to apply the medication only in the direction of hair growth, and not in a circular motion. Acne and dermatitis can be minimized by starting with a low concentration of coal tar. To prevent sunburn and photocontact dermatitis, unless the dermatologist has specified otherwise, consumers should be warned to avoid excessive sunlight or to apply a sunscreen with a high sun protection factor. Pre-existing folliculitis, severe acne or concomitant administration of other photosensitizing drugs are possible contraindications to coal tar use. (For more information see the *Sunscreens and Tanning Products* chapter.)

CORTICOSTEROIDS

Corticosteroids have complex anti-inflammatory and immunomodulatory effects. When applied to inflammatory skin lesions, they relieve redness, warmth, swelling and pain as well as pruritus. Topically, they are useful for the local control of many types of inflammatory, allergic and pruritic dermatoses, including atopic dermatitis, irritant and allergic contact dermatitis, dry skin and seborrheic dermatitis.

Percutaneous absorption of corticosteroids depends on the patient, the use of occlusive dressings, the area in which it is applied, the concentration of the corticosteroid and the vehicle. Corticosteroid absorption is greater through damaged than through intact skin, although absorption is low: only 2% of topically applied hydrocortisone is absorbed through damaged skin. Corticosteroid penetration can be enhanced 10-fold by following application with an occlusive dressing. Penetration is greater when corticosteroids are applied to the scrotum, axilla, eyelid, face and scalp as compared to the extremities, palms and soles. Prolonged absorption can occur even after washing, possibly because a drug reservoir is formed in the stratum corneum. Absorption is enhanced in children under 18 months of age; therefore, nonprescription hydrocortisone products are not intended for young children.

Topical hydrocortisone 0.5% is available without a prescription in ointment, cream or lotion. Ointments are more occlusive and thus preferred for dry, scaly or lichenified lesions, or those on areas more resistant to absorption (e.g., palms and soles, extremities, trunk). Creams can be used in intertriginous or moist areas because they are more drying. Lotions are useful on the scalp and other hairy areas. They may be more convenient for large areas when a minimal application will suffice.

Because a reservoir of drug is formed in the stratum corneum, frequent application is not required. Adults and children over 2 years of age should apply the product to the affected area 3 to 4 times a day. Once the condition is under control, the frequency of application can be reduced to a minimum that will maintain control. The amount of drug that can be absorbed into the stratum corneum at any time is limited; thus, there is no benefit to applying corticosteroids liberally. Applying topical corticosteroids sparingly will reduce the risk of side effects while providing economic benefit.

Topical 0.5% hydrocortisone is safe when used properly. The most common adverse drug reactions are local, including contact dermatitis, allergic reactions, pain and pruritus. Contact dermatitis and allergic reactions are most likely secondary to sensitizing additives, including stabilizers and preservatives. Adverse reactions reported with topical fluorinated steroids, such as striae, thinning of the skin or adrenocortical suppression from systemic absorption do not appear to be a problem with topical 0.5% hydrocortisone when it is used properly. Tolerance to the anti-inflammatory effects of corticosteroids has occurred with continued use. Withdrawal of the drug for a few days or substitution with a prescription steroid may restore responsiveness. Nonprescription topical corticosteroids are intended for temporary relief of inflammation and pruritus. If the skin lesions worsen or symptoms persist more than 7 days despite hydrocortisone use, the patient should consult a physician.

CYTOSTATIC SHAMPOOS

Selenium sulfide, zinc pyrithione and ketoconazole shampoos are used to reduce scale in seborrheic dermatitis and dandruff. They have a cytostatic effect that slows cell turnover and an antiyeast effect against *P. ovale*. Ketoconazole impairs the synthesis of a component in fungal and yeast cell membranes. The patient should apply the medicated shampoo after a cleansing shampoo with a nonmedicated product. The medicated shampoo should be left on for at least 5 minutes to penetrate the affected skin. Remind the patient that the scalp, not the hair, is being treated. If the odor of the medicated shampoo is offensive, the patient can finish with a regular shampoo.

Zinc pyrithione has few reported side effects. However, numerous precautions must be taken with selenium sulfide. Patients must remove all jewelry before its use, and wash hands thoroughly afterward. It should not be used within 2 days of applying hair tints or perm solutions. Selenium sulfide may stain blond or grey hair if rinsed inadequately. Selenium-containing shampoos do not remove oil well, and may lead to oily hair and hair loss with excessive use. Pretreatment with a nonmedicated shampoo may help minimize this problem. Selenium sulfide should not be applied to inflamed or damaged skin and its use should be discontinued if skin irritation, conjunctivitis or hair loss occurs. It is toxic if ingested orally and must be kept out of reach of children. Ketoconazole should not be used within 2 weeks after treatment with topical corticosteroids. Otherwise it is well tolerated. Adverse effects have included dry or greasy scalp or hair and mild scalp irritation.

EMOLLIENTS

Emollients and moisturizers are bland oleaginous substances that are applied to the skin by rubbing. They are used to replace natural skin oils, cover tiny fissures in the skin and provide a soothing protective film. They give the impression of softening and smoothing of the skin surface. While they are unable to hydrate the skin—only water can do that—some may slow evaporation of moisture from the skin and maintain hydration if applied immediately after bathing. Emollients are commonly used as vehicles for topically applied medications. When recommending an emollient product for a skin condition consider the dosage form as well as the additives. Emollients and moisturizers may be ointments, creams, gels or lotions. Active ingredients may include occlusives, humectants, emollients and proteins.

Dosage Forms: Ointments are semisolid preparations that contain a high proportion of oleaginous material. They may be water repellent, such as lanolin or petrolatum, emulsifiable, such as hydrophilic petrolatum or hydrophilic lanolin, or contain water in a water-in-oil emulsion base. Ointments spread easily, form a protective film over the skin, and act as a lubricant and vehicle for medications. Because they are occlusive they are most useful in conditions where dry skin predominates. Ointment bases generally provide better penetration of incorporated drugs because they are occlusive. They should be avoided in intertriginous or hairy areas as they tend to trap heat and sweat and lead to maceration. In addition, they should not be used on oozing lesions. Because they are greasy and often difficult to wash off, they may be cosmetically unappealing.

A cream is a soft, water-miscible preparation that is less greasy than an ointment. Dermatologists use the term cream to denote an oil-in-water emulsion. Although some water-in-oil emulsions are soft and cream-like they are not water miscible. Creams are intended to be rubbed in well until they disappear. If the cream can be seen on the skin after application, the patient has applied too much or has not rubbed it in fully. In general, 1 g of cream should cover a 10 cm^2 area. Table 4 lists average amounts of cream needed to cover various parts of the body when applied sparingly. Patients prefer products without a greasy feel; however, the thin film

TABLE 4: Average Amounts of Cream Needed for Application to Various Body Parts (Adults)

Body Area	Single Application	Amount Needed For 1 Week (applied 3x/day)
Both hands Head Face Genital/anal	2 g	45 g
Each arm Front of trunk Back of trunk	3 g	60 g
Each leg	4 g	90 g
Whole body	30–60 g	700–1,500 g

Adapted with permission from Bond CA. Skin Disorders I. In: Koda-Kimble MA, Young LY, eds. Applied Therapeutics: The Clinical Use of Drugs. 5th ed. Vancouver, WA: Applied Therapeutics, Inc., 1992:64.1–64.16.

provides inadequate protection against transepidermal water loss. Water-in-oil emulsions are suitable for chronic, dry, scaly dermatoses. Oil-in-water emulsions are suitable for a less serious condition or the resolving stage of oozing dermatitis. Lotion-like oil-in-water emulsions are cosmetically appealing and easy to rub in. However, lotions contain a higher proportion of water and are more drying than creams. They may be useful as a regular moisturizer in mild cases of xerosis, but generally lotions are not advised in dry skin because of their drying effect.

Gels are a form of ointment containing propylene glycol and alcohol, acetone or water. They are clear, nongreasy, nonstaining and quick drying but are not occlusive or moisturizing. They are too drying for use in dry skin conditions. They are most useful as a vehicle for medications to be applied to hairy areas. Application to abraded skin will produce irritation and stinging because of the alcohol content.

Active Ingredients: Occlusives are substances that physically block transepidermal water loss from the stratum corneum. Petrolatum in a minimum concentration of 5% is the most effective occlusive, especially if it is applied immediately after soaking to maintain hydration of the skin. Unfortunately it is greasy and cosmetically unappealing, and it can stain clothing. Its occlusive effect can be too pronounced, leading to sweat retention and maceration or folliculitis, particularly in hot or humid conditions. As a result compliance may be a problem, and it is rarely used to treat dry skin conditions.

Humectants attract water when applied to the skin and theoretically improve hydration of the stratum corneum. However, the water drawn to the skin is transepidermal water, not atmospheric water. Continued evaporation of water from the skin can actually result in increased transepidermal water loss, which can exacerbate dryness. Humectants include glycerin, sorbitol, urea, alpha-hydroxy acids (e.g., lactic acid) and sugars.

Emollients, such as mineral oil, lanolin, fatty acids, cholesterol and squalene, smooth rough skin by filling spaces between skin flakes with drops of oil. They are usually not occlusive unless applied heavily. When combined with an emulsifier, they may help hold oil and water together in the stratum corneum. Vitamin E is a common additive to moisturizers that appears to have no effect other than as an emollient.

Moisturizers containing collagen or other proteins (e.g., keratin, elastin) claim to rejuvenate the skin by replenishing essential proteins in the skin. This is unlikely to occur, however, since protein molecules are too large to penetrate the epidermis. Protein additives provide temporary relief of dry skin by filling irregularities on the skin surface like emollients. When they dry, they shrink slightly, leaving a protein film that appears to smooth the skin and stretch out some of the fine wrinkles.

In addition to their humectant properties, urea and lactic acid are keratolytic. Urea is humectant in lower concentrations (10%) but in higher concentrations (20 to 30%) it is mildly keratolytic by disrupting hydrogen bonds of epidermal proteins. Keratolytic concentrations of urea may be helpful to remove scales in chronic scaly atopic dermatitis or xerosis. Urea preparations can irritate inflamed skin or oozing lesions and should not be used on open skin areas. Alpha-hydroxy acids such as lactic acid, citric acid and glycolic acid appear to increase cohesion of stratum corneum cells, reducing the roughness and scaling in xerosis and hyperkeratotic conditions. Concentrations of 2 to 5% are preferred, since higher concentrations may be irritating. Higher concentrations of lactic acid (12%) and glycolic acid (10%) have proven effective in dry skin.

KERATOLYTICS

Keratolytics loosen bonds between keratinocytes in the stratum corneum and facilitate desquamation. Mild keratolytics such as urea or lactic acid may be useful in dry skin conditions because they also have a humectant effect that can help hydrate the stratum corneum. Salicylic acid, sulfur and resorcinol-containing shampoos may be useful in resistant cases of seborrheic dermatitis to soften and detach keratin flakes. They should not be used in atopic dermatitis because they are too irritating. Available nonprescription products include salicylic acid 2 to 3%, sulfur 3 to 5% and resorcinol 1 to 2%. Higher concentrations may produce faster results, but proportionally more irritation. As with other medicated shampoos, contact time of at least 5 minutes is recommended to allow the agent to soften and loosen the scale.

SOAKS

Water cools and dries the skin through evaporation. The resulting vasoconstriction alleviates erythema and warmth by reducing the increased local blood flow present in inflammatory lesions. Soaking can also cleanse the skin of exudates, soften crusts for removal and aid in débridement. It is indicated for acute inflammatory states with oozing, weeping and crusting. Soaking also restores water to the stratum corneum and is indicated for hydration in some dry skin conditions. Wet dressings or compresses are normally used on small areas such as the scalp and extremities, or when the cooling effect is important. Immersion or bathing is easier for large areas or hands and feet. Bathing is less drying and cooling because evaporation from the skin is reduced.

There are two types of wet dressings: soaks and compresses. Soaks are used to remove dry, crusted areas. To prepare a soak, soak gauze or a cloth in warm tap water and gently squeeze out the excess water until it is wet but not dripping. Wrap the affected area and cover with a dry towel. Leave in place for 10 to 20 minutes, rewetting as necessary. If the dressing is allowed to dry, crusts will adhere to it and be removed with the dressing. This is painful and can cause tissue damage. Soaks can be used up to 3 to 4 times a day. Compresses are useful for acute eczematous lesions. Apply moistened gauze squares, *J-cloth* or other thin cloth to the affected area with or without a fan. Alternatively, apply intermittently: on 1 minute, off 1 minute. The goal is to promote evaporation and drying. Overuse of wet dressings leads to excessive drying or cooling. To prevent hypothermia, especially in children, apply wet dressings to no more than 30% of the body surface at one time. Warm baths are preferred to soak large areas.

Astringents reduce exudates by precipitating protein and can be added to the soak water to dry oozing, weeping lesions. Burow's solution is usually diluted to a 1:10 to 1:40 solution for use as a wet dressing, soak or bath. Refer to the product instructions for specific dilution guidelines.

RECOMMENDED READING

Bond CA. Skin disorders Part 1. In: Young LY, Koda-Kimble MA, eds. Applied Therapeutics: The Clinical Use of Drugs. Vancouver, WA: Applied Therapeutics Inc., 1992;64.1-16.

Fisher AA. The role of nonsensitizing alternatives in the management of allergic contact dermatitis. Semin Dermatol 1986;5:263-72.

Hogan DH. Contact dermatitis. Med North Am 1989;31:5740-46.

Kligman AM, Leyden JJ. Seborrheic dermatitis. Semin Dermatol 1983;2:57-59.

Sampson HA. Atopic dermatitis. Ann Allergy 1992; 69(6):469-79.

Wehr RF, Krochmal L. Considerations in selecting a moisturizer. Cutis 1987;39(6):512-15.

8

EAR CARE PRODUCTS

Lynn Torsher

CONTENTS

Anatomy and Physiology 149

General Disorders of the Ear 151
- Hearing Loss
- Discharge From the Ear
- Ear Pain
- Tinnitus/Vertigo

Disorders of the External Ear 153
- Auricle
- External Auditory Canal

Pharmaceutical Agents 159

Recommended Reading 161

ANATOMY AND PHYSIOLOGY

There are three distinct parts to the ear: external, middle and inner (Figure 1). The external portion includes the auricle or pinna, the question-mark shaped appendage found on the side of the head, and the auditory canal, which extends from the centre of the auricle inward to the tympanic membrane, or ear drum. The auricle is elastic cartilage, except at the tip (ear lobe), which is primarily fat and covered with skin. The auditory canal is about 24 mm in length, and the outer third is cartilage, lined with skin, hair and cerumen (ear wax) glands. The inner two-thirds is bone, lined with a thin epithelial layer. The tympanic membrane is a cone-shaped fibrous layer covered on the outer side by epithelium and on the inner side by mucous membrane. It is nearly circular in shape and measures about 9 mm by 8 mm.

The middle ear, the area between the tympanic

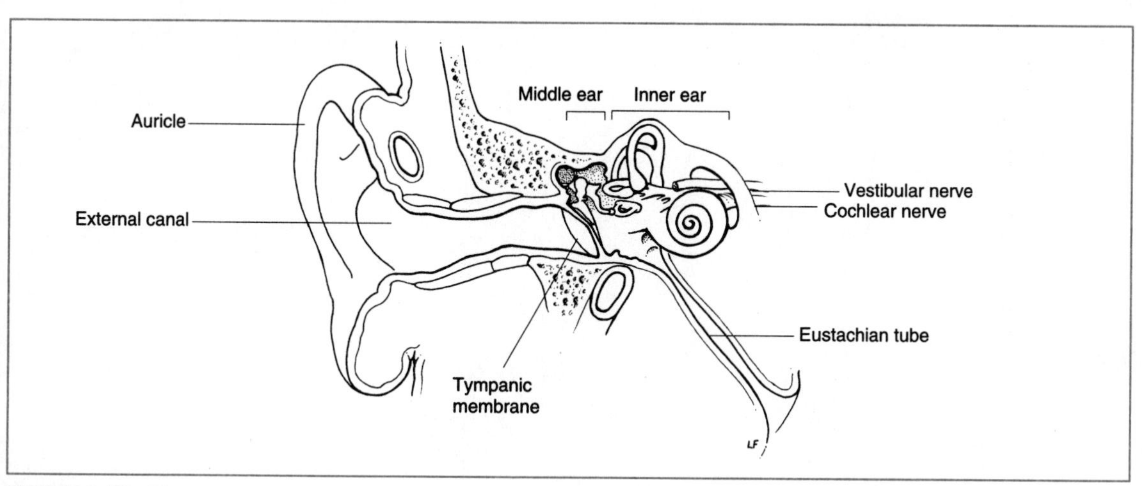

FIGURE 1: The Ear

Anatomy and Physiology

membrane and the oval window, contains the ossicles: three tiny bones named the malleus (hammer), incus (anvil) and stapes (stirrup). The handle of the malleus is embedded in the tympanic membrane, and the head touches the incus, which in turn rests against the stapes. The foot plate of the stapes is attached to the oval window. The eustachian tube passes from the nasopharynx into the middle ear cavity and allows middle ear pressure to be equalized by opening with swallowing.

The inner ear is housed within the skull and includes the cochlea, which is a system of coiled, fluid-filled tubes, the organ of corti and the vestibular apparatus.

Sound waves conducted through the air are captured by the auricle, move down the auditory canal and cause the tympanic membrane to vibrate, which initiates movement through the ossicular chain that results in an in-and-out movement of the oval window membrane. This in turn displaces fluid within the cochlea and creates a waving motion of hair cells located on the organ of corti. These hair cells move in patterns specific to the frequency of the fluid waves passing over them and synapse directly with the cochlear nerve, ultimately transmitting impulses to the brain that are interpreted as sound. Sound waves can also be conducted through the bones of the skull directly into the cochlea.

The vestibular apparatus is made up of the utricle, saccule and three semicircular canals. The three semicircular canals are at right angles to each other and represent all planes in space. Fluid within these structures moves in response to movements of the head and body, in turn stimulating hair cells that synapse with the vestibular nerve, ultimately informing the brain of the body's orientation and equilibrium status. The cochlear and vestibular nerves combine to form the eighth cranial nerve, which links the ear to the brain stem.

GENERAL DISORDERS OF THE EAR

HEARING LOSS

A loss of hearing may result if sound is unable to reach the inner ear due to occlusion of the ear canal by cerumen, foreign bodies, swelling, a build-up of fluid or rupture of the ear drum. Known as conduction deafness, it is temporary and correctable in most cases. Hearing loss may also occur because of damage to the cochlea or organ of corti. This is known as nerve deafness and may result from exposure to intense noise, drugs, disease or aging (Table 1). The degree of damage to the organs determines whether the loss is permanent.

DISCHARGE FROM THE EAR

The most common ear discharge is cerumen or ear wax. It is a pale yellow to brown oily substance and is a normal component of the auditory canal, where it serves as an antibacterial lubricant. It naturally migrates out of the canal, aided by jaw movements, such as chewing or swallowing. Substances other than cerumen that may drain from the ear include serum, pus, cerebrospinal fluid and blood. Any of these is an indication of disease, and a physician should be consulted promptly.

EAR PAIN

Pain in the area of the ear may be the first symptom of an infection or injury to the ear. Rupture of the ear drum produces sudden sharp pain, often accompanied by bleeding. It may result from direct trauma, such as a puncture with a cotton-tipped swab, or from extreme pressure due to an explosion or slap to the head. Sudden changes in atmospheric pressure, which can occur while flying or diving, can also result in ear pain or perforation of the drum. This occurs if swelling or obstruction of either the external canal or eustachian tube prevents equalization of pressure on both sides of the tympanic membrane.

Several cranial and cervical nerves lie near the ear and can transmit impulses that are incorrectly interpreted as ear pain by the brain. Pain may be referred to the ear in dental infections, ulcers of the mouth or throat, tonsillitis, tumors of the sinuses, throat, tongue, mouth or esophagus, or neuralgias of the head and neck.

Mild ear pain is best treated with oral analgesics such as acetaminophen, ASA or ibuprofen. Pain that is severe, persists longer than 24 hours or is accompanied by discharge should be evaluated by a physician.

TINNITUS/VERTIGO

Tinnitus is a ringing sound in the ear. Vertigo is a sensation of whirling. A number of drugs can cause tinnitus; however, either of these conditions may be indicative of a variety of other inner ear disorders and should be evaluated by a physician.

ADVICE FOR THE PATIENT

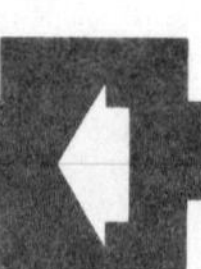

Tips for Preventing Ear Pain While Flying

- Just before landing, chew some gum or suck on a hard candy or mint. If none are available, try swallowing or yawning or other similar movements of the jaw to equalize pressure on the ear drum.
- Infants should be given something to drink during landing.
- Avoid flying when you have a cold. If you must fly with a cold, take an oral decongestant such as pseudoephedrine about 1 hour before descending, or use a nasal decongestant spray about 15 minutes before landing.

TABLE 1: Some Ototoxic Drugs

High Relative Risk Agents	Type of Toxicity	Comments
Aminoglycosides		
amikacin gentamicin tobramycin streptomycin neomycin	Hearing loss or vertigo	May onset after drugs are stopped Degree of damage dependent on dose and duration
Loop diuretics		
furosemide ethacrynic acid bumetanide	Hearing loss	High doses (usually parenteral use) Potentiated by aminoglycosides Generally reversible Risk increases in presence of renal or hepatic dysfunction
Antineoplastics		
cisplatin carboplatin	Hearing loss, tinnitus	Degree of damage dependent on dose and duration May be irreversible
vincristine vinblastine	Hearing loss	Degree of damage dependent on dose and duration May be irreversible
nitrogen mustard	Vertigo	Degree of damage dependent on dose and duration May be irreversible
Low Relative Risk Agents	**Type of Toxicity**	**Comments**
Antibiotics		
minocycline	Vertigo	Generally reversible
erythromycin	Hearing loss or vertigo	High doses Generally reversible
vancomycin	Hearing loss	If used with aminoglycosides Little evidence of toxicity if used alone
NSAIDS		
ASA	Tinnitus, hearing loss or vertigo	High doses Generally reversible
naproxen	Hearing loss	May be irreversible
indomethacin	Tinnitus	Generally reversible
Antimalarials		
quinine	Tinnitus, hearing loss, or vertigo	Large doses Generally reversible
chloroquine	Tinnitus or hearing loss	Usual doses over long term May be irreversible
Others		
deferoxamine	Hearing loss	High doses over long term May be irreversible

DISORDERS OF THE EXTERNAL EAR

AURICLE

Disorders of the auricle that are amenable to self-treatment include minor, traumatic injuries (e.g., burns, frostbite or lacerations), dermatitis and minor infections. With the exception of minor infections, appropriate self-treatment for these conditions may be found elsewhere in this book.

Disorders of the auricle that should be referred to a physician for treatment include carcinoma, keloid, hematoma and viral infections, such as herpes zoster (Table 2).

Infections

Infections of the auricle usually occur secondarily to traumatic injury or dermatitis, and are usually bacterial in origin. Viral and fungal infections may also occur. Ear piercing is a deliberate injury that carries a 30 to 40% complication rate. Allergy to nickel or gold earrings, or infections are the most common complications; however, systemic illnesses such as hepatitis, tuberculosis, or HIV infection, and ear-lobe deformities have occurred when poor technique was used.

TABLE 2: Differential Assessment of Disorders of the Auricle

	Signs and Symptoms					
Condition	**Redness**	**Warmth**	**Swelling**	**Discharge**	**Pain**	**Other**
Minor infection	Localized	Slight	Localized	Possibly pus	Mild	History of recent trauma
Perichondritis	Significant, often entire auricle involved	Significant	Significant, often entire auricle involved	Possibly pus/serous	Moderate-severe	Recent trauma or infection common; neck and cervical lymph node swelling possible
Herpes zoster	Localized	Possibly	Possibly	Possibly serous	Severe	Crusted lesions appear on auricle or in canal; often facial nerve paralysis and generalized illness
Keloid	No	No	Hard, nodular, scarlike	No	Mild or none	Hyperimmune response to injury; most common in blacks, Asians
Basal cell carcinoma	No	No	No	No	None to mild	Waxy, raised, brown wart-like lesion; history of prolonged sun exposure
Squamous cell carcinoma	Possibly	No	Possibly	Possibly blood	None to moderate	Rough, thickened, scaly; history of prolonged sun exposure
Seborrhea	Possibly	Possibly	No	No	Itching or moderate burning pain	Oily, scaly lesions; usually also present elsewhere
Allergic dermatitis	Significant	Frequently	Possibly	No	Itching or burning pain	Usually associated with chemical or metal contact
Hematoma	No	Possibly	Probably	No	Mild to severe	Bruising; bluish, round blood filled lesions

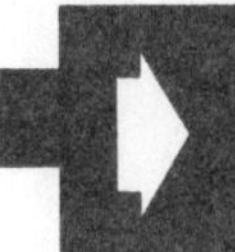

ADVICE FOR THE PATIENT

Guidelines to Reduce Risk of Ear Piercing Complications

- Piercing should be done only by individuals with proper training and sterile equipment. Home-pierced ears have a higher rate of infection and complication.
- Do not pierce the ears of children under 5 years of age. Earrings tend to get caught during play, and proper hygiene is difficult.
- Individuals with valvular heart disease, diabetes, glomerulonephritis or a history of rheumatic fever should not have their ears pierced, as the risk for systemic infection is increased.
- Individuals with a history of keloid formation should not have their ears pierced.
- Examine ears carefully following the procedure, watching for signs of dermatitis or eczema, and feel lobes for cysts or nodules. Consult a physician promptly if any of the above develop.
- Avoid the use of gold in newly pierced ears, and earrings containing nickel altogether, to reduce risk of allergic dermatitis.
- Studs should be made in a single piece from surgical grade stainless steel.
- Before the procedure, earlobes should be cleaned with alcohol and allowed to dry, or cleansed with chlorhexidine soap.

Perichondritis is a complication of an external ear infection or traumatic injury, in which infection spreads to the cartilage of the auricle. It is usually caused by *Pseudomonas* or *Staphylococcus* organisms, and prompt referral to a physician is necessary to prevent serious disease or ear deformity.

SYMPTOMS

The affected area may appear warm, red, tender, or swollen. Pus or serous discharge may be present.

TREATMENT

Nonpharmacological Treatment

Wash with an antibacterial soap. Apply warm compresses for 20 minutes every 6 to 8 hours. Remove earring if present.

Pharmacological Treatment

Antibiotic ointment may be applied. Consult a physician if condition worsens, or if no improvement after 2 days.

EXTERNAL AUDITORY CANAL

The external auditory canal is subject to a number of disorders, including obstruction by a foreign body, impacted cerumen, boils or infection. Infections may be bacterial, viral or fungal by nature. Self-treatment is useful for impacted cerumen, and prevention and treatment of mild infections. Foreign body removal and treatment of advanced infections or boils in the ear canal is best referred to a physician. Otitis media (infection of the inner ear), bullous myringitis (infection of the ear drum) and ruptured ear drum are middle ear conditions that may present with similar symptoms but are not amenable to self-treatment and must be ruled out before any nonprescription therapy is begun (Table 3).

Impacted Cerumen

Some individuals produce large amounts of cerumen or ear wax, and normal mechanisms to promote its migration out of the ear canal are inefficient, resulting in a wax plug. Secondary infections may occur as the occlusion of the ear canal promotes moisture retention, leading to skin breakdown and growth of microorganisms.

SYMPTOMS

Individuals may experience diminished hearing, a sudden hearing loss, or a pressure sensation in the ear. Ear pain may or may not be present.

TREATMENT

Nonpharmacological Treatment

Clean water is an effective softener of ear plugs, and olive or mineral oils have traditionally been used as softening agents, although their efficacy has never been definitively shown. A few drops of oil or water placed in the ear canal twice daily for 2 to 3 days may result in softening of the wax plug such that instillation of warm water with an ear syringe will flush it out. Liquids should **never** be instilled into the ear canal if there is any possibility that the tympanic membrane is not intact.

Pharmacological Treatment

Carbamide peroxide is suitable occasionally to soften and loosen ear wax. Five drops may be instilled into the affected ear and allowed to remain for 15 minutes, followed by a gentle syringing of the ear canal. Docusate liquid has also been shown to safely and effectively soften ear wax prior to removal. Other cerumenolytic agents such as triethanolamine polypeptide oleate, or chlorobutanol may cause irritation, and are not recommended.

Otitis Externa

Also known as swimmer's ear, this occurs most commonly during the summer months, although it may be seen at any time in diabetics or other individuals with compromised immune systems. It is caused by moisture in the ear canal, which produces softening and breakdown of the tissues, and neutralizes the normally acidic environment allowing microorganisms to flourish. *Pseudomonas*

TABLE 3: Differential Assessment of Disorders of the External Ear Canal

	Signs and Symptoms				
Condition	**Pain**	**Itching**	**Discharge**	**Hearing Loss**	**Other**
Impacted cerumen	Rarely, unless also infected	Frequently	Rarely, unless also infected	Frequently, often acute loss of hearing	
Bacterial otitis externa	Frequently; worse with movement of auricle	Sometimes	Frequently; serous/pus	Sometimes	Recent swimming or attempt to scratch ear canal
Fungal otitis externa	Sometimes; worse with movement of auricle	Frequently	Rarely	Sometimes	Recent swimming
Necrotizing otitis externa	Severe, constant; deep within head	Rarely	Sometimes; serous or pus	Frequently	Facial nerve paralysis possible; recent history of otitis externa; usually diabetics or immune compromised
Otitis media (middle ear infection)	Frequently; full or hollow feeling to constant, sharp pain; pain relieved if drum ruptures	Rarely	Sometimes; serous/pus; blood if ear drum perforated	Frequently	Recent upper respiratory infection; fever; usually child
Rupture of ear drum	Sudden sharp, short duration; often dizziness	Rarely	Frequently; pink, serous	Frequently	Recent infection of middle ear, or history of trauma or flying/diving
Boil	Frequently; constant, sharp	Rarely	Rarely except if ruptures; pus	Rarely	Infected hair follicle
Bullous myringitis	Frequently; constant sharp; sudden relief upon rupture of blister	Rarely	Sometimes—if rupture; pink, serous	Frequently	Recent respiratory tract infection; blood filled blisters on ear drum
Foreign object	Frequently, especially with chewing	Sometimes	Sometimes, if also infected	Frequently	Usually young child; if adult—history of something in ear
Dermatitis	Frequently; stinging or burning	Frequently	Sometimes, if also infected	Rarely	Dermatitis or seborrhea elsewhere

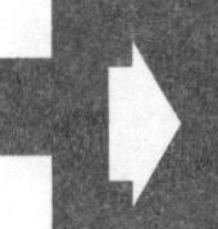

ADVICE FOR THE PATIENT

Ear Syringing Techniques

- Fill ear syringe with luke warm water. Test temperature on inside of wrist.
- Have subject hold a basin just below the ear to catch the outflow.
- Straighten the ear canal by gently pulling upwards and backwards on the auricle (in a child pull downwards and backwards).
- Insert ear syringe just into the opening of the ear canal.
- Direct stream of water along the upper surface of ear canal such that the returning flow pushes cerumen out from behind.
- Never attempt to flush out the ear canal if there is any possibility the ear drum is not intact.
- It is difficult to perform this procedure on one's self; you may wish to get help from a friend.

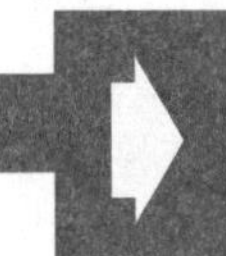

ADVICE FOR THE PATIENT

Care of the Ears Following Piercing

- Wipe twice daily with rubbing alcohol for the first 6 weeks. Be sure to get between stud and skin on the front, and between earring back and skin on the back of the lobe.
- Chlorhexidine soap may be used in place of alcohol to prevent drying and cracking of earlobes.
- Do not turn or twist earrings, this increases the risk of infection.
  Leave studs in place for 6 weeks.
- Ensure all shampoo is rinsed well from ear areas, and avoid use of hair sprays and perfumes until lobes are well healed.
- At end of healing period, the earlobe may be lubricated with soap and water to allow easy removal of the stud.
- Once earlobes are healed, wash daily with soap and water, just as one would wash the face.
- Earrings should be washed with soap and water prior to each use.

is the most common pathogen isolated, but *Staphylococcus, Streptococcus, Proteus,* or fungus may also be seen.

Necrotizing (or malignant) otitis externa is a complication of otitis externa in which infection spreads into the mastoid space or temporal bones of the skull. It is most frequently seen in patients with compromised immune systems, including those with diabetes or HIV, the elderly, or those receiving chemotherapy or steroids. Prompt medical treatment is necessary. Because diabetics in particular are at risk for serious complications from otitis externa, "Are you diabetic?" should be the first question asked by the health professional when consulted about an ear problem. If the answer is yes, prompt referral to a physician is necessary.

SYMPTOMS

The individual may complain of itching or pain, especially with movement of the auricle or jaw. The ear will feel plugged, and may discharge a cheesy substance.

TREATMENT

Nonpharmacological Treatment

Mild cases can be treated by instilling a mixture of 2/3 isopropyl alcohol and 1/3 white vinegar. Commercial products are also available that contain acetic acid or aluminum acetate. If the condition worsens or shows no improvement after 2 days, a physician should be consulted.

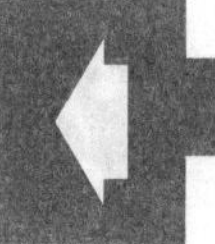

PREVENTION

Healthy ear canals can be effectively dried after swimming or showering by the instillation of rubbing alcohol. Use enough alcohol to fill the canal, allow it to sit for a minute, then tilt head down to drain it out. Alternatively, acetic acid or aluminum acetate ear drops may be used after showering or water sports. Five drops of solution in each ear will restore the normal acidic pH and discourage bacterial or fungal growth.

ADVICE FOR THE PATIENT

How to Administer Ear Drops

- Wash the hands thoroughly.
- Drops may be warmed by rolling the container between the palms of the hands. Do not place the container in hot water, or use any other means to warm the solution.
- Tilt the head sideways, with the affected ear upwards.
- Place the required number of drops (usually 5 to 10) into the ear canal.
- Do not allow the dropper tip to touch the ear canal or any other surface.
- Keep the head tilted for several minutes.
- Insert cotton plug *only if recommended by your physician*. This must be placed gently in opening of the ear canal. Do not push it too far inside.
- You may wish to get help from a friend.

Disorders of the External Ear

PATIENT ASSESSMENT QUESTIONS

Q Do you have an ear ache? Is it worsened by movements of the jaw, or auricle?

Pain due to inflammation or infection of the external canal (e.g., boils, otitis externa) or otitis media tends to be constant, and can be severe. Pain that worsens with manipulation of the auricle or movement of the jaw is often associated with a problem of the external ear (but does not completely rule out involvement of the middle ear). Pain that occurs only with movement of the jaw implies a problem with the temporomandibular joint, or the teeth. Oral analgesics may be recommended for mild pain, and a physician should be consulted if it continues beyond 2 days.

Q Have you recently been swimming?

Otitis externa occurs 24 to 72 hours after swimming or water sports. Commercial acetic acid or aluminum acetate otic drops or a solution of 2/3 isopropyl alcohol and 1/3 white vinegar may relieve the symptoms. If the problem has not improved after 2 days, a physician should be seen. Diving without equalizing pressure in the middle ear can cause rupture of the tympanic membrane. If this is a possibility, nothing should be put into the ear, and a physician should be consulted.

Q Is the ear itchy?

Itchy ears may be caused by dermatitis of the ear canal, or by irritation caused by a build up of ear wax. *Buro-Sol Otic*, aluminum acetate and benzethonium chloride solution, may be used to relieve itchiness due to dermatitis. More severe cases may require referral to a physician and use of corticosteroids. Docusate liquid, a stool softener usually used for treatment of constipation, has been shown to soften ear wax. Although efficacy is unproven, olive or mineral oils have traditionally been used. Clean water is also effective. The softening agent should be instilled into the ear twice daily for 1 to 3 days. This should be followed by flushing of the ear with warm water to remove any debris. Attempts to scratch the ear with cotton tipped applicators, hair pins, etc, may result in injury to the ear canal. Patients should be cautioned against putting anything smaller than their baby finger in their ears.

Q Is there any discharge from the ear?

Discharge other than cerumen may indicate trauma or infection. Discharge of blood or pus, followed by sudden pain relief may indicate a ruptured boil, or rupture of a blister on the tympanic membrane. A referral to a physician is necessary.

Q Did your hearing difficulty occur suddenly?

Sudden hearing loss may indicate the presence of a foreign body, a wax plug, a perforation of the tympanic membrane or serious infection. A gradual loss of hearing occurs primarily as a result of aging, autoimmune disorders, or with some drugs. Ototoxic drugs include furosemide, aminoglycosides, chloramphenicol, cisplatin, nitrogen mustard, salicylates, and quinine, as well as many others. The degree of hearing loss is a function of the blood level of the drugs in most cases, and may be reversible (e.g., salicylates, ethacrynic acid). Two ototoxic drugs used together will result in impairment greater than would be suggested by blood levels of the individual agents.

Q Do you feel dizzy, or have a ringing sensation in your ears?

Many of the drugs mentioned above can cause tinnitus, or ringing in the ears, which is indicative of an irritation of the cochlea in the inner ear. Patients with this complaint should be advised to consult a physician, and stop use of salicylates if they are taking them. Dizziness may be associated with middle ear infection. True vertigo is a sensation of whirling or falling, and indicates a disorder of the vestibular system. Patients with this complaint should be referred to a physician.

PHARMACEUTICAL AGENTS

Acetic Acid: When diluted to 1 to 5%, acetic acid has antibacterial properties that are a function of its acidic pH, small molecular size and lipid solubility. Household vinegar is 5% acetic acid. Topically, it is well tolerated and does not promote the growth of resistant organisms. It can be safely and effectively used for the prevention of swimmer's ear.

Aluminum Acetate: This is a clear, colorless solution that contains about 5% aluminum acetate stabilized with boric acid. It provides antibacterial activity as a function of its acidic pH, and anti-inflammatory effects as a result of the astringent properties of aluminum salts. It forms a protective layer on the surface of the skin, and is poorly absorbed systemically. It is used topically at concentrations of 1:10 to 1:40 for the prevention of swimmer's ear, and treatment of otitis externa. Aluminum acetate solution can also be used as a compress for treatment of dermatitis of the auricle.

Antipyrine: Also known as phenazone, this ingredient has traditionally been included in ear preparations as an analgesic and antipyretic agent. It is a weak antiseptic, causes vasoconstriction, and impairs sensory nerve conduction when applied topically. It is no longer recommended for use.

Benzocaine: This is an ester type local anesthetic agent that produces reversible loss of local sensation by reducing the conduction of sensory nerve impulses. It is readily absorbed through mucous membranes and damaged skin. It should not be used in children under 2 years of age, as systemic absorption of benzocaine has been associated with methemoglobinemia. It has also been associated with severe hypersensitivity reactions. Its use should be immediately discontinued if a rash or skin irritation develops. The use of benzocaine in nonprescription ear products is generally discouraged. Serious complications may result if this agent is used when the tympanic membrane is perforated, and it may mask signs of infection that, if left untreated, may also result in serious complications.

Systemic analgesics are considered safer and more effective, and are preferred.

Benzethonium Chloride: This is a tertiary amine compound included in some otic preparations for its anti-infective and astringent properties. Its effectiveness is reduced in the presence of organic matter or soaps, and it can cause irritation or dermatitis.

Camphor: This ingredient has traditionally been used as a mild antiseptic, antipruritic, and rubefacient on the skin. The rubefacient effects make patients feel better, but do not actually have any healing effects. Its value in ear preparations is questionable.

Carbamide Peroxide: This compound is composed of one molecule of urea with one molecule of hydrogen peroxide. Upon contact with moisture, the compound dissociates. Urea acts as a keratolytic, and hydrogen peroxide undergoes a reaction with catalase enzymes to produce oxygen, which results in a foaming action. The physical effects of the reaction provide a mechanical means of dislodging ear wax plugs. Clinical studies have found it to be more effective than glycerin alone for softening ear wax, but it could not be shown either more or less effective than triethanolamine polypeptide oleate, or chlorobutanol-containing products. For facilitating the removal of ear wax, carbamide peroxide should be instilled into the affected ear twice daily for up to 4 days, and followed by syringing of the ear. Frequent or prolonged use can cause maceration of the ear canal, and delay healing. It should never be instilled into the ear if there is a possibility that the tympanic membrane is not intact, or in the presence of pain or drainage from the ear.

Chlorobutanol: This is a crystalloid substance with an odor and taste similar to camphor. It has antimicrobial and antifungal activity and is used as a preservative in pharmaceutical products.

Glycerin: This is a colorless, odorless liquid with a sweet taste, and a slightly acidic pH. Topically, it is used as a lubricating and softening agent, and can be used as a solvent or vehicle for oral medications. In the ear, it has been utilized as an emulsifier to facilitate the removal of impacted cerumen. Although it is well tolerated, it has been shown less effective than other agents for softening ear wax plugs.

Gramicidin D: This polypeptide antibiotic interferes with bacterial cell metabolism, and is effective primarily against gram-positive organisms. It is useful topically, and systemic absorption is minimal

Pharmaceutical Agents

because it is inactivated by serum. It is available in combination with other antibiotics in various products. It should only be used when the diagnosis of infection is certain, and complications such as ear drum perforation or other serious conditions have been ruled out. If symptoms have not improved after 2 days, a physician should be consulted.

Isopropyl Alcohol: This agent is used for its antiseptic properties, and as a vehicle or solvent for other drugs or chemicals. It is very effective for drying of the ear canal, and may be used undiluted on intact skin, or diluted with acetic acid as an antimicrobial agent.

Lidocaine: This is an amide type local anesthetic agent with actions like those of benzocaine. It also is readily absorbed through mucous membranes and should not be applied to damaged skin. Its use should be immediately discontinued if a rash or irritation develops. Serious complications may result if this agent is used when the tympanic membrane is perforated, and it may mask signs of infection that, if left untreated, may also result in serious complications. Systemic analgesics are considered safer and more effective, and are preferred.

Paradichlorobenzene: This chemical is an insecticide and fumigant used to combat clothes moths. It causes irritation to mucous membranes and can cause liver toxicity with prolonged exposure. There is no justification for its use in otic preparations.

Polymyxin B Sulfate: This is a bactericidal agent effective against most gram-negative organisms. It destroys bacterial cell membranes by binding to phosphate groups in the lipid structure. Resistance develops rarely, and absorption through the skin is minimal. It is available in combination with other antibiotics but should only be used when the diagnosis of infection is certain, and complications such as ear drum perforation or other serious conditions have been ruled out. If symptoms have not improved after 2 days, a physician should be consulted.

Propylene Glycol: This is a clear, colorless, odorless, viscous, hygroscopic liquid with a sweet taste. It is used primarily as a solvent, or preservative for medications. It has mild bacteriostatic and antifungal properties. Contact dermatitis has been associated with prolonged use.

Triethanolamine Polypeptide Oleate: This is a soap composed of an amine base and a fatty acid (oleic acid). Its principle use is as an emulsifying agent, and it has been used to soften ear wax plugs. Although clinical studies have shown it to be equal in efficacy to carbamide peroxide and olive oil for this purpose, it has been associated with severe hypersensitivity reactions. For this reason, it is recommended only for use under the supervision of a physician. It should never be allowed to remain in the ear canal longer than 30 minutes, and should never be instilled if there is any possibility that the tympanic membrane is not intact.

RECOMMENDED READING

Guyton AC, ed. Textbook of Medical Physiology. 8th ed. Philadelphia: WB Saunders, 1991:570-84.

Ballenger JJ. Diseases of the Nose, Throat, Ear, Head, and Neck. 14th ed. Philadelphia: Lea and Febiger, 1991:1069-118.

Strome M, Kelly JH, Fried MP, eds. Manual of Otolaryngology: Diagnosis and Therapy. 2nd ed. Boston: Little, Brown and Company, 1992: 49-106.

9

EYE CARE PRODUCTS

LYNN R. TROTTIER / DAVID S. WING

CONTENTS

Anatomy and Physiology of the Eye 163

Disorders of the Eyelids 167
- Blepharitis
- Hordeolum (Stye)
- Chalazion (Cyst)

Disorders of the Conjunctiva 170
- Bacterial Conjunctivitis
- Viral Conjunctivitis
- Allergic Conjunctivitis
- Chemical or Irritative Conjunctivitis
- Subconjunctival Hemorrhage

Dry Eye 177
- Symptoms
- Treatment

Trauma 181

Contact Lens Care 188
- Types of Contact Lenses
- Contact Lenses and Drugs
- Compliance

Ophthalmic Product Information 199
- Anesthetics—Local
- Antihistamines
- Anti-infectives
- Artificial Tears (Demulcents)
- Astringents
- Decongestants (Eye Whiteners, Vasoconstrictors)
- Preservatives
- Miscellaneous Ingredients
- Formulations

Contact Lens Product Information 207
- Routine Care of Contact Lenses
- Cleaning Solutions
- Disinfection
- Wetting and Viscosity Agents
- Multifunction Solutions
- Accessory Solutions
- Buffers
- Preservatives (Antimicrobial Agents)
- Mixing Solutions

Recommended Reading 222

ANATOMY AND PHYSIOLOGY OF THE EYE

Figure 1 illustrates the major structures of the eye. The cornea is transparent, avascular, and refracts light into the inner eye. The lens, also avascular and transparent, focuses incoming light to the retina. The sclera is the fibrous outer protective coating of the eye, and the iris a circular pigmented tissue behind the cornea. The retina, at the back of the eye, contains the rods and cones necessary for vision.

Eyelids

The eyelids are thin, movable "curtains" of skin that cover the exposed anterior surface of the eyeball (Figure 2). If any loud noise, sudden movement or excessive light is interpreted as potentially harmful, an involuntary blink reflex closes the lids. Blinking spreads the tear film over the cornea and conjunctival surfaces keeping the mucous membrane moist. The lids are very flexible as the skin is extremely thin and elastic. Loose areolar tissue (e.g., tissue containing minute spaces) beneath the eyelid and periocular skin is capable of massive edematous distention. Dense fibrous tissue (tarsal plates) gives the eyelids their relative shape. A number of glands are contained within the eyelids (Figure 1 and Table 1). Eyelashes protect the eye from dust and perspiration.

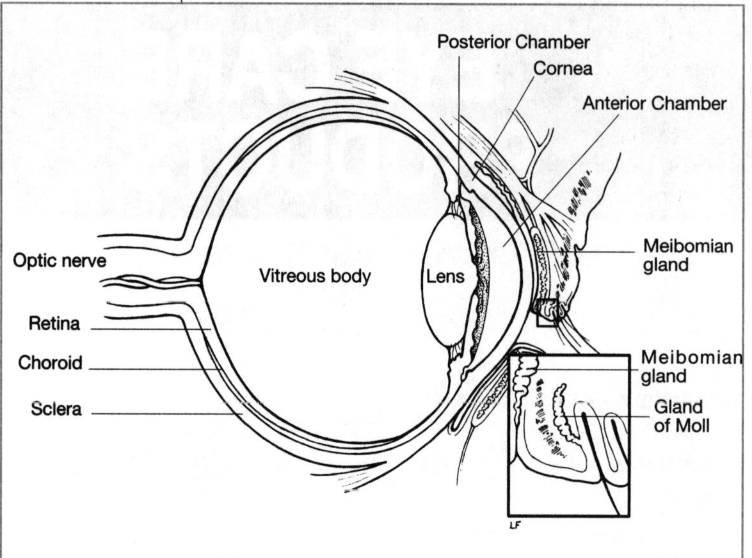

FIGURE 1: Anatomy of the Eye

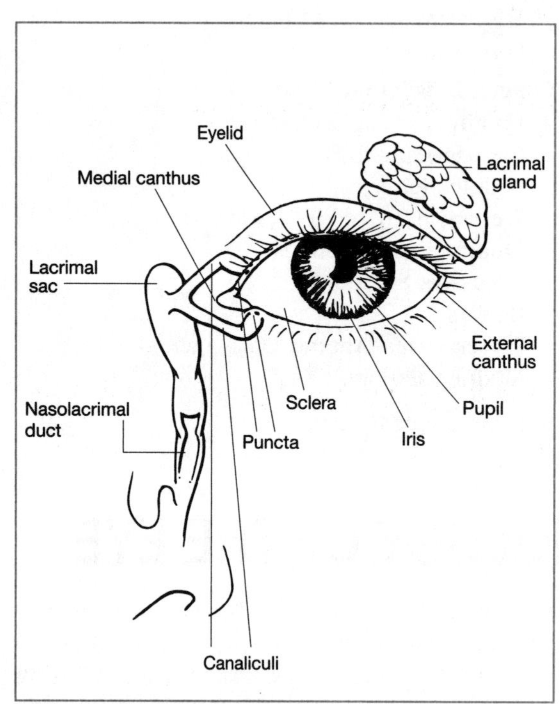

FIGURE 2: Lacrimal Apparatus and External Landmarks of the Eye

Conjunctiva

The conjunctiva, a thin, transparent mucous membrane with an extensive vascular network, lines the anterior surface of the eyeball (except for the cornea) and the posterior surface of the eyelid. Because of its exposed position, the conjunctiva is susceptible to invasion by microorganisms and to damage by environmental stressors. Being a mucosal surface, it is predisposed to systemic diseases involving the skin and mucous membranes.

Several processes protect the conjunctiva. The wiper-like action of the lids spreads the tears and continually flushes the conjunctiva; the aqueous layer of tears dilutes potential pathogens and allergens; the mucous layer of the tears traps debris; and lysozymes and antibodies in the tears serve as antimicrobial agents.

Tear Film and Lacrimal Apparatus

The tear film, which covers the corneal and conjunctival surfaces, has three layers that completely cover the most superficial cells (epithelial cells) (Table 2). The thickest layer, the aqueous tear fluid, contains water soluble substances (e.g., salt, proteins) and is produced by the lacrimal gland located at the upper, outer angle of the lid and by the accessory lacrimal glands located in the palpebral conjunctiva. An oily (lipid) film, produced mainly by the Meibomian glands, covers the surface of the aqueous layer; it is thought to reduce the evaporation rate of tears and form a water-tight seal when the lids are closed. Between the aqueous layer and the epithelial cells of the eye is the mucoid layer. Principally produced by special conjunctival cells, this layer helps spread the aqueous tear film over the lipoprotein epithelial cells of the conjunctiva and cornea. It may also help stabilize the tear film, which serves several functions (Table 3).

Tears have an average pH of 7.35 and under normal conditions are isotonic. Ten per cent of the tear film is lost by evaporation, the remainder

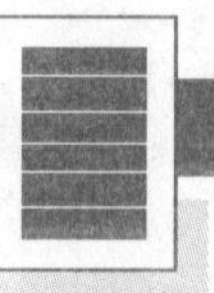

TABLE 1: Glands Contained Within the Eyelids
Meibomian glands (modified sebaceous glands on the posterior margin)
Glands of Zeis (modified sebaceous glands on the anterior margin at the base of the eyelashes)
Glands of Moll (modified sweat glands on the anterior margin near the base of the eyelashes)

constantly drained from the eye via two lacrimal puncta (orifices at the nasal side of the upper and lower lids). The tears are carried via lacrimal canaliculi to the lacrimal sac. They exit through the nasolacrimal duct and are discharged as part of the nasal secretions (thus, the runny nose associated with crying) (Figure 2). Eye drops or eye ointments can be absorbed into the body via this route either by absorption through the nasal mucous membrane or by swallowing into the gastrointestinal tract. They can also be absorbed via the vascular system in the conjunctiva. (When absorbed via the nasal mucosa or conjunctiva, they avoid first-pass metabolism.)

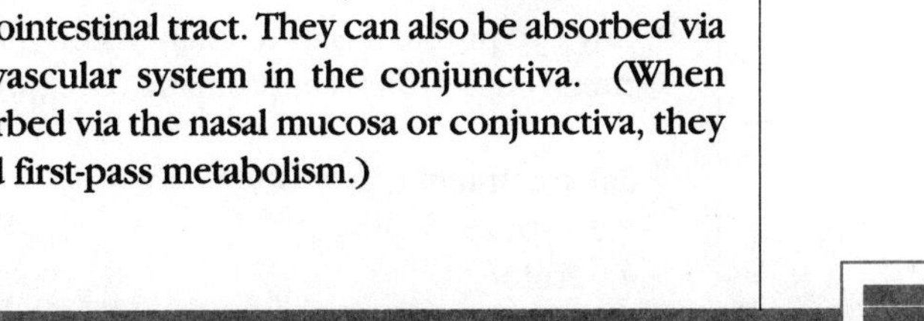

TABLE 2: The Three Layers of the Tear Film
Oily or lipid (outer) layer
Aqueous (middle) layer
Mucoid (inner) layer adhering to the surface of the eye

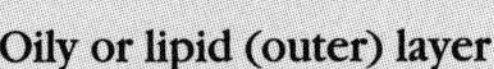

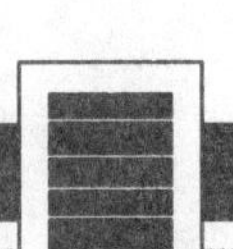

TABLE 3: Functions of the Tear Film
Formation of an almost perfectly smooth optical surface on the cornea
Lubrication for the eyes and lids
Protective antibacterial action (e.g., lysozyme destroys bacteria; IgA assists in controlling infection; lactoferrin is a bacteriostatic agent)
Mechanical flushing of microorganisms, debris and antigens
Moistening, oxygenation and nutrition of the cornea

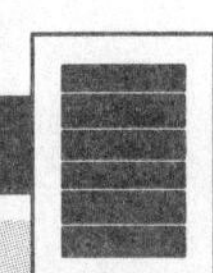

TABLE 4: Ocular Conditions Associated with Red Eye
Eyelid problems
Conjunctival problems
Dry eyes
Corneal or internal eye disorders
Glaucoma
Trauma

Self-treatment Guidelines for Eye Disorders

➤ Any eye problem is potentially vision-threatening. In general, nonprescription ophthalmic medications offer symptomatic relief; they are not curative.

Self-treatment is appropriate for:
- eyestrain
- burning
- itching
- stinging
- mild tearing
- mild, diffuse, redness of the conjunctiva

Referral to an eye care professional is essential for:
- pain
- photophobia (sensitivity to bright light)
- altered vision
- redness immediately around cornea
- severe redness of the conjunctiva or eyelids
- excessive discharge
- abnormal pupils (e.g., constricted, semi-dilated, oval-shaped, unequal size)
- floating spots (sudden appearance)
- trauma (to or near the eye)
- headache
- a child or elderly individual
- underlying medical condition (e.g., diabetes)
- self-medication longer than 48 hours (with anti-infectives) or 72 hours (with other agents) when the condition is nonresponsive or worsens
- untreated conditions lasting longer than 48 hours

➤ Perhaps the most frequent ocular problems that individuals seek help for involve red eye (Table 4), which must be properly diagnosed, as they can range in severity from insignificant to threatening vision permanently.

➤ When moderate to severe infectious disease processes are suspected, especially if the condition is recurrent, or if the individual has an underlying systemic disease (e.g., diabetes), the individual should be referred to an eye care professional. Although most bacterial and viral infections of the external eye are self-limiting and pose a minor risk to vision, there is always the possibility of vision-threatening, severe bacterial disease (pseudomonas infection), viral disease (herpetic keratitis) or fungal infection (*Acanthamoeba*).

➤ Self-treatment of conjunctival disorders (conjunctivitis) carries a greater risk than self-treatment of eyelid disorders (blepharitis, hordeolum or chalazion).

➤ Chronic use of any nonprescription eye product should be supervised by an eye care professional to reduce the risk of ocular damage caused by both the underlying disorder and the medication. If in doubt, refer the individual to an eye care professional.

DISORDERS OF THE EYELIDS

Many health professionals are responsible for the health of the eye (e.g., family practice physician, ophthalmologist, optometrist). For the purposes of this chapter, they will be collectively named eye care professionals.

BLEPHARITIS

Blepharitis, an acute or chronic inflammation of the eyelid margin, is one of the most common causes of eye disease. It may begin in early childhood, and if not treated appropriately, an acute episode may become chronic and continue for months or years.

Etiology

Staphylococcus aureus, *Staphylococcus epidermidis* or seborrhea, alone or in combination can cause blepharitis. Mixed (combination) blepharitis is probably the most common. *Pityrosporum ovale* is associated with, but not a proven causative pathogen for seborrheic blepharitis. Dysfunction of the sebaceous glands is also associated with seborrheic blepharitis. Meibomian gland dysfunction may play a role in chronic blepharitis (e.g., blockage may cause an accumulation of secretions with secondary infection).

Staphylococcus aureus can cause ulceration of the lid margin. If improperly treated, the lashes may become distorted, grow inward to irritate the cornea or fall out. Both staphylococcal and seborrheic blepharitis predispose an individual to recurrent conjunctivitis.

Pubic lice (crabs), which have a predilection for widely spaced hair, can thrive in the eyelashes. The nits attach to the lashes and cause an irritative blepharitis. The condition develops through sexual or close bodily contact.

Irritant, chemical or allergic blepharitis may be provoked in numerous ways (Table 5). Allergic blepharitis is often a contact rather than an atopic reaction (Table 6).

Symptoms

The primary symptoms of blepharitis include unsightly hyperemia along the lid margins (red rims) as well as burning, irritation and itching. There may be edema and photophobia, but vision usually remains normal. In chronic blepharitis many patients have symptoms of dry eye.

With *Staphylococcus aureus* colonization, dry fibrin exudate encircles the lashes, and the individual often complains the lashes are stuck together on awakening. Many dry and flaky scales can be

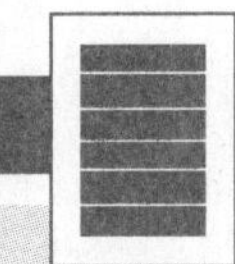

TABLE 5: Substances That May Provoke Irritant, Chemical or Allergic Blepharitis

Smoke	Plants (e.g., poison ivy)
Drug (e.g., atropine, neomycin, pilocarpine, tetracaine, timolol)	Metal (e.g., nickel eyeglass frames)
Cosmetics	Rubbing the eyes (e.g., in response to local irritation, congestion or attempts to clear vision)

TABLE 6: Types of Ophthalmic Hypersensitivity Reactions

Atopic (Type I)	Contact (Type IV)
e.g., acute allergic conjunctivitis, atopic dermatitis, allergic rhinitis	e.g., contact dermatitis
Immediate hypersensitivity	Delayed hypersensitivity
Generally rapid onset after exposure to antigen and short-lived (but there may be a late phase reaction)	Generally occurs at least 24 hours after exposure to antigen
Antibody mediated (mainly IgE)	T lymphocyte mediated
Degranulated mast cells and basophils release mediators (e.g., histamine)	Sensitized T lymphocytes release lymphokines

seen attached to the lashes; the lids are red with tiny ulcers on the margins. If untreated, the lashes may fall out.

With the seborrheic type, the scales are yellow and greasy, and the tear film may appear oily due to altered Meibomian gland activity, but there are no ulcers, and the lid margins are not as red.

In a combination type, both dry and greasy scales can be seen with red margins and ulcers.

In pubic lice infestations and allergic blepharitis, the dominant symptom often is pruritus. With lice, there may also be crusting of the lid margin and nits (or occasionally adult lice) attached to the eyelashes.

Treatment

Nonpharmacological Treatment

When treating infectious or seborrheic blepharitis, thorough cleansing of the lids is essential. Warm moist compresses (using a clean facecloth or gauze pads) applied for 5 to 15 minutes, up to 4 times a day, tapering to once daily, soften crusts. A cotton-tipped applicator or cotton pledget dipped in warm water or baby shampoo (diluted 1:1 or 1:5 with tap water) effectively removes scales and crusts. The mainstay of treatment is lid hygiene at least twice a day. It is particularly important following sleep as debris collects and builds up on the lids while the eyes are closed. If recurrences are a problem, daily lid cleaning for at least 1 month will help to minimize them.

With irritant, chemical or allergic blepharitis it is critical that the offending agent (Table 5) be removed. Cold compresses saturated with normal saline (or Burow's solution 1:40) may be soothing. A facecloth moistened with cold water and applied to the eyelids for several minutes can also be used as a cold compress.

Pharmacological Treatment

Nonprescription lid cleansers are available for removing the scales and crusts of infectious or seborrheic blepharitis.

The agent of choice for self-medication of infectious blepharitis is bacitracin ophthalmic ointment, although gramicidin/polymyxin can also be used. Bacitracin is preferred because of its selective effectiveness against gram-positive organisms. It should be applied 3 to 5 times daily for 1 week. Chronic or recurrent blepharitis may require initial acute treatment, then maintenance treatment at bedtime for 4 to 8 weeks. Ophthalmic ointments are the most effective dosage form for blepharitis.

For seborrheic blepharitis, one drop of an artificial tear 2 to 4 times daily may provide comfort and reduce debris and oil on the tear film. If seborrhea of the scalp coexists, an antiseborrheic shampoo, such as selenium sulfide should be used once or twice weekly; ocular contact must be avoided as it may result in toxic conjunctivitis. When the scalp is treated, the seborrheic blepharitis often resolves.

Treatment of pubic lice infestations of the eyelashes is discussed in the Antiparasitic and Anthelmintic Products chapter.

HORDEOLUM (Stye)

Hordeolum, or stye, an acute, pus-producing inflammation, begins in the follicle of an eyelash or in one of the eyelid glands. If a Meibomian gland is involved, the swelling can be massive; while if the glands of Moll or Zeis are involved, there is less, and more superficial swelling. The causative organism is usually *Staphylococcus aureus*. Styes are often associated with lowered resistance (e.g., debility or diabetes) or local predilection (e.g., concomitant blepharitis or acne vulgaris).

Symptoms

Initial symptoms are tenderness, edema and redness, which may be diffused over the lid. In a few days, a small collection of pus appears along the eyelid margin. Until the pustule ruptures, usually in 3 to 4 days, the individual may experience considerable pain. The greater the swelling, the more intense the pain. Sometimes the stye spontaneously resolves without discharging its contents. As the infection may spread along the lid margin, directly or via fingers, styes often appear in "crops." If this condition is not appropriately treated, particularly in a severely debilitated individual, the infection can be internalized to produce orbital cellulitis which is considered a medical emergency.

Treatment

Nonpharmacological Treatment

The application of warm, moist compresses 3 or 4 times a day for 10 to 15 minutes, encourages drainage by opening the glands or eyelash folliculi. The warmth also draws more blood to the area, increasing the number of inflammatory and repair mediators. These mediators close off and clean up the infection. Light massage over the lesion several times a day may help. *The lesions should not be squeezed as this may spread the bacteria and cause cellulitis.*

Pharmacological Treatment

Nonprescription antibiotic eye ointment applied following the heat treatments is unlikely to cure the stye, but it may reduce the possibility of spreading the infection further along the lid. The agent of choice for self-medication of a stye is bacitracin ophthalmic ointment, although gramicidin/polymyxin can also be used. Bacitracin is preferred because of its selective effectiveness against gram-positive organisms. If warm compresses are ineffective, if the stye does not improve after 48 hours, if there are multiple styes or if there are other complicating medical conditions, the individual should be referred to an eye care professional.

CHALAZION (Cyst)

Chalazion (Meibomian or tarsal cyst) is a chronic, granulomatous inflammation of a Meibomian gland due to retention of normal secretions. It is not an infection. It may occur spontaneously or it may be associated with seborrhea or acne rosacea.

Symptoms

The cyst develops over several weeks. It most commonly occurs in the upper lid and feels like a small pebble. It bulges externally but points toward the conjunctival side of the eyelid. Usually, the lid margin is not involved. The lesion is often painless, but is cosmetically embarrassing. The conjunctiva may be slightly reddened. If the chalazion is large enough, it may result in inadequate lid closure and dry eye. Sometimes it resolves spontaneously. Secondary infection can occur. Recurrent chalazia may be indicative of a serious disease and require medical attention.

Treatment

Management of a minor chalazion usually involves use of warm, moist compresses 4 times a day. If the chalazion persists, management by an eye care professional may be necessary. In severe or recurrent cases, excision or injection of corticosteroids may be performed by an ophthalmologist. To prevent secondary infection, the agent of choice for self-medication of chalazion is bacitracin ophthalmic ointment, although gramicidin/polymyxin can also be used. Bacitracin is preferred because of its selective effectiveness against gram-positive organisms. The ophthalmic ointment should be applied to the lid for 3 to 4 weeks.

DISORDERS OF THE CONJUNCTIVA

Inflammation of the conjunctiva, conjunctivitis, is the most common eye disorder. The severity can range from mild hyperemia (redness) with tearing to severe hyperemia with copious purulent discharge. Causes of conjunctivitis are numerous (Table 7). Accurate diagnosis is very important as some types may resemble serious ocular conditions (e.g., keratitis, glaucoma—Table 8) or may be associated with severe systemic disease (Table 7).

Conjunctivitis is characterized by diffuse redness in both eyes that may first appear in only one eye. The redness is more marked at the outer aspects of the eye and is less around the cornea. Redness in a ring immediately around the cornea suggests potentially vision-threatening disorders of the cornea or deeper structures. The individual may also complain of discharge, burning, stinging, scratching, a gritty or foreign body sensation, a sensation of fullness around the eyes, itching and photophobia.

The following discussion focuses on the more common types of conjunctivitis: bacterial/viral, allergic and chemical (Table 9).

TABLE 7: Some Causes of Conjunctivitis

INFECTIOUS
(Partial listing of potential pathogens)

Bacteria
Haemophilus influenzae
Neisseria gonorrhoeae
Neisseria meningitidis
Pseudomonas aeruginosa
Staphylococcus aureus
Staphylococcus epidermidis
Streptococcus pneumoniae

Chlamydial
Chlamydia oculogenitalis
Chlamydia trachomatis

Viral
Most adenovirus strains
Herpes simplex type 1 and type 2
Varicella-zoster
Measles

Fungal *(rare)*
Candida

Parasitic *(rare)*
Pediculosis pubis

IMMUNOLOGIC
Immediate Hypersensitivity Reactions *(Allergic)*
Acute allergic conjunctivitis: seasonal (e.g., grass, pollens) or perennial (e.g., animal dander, dust mites)
Vernal keratoconjunctivitis
Giant papillary conjunctivitis
Atopic keratoconjunctivitis

Delayed Hypersensitivity Reactions
Mild conjunctivitis secondary to contact blepharitis

Autoimmune Disease
Cicatricial pemphigoid
Keratoconjunctivitis sicca associated with Sjögren's syndrome

CHEMICAL OR IRRITATIVE
Alcohol
Iatrogenic (medications)—Table 10
Occupational/environmental
Acids
Alkalies
Air pollutants (e.g., fumes)
Chlorine (e.g., in swimming pools)
Dry environment
Dust
Heat
Poor ventilation
Smoke
Ultraviolet light
Wind
Eyelid Anatomical Abnormalities

ASSOCIATED WITH SYSTEMIC DISEASE
Rheumatic disorders
(e.g., Reiter's syndrome, rheumatoid arthritis)
Skin diseases
(e.g., acne rosacea, psoriasis, atopic dermatitis)
Other (e.g., polycythemia, gout, thyroid disease, tuberculosis, syphilis)

SECONDARY TO DACRYOCYSTITIS OR CANALICULITIS

SECONDARY TO TUMORS OF CONJUNCTIVA OR LID MARGINS

Adapted with permission from: Vaughan D, Asbury T, Riordan-Eva P, eds. General Ophthalmology. 13th ed. Connecticut: Appleton & Lange, 1992.

TABLE 8: Differential Diagnosis of Common Causes of Inflamed Eye

	Acute Conjunctivitis	Acute Iritis*	Acute Glaucoma†	Corneal Trauma or Infection (Keratitis)
Incidence	Extremely common	Common	Uncommon	Common
Discharge	Moderate to copious	None	None	Watery or purulent
Vision	No effect on vision	Slightly blurred	Markedly blurred	Usually blurred
Pain	None	Moderate	Severe	Moderate to Severe
Conjunctival injection‡	Diffuse; more toward fornices	Mainly circumcorneal	Diffuse	Diffuse
Cornea	Clear	Usually clear	Steamy	Change in clarity related to cause
Pupil size	Normal	Small	Moderately dilated and fixed	Normal
Pupillary light response	Normal	Poor	None	Normal
Intraocular pressure	Normal	Normal	Elevated	Normal
Smear	Causative organisms	No organisms	No organisms	Organisms found only in corneal ulcers due to infection

* Acute anterior uveitis.
† Angle-closure glaucoma.
‡ Term used to mean congestion of ciliary or conjunctival blood vessels.
Adapted with permission from: Vaughan D, Asbury T, Riordan-Eva P, eds. General Ophthalmology. 13th ed. Connecticut: Appleton & Lange, 1992.

TABLE 9: Differential Diagnosis of the Common Types of Conjunctivitis

Clinical Findings and Cytology	Bacterial	Viral	Chlamydial	Atopic (Allergic)
Itching	Minimal	Minimal	Minimal	Severe
Hyperemia	Generalized	Generalized	Generalized	Generalized
Tearing	Moderate	Profuse	Moderate	Moderate
Exudation	Profuse	Minimal	Profuse	Minimal
Preauricular adenopathy	Uncommon	Common	Common only in inclusion conjunctivitis	None
In stained scrapings and exudates	Bacteria, PMNs*	Monocytes	PMNs, plasma cells, inclusion bodies	Eosinophils
Associated sore throat and fever	Occasionally	Occasionally	Never	Never

* Polymorphonuclear cells.
Adapted with permission from: Vaughan D, Asbury T, Riordan-Eva P, eds. General Ophthalmology. 13th ed. Connecticut: Appleton & Lange, 1992.

BACTERIAL CONJUNCTIVITIS

Etiology

A wide variety of organisms are responsible for this disease (Table 7). The most common are *Staphylococcus aureus, Staphylococcus epidermidis, Streptococcus pneumoniae* and *Haemophilus influenzae*. Although less common, conjunctivitis may be due to *Neisseria gonorrhoeae, Pseudomonas aeruginosa* or *Proteus* species.

Symptoms

With the acute form, onset is abrupt and frequently characterized by purulent or mucopurulent discharge. The lids may be edematous and stuck together on awakening. Some acute bacterial forms are self-limiting and often resolve spontaneously in 7 to 10 days. It is considered a chronic infection when it lasts for more than 2 weeks. Some forms of purulent acute conjunctivitis (e.g., *Neisseria* species), if not treated early, may result in serious complications. Mucopurulent forms (e.g., *Streptococcus pneumoniae*—known as pink eye in temperate climates) often occur in epidemics. Subacute conjunctivitis (e.g., *H. influenzae*) is characterized by thin, watery or flocculent (containing flaky masses) exudate.

Treatment

Although bacterial conjunctivitis does not usually result in serious disease, moderate to severe bacterial conjunctivitis should be assessed and managed by an eye care professional.

Nonpharmacological Treatment

Particularly if there is excessive purulent discharge, the eyes should be cleaned with gauze compresses or lid cleanser prior to instillation of ophthalmic

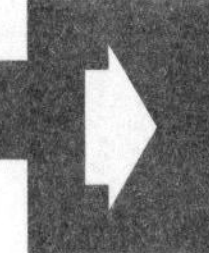

ADVICE FOR THE PATIENT

Infections of the Eyelids or Conjunctiva

(infectious blepharitis or infectious conjunctivitis)

➤ See your eye care professional if:
- you have pain, altered vision or severe redness;
- this is a recurrent condition;
- you have an underlying disease (e.g., diabetes);
- self-treatment longer than 48 hours (with anti-infectives) or 72 hours (with other agents) does not clear up the condition or the condition worsens;
- without treatment the condition has lasted longer than 48 hours.

➤ Use separate facecloths, towels, pillows and sheets from other family members since the infection may be transmitted.

➤ Do not use an eye patch unless recommended by your eye care professional.

➤ Do not use an eyecup as they can become contaminated and spread the infection.

➤ Cosmetics (e.g., mascara) can be a source of reinfection.

➤ Frequently wash your hands particularly before and after touching your eye(s).

➤ For eye infections, it is important that the eyes are cleaned, especially before applying any medication. This is particularly true when there is:
- an eyelid infection (the lids must be thoroughly cleaned);
- sticky discharge.

preparations. Eye patches must be avoided as they produce an incubatory environment.

Pharmacological Treatment

Although bacterial conjunctivitis is generally self-limiting, treatment with antibiotic ophthalmic preparations can reduce the duration of infection to 2 to 3 days. Sometimes a broad spectrum ophthalmic antibacterial will be used empirically or until the causative organism has been identified. For mild to moderate bacterial conjunctivitis, a broad spectrum nonprescription ophthalmic antibacterial (e.g., polymyxin/gramicidin/bacitracin) can be administered 4 times daily for 5 to 7 days; for severe conjunctivitis, prescription ophthalmic antibiotics are usually administered.

Eye drops are usually preferred, but ointments can be used for the nighttime dose to prolong contact or to control morning stickiness. Ointments may also be preferred for the treatment of younger children who cry after the instillation of eye drops.

VIRAL CONJUNCTIVITIS

Viral conjunctivitis may be associated with or follow an upper respiratory tract infection, particularly in children, or it may be limited to infection of the corneal and conjunctival epithelium.

Symptoms

Symptoms and contagion vary according to the virus. Severity ranges from mild to severely disabling and potentially sight-threatening. Some adenoviruses produce a watery discharge and the preauricular lymph nodes may become enlarged. Acute infections may last 1 to 4 weeks. Viral conjunctivitis may be accompanied by systemic symptoms (e.g., sore throat and fever).

Treatment

Nonpharmacological Treatment

Cold compresses may provide some symptomatic relief for mild viral conjunctivitis.

Pharmacological Treatment

Moderate to severe viral conjunctivitis should be assessed and managed by an eye care professional. Artificial tears may provide some symptomatic relief.

ALLERGIC CONJUNCTIVITIS

Several categories of immunologic conjunctivitis exist (Table 7), the most common allergic conjunctivitis. It may exist alone or be a part of a more widespread allergic condition (e.g., atopic dermatitis/eczema) and may be associated with a genetic predisposition. There are four major categories of allergic conjunctivitis: acute allergic conjunctivitis, vernal keratoconjunctivitis, giant papillary conjunctivitis and atopic keratoconjunctivitis. In contrast to acute allergic conjunctivitis, the last three categories are potentially serious ocular disorders. The differences in severity and manifestation between these disorders may be explained by the difference in pathogenesis. Although they are all immediate hypersensitivity reactions (Table 6), each condition is characterized by a particular cellular and mediator profile. There are differences in the types and numbers of inflammatory cells involved and the chemical mediators released.

Acute Allergic Conjunctivitis

Acute allergic conjunctivitis may be a seasonal disorder, known as hayfever or *seasonal allergic conjunctivitis*, or it may be a year round disorder known as *perennial allergic conjunctivitis*. The seasonal form is the most common, accounting for 90% of all allergic conjunctivitis disorders. Acute allergic conjunctivitis can occur at any age, although onset of the perennial form is usually in infancy while the seasonal form usually appears between the ages of 20 and 40. The seasonal form is induced by airborne allergens such as ragweed and pollen, while the perennial form is induced by antigens such as dust, mites, animal dander and feathers. Patients with dry eyes may be more susceptible as the tear film, the natural barrier to antigens, is deficient (Table 3).

Symptoms

With acute allergic conjunctivitis, patients present with complaints of itchy eyes, frequently accompanied by a burning sensation and watery discharge. The itching is low grade. There is mild conjunctival inflammation (redness). There may be foreign body sensation and swelling of the lids. It is often associated with rhinitis. With the perennial form, symptoms are present throughout the year (although 79% of patients may have seasonal exacerbations), while the seasonal form appears during pollen season. Clinical features include exacerbations and remissions depending on allergen contact. For example, with seasonal allergic conjunctivitis, weather (e.g., worse when warm and dry), time of year or time of day (e.g., ragweed pollen counts are usually worse from 9 a.m. to noon), and environment (e.g., worse when outdoors during pollen season) influence symptoms. Acute allergic conjunctivitis is rarely a sight-threatening disease although patients complain of extreme and annoying discomfort. The frequency and severity of attacks tend to lessen as the patient ages.

Differential Diagnosis

Other forms of allergic conjunctivitis, such as vernal keratoconjunctivitis, giant papillary conjunctivitis and atopic keratoconjunctivitis should be differentiated from acute allergic conjunctivitis.

Vernal keratoconjunctivitis, also known as spring catarrh or warm weather conjunctivitis, is not common. It is a potentially serious condition as it can damage the cornea. It is usually a disease of young people beginning before age 10, burning out after 2 to 10 years. Males are affected twice as often as females, and there is often a family or personal history of an atopic condition such as asthma, eczema or seasonal rhinitis. It is more common in warm, dry (versus temperate) climates and almost nonexistent in cold climates. It usually presents from early spring until the fall. Specific allergens are difficult to identify, but these patients sometimes have additional pollen-related symptomatology (e.g., seasonal rhinitis).

The patient complains of severe, continuous itching and a thick, elastic, ropy discharge. There can also be burning, tearing and severe photophobia. The conjunctiva lining the upper eyelids has large inflammatory nodules that can have a cobblestone appearance.

Giant papillary conjunctivitis is usually associated with contact lens wear but can also be induced by other types of trauma to the conjunctiva lining the eyelids, such as plastic artificial eyes or post-operative sutures in the conjunctiva or cornea. The condition may also involve the cornea. The incidence is greater in individuals wearing soft (hydrophilic) contact lenses. The cause is unknown but is generally considered to include hypersensitivity (allergic) reactions to deposits on the lenses, mechanical trauma induced by the lens edge, or reactions to the lens material itself or to the components of lens care solutions (e.g., cleansing agents or preservatives).

Early symptoms may be minor such as lid discomfort or pain when contact lenses are removed, slightly blurred vision due to deposits on the lenses, mucus accumulation, mild tearing and mild itching. In the early stages it may resemble seasonal allergic conjunctivitis or early infectious conjunctivitis. As the disease progresses, there are large amounts of mucus discharged, the patient complains of foreign body sensation while wearing the lenses and upper lid "grabbing" of the contact lens (the contact lens may actually be pulled off the cornea onto the lid). There can be a mucous, milky discharge covering giant papillae, large inflammatory nodules on the underside of the upper lids. The giant papillae are smaller and flatter than those of vernal keratoconjunctivitis and generally do not have a cobblestone appearance.

Atopic keratoconjunctivitis may begin in the late teens, and peak incidence is in the 30 to 50 age group. Males are more affected than females. It is often associated with atopic dermatitis (eczema) beginning in childhood and with asthma. There is usually a family history of allergy. Seasonal variation and association with hot climates is less than with vernal keratoconjunctivitis although there may be exacerbations in either summer or winter in many patients. Many individuals report that animals, dust or foods may precipitate symptoms.

Atopic keratoconjunctivitis is characterized by moderate to severe itching, a burning sensation, swollen eyelids, a mucous discharge, photophobia, lid edema and loss of eyelashes. There may be potentially blinding damage to the cornea. The lid margins are red and the conjunctiva appears milky. Unlike vernal keratoconjunctivitis and giant papillary conjunctivitis, the inflammatory nodules are not giant sized and usually are enlarged on the lower rather than the upper underside of the eyelid. There may be secondary skin (e.g., eyelid) or corneal infections; severe dry eyes may also develop.

Treatment

Nonpharmacological Treatment

Management for acute allergic conjunctivitis is environmental control—the identification, then elimination of the causative antigen. Generally, this strategy is more successful for perennial rather than seasonal allergic conjunctivitis.

In perennial allergic conjunctivitis, if the causative agent is dust or animal dander, the removal of textile items (e.g., carpets, upholstered furniture, mattresses, stuffed animals) and regular vacuuming is beneficial. However, if dust mites are the culprit, special cleansing agents (e.g., acaracides such as benzyl benzoate compounds) may be needed to exterminate the mites. There are preliminary experiments suggesting that exposure (e.g., 3 to 6 hours) of carpets (pile side down on a concrete slab) to the direct summer sun may create a microenvironment of low humidity and high temperature that will kill both live mites and their eggs. It is thought that keeping items (e.g., plush toys wrapped in a bag) in the freezer for several days can also kill the mites.

Symptoms of seasonal allergic conjunctivitis may be reduced by modifying the environment (e.g., moving to a cooler, damper climate; staying indoors on hot, dry days or during high pollen count times of the day or year.)

For the mildly symptomatic patient, cool, moist compresses are often effective, as the vasculature and tissues affected are so superficial. Irrigation with an eye wash twice a day may also be helpful. Wearing cotton gloves may prevent rubbing and scratching.

During the allergy season, contact lenses may be poorly tolerated, and the individual may need to temporarily stop wearing them.

Pharmacological Treatment

Treatment of acute allergic conjunctivitis—seasonal and perennial—is primarily symptomatic.

For mild symptoms, artificial tears administered 4 to 6 times per day may provide relief as they keep the eye lubricated and augment the tear film to reduce allergen contact with the conjunctiva. Controlled clinical trials demonstrate a strong placebo effect when artificial tears are used for management of seasonal allergic conjunctivitis.

For more bothersome symptoms, an ophthalmic antihistamine and/or short-term use (< 4 days) of an ophthalmic decongestant may be useful. A combination ophthalmic product (e.g., a decongestant and antihistamine) may be more effective than either agent alone. They can successfully alleviate itching, redness and swelling. Oral antihistamines can also be helpful. With recurrent and/or moderate to severe cases of acute allergic conjunctivitis, individuals should be referred to an eye care professional. Prescription therapy may include the use of mast cell stabilizers (e.g., sodium cromoglycate, lodoxamide), oral or ophthalmic H_1-antihistamines (e.g., levocabastine), or nonsteroidal anti-inflammatory drugs (e.g., diclofenac ophthalmic drops). In chronic cases, corticosteroids (e.g., prednisolone or fluorometholone ophthalmic drops) may be needed.

CHEMICAL OR IRRITATIVE CONJUNCTIVITIS

Etiology

Numerous chemical substances can cause toxicity or hypersensitivity in the conjunctiva. These can include ophthalmic medications or preservatives (Table 10), personal hygiene items (e.g., soaps, deodorants, hair sprays, cosmetics), occupational hazards (e.g., acids, alkalies, fertilizers, fumigating agents, dry cleaning solutions, etc.) or environmental factors (e.g., wind, smog, tobacco smoke, chlorine in swimming pools).

Symptoms

Symptoms may occur minutes to hours after exposure or be delayed 1 to 2 days. The skin on the eyelids or around the eyes may be involved. Symptoms may vary from mild to severe with redness, irritation, tearing and a gritty foreign body sensa-

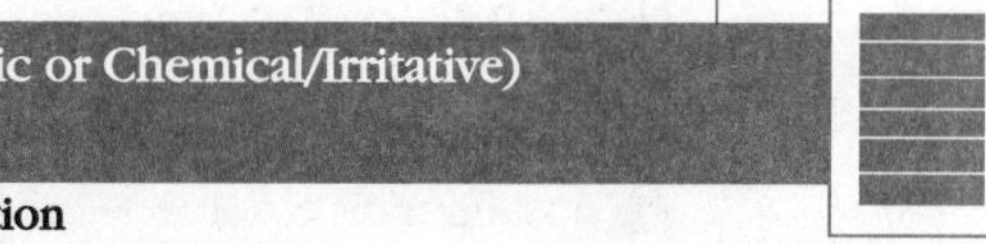

TABLE 10: Ophthalmic Preparations That May Cause Iatrogenic (Allergic or Chemical/Irritative) Conjunctivitis

Nonprescription	Prescription
Antihistamines	Glaucoma medications (e.g., timolol, pilocarpine)
Decongestants (prolonged instillation)	Anti-infectives (e.g., gentamicin, neomycin, sulfonamides, idoxuridine, trifluridine)
Miscellaneous ingredients (e.g., boric acid, lanolin)	Anesthetics (e.g., tetracaine)
Preservatives (e.g., benzalkonium chloride, thimerosal—in contact lens solutions)	Cycloplegics (e.g., atropine)

tion. With prolonged exposure to any chemical or acute exposure to a particularly noxious substance (e.g., acid, alkali) there may be permanent corneal and conjunctival damage. With some substances, signs and symptoms may persist for weeks or months. Acute exposure to noxious chemicals should be treated as a medical emergency (see the Trauma section).

Treatment

For chemical/irritative/allergic conjunctivitis associated with contact lens wear, see the Contact Lens Care section.

Nonpharmacological Treatment

The mainstay of therapy is to eliminate the offending substance. Cool compresses may provide symptomatic relief.

Pharmacological Treatment

For minor irritations (e.g., loose foreign material, exposure to smog or chlorinated swimming pool water) an eye wash will promote removal of the chemical or irritant. For other minor irritations (e.g., minor exposure to wind, sun) artificial tears will provide temporary symptomatic relief. The patient should be informed that symptoms may persist for several days even after the causative agent is eliminated. Use of ophthalmic decongestants is discouraged as they may mask symptoms of continuing toxic reactions. Antihistamines appear to be of little value in this type of reaction as it is usually not an immediate hypersensitivity reaction. If inflammation is severe or nonresponsive within 48 hours, the individual should be referred to an eye care professional.

SUBCONJUNCTIVAL HEMORRHAGE

Subconjunctival hemorrhage appears when a conjunctival vessel ruptures. This can occur in any age group from numerous causes (Table 11).

Symptoms

A bright red patch appears on the sclera, usually in only one eye.

Treatment

The individual should be referred to an eye care professional to rule out serious disorders. In most instances, no treatment is required; the hemorrhage gradually fades over a period of 2 to 3 weeks.

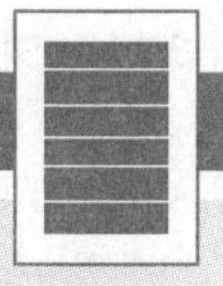

TABLE 11: Some Causes of Subconjunctival Hemorrhage
Severe or minimal trauma (e.g., following a severe blow or after rubbing the eye)
Sudden rise in venous pressure, particularly in the elderly (e.g., coughing, straining, sneezing, vomiting)
Systemic disease (e.g., hypertension, blood dyscrasias)
Adenovirus/bacterial conjunctivitis
Spontaneous (unknown cause)

DRY EYE

Dry eye can be a serious problem, the result of deficiency of any of the tear film components or defective spreading of the tear film (Table 12). This can cause tear film instability, which may have mild consequences initially but progress to potentially vision-threatening ocular surface damage.

SYMPTOMS

Individuals with dry eye most frequently complain of a sandy, gritty sensation that may have remissions and exacerbations. Other common symptoms include redness, itching, inability to produce tears, burning sensation, excessive mucus secretion, photosensitivity and difficulty moving the eyelids. The eye may appear normal in mild cases. Ophthalmic examination is necessary to determine the cause of dry eye (e.g., tear production deficiency, unstable tear film, etc.). Initially, vision may be slightly impaired (optical properties of tear film are disrupted), and the person may be mildly uncomfortable. Eventually it may result in corneal ulceration/scarring, severe discomfort and secondary bacterial infection.

TREATMENT

Mild to moderate cases of dry eye generally respond well to artificial tears and lubricants. Treatment of severe dry eye is chronic and complete relief is probably not achievable.

Nonpharmacological Treatment

Cool, moist compresses may give symptomatic relief to burning, dry eyes. Environmental changes

TABLE 12: Some Causes of Dry Eye

Cause	Examples
Aqueous deficiency Caused by hypofunction of the lacrimal glands	Aging Medications - anticholinergics (e.g., atropine, tricyclic antidepressants) - antihistamines - cardiovascular drugs (e.g., diuretics, beta-blockers) Sjögren's syndrome (a chronic connective tissue disease that occurs predominantly in middle-aged women and is characterized by dry mouth, dry eyes with or without rheumatic disorder) Excessive evaporation (dry climate or lipid deficiency)
Lipid deficiency Caused by hypofunction or loss of sebaceous glands	Lid margin scarring Blepharitis
Mucin deficiency Caused by hypofunction or loss of special conjunctival cells	Stevens-Johnson syndrome Chemical burns Chronic conjunctivitis Avitaminosis A
Impaired spreading of the tear film	Altered blink reflex - thyroid disorders - medications (eg., sedatives, muscle relaxants, antihistamines) Lid closure abnormalities Contact lens wear Altered corneal surface

(e.g., reduction of room temperature, use of room humidifiers, wearing of protective eyeglasses with side pieces, swimming goggles) may be beneficial.

Pharmacological Treatment

Tear film supplementation or eye lubrication are the basis of management. Frequent instillation of artificial tears (up to 6 times daily) can be tried. For more frequent use, preservative-free unit dose artificial tears should be used. In moderate to severe cases, artificial tears in combination with nighttime use of a bland ophthalmic lubricant ointment can be effective. If these procedures are unsuccessful or if the condition persists for more than 72 hours, the individual should be referred to an eye care professional. Long-term use of artificial tears should be under the supervision of an eye care professional to reduce the risk of irreversible ocular surface damage.

FIGURE 3

Suggested Approach for Treating Blepharitis/Conjunctivitis/Dry Eye

Condition	Basic Care	Self-Treatment	Referral to Eye Care Professional
Pain, photophobia, altered vision, redness immediately around cornea, severe redness of the conjunctiva or eyelids, excessive discharge, abnormal pupils, floating spots (sudden appearance), trauma, headache, patient is a child or elderly person, severe underlying medical conditions, nonprescription medication does not clear up the problem within 48–72 hours, conditions generally lasting longer than 48 hours			Yes (immediately)
Blepharitis due to infection and/or seborrhea	• warm, moist compresses for 5–15 minutes, 4 times daily • lid cleansing, at least twice daily • separate towels from other family members	• if co-existent seborrhea, use anti-seborrheic shampoo 1–2 times weekly (avoid ocular contact), and artificial tears 2–4 times daily • nonprescription anti-infective eye ointment (e.g., bacitracin) 3–5 times daily for 1 week (for chronic condition, acute treatment then maintenance treatment at bedtime for 4–8 weeks)	if ineffective → Yes
Blepharitis associated with initial occurrence of single stye	• warm moist compresses for 10–15 minutes 3–4 times daily • separate towels from other family members • do not squeeze	• nonprescription anti-infective eye ointment (e.g., bacitracin) may prevent spread	if ineffective → Yes
Blepharitis associated with multiple styes or stye persisting for longer than 48 hours			Yes
Blepharitis associated with minor chalazion	• warm, moist compresses 4 times daily	• nonprescription anti-infective eye ointment may prevent secondary infection	if ineffective → Yes
Blepharitis associated with severe or recurrent chalazion			Yes
Blepharitis due to irritant or allergen	• eliminate cause • cool, moist compresses for several minutes several times daily		if ineffective → Yes

FIGURE 3 *(cont'd)*

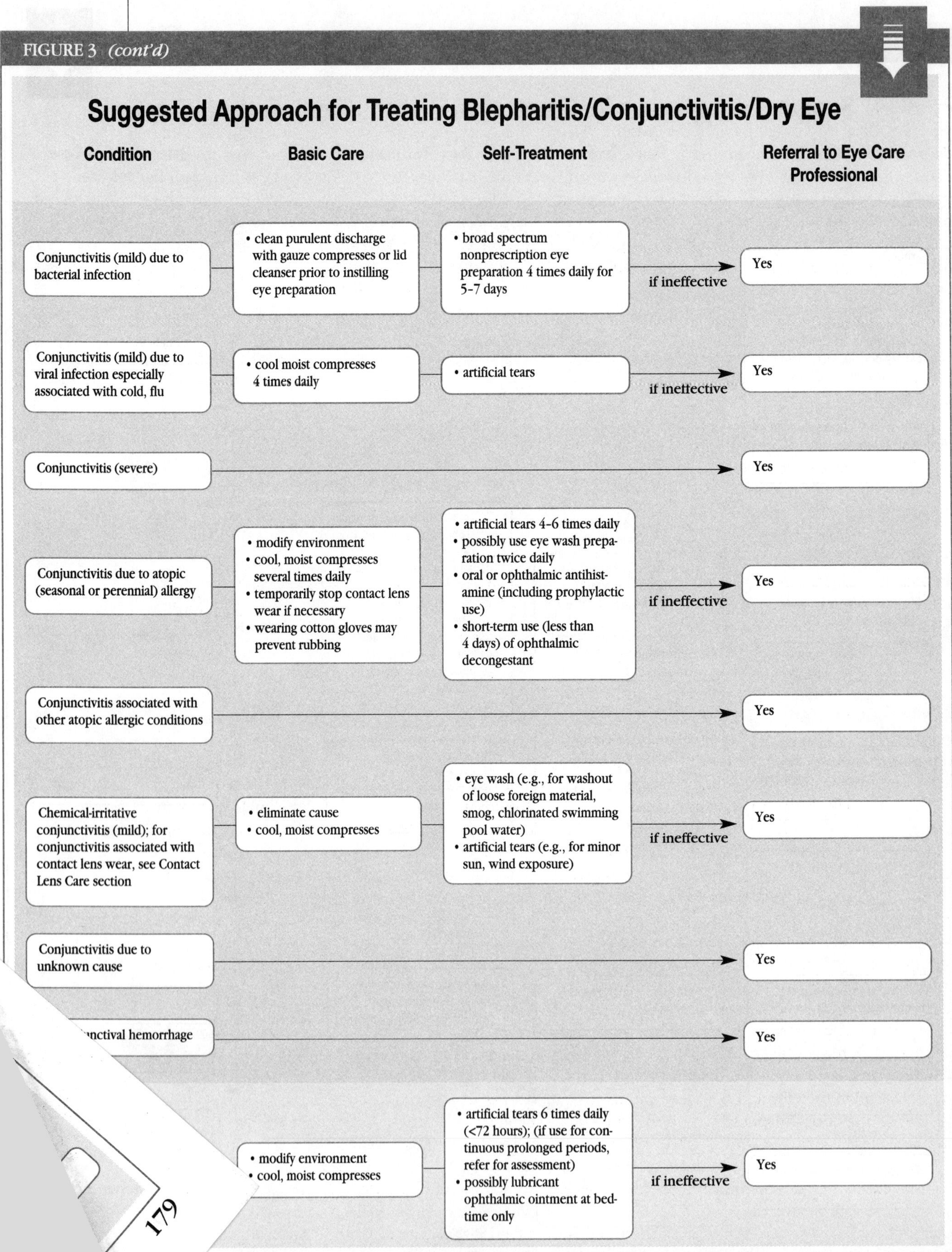

TRAUMA

Trauma to the eye may require immediate attention. Bleeding, pain, photophobia and decreased vision indicate serious eye injury. Immediate steps should be taken to implement appropriate first-aid measures that may prevent blindness. A shield (e.g., bottom third of a paper cup) taped over the eye may help to prevent further damage during transport to a hospital or emergency clinic.

Contusion from a blunt instrument (e.g., fist, baseball, hockey puck, golf ball, squash ball or champagne cork) is characterized by the familiar black eye (edema, lid discoloration, lid closure) and sometimes double vision. Immediate ocular examination is necessary to rule out severe underlying damage. During transport to medical aid, cold compresses can reduce the swelling and provide comfort. Pressure must not be applied, particularly if there is obvious rupture of the eye.

Laceration caused by high-velocity blunt objects (e.g., car steering wheel) or sharp objects (e.g., a knife, a pencil or flying metal from using a hammer and chisel or power tool) is a medical emergency. With these injuries, it is important to avoid applying pressure as this can further damage the eye. Even wiping away tears or blood may increase the damage. Protruding objects (e.g., a fishhook) should not be removed. The individual should be immobilized and transferred to the nearest emergency clinic or ophthalmologist. The longer the delay, the greater the risk of damage and infection.

Foreign body damage varies in severity. If the particle is on the conjunctiva, blinking and tearing may be enough to remove the object. If these processes are ineffective, the particle may be wiped out using a spindle of facial tissue or moistened cotton-tipped applicator, or washed out using an eye wash or normal saline solution. The individual should avoid rubbing the eye, because rubbing may embed the particle further. If the pain continues, if there is still a foreign body sensation or if the particle is seen on the cornea, there may be corneal abrasion. A foreign object must only be removed from the cornea by an eye care professional. Continued abrasion by a foreign body can predispose the eye to infection—especially by opportunistic pathogens that cause severe corneal ulceration (e.g., *Pseudomonas*). The eye must be lightly covered, and the person transferred for ocular examination and treatment.

Chemical burns require emergency first aid as soon as possible. They may result from splashing household or industrial products (e.g., plaster, dishwasher granules, bleach, toilet cleansers, ammonia) into the eye. An antidote should not be used. Immediate, prolonged (20 to 30 minutes) irrigation of the surface of the eye prevents permanent scarring more effectively than any other treatment. This washing is best achieved by having the individual lie down and firmly holding the eye under a slow, steady stream of cool water (or sterile normal saline) while the individual blinks. (A bowl can be held next to the face to try to catch the irrigant.) Such washing is uncomfortable and gradually produces a numbing coldness of the eye. The washed eye will likely be bloodshot after the washing. Any particulate matter needs to be removed. After copious washing (e.g., with 2 L of fluid) for at least another 20 minutes, further medical attention is essential. Watch for respiratory distress as there may be swelling of the soft tissues of the upper airway as a result of systemic absorption.

Thermal burns most commonly damage the eyelids but may also damage the cornea, iris or retina. Ultraviolet (UV) radiation can injure the cornea, resulting in pain, photophobia, tearing, blurred vision and foreign body sensation 6 to 12 hours after exposure. Welders refer to the condition as arc-eye or flashburn and snow-skiers call it snow-blindness. Other sources causing UV ocular damage include sunlamps and reflections from bright sand or sea when protective sunglasses are not worn. The condition is self-limiting but requires the attention of an eye care professional. Treatment may include instillation of antibiotic eye drops (to reduce the risk of infection), the use of drugs that relax the muscles inside the eye (to provide comfort, especially from photophobia), as well as administration of oral analgesics and use of eye patches.

Other types of radiant energy damage occur on exposure to infrared radiation (e.g., watching a total eclipse of the sun without eye protection) or excessive x-ray radiation. The individual should be referred to an eye care professional.

Hard (PMMA) contact lenses worn for periods in excess of suggested routines (e.g., overwear syndrome) may cause severe pain and photophobia several hours after the contacts are removed (see the Contact Lens Care section). The individual should be referred to an eye care professional. The contact lenses should not be reinserted for at least a day or two afterward, and preferably only after a complete eye and lens examination.

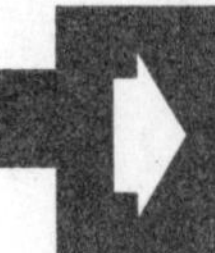

ADVICE FOR THE PATIENT

Instillation of Ophthalmic Solutions

- Wash hands thoroughly.
- Carefully remove the bottle cap and avoid contaminating the rim or inner side of the cap (lay it on its side on a clean, dry tissue).
- Tilt head back or lie down.
- If the medication is a suspension, shake before using.
- While eyes are open, grasp the lower lid below the eyelashes and gently pull the lid away from the eye to form a pouch. (If you cannot make a pouch, gently pull down on the lower lid.)
- Approach the eye from the side, with the long axis of the dropper or bottle parallel to the lid margin. This reduces the risk of accidentally hitting the eye with the container tip.
- Hold the tip near the lid, but at least 2.5 cm (1 inch) away. Do not touch the lids or lashes.
- Look toward the ceiling. Looking up moves the cornea away from the instillation site, minimizing the blink reflex.
- Instil 1 drop into the pouch. Hold this position to let the drop fall as deep as possible into the pouch.
- Look down for several seconds and then slowly release the lower lid. Looking down brings the cornea into maximum contact with the instilled drug. (This is especially important for infections of the cornea.)
- Gently close (do not squeeze) the eyes for at least 30 seconds (up to 5 minutes). A tissue may be used to blot around the eye, but do not rub. Closing the eye helps prevent loss and reduces the rate of systemic absorption of the solution caused by blinking. If the eye is closed too tightly, the medication may be expelled.
- Applying gentle pressure across the bridge of the nose with your thumb and forefinger may also help prevent loss and systemic absorption via the nasolacrimal duct. If you have recently undergone eye surgery, ask your ophthalmologist whether pressure should be applied to the bridge of the nose.
- Before opening the eye, blot away excess medication. Do not rub the eye. Try not to blink.
- Do not rinse the eye drop container tip. Replace the bottle cap.
- Wash hands thoroughly.
- If multiple drops are prescribed, wait 3 to 5 minutes between the instillation of each drop. This ensures the first drop is not flushed away and the second drop is not diluted by the first.
- If multiple medications are used, wait 5 to 10 minutes between medications.

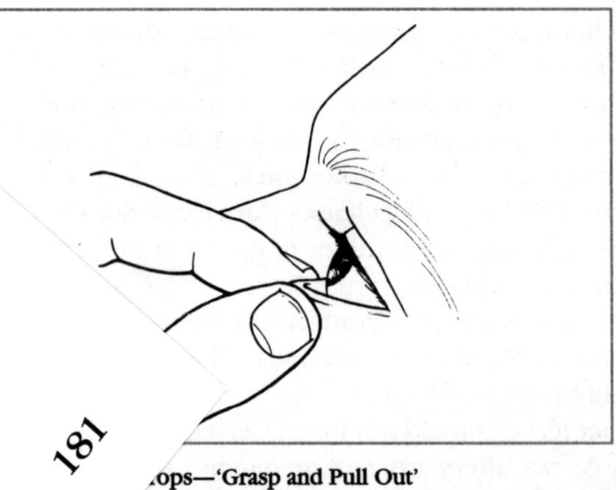

…ops—'Grasp and Pull Out'

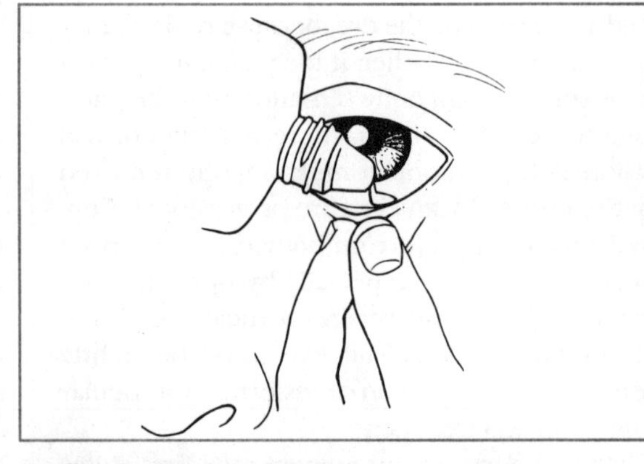

Instilling Eye Drops

181

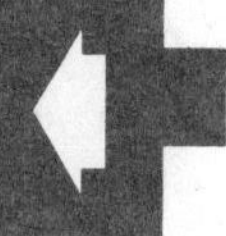

ADVICE FOR THE PATIENT

Special Considerations

- If you have problems with balance or dizziness, while using your eye product, lie down or sit down in a very stable position to reduce the risk of falling.
- If you have tremors or arthritis, devices are available that can help you administer eye drops. Discuss this with your pharmacist or eye care professional.

Special Advice for Instilling Eye Drops in Children

- Wash your hands thoroughly.
- **Positioning:**
  Have the child lie down and close the eyes.

  Alternate Method
  For infants and small children who may not cooperate, an alternative method can be tried. Sit on the floor and have the child sit on your lap—legs astride yours—facing you. While supporting the back and head, gently lower the child backward until he or she is lying along your legs. You have the option of having your own legs at an angle toward your body. Several options are then available, according to the control desired. With the child supine, hold the head with one hand and instil drops with the other on the side you are holding. In very resistant cases, the child's head may be gently clamped between your legs, and the feet wedged against your body under your arms. Either procedure can be done with the assistance of a third individual.
- **Instillation:**
  Approach the eye holding the long axis of the container parallel to the lid margin, resting the hand on the child's cheek to prevent injury to the eye if the child moves suddenly.
  Instil the drops as previously discussed.

  Alternate Methods:
  1. Use the *closed eye method*: Place the drop on the eyelid in the inner corner of the eye, then have the child open the eye so the drop falls in by gravity. (This method is also useful for adults with a strong blink reflex.)
  2. Pull the lower lid down and instil the drop through the lashes, avoiding touching the bottle to the lashes.
  3. If the instillation of drops or ointment application is important (e.g., to deal with an infected eye), it is better, although not ideal, to get some drops or ointment on the lids and lashes (keeping the lids closed momentarily) and allow the preparation to seep onto the surface of the eye, than for no drops or ointment to be used at all.

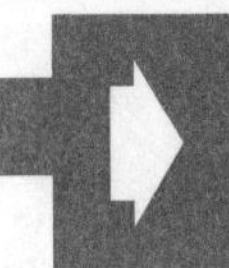

ADVICE FOR THE PATIENT

Administration of Ophthalmic Ointments

- Wash hands thoroughly.
- Hold the tube in your hand for a few minutes to warm the ointment and facilitate flow. Remove the container cap (lay it on its side on a clean, dry tissue).
- When opening the tube for the first time, squeeze out and discard the first 0.25 cm of ointment as it may be too dry.
- Tilt head back or lie down.
- While your eyes are open, grasp the lower lid below the eyelashes and gently pull the lid away from the eye to form a pouch. (If you cannot make a pouch, gently pull down on the lower lid.)
- Approach the eye from the side, with the long axis of the tube parallel to the lid margin.
- Hold the tip near the lid. Do not touch the lids or lashes.
- Look toward the ceiling. Looking up moves the cornea away from the instillation site, minimizing the blink reflex.
- Place 0.5 to 1 cm (¼ to ½ inch) of ointment into the pouch. It is not necessary to place the ointment along the entire length of the pouch.
- Gently close the eye for 1 to 2 minutes and roll the eyeball in all directions.
- Replace the container cap.
- After the ointment is used, vision may be blurred for a few minutes; do not drive or operate machinery until blurriness disappears.
- Using a clean tissue, remove excess ointment from the lid margins.
- Wash hands thoroughly.
- If both an ointment and solution are used, use the solution first. Wait at least 5 minutes before using the ointment.
- If different types of ointments are to be used, wait about 10 minutes before using the second one.
- If ointments are to be applied to the outer eyelids, place the ointment on a sterile cotton-tipped applicator and apply to the lid.

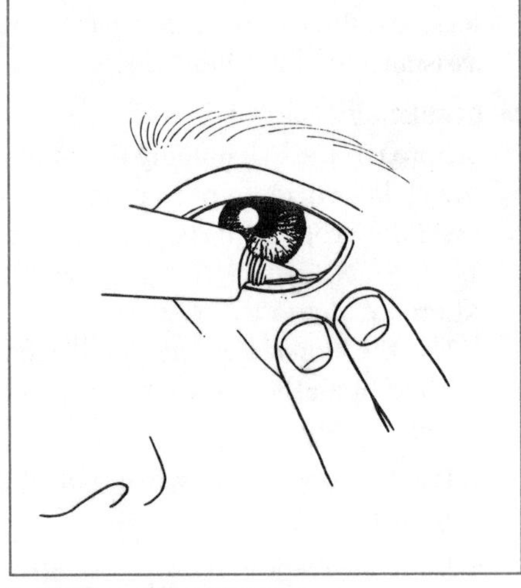

Instillation of Eye Ointment

ADVICE FOR THE PATIENT

Use of Ophthalmic Products

- For external use only.
- Never share your eye products with another person.
- Tightly close containers.
- Store in a cool, dark place.
- Discard the product:
  - if it changes color;
  - if it changes and becomes cloudy (or if particles appear);
  - if it was opened more than 1 month ago;
  - immediately after use if it is a single (or unit) dose package (without preservatives); it is intended for a single use only—do not reuse leftover product.
- Keep out of reach of children.
- If you are having difficulties administering your eye product, have a family member or friend assist you.
- Thoroughly wash hands before and after using the product.
- Never contaminate the container tip by allowing it to touch the eyes, eyelids, eyelashes, fingers or counter surface. This applies to the cap of the container as well. Replace the cap as soon as possible.
- Use only as directed.
- Some products may temporarily blur vision; therefore, be cautious while driving or performing other hazardous tasks.
- Discontinue the medication and see your eye care professional if:
  - you experience eye pain;
  - your eyes are sensitive to light;
  - you experience visual changes;
  - the eye irritation and redness continues;
  - self-medicating for more than 48 hours (with anti-infectives) or 72 hours (with other agents) does not clear up the condition or the condition worsens;
  - without treatment the condition has lasted longer than 48 hours.

PATIENT ASSESSMENT QUESTIONS

Q ***Is this problem with your own eyes, or another person's eyes?***
Age is important, particularly in the case of an infant (due to the possibility of congenital disorders or low resistance to infection) or an older individual (due to the increased risk of angle-closure glaucoma). These individuals may also be more sensitive to ophthalmic decongestants.

Q ***How are your eyes bothering you?***
Ask the consumer to describe the problem using their own words. Depending on the reply, the following questions may be applicable.

Q ***Is there pain or photophobia? Does it feel as though something is in your eye (foreign body sensation)?***
Pain or photophobia (eye discomfort induced by bright lights) may indicate a severe disease process. Superficial foreign body sensation may indicate a lesion on the eyelid, something on the conjunctiva or cornea, or inflammation of the conjunctiva or cornea. Sharp pain is usually associated with corneal disease; dull, severe aching pain can be associated with disease or other severe disorders of the inside of the eye. All these conditions require medical attention. Herpes simplex keratitis is an exception, because recurrent infection may reduce corneal sensation so pain is not a prominent symptom. Untreated, it can cause blindness.

Eye drops may be requested for ocular pain associated with headache, blurring vision, redness of the eyes and colored halos around lights. Consumers may associate these symptoms with tired eyes. Nausea, vomiting and sweating can also occur. On questioning, individuals may admit to ocular discomfort in the evening, when watching television or a movie in a darkened room, or during periods of anxiety. This history suggests the patient may have experienced an attack of angle-closure glaucoma. These attacks of ocular discomfort may be self-limiting, especially when the person is exposed to light. For example, an individual may have ocular pain while watching television, but the symptoms are relieved upon entering a well-lit room. The ocular discomfort probably has subsided by the time the person seeks help, but a product for future use may be requested. The patient must be referred to an eye care professional.

Q ***Are your eyes burning and itchy?***
Burning, stinging and an uncomfortable feeling in the eye are seldom characteristic of serious eye disease. Usually these symptoms are only annoying and may be treated with nonprescription medications; however, infectious conjunctivitis requires medical treatment.

Itching may be a sign of ocular allergy. If the symptoms are mild, nonprescription medications can provide symptomatic relief.

Q ***Is your vision normal? Blurred? Double? Spotty?***
Vision may be normal in blepharitis, conjunctivitis and systemic disease. Sudden or gradual vision loss can indicate ocular disease (e.g., hemorrhage, infection, glaucoma or cataracts) or systemic disease (e.g., diabetes, hypertension, transient ischemic attacks, cerebral artery occlusion or blood dyscrasias). Double vision indicates the eyes are not pointing in the same direction (e.g., in ocular muscle disorders or following trauma). Spotty vision may indicate the presence of debris in the vitreous humor (floaters), which may be due to serious disease (e.g., retinal detachment). The individual should be referred for an eye examination, particularly if elderly.

Q ***Are your eyes red?***
Depending on the characteristics and location of redness, the problem may be extremely serious. Except for temporary, mild cases of irritative conjunctivitis, seasonal or perennial allergic conjunctivitis or dry eyes, medical attention is necessary.

Q ***Is there discharge? Excessive tearing?***
Discharge that is purulent (eyelashes may be stuck together on awakening), foamy or stringy may signify bacterial infection or severe allergic conjunctivitis. Clear, watery discharge may indicate viral infection.

?

PATIENT ASSESSMENT QUESTIONS (*cont'd*)

Excessive tearing appears in most inflammatory (e.g., uveitis) and allergic conditions of the eye. It also accompanies photophobia. Tear overflow can result from blockage of the lacrimal drainage system or abnormality of the eyelid.

Q ***Do you have dry eyes?***
Chronic alteration of the tear film may result in permanent scarring of the external surfaces of the eye. An individual with persistent dry eyes should be referred to their eye care professional.

Q ***Are the pupils of the eyes normal?***
Constricted pupils can be a sign of inflammation inside the eye (e.g., iritis). Semi-dilated or oval-shaped pupils may accompany acute stages of glaucoma. Unequal pupils may indicate injury to the pupil or a head trauma.

Q ***Where were you and what were you doing when you first noticed the symptoms?***
The person may have been exposed to pollutants (dust or wind), may have splashed a chemical in the eye, may have had a small piece of metal penetrate the eye or may have been exposed to excessive ultraviolet radiation (skiing or welding-arc flash). The last three are all medical emergencies.

Q ***Do you wear contact lenses? Which contact lens products do you use?***
Some contact lenses, when worn for prolonged periods, may cause pain and photophobia several hours after they are removed. Many nonprescription ophthalmic medications should not be used when lenses, particularly soft lenses, are in the eye. Some people may be sensitive to ingredients in the contact lens products. (See the Contact Lens Care section.)

Q ***Do you have any allergies?***
Anyone who suffers from hayfever may have accompanying acute allergic conjunctivitis. The person may be sensitive to cosmetics and have an allergic blepharitis. Components of nonprescription ophthalmic products may cause allergic reactions.

Q ***Have you had similar episodes before?***
If this problem is recurrent, it may have serious complications and should be referred to an eye care professional.

Q ***How long have you had the problem? Have you used any medications for it? Which one(s)?***
In general, any condition that persists for more than 48 hours should be examined by an eye care professional. The individual may have rebound conjunctival hyperemia due to overuse of ophthalmic decongestants.

Q ***Are you under the care of a physician for any medical conditions (e.g., diabetes, cardiovascular disease, high blood pressure, hyperthyroidism, glaucoma)? Are you pregnant?***
The person may have lowered resistance to infection. These conditions may place limitations on self-treatment.

Q ***Are you taking other medications (prescription or nonprescription)?***
Numerous prescribed medications can cause ocular or visual problems (e.g., oral antihistamines: blurred vision, reduced tear volume and decreased blink reflex; antidepressants: blurred vision; digoxin: blurred or yellow vision).

CONTACT LENS CARE

Pathophysiology

Tears constantly bathe the cornea supplying oxygen. Contact lenses are foreign bodies that sit on a tear cushion and do not actually contact the eye, as implied by their name. All contact lenses act as physical barriers, interfering with the supply of oxygen from the tears to the cornea, producing progressive hypoxia and edema. Whether clinical symptoms result depends on duration of wear, compliance with care regimen, lens materials, lens design and fit.

Indications

Contact lenses can correct hyperopia, myopia, astigmatism, presbyopia and aphakia. Hyperopia and myopia are errors in refraction where parallel rays of light do not focus properly on the retina. In hyperopia (farsightedness), light focuses behind the retina, causing near objects to be blurry while distant objects are focused. In myopia (nearsightedness), light focuses before reaching the retina, causing near objects to be focused and distant objects to be blurry (Figure 4). In astigmatism, the shape of the eye or cornea is oval or elliptical, causing parallel rays of light to intersect at two different points. Presbyopia is part of natural aging where control of the state of contraction of the ciliary muscle for accommodation is decreased, resulting in progressive decline in clear vision for near objects. In aphakia, the lens is absent, either congenitally, or more likely, due to surgery for removal of a cataract (loss of transparency of lens). Aphakic individuals have reduced near and far vision.

TYPES OF CONTACT LENSES

(For a summary of the advantages and disadvantages of hard, gas permeable and soft contact lenses, see Table 13.)

Hard (PMMA) Lenses

Hard, polymethylmethacrylate (PMMA) contact lenses are almost obsolete in Canada. The two types are corneal (small), which make up the vast majority of hard lenses, and scleral (large).

Gas Permeable Lenses

The rigid gas permeable (RGP) lens was developed to combine the optical qualities and durability of PMMA with the oxygen permeability and comfort of soft contact lenses. These lenses have a sufficiently high oxygen permeability to prevent clini-

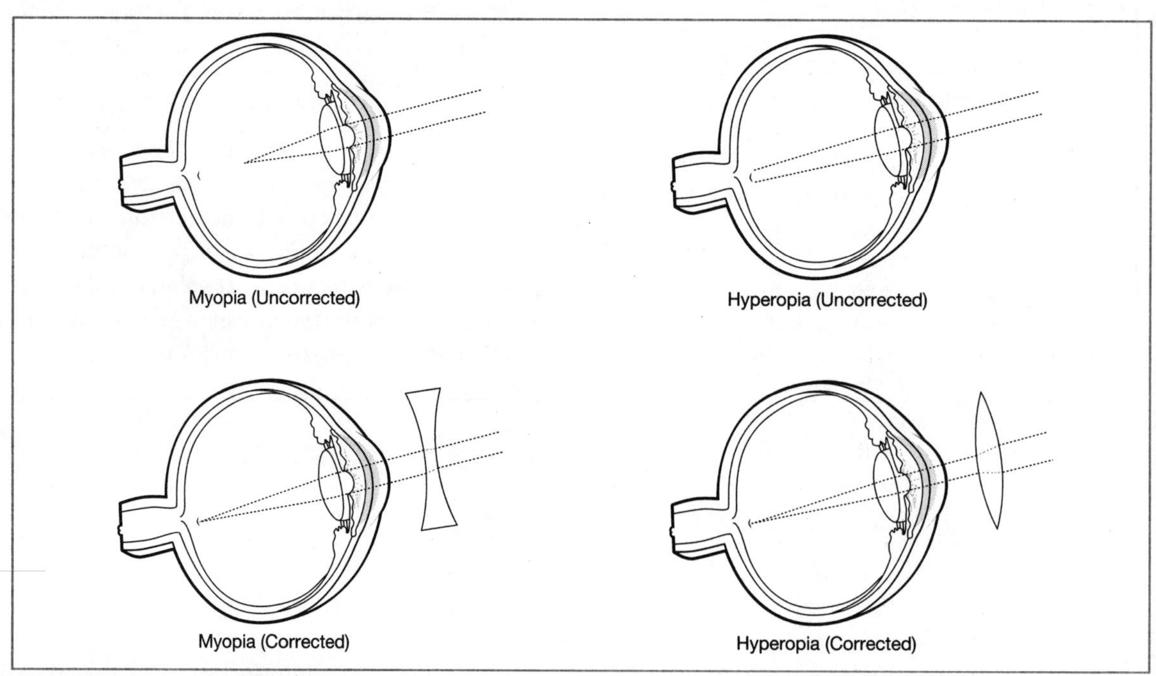

FIGURE 4: Hyperopia and Myopia

cally observable corneal edema in normal wear, leading to fewer complications and, in general, better long-term visual acuity than either hard (PMMA) or soft lenses. The two main types are: silicone/acrylate and fluorinated silicone-acrylate. The major difference is the fluorine that allows even greater oxygen permeability, surface wettability and flexibility.

Soft (Hydrogel) Lenses

Soft contacts are made of a flexible polymeric material, hydroxyethylmethacrylate (HEMA), with a high capacity for water absorption. Increased comfort is the main advantage and is due to flexibility (which increases with greater water content), soft thin edges, hydrophilic nature, and large diameter. In addition to correcting refractive errors, these lenses are used to protect the cornea (e.g., exposure keratitis), prevent corneal scarring (e.g., following chemical burns) and administer drugs (e.g., pilocarpine for glaucoma).

Soft lenses have a short adaptation time (Table 13). Unfortunately, their open matrix concentrates ophthalmic preparations, environmental pollutants, chemical vapors, oil and dust from fingers, cosmetics and some contact lens solution preservatives, all of which can lead to ocular irritation. These materials also tend to develop lens deposits more rapidly than hard or gas permeable materials.

Silicone Lenses

Silicone lenses have a high permeability for oxygen and other gases. Due to production and maintenance problems that led to poor demand, silicone lenses were discontinued in 1985. The lens is still available on a limited basis for certain aphakic conditions.

Flexible Wear

Extended wear is defined as wearing a contact lens for 24 hours or more. The lenses are usually soft and vary in thickness relative to the water content.

Early uncontrolled trials suggested that the rate of serious complications with extended wear was not excessive and many wearers adopted them. Unfortunately their tremendous growth was associated with reports of microbial keratitis, with *Pseudomonas aeruginosa* being the most frequent isolate, which caused some patients to lose vision and possibly their eyes. *Pseudomonas aeruginosa* is environmentally widespread and has been found in high concentrations in contact lens storage solutions. It has been suggested that contamination of lenses from poor hygiene and handling is responsible for transferring *Pseudomonas* to the eye. The risk increases incrementally with length of extended wear. More careful lens hygiene lowers the risk. With extended wear, solutions became contaminated because they are used up very slowly. There was a 22% contamination rate of solutions used for extended wear lenses compared to 6% with daily wear. For extended wear, solutions should be discarded after 21 days, and lens containers thoroughly cleaned before each use. The increased risk of extended wear may be due to the combination of hypoxia from overnight wear, poor hygiene, build-up of lens deposits, constant exposure of the cornea to pathogens bound to the lens and the breakdown of the epithelial barrier from physiological, chemical and/or mechanical stress. Table 14 summarizes the relative risk of ulcerative keratitis according to type of lens and wear. To decrease the frequency of infection, the U.S. Food and Drug Administration (FDA) recommended that extended wear soft lenses be worn from 1 to 7 days before removal for cleaning/disinfection or disposal. Most practitioners encourage daily wear (e.g., 10 to 12 hours/day at most). Frequent lens removal and replacement should help minimize the incidence of complications. A 2,400 patient study found that users of extended wear disposables are just as likely as users of conventional extended wear lenses to develop corneal ulcers. However, patients using disposables typically experienced small peripheral ulcers while those using conventional lenses almost always developed central ones. The major advantage of disposable lenses is a lower incidence of giant papillary conjunctivitis.

Some wearers, who have encountered problems with soft lenses (e.g., lens deposits and side effects), have tried gas permeable lenses for extended wear. Recent data indicate they can be worn safely for extended periods. These lenses may have fewer risks than soft lenses and offer superior vision.

Disposable Contact Lenses

Unlike conventional extended wear lenses, which are cleaned and disinfected, disposable lenses are worn once, discarded and replaced by a new lens at intervals determined by the manufacturer. The need for daily cleaning and weekly enzyme cleaning is eliminated or reduced if these lenses are worn on an extended wear basis. However, daily cleaning is essential if the disposable lenses are worn on a daily wear basis. Disposable lenses are expected to eliminate or decrease the problems associated with lens deposits and allergic reactions to solutions, but side effects such as sterile corneal infiltrates, corneal ulcers and pseudomonas keratitis have been reported. Compliance is expected to be easier, but case reports exist of the development of keratitis in noncompliant wearers (reinserting disposable lenses without disinfection, absence of daily cleaning, or inadequate disinfection). The increased cost of disposable lenses has prompted some consumers to wear them longer than recommended. A recent study indicates that disposable

TABLE 13: Comparison of the Different Types of Contact Lenses

Characteristics	Hard (PMMA)	Gas Permeable	Soft
Composition	Polymethylmethacrylate (PMMA)	Silicone/acrylate, fluorinated silicone-acrylate	Hydroxyethylmethacrylate (HEMA) is the most common polymer
Water content	Up to 1.5%	2–3% (only slightly greater than PMMA lenses)	29–85%
Life expectancy*	About 5 yrs	About 2–4 yrs (if there is no warping)	1 wk–2 yrs
Solution requirements	Hard lens solutions	Gas permeable solutions	Soft lens solutions
Advantages	Excellent visual acuity; can be polished if surface is scratched; may last 15 to 20 years; relatively inexpensive to replace and maintain; both hard and gas permeable lenses are able to correct some vision problems (e.g., keratoconus, astigmatism) better than soft lenses	*Over hard (PMMA) lenses*: increased comfort; increased wearing time; elimination of overwear syndrome; rapid adaptation to glasses after lens removal; decreased risk of lens loss *Over soft lenses*: superior optics; increased durability; decreased risk of lens discoloration with various chemicals; less likely to be contaminated; easier to care for; more prescriptions are possible; rigidity is advantageous in keratoconus	Flexibility allows easy insertion and removal; large size facilitates easy fitting and decreased risk of lens loss; close fit prevents entry of wind and dust which can scratch cornea; useful for athletes and children since they do not pop out easily; maximum wear time is achieved within days of fitting; ideal for occasional use because of short adaptation period; alternating with glasses is not a problem
Disadvantages	Gas impermeable material, may warp, crack or chip requiring replacement; short wear time; small size and relative rigidity can lead to popping out and subsequent loss; blurred vision from corneal swelling for about 1 hour when glasses are used after lens removal; corneal abrasion can occur if dust or other particles are caught underneath lens; up to 1 month may be required to gradually establish maximum wearing time; hydrophobic; overwear syndrome	Hydrophobic-wetting required for compatibility with the eye; possibly less comfortable than soft lenses; less durable and more susceptible to protein deposits than PMMA lenses; cannot be tinted as readily as hard or soft lenses	Compared to hard lenses they are more fragile (easily torn by fingernails) and more susceptible to protein and calcium deposits from tearfilm (due to "open matrix"); are only suitable for about 80% of potential wearers; high altitude and low humidity can decrease visual acuity; low oxygen pressures can decrease the oxygen received by cornea, resulting in corneal swelling and decreased vision; low humidity can increase the rate of tear evaporation causing lenses to dry and become uncomfortable; risk of microbial contamination

*When soft or gas permeable lenses are used for extended wear, the lens life averages 8–10 months although the individual life is highly variable and is dependent on length of time between cleanings, amount of ocular secretions, user handling and fragility of the lens.

soft lens users are three times more likely than conventional daily wear users to develop ulcerative keratitis. This is thought due to those who wear their disposable lenses overnight more often than conventional daily wearers. The vast majority of patients use their disposable lenses for the recommended period of time.

Acanthamoeba keratitis has become more common, likely due to the popularity of contact lenses. *Acanthamoeba* is widespread in the environment making avoidance impossible. It adheres to soft lenses and has been found in the lens cases of asymptomatic wearers. Serious infections may require penetrating keratoplasty or enucleation. The organism exists as either a rapidly growing trophozoite or when conditions become unfavorable for growth, a protective cyst that can survive extremes of temperature and pH.

Current literature supports a lower risk of ulceration in patients who use extended wear disposables compared to conventional extended wear lenses. The risk of ulceration is lower for disposables worn on a daily wear basis than for conventional daily wear lenses. The risk of ulceration is always higher with an extended wear regimen.

Planned Replacement Programs (PRPs)

Also known as disposable or frequent replacement programs (D/FRP), this development occurred because of poor compliance with extended wear lenses. In a PRP, a wearer will wear lenses on a daily basis and dispose of them either monthly or quarterly, depending on lens type. Many PRP lenses are the same as those marketed to be disposed of more frequently. They are sold in sets of 4 or 12. Advantages include: regular insertion of a sterile lens, less cost from reduced need for solutions, improved vision, improved comfort, improved compliance, more convenience, fewer problems associated with lost or damaged lenses and fewer complaint-related office visits (reduction in giant papillary conjunctivitis, acute red eye, and infective or inflammatory keratitis). In addition to supplied lenses, a disposable system that includes solutions and storage cases, which are replaced at regular intervals, may decrease the risk of ocular infections. Most disposable lenses in Canada are prescribed for daily wear. Approximately 20% of soft lens wearers are on a PRP. Most wearers can wear a pair

TABLE 14: Relative Complications of Contact Lens Wear

Relative Risk of Developing Ulcerative Keratitis	
According to Lens Type	
Extended wear soft compared to PMMA	10 times
Extended wear soft compared to RGP	5 times
Extended wear soft compared to daily wear soft	5 times
According to Type of Wear	
Extended compared to daily wear	4 times
Extended overnight compared to daily overnight	10–15 times
Relative Risk of Contact Lens Complications of Disposable Lenses	
Daily wear disposable compared to regular daily wear	0.5 times
Extended wear disposable compared to daily wear disposable	1.5 times
Annual Incidence of Ulcerative Keratitis Among Cosmetic Lens Wearers	
Lens Type	**Incidence of Ulcerative Keratitis (per 10,000 per year)**
Hard (PMMA)*	2
Rigid gas permeable	4
Daily wear soft	4.1
Extended wear soft	20.9

* PMMA—polymethylmethacrylate

of disposable lenses for a maximum of 14 days of daily wear.

Traditionally, wearers visited their eye care professional yearly for an eye examination and perhaps a new set of lenses. After the initial contact lens care kit was used up, further supplies were obtained from a pharmacy. With PRPs, wearers return to the eye care professional more frequently. The concept of supplying lens care products in conjunction with regular visits offered advantages. Convenience to the wearer is increased and compliance is easier to monitor.

Experience is limited with daily disposable lenses (e.g., lenses disposed of after a single daily wearing period), but preliminary evidence suggests they would be good for wearers with problems (such as giant papillary conjunctivitis, dry eye, allergies, lens deposits, red eye), occasional wearers, those unhappy with their care systems, travellers and busy professionals. The use of daily disposable lenses may be more costly, but appears to present a smaller risk than extended wear and greater convenience than daily reusable lenses. Advantages of wearer convenience (cleaning and disinfection would no longer be required), compliance, improved vision and physical comfort support this method of lens delivery.

CONTACT LENSES AND DRUGS

Oral Contraceptives

Lens intolerance has been associated with the use of oral contraceptives, but the effect appears to vary and is more likely associated with older, high dose oral contraceptives. Well-fitted contact lens wearers may experience fewer complications than poorly fitted users. Oral contraceptive use may produce two effects: first, the fluid-retaining properties of the estrogen are thought to produce corneal and lid swelling, which increase the wearer's awareness of and sensitivity to the lenses, resulting in reduced wearing time, decreased visual acuity and photophobia. Second, altered tear composition may decrease the lubricating ability of tears: a sticky mucus deposited on the lens can produce allergic conjunctivitis and uncomfortable blurry vision.

After about 3 months of oral contraceptive use, a new hormonal equilibrium is attained. It also takes about 3 months to return to normal when oral contraceptives are discontinued. Reducing the wear time for the first 3 months and cleaning the lens thoroughly may be adequate for a successful transition. If these measures are inadequate, the contact lenses may have to be modified or refitted. If this is not acceptable, contact lens wear may have to be discontinued until the oral contraceptive is discontinued.

Pregnancy or menstruation produce similar effects.

Ophthalmic Medications

Dark discoloration of soft lenses has occurred with repeated use of phenylephrine, epinephrine or tetrahydrozoline, and other readily oxidizable adrenergic-containing solutions. Diagnostic solutions containing fluorescein or rose bengal can produce a yellow green or crimson red discoloration of the lens if it is put into the eye too soon after eye examinations.

Drugs administered locally during contact lens wear can affect tear composition, pharmacologic responses to drugs and the lenses themselves. An eye care professional will instruct the wearer if any local medication is to be used with lens wear. Common ophthalmic medications (e.g., naphazoline, pilocarpine, dipivefrin, prednisolone, dexamethasone, neomycin, polymyxin B) generally should not damage a soft lens. Contact lens wearers usually report initial discomfort on the instillation of local drugs not related to contact lens wear. The response may be due to a pre-existing corneal stress directly associated with contact lens wear. The comfort and successful function of contact lenses is dependent on normal tear dynamics. Most local medication not specifically formulated for use with contact lenses affects tear dynamics. Fortunately, the effect lasts less than 10 minutes after administration.

Temporary lens intolerance and decreased visual acuity can occur with solutions buffered at pH values far from the ideal of 7.4. Abnormally acidic pH can promote lens dehydration and lens steepening; abnormally basic pH has the opposite effect, promoting lens hydration and lens flattening.

Nonprescription products for the eye should not be used without consulting an eye care professional; the ingredients may not be compatible with contact lens solutions. Such incompatibilities may be noted on the labels of eye care products.

Acne medications that contain benzoyl peroxide can cause tinted soft lenses to fade from inadequately washed hands. Distilled or tap water that contains chlorine can also cause fading of tinted lenses, especially if the tint was applied to a preformed contact lens.

Systemic Medications

A good fit of a rigid or hard contact lens depends on the constant supply of oxygen from fresh tears moving under the lens with each blink. With soft lenses, blinking is required to maintain proper lens hydration. If a previously well-fitting hard or soft lens produces irritation and redness, the blink should be investigated. Sedatives, hypnotics and antihistamines can decrease the blink rate in susceptible people. This may lead to incomplete blinking, which can cause problems, especially those related to reduced wearing time.

Decreased tear volume can contribute to corneal drying in hard lens wearers and to annoying irritation and tenacious lens deposits in soft lens wearers. Oral antihistamines, anticholinergics, tricyclic antidepressants, beta-blockers and diuretics have been reported to decrease tear volume, which could promote contact lens sticking or even adherence. Salicylic acid appears in tears after oral ASA administration. Salicylic acid may be absorbed by soft lenses, resulting in an increased incidence of unexplained ocular irritation and redness in ASA users.

Rifampin may cause soft contact lenses to turn orange. Although the effect varies, it might be advisable for rifampin users not to wear soft contact lenses while taking the drug. Other drugs excreted into tears and reported to discolor soft lenses include phenazopyridine, tetracycline, phenolphthalein, nitrofurantoin and sulfasalazine. Contact lens wear will not likely be successful in individuals using isotretinoin since the drug can cause irritative conjunctivitis and possible Meibomian gland dysfunction.

Smoking

Smokers have a higher incidence of pigmented soft lenses than nonsmokers, likely from stimulation of melanin production by nicotine and other aromatic compounds present in cigarette smoke. Initially, pigmentation has little effect on visual acuity, but eventually, the deposits cause the lens to become less flexible, deforming it and giving it a leathery texture. The wearer should be counselled about the potential for lens spoilage. Finger- or smoke-transferred nicotine can reduce the physical and sometimes optical clarity of lenses. Smokers should thoroughly clean their hands before handling contact lenses. They are advised to use the third or the least nicotine-stained finger and the palm of the other hand for lens cleaning and rinsing.

COMPLIANCE

Noncompliance is the greatest threat to eye comfort and lens life. A 1987 FDA survey found that 86% of wearers who experience problems do not immediately contact their eye care professional. A 1990 Bausch and Lomb Consumer Attitudes and Usage survey found that only 46% had their care kit opened and explained. Less than 25% had a full explanation without the kit being opened. Minimal explanation was given to 17% while 8% received no explanation. The remaining 4% could not remember what they were told. With patients retaining 50% or less of the information they are given, it is not surprising there is a potential for misunderstanding and incorrect product use. It has been suggested that more than 50% of adverse reactions are due to noncompliance, such as inadequate cleaning or rinsing before chemical or thermal disinfection. Economizing by using old solutions was the most common form of noncompliance in one practice. Noncompliance can lead to microbial keratitis and corneal ulceration, which likely starts from the inoculation by a pathogenic microorganism. Solution contamination, inadequate lens disinfection, manipulation of the lens in the eye and poor hygiene all increase the exposure of the eye to pathogens. Storage solutions are often implicated as the source of infection as cultures from the eye and solution yield the same pathogen. The source of acanthamoeba keratitis appears to be a homemade saline solution or tap water used for rinsing lenses. It has been documented through epidemiologic studies that poor compliance with the care regimen increases the risk of this infection. A recent compliance study of daily wear found a 40% noncompliance rate. Noncompliance was more frequent in individuals 10 to 30 years of age, greater than 50 years of age, and in those consumers wearing lenses for more than 2 years. It was also noted that noncompliance was more common in those wearers who were not indoctrinated by the researchers. Compliance was defined as: hand washing before lens handling, correct use of an approved (FDA) care system and adherence to a recommended wear schedule. Another study found a 46% noncompliance rate. Those under the age of 30 and wearing lenses for convenience or cosmetic reasons were the two factors statistically associated with noncompliance.

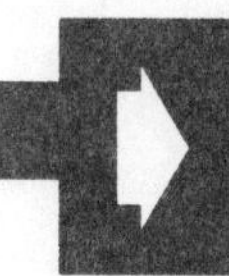

ADVICE FOR THE PATIENT

Contact Lens Care

- Follow exactly the care regimen prescribed for you.
- Follow exactly the directions for using contact lens care solutions.
- If you suspect problems or have questions, contact your eye care professional.

Hard and soft lenses:

- Each solution is formulated for a special purpose. Use hard lens solutions for hard lenses only, and soft lens solutions for soft lenses only. Never use chemical disinfecting solutions for thermal disinfection.
- Thoroughly wash using oil-free soap and dry your hands before handling your lenses. Debris on your hands can be transferred to your lenses.
- Keep your fingernails short to prevent tearing and scratching of your lenses.
- If you remove lenses over a sink, close or cover the drain to prevent possible lens loss.
- Do not wear lenses while swimming, they may wash out. Soft lenses can stick to the eye due to the hypertonicity of swimming pool water.
- Wear protective eyegear if you participate in contact sports.
- Do not wear lenses if your eyes are red or irritated.
- Do not use any household products, such as detergents, soaps, shampoos, skin cleansers or toothpaste, to clean your lenses.
- Do not use solutions from different manufacturers, unless your eye care professional recommends otherwise, since the solutions may not be compatible with each other.
- Do not use contact lens products beyond their expiry date.
- Keep all contact lens products out of the reach of children.
- Thoroughly clean and rinse lenses after removal and prior to disinfection. The vast majority of microorganisms are removed with this step.
- Thoroughly rinse off cleaners or disinfectants before inserting the lens into the eye. Residues can produce adverse effects on the eye and lens.
- Contact lenses should not be worn to the beauty salon. If worn under a hair dryer, the hot air will cause mucus and tears to dry and harden on the lenses.
- Change disinfecting (soaking) solutions daily.
- Avoid contamination of bottle tips.
- Thoroughly clean, rinse and air dry the contact lens case each morning after lens insertion. The case should be cleaned occasionally with lens cleaner and replaced at least every 3 months.
- Daily wear lenses should not be overworn.
- Extended wear lenses should be removed daily.
- If wearing daily wear lenses, visit your eye care professional at least once every 6 months.
- If wearing extended wear lenses, visit your eye care professional at least once every 2 to 3 months.
- Contact your eye care professional if there is redness, swelling, pain or irritation.

Contact lenses with cosmetics:

- Do not apply cosmetics if eyes are swollen, red or infected.

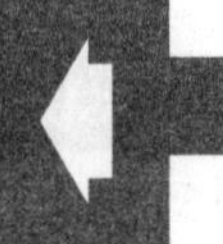

ADVICE FOR THE PATIENT (*cont'd*)

- Use a good quality water-resistant mascara that does not flake off. Problems occur from mascara on or underneath lenses.
- Use oil-free and fragrance-free eye makeup.
- Apply eye makeup sparingly and remove it all daily.
- Warn your cosmetologist that you wear contact lenses.
- Never share eye cosmetics; another person's bacteria may be dangerous to your eyes.
- When using hair dyes, bleaches, perm lotions or medicated shampoos, remove lenses.
- Spray deodorants and hairsprays can irritate your eyes. Particles accumulating on your lenses may cause discomfort, and lens replacement may be necessary. Protect your lenses by closing your eyes when you spray, and walking away from the area. Use pump sprays if possible.
- You can prevent smearing of eye makeup if lens removal is necessary by tilting your head to one side after reinsertion of your lenses. Tears then run to the side of the eye.
- Before handling lenses, scrub your hands and fingers thoroughly to remove all cosmetics, including nail polish, nail polish remover, perfumes, colognes, lotions and suntan oil.
- Apply cosmetics after inserting lenses.
- Remove lenses before removing makeup.

Hard lenses:

- Never rub your eyes when lenses are in place. Do not rinse your lenses under hot water, to avoid warping, especially in gas permeable lenses.
- Never use saliva to wet your lenses; it contains bacteria that can cause infection.
- Never rinse with tap water after your lenses have been cleaned or disinfected.

Soft lenses:

- Rinse hands thoroughly after washing. Soap residues can bind to soft lenses.
- Change boiling solutions regularly.
- Commercially preserved solutions should be discarded within 2 months.
- Do not use discolored enzyme products.
- If you wish to change solutions, contact your eye care professional.
- Remove your lenses before applying ophthalmic preparations. Do not reinsert your lenses for at least 1 hour unless otherwise instructed by your eye care professional.
- When storing, carefully centre the lenses in the case and close lid tightly.
- Do not mix chemical and heat methods of disinfection.
- If your lenses become stuck, moisten with saline or daily cleaner before sliding them apart.
- If a lens tears, save the pieces as your eye care professional will want to ensure none of the pieces have become lodged in your eye. Some companies may replace torn lenses.
- If you fall asleep with your lenses on, moisten them with lubricating drops before removing them.
- Wait 1 hour before reinserting your lenses if you have been swimming.
- Soft lenses exposed to contaminated saline or water should be thermally disinfected as current chemical disinfection solutions are ineffective against *Acanthamoeba*.

FIGURE 7

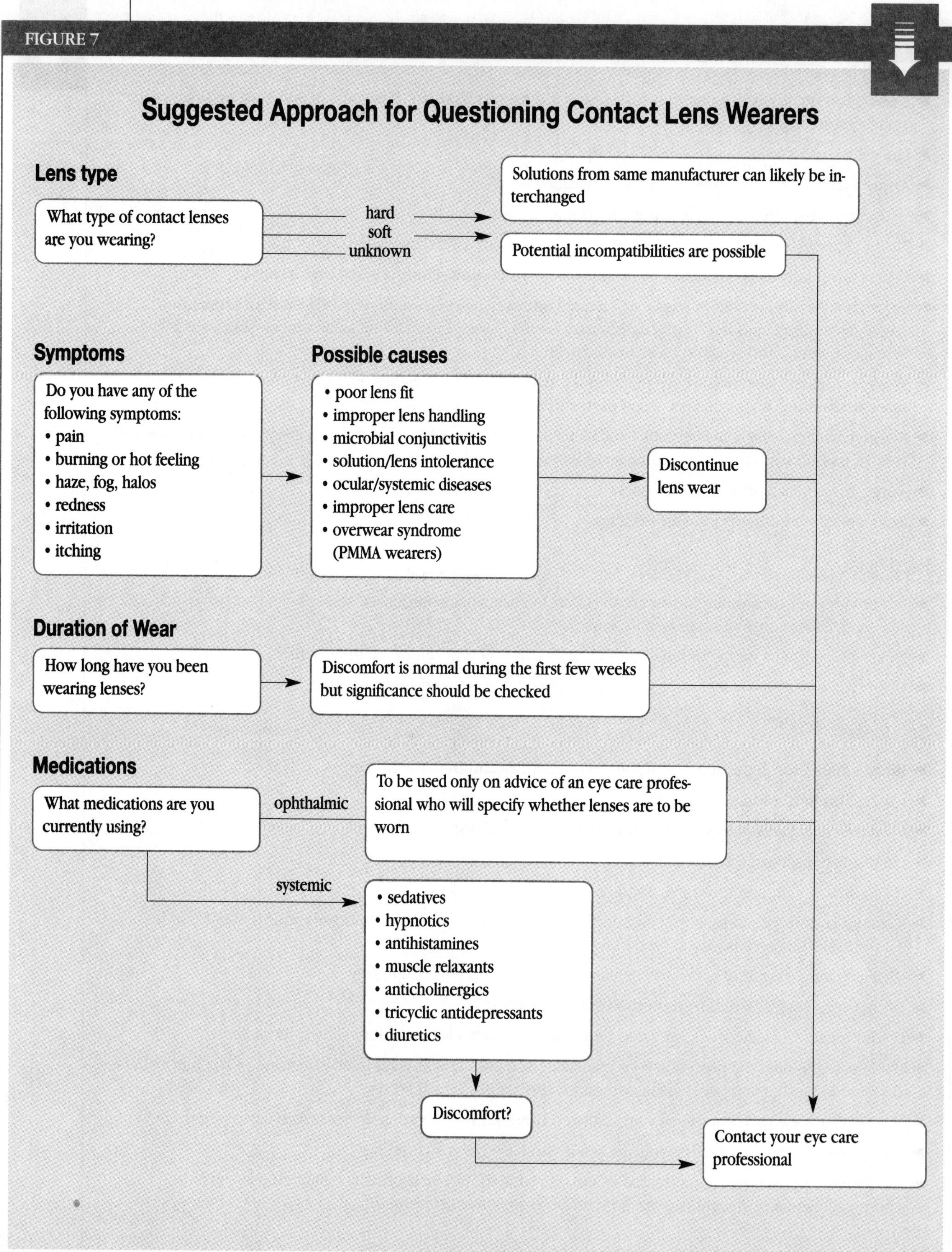
Suggested Approach for Questioning Contact Lens Wearers
Lens type
What type of contact lenses are you wearing?
hard
soft
unknown
Solutions from same manufacturer can likely be interchanged
Potential incompatibilities are possible
Symptoms
Possible causes
Do you have any of the following symptoms:
• pain
• burning or hot feeling
• haze, fog, halos
• redness
• irritation
• itching
• poor lens fit
• improper lens handling
• microbial conjunctivitis
• solution/lens intolerance
• ocular/systemic diseases
• improper lens care
• overwear syndrome (PMMA wearers)
Discontinue lens wear
Duration of Wear
How long have you been wearing lenses?
Discomfort is normal during the first few weeks but significance should be checked
Medications
What medications are you currently using?
ophthalmic
To be used only on advice of an eye care professional who will specify whether lenses are to be worn
systemic
• sedatives
• hypnotics
• antihistamines
• muscle relaxants
• anticholinergics
• tricyclic antidepressants
• diuretics
Discomfort?
Contact your eye care professional

FIGURE 7 *(cont'd)*

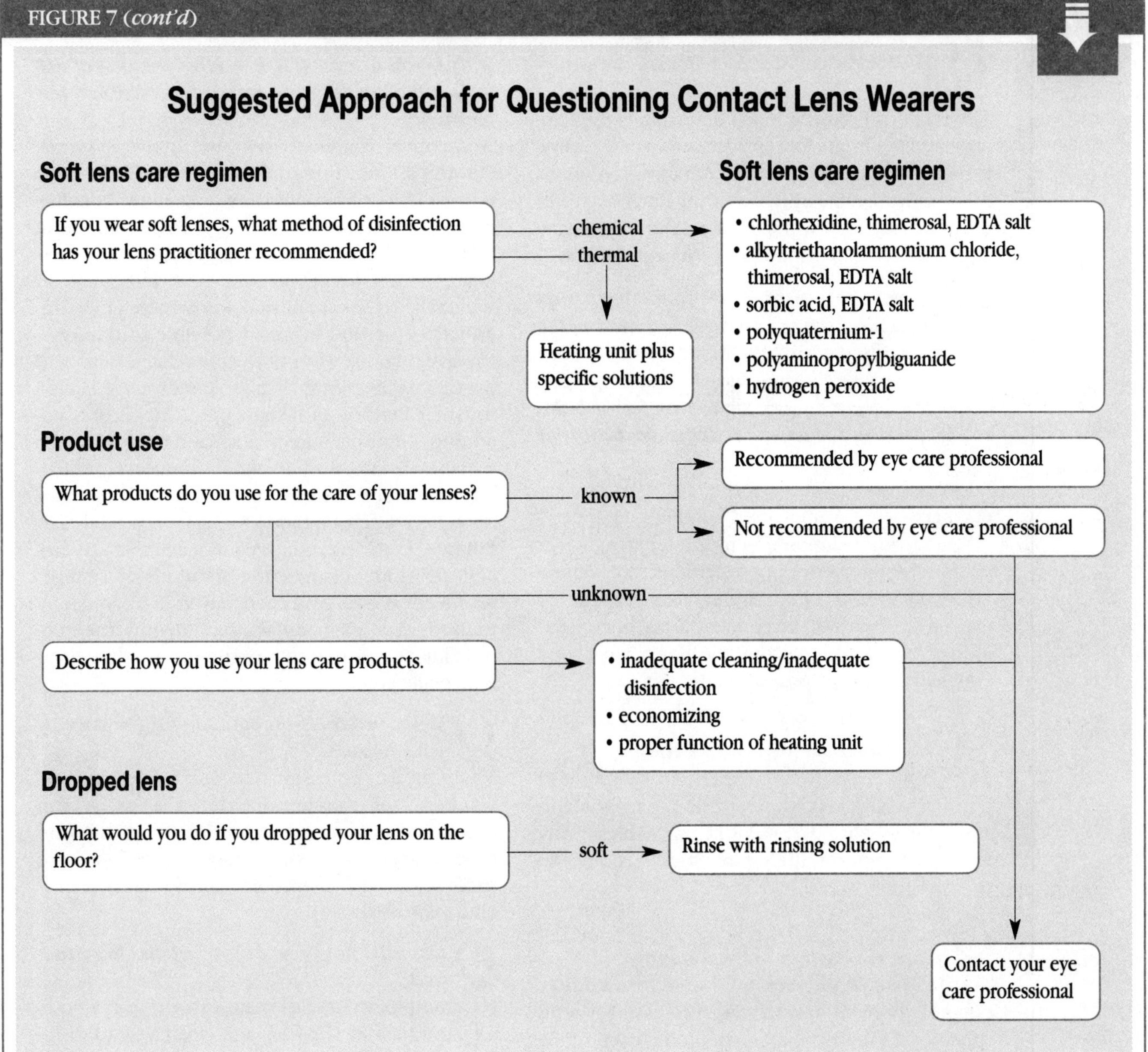

PATIENT ASSESSMENT QUESTIONS

Q What type of contact lenses are you wearing?
The lens type (hard or soft) determines the care regimen. Solutions for hard lenses from the same manufacturer can likely be interchanged. Solutions for both hard and soft lenses from a manufacturer other than the one who produced the lens may be incompatible. Consult an eye care professional.

Q Do you have any of the following symptoms: pain when inserting or wearing the lenses or after wearing them; burning that causes excessive tearing; inability to keep your eyes open; severe or persistent haze, fog or halos while wearing the lenses; redness, irritation or itching?
These symptoms may be due to poor lens fit, damaged lenses, improper handling, microbial conjunctivitis, solution or lens intolerance, ocular or systemic disease, or improper lens care. Painful lid swelling and photophobia may be due to overwear. If any of these symptoms occur, the individual should discontinue lens wear and contact an eye care professional.

Q How long have you worn lenses?
Every contact lens wearer experiences discomfort during the first few weeks while the eyes adapt. Since it may not be obvious at first which problems are significant, the wearer should contact an eye care professional.

Q What medication are you taking?
Any ophthalmic preparation should be used only on the advice of an eye care professional who specifies if the medication should be used while the lens is in place. Other drugs, such as phenylephrine, epinephrine and tetrahydrozoline, can discolor soft lenses. Products may not be compatible with contact-lens-solution ingredients. Almost all ophthalmic preparations not specifically designed for use with contact lenses cause temporary discomfort. Numerous systemic medications may alter eye dynamics sufficiently to warrant therapeutic intervention. Sedatives (including alcohol), hypnotics, antihistamines and muscle relaxants can affect the eyelid, producing incomplete blinking or a decreased rate of blinking. Antihistamines, anticholinergics, tricyclic antidepressants and diuretics can decrease tear volume, leading to significant discomfort.

Q If you wear soft lenses, what method of disinfection did your eye care professional recommend?
A chemical regimen uses one of five systems: chlorhexidine, thimerosal and an EDTA salt; polyquad; polyaminopropylbiguanide; alkyltriethanolammonium chloride (AKTAC), thimerosal and an EDTA salt; and hydrogen peroxide. A thermal regimen uses a heating unit and saline in which the lenses are heated. Knowledge of the disinfection method makes it possible to reinforce the instructions of the eye care professional and prevent wearers from using solutions not designed for their method of disinfection. Chemical disinfecting solutions sometimes cannot be used for thermal disinfection. If such a solution is repeatedly used for thermal disinfection, the lenses can become white or opaque. Counsel the wearer to follow specific product recommendations. Hydrogen peroxide disinfection requires two steps: disinfection with hydrogen peroxide 3% and neutralization. Most manufacturers identify the neutralizing solution with a predominantly green or blue package.

Q What products do you use for the care of your lenses?
The eye care professional recommended specific products for the lenses. The pharmacist can determine and correct inappropriate substitution of products. Refer the wearer to an eye care professional if any products are not known or if confusion arises.

Q Describe how you use your lens care products.
Noncompliance is the greatest threat to eye comfort and lens life. Inadequate cleaning and disinfection cause about 50% of all problems associated with contact lenses. The attempt to economize by using solutions that should have been discarded was the most common form of noncompliance in one practice. Some consumers even forget to plug in their heating unit. To determine noncompliance, ask wearers to describe their care regimen.

Q What measures do you take before insertion if you drop your lens on the floor?
Frequently, the lens is picked up and promptly inserted along with whatever the lens has collected. Rinse hard (PMMA or gas permeable) lenses with an aerosol saline solution. Rinse soft lenses thoroughly with an appropriate rinsing solution.

OPHTHALMIC PRODUCT INFORMATION

ANESTHETICS—LOCAL

Local anesthetic ophthalmic solutions and ointments (e.g., tetracaine and proparacaine) are available without a prescription in some provinces. These medications are used by eye care professionals during certain eye examinations. Individuals should never self-medicate with these preparations because of their inherent toxicities with long-term or inappropriate use. Generally, with normal use in diagnostic environments, local anesthetics have transient, mild side effects. There is relatively low systemic and ocular toxicity.

The following problems may arise from instillation of a local anesthetic in the eye: self-inflicted corneal damage to the open eye, caused by loss of the blink reflex combined with a numbing sensation—patients must be warned not to touch or rub the eye after instillation; local allergic reactions, particularly with proparacaine; corneal edema; blurred vision; increased rate of tear evaporation; and mild to intense ocular pain if instillation is repeated. Additionally, with decreased reflex secretion of tears and resulting increased length of time required for tear washout, anesthetics allow topically applied agents to be in contact with the eye for a prolonged period of time.

Tetracaine (amethocaine 0.5%) and **proparacaine** (proxymetacaine 0.5%) are commonly used ester-type local ocular anesthetics. They are approximately equipotent, although proparacaine does not penetrate the cornea or conjunctiva as well as tetracaine. Onset of action is about 20 seconds and duration is approximately 15 minutes; the ointment formulation causes prolonged anesthesia. Proparacaine is used more commonly in clinical practice, as it may produce less irritation than tetracaine when instilled; tetracaine may cause considerable stinging for 30 seconds after it is instilled into the conjunctival sac. Conjunctival redness may also occur. Proparacaine usually produces little irritation on instillation, but irritation and stinging may occur several hours after. Rarely, there may be tearing, photophobia or allergic reactions, including contact dermatitis. When tetracaine, a para-aminobenzoic acid ester, is metabolized, it may inhibit the action of sulfonamide (antibacterial) drugs; if only 1 or 2 drops of tetracaine are used for a local procedure, this effect is probably minimal. Due to delayed metabolism, circulating blood levels of these local anesthetics may be increased in individuals using anticholinesterase drugs such as echothiophate.

Amylocaine and **butacaine** are less commonly used ester-type local anesthetics.

ANTIHISTAMINES

During allergic reactions, various chemical mediators (including histamine) are released. As with inflammation, these mediators alter blood vessels, causing redness and edema; stimulate nerve endings, causing itching; and directly stimulate lacrimal glands, causing tearing. Antihistamines bind to histamine receptor sites, blocking the actions of histamine. Some antihistamines may also inhibit mediator release and have an anticholinergic effect. The effect of antihistamines depends on the role of histamine in the allergic process. It is thought that H_1-receptors primarily mediate itching and H_2-receptors vasodilation, although these roles may not be as distinct as previously believed. Antihistamines are of value in immediate-response allergies (e.g., acute allergic conjunctivitis—seasonal or perennial allergic conjunctivitis) where histamine is released from mast cells. Antihistamines produce vasoconstriction and provide symptomatic relief.

In immediate-response allergies, H_1-blocking antihistamines can be particularly effective in reducing the itching and may help reduce vasodilation (redness). Treatment prior to an anticipated exposure may prevent an acute episode of acute allergic conjunctivitis. Ophthalmic antihistamines, particularly when used in combination with a decongestant, can effectively alleviate symptoms of acute allergic conjunctivitis, especially mild to moderate disease. The combination is more effective than either drug alone. Ophthalmic antihistamines have an immediate effect unlike oral antihistamines, which exert their effect in 1 to 3 hours. Oral antihistamines have demonstrated effectiveness in treatment of rhinoconjunctivitis, but they may be more effective in treatment of nasal rather than ocular symptoms. Oral antihistamines may be of value to those patients with more severe symptoms or those associated with nasal or pharyngeal complaints.

Oral antihistamines (for more information see the Allergy and Cold Products chapter), particularly the first generation agents, are associated with CNS effects such as drowsiness. The newer third generation agents are much less likely to be associated with troublesome CNS effects; however, there is concern because of the rare occurrence of cardiac arrhythmias. Oral antihistamines may also cause blurred vision, reduced tear volume and decreased blink reflex.

Ophthalmic antihistamines may cause contact dermatitis of the eyelids or periocular skin; individuals sensitive to an antihistamine may exhibit cross-sensitivity to other antihistamines. Ophthalmic antihistamines, like ophthalmic decongestants may dilate the pupils causing photophobia and, in patients predisposed to angle-closure glaucoma, may precipitate an acute attack.

Clinical experience suggests that prolonged use of antihistamines may lead to tolerance and reduced response; for those cases, a different class of antihistamine may be beneficial.

Topical antihistamines marketed in nonprescription ophthalmic preparations include antazoline, pyrilamine maleate and pheniramine maleate. They are available commercially in combination with the decongestant drugs discussed above. Their safety in children, pregnancy and lactation has not been established.

Antazoline, an ethylenediamine antihistamine, appears to be less sensitizing than other topical antihistamines. Upon instillation, there may be mild stinging. Symptomatic relief and vasoconstriction should be provided in minutes, especially if combined with a decongestant. The drug has a short duration of action and is usually instilled every 3 to 4 hours as required. Antazoline is often combined with the decongestant naphazoline.

Pyrilamine maleate, another ethylenediamine antihistamine, is as efficacious as antazoline. It is used in low concentration (0.1%).

Pheniramine maleate, an alkylamine antihistamine, is as efficacious as antazoline.

ANTI-INFECTIVES

Indiscriminate use of nonprescription ophthalmic anti-infectives is unwise. Their use may delay proper diagnosis resulting in serious ocular damage. Generally, their safety in children, pregnancy and lactation has not been established.

Boric acid and sodium borate solutions, used as buffers in ophthalmic preparations, are also weak bacteriostatic and fungistatic agents. Sodium borate has also been used as a mild astringent; however, efficacy has not been established. These agents are used in some external ophthalmic irrigating solutions (e.g., eye washes) to relieve irritated eyes or to flush loose foreign bodies/allergens/pollutants from the eye. Generally these agents are well-tolerated provided individuals are not allergic to them.

One author recommends that solutions for topical use not exceed a concentration of 2%, as greater concentrations exert a phagolytic effect that may depress a primary defence mechanism against bacterial invasion. Since absorption of boric acid through extensive areas of broken skin or through inadvertent oral ingestion may result in potentially fatal poisoning, commercial preparations (particularly large volume ones) must be kept out of reach of children.

Some commercial boric acid/sodium borate products (e.g., eye washes) are marketed with an eyecup; care must be taken to clean the eyecup thoroughly to prevent contamination and to avoid washing skin bacteria into the eye. For these reasons, use of an eyecup is generally discouraged.

Boric acid is incompatible with polyvinyl alcohol (contained in some ophthalmic and contact lens solutions).

Salicylic acid, found in some commercial products, has a slight antiseptic action. It may cause irritation when instilled. Its efficacy in ophthalmic preparations has not been assessed.

Bacitracin, gramicidin and polymyxin B are available without prescription. When combined, these bactericidal polypeptides have broad-spectrum activity. With ophthalmic use of these antibiotics, hypersensitivity and side effects are rare.

Bacitracin is available as an ophthalmic ointment alone or in combination with another antibiotic. It is active primarily against a variety of gram-positive organisms (e.g., *Staphylococcus aureus* and *Streptococcus pneumoniae*). Bacterial resistance develops slowly if at all. The action of bacitracin is not affected by blood, pus, necrotic tissue or bacterial enzymes. It rarely causes hypersensitivity. It does not readily penetrate the intact cornea in therapeutic amounts. As bacitracin solutions are unstable, only nonprescription ophthalmic ointments are available commercially.

Gramicidin is available in combination ophthalmic antibiotic preparations. Like bacitracin, it acts against common gram-positive ocular pathogens. It must not be used on recently traumatized areas; bleeding may recur due to hemolysis.

Polymyxin B is available as either an ophthalmic ointment in combination with bacitracin or as an ophthalmic solution in combination with gramicidin. Polymyxin is active against numerous gram-negative organisms, including *Pseudomonas* *aeruginosa, Escherichia coli, Klebsiella pneumoniae, Enterobacter aerogenes*; it is not active against *Proteus vulgaris* or most strains of *Neisseria* and *Serratia*. Bacterial resistance is infrequent. Polymyxin B does not readily penetrate an intact cornea. Hypersensitivity reactions are rare.

ARTIFICIAL TEARS (Demulcents)

Many agents, particularly water-soluble polymers, have been introduced over the past 40 years as potential tear substitutes or supplements (Table 15). They add volume to the tears and promote tear film stability. They are used in numerous ocular conditions (Table 16), particularly as the primary symptomatic treatment for dry eyes.

When artificial tears were first introduced, the main problem was the short duration of action. Initially, researchers thought retention and contact time was prolonged by higher concentrations of the polymers. Researchers now believe one of the critical factors increasing duration of action is the adsorptive property. Long chain polymers have multiple points where they can adsorb to the cornea rendering them more wettable (similar effect to that of the mucin layer of the tear film, e.g., mucomimetic or lacriphilic).

Some cellulose derivatives and polyvinyl alcohol provide symptomatic relief for 30 to 45 minutes. Some combination products (e.g., cellulose derivatives plus povidone or cellulose derivatives plus dextran) may have effects lasting up to 90 minutes.

Product Selection

Preparations promoted as having mucomimetic activity (e.g., *Celluvisc, Teardrops, Tears Naturale II, Tears Plus*) may be beneficial in mucin-deficient dry eye conditions. Some patients may prefer a hypotonic solution (e.g., *Hypotears*) that may help balance the hyperosmotic tear film that results from frequent instability (e.g., as associated with keratoconjunctivitis sicca). Preservative-free preparations are recommended for patients who are sensitive to preservatives or who need to apply tear substitutes more frequently than 6 times daily. (Frequent exposure to some preservatives, e.g., benzalkonium chloride, may be mildly toxic to the dry eye and thus make the condition worse.)

Patients who require frequent instillation of artificial tears (e.g., every 2 to 4 hours) may benefit from ophthalmic inserts of polymers (e.g., *Lacrisert*). These inserts are water soluble (hydroxy-

TABLE 15: Polymers Used in Artificial Tears
Cellulose derivatives (e.g., carboxymethylcellulose, hydroxypropyl methylcellulose, methylcellulose)
Dextran polymers
Hyaluronic acid
Polyesters (e.g., polyethylene glycol, polysorbate 80 [poloxamer])
Polyvinyls (e.g., polyvinyl alcohol, polyvinylpyrrolidone [povidone])

TABLE 16: Some Indications for Artificial Tears

Indication	Function
Dry eyes	Alleviates symptoms Prevents corneal damage
Blepharitis Chronic seborrheic	 Reduces debris and oil in the tear film
Conjunctivitis Irritant Allergic	 Temporary relief of discomfort and dryness Temporary relief of discomfort Deterrent to allergen (e.g., serves as a barrier and helps dilute the allergen)

Ophthalmic Product Information

propyl cellulose) and dissolve slowly over 6 hours. They may be effective for several hours or most of a day. They are placed in the lower conjunctival pouch once or twice daily. They may be more beneficial in younger patients, with mild to moderate dry eyes, who still have enough tears to help dissolve the inserts, the manual dexterity to insert them, and whose eyelids have sufficient tonus to keep the insert in place. A special device is needed to place them in the lower eyelid pouch.

Although in vitro testing may suggest one product is preferable to another, the testing does not necessarily parallel clinical effectiveness. Detailed clinical analysis and comparison is not readily available. Clinically, user acceptance varies widely and the individual may end up selecting the most suitable and least irritating preparation by trial and error. No one preparation is consistently more efficacious and better tolerated; individual preferences may change, probably reflecting the fluctuating nature and different etiologies of dry eyes. Clinically, practitioners tend to distinguish between the different formulations searching for effective treatment: mucomimetic or lacriphilic drops, hypoallergenic drops, and hypoosmolar drops. Some products with a variety of other ingredients periodically gain brief popular use, but the mainstay of therapy is based on the polymers.

Side Effects

Artificial tears generally do not have significant side effects. Viscous preparations have a tendency to form crusts at the lid margins if allowed to dry, causing discomfort. The main disadvantages of artificial tears are short duration of action, development of sensitivity to the preservatives (e.g., thimerosal), and possible corneal epithelial damage associated with the use of preservatives (e.g., possibly benzalkonium chloride if used more than 6 times daily). Polymer inserts may cause blurred vision and irritation after a few hours. Some people have difficulty applying and retaining the insert in the eye. Correct insertion techniques should be supervised by an eye care professional; a drop of saline or artificial tear instilled immediately after placement of the insert, may help wet it and alleviate discomfort.

Dosage

For the person who complains of dry or irritated eyes, the short-term use of artificial tears (e.g., 72 hours) can be recommended. It is generally not advisable to use these eye drops more than 6 times a day. If this treatment is ineffective or if the condition persists, the individual should consult an eye care professional; more elaborate treatment may be required to prevent irreversible ocular damage (e.g., hydrophilic bandage lenses, eye drops containing mucolytic agents or surgical alterations).

Other Products

Ocular lubricant (emollient) ointments—containing petrolatum, mineral oil and lanolin derivatives—are commercially available, although not advocated as tear substitutes. These constituents are in most ophthalmic ointment bases. The products are promoted for lubrication following surgery, removal of a foreign body and sun/wind exposure. They help to reduce tear evaporation. Some practitioners prescribe these ointments for use at bedtime as an adjunct to treatment with artificial tears. They should not be used during the day as they may further aggravate the dry eye condition—blinking spreads the ointment over the tear film, disrupting the film and causing formation of dry spots. Major disadvantages are blurred vision, poor mixing with the hydrophilic tears and formation of a coating on contact lenses. There is also a case report of aspiration-induced lipoid pneumonitis associated with bedtime use of an ocular lubricant ointment; if a cough develops, this potential complication should be considered. If ocular irritation occurs, the ointment should be discontinued.

ASTRINGENTS

Astringents, by precipitating protein, may help to clear mucus from the outer surface of the eye.

Allantoin, an xanthine alkaloid, has astringent properties. Its efficacy in ophthalmic preparations is unknown.

Zinc sulfate (0.25%) is a mild astringent and weak antiseptic. In concentrations used in nonprescription products, it has little ability to penetrate tissues, so is considered safe for use in the eye. A solution of zinc sulfate 0.25% may clear mucin from the outer surface of the eye and may provide subjective relief from minor eye irritations. Zinc sulfate does not produce vasoconstriction of conjunctival blood vessels. Side effects include transient stinging and burning.

Boric acid and sodium borate—see the Anti-infectives section.

DECONGESTANTS (Eye Whiteners, Vasoconstrictors)

Ocular congestion (diffuse redness of the white of the eye) indicates the presence of abnormal amounts of blood in the vessels of the eye. Also known as hyperemia, it can occur during inflammatory and allergic reactions.

During inflammation, the body attempts to counteract and remove any irritants as well as repair damage. This process can be elicited by disease (e.g., microbial infection) or injury (e.g., chemical, radiant energy or mechanical). Disease or injury traumatizes ocular tissue, causing release of various mediators. The principal mediators are thought to be natural substances produced by the body, such as histamine and prostaglandins that primarily result in two changes. The first change, vascular, occurs as blood vessels and capillaries dilate, providing greater blood flow to the damaged area, which then becomes red and hot. Increased vessel permeability allows various constituents to enter the irritated tissue. The second change involves formation of an inflammatory exudate of plasma and white blood cells. The exudate causes swelling, and the tension exerted on the surrounding tissue stimulates pain receptors.

Ophthalmic decongestants act both in inflammatory and allergic conditions by reversing dilation of blood vessels (e.g., causing vasoconstriction), which decongests and whitens the conjunctiva (thus leading to the term eye whitener). Minor, temporary ocular irritations can be relieved, but generally use of decongestants for these conditions is discouraged as they may mask symptoms of continuing toxic reactions (e.g., minor, temporary conjunctival response to smog, swimming pool chlorine). Decongestants may be useful, particularly when combined with an antihistamine, for treatment of acute seasonal or perennial allergic conjunctivitis. Their effectiveness for prophylaxis in acute allergic conjunctivitis is limited. They can be useful for short-term treatment before initiation of more potent medications (e.g., anti-inflammatories) to improve delivery of these agents.

Decongestants are used for symptomatic relief as well as cosmetic reasons, generally only short-term (3 to 5 consecutive days). Treatment beyond this time should be under the direction of an eye care professional. Overuse of decongestants may mask potentially serious disorders (e.g., infections, continuing toxic reactions) and delay appropriate treatment.

Sympathomimetic (epinephrine/adrenaline-like or adrenergic) drugs are used as ophthalmic decongestants (vasoconstrictors) (Table 17). They stimulate alpha-adrenergic receptors in the conjunctival blood vessels to produce vasoconstriction and to symptomatically relieve redness and swelling. In general, because of the low concentrations used, nonprescription ophthalmic decongestants are considered safe. However, these drugs are potentially capable of causing ocular problems (Table 18). Nonprescription sympathomimetics should not be used in individuals with angle-closure glaucoma, because even in small doses, they may cause pupillary dilation, particularly if the cornea is diseased or damaged (e.g., dry eye, keratitis, trauma or surgery).

A controversial ocular problem associated with the use of ophthalmic decongestants is rebound (or reactive) hyperemia. With too frequent or prolonged use, hyperemia may become worse. The preparation may continue to whiten the eye when the drops are instilled, but the redness quickly returns and the individual instills more solution. If this pattern continues and the condition worsens, the medication must be discontinued. When discontinued, the reaction subsides. Additionally, after instilling decongestants, some individuals may develop red eye resulting from an allergic reaction to the preservative or other ingredient.

TABLE 17: Ophthalmic Decongestants

	Usual Concentration (%)	Onset (Minutes)	Duration (Hours)
Phenylephrine	0.12	Rapid	0.5-4
Imidazole Derivatives			
Naphazoline	0.01-0.03	Rapid (5-10)	2-6
Oxymetazoline	0.025	Rapid (5-10)	6-12
Tetrahydrozoline	0.01-0.05	Rapid (5-10)	2-8

Ophthalmic Product Information

Since these decongestants are sympathomimetic amines, they can elicit systemic effects associated with elevation of epinephrine when absorbed into the systemic circulation (e.g., via conjunctival blood vessels or via absorption following drainage through the nasolacrimal system). Usually the concentrations used in nonprescription eye drops are insufficient to cause serious problems, but precautions must be taken for certain individuals (Table 19). They may cause headache, nausea, hypertension, arrhythmias, nervousness, dizziness, weakness, and/or sweating. Safety in pregnancy, lactation and children has not been established.

Phenylephrine, a direct-acting sympathomimetic drug, can cause transient stinging when instilled. Allergies may develop and there may be cross-sensitivity with epinephrine. It may cause rebound miosis and decreased mydriatic response to glaucoma therapy in older persons. It may also cause temporary blurred or unstable vision so patients should be warned to be cautious while driving or performing other hazardous tasks. Solutions of phenylephrine may oxidize on exposure to air and bright light, resulting in greatly reduced efficacy. Sometimes a sulfite antioxidant is used as a stabilizer in these products, which may be a problem for those individuals (e.g., asthmatics, nonasthmatic atopic individuals) who are susceptible to severe sulfite sensitivity. Repeated use of phenylephrine solutions may cause a brown discoloration of some soft contact lenses.

Naphazoline, oxymetazoline and **tetrahydrozoline** are imidazole derivatives, structurally different from phenylephrine but similar in effectiveness. In general, oxymetazoline and tetrahydrozoline have a longer duration of action than naphazoline. The imidazole agents are more stable in solution, have a longer shelf-life and a longer duration of action than phenylephrine. They can cause stinging on initial instillation, and redness and irritation have

TABLE 18: Potential Ocular Problems Associated with the Use of Ophthalmic Decongestants

Problem	Comments
Mydriasis (dilation of the pupil) leading to:	Mydriasis is possible, especially if the products are used frequently and/or if there are corneal defects (e.g., trauma, surgery, dry eye, keratitis) which allow penetration through the cornea
a) Photophobia	Caused by mydriasis
b) Angle-closure glaucoma	Caused by mydriasis Susceptible individuals include those with angle-closure glaucoma prior to peripheral iridectomy and those with a predisposition to angle block (e.g., family history of angle-closure glaucoma, over 50 years of age, far-sighted, current drug therapy with systemic medications causing pupillary dilatation)
Masking of potential serious ocular disorders (e.g., infection, angle-closure glaucoma, continuing toxic reactions)	There are case reports where blindness resulted when patients suffered acute angle-closure glaucoma and misused eye drops in an attempt to whiten the eye

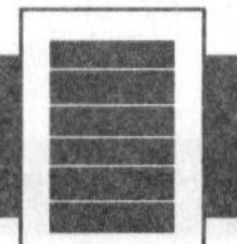

TABLE 19: Populations for Which Ophthalmic Sympathomimetic Decongestants Must be Used Cautiously Due to Systemic Effects

Chronic disease states (e.g., severe hypertension, hyperthyroidism, cardiac disorders, diabetes, asthma or emphysema where cardiac disease has developed, cerebral arteriosclerosis—including a family history of stroke)

Medication usage (e.g., tricyclic antidepressants, MAO inhibitors, adrenergic beta-blocking agents, reserpine, guanethidine, methyldopa, cardiac glycosides, local anesthetics)

Pediatric or geriatric groups

Lactation and pregnancy

Prior to surgery (e.g., anesthetics such as cyclopropane or halothane may sensitize myocardium to sympathomimetics)

been reported. There have also been reports of sedation (especially in children), headache, nausea and dizziness. With oxymetazoline, lid retraction has occasionally been observed; with tetrahydrozoline, blurred vision reported.

PRESERVATIVES

Preservatives are used to maintain sterility of eye preparations after the container is opened. This precaution prevents instillation of microbiologically contaminated drugs into the eye.

The organism most frequently implicated in reports of contaminated ophthalmic solutions is *Pseudomonas aeruginosa*, an organism that can destroy the eye within 24 to 48 hours. Preservatives currently used in Canada include benzalkonium chloride (BAC); disodium edetate (EDTA); chlorobutanol; organomercurials such as phenylmercuric acetate (PMA), phenylmercuric nitrate (PMN) and thimerosal; and parabens (methylparaben and propylparaben). Most nonprescription ophthalmic products are preserved with BAC or chlorobutanol. If use of these ophthalmic preservatives (e.g., artificial tears for treatment of dry eye) exceeds 6 times per day, preservative-free products should be considered if there are any signs of irritation or toxic keratitis.

Benzalkonium chloride, a quaternary ammonium surfactant, is used as a preservative in a concentration of 0.004 to 0.01%. It acts rapidly against organisms, but its effect against *Pseudomonas* is limited.

Adverse reactions (e.g., irritation) may occur but are usually reversible when the preparation is discontinued. BAC is not used in soft contact lens solutions as it binds to the soft lenses after prolonged exposure and may result in toxic levels of BAC at the cornea.

EDTA potentiates the activity of BAC by chelating divalent calcium and magnesium ions, which compete with BAC for sites on the organism. EDTA itself has some antimicrobial effect. It may be a weak sensitizing agent.

Chlorobutanol in a concentration of 0.5% has bacteriostatic activity against gram-negative and gram-positive organisms; it also inhibits *Pseudomonas* and fungi. Its major disadvantage is its slow action. Allergic reactions are uncommon with topical use. Chlorobutanol may sting on application but does not have major toxic effects. It adsorbs to soft contact lenses.

Organomercurials are normally used at concentrations of 0.002 to 0.004%. They have slow, weak antibacterial and antifungal action but are active against *Pseudomonas aeruginosa*. PMN is considered by some to be more active and less irritating than PMA and thimerosal. Contact sensitivity can be a problem, particularly with thimerosal. The action of thimerosal is potentiated by EDTA.

Parabens are generally used in ointments and are more effective against molds and fungi than against bacteria; they are considered slow and ineffective bacteriostatic agents. They may also cause painful ocular irritation and allergic reactions.

MISCELLANEOUS INGREDIENTS

Antipyrine, a pyrazolone derivative used locally, may act as a mild anesthetic, weak antiseptic and mild styptic (constricts superficial blood vessels). An anesthetic effect, no matter how slight, may mask symptoms of serious ocular disorders and may ultimately injure the eye.

Hamamelis (witch hazel) is used well-diluted in some eye wash products. It has mild astringent properties.

Hydrastine and **berberine** are alkaloids obtained from the hydrastis plant and are included in some eye preparations. Their use in conjunctivitis is based entirely on empirical observation.

Lanolin or **cetyl alcohol** 5% is often added to emulsify ointment formulations, thus increasing the absorption of water-soluble drugs and water. Purified lanolin also helps distribute the drug throughout the ointment base.

Methylene blue is a thiazine dye with weak antiseptic and tissue-staining properties. There is little documentation on the efficacy and side effect profile when used in ophthalmic preparations.

Mineral oil, when added to white petrolatum during formulation of an ointment base, allows the vehicle to melt at or below conjunctival temperature.

Sodium bisulfite is used as an antioxidant (e.g., for solutions of phenylephrine).

Other ingredients are used as tonicity agents (e.g., sodium chloride) or buffers (e.g., phosphates, citric acid, sodium borate, boric acid). Ophthalmic solutions can be buffered at a pH of approximately 7.4 (tear pH), although the eye can usually tolerate the slightly acidic character (pH 6.2 to 6.5) of many nonprescription eye drops. This acidity may be partly responsible for the transient stinging on instillation.

Ophthalmic Product Information

FORMULATIONS

Advantages and disadvantages are associated with the use of ophthalmic solutions and ointments (Table 20).

Although systemic effects may occur, they are lessened with ointments because conjunctival absorption is slower than with drops, and nasolacrimal drainage is minimal.

Animal and clinical studies have not indicated that commercial ointment bases interfere with wound healing of corneal or conjunctival surfaces (after infections, etc.). Current ointment bases differ from those used in the past, as they are nonemulsive, do not contain the stiffer grades of petrolatum and are less viscous. Also, the base melts rapidly and floats above the tear film, so epithelial mitosis continues without interference.

Ophthalmic ointments are preferred when treating eyelid inflammation (blepharitis) and may be used to control morning stickiness associated with bacterial infection of the conjunctiva. They may also be used for children to prevent "crying out" of the medication.

The Pharmaceutical Codex recommends discarding multidose ophthalmic solutions for home use 4 weeks after opening. Writing the date on the container when it is opened facilitates this practice. Nonpreserved single dose or unit dose preparations must be discarded immediately after opening; leftover opened product must not be saved for future use under any circumstances.

For nonresidential use, the Codex also recommends these solutions be used for not more than 1 week in hospital wards. New containers should be used pre- and postoperatively. Single dose forms are required in all circumstances in which the dangers of infection are high. For clinics and emergency departments dealing with external eye disorders, single dose containers or one application of a multidose product is recommended. Multidose containers used in outpatient clinics should be discarded at the end of each day. First aid irrigating agents without preservatives should be used for a maximum of 24 hours, and residual contents then discarded.

Although products may have the same type and concentration of active ingredients, variation in tonicity, pH or preservatives may produce different effects. For example, if one product produces discomfort on instillation, there may be tearing, and the active ingredient may be washed away.

TABLE 20: Comparison of Characteristics of Ophthalmic Solutions vs Ophthalmic Ointments

Characteristic	Solutions	Ointments
Instillation	Easier	More difficult
Frequency of instillation*	More	Less
Contact time†	Shorter	Longer (slower movement through nasolacrimal drainage)
Irritation on instillation‡	Frequent	Rare
Discharge retention§	No	Yes
Skin reactions	Few	More frequent (contact dermatitis)
Blurred vision	No	Yes (film spreads over eye)
Systemic reactions	More frequent	Less frequent
Inhibition of corneal epithelial regeneration	No	Unlikely
Readily contaminated (requires preservatives)	Yes	Less likely
Stability a problem with storage#	Yes	Less likely

* Polymers in solution enhance contact time (see Artificial Tears). Ointments have traditionally been used for bedtime therapy to avoid instillation during sleeping hours; since ointments are less readily washed out with tears, they are also valuable in children.
† Generalization.
‡ Stinging, burning.
§ Discharge experienced with bacterial infection.
\# Hydrolysis, oxidation, heat degradation.

CONTACT LENS PRODUCT INFORMATION

When contact lenses are purchased, the eye care professional usually gives the wearer a starter kit containing a complete lens care system. Once the sample kit is used up, wearers tend to replace their solutions with the same brand. Consequently, the solutions carried by individual pharmacies tend to be based on the recommendations eye care professionals make to their wearers. They choose products from clinical experience, recommendations in the clinical articles in eye care literature, advertising, advice from colleagues and user preference. Four important factors are safety, efficacy, cost and simplicity. Comparisons are often outdated because manufacturers reformulate their products frequently. In the past, the number of contact lens solutions seemed to increase each year but due to Planned Replacement Programs (PRP) and multifunction (all purpose) solutions, this appears to be no longer true.

Most solutions contain more than 95% purified water. Solution functions are determined by adding preservatives, wetting agents, buffers, surfactants, cleaners and disinfectants. New solutions can be made up of different combinations and concentrations of the same components. Although the efficacy and adverse effects of each component are discussed, individual wearer characteristics may be the deciding factor. Proper compliance, responsible use and wearer education needs to be improved to optimize contact lens safety. Product substitution is not recommended unless directed by the eye care professional. In addition, cost must be considered in long-term use of solutions.

ROUTINE CARE OF CONTACT LENSES

Figures 5 and 6 summarize the recommended steps for the routine care of contact lenses. The importance of each step performed in the proper sequence is vital to maximize eye safety.

The hydrophilic nature of soft lens material requires extra attention to cleaning and disinfection. Compared to gas permeable and hard (PMMA) lenses, soft lenses are more susceptible to protein deposits from tear film and also tend to concentrate ingredients from cosmetics and ophthalmic preparations more readily. Soft lenses are more comfortable for some people but have a higher risk of infection.

The care regimen for soft lenses is more complex than for hard lenses. Increased susceptibility to protein deposits requires weekly use of an enzyme cleaner. For disinfection, wearers can choose one of five chemical regimens or a thermal regimen. Benzalkonium chloride and chlorobutanol should not be used in solutions for soft contact lenses because of adsorption by the HEMA polymer and subsequent rapid release, which causes ocular tissue damage.

CLEANING SOLUTIONS

Cleaning is the most important step in the proper care of all contact lenses. It optimizes visual acuity, comfort, wearer health, lens life, and both wearer and eye care professional costs. Debris from numerous sources collects on the lens surface almost from the moment of insertion (Table 21). Extended wear lenses quickly develop a thick coating because they are worn constantly. The longer the interval between cleaning, the greater is the risk of complications such as ulcerative keratitis and acanthamoeba keratitis. Despite claims that certain contact lens materials collect certain types of debris, a mixture of debris types is usually found, independent of lens composition. The proper use of surfactants reduces lens coatings, which can contribute to ocular infections. Enzyme cleaners are usually recommended for soft lenses but hard (PMMA and gas permeable) lenses will also benefit from their use.

Surfactant Cleaners

Since many contact lens contaminants are not water soluble, rinsing the lens does not remove all the debris. As the preservative may be inactivated by debris, the lens should be thoroughly cleaned with a surfactant before disinfecting and storing. Surfactants also emulsify and suspend organisms, reducing contamination and facilitating disinfection. Proper cleaning and rinsing can remove more than 99.9% of the contaminants prior to the disinfection step. Since most lens pathogens use organic deposits as food, removal of the food source by effective cleaning can reduce the viability of any surviving pathogens.

FIGURE 5

Hard/Gas Permeable Contact Lens Care

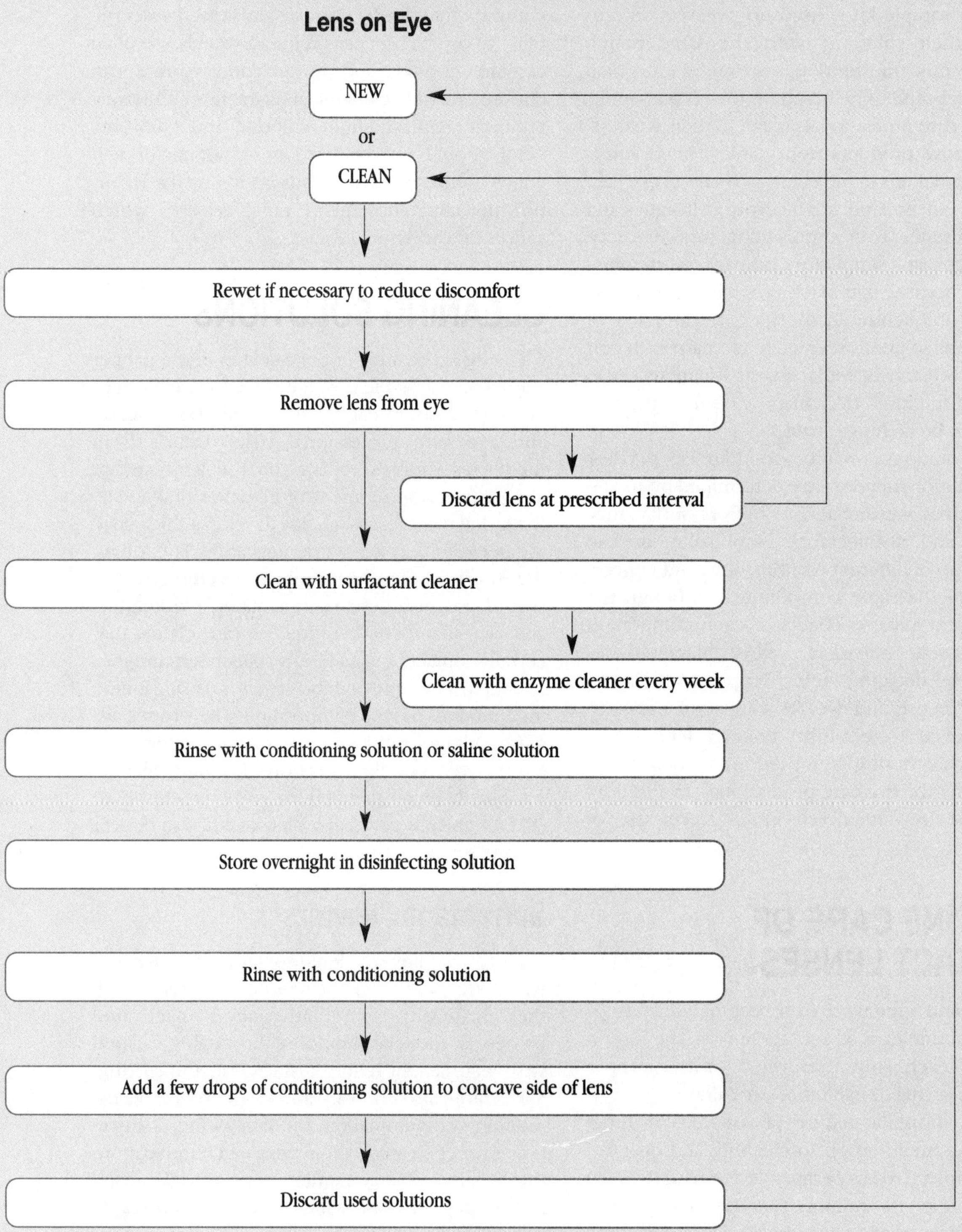

Lens on Eye

NEW
or
CLEAN

↓

Rewet if necessary to reduce discomfort

↓

Remove lens from eye

→ Discard lens at prescribed interval (→ NEW)

↓

Clean with surfactant cleaner

→ Clean with enzyme cleaner every week

↓

Rinse with conditioning solution or saline solution

↓

Store overnight in disinfecting solution

↓

Rinse with conditioning solution

↓

Add a few drops of conditioning solution to concave side of lens

↓

Discard used solutions (→ CLEAN)

FIGURE 6

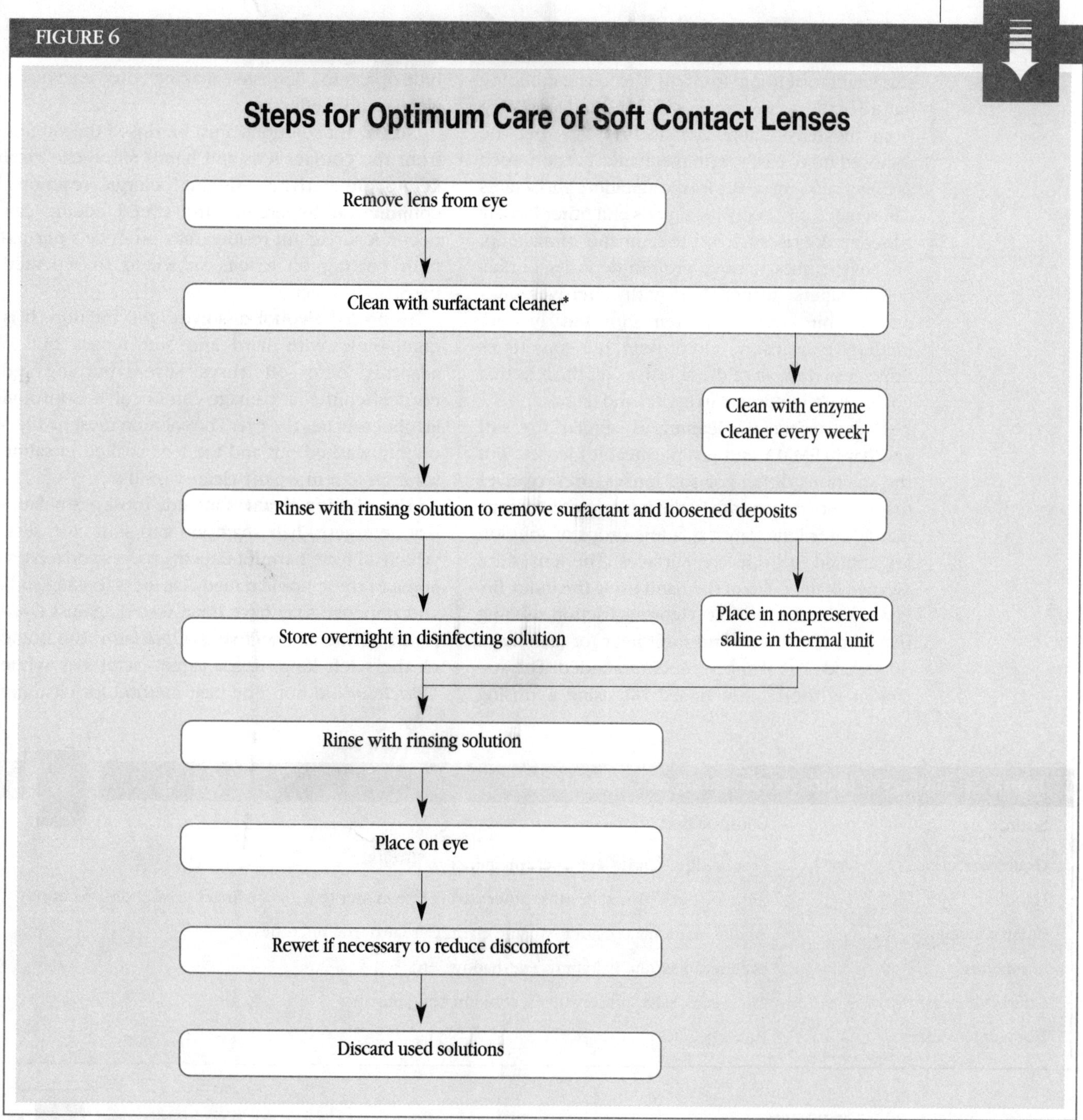

* It is important to rub the lens on the periphery first, since this is where the debris begins to accumulate, then work towards the centre; both sides should be done for at least 20 seconds each.

† The addition of this step to chemical disinfection has decreased the incidence of red eyes, limbal injection, and discomfort in one study. This step has been incorporated into the recommendations of most manufacturers. Regular papain tablets are not recommended for extended wear lenses, but subtilisin tablets can be used.

Both surfactants and debris have hydrophilic and hydrophobic components. The process of the surfactant orienting itself to the corresponding nature of the debris causes softening and loosening from the lens (Table 22). Debris can then be removed more easily with mechanical action, such as finger rubbing or automatic agitation. Surfactants can remove oily deposits, mucus and other loosely adherent debris, such as the remnants of makeup, but they cannot remove protein deposits. Surfactant cleaners formulated with abrasives may remove thin layers of protein film, but they are ineffective against bound protein. It is sometimes difficult to rinse all of the abrasives off the lens that could result in corneal irritation and damage.

Daily surfactant cleaning is similar for soft and hard (PMMA and gas permeable) lenses, but the solutions differ. For soft lenses, preservatives that do not concentrate in the lens are used. Immediately after lens removal, a few drops of solution are applied to both lens surfaces. The lenses are cleaned in the palm of the hand using the index finger in a circular motion. Vigorous friction rubbing between the thumb and forefinger for as long as 30 seconds has also been recommended. The surfactant is thoroughly rinsed off using a rinsing solution before disinfection. The surfactant is used before the enzyme as it acts on the lipids that may hide protein deposits making the enzymatic cleaner more effective.

Surfactant solutions must be rinsed thoroughly from the contact lens and hands since chemical keratoconjunctivitis, stinging, allergic reactions, conjunctival hyperemia and eyelid edema can occur. A surfactant residue may produce a permanent coating on a lens subjected to repeated thermal disinfection.

Isopropyl alcohol dissolves lipid buildup. It is compatible with hard and soft lenses but is adsorbed onto soft lenses. Severe burning and corneal epithelial damage can occur if isopropyl alcohol touches the eye. The solution must be thoroughly washed out and the lens soaked in saline solution to remove the cleaner residue.

Unorthodox cleaners include toothpaste, laundry detergent, hair shampoo and skin cleansers, which all have harmful effects on eyes and lenses. Some of these home remedy cleaners (baking soda and popcorn salt) have been tested against *Opticlean*. While as effective as *Opticlean*, the home cleaners left long, deep, jagged scratches while *Opticlean* did not. The best method for cleaning

TABLE 21: Etiology of Debris Accumulating on Contact Lenses

Source	Composition
Ocular secretions (e.g., tears)	Protein, lipids, salts, enzymes, pigments
Handling	Protein, oils, cosmetics, salts, other particulate matter (e.g., soap, finger grease, dirt, nicotine)
Environmental	Smoke, particulate matter, volatile chemicals, airborne microbes
Cosmetics	Eyeliner, mascara, hairspray, eyeshadow, etc.
Contact lens solutions	Chemicals, salts, preservatives, solution contaminants
Contact lens cases	Bacteria, salts

TABLE 22: Classification of Surfactants

Type	Charge	Examples	Comments
Nonionic	None	Poloxamer 407	Effective, compatible and generally the least toxic
Amphoteric	Positive and negative	Miranol	Depends on pH for maximum effectiveness
Cationic	Positive	Benzalkonium chloride	Effective, but limited in usefulness, especially with soft contact lenses
Anionic	Negative	Sodium lauryl sulfate Soaps	Effective, but generally not used because of high potential for eye irritation and incompatibility with many ingredients; are generally less stable than nonionic surfactants

lenses is a sterile regimen of known surfactants recommended by the eye care professional.

Enzyme Cleaners

Protein begins accumulating from the first day of wear, even in users who may be asymptomatic. Eventually, wearers may develop giant papillary conjunctivitis. The incidence can be reduced significantly by weekly enzymatic cleaning. If deposits are allowed to form, bacteria can adhere, leading to ulcerative keratitis. Most eye care professionals recommend weekly prophylactic cleaning with enzymes although a recent study suggests that it may not be necessary in a PRP.

Most enzyme cleaners contain papain, pancreatin or subtilisin. Enzymes are used to remove protein deposits and prevent their buildup. Enzymes catalyze the natural breakdown of debris into simple compounds, which become softer and easier to remove by mechanical action or rinsing. The lens must be rubbed to effectively remove the broken down protein molecules. Enzymes cannot replace surfactants for cleaning efficiency. Furthermore, their action is slow, requiring 6 to 12 hours. However, regular use of even short soaking times can effectively prevent protein buildup. This is especially useful for high water lenses, which can take up enzyme into the lens matrix with prolonged soaking periods, sometimes resulting in irritation. Subtilisin has little capacity to bind to the lens and was thought safe for long soak times even with high-water content lenses. A comparison of subtilisin and pancreatin using different soak times found no difference in efficacy or comfort. Longer soak times improved visual clarity but was more likely to cause discomfort. A comparison of papain, pancreatin and subtilisin found all enzyme cleaners to be effective but subtilisin-soaked lenses consistently had the least deposit. Enzyme tablets should be dissolved only in sterile saline. Using another solution (such as wetting) could produce a firm gel or other type of new reaction.

The use of enzymes does not replace the need for daily surfactant cleaning, since nonprotein deposits are not removed. Enzymes are specific, so other debris mixed with or covering protein renders enzymes useless. A surfactant removes this nonprotein debris and enables the enzyme to exert its effect. Optimal lens cleaning involves daily use of a surfactant followed by weekly treatment with an enzyme cleaner although deposits are not completely removed. Without enzymes in the cleaning regimen, visual acuity can decrease. Protein accumulation may lead to allergic conjunctivitis as the protein acts as an antigen. It has also been demonstrated that *Pseudomonas aeruginosa* adheres more readily if a soft lens has a mucin or mucin and protein coating.

Papain is a protease (an enzyme that acts on proteins) obtained from the papaya plant. Cysteine is added as a stabilizer and reportedly aids in protein removal. Cysteine imparts the unpleasant odor associated with papain. Papain does not affect the lens matrix. It may be more effective when used with heat disinfection since heat (40 to 60°C) denatures protein more easily than chemical disinfection. Papain can then more readily attack the denatured protein. An enzyme cleaner added to a chemical disinfection regimen is more effective than chemical disinfection alone in preventing protein deposits. It also helps prolong lens life. Enzyme removal of protein is not the same as disinfection. Papain and pancreatin are equally effective at removing protein deposits after 24 hours although pancreatin appears to work faster.

Papain can adsorb onto HEMA lenses and cause burning, pain, photophobia, conjunctival hyperemia, punctate keratitis, corneal edema and conjunctival edema. Local ocular anaphylaxis has been reported. Thorough rinsing of the lens after enzyme cleaning is imperative. Pancreatin has been used successfully by people sensitive to papain but must also be rinsed thoroughly from the lens prior to application to prevent ocular irritation.

Pancreatin is derived from pork pancrease. It is a mixture of protease, lipase and amylase that catalyzes the breakdown of proteins, fats, phospholipids, starch and polysaccharides. An effective surfactant has the same spectrum except for the protein.

Subtilisin is a protease derived from the *Bacillus* bacteria. It is reported to have less specific binding characteristics and be capable of breaking more types of protein bonds than either papain or pancreatin.

DISINFECTION

Disinfecting solutions are designed to disinfect and maintain a disinfected lens, to maintain the hydrated equilibrium of the lens while it is not being worn and to prevent debris from remaining after cleaning. Disinfection destroys all vegetative bacterial cells except spores; sterilization destroys all microbial activity. Contact lenses require only disinfection. Many studies have been performed comparing the efficacy of various products. It is usually difficult for nonmicrobiologists to interpret these studies. To put them into perspective, it should be remembered that all disinfection regimens approved for sale in Canada are effective for their label claims. Extensive testing is required by the Health Protection Branch to support label claims before approval is granted. Therefore, arguments concerning relative efficacy are irrelevant.

A disinfectant actively kills bacteria on lenses; a preservative maintains the sterility of a solution against outside insult. A preserved saline solution does not disinfect unless used for thermal disinfection. Most soaking solutions contain disinfectants and preservatives. Some also contain surfactants but in a lower concentration than in cleaning solutions, so soaking does not replace daily cleaning.

Soaking or Storage Solutions

Organomercurials

Organomercurials kill bacteria and fungi slowly, probably by inhibiting sulfhydryl enzymes. They are incompatible with rose bengal and benzalkonium chloride in certain concentrations and are inhibited by EDTA and inactivated by rubber. Adverse effects include allergy, chemosis (conjunctival edema), keratitis, conjunctival hyperemia, burning, irritation and lens vacuoles.

Thimerosal, the most popular organomercurial, is generally used at 0.001 to 0.004%. The maximum concentration is 0.01%. Thimerosal alone successfully passes all the tests required by the US FDA to qualify as a preservative in contact lens solutions, and its combination with chlorhexidine or alkyltriethylammonium chloride yields an effective broad spectrum disinfectant. Its usefulness combined with chlorhexidine is discussed in the chlorhexidine section.

Thimerosal can be inactivated by corneal fluids and must be used in neutral or slightly alkaline conditions. The amount of thimerosal retained by HEMA lenses correlates with the water content of the lens. Storage equilibrium is reached after 1 hour, and when the lens is inserted, the thimerosal leaves the lens just as rapidly. Thimerosal can cause gray to black lens discoloration in thermal disinfection regimens.

Phenylmercuric nitrate is the other organomercurial preservative in contact lens solutions. The maximum concentration for use in the eye is 0.004%. It should not be used with soft lenses because it binds to the lenses and is precipitated by halide ions (present in debris).

Chlorhexidine

Chlorhexidine is effective against gram-negative and gram-positive bacteria, although less effective against the latter. It is more effective than thimerosal, but at low concentrations (e.g., 0.005%), clinical efficacy varies. It is more toxic to ocular tissues than thimerosal. The best results are obtained when chlorhexidine is combined with thimerosal (for its antifungal effect) and EDTA (for antimicrobial effect). This combination is effective against acanthamoeba cysts, but some chlorhexidine formulations may not be. Disinfection requires at least 4 hours, preferably overnight.

Chlorhexidine is compatible with most ophthalmic products but incompatible with soaps, anions and fluorescein solutions and is inactivated by cork, starch, magnesium, zinc and calcium compounds. It binds strongly to HEMA lenses, especially in the presence of other adjuvants (such as electrolyte or hydrophilic polymers). Soft lenses store chlorhexidine, which leaves slowly after insertion, exposing the eye to a decreasing concentration. The binding capacity of chlorhexidine is about one-sixth that of benzalkonium chloride and a large percentage is absorbed by tear proteins. The presence of protein can increase the concentration of chlorhexidine in the lens, so it is important to remove protein regularly with an enzymatic cleaner before soaking the lenses in chlorhexidine. Lenses saturated with chlorhexidine become hydrophobic and adsorb lipids to their surfaces. Chlorhexidine can eventually cause lens filming, yellowing and decreased wettability. Solutions should be discarded if they have a greenish tinge.

With extended use, a solution of 0.005% appears nontoxic to eye tissue, but skin sensitivities, eye discomfort and irritation of the conjunctiva have been reported. Direct application to the eye may cause conjunctivitis.

EDTA

EDTA and its salts edetate, disodium edetate and trisodium edetate break down the bacterial cell wall with a detergent action. It is not a preservative, but its presence enhances the activity of preservatives. EDTA also acts as a buffer.

The usual concentrations of EDTA range from 0.01 to 0.1%. These concentrations cannot prevent or remove inorganic calcium deposits from lenses, which requires concentrations of 0.35 to 1.85%. EDTA enhances the activity of benzalkonium chloride, chlorobutanol, chlorhexidine and thimerosal by chelating calcium and magnesium ions, which compete with preservatives for sites on the organism. Conjunctival edema, hyperemia and irritation are possible.

Lens Storage

Contact lenses should be stored in contact lens cases. They should be completely covered by the soaking solution when not worn, as they can dry out, changing the lens parameters slightly. Soaking maintains hydration, making it wet more readily. A hard (PMMA and gas permeable) lens dries out in just 12 hours (changing the lens parameter), but it requires about 72 hours to fully hydrate again. Storage cases must be kept clean by routinely boiling them in water. The lens case is allowed to cool 30 to 45 minutes before replacing the lenses. Some types of lens cases that cannot withstand boiling should be replaced at least monthly. To optimize disinfection and minimize potential irritation, lenses should be cleaned with a surfactant cleaner before disinfecting and soaking. The soaking solution should be replaced daily and the case flushed of old solution before adding new solution. Some manufacturers and researchers now recommend regular replacement of contact lens cases due to the risk of contamination from biofilm buildup. A new method being investigated for cleaning cases is to microwave the case for 30 seconds or less, first removing the lenses.

Chemical Disinfection Products

Chemical disinfection of soft lenses is similar to the soaking process for hard (PMMA and gas permeable) lenses: they are soaked (or stored), usually overnight, in a chemical disinfecting solution. With the appropriate solutions, chemical disinfection can be used for all soft contact lens materials. Unlike hard lens soaking solutions, disinfecting solutions for soft lenses must be rinsed off (with at least 25 mL of rinsing solution)—except for some multifunction solutions—before the lenses are inserted in the eyes. With hard lenses, saline solution or the disinfecting solution is used for rinsing. With all lenses, tap water is not recommended because of potential accumulation of minerals on the lens and possible contamination (e.g., acanthamoeba keratitis). Normal saline is generally used as the rinsing solution for soft lenses, which is required after soft lens cleaning, before lens disinfection.

There are five chemical disinfection systems in Canada for soft contact lenses: chlorhexidine, thimerosal and an EDTA salt; alkyltriethanolammonium chloride (AKTAC), thimerosal and an EDTA salt; polyquaternium-1 (polyquad); polyaminopropylbiguanide; and hydrogen peroxide. Hydrogen peroxide systems must be inactivated after disinfection before the lens is worn. Sorbic acid (or potassium sorbate) combined with an EDTA salt is not a chemical disinfection system but rather a soaking and rinsing system. Sorbic acid is gradually replacing thimerosal in these systems.

The advantages of chemical disinfectants are: ease of use (fewer products, fewer steps); greater compliance due to ease of use; lower overall cost; and no chance of forgetting to neutralize the disinfectant. Most literature on chemical disinfection concerns the first two systems.

Failure rates for chemical disinfection vary from 0.63 to 40.5%. This wide range may be due to quality of user instruction, user selection or lens condition. Two major causes of the high rates of failure with chemical disinfection have been suggested: failure to rule out extremely fair-skinned, light-eyed users with a history of sensitivity to sun and chemicals, and improper and inadequate lens cleaning by the user. More than 95% of wearers can successfully use chemical disinfection if wearers are carefully selected and instructed on the importance of thorough cleaning.

The disadvantages of chemical disinfection solutions are adverse effects from solution components, difficulty differentiating between changes produced by solutions and by lenses, and incompatibilities between chemical and thermal disinfection systems.

In addition to the preservatives for both hard (PMMA and gas permeable) and soft lenses, AKTAC and sorbic acid are used for soft lenses.

Alkyltriethanolammonium chloride (AKTAC, Quaternium 16) is a quaternary ammonium like benzalkonium chloride. Its antimicrobial effect outweighs its surfactant effect. Disinfection is slow but effective. It is not as effective against bacteria and fungi as chlorhexidine, and probably not effective against *Acanthamoeba*. A 0.03% solution alters the physical parameters of a soft lens minimally over a year, but these changes are reversible with saline soaking. Reactions similar to those of thimerosal can occur in 10 to 15% of wearers. AKTAC cannot be used with CSI (glyceryl methacrylate) lenses due to the development of adverse corneal and conjunctival responses.

Sorbic acid (or potassium sorbate) has limited antimicrobial activity, with weak activity against fungi and *Acanthamoeba*. It is most effective at a pH of 4 or less, which is enough to cause some ocular irritation. However, if the pH is raised even up to 6.5, sorbic acid loses its effectiveness as a preservative. Its use in soaking and wetting solutions may not be justified since the pH of these solutions is about 7. Preserved saline solutions containing sorbic acid are used only as a preservative and not for disinfection.

Sorbic acid's fungistatic activity is increased by acids and sodium chloride; effective concentrations are 0.1 to 0.2%. Concentration in HEMA lenses is minimal, and it diffuses freely from the lens to the surrounding fluids. It is compatible with nonionic surfactants and is relatively nontoxic, although eye irritation and allergic dermatitis have been reported.

Sorbic acid combined with lens deposits has been implicated in lens discoloration. Lenses should not be stored in these solutions for more than 1 or 2 weeks because of discoloration (usually brownish). Minimizing the formation of deposits and following the recommendations of the eye care professional minimizes lens discoloration. High water content lenses (55% or greater), if heated with a sorbic acid system, yellow over time since they absorb significant amounts of protein, which reacts with heat. Gray-green discoloration has been reported when heat was used with a sorbic acid concentration greater than 0.15%.

Two new disinfectants are **polyquaternium-1** and **polyaminopropylbiguanide**. The antimicrobial activities of three new nonperoxide soft contact lens disinfection systems, *ReNu Multi-Purpose Solution* (0.00005% polyaminopropylbiguanide), *Opti-Soft Disinfecting Solution* (0.001% polyquaternium-1), *Opti-Free Rinsing, Disinfecting and Storage Solution* (0.001% polyquaternium-1), were compared to *Soft Mate Disinfecting Solution* (0.005% chlorhexidine digluconate) versus the organisms specified by the FDA for evaluating microbiological effectiveness of soft lens chemical disinfection solutions. All demonstrated excellent activity against *Pseudomonas aeruginosa* and *Staphylococcus epidermidis* with complete disinfection in 4 hours. Only *Soft Mate* disinfected *Serratia marcescens* and *Candida albicans* in 4 hours and reduced the spore count of *Aspergillus fumigatus*. The others reduced *Candida albicans* only slightly and had virtually no activity against *Aspergillus fumigatus*. Against *Serratia marcescens*, they were marginally effective. For newer chemical disinfection systems, diligent cleaning and rinsing are the most important steps. Polyaminopropylbiguanide and polyquaternium-1 are less effective than thimerosal/chlorhexidine against *Acanthamoeba* cysts.

Oxidizing agents include peroxides (hydrogen peroxide and sodium peroxide), peroxy salts (sodium perborate) and chlorine-related compounds (sodium hypochlorite); the only one used in Canada is hydrogen peroxide. Oxidizing agents are inherently unstable and, in the presence of organic debris, form free radicals that attack and disperse debris. The effervescence is a secondary means of removing debris from the lens matrix. They also act as germicides by releasing newly formed oxygen.

All oxidizing agents have a strong cleaning action independent of the nature of debris. However, all manufacturers who market hydrogen peroxide systems, recommend the use of daily cleaners and weekly enzyme cleaners. They do not affect the tint of soft lenses. Reports conflict on whether hydrogen peroxide damages lenses. Warping may result if hydrogen peroxide is used with gas permeable lenses. The safety of hydrogen peroxide systems relies entirely on adequate neutralization of the hydrogen peroxide. Neutralization methods include the use of a platinum catalyst, sodium pyruvate, catalase or rinsing and dilution. These systems are either one-step, where neutralization occurs automatically, or two-step, where the consumer initiates neutralization after disinfection. Keratopathy, which developed in consumers using the one step-catalytic neutralization, resolved when switched to a hydrogen peroxide system using a second catalase neutralization step. Although instillation of hydrogen peroxide (3%) 3 times a day for 5 days produced no ocular damage, lenses should be thoroughly rinsed of hydrogen peroxide to prevent potential eye irritation. No permanent corneal damage due to hydrogen peroxide has been reported. However, insertion of a soft lens inadvertently stored in 3% hydrogen peroxide produced an immediate, painful reaction that took 48 hours to clear. Exposure of the eyes to 3% hydrogen peroxide from disinfection systems can result in stinging, tearing, hyperemia, blepharospasm, edema and possibly permanent corneal damage. No adverse effects have been observed with ocular hydrogen peroxide levels used in the routine proper use of hydrogen peroxide systems. Cleaning the lens with a surfactant followed by thorough rinsing and a 2- to 3-hour soak in 3% hydrogen peroxide disinfects the lens. This time is required to eradicate

Acanthamoeba, which is well within the recommendation of a 6-hour disinfection with some products. Other systems recommend disinfection times of 10 to 20 minutes. Fungi require 1 to 2 hours. Oxidizing agents destroy pigments and remove color from the lens. When the pigment is oxidized and soluble, small voids remain in the lens matrix, resulting in a spongy layer at the site of pigment deposition. Oxidizing agents work most efficiently when combined with heat.

Generic hydrogen peroxide is not recommended, as it is designed for topical use and meets less strict standards than ophthalmic hydrogen peroxide. Some generic hydrogen peroxide contains impurities, stabilizers or other additives that irritate ocular tissue or discolor the lenses.

Allergic Reactions

Agreement is lacking on the proportion of chemical disinfection users who develop a sufficiently severe eye reaction to warrant cessation of the regimen. Depending on the study, the incidence ranges from 0.5 to 73%, although 5 to 10% appears to be the most frequent estimate. Some reports do not rule out the possibility of a reaction to chlorhexidine, EDTA or sorbic acid. Due to patient sensitivities to thimerosal and chlorhexidine, most solutions no longer contain these compounds.

Nonallergic reactions are possible since many components can act as primary irritants. Contact lens solution components are unlikely to provoke an allergic response directly due to their small molecular size. These components can act as haptens or incomplete antigens, which bind to body proteins to form complexes that stimulate an immune reaction against the component. An allergic response is facilitated by large amounts of antigen and the antigen persisting at the reaction site. Daily use of lenses stored in an allergy-causing solution provides ideal conditions for the continuous availability of antigen to produce an allergic reaction in susceptible users, especially if a protein coating increases the amount of antigen bound to the lens.

An adverse ocular response due to allergy or toxicity encompasses a wide range of signs and symptoms. Since redness is usually present, the reaction has been called red eye or the red eye syndrome. Other symptoms include discomfort on lens insertion, decreased wearing time, stinging, burning, dryness, itching, irritation, tearing, discharge, swelling, blurring and nasal fullness. Signs include conjunctival hyperemia and edema, papillary follicular hypertrophy, corneal edema, pseudocysts, fluorescein or rose bengal staining, sloughed epithelial cells, limbal follicles, and ulceration and infiltrates. Tears may be excessive or excess mucus secretion may develop with excessive lipid-contaminated mucus threads. The lids may become swollen, and, in extreme cases, the facial derma affected. Corneal opacities have been reported with the use of some preserved saline solutions.

An allergic reaction to solution components, particularly preservatives, may take days to months to develop before the onset of keratoconjunctivitis. Users who experience a reaction soon after exposure to a solution may have had a pre-existing but unrecognized sensitivity. In other users, sensitization or toxicity may have come from repeated application of exposed soft lenses to the cornea. Factors that increase the risk of developing an allergy include: allergy to intravenous pyelogram (IVP) dyes or povidone-iodine, penicillin allergy, diabetic relatives, concurrent tetracycline treatment. It has been postulated that tetracycline chelates the mercury in thimerosal, precipitating the response. Discontinuing the tetracycline or the thimerosal-containing solution has cleared the reaction. The easiest and possibly the best way to predict which wearers may react to preservatives is to take a careful history. People with a history of atopic problems tend to have more severe reactions than other users.

Allergic reactions are best treated by removing the source of antigen. A mild response may be resolved by rinsing lenses well before insertion, using more thorough surfactant cleaning techniques, rinsing the lenses well after surfactant cleaning and soaking the lenses for 5 minutes in saline before insertion. If these procedures fail, a multipurge procedure must be performed to remove surface deposits or chemicals. An alternative system can be initiated using different chemical disinfectants and preservatives or a thermal nonpreserved system. If symptoms persist, a lens reaction should be considered.

In addition to user noncompliance, numerous other causes of adverse reactions have been postulated. These include the types, combinations or concentrations of preservatives; the chemical changes in residual chemicals left on lenses from thermal disinfection; cross-usage of systems in going from thermal to chemical disinfection (denatured proteins adsorb chemicals, which then become severe irritants); poor fit; defective lenses;

extraneous lens deposits; environmental factors; sensitivities; allergies; incomplete care regimens; and solution-related and bacterial problems.

Thermal Disinfection

Thermal disinfection uses an elevated temperature to kill heat-sensitive microorganisms. It is probably the strongest disinfecting system available. Only heat has been shown completely effective against *Acanthamoeba* cysts. It applies only to soft and pure silicone lenses as other lens types cannot withstand the temperatures required. Thermal disinfection is nonspecific and works by gross protein denaturation of microorganisms. The lenses are placed in a specially designed case that is then filled with isotonic saline and placed in a heating unit. Most units heat the lenses to 80°C for 10 minutes before automatically shutting off. This time and temperature kills bacteria and fungi of potential hazard to the eye (e.g., *Pseudomonas aeruginosa*, *Staphylococcus aureus*, *Escherichia coli*, *Candida albicans*, and *Aspergillus niger*) and *Acanthamoeba*. Sterilization requires 120°C for 15 minutes and 103.43 kilopascals. Since the lenses are disinfected rather than sterilized, spores can germinate if the lenses are stored for a prolonged period. The lenses should be disinfected before wearing after prolonged storage. Saline intended for thermal disinfection should not contain chlorhexidine, since lenses stored in such solutions become opaque after a few boiling cycles. Thermal disinfection is not used with high water content lenses (55% or greater) as this system may discolor lenses and reduce performance.

Numerous disadvantages of thermal disinfection have been cited. The initial cost of purchase is relatively high, although the yearly cost is the lowest of all systems. Microorganisms can accumulate if the procedure is not performed daily and if fresh saline is not prepared daily. If heating is not performed daily to destroy vegetative forms of the bacteria, spores may survive to cause lens damage. Repeated heating may decrease lens life. It has been suggested that the lens loss rate doubles from chips, rips and cracks, but in one study, no adverse effects from thermal disinfection occurred for 30 months. Microorganisms on the lens surface may cause lens discomfort, loss of transparency, loss of acuity, lens discoloration, conjunctival hyperemia, change in lens fitting and reduced lens porosity. If microproteins and surfactants are not adequately removed, they are baked onto the lens, decreasing lens life. With proper cleaning, the lens life with hydrogen peroxide and thermal disinfection is similar. Regular omission of cleaning before heating causes deposits to build up, decreasing visual acuity and creating discomfort. Multiple reuse of thimerosal-containing solutions with heat disinfection, may result in gray-black mercurial deposits on the lens. Usually, these deposits are first found in the lens case.

Thermal disinfection is inconvenient and likely to be neglected. Electricity is required, and saline problems and mechanical failure can occur. Due to these potential problems, chemical disinfection is preferred by most wearers. Newer heat disinfection units are small, lightweight, cordless and accept various power requirements. Although popularity has dropped for these systems, thermal disinfection is still as effective as any other system.

Microwave and ultraviolet sterilization of soft lenses is still under study.

Saline is available in two forms: preserved saline solutions and unit dose or multidose unpreserved saline. Salt tablets are no longer marketed by any manufacturer in Canada.

Preserved saline minimizes the risk of contamination during repeated use, and the correct concentration is controlled by the manufacturer. The cost is significantly higher than for salt tablets, but safety and convenience are greater. Unfortunately, many users of preserved saline develop preservative sensitivity. The introduction of sorbic acid and polyaminopropylbiguanide preserved saline should decrease the incidence of sensitivity reactions. The introduction of thimerosal-free saline in a 120 mL unit dose size or a multidose aerosol form should also help overcome potential sensitivity reactions. Aerosol and other salines should be buffered to ensure that pH stays within the ocular comfort range.

Unpreserved unit dose saline overcomes potential mixing errors by the user and potential sensitivity reactions, but microbial contamination can occur if the solution stands longer than the recommended time or if used improperly. However, multidose aerosol preserved saline is equally effective in preventing sensitivity reactions and remains sterile for the life of the product because of the aerosol mechanism at the top of the can. Before each use, a small amount of saline should be discharged. The saline inside the mechanism is open to the outside environment and may be contaminated.

Table 23 summarizes chemical and thermal disinfection regimens. Protein films are more of a problem with thermally disinfected lenses; inorganic deposits are more frequent in chemically disinfected lenses. However, any enzyme cleaner minimizes the potential buildup of protein deposits. A switch to chemical disinfection may be valuable for wearers with pigment deposit, mercurial deposit or rust deposit problems or microbial growth.

Very few wearers use heat disinfection. Almost all new patients use a chemical regimen. The advantages and disadvantages of each should be explained to the consumer. A careless person may be a better candidate for thermal disinfection since most of the work is done by the heat; however, deposits or solutions may be baked onto the lens. Sloppy technique with chemical disinfection often produces problems.

WETTING AND VISCOSITY AGENTS

Wetting Agents

Hard (PMMA and gas permeable) lenses require wetting to reduce the foreign body sensation on insertion. Natural saliva is an excellent wetting solution but contains many potential pathogens and should never be used.

Wetting agents reduce surface interactions between tears and the contact lens or between tears and the cornea, allowing the tears to spread evenly. They generally contain large polymers that increase the tear flow over a hydrophobic lens surface and provide a brief cushion between the lens and cornea.

A hydrophobic hard (PMMA and gas permeable) lens must be wet to avoid discomfort and possible damage to the eyes. The mucin layer of the tear film contains highly hydrated polysaccharides that wet the lens, but this deposition can take up to 15 minutes to develop, during which the wearer is uncomfortable. A wetting and cushioning solution minimizes the transitional discomfort until the eyes adjust. The solution is applied to the concave side of the lens immediately before insertion.

The wetting solution serves other functions. It protects the lens surface with a viscous coating, thus avoiding direct contact with the finger during insertion. It lubricates the lid and lens surface, which cushions the lens on the cornea. It aids in lens cleaning after removal from the eye. It facilitates lens insertion by stabilizing the lens on the fingertips.

Wearers who have surface drying of their contact lenses report blurry vision, lens dryness, scleral hyperemia and itching. Properties such as pH, osmolarity and wetting angle, are usually not included on the product label. Although irrelevant to the average wearer, these properties may be important for the atypical user with problems. When the three properties were evaluated with 10 hard lens solutions (most were for wetting), no two solutions had similar properties.

TABLE 23: Pros and Cons of Chemical and Thermal Disinfection of Soft Contact Lenses

Factor	Chemical	Thermal
Efficacy	High	High
Convenience	High	Moderate
Restrictions on type of lens	No	Yes
Special apparatus and power required	No	Yes
Cost	Cheaper initially	May be cheaper eventually
Lens life	about 2.5 yr	about 1 yr
Time required	6–8 hr	about 1 hr
Debris buildup	Low to moderate	High
Compliance	Similar	Similar
Acceptability	High (85%)	High (95%)
Extended wear lenses	Tolerated better	Not tolerated well

Examples of wetting agents found in hard contact lens solutions include polyvinyl alcohol, poloxamer 407 and polysorbate 80.

Viscosity Agents

Viscosity agents are large colloidal molecules that increase resistance to flow and are used to hold tears in the eyes. They produce a cushioning and lubricant effect between the lens and the eyelid and the lens and the cornea (Table 24). They are not recommended in soaking solutions since they can retard diffusion of lens contaminants into the solution. They are not wetting agents, so they do not enhance the spread of tears over the cornea. The pH of lubricating solutions changes after the expiration date and, if used, may cause burning or stinging.

Rewetting Agents

Lubricating and rewetting drops are applied directly to relieve dry eyes when wearing a hard (PMMA and gas permeable) or soft lens. These solutions usually contain saline, preservatives and a viscosity agent for cushioning. In extended wear, they are also used as flushing agents before sleep and immediately upon awakening to remove debris accumulated under the lens. Most rewetting solutions designed for soft lenses are also compatible with hard (PMMA and gas permeable) lenses, but the reverse may not be true (Table 25).

Soft contact lenses are hydrophilic and do not require a wetting solution to adapt to the eye. However, they do tend to dry out through the day, especially in a dry or polluted environment. Up to 75% of soft lens wearers experience this symptom. One or more of the following can contribute to dry eye symptoms: diuretics, hormones (e.g., oral contraceptives) and lack of adequate tearing due to age, certain illnesses, air conditioning or low humidity. Rewetting solutions, artificial tears preserved with chemicals compatible with soft lenses, rehydrate the lens but should be limited to 1 drop every 4 to 5 hours. If drops are used more frequently, the user may develop red, irritated eyes and a foreign body sensation. Other artificial tears should not be used for rewetting soft contact lenses since most contain preservatives (e.g., benzalkonium chloride) that are incompatible with soft lenses. No one product is consistently superior to any other, although nonpreserved solutions generally yield the higher comfort scores. In addition, lubricants have not been found significantly superior to saline.

Rewetting solutions can be used several times daily to relieve the discomfort of dehydration and partly to clean the lens. If the rewetting period is too short, the lenses may have to be removed once daily for surfactant cleaning and saline rinsing to increase lens wettability.

MULTIFUNCTION SOLUTIONS

For hard lenses, the eye care professional can recommend as many as five single-purpose products or as few as one all-purpose product. For convenience, numerous products combine two or

TABLE 24: Viscosity Agents

Agent	Properties	Adverse Effects
Methylcellulose (actually hydroxypropyl methylcellulose in most solutions)	Viscosity range is 10 to 15,000 centipoises for 2% solutions.	Cellulose derivatives have few side effects, although granulation on the eyelids and conjunctiva is possible under dry conditions.
	Nonionic and therefore stable over a wide pH (2–12); at pH less than 2, viscosity decreases; temperatures greater than 50°C cause precipitation in water; nearly inert chemically and is entirely compatible with the drugs commonly used in the eye; will form complexes with most of the hydroxybenzoates; does not support growth of microorganisms.	Corneal edema has been reported with methylcellulose instillation.
Ethylcellulose (actually hydroxyethylcellulose in most solutions)	Viscosity is not affected by pH changes between 5 and 10. Like methylcellulose, it is nonionic and water-soluble; unlike methylcellulose, it is not precipitated from water by an elevated temperature.	

TABLE 25: Wetting Agents		
Agent	**Properties**	**Adverse Effects**
Polyvinyl alcohol (PVA)	Has some viscosity building effect and, unlike some viscosity agents (e.g., methylcellulose), does not retard regeneration of corneal epithelium. Some wetting solutions are adjusted to pH 5 to 6 since acetylated PVA can decompose in alkaline pH into polyvinyl alcohol and acetic acid which can irritate the eyes.	All wetting agents are fairly inert, but they may slightly retard healing of the corneal epithelium. Allergic reactions to PVA have been reported.
Polyvinylpyrrolidone (povidone)	Reduces the chemical binding characteristics of soft lenses without reducing antibacterial activity. Wetting capacity is less than PVA.	
Adsorbobase povidone	Exact structure has not been released.	

more functions in a single solution. Controversy surrounds the extent of compromise of the primary functions, especially cleaning, with multifunctional solutions for hard lenses. Clinical evaluation of a nine-ingredient, all-purpose hard lens solution (clean, wet, disinfect, cushion and rewet) found consumers readily accepted the solution and it cleaned as well as single-purpose solutions. Comparative studies with single-purpose solutions in a clinical setting are required to substantiate this study.

With soft lenses, inattentive young people and older individuals often have difficulty with a regimen consisting of many solutions. Most noncompliance problems result from using several solutions in a certain sequence. User noncompliance (inadequate cleaning and disinfection) caused about half the problems in a large study of soft lens wearers. Preliminary investigations with a multifunction solution for soft lenses have found improved compliance and good user acceptance. A recent comparison of a single product system versus three multiproduct systems showed no significant differences in visible protein. Multifunction solutions may be indicated where improved wearer compliance is the primary factor. For soft lenses, multifunction solutions can no longer be considered a compromise. Multifunction soft lens care products are the fastest growing segment of the contact lens care market.

Multifunction solutions do not guarantee increased compliance. Eye care professionals must continuously stress lens hygiene and periodically have wearers demonstrate their lens care technique.

ACCESSORY SOLUTIONS

Accessory solutions include any combination of rewetting, lubricating and cushioning solutions. Solutions in this class have all three properties in varying degrees despite their label claims, but the clinical significance of these differences is not known.

An unusually dry environment, such as one caused by air conditioning or central heating, may cause the eye or lens to dry out during wear. A few drops of rewetting solution placed in the eye every hour often relieves the discomfort.

A study of eight solutions found that no two were alike in terms of viscosity, osmotic balance, acidity, buffering capacity and wetting angle. With such knowledge, the solution can be individualized to the wearer; certain viscosities may be more appropriate for the dry-eyed user versus the user with a thin watery tear; a more alkaline solution can be recommended for the acid-sensitive eye. The selection may be based on preservative content if the wearer is allergic to specific preservatives.

Artificial tears, also known as tear substitutes, moisturizing drops, lubricants and soothing agents, are recommended for wetting the surface of the eye once the lens is removed. They are not recommended for lubricating the lens while it is in the eye.

Cushioning agents provide an additional buffer layer between the lens, cornea and eyelid.

Tap water is not recommended as a rinsing solution due to the increasing number of cases of acanthamoeba keratitis in rigid lens wearers.

BUFFERS

Buffers resist changes in pH from additions of small amounts of acid or base. In contact lens solutions, buffers stabilize components and improve comfort on instillation. Normal tears have a pH of about 7.3 and a high buffering capacity due to their protein content. Placing 1 or 2 drops of solution into the eye stimulates tear flow and rapid neutralization of excess hydrogen and hydroxyl ions within the buffering capacity of the tears. Solutions of pH 6 to 9 generally can be tolerated. Solutions that are acidic or alkaline for ingredient stability should not be buffered, or should be minimally buffered, so rapid neutralization by tears can occur on instillation. It has been recommended that buffered solutions be used to ensure eye comfort unless contraindicated.

Buffers include: sodium carbonate, boric acid, sodium borate, sodium bicarbonate, sodium phosphate and disodium phosphate. Borate buffers react with polyvinyl alcohol (contained in artificial tears) to form a thick, filmy coating on lenses. Solutions with these components should not be mixed.

PRESERVATIVES (Antimicrobial Agents)

Benzalkonium and chlorobutanol are used in solutions for hard (PMMA and gas permeable) lenses only.

Benzalkonium chloride probably changes the permeability of the cell membrane of the organism. It is effective against gram-negative and gram-positive bacteria. Most lens care solutions use concentrations of 0.003 to 0.01%. Excessive concentrations may damage the corneal and conjunctival epithelium, but weak concentrations may be ineffective. Other antibacterial agents, such as EDTA or chlorobutanol, are combined with benzalkonium chloride to produce a synergistic effect. Benzalkonium chloride with EDTA is perhaps the best combination for hard contact lens solutions. It has surfactant properties and can also enhance transcorneal drug penetration.

PMMA does not carry a charge in water, so the ionic characteristics of solution components (such as benzalkonium chloride) are not important. It is absorbed by soft lenses that subsequently release benzalkonium chloride at concentrations sufficient to produce side effects. Due to benzalkonium chloride's ionic nature, numerous drug interactions are possible (e.g., nitrate, salicylate, fluorescein solutions and some sulfonamides). The bactericidal activity decreases in the presence of cotton, methylcellulose, soaps, metallic ions and rubber. To maintain optimal activity, contact lens cases should be thoroughly rinsed of soap. Rubber ring case liners should be avoided.

Adverse reactions have been reported even with low concentrations. Although benzalkonium chloride can retard epithelial regeneration, most reactions (e.g., epithelial damage or conjunctivitis) are superficial and reversible upon drug cessation. Corneal irritation has been reported and may be related to adsorption by RGP material. There has been an increased incidence of contact lens-associated conjunctivitis and keratitis from *Serratia marcescens*, a rare gram-negative bacteria thought to be of relevance only in the hospital setting. Although the most common causes of contact lens-associated ulcers are *Pseudomonas* or *Staphylococcus*, the most common isolate from rigid gas permeable lenses is *Serratia*. It has been suggested that *Serratia* has developed resistance more readily to rigid gas permeable lens disinfection systems that employ benzalkonium chloride/chlorhexidine than to disinfectants used for soft lenses.

Chlorobutanol above 0.35% is bacteriostatic against fungi and gram-positive and gram-negative bacteria. It is bactericidal only when exposure exceeds 24 hours. It is effective only after it penetrates the bacterial cell, where it is converted to a lethal epitoxoid by the organism. It is incompatible with silicone lenses.

Chlorobutanol has no advantage over benzalkonium chloride. Due to its volatility, solutions exposed to air may fall below effective concentrations. It is synergistic with phenols and quaternaries, such as benzalkonium chloride, but requires a pH less than 6 or it breaks down to hydrochloric acid and other hydrocarbons. It does not appear to reduce the pharmacologic activity of other ophthalmic medications. It is concentrated in soft lenses and may cause a mild conjunctivitis. No allergic reactions with topical use have been reported.

MIXING SOLUTIONS

Solutions from different manufacturers should not be used unless recommended by an eye care professional. Manufacturers formulate each component solution of a care regimen to be compatible with each of the other components. Preclinical and ongoing research ensures their compatibility and efficacy. The effect of substituting even one solution from a different manufacturer is not predictable even if it has the same active ingredients in the same concentration. About the only solution that can be substituted by the consumer is aerosol saline.

Mixing solutions from different manufacturers is hazardous due to the proliferation of lens care products and contact lens materials. In the never ending quest to improve comfort and wear time, researchers experiment with newer and more complex lens polymers. This diversity of materials with their own individual cleaning and disinfecting requirements has stimulated manufacturers to become more specific in the design of solutions. If the wrong solution got into a lens that required specific solutions, the lens could be ruined.

RECOMMENDED READING

Eye Disorders

Abelson MB, George MA, Garofalo C. Differential diagnosis of ocular allergic disorders. Ann Allergy 1993;70:95-109.

Abelson MB, Schaefer K. Conjunctivitis of allergic origin: immunologic mechanisms and current approaches to therapy. Surv Ophthalmol 1993; 38(suppl):115-32.

Bartlett JD, Ghormley NR, Jaanus SD, et al, eds. Ophthalmic drug facts. St Louis: Facts and Comparisons, 1994.

Bartlett JD, Swanson MW. Ophthalmic products. In: Handbook of Nonprescription Drugs. 10th ed. Washington: American Pharmaceutical Association, 1993.

Bennett DR, ed. Drug Evaluations—Annual 1994. Chicago: American Medical Association, 1993.

Ciprandi G, et al. Drug treatment of allergic conjunctivitis. Drugs 1992;43(2):154-76.

Doughty MJ. A practical guide to therapeutic drugs for primary eye care in Canada. Can J Optom 1994;56(3):133-46.

Ophthalmic drug products for over-the-counter human use; final monograph; final rule. Federal Register 1988;53(43):7076-93.

Reese RE, Betts RF, eds. A Practical Approach to Infectious Diseases. Boston: Little, Brown, 1991.

Sanford JP, Gilbert DN, Gerberding JL, et al, eds. Guide to Antimicrobial Therapy. Dallas: Antimicrobial Therapy Inc, 1994.

Schachat AP, ed. Current Practice in Ophthalmology. St. Louis: Mosby, 1992.

Vaughan D, Asbury T, Riordan-Eva P, eds. General Ophthalmology. 13th ed. Connecticut: Appleton & Lange, 1992.

Contact Lenses

Schein OD, Glynn RJ, Poggio EC, et al. Microbial Keratitis Study Group. The relative risk of ulcerative keratitis among users of daily-wear and extended-wear soft contact lenses. A case-control study. N Engl J Med 1989;321:773-78.

Gellatly KW. Disposable contact lenses: a clinical performance review. Can J Optom 1993;55: 166-73.

Marshall EC. Disposable vs non-disposable contact lenses—the relative risk of ocular infection. J Am Optom Assoc 1992;63:28-34.

Gordon KD. Disinfection efficacy of soft lens care systems. Prac Optom 1991;2:149-151.

International Committee on Contact Lenses. Contact lens maintenance systems. Int Contact Lens Clin 1992;19:153-56.

Persico J. Keep the bugs out. Optom Mgtmt 1993;Feb:59-64.

Trick LR. Patient compliance—don't count on it! J Am Optom Assoc 1993;64:264-70.

10

FIRST AID PRODUCTS

KIMBERLEY ROWAT WHITE

CONTENTS

The Skin 223
Minor Cuts and Wounds 224
- Wound Classification
- Wound Healing
- Treatment

Skin Infection 228
- Pathophysiology
- Bacterial Skin Infections
- Fungal Skin Infections
- Viral Skin Infections

Burns 235
- Burn Wound Pathology
- Burn Wound Classification and Appearance
- Treatment

Frostbite 238
Poisoning 239
Insect Bites and Stings 241
- Prevention
- Treatment

Pharmaceutical Agents 248
- Anesthetics
- Antibiotics
- Antifungals
- Antipruritics
- Antiseptics
- Astringents
- Cleansers
- Corticosteroids
- Dressings
- Insect Repellents
- Ipecac

Recommended Reading 259

THE SKIN

The skin is the largest organ in the human body. It makes up part of the integumentary system that includes the skin, hair and nails. The skin's functions are to protect the underlying structures of the body, provide sensation, prevent dehydration, act as a barrier to infection, assist with temperature regulation and the production of vitamin D, and store minerals.

Injuries to the skin break the protective barrier of the body, letting out vital fluids and providing access for microbes that can lead to infection. The skin has two major layers, the epidermis and the dermis, separated by the basement membrane. The epidermis, which is outside, is avascular and has five layers, the outermost a dead layer called the stratum corneum.

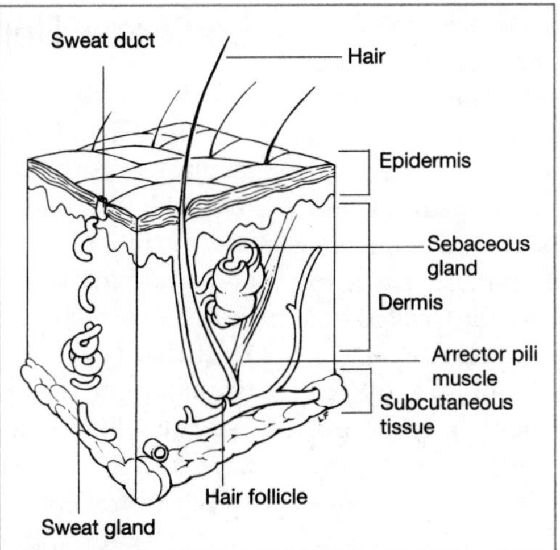

FIGURE 1: Skin

Epidermal cells also form a thin layer under, within or along the surface of epidermal appendages (nails, hair follicles, sweat and sebaceous glands).

The dermis, the thickest skin layer, has few cells: the fibroblasts that manufacture dermal proteins, collagen and elastin. Collagen is the major structural protein of the skin, giving it its tensile strength, elastin its elastic recoil. The dermis layer gives rise to the sweat and sebaceous glands.

Beneath the dermis is a layer of loose connective tissue called the hypodermis or subcutaneous layer. Both the dermis and hypodermis contain blood vessels and nerves. Blood circulation in the dermis supplies oxygen and nutrients to the epidermis. See Figure 1.

MINOR CUTS AND WOUNDS

WOUND CLASSIFICATION

A wound is an injury to a soft tissue. An open wound involves a break in the skin, a closed wound damage to the soft tissues beneath. Bruises and frostbite are closed wounds; abrasions, lacerations, avulsions, punctures and burns are open wounds.

A bruise, also called a contusion, is the most common closed wound. Bruises result from excess force to the skin that causes bleeding in the soft tissues and vessels beneath. Other fluids leak into the area causing swelling.

Open wounds can be divided into four categories: abrasions, lacerations, avulsions and punctures. The most common open wounds are abrasions or scrapes. A laceration is a cut to the skin with smooth or jagged edges, an avulsion when a piece of skin or soft tissue is torn away. A tear that produces a flap of skin that remains attached is classified as a partial avulsion. When a pointed object, such as a nail, splinter, glass, knife or bullet, pierces the skin, it is a puncture wound, which can be dangerous because bacteria can be introduced deep into the tissues.

Wounds to the skin can also be classified according to their depth. Superficial wounds involve loss of the epidermis. Partial thickness wounds involve both the epidermis and dermis. Full thickness wounds extend into the subcutaneous layer or further into muscle or bone. Minor cuts and wounds are limited to the epidermis or extend superficially into the dermis.

Another way to classify wounds is by the Black, Yellow, Red (BYR) color concept that describes healing stages of the surface of an open wound regardless of the tissue layers involved. A black wound is covered with black necrotic tissue, called an eschar. Once this is removed by debridement, the wound begins to form a yellowish-colored fibrous granulation tissue as it heals, called the yellow stage. As granulation tissue matures and becomes vascular, it appears beefy red and shiny and is ready to permit avascular epithelial tissue to grow over the top (re-epithelialization), called the red stage. The goal of therapy with a black wound is to remove the surface to get to the healthy red tissue underneath (e.g., remove necrotic tissue and exudate). Sloughed tissue or exudate may appear yellow and should be removed, but yellow fibrous granulation tissue should be left in place. There are healthy and unhealthy shades of red. Healthy granulation tissue is usually described as beefy, red, and shiny, which reflects new blood vessel formation (neoangiogenesis) as well as good hydration and oxygenation.

WOUND HEALING

Wounds heal differently depending on whether they are superficial, partial thickness or full thickness wounds. Superficial wound healing involves re-establishment of the epidermal layer. Unlike the dermis layer, the epidermis is able to regenerate itself. The dermis layer repairs itself with connective tissue called scar tissue. In partial thickness wounds where only part of the dermis has been removed, endothelial cells (epithelium), which line the epidermal appendages, remain intact in the wound bed. These epithelial cells from the appendages and from the wound edges re-epithelialize the wound while connective tissue is being repaired (dermal layer). Deep partial thickness wounds, and full-thickness wounds where the dermal layer and epidermal appendages have been completely removed, are only able to form scar tissue. Epidermal cells from the wound edges can generally migrate only 3 cm. Skin grafting used for these wounds provides epidermal cells to help re-epithelialize the wound. A moist environment is now known to assist this healing process and is considered superior to dry wound healing.

Partial thickness wounds heal in stages: an initial inflammatory response, epithelial proliferation and migration, re-establishment of the epidermal layers.

Epidermal Repair

Initial injury to tissue triggers an inflammatory response. There is edema and a serous exudate containing leukocytes and enzymes. This stage lasts less than 24 hours, during which epithelial proliferation and migration will begin from the wound edges and epidermal appendages. If the wound is kept moist, this migration will begin within 8 hours. Epithelial cells can only migrate across a moist wound. If the wound is allowed to dry, the serous exudate will form a scab. The epithelial cells then have to tunnel down seeking moisture under the scab. The epidermal cells then secrete collagenase to dissolve the scab so they can migrate under it in the moist environment. If wounds are kept moist, a scab will not form, and re-epithelialization will be complete in approximately 4 days compared to 6 to 7 days for a dry wound. Once the wound bed is re-epithelialized, the cells migrate upward to restratify.

Dermal Repair

Partial thickness wound repair involves dermal and epidermal repair.

Dermal repair includes granulation, contraction, and re-epithelialization. Granulation means the formation of new connective tissue, including blood vessels (neoangiogenesis) and collagen. Collagen is synthesized by fibroblasts, which begin to proliferate during this phase and are abundant 7 days after the injury. If the wound has been kept moist, granulation will begin only 3 days after the injury, usually continuing for about 10 to 15 days, but can continue for months. Contraction of the new connective tissue occurs simultaneously with granulation. For those partial thickness wounds that have intact epidermal appendages, dermal and epidermal repair are simultaneous.

Tissue Oxygenation

Hypoxia in a wound can act as an initial stimulus for neoangiogenesis and fibroblast proliferation. However, continued fibroblastic proliferation, collagen synthesis, epithelial proliferation and migration, and the bactericidal action of leukocytes are all dependent on adequate tissue oxygenation. This does not mean that wounds should be kept open to air. Wounds obtain their oxygen from blood within tissues, not from the air.

TREATMENT

Treatment of Minor Closed Wounds

Most minor closed wounds can be treated with a few simple steps. Immediately after a closed wound injury occurs, apply pressure to the area to reduce bleeding. Keep the area elevated and apply ice or a cold pack to help reduce swelling and decrease pain. Wrap the ice or cold pack in a towel or other cloth and hold to the wound for 15 minutes once every hour for as long as the pain continues.

Treatment of Open Wounds

Depending on the depth and classification of an open wound, topical products and dressings will differ somewhat. For a superficial abrasion, cleansing and application of a moist dressing or bandage is all that is required. To treat the pain of minor open wounds, oral analgesics should be used whenever possible. There is a risk of sensitization with topical anesthetics. Current principles of cleansing, debridement, topical products and dressings for open wounds are discussed in depth below.

Topical Therapy: Topical wound therapy can alter the surface environment and help or hinder the healing process. The goal is to enhance the healing process.

When treating wounds with topical products, one principle should always be kept in mind: never put anything in a wound that you would not put in your eye.

Historically, the focus of wound care was to prevent infection. This involved aggressive cleansing, use of antiseptics, application of antibiotics and keeping the wound dry through air exposure and using dry dressings. Current research shows moist wound healing to be superior.

Choosing Wound Dressings

Superficial wounds and partial thickness wounds involving the loss of only a small amount of dermis require only the basics of wound healing: a moist wound surface, thermal insulation and protection against trauma and bacteria. Partial thickness wounds that involve a greater loss of the dermis will require absorption of moderate amounts of exudate.

Dressings that can be used to treat partial thickness wounds include hydrocolloid dressings, transparent adhesive dressings, sheet form of gel dressings, synthetic barrier dressings, and emollient dressings with a secondary nonadhesive dressing.

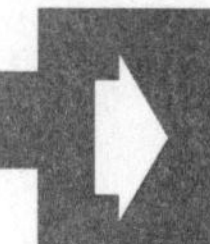

COUNSELLING TIPS

General Principles for the Care of all Open Wounds

Step 1: Cleansing and Debridement

The first step in wound management is removal of necrotic tissue and foreign particles (except in ischemic wounds), which serve as a medium for bacterial growth. Cleansing removes bacteria and contaminants such as wound exudate. Wound cleansing does not mean wound disinfection and should not be thought of as the same procedure. Necrotic wounds must be debrided while non-necrotic wounds require cleansing only, which may be done by the patient. Debridement of wounds with dressings should only be done by a health care professional, and surgical debridement must be performed by a physician.

- ***Cleansing:*** The procedures and products for cleansing a wound differ depending on whether the wound is clean and proliferating (non-necrotic) or necrotic and infected.

  For cleansing a wound, irrigation is now considered the method of choice. Irrigation dislodges contaminants and decreases bacterial colonization. Sodium chloride 0.9% in sterile water (normal saline) is the preferred agent because it is not cytotoxic, therefore does not interfere with the healing process. Nonionic surfactant cleansers may also be used but are more costly.

  Mechanical cleansing with cotton wool is not recommended because the fibres shed on the wound surface and serve as a nidus for infection. Also, a foreign body reaction could occur to the fibres and delay wound healing. Mechanical cleansing of wounds can cause redistribution of bacteria rather than decreasing the count. If mechanical cleansing is done, gauze pads should be used because they do not shed.

- ***Clean Proliferative Wounds:*** The goal with clean wounds is to gently flush the wound to remove debris but not disturb the wound surface. Clean wounds are covered with a proliferative layer containing growth factors and nutrients. For these wounds, normal saline is the ideal cleanser because it is noncytotoxic. Nonionic surfactants may also be used. The wound can be gently flushed using a syringe plunger without a needle. Antiseptics should not be used on clean wounds because they are nonselectively cytotoxic (see Antiseptics), toxic not only to bacteria but also to cells needed for wound repair. A wound can be colonized with bacteria, but this does not mean it is infected. Colonization of skin flora over a wound surface is normal and does not seem to interfere with wound healing. Antiseptics may be applied to the tissue surrounding a wound but not to the wound surface.

- ***Infected or Necrotic Wounds:*** Unlike clean proliferating wounds, infected or necrotic wounds are heavily contaminated and require thorough irrigation of the wound surface. For wounds that appear heavily infected or necrotic, referral to a physician is required. High-pressure irrigation using a syringe with a 19-gauge needle attached or hydrotherapy by or under the supervision of a medical professional can be used to cleanse these types of wounds. Nonionic surfactant cleansers or normal saline may be used, but the use of antiseptics for cleansing infected or necrotic wounds is controversial (see Antiseptics).

- ***Debridement:*** Debridement with the body's own immune system involves the macrophages and leukocytes. This autodebridement is also known as autolysis and is enhanced by a moist wound environment. Dressings can be used to enhance autolysis, which is discussed later in the chapter under Dressings. Debridement may also be achieved enzymatically. Nonprescription products contain fibrinolysin-desoxyribonuclease (*Elase*) and collagenase (*Santyl*), while prescription products contain sutilains (*Travase*). While these products are effective debriding agents, their effects on granulation and re-epithelialization are relatively unstudied. The autolytic dressings permit the other stages to begin simultaneously and are therefore generally preferred. Debridement can also be achieved by surgically removing the eschar.

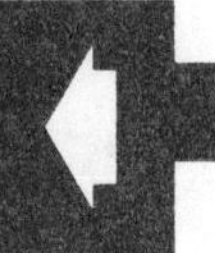

COUNSELLING TIPS (*cont'd*)

Step 2: Identification and Elimination of Infection

Ideally, treatment of wound infections should be based on culture results. However, infections of minor wounds may be self-treated empirically, based on the most likely involved bacteria. Cultures are usually done only if the minor wound infection is unresponsive to treatment. Bacteria compete with fibroblasts for oxygen thereby delaying collagen synthesis. Infection prolongs the inflammatory stage, prevents epidermal migration and causes additional tissue damage.

Step 3: Obliteration of Dead Space

Dead space exists in a wound where there is tissue destruction underneath intact tissue. This can be obliterated by lightly packing it. If not packed, the wound may heal over enclosing a fluid-filled pocket where bacteria can grow, leading to abscess formation.

Step 4: Absorption of Excess Exudate

Although a moist wound is ideal for wound healing, too much moisture can macerate surrounding tissues and dilute the wound healing factors. Also, the wound exudate contains bacteria that can impede the healing process.

Step 5: Maintaining a Moist Wound Surface

Moisture prevents cell death and promotes epidermal migration and granulation. It encourages auto-debridement by enhancing leukocyte migration into the wound and accumulation of enzymes.

Step 6: Providing Thermal Insulation to the Wound

Maintaining normal tissue temperature facilitates a good blood supply and epidermal migration.

Step 7: Protecting the Wound Against Trauma and Bacterial Invasion

Trauma damages the newly formed tissues. Uncovered wounds are open to bacteria and infection.

SKIN INFECTION

PATHOPHYSIOLOGY

The skin can protect itself against assaults from water, chemicals, bacteria and viruses. Its barrier to bacteria and viruses includes the stratum corneum, sebum, the normal skin flora and the skin's immune system. The stratum corneum is a physical barrier, but must be intact to do so, and its constant shedding prevents invasion by microbes.

The sebum is an acidic oily substance secreted by the sebaceous glands that coats the skin. This environment (mean pH 5.5) is not conducive to microbial growth. The sebum also contains antibacterial substances. The skin's immune system involves the Langerhans' cells in the epidermis and the macrophages and mast cells in the dermis.

Resident bacteria on the skin (normal skin flora) include *Staphylococcus epidermidis*, *Streptococcus, Corynebacterium, Diphtheroids, Propionibacterium, Peptococcus, Brevibacterium, Neisseria*, and *Acinetobacter*. Resident bacteria keep pathogenic bacteria in check.

Infected wounds without necrotic tissue usually involve aerobic bacteria, such as *Staphylococcus aureus* and group A *Streptococcus* and *Pseudomonas*. Wounds that contain necrotic tissue often involve both aerobic and anaerobic bacteria. Infection not only prevents wound healing but also causes additional tissue destruction.

Adequate oxygenation of wound tissues is required to allow leukocytes to kill bacteria, especially important with bacteria such as *Staphylococcus aureus* and *Enterobacteriaceae*.

BACTERIAL SKIN INFECTIONS

Wound Bacteria

All patients who have penetrating wounds or burns should be advised to see a physician to receive prophylaxis against tetanus (*Clostridium tetani*) if there is any doubt as to their immunization status. Tetanus boosters are now preferentially combined with diphtheria toxoid vaccine (Td).

Bacterial involvement varies depending on the type of wound. Infected traumatic wounds of the extremity most commonly involve *Staphylococcus aureus*, group A and anaerobic *Streptococcus, Enterobacteriaceae* (e.g., *Klebsiella, Proteus, Enterobacter*), *Clostridium perfringens*, *Clostridium tetani* and *Pseudomonas* if there has been water exposure. Post-operative wounds most commonly involve *Staphylococcus aureus*, group A *Streptococcus, Enterobacteriaceae* and *Pseudomonas*.

Microorganisms proliferate rapidly in the burn wound. Initially, the normal skin flora contaminate the wound. They are mostly gram-positive, particularly *Streptococcus*, especially beta-hemolytic *Streptococci*, and *Staphylococcus aureus*. By the fifth day after the injury, gram-negative organisms predominate, especially *Pseudomonas aeruginosa*. Other gram-negative bacteria commonly found in burn wounds are *Enterobacteriaceae, Serratia* and *Providencia. Aspergillus* (fungus), *Herpes simplex* virus and *Cytomegalovirus* may also be involved in burn infections. If the burn becomes infected, tissue destruction occurs converting the burn wound to a deeper one.

Infected decubitus ulcers are usually polymicrobic and can involve groups A,C,D, and anaerobic *Streptococcus, Enterobacteriaceae, Pseudomonas, Bacteroides* (an anaerobic bacteria) and *Staphylococcus aureus*.

Identifying Infection

An open wound can be assessed for infection by its color and by the type of exudate. Extremely odorous and purulent exudate usually suggests an anaerobic infection. Wounds that are black or necrotic are frequently infected with both aerobic and anaerobic bacteria.

All open wounds contain bacteria. The difference between contamination of a wound, which is normal, and infection is in the colony count of the bacteria. A bacterial colony count greater than 100,000 organisms per mL or, in S.I. units, greater than 100 million colony forming units per litre (>100 M CFU/L) indicates infection. However, clinical infections can occur with beta-hemolytic *Streptococcus* counts <100 M CFU/L.

The clinical signs of infection may include erythema (redness), edema (swelling), induration (abnormal firmness with a definite margin), purulence (thick fluid exudate containing leukocytes, bacteria and cellular debris; pus) or very foul smelling drainage, pain or crepitance (crackling sound). Another sign of possible infection is a wound that will not heal despite appropriate therapy. A wound with a "silent" infection may appear uninfected but on culture, may grow >100 M CFU/L. Because infection prevents epithelial migration, these silent infected wounds may present with hypertrophic granulation tissue facilitated by moist dressings, but with no epithelialization. Streptococcal skin infections usually present with lymphangitis, and staphylococcal infections present with excess pus.

A patient with a systemic infection from a wound will present with a fever and leukocytosis (increased white blood cell count).

Impetigo

Impetigo is the most common superficial bacterial skin infection, and the majority of cases occur in children. It is caused most often by *Staphylococcus aureus* but also by group A beta-hemolytic *Streptococci* such as *S. pyogenes*. Bullous impetigo (blistering) is usually caused by *S. aureus* and often involves a single area of the skin, such as the face. Single blisters may occur and be confused with herpes simplex lesions. The usual presentation of impetigo is pustular lesions that may rupture and form a golden brown crust when the purulent discharge dries.

Treatment: If the impetigo is not extensive, the condition may be treated topically. Treatment involves frequent cleansing, gentle debridement of the crusted lesions, and application of topical antibiotics, such as bacitracin, gramicidin (only marketed in combination with polymyxin B) and mupirocin. Mupirocin is generally the agent of choice. For extensive impetigo, oral antibiotics are required. Patients should be advised to avoid scratching the lesions as this can spread the infection. Epsom salt baths and compresses have also been used adjunctively in the treatment of impetigo. For method of use, see Furuncles and Carbuncles.

Ecthyma

Ecthyma is a more severe form of impetigo that spreads through the epidermis into the dermis. Lesions are often irregular and located on forearms and lower extremities such as the shins. This is most common in children and the elderly or debilitated patients. The lesions present as shallow ulcers covered by greenish yellow crusts. Treatment is the same as for impetigo.

Erysipelas

Erysipelas is a more severe bacterial skin infection than impetigo. It involves deeper layers of the skin and is intracutaneous in nature. Most common in the very young and the elderly, it is caused by group A *Streptococci,* and rarely by other *Streptococci*, and *S. aureus*. Erysipelas occurs most commonly on the cheeks and bridge of the nose, and presents with an acute fiery red skin color, which distinguishes it from cellulitis.

Erysipelas infection is painful, has a sharply demarcated border with a palpable edge, vesicles or bullae may develop, and a butterfly formation (such as seen with systemic lupus erythematosus) may be present. Systemic symptoms occur abruptly (malaise, fever and chills). The individual should be referred to their physician for diagnosis and treatment.

Treatment: Requires oral antibiotics; for more severe infection, intravenous antibiotics are required.

Cellulitis

Cellulitis is a deeper infection of the skin than erysipelas, and is a spreading infection that involves the skin, subcutaneous tissues and sometimes deeper connective tissues. With cellulitis, a watery exudate forms and spreads through the tissues and interstitial spaces. Ulceration and abscess can occur. Cellulitis presents as a diffuse (no palpable edge) acute inflammation of the skin with edema, hyperemia (increased blood flow), white blood cell infiltration, and possible erythema. Prompt medical attention is required.

Treatment: Requires oral antibiotics; more severe and invasive cellulitis requires intravenous antibiotics and possibly surgical debridement.

Folliculitis

Folliculitis is an infection within the hair follicles most commonly caused by *Staphylococcus aureus*. It presents as small erythematous papules (2 to 5 mm), often with central pustules, which are sometimes pruritic occurring most commonly on the buttocks, hips and axillae. Scarring is rare and healing usually occurs spontaneously within 5 days.

Treatment: Includes application of saline compresses and topical antibiotics. Occasionally, a folliculitis papule can develop into a furuncle.

Furuncles and Carbuncles

Furuncles usually develop from folliculitis papules that have spread deeper into the dermis layer. Carbuncles are more severe and extend into the subcutaneous fat.

Like folliculitis, furuncles and carbuncles are caused most often by *Staphylococcus aureus* in areas subject to irritation from friction or perspiration, such as the neck, face, buttocks and axillae. Carbuncles occur most often on the neck, back and thighs.

Risk factors for the development of furuncles and carbuncles are immunosuppression (e.g., use of corticosteroids, impaired neutrophil function, diabetes mellitus) or obesity.

Treatment: Basic treatment involves local application of moist warm saline compresses to encourage drainage of pus from the hair follicles. Epsom salt compresses and baths have also been used. A 20% compress solution can be made by dissolving 200 mL of epsom salts in 1 L of warm water. The soaked cloth can be held over the lesion for 15 to 20 minutes up to 6 times daily. To keep the compress moist and warm, the cloth should be resoaked every 5 to 10 minutes. The solution should be made fresh prior to each use, and never reused. An epsom salt bath can be made by adding 2 to 4 cups of salt to a bathtub of warm water. Patients should wash the areas with soap and water or sudsy chlorhexidine 4% at least twice daily to decrease the external *S. aureus* colony counts. They should be advised to avoid manipulation of the lesions to decrease the risk of spreading the infection, and developing cellulitis and systemic infection. Lesions should be covered with sterile dressings to prevent the patient from touching them. Towels and washcloths should not be shared with other individuals and should be washed in hot water after each use. Bed sheets, underwear, or any clothing that comes in contact with the lesions should be changed daily.

Patients should be referred to a physician if the lesions are not draining, are present on the face, or if the erythema is spreading or the patient has a fever. In these cases systemic antibiotics are required to ensure adequate penetration into the lesions.

FUNGAL SKIN INFECTIONS

Superficial fungal infections of the skin are classified as either dermatophytes or yeast infections. Dermatophyte infections are also known as ringworm or tinea. The word tinea means fungus but does not refer to all fungal infections. Dermatophyte infections include tinea pedis, tinea capitis, tinea cruris and tinea corporis. Yeast infections include candidiasis (also called moniliasis) and tinea versicolor.

Dermatophyte infections of the skin are caused by species of *Trichophyton, Microsporum* or *Epidermophyton* and are named for the area of the body they affect rather than the fungal species causing the infection. Dermatophytes infect the superficial layer of the epidermis, the keratin layer. Mucosal areas of skin are spared from dermatophyte infections because they do not have a keratin layer that dermatophytes need to survive.

Dermatophyte infections can be difficult to diagnose visually and can be confused with eczema, superficial bacterial infections and contact dermatitis. Dermatophyte infection should be considered whenever scaling is present with or without erythema.

The classic presentation is an annular or ringlike lesion with a border that is erythematous (red), scaling and slightly raised, hence the name ringworm. Although the term ringworm describes a broad category of dermatophyte infections, it is most commonly used to refer to tinea corporis.

Confusion occurs in diagnosis when the ring is not evident since inflammation may or may not be present with dermatophyte infections. When inflammation is present and severe, vesicles may develop along the active border. Topical corticosteroids should never be applied to possible fungal infections until accurate diagnosis has been made, and they are used concurrently with appropriate antifungals. Topical corticosteroids can cause local immunosuppression exacerbating the infection and make diagnosis difficult by masking the inflammation.

Tinea Pedis

Tinea pedis, also known as athlete's foot is a dermatophyte infection of the foot caused by either *Trichophyton rubrum* or *Trichophyton mentagrophytes* or less commonly *Epidermophyton floccosum*, found more often in men than women. See the Foot Care Products chapter.

Tinea Cruris

Tinea cruris (jock itch) is a dermatophyte infection of the groin usually caused by *Trichophyton rubrum, Trichophyton mentagrophytes* or *Epidermophyton floccosum*. It occurs mainly in young men (see the Men's Health Care Products chapter).

Tinea Corporis

Tinea corporis, also referred to as ringworm, most commonly affects the trunk or legs and may produce little to no itching. Tinea corporis most often affects people in humid climates and is uncommon in temperate climates. Tinea corporis is caused by species of *Trichophyton* and *Microsporum*. Tinea corporis lesions usually begin as flat scaly lesions that develop raised scaly margins and spread outward. The centre area may become brown or hypopigmented compared to the border.

When *T. rubrum* infection occurs on the lower legs (most common in women who shave), the infection may spread into the hair follicles, producing nodules. *T. rubrum* infection can be differentiated from erythema nodosum by the classic ringlike scaling margin.

Treatment: Mild tinea corporis can be self-treated topically with an imidazole antifungal cream (clotrimazole 1% or miconazole 2%) or tolnaftate cream. Lesions usually begin to respond to topical antifungal treatment within 2 weeks, but therapy should continue for at least 1 week after resolution of the lesions, usually at least 4 weeks.

After gentle but thorough cleansing of the area with a mild cleanser, patients should be advised to apply the chosen antifungal cream using sufficient quantities to cover the entire affected area and into the surrounding skin and to gently massage the cream in, until it disappears. It should be applied this way, twice daily, in the morning and evening.

Toxicity with these preparations is low although local irritation and stinging have been reported infrequently when applied to open areas of the skin. Occlusive dressings should not be used, but loose porous dressings, such as gauze, may be applied over the treated areas. Patients should be advised to wear loose clothing to avoid occlusion.

Individuals with deeper or more wide-spread tinea corporis should be referred to their physician. Oral prescription antifungals may be required.

Tinea Capitis

Tinea capitis is a dermatophyte infection of the scalp caused by many different species of *Trichophyton* and *Microsporum*; *T. tonsurans* is the most common, followed by *M. canis*. It occurs most commonly in children 4 to 6 years of age, and rarely affects adults. The overall incidence in children is 4% (U.S. data) with the highest incidence in female African-American children (12.7%), thought to be secondary to the tight-braided hairstyles worn and the occlusive pomades used.

Tinea capitis usually starts with a small patch of scaling skin with hair loss in the lesion, which is often itchy. The degree of inflammation varies but is usually minimal. Tinea capitis commonly presents as a single lesion or multiple small lesions.

The classic sign of tinea capitis is alopecia. Hairs may break off a few millimetres above the skin surface or at the surface, producing a black dot appearance called black dot ringworm. Inflammation may be intense in some cases, and the affected area may develop pustules with purulent crusted exudate or thick scale. If inflammation is severe, a hypersensitivity reaction to the fungus may develop, called a kerion, which is an indurated inflammatory mass that is purulent. A high degree of inflammation also increases the chance of spontaneous resolution because the inflammatory reaction helps kill the fungus and increase shedding of the infected stratum corneum. Cases of tinea capitis with mild pruritus, minimal or diffuse scaling and flaking, and none or only a few broken hairs may be mistakenly diagnosed as seborrheic dermatitis, atopic dermatitis, or dandruff. In these noninflammatory cases where there is no alopecia, the disease can remain undiagnosed for years. Diagnosis and differentiation from severe dandruff and seborrheic dermatitis can be determined by cytology and culture.

Up to 30% of family members may have an asymptomatic infection. Relatives and close contacts should frequently check themselves carefully for development of infection and be referred to a physician to rule out asymptomatic infection. If one family member is infected with *T. tonsurans*, some clinicians believe all family members should be treated.

T. tonsurans is not only spread from person to person, but also by fomites (inanimate objects on which fungus remains viable). A common source for spread of *M. canis* is cats. Fomites include combs, brushes, bed clothing, floors, and telephones. A method proven to eradicate the fungus from fomites remains to be determined. However, patients should wash combs and brushes frequently (suggest at least daily) in hot water and should not share them with family members or friends. Bed clothing should be washed frequently in hot water, especially pillow cases. Floors should be mopped with a strong disinfectant, all washable objects laundered, and nonwashable objects vacuumed. Spraying and wiping the telephone with 70% isopropyl alcohol after each use will also help control the spread of infection.

Treatment: Patients should be referred to their physician for diagnosis and treatment of tinea capitis, generally with oral prescription antifungals. If a kerion is present, systemic corticosteroids may be required to prevent scarring alopecia and decrease the pain of inflammation. Topical preparations can be used adjunctively, but additional benefit may be minimal because they do not adequately penetrate infected hairs or reach deep within the hair follicles. Shampoos containing salicylic acid may help with scale and spore removal. Selenium sulfide 2.5% shampoo is sporicidal and when used twice weekly may decrease shedding of the fungal spores and infectivity. Treatment should be continued twice weekly, for 4 weeks.

Tinea Versicolor (Pityriasis Versicolor)

Tinea versicolor is a fungal infection of the stratum corneum layer of the skin caused not by a dermatophyte but by the yeast *Malassezia furfur*. *M. furfur*, previously known as *Pityrosporum orbiculare* or *Pityrosporum ovale*, is now known to be the same yeast in different growth stages. *M. furfur* is part of the normal skin flora, but in certain conditions can overgrow, such as in immunosuppression, use of corticosteroids or oral contraceptives, pregnancy, malnutrition, burns, excess heat and humidity, genetically oily skin and with application of oils to the skin. *M. furfur* is present in the greatest numbers on areas of the skin with the greatest sebaceous activity. The infection is usually found on the neck and upper trunk and often spreads to the upper arms and abdomen. It can also spread to the face, back of the hands, and legs. Tinea versicolor is most common in adolescents and young adults because of increased sebaceous activity. Untreated infection with tinea versicolor may vary in activity for years but is eventually self-limiting and disappears with advancing age.

Tinea versicolor lesions usually begin as small macules (flat discolored patches) that are white, pink, or brown and expand radially. They are usually asymptomatic with little to no inflammation. *M. furfur* produces dicarboxylic acids and toxic lipoperoxidases that can result in hypomelanosis and hypopigmentation, explaining the white lesions. White lesions may not be noticed on fair-skinned individuals, especially in winter, but they become obvious when surrounding skin is tanned. Uncommonly, when inflammation is present, the lesions may present as macules, patches or follicular papules that appear red to fawn colored, and may be itchy. Infection of hair follicles (pityrosporum folliculitis) may be misdiagnosed as acne. Occasionally toxicity to melanocytes from *M. furfur* infection can increase distribution of melanin to keratinocytes, resulting in hyperpigmented, or brown tinea versicolor lesions, most commonly in black individuals. It is not known if tinea versicolor infections are contagious.

Treatment: The individual should be referred to their physician for diagnosis and treatment of tinea versicolor, generally for cosmetic purposes only. Tinea versicolor can be treated with topical imidazole antifungals (clotrimazole or miconazole), selenium sulfide 2.5% suspension, sulfur 2%/salicylic acid 2% combination shampoo or zinc pyrithione 1% shampoo. Imidazole creams are used twice daily for 2 weeks. Selenium sulfide 2.5% is recommended for more extensive tinea versicolor infections and can be used in one of two ways. The first is application of the suspension to the affected and surrounding area for 10 minutes daily for 7 consecutive days. The second is to apply the suspension to the affected area at bedtime, leave it on overnight and rinse it off in the morning, repeated once weekly for 1 to 4 weeks depending on the severity of the infection. The sulfur/salicylic acid shampoo should be applied as a lotion to the affected area daily at bedtime and rinsed off in the morning for 7 consecutive days. Zinc pyrithione 1% shampoo can be scrubbed into the affected area with a bathtub brush and the lather left on the affected areas for 5 minutes before showering, repeated daily for 14 days.

Once effectively treated, repigmentation of the affected areas may take several months. Periodic use of sulfur/salicylic acid combination soap may prevent recurrence of tinea versicolor, but it is very drying.

Refractory or recurrent infections can be effectively treated with oral prescription antifungal medications.

Candidiasis

Candida species are yeastlike fungi that, unlike dermatophytes, are not restricted to superficial skin involvement and can lead to systemic infections.

Candida skin and mucous membrane infections involve only the outer layers of the skin, almost always in moist areas or in skin folds. Candidal overgrowth can cause vulvovaginitis (see the Women's Health Care Products chapter), oral candidiasis (see the Oral Health Care Products chapter), diaper rash (see the Dermatitis, Seborrhea, Dandruff and Dry Skin Products chapter) and cutaneous candidiasis of intertriginal skin folds (apposing skin folds).

Cutaneous and Intertriginal Candidiasis

Cutaneous candidal infections occur in skin folds because the moisture and heat in those areas provide an ideal environment for growth. Predisposing factors are those that encourage heat and accumulation of moisture, such as tight or occlusive clothing, hot and humid weather and poor hygiene. Also, inflammatory skin conditions, such as psoriasis or atopic dermatitis, tend to encourage yeast overgrowth.

Skin fold areas most commonly involved are underneath the breasts, the groin and rectal areas, the axillae, and in between the fingers and toes (on the webs).

Candidiasis of the large folds can present in two ways. One is multiple small red papules, each papule margined with a scale that is moist within the area of the apposing folds. If the infection has spread beyond the folds, the lesions will be present as pustules rather than papules due to lack of maceration. The second way is one large, moist erythematous plaque, again with a border of scale. Fissures may be present. Again, small individual pustules may be present outside the area of the apposing folds of skin. In both cases, the satellite pustules are a classic sign of candidiasis.

Candidiasis of the finger and toe webs develops most commonly in people whose jobs keep these intertriginous areas moist, such as dishwashers and dentists, or in predisposed people whose footwear is occlusive. The skin looks macerated and white with splits or erosions revealing moist pink skin underneath. Untreated infection can lead to secondary bacterial infection.

Treatment: Candidiasis of skin folds can be prevented by keeping the predisposed areas cool and dry, loose clothing (avoid pantyhose), manually drying the areas when moisture does accumulate and applying nonmedicated powders (preferably nonperfumed to avoid irritation). Treatment of the infection requires application of topical antifungals. The imidazole antifungals (miconazole or clotrimazole) are the drugs of choice. In chronic or severe cases, or when a systemic infection is also involved, oral or intravenous prescription antifungals will be required.

After cleansing with a gentle cleanser, miconazole or clotrimazole should be applied in sufficient quantities to cover the affected area and surrounding skin twice daily for 2 weeks. Nystatin should be applied 3 to 4 times daily for 2 weeks. Creams should be massaged in well to avoid maceration.

In addition to preventive measures and specific antifungal treatment, topical astringent soaks, such as wet Burow's (aluminum acetate) solution, may be applied to weeping or macerated fungal lesions to help dry them and temporarily decrease inflammation and itching. Burow's solution compresses can be applied for 20 to 30 minutes 2 to 6 times daily. Compresses should be discontinued as soon as the lesions or rash have dried adequately. Astringent solutions should not be used on open wounds or rashes with fissures or breaks in the skin.

VIRAL SKIN INFECTIONS

Viral skin infections include warts, molluscum contagiosum, herpes simplex, varicella zoster, herpes zoster and hand, foot and mouth disease. In this chapter, only varicella zoster (chickenpox) will be discussed.

Varicella Zoster (Chickenpox)

Chickenpox is a highly contagious self-limiting viral infection that affects the epidermis layer of the skin and mucous membranes. Most individuals have been infected by the time they reach adulthood. The disease is usually mild in immunocompetent children and increases in severity in neonates, adolescents and adults. Chickenpox can be fatal in immunocompromised individuals.

After an incubation period of approximately 17 to 21 days, lesions begin to erupt, usually starting on the scalp or trunk of the body, then newer lesions begin to erupt on the extremities.

An individual chickenpox lesion develops a small red papule (2 to 4 mm diameter) that develops into an irregular shaped vesicle or blister with erythema. The presence of vesicles is a diagnostic feature of chickenpox. In the next stage, the vesicles become cloudy with an indented centre, and rupture in 8 to 12 hours. It is the contents of the ruptured vesicles that is infectious through contact or airborne droplets. During the vesicular stage, the lesions are mildly to intensely itchy, and there is mild fever and pain. After the vesicles have ruptured, the lesions form a crust, and the erythema disappears. The crust usually falls off in about 7 days. Chickenpox lesions typically develop, erupt and are present in all stages of development during the first 5 days of the disease. The presence of pruritus, mild fever, pain, vesicles and lesions in different stages of development are all diagnostic symptoms of chickenpox. New lesions do not usually develop after the fourth day. In some cases, lesions may be present in such small numbers that the disease may be unnoticed, while in other cases, lesions are too numerous to count. A complete course of chickenpox lasts 10 to 14 days and usually confers life-long immunity. There is no scarring unless the lesions have been scratched and excoriated or a secondary bacterial infection developed. The presence of large or painful lesions may indicate secondary bacterial infection, and patients should be referred to a physician. Complications of chickenpox are uncommon but may include pneumonia (most common in adults), myelitis (inflammation of the spinal cord or bone marrow), aseptic meningitis, encephalitis, Reye's syndrome, myocarditis, and Guillain-Barré syndrome. Patients should be immediately referred to a physician if signs of encephalopathy occur, such as ataxia (incoordination), nystagmus, or tremors, or signs of Reye's syndrome, such as vomiting and rapid neurologic deterioration. In the majority of cases, however, complications do not occur, and treatment is symptomatic.

Treatment: Treatment of uncomplicated chickenpox includes gentle cleansing of the lesions, management of fever, pain and pruritus and prevention of secondary complications, such as bacterial superinfection and scarring.

Cleansing should be done with a gentle cleanser being careful not to prematurely remove scabs or crusts. Fingernails should be kept short and mittens applied to the hands of infants and small children to decrease excoriation from scratching and avoid removing crusts. Older patients should be advised not to scratch but keeping nails short will help prevent secondary bacterial infection if scratching does occur, by reducing the breeding ground for bacteria under the nails. Also to help decrease the risk of secondary infection, bed sheets, pillow cases and underclothing should be changed daily.

To treat the pain and fever of chickenpox, acetaminophen is the drug of choice. Products that contain ASA should never be used in patients with chickenpox (or flu) because of the risk of Reye's syndrome, an acute inflammatory encephalopathy. Normally 20 to 30% of all cases of Reye's syndrome occur postvaricella infection, but an increased risk has been linked with ASA use. Ibuprofen has not been linked to increased risk of Reye's syndrome in children with chickenpox, but it is probably safest to use acetaminophen.

Treatment for pruritus includes oral antihistamines, such as diphenhydramine or chlorpheniramine, and topical cream or lotion astringents, such as plain calamine lotion or zinc oxide cream. Colloidal oatmeal bath oil may also help to relieve the pruritus associated with chickenpox through its emollient effect. The bath oil should be shaken well and 1 to 2 capfuls of oil added to the bath. The child or affected person may soak in the bath for 10 to 20 minutes and the skin gently patted dry with a soft clean towel to avoid disrupting the vesicles and crusted lesions. Cornstarch baths have also been used to relieve pruritus associated with chickenpox. They are prepared by mixing 2 cups of cornstarch with 4 cups of water, then adding the mixture to a bathtub full of water.

Topical antihistamines are not recommended because of the risk of sensitization and increased systemic absorption when applied to chickenpox lesions, especially applied to large body areas. Given orally, 40 to 60% of the dose is eliminated through first-pass metabolism. However, when applied topically, the first-pass elimination is bypassed so more drug reaches the systemic circulation. Overdosage from topical application of large amounts of diphenhydramine to large body surface areas has occurred in children, resulting in changes in mental status, including bizarre behavior and visual and auditory hallucinations that may mimic varicella encephalitis. This risk of overdose increases when oral antihistamines are used concomitantly. When antihistamines are used, they should only be given orally to treat chickenpox that affects large areas so the dose can be accurately controlled. Because of the case reports of overdosage from topical application of diphenhydramine in children, the manufacturer of a calamine-diphenhydramine combination product now contraindicates its use in children under 6 years of age.

In addition to acetaminophen and antipruritics, affected individuals should stay well-hydrated by drinking plenty of fluids. Children should be offered frequent fluids including popsicles and gelatin.

The use of oral acyclovir (by prescription only) to treat uncomplicated chickenpox in immunocompetent children is controversial, but generally felt to be unnecessary.

Pregnant women not previously infected with chickenpox should avoid contact with infected individuals. Varicella zoster infection (chickenpox) in nonimmune pregnant women in the first half of pregnancy has resulted in harm to the fetus.

BURNS

About 200,000 Canadians are burned each year. The majority (95%) are minor and can be treated on an outpatient basis. Burns can be caused by exposure to hot liquids, steam, flammable substances, electricity, hot solid materials (e.g., molten metal), caustic chemicals, excess ultraviolet light or severe cold (e.g., liquid nitrogen). Burn severity is determined by the surface area involved and the depth of the burn.

A minor burn is a superficial (epidermal) to moderate-depth, partial thickness wound that affects less than 20% of total body surface area (TBSA), and is not life threatening. This definition holds true except in those younger than 5 years of age or older than 55, in whom the dermis layer is much thinner, so the severity of a burn can be greater. Burns that occur to critical areas of the body, such as the face, eyes, ears, hands, feet and perineum should not be considered minor.

To estimate total body surface area (TBSA), the Wallace rule of nines can be used. In adults and children over 10 years of age, the head and each arm is 9% of TBSA, each leg and the anterior and posterior trunk are each 18% of TBSA, and the perineum is 1%. The percentage of TBSA of the head and legs of a child under 10 years of age is different than that of an adult. A child's head at birth represents 20% of the TBSA, and the legs are each 12 to 13% TBSA. With each added year of age until age 10, a child's head decreases by 1% TBSA, and each leg increases by 1% TBSA.

BURN WOUND PATHOLOGY

As with other types of wounds, the initial step in the healing of burns is the inflammatory stage that initiates and directs wound healing. In partial thickness burns, this inflammation causes leakage and sequestering of extracellular fluid in the burn, which forms blisters or a sticky yellow eschar. In all burns, the inflammatory response can be extensive and self-perpetuating, and progressive thrombosis can occur, resulting in destruction of the normal tissue surrounding the wound by inflammatory mediators. For this reason, burns often cannot be classified for 2 to 3 days after the injury, as they can become more severe than they appear initially.

BURN WOUND CLASSIFICATION AND APPEARANCE

Burns are classified by depth. Superficial burns appear red and blanch with pressure. Partial thickness wounds are very painful wounds because of extension into the dermis, which contains nerve endings, but the nerve endings remain intact. They appear salmon-pink, wet, and blanch with pressure. Deep partial thickness burns (more dermis removed) are usually a speckled combination of wet pink (dermal vessels) and chalky white, and are less painful than moderate partial thickness wounds because more nerve endings are destroyed. Partial thickness burns classically form blisters. However, this can be misleading in classifying a burn because blisters can sometimes overlie small full-thickness burns. Full thickness burns are dry, chalky white or charred with visible thrombosed vessels, and are painless because the nerve endings have been destroyed. These wounds feel deep pressure sensation only.

How Did the Burn Occur?

Knowing how a burn occurred can aid in determining its severity. Excessive exposure to sunlight usually causes superficial burns that blister within 24 hours. Electrical burns usually appear less severe than they really are. Electrical burns appear superficial on the surface but have deep underlying tissue damage that may not be evident for a few days.

Flash burns from flammable substances, such as propane, usually cause partial thickness burns. Scalds can cause full thickness burns but may appear as partial thickness because of the redness from fixed hemoglobin in the burnt tissue (thrombosis).

TREATMENT

Good burn management requires assessment of burn severity, control of pain, cleansing and debridement, and prevention of infection. The initial treatment of a burn after removal of the heat source is to apply cool (not cold) moist compresses to relieve pain and remove residual heat. Because

Medical Referral: Open Wounds and Burns

Patients with serious soft tissue injuries must be referred to a physician. Signs and symptoms include heavy bleeding, severe swelling or discoloration, severe pain or the patient's inability to move the injured body part, or signs of infection. A wound may be infected if the area around the wound is red, swollen and warm, or if the wound throbs with pain. Other signs of infection are red streaks extending outward from the wound or pus discharge. A person with an infected wound may also show signs of systemic toxicity, such as fever and feeling generally unwell. Individuals with puncture wounds must be referred to a physician if they have not had, or are unsure if they have had, up-to-date tetanus immunization.

For those with minor wounds, such as lacerations, stitches may be required: usually any wound longer than 2 cm or any laceration on the face or hands when the edges of the skin do not fall together. Immediate referral is required as the chances of infection and scarring are decreased the sooner the wound is stitched.

Patients should be referred for medical attention for burns, if it is a child or if the burn is anything but superficial (epidermal involvement only), or has occurred on one of the critical areas of the body (hand, face, ears, eyes, feet, or perineum). Patients with burns may require tetanus immunization. Patients who develop blisters should seek medical attention because blisters are the cardinal sign of partial thickness burns (or higher grade). Patients who have had electrical burns should always be referred to a physician because underlying deep tissue damage is not visually apparent, and these patients are at risk of cardiac arrhythmias for 72 hours postexposure.

Hospital admission may be required for patients of all ages who have had partial thickness burns of 5% TBSA or who have any full thickness burns. Hospital admission is usually required for partial thickness burns involving 15% TBSA in adults or 10% TBSA in children. Patients referred to a physician may need to return to the physician in 2 to 3 days for re-examination as thermal injury can progress over this period.

Once the burn has been accurately diagnosed, the treatment of minor burns can usually be managed on an outpatient basis and is limited to the care of the wound. Patients should be advised to observe their burns and to see a physician if there are signs of infection, pain worsens, or blisters or fever develop.

soft tissue can continue to burn for a few minutes after removal of the heat source, the burned area needs to be cooled immediately. Immersing it in cool water is best but soaked towels, sheets or clothes can also be used. If a burn involves a large percentage of TBSA, do not try to cool the burn excessively because patients with large burns are prone to hypothermia.

Cleansing of Burn Wounds

Analgesia, orally or parenterally, may be required prior to cleansing and debriding burns, depending on their severity. As with other open wounds, burns are best cleansed with normal saline, although nonionic surfactant cleansers may be used but are more costly. Irrigation is the best method of cleansing. Cleansing burns with antiseptics is not necessary and may delay wound healing, (e.g., the use of half-strength povidone-iodine). Keeping in mind the rule of not introducing anything into a wound that would not be permitted in the eye, if an antiseptic is used to clean a burn, a dilute solution of chlorhexidine (e.g., 0.05% solution) is probably the least cytotoxic. If chlorhexidine is used, the burn should be irrigated with copious quantities of saline after the cleansing to prevent damage caused by residual chlorhexidine. Since antiseptics must remain in contact with bacteria for a significant time to be effective, the risk-benefit ratio of the chlorhexidine must be evaluated.

If debridement is necessary to remove embedded materials, necrotic tissue, or loose tissue from ruptured blisters, irrigation can be done with a syringe or a *Water Pik* device to create some force. Saline soaked gauze pads may also be used to debride by continuous wetting and wiping of the wound in the same direction.

All patients who develop blisters on burns should be referred to a physician. Whether or not intact blisters should be ruptured and debrided is a controversial issue. Some clinicians believe that blisters provide a barrier to bacteria, such as *Staphylococcus aureus*. Research indicates that blister fluid provides a good medium for bacterial culture, escalates the inflammatory response and impairs leukocyte function and fibrinolysis. Clean blisters (clear fluid) may be left intact unless rupture appears imminent, then the roof should be left intact by withdrawing the fluid from the blister with a sterile needle and syringe. Blisters containing cloudy fluid should be ruptured using a sterile needle, cleansed and debrided by a health professional. Blisters that are suspected of covering a full thickness burn also need to be removed in the appropriate medical setting. The yellow eschar on second degree burns should not be removed because it is painful and causes bleeding. Outpatient management of burns by the patient involves once or twice daily cleansing and application of a dressing.

Dressings for Burns

Dressings are applied after the wound has been cleansed. Superficial burns (epidermal involvement only) require minimal treatment. Simple moisturizers provided as oil-in-water lotions or creams should be recommended because they are easy to remove and provide a moist environment for healing. A dressing overtop may not be required for very small burns, but a simple gauze dressing will provide more protection against trauma and bacteria. Butter and other greasy home remedies should never be used on burns because they are not clean and their application can introduce bacteria into the wound. A topical antibiotic is not required for prevention of infection. If a burn develops blisters, the patient should be referred to a physician. Partial thickness and full thickness burns require dressings. Current research indicates that occlusive dressings may be used on burns provided the wound is not infected. Occlusive hydrocolloid dressings may decrease the risk of infection by preventing bacterial invasion from the environment. For burns that have greater evaporative water loss, semipermeable dressings such as transparent adhesive dressings are better because they allow some of the water to escape (thus avoiding maceration) while still providing a barrier against external bacterial invasion.

Dressings for burns are continued until complete healing has occurred. Partial thickness burns should heal within 3 weeks. If not healed, referral to a surgeon will be required for grafting. The burned area is often dry and itchy for several months after healing. Healed burns require 6 months to 2 years to completely mature. A light moisturizer should be routinely applied to the area during this time. Moisturizers should be tested on normal skin first and those containing high percentages of lanolin avoided to decrease risk of irritation. For persistent itchiness in a healed burn, oral antihistamines and topical astringent soaks may be used. A healed burn should not be exposed to the sun without sunscreen for 1 year.

Topical Anesthetics and Topical Antihistamines for Burns

Topical anesthetics and topical antihistamines should not be used on burns because of the risk of sensitization and further injury.

FROSTBITE

Frostbite is the freezing of tissues exposed to such extreme cold that the body is unable to supply enough heat to the affected area. It most commonly affects the extremities, such as the fingers, hands, toes, feet, ears and nose. Frostbite occurs when the water in the cells and interstitial spaces of the tissues freezes and forms ice crystals that swell, damaging or destroying the cells. Frostbite can be superficial if it involves only the skin, or deep if the tissues beneath the skin have also been frozen. Frostbite is very dangerous and can lead to death of the affected body part, requiring amputation.

The signs and symptoms of frostbite include lack of feeling in the affected area, skin that is cold to the touch and appears waxy, and skin that is discolored to white, yellow, or blue or has a flushed appearance.

Frostbite may also occur with hypothermia, which is more serious and life-threatening. Signs and symptoms of hypothermia include shivering in the early stages, numbness, lack of coordination, confused or unusual behavior, and body temperature below 35°C.

Treatment

Hypothermia should be treated before frostbite. Hypothermia is a medical emergency and the EMS (Emergency Medical System) should be called as the first step in the care of the patient. After the EMS has been called, first aid treatment begins with the removal of any wet clothing. The patient should then be dried and warmed by wrapping in blankets or putting on dry clothing. The patient should be moved to a warm environment but not put into a warm bath, because rapid warming can cause heart problems. However, other heat sources may be used, such as a hot water bottle (wrapped in a towel), body heat, or heating pads if the patient is dry. The patient can be given warm liquids to drink, such as plain warm water or lemon water, but not caffeine or alcohol. Contrary to popular belief, tea, coffee and alcohol do not warm you up, but hinder the body's ability to produce heat because they cause vasodilation and heat loss. In severe cases of hypothermia, the patient may become unconscious, the pulse slow and irregular and may take up to 45 seconds to detect. If a pulse cannot be detected within 45 seconds, Cardiopulmonary Resuscitation (CPR) may be required until EMS arrives.

For treatment of frostbite, the affected area should be covered to keep it warm and handled gently. Frostbitten tissue should not be rubbed because this can lead to further damage. To gently warm the area, it may be immersed in comfortably warm, not hot, water. The ideal water temperature is 40.5°C, measured with a thermometer if possible. The frostbitten area should be immersed until it looks red and edematous and feels warm. If the skin does not become red and warm but remains cool and pale, it indicates a full thickness injury. The area should then be covered with a dry, sterile dressing to keep it warm, cotton or gauze placed between affected fingers or toes, and the patient taken to a physician as soon as possible.

POISONING

Poisons can enter the body by inhalation, absorption through the skin, and ingestion. Many substances that are not poisonous in small amounts can become toxic in larger amounts.

General Guidelines

Even if the type of poisoning or exact substance causing a poisoning is not known, general guidelines can be followed. Drug and Poison Information Centres (DPIC) in all provinces can be telephoned and will provide information on what to do. The number of the poison information centre in your province should be kept by the telephone.

Treatment

Emergency Action Principles for Poisonings (The Canadian Red Cross Society. First Aid: The Vital Link. 1994)

1. Survey the scene to ensure no danger.
2. Check the casualty for unresponsiveness. If the person does not respond, call the Emergency Medical System (e.g., 911).
3. Do a primary survey and care for life-threatening problems. Call EMS for help if necessary.
4. Do a secondary survey, if needed, and care for other problems.
5. Keep monitoring the patient and possible life-threatening problems until EMS arrives.
6. Help the casualty rest in the most comfortable position and give reassurance.

(For more information see The Canadian Red Cross Society. First Aid: The Vital Link.)

Inhaled Poisons

Inhaled poisons include gases and fumes. Examples include carbon monoxide from car exhaust or a faulty heater or furnace, nitrous oxide, chlorine gas, such as in commercial swimming facilities, and fumes from industrial products, such as glues, paints, and cleaning solvents.

General Guidelines

As soon as possible after inhalation of the poison, the victim should be removed to fresh air (for oxygen) provided it is safe enough for the helper to do so. The Emergency Medical System should be called if necessary, and the Emergency Action Principles for Poisonings (Canadian Red Cross Guidelines) followed.

Absorbed Poisons (Dermal Poisons)

Dermal poisons enter the system via absorption through the skin. Examples include plants such as poison oak, poison ivy and poison sumac, and lipid-soluble chemicals, such as solvents, paint strippers and insecticides.

General Guidelines

After contact with a dermal poison, such as a poisonous plant, remove the contaminated clothing (being careful to avoid contact with the affected area of clothing) and wash the affected area of skin as soon as possible with soap and water. If a mild rash develops, a simple moisturizer will help soothe the itch and keep the area moist, which enhances wound healing. An astringent such as calamine lotion, zinc oxide ointment, witch hazel or aluminum acetate solution (Burow's solution) may be used to provide temporary relief of inflammation and itching provided the rash is relatively intact. Astringents should not be used if the area is open or raw. They also are drying and should be replaced as soon as possible with moisturizers to create a moist environment to enhance wound healing. For very itchy or weeping rashes, an oral antihistamine, such as diphenhydramine or chlorpheniramine, may be required. If blisters develop or if a very large area is affected, the patient should be referred to a physician.

After contact with a poisonous dry or wet chemical, call the Poison Information Centre and follow their instructions. In most cases the area should be flushed with copious amounts of continuous running water to remove the chemical from the skin. This may be advised even for dry chemicals that are activated by water because the continuous flushing of the water will remove the chemical quickly. In areas where running water is not immediately available, dry chemicals should be brushed off the skin. In all cases, the helper and the victim should protect themselves from further contact with the chemical by wearing gloves or protective face gear, such as glasses, or a dust mask, in the case of dry chemicals.

Ingested Poisons

Ingested poisons are those that enter the system by swallowing or coming in contact with the mouth or lips. Approximately 80% of all poisonings are caused by ingestion, commonly medications, cleaning products, pesticides and plants. Never give a poison victim anything to eat or drink unless directed by the Poison Information Centre. If a patient exposed to an unknown poison vomits, saving some of the vomitus for medical personnel will help with later diagnosis.

Gastric Contamination

Traditionally, poisonings such as drug overdoses have been treated with gastric-emptying, emesis or gastric lavage, followed by administration of activated charcoal and a cathartic agent. Based on current research, the consensus is that activated charcoal alone is as effective as, or more effective than, emesis or lavage with or without activated charcoal. Gastric emptying may provide additional benefit if the emesis or lavage is begun soon after the poisoning has taken place. Certain poisons are not adequately absorbed by charcoal, including methanol, lithium, and iron, then gastric emptying is necessary. Neither emesis nor lavage is of benefit if treatment is delayed because the stomach will have emptied into the small intestine making the toxin inaccessible.

The superiority of gastric lavage over ipecac-induced emesis for gastric emptying is controversial. Recent studies have demonstrated that gravity-flow gastric lavage using a large-bore tube and adequate fluid volume is superior to ipecac-induced emesis, especially for highly toxic poisonings.

Some clinicians feel the benefits of syrup of ipecac are limited but may be useful when medical care is more than 30 minutes from home. These clinicians feel ipecac is an impediment to therapy because activated charcoal cannot be administered until emesis is complete. One study found that ipecac decreased the efficacy of activated charcoal by 16%. However, a role may still exist for ipecac use in the home and in the hospital for small children in whom the small diameter of the lavage tube required limits the effectiveness of lavage.

General Guidelines

Call the poison centre and follow directions. The poison centre may advise the patient to drink water to dilute the poison in the stomach. For certain poisonings, such as drug and poisonous plant ingestions, the poison centre may advise the administration of syrup of ipecac to induce vomiting. Vomiting should never be induced if the patient:

- is already unconscious or is very drowsy and may become unconscious before emesis occurs;
- is having convulsions or has ingested substances that cause rapid onset of seizures, such as strychnine or camphor; *
- is pregnant;
- has ingested a corrosive substance (an acid or an alkali) or a petroleum product** (such as kerosene or gasoline);
- has heart disease;
- has an absent or impaired gag reflex;
- is a baby less than 6 months of age.

*Ipecac-induced emesis is relatively contraindicated for substances that can cause seizures, such as tricyclic antidepressants and isoniazid, or those that may cause dystonic reactions, such as phenothiazines.

**Ipecac-induced emesis for patients who have ingested petroleum distillates, such as gasoline and kerosene, or pesticides is controversial.

INSECT BITES AND STINGS

Insects can be commonly categorized as biters, chewers, or stingers. Mosquitoes and blackflies are both species of the Diptera order of insects and are categorized as biters. Biters attack the skin of their victims with mandibles to extract nourishment, or a blood meal, at some stage during their development. When mosquitoes and blackflies bite their victims they release acidic venom into their skin that contains allergens, and, in addition to the actual biting, causes most of the swelling and itch. Blackflies also release an anesthetizing substance into the skin as they bite so most of the pain is delayed, but may last 5 to 10 days.

Chiggers are the larvae of mites of the Trombiculidae family in the Arachnida class, and are an example of insects that chew. During the larval stage of the mite, a meal is required to complete the development process. Chewing insects do not feed on blood but rather extract small portions of lymph and epidermal tissue to obtain their nourishment. As they chew they release proteolytic enzymes that dissolve skin cells assisting them in this extraction of tissues. This enzymatic breakdown creates a stylosome or tube through the epidermis, with the enzymes causing an intensely itchy and long-lasting lesion in the skin.

The most common stinging insects are members of the Hymenoptera order, which include the *Apis*, *Vespa* and stinging or imported fire ants. The *Apis* includes honeybees and bumblebees, and the *Vespa* includes hornets, yellow jackets (a species of hornet) and wasps. Bites and stings from these insects can be painful but are rarely fatal. In allergic individuals, however, reactions can be fatal. Hymenoptera insects are most active during daylight hours and are most commonly encountered in and around forests or woodsy settings. They are attracted by white or brightly colored clothing (especially blue) and perfumes.

Honeybees (Apis)

Bees are vegetarian in that they feed on flowering plant products. The majority of honeybee stings occur when the person walks barefoot on clover-covered ground. Bees usually only sting when provoked.

The honeybee is unique in the Hymenoptera order because of the nature of its stinging apparatus. Its stinger contains a barb that holds the stinger in the victim. Once the victim is stung, the bee disengages, leaving behind its stinger and the venom sac, which results in the bee's death. The venom sac can be seen in the skin of the victim. The major venom fractions from the honeybee include phospholipase A_2, hyaluronidase, acid phosphatase and mellitin.

Hornets (Vespa) and Wasps (Polistes)

Hornets are carnivorous, feeding on smaller insects and worms. They are attracted to fruit and decaying matter, gravitating toward trash cans, especially trash with sugar debris, such as old pop cans and candy wrappers. Wasps tend to be found near their hives in the eaves of houses and crevices of buildings, while yellow jackets nest in the ground under logs, or in walls, and hornets have hanging nests in trees and shrubs.

Unlike bees, hornets and wasps do not leave their stinger in the victim, so they may sting repeatedly throughout their lifetime.

Hornet venom contains phospholipases and what is known as hornet kinins and other antigens. Recently hornet antigen 5 has been DNA coded, which is promising for the development of specific venom immunotherapy.

Wasp venom contains phospholipases, hyaluronidase and wasp kinins. Research has shown these kinins behave the same as bradykinin, a potent vasodilator that increases vascular permeability and stimulates pain receptors.

Ants (Imported Fire Ants; Solenopsis)

Ants are social insects and usually attack in swarms, most often those who inadvertently choose an ant mound to sleep on. Ants may move their mounds 3 to 4 times daily.

The method of stinging by ants, a two-part process, is unique among the Hymenoptera. They attach two pinching jaws to the skin, stinging the victim in a circular pattern around the point of attachment by swivelling around their head. Ants sting with an ovipositor apparatus that is on their abdomen. Ant bites can usually be recognized by the circular arrangement of papules or wheals that form within 24 hours around the two red puncta sites. The wheals may be filled with clear fluid or pus that is usually sterile.

Insect Venom

The venom of bees, hornets, and wasps contains up to 50% proteins (dry weight), many of which are highly immunogenic. Ant venom is different from other Hymenoptera venom because it contains only 1 to 5% proteins (dry weight) and has a lower antigenicity.

The usual reaction to an insect sting includes local pain, erythema (redness) and swelling. Unlike stings, insect bites do not cause pain. The reaction to insect bites and stings is usually only local, subsiding in 1 or 2 hours.

Occasionally, there are large local reactions to insect stings: extensive swelling around the sting site, usually peaking at 48 hours. These reactions may last as long as 1 week, and fatigue and nausea may occur.

Ticks (Ixodes) and Lyme Disease

Ticks belong to the Arachnida class of insects, are relatively long-lived and develop into adults over a 2-year period. The tick life-cycle has three stages, the larval, the nymphal and the adult. The nymphal and adult tick have 8 legs (4 pairs) and no antennae. Ticks detect potential hosts using sensory organs on their front legs. They then drop from leaves or shrubs or crawl from blades of grass onto the host. Tick bites are most common in forests and wooded areas but may occur in other areas where hosts, such as the mouse and deer, live.

Ticks bite using cheliceral digits (one of the first pair of appendages near the mouth) to cut into the skin of the host, then penetrating the skin until they find capillary blood on which to feed. Larger "teeth" on the tick are then used to hold the tick in place. Once attached, it secretes a cement-like substance, anticoagulants and immunosuppressants to facilitate feeding.

Ticks prefer to penetrate warm skin folds of their victims and bites are usually painless. Ticks can become infected with a spirochetal bacteria (*Borrelia burgdorferi*) by ingesting the blood of hosts that carry the bacteria, including many animals and birds. This bacteria can then be transmitted to humans through bites causing Lyme disease. Tick season is April through September. The majority of tick bites in humans are caused by nymphal ticks in early May to July, the remainder by adult ticks in early spring or fall. The ticks reported to transmit Lyme disease to humans are the deer ticks (*Ixodes dammini*) in Eastern Canada, and *Ixodes pacificus* and *angustus* in Western Canada. In Western Canada, only 1% of ticks carry *Borrelia burgdorferi*. The most common vector is *Ixodes dammini*. Up to 50% of *Ixodes dammini* ticks in Eastern Canada (especially Point Pelee Park and Longpoint) carry *Borrelia burgdorferi*. This tick is relatively small compared to other ticks, measuring about 3 mm as an adult. They are dark brown but become reddish-brown when full of blood after feeding.

Studies have shown that once a tick has attached to the skin, disease transmission can take up to 24 hours. If a tick is removed correctly soon after attachment, disease transmission may be prevented. Because tick bites are painless, it is important to check oneself, children and pets frequently during and after walks through wooded areas and brush, especially deer and mice habitats. If the tick was attached longer than 24 hours before removal, referral to a physician is necessary, as oral antibiotic prophylaxis may be required. In all cases of tick bites, patients should be advised to watch for the development of a bulls-eye rash within 3 to 32 days after the bite (Stage I of Lyme disease).

The bulls-eye rash is ring-shaped (erythema chronicum migrans), surrounds the bite and expands over days to weeks. The centre of the rash is blanched, the ring is red and can be raised or flat. Flu-like symptoms in Stage I include fever, chills, arthralgias and myalgias.

If signs or symptoms of Stage I occur, the victim should be seen by a physician promptly for diagnosis. In Stage I, systemic antibiotics are very effective in treating Lyme disease.

PREVENTION

Allergic individuals should avoid situations where stinging insects are likely to be found: wooded areas, outdoor picnics, wearing brightly colored clothing (especially white and bright blue) and wearing perfume.

For prevention of stings and bites in wooded or grassy areas, certain guidelines can be followed:

- wear a long sleeved shirt and pants;
- light-colored (not bright) clothing allows ticks to be seen more easily;
- tuck pant legs into socks or boots;
- tuck shirt into pants;
- avoid perfumes;
- in tick-infested areas, use a rubber band or tape the area where pants and socks meet so nothing can get under clothing and wear tightly woven clothing to make it more difficult for ticks to adhere;

- avoid underbrush and tall grass when hiking; stay in the middle of trails;
- inspect yourself carefully for insects or ticks after being outdoors, especially the back of the neck, the scalp line and hairy areas; check routinely if out for a long time;
- use mosquito netting to provide a physical barrier to mosquitoes and other insects; netting can be placed over tents, baby carriages, strollers and playpens;
- wear skin insect repellent such as DEET 50 to 75% on adults and DEET 10 to 20% on infants and children (not on infants less than 6 months of age);
- spray natural fibre netting, tents, or clothing with a clothing insect repellent such as DEET 30 to 100%.

Insect Repellents

Insect repellents are poisonous and must be used with caution. They should be kept out of the reach of children, as ingestion can be fatal.

Insect repellents can be used to repel mosquitoes, chiggers, ticks, fleas, gnats and biting flies, but none are effective against bees and wasps.

Insect repellents should not be used on children less than 6 months of age because of their large surface area to volume ratio, thus increased absorption and risk of toxicity. When applying repellents to the skin, extreme care must be taken not to get them in the eyes, in any wounds or on the lips. They should not be applied to children's hands if the children put their hands in their mouths. Each application of repellent should be spread over the skin for approximately 10 to 15 seconds.

Repellents should not be applied under occlusive dressings or clothing, on open wounds or irritated skin because of increased absorption.

Long-term use or frequent total-body application should be avoided to decrease the percutaneous absorption, the incidence of systemic toxicity and adverse effects. Insect repellents should be removed from the skin when no longer required by washing with soap and water.

Insect repellents can be sprayed on thin clothing to prevent mosquitoes from biting through. Repellents are safe on clothing made from natural fabrics, but may damage synthetic materials, such as rayon.

Spray forms of repellents should only be used if necessary, such as application to clothing, because of risk of inhalation and toxicity. Sprays should be avoided in children, and lotions, liquids, and stick formulations used whenever possible.

If a suspect adverse reaction occurs, patients should be referred to a physician and told to bring the spray container with them.

Repellents are classified as either **olfactory** repellents, which are volatile and repel insects through smell, or **gustatory**, also called contact repellents, which repel insects through taste.

The olfactory repellents produce a larger area of repellency but evaporate more quickly than the contact repellents and so must be applied more frequently.

The contact repellents provide a more concentrated barrier, but insects must touch the skin to work. The rate of loss from the skin for both kinds of repellents increases with higher temperatures (evaporation), higher wind velocity, sweating, clothing friction, and washing. Both types of repellents must be applied carefully to cover all exposed surfaces, because some insects, such as mosquitoes, are able to detect repellent-free areas.

The contact insect repellents are further classified as **skin repellents** such as DEET (N, N-diethyl-m-toluamide ≤75%), DMP (dimethyl phthalate), di-N-propyl isocinchomeronate and n-octyl bicycloheptene dicarboximide, or **clothing repellents**, which in Canada includes only DEET (up to 100%).

TREATMENT

The treatment of normal reactions to insect bites and stings usually only involves removal of insect parts where necessary, and local application of cold compresses and oral analgesics to alleviate the itch and pain. If cold compresses are not effective, application of hot water compresses (49 to 54°C, not hot enough to cause a burn) may decrease itching for up to 8 hours. These must be used with care. The water must be adequately hot, since rebound vasodilation will increase or stimulate itching. For large local reactions, oral anti-inflammatory agents, and oral antihistamines may be required to reduce pain and decrease the inflammatory reaction. In rare cases, for severe local reactions with extensive swelling, a prescription oral corticosteroid may be required.

Most topical agents used to decrease the pain and itching of insect bites and stings are ineffective because of minimal penetration into the centre of the reaction. While topical corticosteroids may not be as effective as astringents and local anesthetics for relief of itching due to insect bites, they are not associated with the sensitizing potential of local anesthetics. They provide an anti-inflammatory effect that increases relief for a bite that is large and

Removal of Insect Parts

Bees

The venom sac left in the skin from a honeybee must be removed manually without applying direct pressure, which can squeeze out the venom causing more pain. Lateral pressure with the blade of a knife is an effective method.

Step 1: Remove the stinger (venom sac) by scraping it away from the skin with a fingernail, knife or plastic card. Do not use tweezers because squeezing the venom sac can extrude more poison into the skin.

Step 2: Wash the bite with soap and water and cover it with a simple dressing, such as a gauze bandage to keep the site clean.

Step 3: Put ice or a cold pack over the area to decrease swelling and pain.

Step 4: Watch the victim for any signs of delayed allergic reaction.

Ticks

Ticks in the skin can be difficult to see, especially the tiny deer tick, which can be as small as the head of a pin. When a tick is found in the skin it should be removed with tweezers. Do not twist, jerk, squeeze or crush the tick because the tick fluids can transmit disease. The tick should be grasped as close to the skin as possible with the tweezers and pulled out slowly with a steady upward pull to avoid breaking it and leaving part behind. If tweezers are not available, the tick can be removed with fingers, making sure to protect them with a glove, plastic wrap or paper. Do not handle a tick with bare hands. A successfully removed tick can be killed by burning it (e.g., campfire), putting it in a container filled with alcohol, or flushing it down the toilet. Hands should be washed immediately to avoid contamination by disease the tick may be carrying.

A tick should not be burned out of the skin, nor should it be covered with petroleum jelly or nail polish, nor pricked with a pin. If the tick cannot be removed or if the mouthparts stay in the skin, the patient should see a physician.

If the tick is removed successfully, the area should be thoroughly washed with soap and water and a simple dressing, such as a gauze bandage, put over the bite to keep the area clean. The bite area should be watched for 1 month for the development of a rash. If a rash occurs, a physician should be seen as soon as possible.

Adapted from: Poisons. In: The Canadian Red Cross Society. First Aid: The Vital Link. 1st ed. St. Louis, MO:Mosby, 1994.

swollen, or one with an allergic component and may be used adjunctively with oral antihistamines. Astringents and local anesthetics may help to temporarily decrease pain and itching.

The astringents are likely the best choice because, although the relief is temporary, they are probably the least harmful to the relatively intact skin. Local anesthetics do provide relief, but the risk of sensitivity must be weighed against the benefit. Topical hydrocortisone may provide some relief for the pain and itching of insect bites and stings although more potent topical corticosteroids are generally more effective. Topical antihistamines are best avoided because the risk of sensitization outweighs the benefit. If an antihistamine effect is required, oral antihistamines are best. None of the topical products above should be applied to open wounds.

Allergy to Insect Bites and Stings

Epidemiologic studies indicate that approximately 0.4 to 4% of the population are allergic to the venom of one or more types of stinging insects (U.S. data). The largest proportion of allergic reactions to insect bites and stings are local, but systemic reactions are the greatest concern.

Of all allergic reactions to insect stings, only 9% are systemic. The venom from imported fire ants appears to be the least antigenic; only 2% of these reactions are systemic.

The other members of the Hymenoptera order of insects are more antigenic than ants and cross-reactivity exists.

Hornet and yellow-jacket venom is extensively cross-reactive but less so with wasp venom. Cross-reactivity of honeybee venom with hornet venom is minimal. Cross-reactivity between hornet and yellow-jacket venom with fire ant venom is very limited.

Systemic allergic reactions can only occur in people who have been previously stung and sensitized. Allergic reactions to insect stings are IgE-mediated. Sensitization occurs in people who develop high IgE antibody titres (antivenom antibodies) after being stung. These IgE antibodies attach to target cells throughout the body (e.g., mast cells and basophils).

With a subsequent sting, the venom attaches to the antivenom antibodies (IgE antibodies), which are attached to the target cells, causing degranulation and release of histamine and other mediators of anaphylaxis. Mediators formed later in the reaction include leukotrienes and prostaglandins. These mediators are chemoattractors of eosinophils and other white blood cells and are responsible for late phase reactions. Anaphylaxis usually occurs within 15 to 20 minutes after the sting but may take up to 72 hours.

Anaphylactic reactions can be limited to the skin (cutaneous) but can also affect the respiratory and cardiovascular systems. Once a person has had an allergic reaction to a sting, the risk of a reaction with subsequent stings is 60%. Also, the risk of more severe systemic allergic reaction increases with subsequent stings. However, long-term studies have shown that in children with systemic reactions confined to the skin only, ≤10% will go on to develop more severe systemic reaction with subsequent stings. Also, as the time interval between the reaction and the subsequent sting increases, the IgE titre decreases, and the likelihood of another reaction decreases.

Cutaneous reactions include flushing, urticaria (hives and wheals), pruritus and angioedema. The leading cause of death is respiratory reactions that include laryngeal edema, laryngospasm and bronchoconstriction. The signs preceding laryngeal obstruction are hoarseness, difficulty talking, and a feeling of choking or throat tightness. Cardiovascular anaphylaxis is the second leading cause of death from anaphylaxis. Clinical features include tachycardia, hypotension, arrhythmia, hypovolemic shock and rarely, myocardial infarction.

Other signs of anaphylaxis include abdominal cramping, nausea, vomiting and diarrhea. Patients taking beta-blockers may have a more severe anaphylactic course because their negative inotropic effect on the heart can worsen hypotension and provide resistance to therapy with epinephrine, and possible worsening of the condition from the unopposed alpha-adrenergic effect of epinephrine.

Treatment of Anaphylaxis

Initial treatment of anaphylaxis prior to hospitalization or during transfer includes administration of epinephrine and H_1-antihistamines. Epinephrine 1:1000 solution is administered subcutaneously or intramuscularly. The dose for children and adults is 0.01 mL/kg (or 0.3 mL/m^2 in children) up to a maximum of 0.3 to 0.5 mL. The dose may be repeated every 15 minutes. In patients with known anaphylaxis to insect stings an additional dose of epinephrine may be injected in the sting site to cause local vasoconstriction and delay systemic absorption of the venom. This dose is half the calculated treatment dose.

After epinephrine has been given, an H_1-antihistamine such as diphenhydramine should be given orally in a dose of up to 50 to 75 mg (adults) and 1 mg/kg (children). Some clinicians also recommend the administration of H_2-antihistamines such as cimetidine and ranitidine to block histamine completely. Immediately after treatment has been initiated, the patient should be transferred to a hospital or the emergency medical system should be contacted, whichever will provide the quickest treatment.

Venom Neutralizers

Papain, the proteolytic enzyme found in meat tenderizers, has been used to break down venom proteins and decrease the pain and inflammation caused by insect bites and stings. However, when applied topically, it probably does not reach the insect venom. One study has shown papain ineffective for the acute treatment of imported fire ant stings, and the authors state that any benefit obtained is probably placebo. Meat tenderizer is not recommended for this use because it is associated with allergic reactions.

Dilute ammonium hydroxide solution (9.5 to 10.5% or less) has commonly been used and is effective in relieving the itching and burning of insect bites and stings. In addition to being a proven counterirritant, ammonia, which is alkaline, may also neutralize the acidic venoms or toxins introduced into the skin by mosquitoes, chiggers, blackflies and Hymenoptera species (bees, wasps, hornets, fire ants). The manufacturer of a product on the market that contains 3.61% ammonia in mineral oil states that because no scientific studies have been done to prove their product neutralizes or denatures insect venom in skin, the company cannot make this claim. However, the company believes the effectiveness of their product is due to its neutralizing effect on the venom. This would explain why, in many cases, the symptoms of itching and burning do not return when the ammonia is applied soon after the bite or sting has occurred. Dilute ammonia solution is recommended for use on adults and children over 2 years of age and may be applied as needed. Ammonia 3.61% in a mineral oil solution usually causes no irritation, but it may cause a slight sting when applied to bites or stings with an open centre. Ammonia solution should

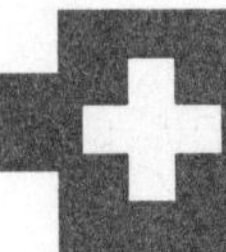

FIRST AID KIT

First aid kits should be kept in locations close to where an injury may occur or anywhere an individual and their family spends a lot of time: the home, cottage, and workplace. The car is also an ideal place because it is usually with the family or individual. First aid kits should be kept in boats and taken hiking, camping or on trips to the beach.

Plastic or metal tool boxes make ideal containers for first aid kits because they are resistant to crushing and protect the contents.

A first aid kit should include:

- first aid manual, such as The Canadian Red Cross Society. First Aid: The Vital Link;
- sterile gauze pads in different sizes (for applying to wounds or cleaning wounds or applying medications);
- adhesive tape (for wrapping or adhering gauze pads);
- adhesive bandages in different sizes;
- moist towellettes (for cleaning small wounds) and ideally 1 or 2 bottles of sterile saline for irrigation or a nonionic surfactant cleanser (for cleaning larger wounds);
- soap (for cleaning hands and intact skin around wounds);
- unscented oil in water cream (for keeping clean wounds moist);
- antibiotic cream or ointment (for treating infected wounds);
- syrup of ipecac (to be used only under the guidance of the regional Poison Control Centre);
- scissors;
- tweezers;
- eye patches;
- flashlight with a new package of batteries;
- coins for pay phone;
- list of emergency phone numbers including the Emergency Medical System, Poison Control Centre and family physician;
- ice packs;
- pencil and paper;
- blanket;
- insect repellent;
- astringent, such as witch hazel, or calamine cream or lotion (with or without pramoxine but not with diphenhydramine) (for decreasing the redness and itch of insect bites and stings);
- oral antihistamines, such as diphenhydramine or chlorpheniramine for allergic reactions to plants or insects;
- epinephrine 1:1000 ampules and syringes or preloaded syringes (and 70% isopropyl alcohol swabs) when an individual or family member has a known history of severe allergy or anaphylaxis with insect bites and stings; the expiry dates on the ampules should be checked routinely;
- tourniquet with the above when an insect bite or sting has occurred on an arm or leg (tourniquet placed between the sting and the body);
- sunscreen.

only be used to treat the itch and burning of insect bites and stings, not applied to open cuts or wounds.

Other Home Remedies Used to Treat Insect Bites and Stings

Other home remedy products applied topically to insect bites and stings include baking soda (sodium bicarbonate), aluminum-containing antiperspirant sticks or roll-ons (aluminum chloride, aluminum zirconyl hydroxychloride, or aluminum chlorohydrate) and liquid antacids. No well-controlled studies have been done using these home remedies, but baking soda and antiperspirants are commonly used to relieve the itch and pain of insect bites and stings and are effective. One theory is that the aluminum in the products penetrates the centre of the sting and denatures and inactivates the proteinaceous venom. The other theory is that these products do not reach the insect venom and so cannot neutralize it, but their effectiveness comes from their astringent action, which provides a temporary topical cooling effect. Baking soda and liquid antacids may also work through a topical astringent effect.

PATIENT ASSESSMENT QUESTIONS

Q What medications have you been applying to the insect bite or sting? Are you allergic to any oral or topical medications?

When patients complain of worsening insect bites and stings, a secondary infection or an allergic component should be ruled out. In general, topical anesthetics should be avoided, especially benzocaine, because of risk of sensitization. A patient allergic to sulfonamides or PABA should not use benzocaine. It is cross-sensitive with sulfonamides and PABA and can greatly increase the risk of an allergic contact dermatitis that will exacerbate the insect bite area.

If a topical anesthetic is greatly desired for an insect bite or sting, products containing pramoxine are the least sensitizing. Local anesthetics should be avoided on open cuts or wounds.

Q What is the topical antihistamine-astringent product being used for?

Topical antihistamines should never be used on chickenpox lesions because of increased absorption that can result in drug overdosage, especially when oral antihistamines are used concomitantly. Symptoms of overdosage, including bizarre behavior and hallucinations, can mimic varicella encephalopathy and lead to unnecessary treatment.

Q What is the antiseptic being purchased for?

Topical antiseptics should not be used for the routine cleansing of open wounds or burns because they are painful and toxic to the skin cells required for wound repair and infection control. Antiseptics are not needed to prevent infection. Bacterial presence does not necessarily lead to infection. Sterile normal saline is the ideal cleanser for open wounds because it approximates physiologic osmolality and is not harmful to healing tissues.

If a wound does become infected, a topical antibiotic cream or ointment is preferred because they are selectively toxic to bacteria, unlike antiseptics, which are nonselectively cytotoxic. Patients should be told never to put anything in a wound that they would not put in their eye.

Sterile normal saline for irrigation or a nonionic surfactant cleanser should be included in a first aid kit rather than antiseptic solution.

Q What does the rash look like? Where is it located? What have you been using to treat it?

Patients who have rashes that are very red, edematous or painful should be asked what topical medications they have been applying. Corticosteroids should never be applied to fungal or bacterial infections without appropriate concomitant antifungals or antibacterials. Applying corticosteroids to undiagnosed rashes risks local immune suppression and suppression of inflammation, which can make diagnosis very difficult: it can eliminate the classic diagnostic red (inflammatory) ring formation of tinea corporis (ringworm), for example. Location of the persistent rash can help diagnosis: a rash in the crural folds of a young man or under the breasts of a woman in the humid summer season could indicate a fungal infection.

Q When did the tick bite occur and how did you remove it?

Ticks can be vectors of Lyme disease, especially in certain areas of Eastern Canada; the incidence in Western Canada is very low. Patients should know how to correctly remove ticks because removal within 24 hours of attachment may prevent disease transmission, especially important for people who do not have access to medical assistance. Patients should be informed that the old tales of using petroleum jelly or burning a tick out of the skin are not appropriate and may actually encourage disease transmission (by injuring the tick). Health professionals should look for a typical bullseye rash that develops 3 to 32 days after the bite of an infected tick, and indicates stage I of Lyme disease. Patients should be promptly referred to a physician for systemic antibiotics.

Q How long have you had flaking of your scalp? What have you been using to treat it? Have you ever had a diagnosis from or a culture of your scalp done by your physician?

Patients who have been using topical dandruff or antiseborrheic shampoo for months or years without success may have undiagnosed tinea capitis. In mild cases of tinea capitis, pruritus and scaling may be minimal and few to no broken hairs present. In more severe cases, areas of hair loss are the classic sign of tinea capitis. The individual should be referred to their physician for an accurate diagnosis.

PHARMACEUTICAL AGENTS

ANESTHETICS

Local anesthetics work by decreasing the permeability of neuronal membranes to sodium ions, which inhibits depolarization and blocks the initiation and conduction of nerve impulses. This membrane stabilizing effect or anesthesia is reversible and very short-lived.

Structurally, the topical local anesthetics can be subgrouped into the ester types (benzocaine and tetracaine), the amide types (dibucaine, lidocaine and prilocaine), and the nonester/nonamide type local anesthetics (pramoxine and dyclonine), which have unique chemical structures.

Topical anesthetics can be sensitizing. The nonester/nonamide type are the least sensitizing, the amide type less sensitizing than the ester type. There is no cross-sensitivity between the three types of local anesthetics (ester, amide, nonester/nonamide), and it is uncommon between different amides but common between different esters. With benzocaine, which is an ethyl ester of para-aminobenzoic acid (PABA), cross-sensitization may occur with sunscreens containing PABA, with paraben preservatives, and with sulfonamides given orally or topically.

Many antipruritic products contain local anesthetics. Some topical antibiotic preparations may also contain local anesthetics intended for relief of pain; however, it is preferable to take oral analgesics.

Drug products that contain a combination of astringents and external analgesics or local anesthetics combine the anti-inflammatory, analgesic and antipruritic effects. Examples include aluminum acetate with menthol and camphor or witch hazel or calamine with pramoxine. These products are promoted to decrease irritation, pain, burning and itching.

A new, nonprescription combination product of topical anesthetics is available as a cream or a single dose patch. *EMLA* (Eutectic Mixture of Local Anesthetics) is a 1:1 oil/water emulsion of a eutectic mixture of lidocaine and prilocaine bases. When a thick layer of the cream is applied to the skin and covered with an occlusive dressing for at least 1 hour, dermal analgesia is achieved for up to 5 hours. The single dose unit patch has a surface area of 40 cm^2 with an active surface area of 10 cm^2. This product is extremely effective prior to surgical procedures such as laser treatment of warts, and tattoos, as well as electrolysis, skin grafting and surgical treatment of local lesions. It is recommended for use on <u>intact skin</u> only and should not be used on open wounds.

Side effects of topical anesthetics include slight stinging and irritation. Topical anesthetics should not be applied to deep or puncture wounds or serious burns because of an increased risk of absorption. Systemic side effects that may occur with excessive dosage and application to open wounds include central nervous system effects, such as excitation or depression, nervousness, tremors, seizures, and cardiovascular effects, such as bradycardia, hypertension and cardiac arrest. Although manufacturers recommend these products not be used for more than 7 days, they should probably be used for a much shorter period until oral analgesia is effective. Topical anesthetics can temporarily mask the signs of local wound infection by causing the skin to blanch, masking inflammation and decreasing pain, another sign of infection. Topical anesthetics (except dibucaine and tetracaine) should not be used on children under 2 years of age without the advice of a physician because a safe dosage has not been determined. Use in children less that 2 years of age, especially under 6 months of age is not generally recommended because of the risk of methemoglobinemia. Infants less that 3 months of age are especially at risk because their levels of the enzyme methemoglobin reductase are much lower than older children and adults. Prilocaine and benzocaine have both been shown to accentuate the development of methemoglobin, and methemoglobinemia has occurred in infants with excessive use. This risk is also increased with concomitant use of other methemoglobin-inducing drugs, such as sulfonamides.

Topical anesthetics are marketed to provide temporary relief of the itching and burning associated with minor cuts and scrapes, minor burns, sunburn, insect bites and stings and other minor skin irritations, but these products should not be put on an open wound. No data could be found to support their safety on delicate wound healing tissues. They are probably safe to apply to intact skin of insect bites and stings but should be avoided on cuts and scrapes.

ANTIBIOTICS

The role of topical antibacterials has not been clearly established. Antibiotics have an advantage over antiseptics in that they are selectively cytotoxic to bacteria. Topical antibiotics may be indicated for wounds that are heavily contaminated. Ideally, a wound culture should be done so the appropriate antibiotic can be used.

Topical antibiotics may be effective in decreasing the number of bacteria on the wound surface, but they do not penetrate nonviable tissue. If an infected wound is necrotic, it must be debrided. In wounds where the infection has invaded the surrounding tissue, systemic (oral or intravenous) antibiotics are required.

Polymyxin B is active against gram-negative bacteria including *Haemophilus influenzae*, *Enterobacter* sp. and *Klebsiella pneumoniae*. It has some activity against *Pseudomonas aeruginosa* but divalent cations (such as calcium) present in wound serum decrease binding of polymyxin B to the *Pseudomonas* cell membrane. Polymyxin is combined with bacitracin or gramicidin for their gram-positive coverage. Gramicidin and bacitracin have similar spectrums of bacterial coverage.

Bacitracin is active against gram-positive bacteria, especially *Staphylococcus aureus* and *Streptococcus pyogenes*. Some strains of *Staphylococcus aureus* have become resistant to bacitracin. Group C and G beta-hemolytic *Streptococci* are less sensitive and group B *Streptococcus* are usually resistant. Bacitracin also covers *Corynebacterium* and *Clostridium*, and gram-negative cocci, such as *Neisseria* (*meningococcus* and *gonococcus*), but gram-negative bacilli are resistant. The activity of bacitracin is not impaired by blood, pus, necrotic tissue, or large inocula of bacteria in wounds.

Gramicidin is also active against gram-positive cocci bacteria. Gram-positive bacilli, such as *Clostridium*, are relatively resistant and gram-negative bacilli are completely resistant to gramicidin.

Gramicidin is combined with polymyxin B in the cream formulation because it is water insoluble and is most stable in cream. Bacitracin is most stable in oil and so is combined with polymyxin B in the ointment form. Bacitracin is also available as a single component in ointment form. The cream is recommended for moist, weeping wounds because it is less occlusive than the ointment and so allows some of the wound moisture to evaporate, preventing maceration. The ointment is recommended for drier wounds. With dry wounds, there is less risk of maceration from the occlusion, and because of its better adherence than cream, ointment will keep the dry wound moist. Because of ointment's greater adherence, it is also recommended for more severely infected wounds. However, it is not recommended for use on burns.

Mupirocin is most active against gram-positive bacteria including *Staphylococcus aureus* and *Staphylococcus epidermidis*, and methicillin-resistant *Staphylococcus aureus (MRSA)*. Mupirocin is also active against *Streptococcus*, including *Streptococcus pneumoniae*, group A beta-hemolytic *Streptococci*, and group B, C and G *Streptococci*. Some gram-negative aerobic bacteria are susceptible, including *H. influenzae* and *Branhamella catarrhalis*, but most *Enterobacteriaceae* (*Klebsiella, Proteus, Enterobacter*) *E. coli* and *Pseudomonas aeruginosa* are resistant. To avoid development of resistance to this valuable topical agent, it should be reserved for use in demonstrated MRSA infections or against *Staphylococcus aureus*, which has become resistant to bacitracin and gramicidin. The polyethylene glycol base of this product may cause stinging and irritation especially on mucous membranes.

ANTIFUNGALS

For an in-depth discussion of specific antifungal agents please refer to the following chapters: Women's Health Care Products, Men's Health Care Products, Foot Care Products and Oral Health Care Products.

ANTIPRURITICS

Antihistamines: Antihistamines used topically include diphenhydramine and tripelennamine. Topical antihistamines are used to treat histamine-mediated pruritus. However, they may not be effective for this indication because the low concentrations of the antihistamines and the salt forms in the products prevent adequate drug penetration into the skin. Some antipruritic effect may occur from the weak local anesthetic effect of the antihistamines. The cooling effect on the skin from the propellant in some aerosol products may provide more relief than the antihistamine.

The use of topical antihistamines is generally not recommended because of the risk of sensitization and subsequent worsening of the rash. The biggest disadvantage of the development of hypersensitivity is that cross-sensitivity, manifested as systemic contact dermatitis, can then occur when any structurally related drugs are given orally. If itching from the insect bites and stings is troublesome, oral antihistamines are more effective and preferred because they are much less likely to initiate sensitivity reactions. Antihistamines should not be used topically on children with chickenpox because of the increased absorption and risk of systemic toxicity secondary to overdosage. When given orally, 40 to 60% of the dose of diphenhydramine is eliminated through first-pass metabolism. When diphenhydramine is applied topically, the first-pass metabolism is bypassed. Overdosage has resulted in changes in mental status, which can be misdiagnosed as varicella encephalopathy. Behavior has returned to normal 24 hours after removal of the topical antihistamine.

Other Antipruritics: Colloidal oatmeal is used in baths for its antipruritic effect. Classified as an emollient (skin softening agent), oatmeal may also have some astringent activity. The bath oil is commonly used to relieve the pruritus associated with chickenpox.

Chamomile extract has been shown in some studies to have a mild anti-inflammatory activity. Primrose oil, which contains linoleic and linolenic acid, may reduce pruritus when used orally, but only after several weeks of continued use, so is not of use treating the acute pruritus of insect bites and stings. One study showed improvement in itch and scaling of eczema in patients who took 6 to 12 capsules of evening primrose oil orally twice daily for 12 weeks.

ANTISEPTICS

Antiseptics and disinfectants are used to kill organisms. Antiseptics differ from disinfectants: antiseptics are used on living tissue while disinfectants are used on inanimate objects, such as surgical instruments. Antiseptics and disinfectants are nonselectively cytotoxic, unlike antibiotics, which are selectively toxic to bacteria. Antiseptics are toxic to cell membranes of all cells including those of bacteria and the cells required for wound repair, such as white blood cells and fibroblasts. Therefore, antiseptics may actually impair the defenses against infection. Antisepsis is not necessary for the wound itself. If used at all, antiseptics are best used on the tissue surrounding a wound. In addition to being cytotoxic, antiseptics may have no advantage over normal saline for controlling infection during cleansing because they are rapidly inactivated by body fluid. Large volumes of the antiseptic would have to be used to overcome this, causing not only cytotoxicity, but irritation, pain and edema.

Antiseptics should never be used prophylactically on clean proliferating wounds. They may be acceptable for use on heavily contaminated wounds, although this is controversial. Some clinicians feel they should never be used. Heavy bacterial contamination of a wound is best reduced by removing necrotic tissue and foreign particles and by frequently irrigating with normal saline.

Antiseptics available today include chlorhexidine, sodium hypochlorite solutions, povidone-iodine, hydrogen peroxide, isopropyl alcohol and acetic acid.

Chlorhexidine: Chlorhexidine is considered the least toxic of the antiseptics commonly used. Current research indicates that chlorhexidine is less damaging to host tissues than are hypochlorite and iodine solutions.

Chlorhexidine is active against many gram-positive and gram-negative bacteria, fungi and viruses. Chlorhexidine is cationic and binds strongly to skin and mucosa. This strong binding prevents its absorption systemically.

Chlorhexidine is available as chlorhexidine gluconate in different strengths with and without alcohol, and in sudsing and nonsudsing forms. Chlorhexidine solutions in water require low concentrations of isopropyl alcohol for preservation purposes only.

The strongest chlorhexidine ready for use is 4% in sterile water sudsing formulation (e.g., *Hibitane*). This formulation is routinely used as a presurgical scrub. The 2% sudsing formulation (*Hibitane 2%*) may be used in noncritical areas, such as hand washing prior to wound care. Both of the sudsing formulations contain a mild detergent and 4% isopropyl alcohol as a preservative. These solutions are used to decrease skin flora count. They may also be used to treat skin infections caused by bacteria, such as *Staphylococcus* and *Streptococcus*. Because of the high concentrations of these solutions they must be rinsed thoroughly with water or saline after use to prevent toxicity to skin cells.

Chlorhexidine 0.5% in 70% isopropyl alcohol solution (e.g., *Hexirub*) should only be used on intact skin. This concentration does not have to be rinsed off. It is used as an adjunct to the chlorhexidine sudsing skin cleaners and also for preparing surgical sites on skin. The high concentration of isopropyl alcohol (70%) is used as an antiseptic for instant kill of microbes while the chlorhexidine prevents regrowth of microorganisms.

Chlorhexidine 0.05% in sterile water with and without 4% isopropyl alcohol as a preservative (e.g., *Hibidil*) is the most dilute of the manufactured chlorhexidine solutions and is the concentration used for cleansing and irrigating wounds, including burns. The large multidose containers contain 4% isopropyl alcohol as a preservative. Chlorhexidine 0.05% is also available without alcohol in 30 mL ampules for single use.

This solution does not have to be rinsed off, according to the manufacturer, but many clinicians recommend irrigation with saline to remove all traces to prevent toxicity to wound repair cells, especially on burns.

There is no literature that supports a difference in outcome between wound irrigation with normal saline vs. chlorhexidine 0.05% in sterile water.

Hypochlorite Solutions: The active ingredient of hypochlorite solutions is available chlorine. These solutions all contain differing percentages of sodium hypochlorite. The activity of these solutions is decreased by organic matter and an alkaline pH.

Hypochlorite dissolves necrotic tissue and controls odors. It is effective against the bacteria *Staphylococcus* and *Streptococcus* but is also toxic to fibroblasts in the normal dilutions used. The intact skin around the wound must be protected to prevent breakdown.

Studies have shown that 0.5% sodium hypochlorite solutions exhibit marked fibroblast toxicity, and significantly decrease wound epithelialization. Even solution concentrations as low as 0.025% and 0.00025% inhibit neutrophil migration and damage fibroblasts and endothelial cells. Some researchers have suggested it should never be used on open wounds. If a sodium hypochlorite solution is to be used, the concentration should not exceed 0.0625% to minimize the deleterious effects on neovascularization and epithelialization.

Sodium hypochlorite solutions are sometimes referred to as Dakin's and Eusol solutions. The commercially available sodium hypochlorite solution (*Hygeol*) contains 1% available chlorine. Dakin's solution is a 1:1 ratio of the 1% solution and water (e.g., *Hygeol* ½ or sodium hypochlorite 0.5%), and Eusol solution is a 1:3 ratio of the 1% solution and water (e.g., *Hygeol* ¼ or sodium hypochlorite 0.25%).

Povidone-iodine: Povidone-iodine is iodine bound to povidone. Povidone-iodine 10% solution contains 1% available iodine. Available iodine does not mean free iodine. Povidone-iodine 10% contains 1 ppm of free iodine, which is the active ingredient. Iodine is active against bacteria, viruses, fungi and *Trichomonas*. Povidone-iodine, unlike iodine, is nonstaining to fabrics. Povidone-iodine is said to have broad spectrum effectiveness when used on intact skin or small, relatively clean wounds. Its ability to penetrate infected or necrotic tissue is questionable. Half-strength povidone-iodine solution (5%) has been used to cleanse burn wounds, but this is no longer recommended because it is cytotoxic, painful and it toughens and dries eschar on burn wounds. It is toxic to wound repair cells, such as fibroblasts, in the concentrations normally used. Some clinicians state 1 ppm of free iodine is not strong enough to be bactericidal. However, higher concentrations are extremely toxic to all cells. Any concentration greater than 0.001% povidone-iodine will kill wound tissue. Some clinicians feel iodine should never be used in wounds because it is a poison and is absorbed systemically. Over time it can cause elevation in thyroid function tests. If used in large amounts it can cause iodine toxicity. Povidone-iodine solution should be rinsed off after use to prevent cytotoxicity to wound repair cells. Other formulations of povidone-iodine are also available and their use on open wounds may also not be advisable.

Hydrogen Peroxide: Traditionally hydrogen peroxide has been used as a cleansing antiseptic and for debridement by its effervescent activity. It should not be used by forceful irrigation to debride because it can cause subcutaneous emphysema that mimics gas gangrene.

Hydrogen peroxide is toxic to fibroblasts. It can ulcerate newly formed repair tissue. It should never be used to pack sinus tracts because it can produce subcutaneous gas, which can lead to air embolisms. Research shows that hydrogen peroxide disturbs new blood vessel formation (neoangiogenesis) in granulation tissue.

Isopropyl Alcohol: Alcohol removes the skin's protective lipid coating and dehydrates the skin. It is toxic to all cells and should never be applied to open wounds.

Acetic Acid: Acetic acid is effective against *Pseudomonas aeruginosa* in superficial wound beds but is ineffective against other gram-negative bacteria. It does not cover gram-positive bacteria. Acetic acid is toxic to fibroblasts in concentrations usually used.

ASTRINGENTS

An astringent is a drug product that is applied to the skin or mucous membranes for a local and limited protein coagulation effect. Astringents are classified as skin protectants. They have low cell penetrability and so the protein coagulation or precipitation is limited to the cell surface and interstitial spaces.

Astringency decreases the permeability of the cell membrane altering the cell's ability to swell and hold water. The tissues contract and wrinkle and capillary endothelium hardens decreasing transcapillary protein movement. The result is tissue blanching, and inhibited local edema, inflammation and exudation. Astringents are acidic, mildly antiseptic and dry the skin. They are used to stop hemorrhage (styptic action), reduce inflammation, toughen the skin and decrease sweating by coagulating protein in the sweat ducts. Antiperspirants are astringents. Astringents are applied to insect bites and stings to relieve the irritation and burning. They are also used in skin fresheners and cleansers to contract the skin surface for a temporary, overall smoother appearance.

The most commonly used astringents are calamine, zinc oxide, zinc sulfate, aluminum acetate, alum and aluminum sulfate, and witch hazel. These products are for external use only and should not come in contact with the eyes.

Aluminum Acetate: Aluminum acetate is used as a 0.13 (0.125) to 0.5% solution. It is indicated for the temporary relief of minor skin irritations and itching due to poison ivy, poison oak, poison sumac, insect bites, athlete's foot, or rashes caused by soaps, detergents, cosmetics, or jewelry. It is also used as a drying agent for wet or weeping eruptions.

Aluminum acetate solution is used as a compress, wet dressing or soak. To use as a compress or wet dressing, saturate a clean soft white cloth, such as a diaper or torn sheet, in the solution. Squeeze out the excess and apply loosely to the affected area. Saturate the cloth in the solution every 15 to 30 minutes and apply to the affected area. Repeat as often as necessary. The compresses should be kept wet and solutions should not be left to sit to avoid concentration, increasing the risk of irritation. Aluminum acetate compresses should not be used under occlusive dressings or covered with plastic to prevent evaporation.

To use as a soak, the affected area can be left in the solution for 15 to 30 minutes, repeated 3 times daily. Whether for compresses, dressings or soaks, the solution should be made fresh before each application and discarded after each use, never reused.

Aluminum acetate solution can be prepared from tablets, powders, or liquid solutions. Burow's solution contains aluminum acetate 5% and boric acid as a buffer. It is further diluted to a 1:10 to 1:40 solution prior to use (0.13 to 0.5% aluminum acetate solution).

Zinc Oxide: Zinc oxide is relatively inert but has mild astringent, antiseptic and protective action. Insoluble in water, it is used in a 15 to 25% concentration in ointments and pastes. It is also an ingredient in Calamine Lotion (USP), which contains 8% w/v each of zinc oxide and calamine powder in suspension. Zinc oxide may temporarily decrease inflammation and relieve pruritus associated with insect bites and stings (due to its astringent effect). Zinc oxide may be applied as required.

Calamine: Calamine is a mixture of zinc oxide with ferric oxide (0.5 to 1%), which gives it its pink color. Insoluble in water, it is available in suspension form in Calamine Lotion (USP), and in cream form combined with other medications. Calamine has the same actions as zinc oxide. Marketed as a skin protectant because of its astringent action, like zinc oxide, it may temporarily decrease the irritation and pruritus of insect bites and stings. The lotion can be applied using a cotton ball or tissue, the cream manually. Calamine may be applied as required.

Alum and Aluminum Sulfate *(concentrated Alum)*: Alum is either aluminum potassium sulfate or aluminum ammonium sulfate and is sometimes used as a local styptic and in astringent lotions. It is used as an astringent in a 0.5 to 5% solution, but concentrations up to 20% may be used on small areas such as insect bites and stings. Aluminum sulfate, also called concentrated alum, is available as 46 to 63% (anhydrous weight) styptic pencils. It is used to coagulate blood (styptic action) and thereby stop the bleeding caused by minor surface cuts and abrasions (e.g., during shaving). Styptic pencils are used by moistening the tip of the pencil with water, touching it to the affected area, drying it after use. There have been no reported toxicities with the use of styptic pencils. They should not be confused with caustic pencils, which are made of silver nitrate.

Witch Hazel: Witch hazel is marketed for the relief of minor skin irritations due to insect bites or minor cuts or scrapes. Witch hazel, currently the official name, is also called Hamamelis water, synonymous with witch hazel water and distilled witch hazel extract. The distilling process removes the tannin.

Tannin has been shown to have anti-inflammatory action secondary to its vasoconstrictor activity. However, witch hazel, or distilled witch hazel extract, has also been shown to have anti-inflammatory activity. Better results may be seen if applied in a phosphatidylcholine cream vehicle that enhances the penetration of witch hazel into the skin.

Witch hazel may be helpful in decreasing the inflammation and pruritus of insect bites and stings and other closed wound irritations. It can be applied as needed.

The distilled extract is commonly used in aftershave lotions, and the nondistilled extract in hemorrhoidal preparations. No data exist to support the use of witch hazel for sunburn, bruises, contusions or sprains or for relieving muscular pains.

CLEANSERS

Any cleanser that you would not put in your eye should not be put in a wound. Wound cleansers are made of two components, the active ingredient and the carrier. Surface active effects are required for cleansing:

- to break the bond between the wound tissue and the foreign particles, such as dirt and bacteria; and
- to decrease the interfacial tension to allow the debris to be rinsed from the wound.

Cleansers are categorized as cationic if they are positively charged, anionic if they are negatively charged, or amphoteric if they have both positive and negative charges on the same molecule. Cleansers that have a full chemical charge (cationic or anionic) increase the permeability of cell membranes, which results in cell death. Therefore, cleansers that are anionic or cationic can be toxic to the repair tissues of wounds and inhibit wound healing.

Products that carry a full chemical charge include soaps and antiseptics.

Products that do not carry a full chemical charge (neutral or amphoteric) include normal saline (0.9% sodium chloride in sterile water) and a chemical group of polymers called nonionic surfactants.

Soaps: Soaps are by definition alkaline in pH. The alkalinity is hard on skin and can decrease the number of cell layers in the stratum corneum, reducing its thickness. Soap emulsifies the acidic lipid layer on the skin and removes it along with the bacteria, which decreases the shield against water loss, increases the risk of irritation and impairs the skin's defences against bacteria.

Saline: Normal saline (0.9% sodium chloride in sterile water) is the ideal cleanser for wounds. With an osmolality of 285 mOsm it approximates physiologic osmolality (280-296 mOsm) and does not harm healing tissues. Saline is safe to put in the eye, which means it is safe to put in a wound. Saline has a low wetting capability (e.g., low surface active effects) and does not soften dry eschar and necrotic tissue to the extent that the new nonionic surfactant cleansers do. If enhanced cleansing capacity is required, the nonionic surfactant cleansers are the best alternative.

Nonionic Surfactants: Like saline, nonionic surfactants are not charged. The nonionic surfactants include a large chemical group of polymers, the majority of which carry enough reactivity to have deleterious effects on skin cell membranes.

A subgroup of the nonionic surfactants are called the Pluronic-Polyols. These polymers are comprised of a hydrophobic core made of oxypropylene, with hydrophilic ends made of oxyethylene groups. Provided the polymer contains at least 80% oxyethylene, it is totally biocompatible (not toxic to cell membranes). Pluronic F68, also called poloxamer 188, is a biocompatible Pluronic-Polyol, and is an ingredient of nonionic surfactant cleansers on the market. These products are biologically inert and nonsensitizing.

The pH and osmolality of these products approximates, or in some cases equals, physiologic pH (7.2 to 7.4) and physiologic osmolality (280 to 296 mOsm). This prevents damage to macrophages and delicate healing tissue. These products pass the Draize eye test meaning they are safe in the eye. They sustain a moist wound environment, and the wetting ability of the Pluronic-Polyols helps to soften eschar and necrotic tissue, which aids in loosening and debridement of the wound. These products may be used on open wounds, burns, mucosa, and periorbital areas. Examples of nonionic surfactant cleansers are *Shur-Clens, Ultra-Klenz*, and *SAF-Clens*.

CORTICOSTEROIDS

Hydrocortisone cream 0.5% (nonprescription strength) has proven anti-inflammatory and antipruritic activity for skin diseases, such as psoriasis and dermatitis. It may be effective in treating the inflammation and itch of insect bites and stings but not as effective for itch as astringents or local anesthetics. It should not be applied to open wounds. Corticosteroids suppress the immune response, mask infection, and can worsen an existing infection if used alone. When used chronically, medium to high potency topical corticosteroids have been associated with skin atrophy, but not hydrocortisone, which is a low potency corticosteroid.

DRESSINGS

Wound dressings today are designed to promote moist wound healing. Wound dressings can be passive or interactive.

Passive dressings protect the wound and provide a moist environment that promotes wound healing. Interactive dressings enhance wound healing by positively interacting with substances in the wound. Research is active in this area.

In choosing a wound dressing, the wound healing principles must be followed. There is no single dressing appropriate for each type of wound. Often there are several dressings in the same category that are equivalent, and choice depends on personal preference. To choose a dressing, the wound must be assessed and one must be aware of the available products. Dressings are chosen based on whether or not the wound requires gentle cleansing (clean proliferative wounds) or debridement (necrotic or infected wounds), whether or not dead space exists for which a light packing will be required, and the amount of exudate present, which determines the required absorptive capacity of the dressing. When choosing among dressings for a specific type of wound, cost and the frequency of dressing changes should be considered.

All dressings need to create a moist environment. A moist wound surface enhances epithelial migration needed for tissue repair. This does not mean a wound should be covered with copious wound drainage, which contains breakdown products of leukocytes and lysed bacteria. Dressings should provide the correct amount of absorptive capacity to remove excessive exudate without drying out the wound surface. They should also provide thermal insulation, protect the wound against trauma and create a barrier against bacterial invasion.

Infected wounds should not be covered with occlusive dressings. In the past, it was believed that occlusion of any wound promoted infection. Current research indicates that occlusive dressings actually decrease the risk of secondary infection when used on clean wounds. Occlusion does not interfere with wound healing as long as the wound edges are adequately oxygenated. Wounds obtain oxygen from tissue not from the air in the environment.

The primary dressing is the dressing against the wound. Some primary dressings require secondary dressings to provide protection and absorption of exudate. See Sidebar "Types of Dressings."

INSECT REPELLENTS

Diethyltoluamide (DEET): DEET is the most effective insect repellent, especially for ticks, mosquitoes and chiggers. It is also effective against gnats, biting flies, and fleas but does not repel wasps or bees. DEET is generally felt to be a safe skin repellent. However, it is lipid soluble and when applied to the skin, up to 50% of the dose is absorbed percutaneously. The majority of the absorbed amount is excreted in the urine within 24 hours. DEET is distributed to liver, muscle and fat and with repeated use can accumulate in fat and in the brain.

Adverse reactions to DEET include dermatitis, erythema and hemorrhagic blistering, allergic responses, and neurotoxicity. Children are at more risk than adults of developing toxic systemic reactions to DEET, most likely due to greater absorption secondary to a larger surface area to body weight ratio.

According to the U.S. Centres for Disease Control Report in 1989, at least 6 cases of toxic systemic reactions from repeated cutaneous application of DEET have been reported since 1961. Neurotoxic reactions occurred, including behavioral changes, ataxia, encephalopathy, seizures and coma. Of these cases, three children died, one of whom was deficient in the enzyme ornithine carbamoyltransferase. Toxic reactions have occurred with varying concentrations of DEET and after as few as three applications. Symptoms of neurotoxicity may be less severe in adults who are exposed to repeated use but have been reported to include confusion, irritability, and insomnia. However, it has been estimated that DEET is used by about 50 to 100 million persons each year, so serious systemic reactions are rare. An exact relationship between the dose of DEET and neurotoxicity has not been determined, although in the U.S., the New York State Department of Health is planning to do epidemiologic studies to evaluate the relationship.

To decrease the risk of systemic toxicity, repellents containing more than 50% DEET should not be used on children, although some clinicians are more stringent and feel it should be no more than 25% DEET. No more than 10 to 20% DEET should be used on infants (older than 6 months of age). No insect repellent should be used on an infant less than 6 months old.

Some clinicians believe that no more than 50 to 55% DEET should be used on adults although higher concentrations are available. The use of 100% DEET is unnecessary on adults because lower concentrations are effective. The lowest effective concentration should be used on adults.

DEET should be applied sparingly while covering all exposed areas since it has no spatial activity. Each application should be spread and rubbed in for approximately 10 to 15 seconds. Under normal conditions, one application should last 4 to 8 hours. However, with conditions causing increased evaporation or loss from the skin, more frequent application may be necessary. Minimizing the frequency of application will decrease the risk of systemic toxicity.

DEET in spray form may also be used as a clothing repellent in concentrations of greater than or equal to 20 to 30% and up to 100%. DEET should be sprayed on natural fabrics only as it will degrade synthetics, plastics, or painted surfaces.

Dimethyl phthalate (DMP): DMP is active against mosquitoes, flies, fleas, chiggers, and ticks, but is less effective than DEET. Adverse cutaneous reactions with DMP have not been reported.

Essential Oils: Before the development of the insect repellents used today (before World War II), many essential oils were used as skin repellents including clove oil, nutmeg oil, oil of wintergreen, pine oil, lavender oil, cedarwood oil, eucalyptus oil, lemongrass oil, peppermint oil and oil of citronella. Essential oils are relatively ineffective.

Oil of citronella was the most widely used agent for repelling insects in the early 1900's but is now known to be relatively ineffective. It is marketed as a repellent for mosquitoes and black flies. Oil of citronella may provide brief activity against mosquitoes. It should not be used for ticks because no information is available to support its use. Oil of citronella 10% is not recommended for use on infants and toddlers.

Avon's *Skin-So-Soft* Bath Oil: *Skin-So-Soft* is a concentrated bath oil that contains di-isopropyl adipate, mineral oil, isopropyl palmitate, and benzophenone-11 as a sunscreen. *Skin-So-Soft* is also available in cream form (with sunscreen) but only the oil has been claimed to be a repellent. One study found *Skin-So-Soft* bath oil effective against biting midges; however, its activity is by trapping the midges in the oily film and not by repelling them. DEET was found to be significantly more effective in this study. This product has been used as a mosquito repellent based on anecdotal reports, but no scientific studies have been done to support this use. In addition, the oil-trapping effect of *Skin-So-Soft* lasts only 10 to 30 minutes at best, so frequent application would be required. Toxicology information on repeated, widespread application is not available, so it should not be used on children for this purpose. It should not be used to repel ticks because no information is available.

Thiamine (vitamin B_1): Oral vitamin B_1 has been used as a mosquito repellent. No controlled scientific studies have been done to support this use, so it cannot be recommended as an effective insect repellent.

IPECAC

Ipecac is a root extract from the South American plants *Cephaelis ipecacuanha* and *Cephaelis acuminata*. Ipecac contains three alkaloids: cephaeline, emetine and psychotrine, which are responsible for its emetic action in decreasing order of potency.

After consultation with the Poison Information Centre or a physician, the use of syrup of ipecac may be advised to induce emesis to remove ingested poisons. The use of ipecac does not preclude the use of other emergency measures to treat poisonings. Its use may be advised as a preliminary measure prior to the delivery of the patient to a hospital. Ipecac should be given as soon as possible after the ingestion and within 1 hour of the ingestion. Ipecac induces emesis by stimulation of the chemoreceptor trigger zone in the brain and by direct irritation of the gastric mucosa. Ipecac is ineffective if the stomach is empty. Ipecac administration must be followed by water to provide volume for vomiting. Milk should not be given after ipecac because it decreases the irritant action of ipecac on the stomach. After oral administration vomiting will usually occur in 15 to 20 minutes. Two or three episodes of vomiting usually occur over a 30- to 60-minute period after a single dose. Twenty-eight to 60% of the ingested toxin will be removed through emesis if ipecac is given within 5 minutes after ingestion of the toxin. If given 1 hour after the ingestion, a maximum of only 30% of the toxin will be removed.

Ipecac should not be given to babies less than 6 months of age because of their poorly developed gag reflex and risk of aspiration. Also, some references suggest ipecac should only be given to children 6 to 9 months of age under medical observation.

Dose of Syrup of Ipecac

Note that ipecac fluid extract is not the same as syrup of ipecac. Ipecac fluid extract is 14 times more concentrated than the syrup.

Adults*: 30 mL followed by 1 to 2 glasses of water

Children 1 to 12 years of age*:
15 mL followed by 1 to 2 glasses of water

Children 6 to 12 months of age:
5 to 10 mL followed by water

* If vomiting has not occurred in 30 minutes, the dose may be repeated in children over 12 months of age and in adults.

Side Effects

The most serious but rare adverse effects reported from the use of ipecac include esophageal tears, pneumothorax, and gastrointestinal hemorrhage. Death has occurred from gastrointestinal hemorrhage but is very rare. Cardiotoxicity can occur with ipecac, but this is clinically not a problem when given in the doses recommended. Some references recommend that ipecac not be used in patients with cardiac disease. Cardiotoxicity and electrolyte imbalance have resulted from using higher than recommended doses and chronic ingestion such as misuse by bulimics for weight loss. The pharmacist should be alert for patients who are purchasing and misusing ipecac for weight loss.

Types of Dressings

Transparent Adhesive Dressings

These are intended for partial thickness wounds, or shallow, full thickness wounds with minimal exudate. These dressings protect, insulate and provide a moist wound surface. Transparent adhesive dressings are semipermeable membranes with a very small pore size. The centre of the dressing is nonadherent and the outer edges are adherent. They should not be used on wounds with friable surrounding skin, and there must be a border of dry intact skin surrounding the wound to which the dressing can adhere. The small pore size of these dressings allows oxygen and water exchange between the wound and the environment, and combined with the hydrophobic surface helps prevent bacterial invasion. Although the pore size allows water vapor to leave the wound, if there is excess wound exudate, it quickly creates a fluid environment. Transparent adhesive dressings are nonabsorptive. The retained moisture supports autolysis. However, these dressings are not intended for exudative wounds. They are intended for shallow wounds because they do not conform to deep wound spaces. The dressings are changed based on exudate accumulation and loss of seal. Examples: *OpSite, Tegaderm*

Hydrocolloid Dressings

These are used for noninfected, partial thickness wounds and shallow, full thickness wounds with minimal exudate. They provide protection against trauma and infection, insulation, a moist wound surface that supports autolysis, and some absorption.

Hydrocolloid dressings are adhesive wafers containing hydroactive particles with a repellent surface. Most are occlusive. Their surface is impermeable to bacteria and environmental contaminants helping prevent infections in clean wounds. These dressings should not be used on infected wounds, especially those at risk of anaerobic infection.

Types of Dressings (*cont'd*)

Some hydrocolloid dressings produce a gel that breaks down fibrin (fibrinolytic). The breakdown products are chemoattractants to endothelial cells, which enhance full thickness wound repair.

Because hydrocolloid dressings only provide moderate absorption, they should not be used on wounds with excessive exudate. They are not recommended for wounds with dry eschar either because the absorptive characteristics will keep the wound too dry and interfere with autolysis.

The edges of these dressings need to be secured with tape. The dressing is changed when there is excess exudate accumulation or if the edges loosen or wrinkle, usually every 3 to 5 days, but may be left on up to 1 week. Examples: *Duoderm, Comfeel Ulcus*

Absorptive Dressings

These dressings are intended for wounds with excess exudate and deep tissue loss, including deep full thickness wounds and wounds with dead tissue. They are designed to absorb large amounts of exudate, fill dead space, and protect the wound from trauma. Absorptive dressings interact with exudate to form a gelatinous mass that wicks moisture out of the wound but maintains a moist wound surface and supports autolysis. These dressings must be packed lightly into wounds because they swell as they absorb exudate. Absorptive dressings may be used alone but a secondary dressing is usually applied over top. Absorptive dressings must be changed once or twice a day by flushing the wound. These dressings do not protect against infection or insulate the wound.

Absorptive dressings include copolymer starch, dextranomer beads, and calcium alginate dressings. Gauze dressings are also absorptive dressings.

Copolymer starch dressings are moist and so can be used on wounds with minimal exudate without risk of drying out the wound. These dressings may be used for wounds with large exudate. Examples: *Comfeel Ulcus Paste and Powder, Duoderm Paste* and *Granules*.

Dextranomer bead dressings come in dry paste form and are only suitable for exudative wounds. Example: *Debrisan*.

Calcium alginate dressings are especially effective in bleeding wounds. The calcium in the dressing exchanges with the sodium in blood and initiates hemostasis. The lower the sodium content in the dressing, the greater the exchange. Examples: *Kaltostat, Algoderm*.

Gauze Dressings

Gauze dressings used to be the mainstay of dressings. Used as is, they create a dry environment. Since moist wound healing is now known to be superior to dry wound healing, dry gauze should be moistened prior to use and kept moist. Gauze may be effective in absorbing exudate and filling sinus tracts. If kept moist with solutions or gels, gauze dressings can also be used to debride wounds by enhancing autolysis. Gauze can also provide a medium for delivering topical substances to the wound, such as antibiotics. Gauze does not protect the wound from trauma or infection, nor insulate or keep the wound moist. Gauze dressings do not have high absorptive capacity and can trap drainage on a wound so need to be changed frequently. Gauze is available in standard sizes or ribbons for filling dead space. Gauze is applied directly against the wound surface. Fine mesh gauze is less likely to traumatize the wound than coarse mesh gauze. Hypertonic gauze may be applied dry to a highly exudative wound. The sodium in these hypertonic gauze dressings helps to draw out exudate. Examples: Plain gauze dressings, *MeSalt* (15% sodium chloride).

Hydrogel Dressings (Gel Dressings)

Gel dressings are designed to keep wounds moist and protect them from trauma. They are not occlusive. They are used to cover partial thickness wounds and to liquify necrotic tissue. Gel dressings contain a high content of water or glycerin and are available in sheet and granulate forms. Both forms enhance autolysis. Granulate gel dressings are used for packing full thickness wounds to fill dead space, and have some absorptive capacity for minimal to moderate exudate. Some gels contain sodium chloride. Gels containing 0.9% sodium chloride are isotonic with body fluids and are intended for use on granulating

Types of Dressings (*cont'd*)

wounds with minimal exudate. Gels containing high percentages of sodium chloride (e.g., 20%) are hypertonic and are intended for debriding exudative wounds. Granulate gels must be changed once or twice daily. Sheet gel dressings are used for partial thickness wounds and do not absorb exudate. The sheets must be cut to fit the size of the wound bed, so as not to cover and macerate surrounding intact skin because of their high percentage of water. Sheet gel dressings can usually be changed every two days, but more frequently if being used to debride a wound. Gel dressings require secondary dressings to insulate and provide a barrier to infection. Examples: *Intrasite Gel, Normal Gel (0.9% sodium chloride), Hypergel (20% sodium chloride)*

Emollient Dressings With and Without Active Ingredients

Emollient dressings include sprays, creams, ointments and liquid gels. Emollients are used to create a moist environment. Active ingredients may be added to the emollients to enhance wound repair. An example of an active ingredient is an antibiotic. Emollient dressings require secondary dressings for absorption of exudate, and to insulate and protect the wound against trauma and bacterial invasion. Examples: *moisturizers (many), barrier creams, e.g., zinc oxide ointment, silicone cream.*

Skin Sealants

Skin sealants are liquid sprays or gels used to create a barrier on intact skin. They usually contain alcohol, are used on healthy intact skin around a wound, never on a wound. Sealants dry to form a transparent seal that provides protection against maceration from wound exudate and irritation from tapes. Examples: *Skin Prep, Hollister Skin Gel*

RECOMMENDED READING

Bryant RA, ed. Acute and Chronic Wounds: Nursing Management. 1st ed. St Louis: Mosby-Year Book, 1992.

The Canadian Red Cross Society. First Aid: The Vital Link. 1st ed. St. Louis: Mosby-Year book, 1994.

Krasner D. Chronic Wound Care: A Clinical Source Book for Healthcare Professionals. King of Prussia, PA: Health Management Publications, 1990.

Rodeheaver G. Controversies in topical wound management. Wounds 1989;1(1):19–34.

11

FOOT CARE PRODUCTS

Betsy Miller

CONTENTS

Athlete's Foot	261
Symptoms	
Treatment	
Corns and Calluses	265
Symptoms	
Treatment	
Plantar Warts	268
Symptoms	
Treatment	
Ingrown Toenails	270
Treatment	
Bunions	271
Treatment	
Pharmaceutical Agents	272
Recommended Reading	274

ATHLETE'S FOOT

Tinea pedis is a specific term for foot infections caused by dermatophytes. It is often used interchangeably with athlete's foot, a more general term used to describe a variety of clinical conditions that present with similar signs and symptoms. The clinical spectrum of athlete's foot ranges from mild scaling and itching to a severe inflammatory process characterized by exudation, fissuring and denudation.

The most common cutaneous fungal infection found in humans, tinea pedis occurs in all parts of the world, but appears to be more prevalent in tropical and temperate climates. In seasonal climates such as Canada's, it seems to flare in the summer and be quiescent in the winter. Occlusive footwear, infrequent changes of shoes or socks, or other conditions that result in hyperhidrosis or maceration of the feet may predispose susceptible individuals to infection.

In some high-risk groups, infections may occur with greater frequency, tend to be more chronic and resistant to treatment and, in rare cases, spread and ultimately become life-threatening. These include the elderly in whom peripheral vascular disease is common, patients with debilitating diseases such as AIDS, patients with diabetes, patients receiving long-term treatment with broad spectrum antibiotics, corticosteroids, radiation or cytotoxic drugs, and immunocompromised patients.

Dermatophtyes (*Trichophyton rubrum, Epidermophyton floccosum* and *Trichophyton mentagrophytes*) initiate the infection by invading and disrupting the horny layer of the skin. Secondary infections may develop when a fissure created by the primary dermatophytic pathogen becomes superinfected by resident skin bacteria. These bacteria induce inflammation and maceration in the presence of a progressively damaged stratum corneum.

It is now recognized that organisms other than dermatophytes can cause athlete's foot. The more severe the clinical symptoms, the more likely yeasts are involved (including *Candida albicans* and other *Candida* species); other saprophytic fungi (including *Aspergillus* species); gram-positive bacteria (such as *Staphylocccus aureus*, and other *Staphylococcus* species); and gram-negative species (such as *Pseudomonas aeruginosa, Proteus mirabilis, Escherichia coli*, and *Enterobacter agglomerans)*.

SYMPTOMS

The term athlete's foot is often used to describe a variety of cutaneous conditions of the feet and toes. A differential diagnosis is important to establish the true etiology and eliminate noninfectious disease that may resemble dermatophytosis, such as contact dermatitis, pustular psoriasis and drug eruptions.

A presumptive diagnosis of dermatophytosis may be reached by reviewing the patient's history, particularly considering risk factors, and assessing the clinical symptoms as part of the initial evaluation of the patient. Clinically there are 4 morphologic variants of tinea pedis (Table 1).

TREATMENT

Nonpharmacological Treatment

In general, proper hygiene will help prevent infections in most individuals and help control them in high-risk groups. Individuals should be counselled to bathe daily and dry feet well between the toes; dust with foot powder, especially between the toes; wear absorbent socks, changed daily or twice daily if the patient is susceptible to hyperhidrosis; wear shoes that breathe (sandals, if possible); change shoes daily and wear different shoes for sports.

Pharmacological Treatment

Selection of drug therapy for athlete's foot depends on a number of factors including:

- the severity of the infection (e.g., intensity of inflammation, presence of vesicles or ulceration);
- duration of infection (e.g., days, weeks, months, years, recurrent);
- responsiveness to previous treatment;
- species of dermatophyte or bacteria;
- patient's age, environment, habits, medical condition and concurrent drug therapy;
- presence of bacterial superinfection;
- patient's preference;
- cost of therapy.

Before recommending nonprescription therapy, the patient should be asked about the following conditions:

- Is the toenail involved? If it is, topical treatment will likely be ineffective. The patient may require oral antifungal therapy. Consultation with a physician is recommended.
- Is there evidence of a secondary bacterial infection such as vesicular eruptions oozing

TABLE 1: Morphologic Variants of Tinea Pedis

Variant	Lesion Morphology	Typical Location	Special Considerations
Chronic interdigital infection	Fissures, scaling or maceration in the interdigital spaces	Very often, the infection is found on the lateral toe webs usually between the fourth and fifth or third and fourth toes. From this area, the infection often spreads to the instep or sole of the foot.	Humidity and warmth worsen this condition. Therefore, patients whose feet are prone to excessive sweating should be encouraged to treat their hyperhidrosis along with the fungal infection.
Mocassin-type infection	Chronic, papulosquamous pattern	Generally found on both feet, it is characterized by a mild inflammation and diffuse scaling on the soles of the feet. Often the toenails are affected (e.g., onychomycosis).	Involvement of the toenails perpetuates the infection such that the toenails must be treated with oral antifungal therapy or surgically removed before the tinea pedis can be successfully treated.
Vesicular	Small vesicles	Near the instep and on the midanterior plantar surface. Skin scaling is also observed in this area and on the toe webs.	Often caused by *T. mentagrophytes.* More prevalent in the summer.
Acute ulcerative disease	Macerated, denuded, weeping lesions	Sole of the foot	Very often, hyperkeratosis and a pungent odor are present. This infection may be complicated by an overgrowth of opportunistic, gram-negative bacteria such as *Proteus* or *Pseudomonas* and for this reason is often referred to as gram-negative athlete's foot or dermatophytosis complex.

purulent material? If so, antibiotic therapy may be appropriate.

- Is the space between the toes foul smelling, whitish, painful, soggy or characterized by erosions, oozing or severe inflammation? If yes, the patient should be referred to a physician.
- Is the foot eczematous with blisters and/or pyoderma (pus-forming)? If yes, refer to a physician.
- How old is the patient? If a child, the patient should be referred to a physician.
- Is the patient in a high risk group or under a physician's supervision for a chronic disease such as diabetes or asthma? If yes, refer to a physician before recommending nonprescription products.

If the infection is acute and superficial, nonprescription antifungal therapy may be safely recommended. Due to the complexity of most infections, treatments that suppress both fungi and bacteria are usually most effective.

While many products are available, not all have had to meet strict approval criteria. In an attempt to classify the various products, the U.S. Food and Drug Administration (FDA) has evaluated the safety and efficacy of nonprescription antifungal products. Although there are some differences between the products available in Canada and those available in the U.S., it is still worthwhile to consider this classification scheme (Table 2).

Miconazole nitrate and clotrimazole are the agents of choice for the treatment of athlete's foot. Both have antifungal activity and weak antibac-

ADVICE FOR THE PATIENT

Athlete's Foot

- Excessive foot sweating contributes to fungal conditions such as athlete's foot. The regular use of absorbent socks and nonocclusive shoes can help prevent the recurrence of athlete's foot.
- Talcum powder, cornstarch or medicated powders containing undecylenates, miconazole or tolnaftate can be used prophylactically. Powders should be dusted inside of regular and athletic shoes, between toes and inside socks.
- For active infection, the infected area should be washed with soap and water and dried thoroughly before application of the antifungal agent. Creams are generally preferred over ointments especially when the area is moist, macerated or oozing, but used sparingly to avoid maceration of the skin. Ointments are preferred when the infected area is dry and scaley.
- In general, antifungal agents should be applied sparingly twice a day. Improvement may not be seen for several days. Complete disappearance of signs and symptoms may require up to 4 full weeks of treatment. Continue application of the drug for about 2 weeks after the condition clears, to ensure the organisms are eradicated.
- If there is no improvement after 4 weeks, consult your physician.

TABLE 2: FDA Classification of Topical Antifungal Nonprescription Ingredients

Generally recognized as safe and effective[a]			
Clioquinol	Haloprogin	Povidone-iodine	Undecylenates
Clotrimazole	Miconazole nitrate	Tolnaftate	
Not generally recognized as safe and effective[b]			
Alcloxa	Camphor	Phenol	Sodium propionate
Alum, potassium	Candicidin	Phenolate sodium	Sulfur
Aluminum sulfate	Chlorothymol	Phenyl salicylate	Tannic acid
Amyltricresols, secondary	Coal tar	Propionic acid	Thymol
Basic fuchsin	Dichlorophen	Propylparaben	Tolindate
Benzethonium chloride	Menthol	Resorcinol	Triacetin
Benzoic acid	Methylparaben	Salicylic acid	Zinc caprylate
Benzoxiquine	Oxyquinoline	Sodium borate	Zinc propionate
Boric acid	Oxyquinoline sulfate	Sodium caprylate	

Reprinted from: (a) Federal Register (U.S.) 1989; 54:51136 and (b) Federal Register (U.S.) 1992; 57:38568.

terial activity against some gram-positive bacteria in vitro, against *C. albicans* and some saprophytic fungi. Anti-inflammatory effects have also been demonstrated.

Tolnaftate is a commonly used nonprescription topical therapy for athlete's foot. It is available as a powder, which may be useful in prophylaxis, or as a solution or cream. While a popular treatment for athlete's foot, its spectrum of activity is limited to dermatophytes, and the recurrence rate is high.

Naftifine is an allylamine antifungal agent available as a 1% cream and 1% gel. It is indicated for dermatophyte infections and has no antibacterial activity. The mechanism of action, while not completely understood, is believed to be somewhat distinct from that of other classes of antifungal agents. It inhibits squalene epoxidase and may have certain anti-inflammatory properties. Naftifine has potent fungistatic and fungicidal activity and good local tolerability. Its novel mechanism of action and effectiveness makes it a useful option in patients with dermatomycoses.

Topical clioquinol, which is bacteriostatic, can also be used for treating fungal infections. Patients should be warned that it can stain fabrics. No studies to determine whether it possesses any anti-inflammatory activity have been done.

Undecylenic acid and its salts have been widely used for the treatment of tinea pedis. This fatty acid has antifungal activity and is reported comparable in efficacy to tolnaftate. Some formulations are available as a zinc salt. The zinc acts as an astringent, which may decrease irritation and inflammation.

Other agents include acids such as salicylic acid with keratolytic action that may facilitate the penetration of antifungal drugs into infected tissues, and drying agents, such as aluminum chloride and aluminum acetate.

CORNS AND CALLUSES

Corns and calluses are common lesions of the feet that develop from prolonged rubbing or frictional pressure that produces a marked thickening of the stratum corneum.

SYMPTOMS

A callus is a diffuse thickening of the skin that may be broad based or have a central core with sharply circumscribed margins. It has definite borders and can range from a few millimetres to several centimetres in diameter. It often appears as an elevated, slightly yellowish lesion and has a normal pattern of skin ridges on its surface. Calluses form on top of joints and on weight-bearing areas, commonly appearing over the metatarsal heads (on the sole), the dorsal aspect of the toes and on the heel.

Calluses often develop as protection against prolonged rubbing, friction or pressure. The most common cause is poorly-fitting shoes. Calluses may also develop in individuals with structural abnormalities that result in improper weight distribution, or in those with biomechanical abnormalities.

A corn (also known as a clavus) is a small, slightly raised, well-defined hyperkeratotic lesion having a central core. It is yellow-grey and ranges from a few millimetres to a centimetre or more in diameter. Triangular in shape with its base on the skin surface, its inward point or apex exerts pressure on the deeper layers of the skin, pressing on nerve endings in the dermis and causing considerable discomfort.

Hard corns are an accumulation of several layers of epidermis over a bony prominence. Typically, they develop on the lateral side of the fifth toe or on the dorsum of the toes where there is no moisture. They appear shiny and polished.

Soft corns are essentially the same lesion as hard corns, but occur between the toes, where the moisture that is always present causes maceration. Soft corns appear as a whitish thickening of the skin and are often mistaken for fungal infections. However, a lesion over nonweight-bearing bony prominences or joints, such as metatarsal heads, the bulb of the great toe, the dorsum of the fifth toe, or the tips of the middle toes, is usually a corn.

Corns are often present but go unnoticed until pain develops. Pressure from ill-fitting shoes is the most frequent cause of pain, which may be severe and sharp (when downward pressure is applied) or dull and discomforting.

Calluses, like corns, are usually asymptomatic, causing pain only when pressure is applied. Individuals who complain of calluses on the sole often compare the discomfort to that of walking with a pebble in the shoe.

ADVICE FOR THE PATIENT

Corns and Calluses

- Always read and follow the instructions on the label of the specific product.
- Soak the affected area in warm water for 10 to 15 minutes to soften the skin. Pat dry.
- If a solution is used, cut a hole in a bandage, apply it to the area so only the lesion appears through the hole, then drop on the solution. Apply 1 drop at a time and allow it to dry or harden. Repeat this procedure until the area is covered. If the solution touches healthy skin, wash it off immediately.
- If a patch is used, trim it to the shape of the corn or callus.
- If a paste is used, apply enough to cover the lesion.
- Cover the lesion with occlusive adhesive tape.
- After 12 to 24 hours, remove the bandage and soak the area in warm water for 10 to 15 minutes.
- Gently remove the soft white tissue by rubbing with a rough towel, pumice stone or callus file, taking care not to rub the adjacent areas.
- Repeat the entire procedure until the corn or callus disappears.
- The condition usually resolves in 10 days. Adhering to the treatment regimen is critical to a successful outcome. Selecting a convenient time for treatment (at bedtime, first thing in the morning or both) may be helpful.
- Do not attempt to hasten the process by using sharp knives or razor blades to cut dead tissue, which may result in infection.

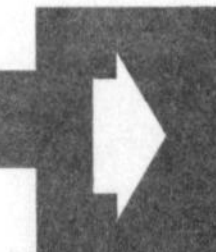

ADVICE FOR THE PATIENT

Proper Footwear

- Select a shoe that is wide enough at the front to allow the toes to extend fully with air circulation between them. Round-toed shoes are obviously a better choice than pointed-toed shoes.
- Avoid shoes with high heels that thrust the front of the foot into the toe of the shoe.
- Be aware that lace-up shoes prevent the front of the foot from pushing into the end of the shoes, which tends to occur with slip-ons.
- Fit shoes with an extra 1.25 cm in length to prevent the toes from banging into the shoe.
- The thicker the sole, the more cushioning the shoe provides. As well, the greater thickness allows some degree of moulding to the shape of the foot.

TREATMENT

Before recommending a treatment, the health care professional must obtain information from the patient about the condition, previous treatments, other medical conditions and current drug therapy. Patients with a history of diabetes mellitus, peripheral vascular disease or serious dermatologic disease should be strongly discouraged from self-treating calluses or corns and referred to a physician or podiatrist.

Nonpharmacological Treatment

Successful treatment of corns and calluses with nonprescription products eliminates the causes: pressure or friction. Advise patients to wear well-fitting, flexible footwear and seek the advice of a physician or podiatrist to correct anatomical foot deformities such as hammertoes, bony spurs and flat feet. In many cases, a change in footwear or correction of the abnormality resolves the corn or callus.

A variety of protective pads made of moleskin, felt and latex foam are available for use in corn and callus prevention and treatment. The pads are made to accommodate the different types, sizes and locations of lesions (aperture pads to circle and protect a specific area, crescent pads to protect around and behind an area, and metatarsal cushions). Moleskin and lambswool sheets are available to construct a pad.

When properly placed, the pad reduces friction and pressure to the irritated area, relieving pain and possibly reducing new lesion formation. Polymer gel cushions have been recently introduced to relieve pain from pressure on the corn or callus. While temporarily beneficial, pads do not treat the cause and should not be recommended for continuous use.

To protect the area from pressure, pads should be made from material as thick as the area to be protected. For example, if protecting a corn, the pad should not be placed over the lesion, but trimmed to surround the area and cushion it from pressure. Pads to reduce friction should be cut to fit the area and placed over it. Padding material with adhesive backing should not be applied over blistered or broken skin. Inserting lambswool in the web spaces may be useful therapy for soft corns, as it separates the toes and decreases friction.

Commercial arch supports intended to support the foot in the ideal natural position may prevent problems from improper weight distribution. These supports are available in standard sizes but may not be suitable for every foot or foot condition. Those made of sponge rubber and other flexible materials adapt freely to the foot and are of limited benefit. More structured and elaborate arch supports are in different widths and sizes, but must be adjusted to ensure maximum benefit. The most effective arch supports are custom fitted to the contours of the foot.

Pharmacological Treatment

Salicylic acid, available in preparations ranging from 10 to 40%, is the only effective agent for corns and calluses. Product selection depends on consumer preference and the condition. No one product has been shown more effective than another in clinical studies. Because of its keratolytic effect, salicylic acid must be applied to the affected area only. It is very important to instruct patients to avoid contact with normal skin. Discourage the use of salicylic acid products in individuals with diabetes mellitus, peripheral vascular disease or serious dermatological conditions.

Soft corns are best treated with products containing low concentrations of salicylic acid (12% as opposed to 40%). Hard corns and calluses are most easily treated with plasters that are generally easier to apply than pastes or collodion products. Plasters and patches are both occlusive and adherent and provide prolonged contact of the drug with the lesion.

Collodion dosage forms are also adherent and occlusive. However, their application requires considerable care to avoid spilling the preparation onto surrounding tissues. Elderly patients and those who are shakey or have poor eyesight probably should avoid these products. Collodions are more useful for treating corns than calluses.

Pastes are the least adherent and occlusive of the three dosage forms available.

Testing for Proper Shoe Size

- With the foot outside the shoe, place the heel of the foot into the heel of the shoe allowing the toes to rest on top of the shoe.
- Notice the overlap of the toes at the front of the shoe; if the overlap is significant, the toes will have to be crammed together.
- Always ensure that the shoe can contain your feet without cramming the toe.

PLANTAR WARTS

The human papilloma virus (HPV) (there are 15 different types) is the cause of all human wart conditions. Type 1 HPV is responsible for solitary plantar warts and type 2 for mosaic plantar warts. Type 1 plantar warts usually appear as deep, painful, solitary growths with a thick overlying epidermal cap. Mosaic warts are much less painful and usually present long before treatment is sought. The cores of these lesions are closely grouped into clusters and may coalesce.

Found on the plantar surface of the foot, these warts occur in about 1 to 2% of the population, but are less frequent than common warts. Peak rates of infection are found in adolescents: some estimates are as high as 25%. Environments such as boarding schools, public pools and the military, where adolescents or young adults live together and bathe in common areas have the highest rates.

The natural history of warts is to resolve spontaneously: 20 to 30% resolution in 6 months and 65% in 2 years. The mechanism is not completely understood. Plantar warts may spread by direct person-to-person contact or by autoinoculation to another body area. Indirectly, the virus spreads through contact with swimming pool or shower floors or other contaminated surfaces. It has been suggested that swimming, especially in warm water with a pH greater than 5, alters the horny skin layer cells on the sole of the foot making the foot more susceptible to infection. The rough surface of pool floors and diving boards abrades tissue and further increases the risk of infection. Since virus particles are contained in the horny layer of the skin, spread of the virus, especially in the heavy traffic areas around the pool, is a particular problem. The incubation period averages between 3 to 4 months, but can be as short as 1 month or as long as 20 months.

ADVICE FOR THE PATIENT

Warts

Since warts are infectious, always:

- Use a clean towel not used by others.
- Use a personal bath mat.
- Avoid walking barefoot (in the doctor's office, public showers, swimming pools and marinas).
- Use a light inner sole material in shoes during treatment and wipe the old sole with alcohol.
- Keep the feet as dry as possible — use chemical drying agents and wear cotton socks.
- If warts recur or persist following treatment for 12 to 14 weeks, the patient should be referred to a physician or podiatrist.

SYMPTOMS

Plantar warts are often very painful. The presenting symptom is usually pain. More than 85% occur over bony prominences, probably the areas of the feet most likely to have small skin breaks. As with calluses, pressure stimulates the growth of the plantar wart resulting in deep involvement in the affected area. In general, pain is proportional to the degree of hyperkeratosis.

Single lesions are thick, hyperkeratotic, with encircling skin ridges. After scraping the lesion, there are multiple capillary tips rising perpendicular to the surface. If the vessels in the capillary tip are thrombosed, they will appear black and are commonly called the "seeds" of the wart. When shaved deeply, the tips will bleed.

While the differential diagnosis encompasses a variety of dermatologic conditions, the most common dilemma is between a keratoma, a callus and a wart. A keratoma may appear as a round homogeneous yellow growth that is difficult to distinguish from a wart without paring. Once scraped, the keratoma has a more diffused border and the skin ridges usually go over rather than around the lesion. Calluses may look similar to a keratoma, but are insensitive to pinprick and semitranslucent, especially when wiped with an alcohol swab. The presence of multiple small black seeds that bleed following scraping of the surface distinguishes plantar warts. Calluses have normal appearing and continuous skin ridge patterns, but papillary lines around a plantar wart are divergent.

TREATMENT

Though natural regression occurs with plantar warts, most practitioners agree that, because of their contagious nature, as the old ones regress, new ones develop.

The ideal treatment should be safe, effective, painless, inexpensive, easily applied, and allow ambulation. It also depends on the age of the patient, the location, depth, size, number, pain and accessibility of the wart. Self-treatment of plantar warts is appropriate if there is no pain.

While products containing podophyllum and cantharidin are available for the treatment of warts in Canada, salicylic acid is the most commonly used nonprescription agent and the only agent recognized as safe and effective by the U.S. FDA Advisory Panel. Lactic acid is often added to the salicylic acid to lower the pH and enhance its action.

In general, nightly application of the selected product is required until all warty tissue is removed. Early discontinuation may result in recurrence of the wart. The rate of involution for warts that are going to resolve has been determined as follows: 30% involute by the end of the first week of treatment, 25% the second week, 25% the third and fourth weeks, and an additional 20% by the end of 2 months. Twelve weeks is usually a reasonable time for a cure if one is going to result.

In a double-blind trial to assess efficacy of treatments for plantar warts, researchers found cure rates of 84% for a 17% salicylic acid collodion preparation, 81% for a 50% podophyllin resin preparation and 66% for a control treatment (collodion) in solitary plantar warts. Overall treatment for mosaic warts was less favorable (58% cure rate compared to 75% for solitary plantar warts). The salicylic acid preparation resulted in the fastest cures. The cure rate for children was higher than for adults. No cases of hypersensitivity or toxicity were reported.

Mosaic warts are particularly resistant to treatment. Because they often cover a large area and care should be taken to avoid scarring, treatment must be somewhat moderate. Rotating the use of different mild products is probably the best approach.

INGROWN TOENAILS

An ingrown toenail occurs when the nail of the toe (most often the big toe) curves under at the sides of the nail so that it grows into the skin. The two most frequent causes are improper cutting of the nails and the wearing of tight shoes. If the nails are cut on a curve with the sides tapered downwards, the nail edges can grow into the skin. Often, a spike of the nail becomes embedded in the soft tissue of the nail bed.

Most ingrown nails do not cause discomfort. However, patients may complain of pain if pressure is applied to the nail or tight shoes are worn. (Toe caps and lambswool padding can be used to reduce the pressure on the affected toe.) In some cases, there is secondary swelling, inflammation and ulceration.

TREATMENT

Proper trimming of nails is probably the best way to prevent ingrown toenails (Figure 1). Nails should be cut straight across so the nail edge slopes down at the centre, not at the corners of the nail. After every shower or bath, patients should use the pads of both thumbs to stretch the skin folds away from the base of the nail.

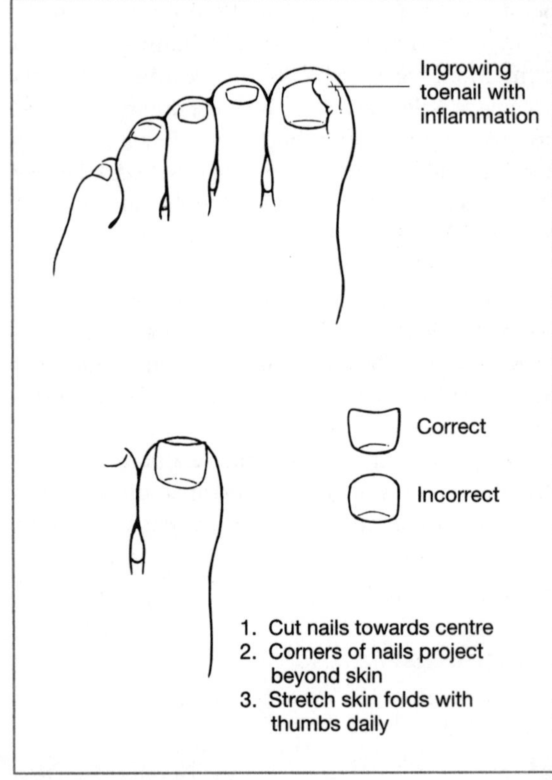

FIGURE 1: Trimming of Ingrown Toenails.

A number of nonprescription products are available to treat ingrown toenails. They contain either sodium sulfide or tannic acid. Sodium sulfide is thought to soften the keratin of the nail and the calloused skin surrounding the nail, relieving the pain and pressure caused by the embedded nail. Tannic acid is thought to harden the skin surrounding the embedded nail and shrink the soft tissue adjacent to it, allowing the nail to resume its normal position. Insufficient clinical data exist to make a definitive statement on the actual effectiveness of these products.

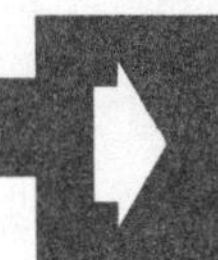

ADVICE FOR THE PATIENT

Ingrown Toenails

- Cleanse affected toes thoroughly.
- Place a small piece of cotton in the nail groove (the side of the nail where the pain is) and wet cotton thoroughly with the solution.
- Repeat several times daily until nail discomfort is relieved, but do not use longer than 7 days.
- Daily foot soaks in warm water may provide some comfort.
- Nonprescription analgesics such as ASA or ibuprofen may relieve the pain and inflammation.
- If there is no improvement after 7 days, see a physician or podiatrist.

BUNIONS

It has long been known that bone can change shape to accommodate the specific needs of the body. Changes in bone structure occur in response to fluctuations in body weight, muscle mass, activity and compensational biomechanics. A good example is the formation of hallux valgus deformities, which develop into a bunion as the surrounding soft tissue becomes inflamed and swells.

The structure of the foot, particularly the inner side and the great toe (also known as the hallux), is essential to the mobility and flexibility required to walk or run. To maintain this mobility and elasticity, certain anatomical disorders are known to occur. Hallux valgus is characterized by a deviation of the great toe toward the outer side of the foot that may result in pressure over the angulation of the metatarsophalangeal joint of the big toe, causing inflammatory swelling of the bursa and a bunion to form.

Bunions are 10 times more common in women than men. Tight-fitting footwear over time is likely a contributing factor. In some cases, there is a congenital predisposition.

TREATMENT

Treatment of bunions depends on the level of discomfort. Usually asymptomatic, bunions that become painful, swollen and tender can limit function and activities.

ADVICE FOR THE PATIENT

Bunions

When using a topical adhesive cushion for a bunion:

- Bathe and dry the foot thoroughly.
- Cut the pad to a shape that conforms to the bunion. To relieve pressure on the bunion, cut it to encircle the bunion (like a donut).
- Avoid constant skin contact with the adhesive-backed pads.
- Do not use pads on blistered or broken skin.
- If the bunion is severe and the padding thick, larger footwear may be necessary.
- If the condition persists, see a physician or podiatrist.

Bunions should not be treated with topical drug therapy, nor should the routine use of nonprescription analgesics be encouraged. The patient should attempt to correct the condition by wearing shoes that allow plenty of room between the forefoot and the inner lining of the front of the shoe. Sandals and athletic shoes that are soft around the toe box are good choices. Bunion guards or topical padding such as moleskin can reduce irritation.

PHARMACEUTICAL AGENTS

Aluminum Salts: Aluminum chloride solutions and aluminum acetate solutions are useful in treating athlete's foot, especially when combined with other topical antifungal drugs. Historically, these products have been used for both the acute, inflammatory state and the wet, soggy type of tinea pedis.

The action and efficacy of aluminum salts is twofold. First, as astringents, they act as drying agents by combining with proteins and altering their ability to absorb water. These agents decrease edema, exudation and inflammation by reducing cell membrane permeability. Second, as antibacterials, aluminum salt solutions (when used in concentrations greater than 20%) directly kill bacteria.

Patients should be instructed to use the appropriate concentration of solution. Aluminum acetate is usually diluted with about 10 to 40 parts water and aluminum chloride is most beneficial in concentrations of 20 to 30%. The foot should be immersed in the solution for 20 minutes up to 3 times a day or the solution applied to the affected area only by using a wet dressing. Prolonged or continuous use may result in necrosis.

Aluminum salts penetrate skin poorly; therefore, their toxicity is minimal. However, deep fissures may be irritated, and the salts may need to be diluted to lower concentrations for initial treatment.

Clioquinol: Clioquinol, previously known as iodochlorhydroxyquin, is effective when used topically for athlete's foot. It has a low level of antibacterial activity. A thin layer of cream or ointment should be applied to the affected area 2 to 3 times a day. Clioquinol has a low incidence of side effects, but may cause itching, redness and irritation. Users should be cautioned that it can stain fabrics. It may also interfere with thyroid function tests.

Clotrimazole: Clotrimazole is an imidazole derivative that has antifungal, antibacterial and anti-inflammatory activity. It acts by inhibiting the biosynthesis of ergosterol and other steroids, and by damaging the fungal cell wall membrane, altering its permeability. It is available as a cream and as a solution. For successful treatment, the cream or solution should be applied regularly (e.g., twice daily) and in sufficient quantities. Adverse reactions have rarely been reported, although cases of mild skin irritation, burning and stinging have occurred.

Miconazole: Miconazole is an imidazole derivative with antifungal, antibacterial and anti-inflammatory activity. It acts against *Candida albicans* and some saprophytic fungi in vitro. It should be used twice daily, once in the morning and once in the evening. Adverse reactions have been reported infrequently and are similar in nature to those reported with clotrimazole.

Naftifine: Naftifine is an allylamine antifungal for topical treatment. In vitro, naftifine has potent fungistatic and fungicidal activity against dermatophytes. Clinical trials have demonstrated improvement in clinical symptoms and overall therapeutic success after a 2- to 5-week course of therapy in a high percentage of patients. Patients should be advised to continue using naftifine for the full treatment period even though symptoms may have subsided and to avoid the use of bandages or wrappings over the affected area.

Salicylic Acid: Salicylic acid is one of the oldest and most commonly used keratolytic agents, available in many strengths (up to 45%) depending on its intended use. It is thought to act on hyperplastic keratin in 2 ways: to reduce keratinocyte adhesion and increase water binding, which results in keratin hydration that causes swelling, softening, maceration and finally desquamation of the stratum corneum. Effectiveness is thought to be enhanced by the presence of moisture and it may be beneficial to soak the affected area in a warm water bath for 5 minutes before applying salicylic acid.

As a corn and callus remover, salicylic acid may be used in strengths of 12 to 40% in a plaster vehicle, or 12 to 17.6% in a collodion-like vehicle. As a wart remover, it may be used in strengths of 17 to 26% in a polyacrylic vehicle, 5 to 17% in a collodion-like vehicle, 17 to 27% in a gel, or 15% in a karaya gum, glycol plaster vehicle.

Patients should be instructed to thoroughly wash and dry the affected area before applying the product. For corns and calluses, the solution is applied once or twice daily as necessary for up to 2 weeks or until the corn or callus is removed. For warts, it should be applied once or twice daily for up to 12 weeks, or until the wart is removed.

To enhance patient compliance, salicylic acid may be delivered to the affected area through a plaster disc or pad, providing direct and continuous contact with the drug. A salicylic acid plaster is a homogeneous solid or semisolid mixture of salicylic acid in an appropriate base, spread on a suitable backing material such as felt, moleskin, cotton or plastic and applied directly to the skin. Alternatively, corn or callus pads that contain small salicylic acid discs can be used. In this case, the patient determines the appropriately sized disc, places it on the skin and covers it with a pad. Application can be simplified with all-in-one products that contain a medicated adhesive pad and a bandage.

For corns and calluses, the plasters or discs are applied and removed within 48 hours with a maximum of 5 treatments over a 14-day period. For warts, the plasters or discs are applied and removed within 48 hours with a maximum treatment period of 12 weeks.

In the past, to prevent absorption of salicylic acid, it was recommended that a film of white petrolatum be applied to the healthy skin surrounding the affected area before applying the salicylic acid product. It is now felt that it is highly unlikely that salicylism will result during corn, callus or wart therapy, and this practice has been largely discarded.

Tolnaftate: Tolnaftate is a commonly used nonprescription antifungal. Despite its popularity, its spectrum of activity is limited to dermatophytes including *T. mentagrophytes* and *T. rubrum* as well as *E. floccosum* and species of *Microsporum*. It works by inhibiting the growth of hyphae, stunting the mycelial growth of the fungi species.

Tolnaftate is available in a variety of formulations including a 1% solution, cream, powder, aerosol powder and 0.072% aerosol liquid. It should be applied sparingly twice daily following cleansing and drying of the affected area. Treatment generally takes 2 to 4 weeks, although some cases may require longer (4 to 6 weeks). The cream formulation should be thoroughly but gently rubbed into the skin. The solution should also be rubbed in well and allowed to dry.

If tolnaftate is used in areas where the skin is thicker than normal (e.g., pressure areas of the foot), concomitant use of a keratolytic agent may be beneficial. Neither keratolytic agents nor wet compresses (e.g., aluminum acetate solution) interfere with the efficacy of tolnaftate. Nevertheless, not all cases of tinea pedis respond to treatment with tolnaftate and the recurrence rate is high. This may be due in part to a bacterial component of the infection. Tolnaftate powder with its cornstarch-talc base is a delivery vehicle for antifungal agents and absorbs moisture, reducing skin maceration. Tolnaftate is most successful in the dry, scaly type of athlete's foot. It is well tolerated with few cases of irritation and hypersensitivity reported.

Undecylenic Acid, Zinc Undecylenate: Undecylenic acid and its salts have been widely used for the treatment of mild superficial fungal infections. It is fungistatic and in mild chronic cases of tinea pedis reported to have comparable efficacy to tolnaftate. It is available as a liquid (10% undecylenic acid) and as an ointment or powder (varying concentrations of undecylenic acid and zinc undecylenate). Zinc undecylenate is thought to liberate undecylenic acid (the active antifungal) on contact with moisture (e.g., perspiration). The zinc component has astringent properties and acts to reduce irritation and inflammation.

The product is applied twice daily following cleansing and drying of the affected area. The treatment period is dependent on the severity of the infection, but if improvement is not apparent after 2 to 4 weeks, the condition should be reassessed and an alternative medication used.

Undecylenic acid preparations are generally nonirritating and sensitization is rarely reported. However, the undiluted solution may cause a transient stinging when applied to broken skin. One drawback to these products is the objectionable odor of the acid, which should not be overlooked when considering patient compliance.

RECOMMENDED READING

Abramson C, McCarthy DJ. Athlete's foot infections. In: Abramson C, McCarthy DJ, Rupp MI, eds. Infectious Diseases of the Lower Extremity. Baltimore: Williams & Wilkins,1991.

Campbell BJ. The treatment of warts. Prim Care 1986;13(3):465-76.

Glover MG. Plantar warts. Foot & Ankle 1990; 11(3):172-78.

Iseli A. The management of ingrown toenails. Aust Fam Physician 1990;19(9):1414-19.

Page JC, Abramson C, Lee WL, et al. Diagnosis and treatment of tinea pedis. A review and update. J Am Podiatr Med Assoc 1991;81(6):304-16.

Richards RN. Calluses, corns and shoes. Semin Dermatol 1991;10(2):112-14.

Silfverskiold JP. Common foot problems. Relieving the pain of bunions, keratoses, corns and calluses. Postgrad Med 1991;89(5):183-88.

12

GASTROINTESTINAL PRODUCTS

PATRICK S. FARMER

CONTENTS

Dyspepsia 275
- Etiology and Physiology
- Symptoms
- Treatment

Gastroesophageal Reflux 282
- Physiology and Pathophysiology
- Etiology
- Symptoms
- Treatment

Gastrointestinal Gas 286
- Etiology and Pathophysiology
- Symptoms
- Treatment

Infantile Colic 289
- Etiology
- Symptoms
- Treatment

Constipation 291
- Anatomy and Physiology
- Etiology
- Symptoms
- Treatment

Diarrhea 297
- Etiology
- Diarrhea in Infants
- Acute Diarrhea in Older Individuals
- Diarrhea during Pregnancy
- Travellers' Diarrhea

Irritable Bowel Syndrome 303
- Etiology
- Symptoms
- Treatment

Nausea and Vomiting 306
- Anatomy and Physiology
- Etiology
- Treatment

Pharmaceutical Agents 310
- Alginic Acid
- Alpha-Galactosidase
- Antacids
- Anticholinergic Agents
- Antidiarrheals
- Antiemetics
- Gripe Water
- Histamine H_2-Receptor Antagonists
- Lactase
- Laxatives
- Oral Rehydration Therapy Solutions
- Simethicone

Recommended Reading 324

DYSPEPSIA

ETIOLOGY AND PHYSIOLOGY

Dyspepsia is defined as episodic or persistent abdominal symptoms, often related to eating, thought to be due to disorders of the proximal portion of the digestive tract. A common complaint, dyspepsia affects up to 40% of the Western population at least occasionally. Patients may describe it variously as heartburn, acid indigestion, sour stomach, or stomach ache.

Dyspepsia may be a sign of an underlying medical condition (Table 1). In a prospective study of 1,540 dyspeptic patients, the most common principal diagnoses were duodenal ulcer (26%), functional dyspepsia (23%), and irritable bowel syndrome (IBS) (15%). Another study found gastroesophageal reflux (GER) disease (24%) to be the most common endoscopically observed cause of upper gastrointestinal tract symptoms; peptic ulcer disease (PUD) and gastroduodenal inflammation were each 20%, and cancer 2%. Functional dyspepsia, with normal endoscopic findings, accounted for the remaining 34%. Although the symptoms of functional dyspepsia may mimic those of PUD or GER disease, the pathophysiology of these disorders is completely different. Duodenal PUD, representing 80% of all PUD, affects 10% of all adults sometime during their lifetime.

The stomach serves as a receptacle in which food undergoes early stages of digestion. The gastric mucosa is adapted to a highly acidic environment. In young adults, normal gastric pH varies typically from 2.0 ± 1.6 (mean fasting) to 3.4 ± 1.8 (postprandial). Hydrochloric acid is secreted by the parietal cells of the fundus of the stomach (Figures 1 and 2). Pepsinogen is released by the chief cells. Reaction of hydrochloric acid with pepsinogen in the lumen of the stomach causes the active proteolytic enzyme pepsin to be released from the pepsinogen structure. A layer of mucus secreted by the mucosal epithelial cells protects the lining of the stomach from autodigestion by pepsin. Prostaglandins E_1 and E_2 stimulate the secretion of mucus and of bicarbonate under the mucus. Disruption of the mucus layer by various factors can result in gastritis or ulceration.

The principal cause of gastritis, duodenitis and duodenal PUD is almost certainly *Helicobacter pylori*, a species of bacteria that resides in the stomachs of approximately 30 to 40% of the adult Western population. The mucosal damage induced by *H. pylori* is perhaps mediated by a reduction in somatostatin activity and a concomitant increase in gastrin secretion and subsequent acid secretion. *H. pylori* isolates have been identified in the stomachs of almost all individuals with chronic active gastritis and 90% of duodenal and 70% of gastric PUD patients. Eradication of *H. pylori* leads to ulcer healing in most individuals, and lesions do not recur unless reinfection occurs. Why more persons infected with *H. pylori* do not develop PUD or upper gastrointestinal inflammation is not known.

Pyloric dysfunction allowing bile to reflux into the stomach has also been associated with gastric PUD. Bile acids exert a detergent effect that can disrupt the protective mucus layer as well as alter the epithelial cells, allowing acid to diffuse back into the cells. Whether this pyloric dysfunction precedes the ulceration or follows it is not known. Its relationship to *H. pylori* infection is not known.

Between 30 and 40% of all gastric ulcers and 15% of duodenal ulcers are induced by ASA and other nonsteroidal anti-inflammatory drugs (NSAIDs). These drugs inhibit the production of prostaglandins, as well as having a direct erosive action on the stomach wall. Use of enteric coated products reduces the incidence of gastric mucosal damage but does not eliminate it. *H. pylori* infection and NSAID use are both associated with an increased risk of peptic ulceration and gastropathy. Furthermore, *H. pylori* exacerbates dyspeptic symptoms in patients receiving NSAIDs. However, *H. pylori* infection has not been shown to potentiate NSAID gastropathy.

Many drugs besides NSAIDs can cause epigastric distress, with or without nausea and without

TABLE 1: Conditions Frequently Associated with Dyspepsia

Structural Diseases of the Gastrointestinal Tract
Cholelithiasis
Chronic pancreatitis
Esophagitis
Gastritis and duodenitis
Gastric and duodenal ulcers
Gastric cancer
Colorectal cancer
Pancreatic cancer
Other intra-abdominal malignancies
Malabsorption syndromes

Structural Disease Involving Other Systems
Ischemic heart disease
Collagen disease

Metabolic Conditions
Diabetes mellitus
Hyper- or hypo(para)thyroidism
Electrolyte disorders

Drugs
Alcohol
NSAIDs
Digitalis
Theophylline
Ampicillin
Erythromycin
Iron supplements
Potassium supplements

detectable mucosal damage. Theophylline, digitalis, ampicillin, erythromycin, other antibiotics, potassium and iron supplements and alcohol are among the most common causes of drug-induced dyspepsia. Alcohol abuse is a risk factor for the development of acute hemorrhagic gastritis.

Cigarette smoking markedly increases the risk of developing PUD, with the heaviest smokers having the greatest risk. Smoking also retards ulcer healing and increases the likelihood of relapse of healed ulcers. Nicotine relaxes the pyloric sphincter, stimulates gastric acid secretion, and inhibits tissue prostaglandins. There is no association between smoking or alcohol consumption and prevalence of *H. pylori* infection, although one recent study by Witteman, Hopman, et al found smoking increased *H. pylori* resistance to metronidazole therapy.

Functional dyspepsia is defined as dyspepsia for which no cause can be found after reasonable investigation has ruled out structural or metabolic disease. While gastritis, duodenal ulcer and gastric cancer are almost certainly causally related to *H. pylori* infection, evidence relating functional dyspepsia to *H. pylori* is less convincing. Nor is functional dyspepsia associated with smoking, alcohol or NSAIDs. Dyspeptic symptoms in many, but not all patients, are associated with disordered gastric motility and emptying. Psychological stress is probably an etiologic factor.

SYMPTOMS

Dyspeptic symptoms are characterized by upper abdominal pain or discomfort, perhaps with anorexia, belching, heartburn and regurgitation, nausea and vomiting. Patients may complain of postprandial fullness and even early satiety or inability to finish a normal meal. Postprandial drowsiness and headache may accompany the gastrointestinal symptoms. In contrast to irritable bowel syndrome (IBS), bowel function of dyspeptic patients usually is normal. Vomiting and retching are much more frequent in alcohol-related dyspepsia than in dyspepsia from other causes. Weight loss accompanying dyspeptic symptoms is predictive of organic disease, especially gastric carcinoma or organic bowel disease, and is a definite indication for referral to a physician. Functional dyspepsia and dyspepsia due to organic disease cannot be differentiated by symptoms alone.

The subdivision of undiagnosed patients with dyspepsia into symptomatic subgroups (ulcer-like, dysmotility-like, reflux-like, and nonspecific) appears to have little clinical utility. More predictive of organic causes for abdominal symptoms are greater age (>40), male gender, pain at night, relief by antacids or food, and previous history of peptic ulcer disease, while younger age, female gender, a short history of frequent upper abdominal pain, no (or sometimes) pain relief with antacid use, and infrequent vomiting were predictive of functional dyspepsia. For example, almost 40% of dyspeptic patients under 25 years of age have normal endoscopic findings (functional dyspepsia) and very rarely have gastric cancer, while the incidence of gastric cancer in patients over 70 years of age whose dyspeptic symptoms warrant upper gastrointestinal endoscopic examination is as high as 33%.

TREATMENT

Nonpharmacological Treatment

The initial step in the management of dyspepsia of any origin is avoidance of precipitating or aggravating factors. Foremost is smoking cessation. Continued smoking retards and often prevents ulcer healing with antisecretory or other pharmacologic agents.

Aside from avoiding foods or beverages the patient can identify as contributing to the symptoms, dietary measures are much less useful. For instance, a bland diet merely increases the psychological and physical discomfort of the patient and may adversely affect compliance with more effec-

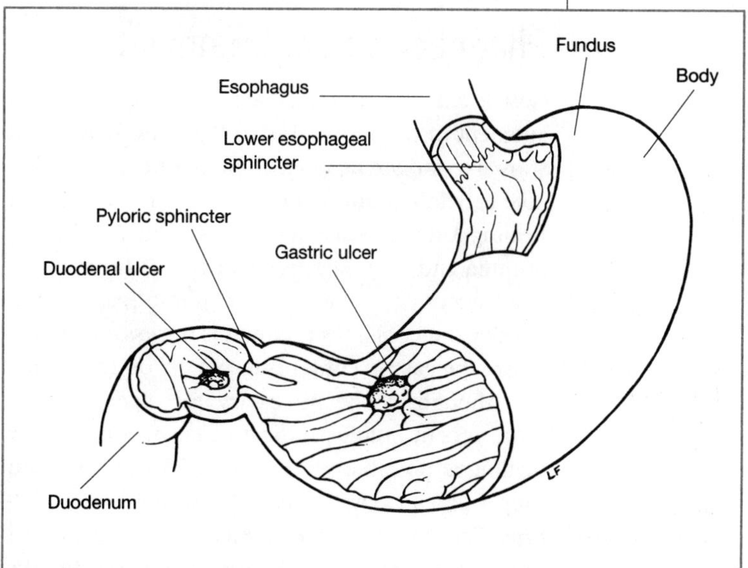

FIGURE 1: Anatomy of the stomach

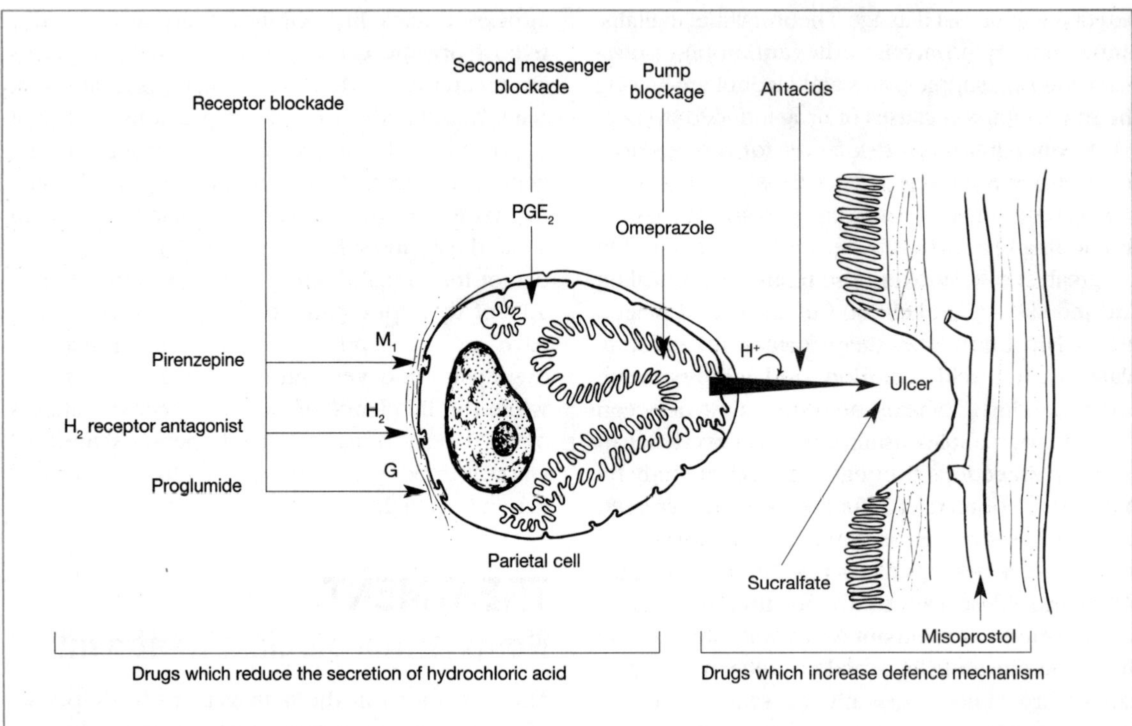

FIGURE 2: Acid Secretion and Sites of Drug Action

tive measures. Milk may temporarily alleviate symptoms, but it is a powerful acid secretogogue, and consumption of large quantities of milk should probably be discouraged. Bran is thought to contain prostaglandin precursors and may provide some benefit as a prophylactic measure, but dietary fibre does not influence symptoms or healing. Bedtime snacks stimulate nocturnal acid secretion and should be avoided.

Pharmacological Treatment

Gastric antacids are effective for symptomatic management of dyspepsia due to PUD and have been shown to induce healing. There has been considerable debate regarding the dose necessary to effect healing. Until 10 years ago, it was believed doses of 80 mEq and 120 mEq, respectively, 7 times a day were necessary to achieve healing of gastric and duodenal ulcers. This regimen is necessary to neutralize the gastric contents to pH 3.5 or 4.0, which was thought to be necessary for ulcer healing. More recent studies indicate that maximal ulcer healing is possible with doses of 50 to 100 mEq only 4 times a day, 1 hour after meals and at bedtime. These regimens resulted in 4-week duodenal ulcer healing rates of over 70%, compared to 30% with placebo, and 6-week gastric ulcer healing rates of nearly 70%, compared to 25% with placebo. These healing rates are almost comparable to those achievable with antisecretory agents or cytoprotective agents, even though such low antacid doses can have only a weak effect on gastric pH. Additional hypothetical mechanisms by which antacids may act include binding/inactivation of pepsin and bile acids, and induction of prostaglandin-mediated cytoprotection.

Nevertheless, patients should be advised not to self-medicate continuing dyspeptic symptoms. Chronic or recurring symptoms should be evaluated by a physician for the detection of possible organic disease. Continuous self-medication can result in so-called silent ulcers: the symptoms are masked but the lesion can continue to develop, leading to complications such as bleeding or perforation. Referral to a physician is particularly essential for patients over 40 years of age, since older patients have a greater risk of developing gastric carcinoma masquerading as PUD and have a higher incidence of *H. pylori*.

The primary treatment for dyspepsia of unknown origin is with antacids. According to an American and British survey, 61% of dyspeptic patients self-medicated with antacids for at least 1 year without consulting their physician. However, double-blind, placebo-controlled studies with antacids, H_2 blockers, anticholinergic agents and sucralfate have failed to show any of these therapies to be of benefit in patients with functional dyspepsia. Many patients with diagnosed functional dyspepsia benefit most from reassurance that they do not have a serious underlying disease, and from advice about avoiding possible offending foods or drugs and smoking.

Selection of a suitable product for an otherwise healthy individual should be governed by the propensity of the agent to promote either constipation (aluminum hydroxide and perhaps calcium carbonate) or diarrhea (magnesium hydroxide) and by cost. Underlying medical conditions of the patient must also be considered. For example, patients with renal failure may accumulate toxic levels of metal cations from chronic use of any antacid. Products containing sodium bicarbonate should be avoided because of their sodium content and systemic effect on the acid/base balance. Sodium-containing antacids are contraindicated in patients with hypertension or congestive heart failure. In healthy patients the regular strength products are suitable for occasional self-treatment of dyspepsia.

In patients under 40 years of age, there is very little risk in postponing a definitive diagnosis of the cause of dyspeptic symptoms for up to 8 weeks. It is therefore reasonable to recommend management of the symptoms for a 2-week period. Patients should be counselled on the proper use of nonprescription products to avoid unnecessary side effects and interactions with other medication. If symptoms do not respond to the nonprescription therapy after a 2-week trial, the patient should be referred to a physician who may wish to try a prescription drug. Older patients should be referred immediately to a physician because of the greater risk of organic disease, including gastric cancer.

For a dyspepsia management algorithm see Figure 3.

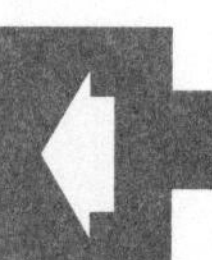

ADVICE FOR THE PATIENT

Dyspepsia

Dyspepsia may be caused or exacerbated by certain lifestyle factors, foods, or drugs:

➤ Where appropriate, reduce or eliminate lifestyle factors that affect dyspepsia:
- quit smoking;
- lose weight;
- limit the intake of alcohol.

➤ Avoid foods that are associated with the symptoms. For example:
- fatty foods;
- coffee and chocolate;
- milk and dairy products;
- spicy foods.

➤ Avoid using nonprescription products containing ASA or ibuprofen.

➤ Keep track of dyspeptic attacks and note anything that might have preceded each one, to help avoid precipitating situations and foods.

➤ Consult a physician or pharmacist about all drug use:
- some prescription drugs can cause dyspepsia;
- self-medication of dyspepsia symptoms should not occur for longer than 2 weeks at a time, and should not be repeated more than twice a year;
- antacids can interfere with the action of many other drugs;
- different antacids have different side effects.

FIGURE 3

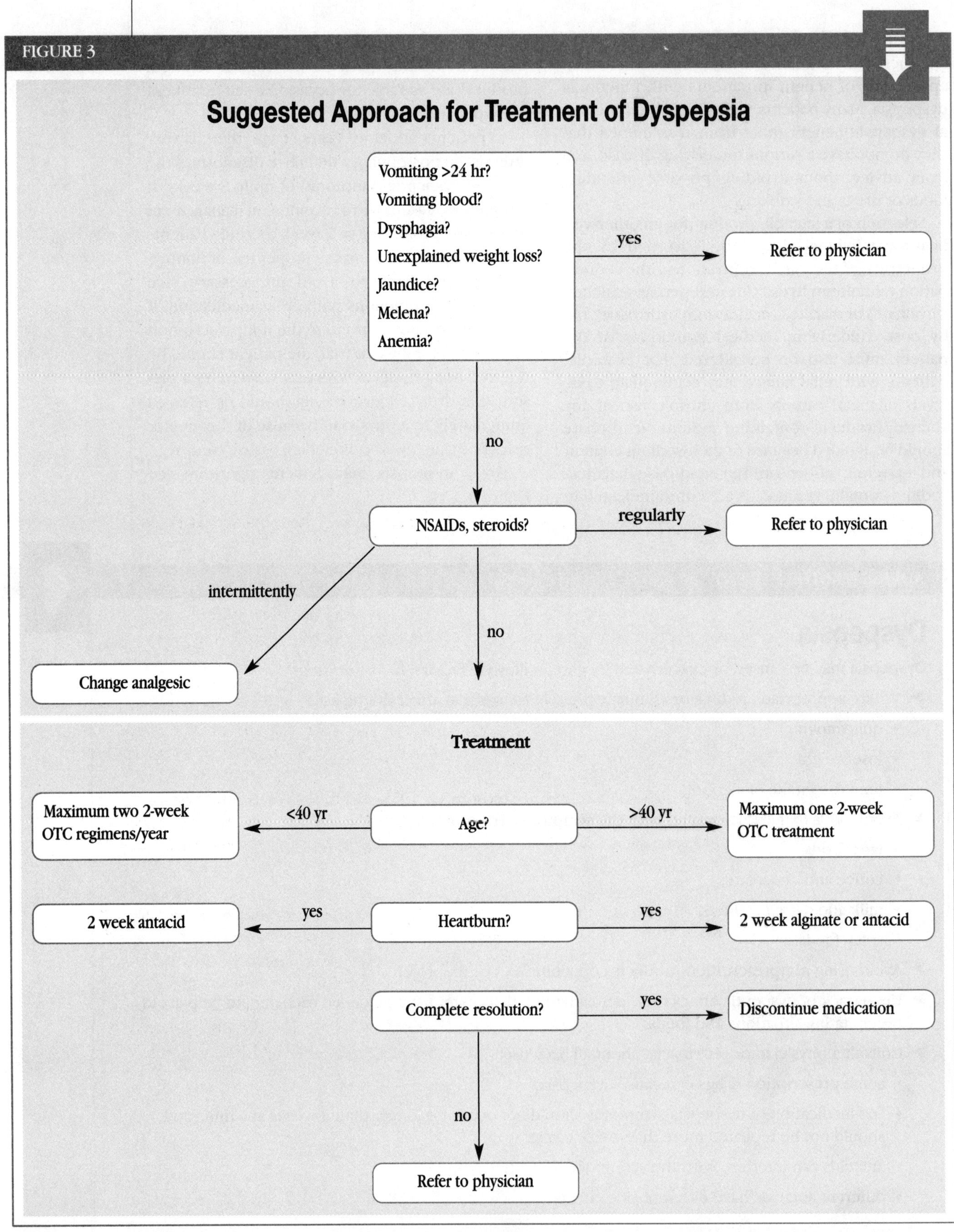

Adapted with permission from: Bond CM. Guidelines for dyspepsia treatment. Pharm J 1994;252(6776):228–229.

PATIENT ASSESSMENT QUESTIONS

?

Q How old is the patient?

In patients over 40 years of age dyspepsia may be the presenting symptom of organic disease such as gastric carcinoma. The patient should be referred to a physician, although one 2-week course of symptomatic remedy may be recommended. Individuals under 40 are much less likely to have a stomach cancer, and occasional short-term (2 weeks) symptomatic management is appropriate. Nevertheless, patients in this younger age group should be advised to see a physician if unexplained dyspeptic episodes occur more frequently than twice a year.

Q Please describe your symptoms.

It is important to establish if the patient is referring to upper gastrointestinal symptoms (dyspepsia). Patients with the following symptoms should be referred to a physician: prolonged vomiting; blood in vomitus or stools; black stools; difficulty in swallowing; sudden or unexplained weight loss; jaundice; anemia; abdominal pain or discomfort associated with exertion or exercise; pain radiating to the back, neck, jaw or arms.

Q How long have you experienced these symptoms?

Abrupt onset of symptoms (unexplained by recent dietary indiscretions) suggests an organic cause that should be evaluated by a physician. Symptoms of more gradual onset are more likely to be amenable to nonprescription management. Self-medication is appropriate for a 2-week period on an occasional basis; if the symptoms are resolved at that time, treatment should be discontinued; if they are not resolved, the patient should be referred to a physician.

Q What have you already tried?

Nonpharmacological measures should be considered first (e.g., cessation of smoking; limiting alcohol use to moderate amounts; avoidance of fatty foods or of foods the patient associates with the onset of symptoms). If the patient has already self-medicated with an appropriate regimen without resolution of the symptoms, or if the symptoms have recurred after a short time, referral to a physician is indicated.

Q Are you using any other medications?

The symptoms may be caused by prescription or nonprescription medication. It may be necessary to consult with the physician or refer the patient to the physician to assess the need to continue the therapy, or consider reducing the dose or changing the therapy. In addition, the potential for any drug interactions with possible nonprescription drug therapy should be evaluated.

Q Do you have any other medical problems or dietary restrictions?

Nonprescription medications may adversely affect other medical conditions of the patient. People with hypertension or congestive heart failure should avoid products with a high sodium content. Magnesium-containing antacids should be avoided by patients with renal failure. People at risk for hypophosphatemia, such as alcoholics or those with gastrointestinal malabsorption syndromes, should avoid aluminum antacids. Persons at risk of hypercalcemia or hypercalciuria, such as those with metastatic malignancies, kidney stones, or using thiazide diuretics or vitamin D supplements, should avoid antacids containing calcium.

Q Do you prefer liquid or tablet medications?

Tablets are usually more convenient and may be more palatable than some liquids. Modern tablet antacid formulations have been shown to be as effective as the corresponding liquids. At the same time, a patient may be convinced that the liquid is superior, and this belief could have an important placebo effect.

GASTROESOPHAGEAL REFLUX

PHYSIOLOGY AND PATHOPHYSIOLOGY

The physiology and pathophysiology of the esophagus belie its apparently simple function as a conduit between the mouth and the stomach. During swallowing, contraction of the pharynx initiates primary peristalsis, culminating in relaxation of the lower esophageal sphincter (LES). This swallow-induced LES relaxation normally lasts less than 5 seconds. The average person swallows about once a minute. Transient LES relaxations lasting 5 to 30 seconds, apparently occur spontaneously and sporadically, unassociated with a peristaltic sequence, and are believed to be normal physiologic events. In healthy individuals, control of transient LES relaxations seems to be subject to the level of consciousness and posture; they are completely suppressed during sleep.

The esophageal mucosa is resistant to injury from brief exposure to gastric acid. Nevertheless, it is not adapted for a continuously acid environment as is the gastric mucosa. The esophageal mucosa is normally at about pH 6. It is protected by peristaltic clearing and by the acid neutralizing capacity of saliva.

Short-lived, asymptomatic reflux of stomach contents after eating occurs commonly. Symptomatic gastroesophageal reflux (GER), on the other hand, is estimated to occur daily in 7 to 10% of adults, and every 3 days in 33% of the population. Over 10% of adults are believed to self-medicate for indigestion at least twice weekly, most of these for heartburn. Fortunately, the vast majority of individuals with GER do not require medical assistance. Untreated, however, chronic reflux can cause inflammation of the esophageal mucosa, perhaps culminating in esophageal ulceration and stricture. Chronic symptomatic reflux esophagitis is referred to as gastroesophageal disease.

The prevalence of GER disease increases with age.

ETIOLOGY

The principal cause of reflux seems to be impaired sphincter control. The majority of patients with chronic GER disease have normal LES pressure, but they are believed to have defective control of transient LES relaxations: 35% of transient LES relaxations in healthy individuals are associated with reflux, 65% in patients with chronic GER disease.

Furthermore, most GER episodes are known to occur during sphincter relaxation unrelated to swallowing. Delayed gastric emptying, as well as large gastric volumes, may contribute to the problem. A recent study of patients with GER disease revealed a significantly higher mean basal acid output than in normal subjects. Reflux of excessively acidic gastric contents may damage the esophageal mucosa. Esophagitis is especially likely to result if the gastric contents include bile. Thus, chronic GER disease may reflect impaired function of both the lower esophageal and pyloric sphincters. A minority of cases of chronic GER disease are thought to be secondary to hiatal hernia. These patients may have defective esophageal peristalsis, with more prolonged swallow-induced LES relaxation during which GER can occur.

Upper GI motility may be reduced by a variety of dietary factors (e.g., fats, chocolate, after-dinner mints, citrus fruit, tomatoes, coffee, or simply large meals). Nicotine is a powerful LES relaxant, and smoking is a major factor in the development of GER disease. Esophageal motility is diminished by various drugs including anticholinergics, beta-adrenergic agonists, calcium channel blockers, nitrates, opiates, progesterone and theophylline. The incidence of GER disease in older individuals correlates with benzodiazepine use. Other drugs, particularly potassium supplements (including enteric coated products), doxycycline and ferrous sulfate, can cause direct esophageal erosion if their transit through the esophagus is delayed. Exercise, especially if intense, causes profound inhibition of esophageal motility, precipitating acute episodes of GER. Factors that affect LES pressure are summarized in Table 2.

SYMPTOMS

The classic symptoms of GER disease are heartburn (intermittent retrosternal burning pain), chest pain, regurgitation of sour, burning fluid and hypersalivation. The pain of heartburn may be a sharp burning sensation and is usually more localized than that of dyspepsia. Sometimes, however, a patient will present with coughing, hoarseness and asthmatic symptoms, perhaps without the classic symptoms of heartburn. Dysphagia, weight loss, or unexplained anemia may indicate severe disease or other conditions such as cancer or achalasia. Serious complications of GER disease include hemorrhage, stenosis (narrowing), aspiration and malnutrition. See Table 3 for medical conditions associated with GER disease.

TREATMENT

Nonpharmacological Treatment

Symptoms of mild reflux disease may be controlled by lifestyle and dietary changes, in conjunction with antacids. The importance of avoiding smoking cannot be overemphasized. Elevation of the head of the bed by about 15 cm significantly increases the nighttime esophageal acid clearance. Eating frequent, small, low-fat meals, excluding chocolate, coffee, alcohol, acidic fruits and antiflatulents is advisable. Late supper hours and eating after supper should be avoided. Reclining immediately after eating may precipitate reflux. Overweight patients seem to have decreased LES tone, and weight loss is usually helpful. These conservative measures also should be encouraged in patients with GER disease complicated with other dyspeptic symptoms.

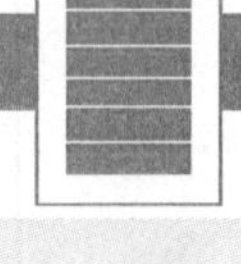

TABLE 2: Factors Affecting LES Pressure

Factors That Decrease LES Pressure	Factors That Increase LES Pressure
Dietary and Behavioral	**Dietary and Behavioral**
Fat	Protein
Whole milk	Skim milk
Citrus juice	Alcohol (low dose)
Tomatoes	Coffee
Chocolate	
Peppermint oil	
Alcohol (>117 mg/100 mL serum)	
Cigarette smoking	
Lying on side or sitting	
Drugs	**Drugs**
β-Adrenergics	Antacids
Anticholinergics	Cholinergic agents
Benzodiazepines	Cisapride
Calcium channel blockers	Domperidone
Opiates	Metoclopramide
Theophylline	
Hormones	**Hormones**
Cholecystokinin	Angiotensin II
Glucagon	Bombesin
Progesterone	Gastrin
Secretin	Motilin
Vasoactive intestinal peptide	Pancreatic polypeptide
	Pitressin

TABLE 3: Medical Conditions Associated with GER Disease

Uncontrolled asthma*
Liver cirrhosis
Portal hypertension
Scleroderma
Pregnancy
Hiatus hernia

*GER may be a causative factor of the asthma, and control of the reflux may improve the respiratory symptoms.

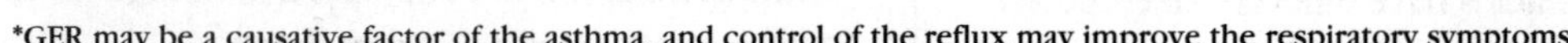

Pharmacological Treatment

Gastric antacids and/or alginic acid are useful adjuncts to the lifestyle modifications. They are especially helpful in controlling daytime symptoms. Besides reducing the acidity of refluxed gastric contents, antacids may increase the pressure. For antacids to be more useful than placebo, they likely must be used in doses large enough to neutralize 140 mEq of acid. That is, 20 to 25 mL or 4 to 5 tablets of high potency antacid formulation must be given 7 times daily, 1 hour and 3 hours after each meal and at bedtime, for 6 to 8 weeks. Such doses are liable to cause side effects and, in any case, are appreciably expensive. Nevertheless, short-term use of antacids for occasional episodes of mild GER is considered safe and appropriate.

An alternative nonprescription agent is alginic acid compound. This agent has no effect on the pH of the gastric contents, nor does it affect the LES pressure. It forms a low density, high viscosity foam that floats raft-like on the stomach contents, creating a physical barrier. Its presence suppresses the occurrence of reflux and, when reflux does occur, the foam acts as a demulcent and buffer between the refluxed material and the esophageal mucosa.

When H_2-blockers become available as nonprescription agents, they will likely become a popular component of conservative therapy although, to be curative, these agents must generally be given in high doses. The present proposal is to approve cimetidine, famotidine and ranitidine in low doses for heartburn and dyspepsia. Even as prescribed drugs, H_2-antagonists are less effective in healing GER disease than they are against PUD. Another class of drugs prescribed for chronic GER disease is prokinetic agents, such as metoclopramide, domperidone and cisapride. These are about equieffective with H_2-antagonists. Combination therapy with prokinetic agents and H_2-antagonists is more effective than either agent alone. A stepwise approach has been advocated, managing mild to moderate GER disease by lifestyle changes aimed at reducing reflux together with antacids and a prokinetic agent, adding H_2-blockers after 2 months when symptoms persisted. Sucralfate, which acts as a mucosal protectant, provides a healing rate comparable with those of other single agents. It is more effective when used in combination with H_2-antagonists. Potent proton pump inhibitors such as omeprazole and lansoprazole provide a high healing rate in 4 to 12 weeks, and are considered by many gastroenterologists to be drugs of choice in severe GER disease, although concerns remain about the safety of their long-term use. The 6-month recurrence rate of chronic GER disease is 50 to 80% without maintenance therapy, and as high as 40% with maintenance H_2-blocker therapy.

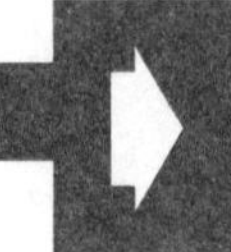

ADVICE FOR THE PATIENT

Gastroesophageal Reflux

To prevent or minimize the occurrence of GER attacks:

- Where appropriate, reduce or eliminate lifestyle factors that affect GER:
  - quit smoking;
  - lose weight;
  - limit the intake of alcohol;
  - eat smaller, more frequent meals;
  - refrain from bending over or lying down shortly after eating;
  - avoid wearing tight clothing;
  - raise head of bed about 15 cm.
- Certain foods may cause GER, and should be avoided:
  - fatty foods;
  - coffee and chocolate;
  - peppermints;
  - other foods the patient may associate with GER attacks.
- Keep track of GER attacks and note anything that might have preceded each one, to help avoid precipitating situations and foods.
- Consult a physician or pharmacist about all drug use:
  - some prescription drugs can cause esophageal injury if not swallowed with sufficient water or if swallowed while lying down;
  - some prescription drugs can increase GER;
  - self-medication of GER disease symptoms should not be used for longer than 2 weeks at a time, and should not be repeated more than twice a year;
  - antacids can interfere with the absorption of many other drugs;
  - different antacids have different side effects.

PATIENT ASSESSMENT QUESTIONS

Q ***Please describe your symptoms. Can you locate the discomfort for me?***

It is important to establish if the patient is referring to upper gastrointestinal symptoms (heartburn). Patients with the following symptoms should be referred to a physician: prolonged vomiting; blood in vomitus or stools; difficulty in swallowing; sudden or unexplained weight loss; jaundice; anemia; abdominal pain or discomfort associated with exertion or exercise; dull or diffuse, crushing chest pain; pain radiating to the back, neck, jaw or arms.

Q ***How long have you experienced these symptoms? Have you had this problem before?***

Occasional indigestion, clearly associated with food intake, may appropriately be treated with lifestyle measures and/or nonprescription medication. If symptoms have been present for more than a few days, or if they frequently recur, referral should be considered. Abrupt onset of symptoms (unexplained by recent dietary indiscretions) suggests an organic cause that should be evaluated by a physician. Self-treatment is appropriate for a 2-week period on an occasional basis; if the symptoms are resolved at that time, treatment should be discontinued; if they are not resolved, the patient should consult a physician.

Q ***Do you smoke?***

Smoking can provoke esophageal reflux and can intensify the symptoms. Drug therapy is less effective in smokers, and relapse is more likely.

Q ***What have you already tried?***

Nonpharmacological measures should be considered first (e.g., cessation of smoking; limiting alcohol use to moderate amounts; avoidance of fatty foods or of foods the patient associates with the onset of symptoms; avoiding lying down after eating; raising the head of the bed). If the patient has already self-medicated with an appropriate regimen, without resolution of the symptoms, or if the symptoms have recurred after a short time, referral to a physician is indicated.

Q ***Are you using any other medications?***

The symptoms may be caused by prescription or nonprescription medication. Potassium supplements, doxycycline and other tetracyclines, iron supplements and NSAIDs are notorious for causing esophageal injury if not swallowed with sufficient water or if swallowed while lying down. Other drugs may affect LES pressure and promote GER. In addition, the potential for any drug interactions with possible nonprescription drug therapy should be evaluated.

Q ***Do you have any other medical problems or dietary restrictions?***

Nonprescription medications may adversely affect other medical conditions of the patient. People with hypertension or congestive heart failure should avoid products with a high sodium content. Magnesium-containing antacids should be avoided by patients with renal failure. People at risk for hypophosphatemia, such as alcoholics or those with gastrointestinal malabsorption syndromes, should avoid aluminum antacids. Persons at risk of hypercalcemia or hypercalciuria, such as those with metastatic malignancies, kidney stones, or using thiazide diuretics or vitamin D supplements, should avoid antacids containing calcium.

GASTROINTESTINAL GAS

ETIOLOGY AND PATHOPHYSIOLOGY

A complaint of too much gas may mean the patient is belching excessively, experiencing abdominal distention or bloating, or is passing excessive rectal gas or flatus.

Excessive gastric gas or belching is almost always due to swallowed air. It most commonly results from gulping air, perhaps as a nervous habit. Many patients suffering from esophagitis, irritable bowel syndrome (IBS) or even angina claim belching provides short-term relief from their discomfort. Chronic belchers should be referred to a physician to rule out such underlying disorders. Other causes include ingestion of carbonated beverages or bicarbonate-containing antacids or chewing gum.

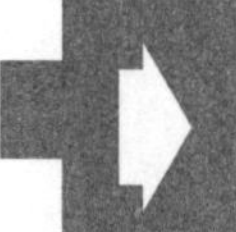

ADVICE FOR THE PATIENT

Gastrointestinal Gas

➤ **Excessive belching**

- Avoid souffles, whipped desserts, carbonated beverages and other ingestibles with a high air content.
- Should the problem continue, it is likely to be due to habitual, probably unconscious, gulping of air.

➤ **Persistent bloating and abdominal distention**, perhaps with gas pains

- If this is the first episode, see your physician for a diagnosis.
- Avoid overeating at a single sitting: eat smaller, more frequent meals.
- A hot water bottle applied to the lower abdomen may alleviate discomfort.

➤ **Flatulence or excessive colonic or rectal gas**

- Avoid gas-producing foods such as legumes and milk products. Pretreatment of these foods with appropriate hydrolytic enzyme preparations may provide some protection against the symptoms.

Bloating and abdominal distention are rarely due to excessive volumes of gas. Rather, the symptoms are probably caused by a gastrointestinal motility disorder (increased visceral sensitivity), and can be considered a variant of IBS. In these patients the intestine apparently responds to gas and liquid by going into spasm. Nevertheless, it must be borne in mind that bloating may also be an early symptom of colon cancer, and patients with persistent complaints should be referred for diagnosis.

Flatulence, or excessive gas in the colon, is due to excessive gas production in the gut. Carbon dioxide and hydrogen result from anaerobic bacterial metabolism of carbohydrates. The delivery of abnormal amounts of fermentable carbohydrates to the colon may be due to dietary factors such as ingestion of legumes, including but not limited to the notorious baked beans, (and to a lesser extent, wheat, oat, potato and corn starches) containing oligosaccharides that are not metabolized in the ileum, or it may be due to a malabsorption syndrome secondary to a deficiency of an enzyme such as lactase. Methane is also produced by colonic anaerobes in about 33 to 50% of the population. The colonic flora of some individuals are able to produce far more gas than the flora of others. These three gases comprise about two-thirds of normal flatus volume, while nitrogen and oxygen from swallowed air account for the remainder. All are odorless. The malodorous gases of flatus are probably mainly sulfur-containing compounds present in small quantities.

SYMPTOMS

Patients complaining of gastrointestinal gas may mean they are belching excessively or passing excessive rectal gas. Most commonly, however, the complaints are likely to refer to gas pains and bloated sensations. The pain is usually in the lower abdomen, although it often moves, and is sensed as a bubble or pocket of gas moving in the intestine. The pain may be dull or sharp, constant or spasmodic. It may cause the patient to bend over or stoop, and it may temporarily immobilize the patient. The abdomen is usually distended; the patient's clothing may feel too tight. Occasionally, abdominal gas pains may be accompanied by sharp stabbing pains in the back or shoulder, perhaps radiating down the arm.

Severe abdominal distress in the absence of a history of abdominal gas or irritable bowel syndrome requires prompt referral to a physician.

TREATMENT

Gastric Gas

The most effective way to control excessive gastric gas and belching is to reduce intake of carbonated beverages and foods containing appreciable amounts of air, and to avoid chewing gum or swallowing air either when gulping food or as a habit. There is no evidence that medications such as simethicone, antacids, histamine H_2-antagonists, anticholinergics, or enzymes are of any value in the treatment of chronic eructation.

Bloating

Similarly, there is little evidence to suggest any of these agents are beneficial in patients with bloating. While anticholinergics, which reduce bowel motility, appear rational and are commonly prescribed, they often aggravate symptoms. Dietary fibre, too, is not superior to placebo, with 50% of patients responding in either group. Since the symptoms seem to be due to abnormal or excessive visceral sensitivity, and since most patients experi-

PATIENT ASSESSMENT QUESTIONS

Q ***Would you please describe your symptoms specifically?***

A complaint of too much gas may mean the patient is belching excessively, experiencing abdominal distention or bloating, or is passing excessive rectal gas or flatus.

Q ***Is your excessive gas related to eating food?***

Intestinal gas usually results from swallowing air or from ingesting gas-producing foods or carbonated beverages. In healthy adults, the frequency of passing rectal gas varies from 5 to 21 times a day. Dietary rather than pharmacological measures are usually more effective in reducing flatulence.

Q ***How long have you experienced bloating and/or gas pains?***

Occasional symptoms may simply be due to dietary indiscretion or overeating. Persistent symptoms suggest a variant of irritable bowel syndrome, but the patient should be referred to a physician to rule out more serious disorders.

TABLE 4: Flatulence Potential of Foods

Normoflatulenic		Moderately flatulenic	Extremely flatulenic
Vegetables	**Carbohydrates**	**Vegetables**	**Vegetables**
Asparagus	Corn chips	Eggplant	Beans
Avocado	Graham crackers	Potatoes	Brussels sprouts
Broccoli	Popcorn		Carrots
Cauliflower	Potato chips	**Fruits**	Celery
Cucumbers	Rice	Apples	Onions
Lettuce		Citrus	
Okra	**Meats**		**Fruits**
Olives	Meat	**Carbohydrates**	Apricots
Peppers	Fish	Bread	Prune juice
Tomatoes	Poultry	Pastries	Raisins
Zucchini			
	Miscellaneous		**Carbohydrates**
Fruits	Eggs		Wheat germ
Berries	Fruit ice		
Cantaloupe	Gelatin desserts		**Dairy**
Grapes	Non-milk chocolate		Milk and milk products
	Nuts		
	Water		

ence the most discomfort after eating large meals, patients should be advised to eat frequent, small meals rather than large meals. Externally applied heat, such as a hot water bottle, may provide some relief, presumably by relaxing the spastic smooth muscle. A patient with colonic gas pain may be able to minimize the discomfort by lying on the left side; perhaps this promotes the distal movement of the offending pool of feces along the transverse colon. Gastroprokinetic agents such as metoclopramide and cisapride, available only by prescription, may be useful.

Flatulence

Many individuals complaining of excessive flatus actually pass gas no more frequently than average, and should simply be reassured that this is normal. It may be of interest to such patients that, in healthy adults, the frequency of passing rectal gas varies from 5 to 21 times a day. Diet rather than pharmacological measures is usually more effective in reducing flatulence. Table 4 reveals the flatulence potential of various foods. A lactose-free diet often is beneficial.

INFANTILE COLIC

ETIOLOGY

Colic is an overused term, but it refers generally to incessant, unexplained crying or screaming with apparent abdominal discomfort, occurring at particular times of the day, usually associated with feeding. Common causes of crying in infants are shown in Table 5.

Autonomic nervous control of the gastrointestinal tract may not be fully developed in some infants before the age of 3 or 4 months. An immature LES will allow frequent regurgitation after feeding. Immature autonomic control of bowel motility may lead to smooth muscle spasms, especially in response to gas, such as from swallowed air.

Colic occurs in 10 to 15% of infants. It is a self-limiting condition, developing during the first few weeks after birth and usually resolving by about 14 weeks.

Infantile colic is generally ascribed to gas trapped in the gastrointestinal tract. A bottle-fed baby may be gulping too fast a flow, swallowing excessive amounts of air. This distends the stomach uncomfortably and gives a premature sense of satiety that might lead to hunger after feeding. Alternatively, the baby may be working too hard at the nipple, again taking in air.

Intolerance to cow's milk can cause symptoms resembling colic, usually accompanied by diarrhea. Similarly, fruit juice, especially apple juice, which contains sugars that infants cannot absorb, can cause diarrhea in infants.

Occasionally factors in the nursing mother's diet may lead to colic: large quantities of caffeine, artificial sweeteners, vitamin supplements or brewer's yeast may contribute to colic. Such foods in the mother's diet as cow's milk, eggs, chicken, fish, citrus fruits, wheat, oats, corn, chocolate and nuts have also been implicated.

SYMPTOMS

A pattern of frantic, persistent crying or screaming after feeding, especially in a bottle-fed infant, is

TABLE 5: Some Common Causes of Infant Crying

Problem	Symptoms	Remedies
Colic	Persistent screaming after feedings, before 14 weeks of age Legs drawn up to abdomen Excessive regurgitation	Use nipple with smaller hole Use collapsible plastic bottle liners Use proper burping technique. Use arm straddle with head higher than feet
Hunger	Crying between feedings Inadequate weight gain	Increase feeding frequency
Overheating	Crying when tightly swaddled Heat rash	Loosen covers, reduce clothing Reduce room temperature
Tired	Crying when handled	Allow baby to sleep
Insomnia	Crying, inability to sleep at bedtime	Avoid excitement, stimulation before bedtime
Inattention or lack of stimulation	Crying, fussiness when left alone	Rocking, cuddling Visual distraction (mobile, etc.) Rhythmic sound distraction (music, vacuum cleaner, clock, etc.)
Ear infection	Crying, with touching the ear Fever may be present	Refer to physician
Teething	Crying, beginning after 5 months of age Excessive salivation Inflamed gums	Teething biscuits, etc.

probably due to colic. A colicky baby usually draws up its legs to its abdomen. Excessive regurgitation is common; sometimes vomiting occurs.

Colicky babies are well-fed. They are happy and healthy between crying spells.

An infant with apparent colic should be examined by a physician initially, to rule out any underlying pathology. This is important to reassure the parents also.

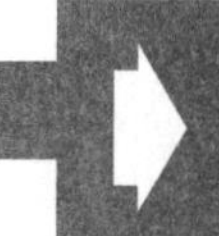

ADVICE FOR THE PARENT

Colic

Babies who are held promptly in response to their crying cried less after 3 months than those babies whose crying was ignored or who received delayed response. On the other hand, feeding in response to crying should be avoided, as overfeeding may lead to bloating and more discomfort. Carrying a fussy infant in a baby carrier positioned in front of the parent's body provides gentle motion and the soothing sound of the heartbeat.

TREATMENT

Nonpharmacological Treatment

A colicky baby may be quietened by laying it astraddle the arm, with its head slightly higher than its feet, and gently rocking it to sleep. The baby may be placed on its abdomen to aid expulsion of gas.

Changing the nipple of the bottle to one with a smaller hole or anticolic design may prevent frequent colic attacks.

Changing the diet of bottle-fed infants to hydrolyzed milk has been shown to be more effective than dicyclomine. Placing the mothers of colicky breast-fed infants on milk-, fish- and egg-free diets was not more effective.

Pharmacological Treatment

Drugs are of questionable benefit and should not be routinely recommended. Because of an association with apnea in infants, dicyclomine is contraindicated in infants less than 6 months of age. Of the pharmaceutical remedies available, simethicone is the only one with any experimental evidence supporting its use.

?

PATIENT ASSESSMENT QUESTIONS

Q ***How old is the baby?***

Colic usually resolves itself by about 14 weeks of age. Teething pain generally begins after 5 months.

Q ***Have you noticed a pattern in the baby's crying time (e.g., following feeding times, between feeds, at bedtime, when left alone)?***

A crying pattern associated with feeding times suggests the symptom is due to either colic or hunger. Crying at bedtime may signify insomnia, possibly due to overexcitement at bedtime. Fussiness when the baby is left alone may reflect a lack of adequate sensory input and might be alleviated by rocking, cuddling or by visual or auditory distractions.

Q ***How long does the baby take to finish feeding?***

A bottle-fed baby should require at least 20 minutes to finish a bottle.

Q ***Have you noticed any other symptoms? (e.g., Are the baby's legs drawn up to the abdomen? Is there excessive regurgitation of food? Is there a fever? Is the baby fingering its ear?)***

Drawn-up legs and excessive regurgitation are commonly associated with colic. Earache due to infection is often manifested by frequent touching of the ear, perhaps accompanied by a fever.

Q ***Is the baby breast-fed or bottle-fed?***

Breast-fed babies may be hungry. The best way to stimulate more breast milk production is to suckle the infant more frequently. At least during the first few weeks, some babies will need to breast-feed every 2 hours. Bottle-fed babies may be working too hard or may be gulping too fast a flow, swallowing excessive amounts of air.

CONSTIPATION

ANATOMY AND PHYSIOLOGY

Normal frequency of bowel movements in healthy orphaned adults is 7.1±3.3 per week, with two-thirds of subjects reporting between 5 and 8. Average daily stool weight is about 100 g (range 35-250 g). Both the frequency and daily stool output are lower for women than men.

The function of the colon is principally as a water absorptive organ. Of the approximate litre of fluid delivered to the colon each day, about 850 mL is reabsorbed. Sodium, chloride and bicarbonate ions are absorbed against high concentration gradients, while potassium ion is secreted. Very little fluid re-enters the lumen in the colon.

Colonic motility consists of several types of smooth muscular movements. Spontaneous contractions of longitudinal muscles are responsible for pendular movements, while contractions of circular muscles produce segmental movements. About 10 contractions of each type pass up and down short segments of the bowel each minute, resulting in a mixing action. Two to four times daily, mass peristaltic contractions of the circular muscles move the contents about one-third the length of the colon. These peristaltic waves are coordinated by the parasympathetic myenteric nerve plexus, sometimes referred to as the gastrointestinal "brain."

The anus has two sphincter muscles, the smooth muscular internal sphincter and the striated, or voluntary, muscular external sphincter. The presence of sufficient feces to distend the rectum causes the internal sphincter to relax. Defecation is voluntarily inhibited by keeping the external sphincter in its normal state of tonic contraction. Defecation is achieved by voluntarily relaxing the sphincter. Reflex contraction of the distended colon, assisted by contracting the abdominal muscles, expels the feces.

The presence of food in the stomach stimulates the gastrocolic reflex, causing contractions of the rectum and the sensation of the need to defecate.

Constipation may be defined as the infrequent and difficult passage of dry stools of low mass. It is experienced occasionally by almost everyone in the Western world. The overall incidence of chronic painless constipation in Western society is 6%, but it rises to 20% among the geriatric population and as high as 40 to 78% among those who are institutionalized. It is more prevalent among women than among men.

ETIOLOGY

Simple or primary constipation may be considered a consequence of lifestyle. Children and young adults, in particular, may suppress the defecation impulse repeatedly until the spinal reflex becomes progressively weaker. This commonly occurs in toddlers undergoing toilet training. Punishment for a soiled diaper or training pants may lead to suppression of defecation on the next occasion. Environmental factors such as inadequate toilet facilities or lack of privacy can also lead to this sort of conditioned constipation in any age group. Travellers and even people in a busy workday also frequently neglect to heed the defecation reflex. Conditioning is probably the single most important cause of simple constipation.

Painful anorectal lesions such as hemorrhoids or fissures may impair sphincter relaxation, as well as causing voluntary suppression of defecation.

Dietary factors represent another aspect of lifestyle that can lead to constipation. Lack of adequate fibre and, perhaps, fluid in the diet is very commonly implicated in simple constipation. Nevertheless, many constipated patients consume as much fibre as nonconstipated persons. Failure to eat breakfast is often suggested as a causative factor, since the gastrocolic reflex is strongest after this meal.

Finally, lack of exercise may contribute to the development of simple constipation. Exercise is thought to improve the tone of the abdominal wall muscles and perhaps to enhance the receptiveness to rectal distention, thereby strengthening the defecation reflex. However, evidence for a beneficial effect of physical activity on colonic function in healthy volunteers is not convincing. While bedridden patients are often constipated, this is not necessarily due to a lack of exercise. The constipation may be a symptom of their underlying disease, or a side effect of their medications.

As indicated above, advancing age is associated with an increased incidence of constipation. The elderly may have decreased smooth muscle tone, although colonic transit time does not necessarily slow with aging. The elderly may also have weakened abdominal wall skeletal muscles. There may be a dulling of the perception of a full rectum. Perhaps environmental factors and complex sociologic influences are most important in the development of constipation in the elderly. They may be nutritionally compromised, eating mostly refined carbohydrates, possibly because of difficulty in mastication or lack of interest in diet. They may simply have difficulty getting to the bathroom. Older individuals are also more likely to be at risk of developing secondary constipation from various pathologies or drugs.

Secondary constipation may be due to a number of etiological factors. It is commonly experienced as a side effect of medication. Drugs that commonly cause constipation are listed in Table 6.

Irritable bowel syndrome is a common cause of constipation. Another motility disorder, described as slow transit, is characterized by intractable, severe constipation with bowel movements every 1 to 4 weeks.

Constipation is a common feature of pregnancy and has a manifold etiology. Hormonal changes, particularly increased production of progesterone and prostaglandins, influence bowel motility. Pressure of the gravid uterus on abdominal and back muscles and on the rectum, together with displacement of the colon may promote constipation. Weakened pelvic floor muscles in multiparous women can increase susceptibility to constipation. Iron supplements, dietary changes, and perhaps lack of exercise also contribute to the problem.

Diverticular disease and colorectal carcinoma cause constipation. The incidence of both these disorders increases with age. The constipation of diverticulitis is often associated with crampy left lower quadrant pain. Danger signs for a cancerous lesion include recent (sudden) onset of constipation, discomfort, gaseousness, anorexia and weight loss, blood in the stool and tenesmus (ineffectual and painful straining at stool).

Other pathologic conditions associated with constipation include endocrine disorders, such as diabetes and hypothyroidism, and neurologic disorders, such as Parkinson's disease and stroke. Chronic constipation in children may be caused by anatomical abnormalities such as anal stenosis and Hirschsprung's disease, or by physiological abnormalities, such as abnormal sphincter response and slow transit.

SYMPTOMS

Constipation means different things to different people. To most people it means difficulty in defecation: excessive, sometimes ineffective straining to pass a stool. Some patients also complain of infrequent defecation. Almost all patients describe an uncomfortable or painful abdominal distention or bloated feeling in association with their constipation. Some patients believe themselves to be constipated if their stool size is too small or if they do not move their bowels each day. Constipation is held responsible by some for such general symptoms as anorexia, headache, lassitude, malaise, even nausea or a bad taste in the mouth.

Simple constipation is generally self-limiting. Diagnosis of chronic functional constipation requires that at least two of the following symptoms be present for at least 3 months: straining at least 75% of the time; hard stools at least 75% of the time; no more than two bowel movements per week.

Fecal impaction and the consequent dilatation of the rectum (in children) or of both rectum and distal colon (adults) leads to reflex relaxation of the internal anal sphincter. The impacted mass acts like a ball valve, and newer soft stool seeps around it, resulting in overflow incontinence (encopresis).

TREATMENT

Nonpharmacological Treatment

If possible, constipation should be managed nonpharmacologically. The individual may be

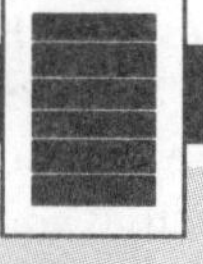

TABLE 6: Drugs That Commonly Cause Constipation
Analgesics and cough suppressants (codeine and other opiates)
Antacids and calcium supplements (aluminum and calcium salts)
Anticonvulsants (e.g., phenytoin)
Antihypertensive agents (e.g., clonidine, reserpine)
Anxiolytic agents (benzodiazepines, e.g., diazepam)
Calcium channel blockers (especially verapamil)
Diuretics
Drugs with anticholinergic properties (e.g., benztropine, trihexyphenidyl, antispasmodics, phenothiazines and tricyclic antidepressants)
Iron salts (ferrous fumarate, ferrous gluconate, ferrous sulfate)
Laxatives (if abused)

encouraged to follow a bowel retraining program to establish a standardized toilet habit. This involves setting aside a fixed time of day, usually shortly after breakfast, to sit on the toilet for a fixed period of time (5 to 30 minutes). Unproductive straining should be avoided. It is difficult to know how effective such programs are, since they have not been evaluated separately.

Mild exercise, such as walking is often advocated as part of a regimen to promote bowel regularity. By improving the tone of abdominal wall muscles, exercise may facilitate voluntary muscle action during defecation. In any case, exercise relieves stress and enhances general well being.

Increasing fluid intake is often included in a lifestyle regimen to combat simple constipation. While it is known that severe dehydration leads to constipation, increasing fluids beyond a normal level is more likely to flush the kidneys than the bowel. In healthy volunteers taking wheat bran, 30 g/day with 600 mL of additional fluid, did not increase stool output any more than bran alone. It has been observed that drinking either regular or decaffeinated coffee on an empty stomach is superior to hot water in stimulating a gastrocolic response.

Increasing dietary fibre is the only lifestyle measure proven to increase stool weights and decrease colonic transit time. This is true both in constipated patients and in healthy volunteers. Compliance with a high fibre diet, consisting of at least 30 g of fibre per day, can be encouraged by gradual introduction over a couple of weeks to minimize flatulence and to accustom the patient to the regimen. It should be given a trial for at least 4 to 6 weeks. Nevertheless, for many patients with simple constipation, increasing dietary fibre alone, or in combination with the above nonpharmacologic measures, is insufficient. This therapeutic failure has been shown not entirely due to noncompliance. Some dietary sources of fibre are described in Table 7.

TABLE 7: Dietary Fibre in Selected Foods

Food	Serving Size	Fibre Content	
		g/serving	g/100 g
Whole bran cereal	30 g	9-10	30-33
Fruit & Fibre	40 g	5.5-6.2	13.8-15.5
Weetabix	35 g	4.6	13.1
Bran Flakes	30 g	4.4-5.3	14.7-17.7
Grapenuts	30 g	3.6	12
Shredded Wheat Spoon Size	30 g	4	13.3
Shredded Wheat Biscuits	25 g	3.2	12.8
Frosted Mini Wheats	30 g	2.9	9.7
Shreddies	30 g	2.7	9.0
Cheerios	30 g	1.5-2.5	5.0-8.3
Captain Crunch	30 g	0.8	2.7
Rice Crispies	30 g	0.3	1
Corn Flakes	30 g	0.8	2.7
Whole wheat bread	2 slices	2.5	4.8
Enriched white bread	2 slices	0.9	1.7
Spinach, cooked, drained	125 mL	10	6
Beans, white, cooked	100 mL	6	7
green or yellow, cooked	125 mL	2	3
Potatoes, cooked in skin	1 long	5	2
peeled, boiled	1 long	2	1
Broccoli, cooked	250 mL	4	4
Peas, cooked	125 mL	3	5
Brussels sprouts, cooked	4	2	3
Carrots, raw	1	2	3
sliced, cooked	100 mL	2	3
Parsnips, cooked, mashed	100 mL	3	3
Tomato, raw, unpeeled	1	2	2
Cabbage, red or green, raw, chopped	100 mL	1	3
Cauliflower, raw, chopped	100 mL	1	2
Celery, inner sticks, raw	3	1	2
Banana	1	3.9	
Orange	1	2.6	
Grapefruit	0.5	0.7	

Pharmacological Treatment

It is appropriate to recommend a suitable laxative for occasional short-term use. Laxatives should not be used for more than 2 or 3 days for simple constipation. The aim should be to achieve the elimination of a soft, formed stool.

Provided the patient does not already have severe constipation with fecal impaction, edible fibre, including bulk-forming laxatives, leads to defecation of soft bulky stools within 1 to 3 days. Milk of magnesia may be used safely for occasional simple constipation, producing its effect within 8 to 12 hours. Cascara, standardized senna and bisacodyl are also suitable for occasional short-term relief of simple constipation, although these agents may cause griping or abdominal spasms in some patients. Bisacodyl commonly gives a watery stool. Taken at bedtime, these laxatives usually lead to defecation after breakfast the following morning. Although as safe and effective as bisacodyl, phenolphthalein products are generally not advisable, largely because they are formulated and marketed in a manner that encourages habitual use.

It is especially important that constipation in pregnancy be managed as far as possible by nonpharmacological means. In particular, pregnant women must avoid castor oil, which may stimulate uterine contractions.

Chronic use of so-called stimulant laxatives and saline laxatives may lead to electrolyte imbalance, while chronic use of mineral oil may lead to deficiency of fat-soluble vitamins.

Chronic constipation in debilitated older individuals or in chronic laxative users (abusers) should be managed with a physician's supervision, using a bulk-forming laxative in combination with low (sublaxative) doses of a stimulant laxative such as standardized senna or bisacodyl. Alternatively, milk of magnesia may be used.

An individual suffering from fecal impaction should be referred to a physician.

Counselling Tips

- Patient education is important.
  - Patients requesting a remedy for constipation should be reassured that normal bowel habits vary from person to person, and that daily stool size and weight vary with the diet.
  - Patients should be given information on the amount of fibre in foods, and be encouraged to ingest at least 15 g of food fibre per day.
  - Normal feces are 75 to 85% water, so adequate fluid intake is essential. The usual requirement is 1.5 to 2 L/day, but this will vary according to a person's size and daily fluid loss, particularly through perspiration.
  - Patients should be taught that the colon is a muscular structure and, as such, must be maintained in a healthy state so that it will respond to activity as required.
  - Patients should be informed that many drugs can cause constipation.
  - Patients should understand that psychological factors such as stress, anxiety and depression are commonly associated with constipation.
  - Patients must understand that past laxative use (or abuse, but they should not be made to feel defensive) may be a causative factor in chronic constipation.
  - Patients should be encouraged to respond to the defecation reflex as soon as practical, to maintain a regular bowel habit.
- Patients must be instructed on proper use of products, and what expectations they should have for their action. Concentrated fibre supplements and saline laxatives must be taken with at least 250 mL fluid, to prevent esophageal or gastrointestinal obstruction in the former case, and to avoid fluid and electrolyte imbalance in the latter.
- The patient should be made aware that failure to produce a bowel movement the day following a complete purgation does not constitute constipation: there is simply nothing left to eliminate.

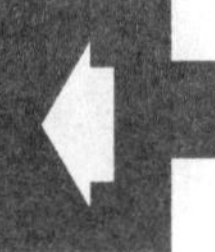

ADVICE FOR THE PATIENT

Constipation

Maintain regular bowel habits. Lifestyle factors that affect bowel function include:

- Dietary measures:
  - ingest at least 15 g of food fibre per day;
  - drink 1.5 to 2 L of fluid per day;
  - eat breakfast.
- Bowel habits:
  - respond to the defecation reflex as soon as practical;
  - allow time for completion of defecation at each sitting;
  - avoid overstaying the visit, or straining unproductively.

Proper use of laxative products:

- Concentrated fibre supplements and saline laxatives must be taken with at least 250 mL of fluid.
- Enteric coated tablets must not be chewed or taken with antacids.
- Enemas are best administered with the individual lying on the left side:
  - the enema reservoir should be only 2 to 5 cm above the hips;
  - an enema should be at body temperature;
  - an enema should be retained as long as possible.
- Proper use of suppositories includes:
  - suppositories must be unwrapped;
  - they may be lubricated with tepid water, but not with oil or grease;
  - they are most effective if used after a meal; the patient should remain reclined for a few minutes after insertion of the suppository to avoid premature expulsion.

PATIENT ASSESSMENT QUESTIONS

***Q** What is the usual pattern of your bowel movements? Has the frequency of your bowel movements or the consistency of your stools changed recently? Do you strain at stool? Have you been examined recently by your physician?*

There is a wide range of frequency of bowel movements among healthy individuals. Stool consistency will help to assess whether the person is truly constipated. An abrupt change in bowel pattern may indicate an underlying bowel disease, including colonic cancer.

***Q** Could you please describe any other abdominal or digestive tract symptoms you have been experiencing? Have you had nausea, vomiting, abdominal pain, rectal bleeding, or black stools?*

Such additional symptoms may indicate a more serious condition such as appendicitis, inflammatory bowel disease, or bleeding peptic ulcer. Laxatives are contraindicated in these circumstances. The patient should be referred to a physician immediately.

***Q** How old is the individual?*

The client may be requesting a laxative for another individual. It is important to know whether the patient is an infant, a child, a pregnant mother or an older individual.

***Q** Do you suffer from any other medical conditions, or are you taking any other medications?*

Drug therapy may cause constipation. Patients with certain medical conditions, such as congestive heart failure, hypertension or chronic renal insufficiency must be made aware of the electrolyte content of some laxative preparations. Pregnant women should avoid any use of castor oil and chronic use of most other laxatives.

***Q** Have you changed your diet or your daily routine recently?*

Dietary changes, travel and other changes in daily routine all can contribute to the development of constipation. The most appropriate management strategy will depend on a knowledge of these factors.

DIARRHEA

ETIOLOGY

Acute diarrhea is a sudden disruption of bowel habits characterized by frequent and numerous liquefied movements. It is a nonspecific intestinal response to an insult such as infections, drugs, inflammatory bowel disease, and ischemia. The most common cause is a viral infection. Bacteria and parasitic agents also cause acute diarrhea. The infection is usually acquired by oral ingestion of the pathogen or of a toxin produced by a microorganism. Fecal contamination of food, water or the hands is the major source of infection. Gastrointestinal defences against pathogenic enteric infection include gastric acid, intestinal motility, and immune mechanisms.

The intestines absorb about 99% of the nearly 10 L of fluid that reach the small intestine each day. In acute diarrhea, intestinal secretion is significantly increased or absorption is impaired. Diarrhea is defined objectively by the loss of more than 200 mL of water in the stool during a 24-hour period.

Active transport of sodium ions by two primary mechanisms in the small intestine causes water to follow passively. Sodium absorption by the first, the Na+/Cl- co-transport mechanism, is inhibited by cyclic AMP, which also stimulates active secretion of chloride. Enterotoxins of certain pathogens (e.g., cholera, *E. coli*) activate the enzyme adenyl cyclase, producing increased amounts of cyclic AMP. The second, Na+/substrate (Na+/glucose or Na+/amino acid) co-transport mechanism, is generally unaffected by infectious organisms.

Other microorganisms may damage the absorptive surface villi of the intestinal mucosa. Still other, so-called invasive pathogens, cause ulceration of the colonic and ileal epithelium, resulting in a bloody diarrhea. A local inflammatory response may contribute further to secretion and fluid loss. Features distinguishing inflammatory from noninflammatory diarrhea are shown in Table 8. Table 9 lists common sources of diarrhea-causing microorganisms.

Next to infections, drugs are the second highest cause of diarrhea. Of particular importance are broad spectrum antibiotics (tetracycline, ampicillin, penicillin, cephalosporins, erythromycin, sulfonamides, cotrimoxazole, chloramphenicol, and clindamycin). Mild, early onset diarrhea associated with antibiotic use is likely to be self-limiting. Diarrhea appearing 2 or 3 days after commencement of antibiotic therapy is probably indicative of a change in the bacterial flora of the gut. Major components of the flora are suppressed by the antibiotic, allowing nonsusceptible enteropathogens to proliferate. Again, this form of diarrhea is usually self-limiting once the offending agent is discontinued. However, use of broad spectrum antibiotics can occasionally lead to a potentially life-threatening condition known as pseudomembranous colitis. The diarrhea associated with this may commence late in the course of antibiotic therapy, or even days or weeks after the conclusion of therapy. Pseudomembranous colitis is caused by *Clostridium difficile*, an enterotoxin-producing organism that is normally a minor component of the gut flora. Clindamycin,

TABLE 8: Inflammatory Versus Noninflammatory Diarrhea

Characteristic	Inflammatory	Noninflammatory
Symptoms	Bloody, small-volume diarrhea Lower left quadrant cramps May be febrile, toxic	Large-volume, watery diarrhea Nausea, vomiting, cramps
Causes	*Shigella, Salmonella,* amebic colitis, *Clostridium difficile*	Viruses, *E. coli,* food poisoning, enterotoxins
Site	Colon	Small intestine
Management	Definite referral	Nonprescription antidiarrheals if mild or moderate

TABLE 9: Common Sources of Enterotoxic Pathogens

Source	Organism
Day care center	*Shigella*, rotavirus, *Clostridium difficile*
Hospital, recent antibiotic or chemotherapy	*C. difficile*
Swimming pool	*Giardia, Cryptosporidium*
Foreign travel	Enterotoxigenic *E. coli, Shigella, Salmonella*
Shellfish	*Vibrio*
Cheese	*Listeria*
Hamburger	*E. coli*
Fried rice	*Bacillus cereus*

ampicillin, cefotaxime and other cephalosporins are the antibiotics most commonly associated with pseudomembranous colitis. The condition requires prompt and diligent management by a physician. Metronidazole and vancomycin are the drugs of choice against *C. difficile*, although relapses or reinfections occur in a significant number of patients.

Other drugs that commonly cause diarrhea are magnesium-containing antacids, laxatives used improperly, nonsteroidal anti-inflammatory drugs (especially mefenamic acid and floctafenine) and antimetabolites.

DIARRHEA IN INFANTS

Dehydration resulting from diarrhea is the major cause of childhood deaths in Third World countries. Even in the United States, diarrhea kills approximately 500 children each year. On average, American and, presumably, Canadian children under 5 years of age experience two episodes of diarrhea per year. Fortunately, most cases are acute and self-limited.

The pathogens are spread rapidly through a day care population by fecal-oral contamination. Frequent and thorough hand-washing by day care workers, particularly after attending children at toileting or changing diapers, and before preparation duties, is essential. Children and child-care workers who have diarrhea, fever, vomiting of infectious origin should be excluded from a day care centre. The risk is highest during the first month of enrollment in day care.

As well as being more susceptible to diarrheal infections, very young children are at higher risk of severe dehydration and inadequate nutrition than older children or nongeriatric adults. Health professionals must be able to recognize the signs of dehydration. A child with mild dehydration will experience loss of up to 5% of body weight, will be thirsty, and perhaps restless. Moderate dehydration is defined by weight loss of 6 to 9%; the child will be thirsty and restless, but also irritable and perhaps lethargic; the eyes will be sunken and the fontanelle depressed; there will be a lack of tears or mucous secretions, and urine output will be decreased; pinched skin will retract slowly (1 to 2 seconds). Severe dehydration is an emergency situation; body weight loss will be 10% or more; a severely dehydrated child will be drowsy, cold and sweaty, with cyanotic limbs; the pulse will be rapid and feeble.

In our society, childhood diarrhea is most commonly caused by viral infections. The illness is usually self-limiting. Rotavirus and enteric adenoviruses usually affect children under the age of 2. Rotavirus gastroenteritis may cause sudden onset diarrhea, vomiting and, usually, a low-grade fever lasting from 2 to 8 days, and may cause dehydration. Adenovirus-associated diarrhea may persist up to 14 days, but vomiting is usually milder and of much shorter duration, and significant dehydration is seen in about half the cases. Many other viruses are known to cause diarrhea variously in toddlers, older children and adults.

Salmonella, Shigella and other bacterial pathogens also cause infantile diarrhea. Both *Salmonella* and *Shigella* are invasive organisms, typically causing fever, malaise, watery diarrhea that may contain blood and mucus. *Salmonella* infection may lead to acute gastroenteritis, nonintestinal infections, bacteremia, enteric fever (including typhoid fever), or an asymptomatic carrier state. Children under the age of 5 may continue to excrete the *Salmonella* organism for several weeks or months after resolution of their diarrhea.

The parasite *Giardia lamblia* also causes childhood diarrhea. Acute giardiasis is characterized by sudden onset watery diarrhea, with foul-smelling, often frothy stools, usually lasting 3 to 4 days. Chronic infection is marked by periodic similar episodes interrupted by asymptomatic periods. This organism is also known to affect growth. It is readily spread in day care centres, as well as via infected food and water.

Other common causes of infantile diarrhea are intolerance to cow's milk or fruit (especially apple) juice.

Treatment

The major sequela of infantile diarrhea is dehydration. Therefore, oral rehydration therapy should be administered to all children with mild to moderate dehydration. Frequent bottles, spoonfuls or sips of oral rehydration solution should be offered over 4 to 6 hours. The WHO and commercial oral rehydration solutions contain sodium, potassium and bicarbonate or citrate ions together with glucose, dextrose or rice syrup solids. The carbohydrate component takes advantage of the Na+/substrate co-transport mechanism, which is generally unimpaired during infectious diarrhea.

Breast-feeding should be continued except in cases of severe diarrhea. In any case, breast-feeding should be resumed or the child placed back on a regular diet, including solids, within the first 24 hours of the diarrheal illness. Early resumption of the normal diet stimulates the production of intestinal disaccharidases, prevents the development of fasting-provoked natriuresis, as well as minimizing the nutritional impact of the diarrheal illness. Although infectious diarrhea is associated with a transient lactase deficiency, human milk is well tolerated during diarrhea and may even reduce the severity and duration of illness. Cow's milk, which actually has less lactose than human milk, may prolong diarrhea slightly. It is recommended that a full-strength lactose-free formula or half-strength cow's milk be used during the first 48 hours, especially in very young bottle-fed infants, gradually reintroducing the patient's regular diet. Heavily sweetened fruit juices and carbonated beverages should be avoided.

Antidiarrheal agents are contraindicated in infants under 2 years of age.

ACUTE DIARRHEA IN OLDER INDIVIDUALS

In the United States, approximately half of deaths resulting from diarrhea occur in patients over the age of 74 years. Residence in a nursing home is the primary risk factor for an elderly person to develop diarrhea. The second most important risk factor is antibiotic treatment, with *Clostridium difficile* being the most important, though not most common pathogen. Refer to Table 10 for other important causes of diarrhea in the elderly.

Diarrhea potentially has more severe consequences in the elderly than for younger adults. The principal risk is dehydration, with consequent poor circulation to vital organs. Atherosclerosis predisposes the patient to dehydration-related morbidity. Diarrhea may also threaten an already compromised nutritional status. Anorexia, malabsorption, increased metabolic demands, or protein-losing enteropathy all may worsen the nutritional state.

Treatment

Prompt oral rehydration is the most important consideration in the management of diarrhea in

TABLE 10: Causes of Diarrhea in Older Individuals

Infection	**Gastrointestinal disease**
Nursing home-acquired	Obstructive lesions
Other	Dysmotility with impaction
	Inflammatory bowel disease
Iatrogenic	Malabsorption
Dietary supplements	Mesenteric atherosclerosis and ischemia
Antacids	Portal hypertension
Osmotic laxatives	
Digoxin, quinidine, methyldopa	**Systemic illness**
	Diabetes mellitus
Neoplastic disease	Thyrotoxicosis
	Uremia

older individuals, to ensure dehydration does not cause infarction of vital organs.

DIARRHEA DURING PREGNANCY

Diarrhea during pregnancy, as at other times, is most often due to viral or bacterial infection. However, especially if associated with a vaginal discharge, diarrhea may be a signal that the pregnancy is at risk. The diarrhea may be caused by relaxin, a placental hormone released to quiet uterine contractions of premature labor.

Treatment

Diarrhea in pregnancy may be treated with locally acting antidiarrheal agents and with safe antibiotics when appropriate. However, fluid replacement is the most important component of management.

TRAVELLERS' DIARRHEA

Persons from developed industrialized countries visiting a developing country risk encountering enteric pathogenic microorganisms for which they have developed no specific immunity. The result is travellers' diarrhea, defined as diarrhea with:

- three loose stools a day;
- a two-fold increase in the number of loose or watery bowel movements;
- more than two loose stools a day in association with a single gastrointestinal symptom such as cramping; or
- one loose or watery stool in association with one symptom of an enteric infection.

It affects up to one-third of those visiting developing countries. Typically, it is mild, with four to five loose or watery stools per day, first appearing 2 to 3 days after arrival, and lasting (untreated) 3 to 4 days. Often the major complaint is abdominal cramps. Malaise, nausea, mild fever and myalgias are also common accompanying symptoms. Attack rates are approximately equal in men and women. Younger travellers are more likely to develop diarrhea than those over age 55. (This may reflect different eating/drinking habits while travelling, or it may reflect different immunities.)

Enterotoxigenic *Escherichia coli* is responsible for 26% to 72% of cases of travellers' diarrhea. *Shigella* is found in about 15% in Mexico, while *Salmonella* is seen more frequently in southern Asia. Relatively few cases are due to intestinal parasites, such as *Amoeba*, *Giardia*, and *Cryptosporidium*.

Achlorhydria, or more than 2 days of therapy with drugs, such as omeprazole or lansoprazole that prohibit gastric acid secretion, is a risk factor of travellers' diarrhea.

Prophylaxis

The most important measure to avoid travellers' diarrhea is best summarized by the dictum: boil it, cook it, peel it or forget it! Travellers to high risk areas should avoid drinking the local tap water or using ice cubes made from tap water. High risk foods, as well as those recommended, are indicated in Table 11. Water can be made safe to drink by treating with tetraglycine hydroperiodide tablets, or by adding 2 drops of chlorine laundry bleach (alternatively, 4 or 5 drops of 2% tincture of iodine) per litre of water and letting stand for at least 30 minutes after mixing. If the water is turbid, these amounts should be doubled. Individuals with thyroid disorders should use iodine with caution. Water may also be sterilized by boiling vigorously for at least 10 minutes (20 minutes at high altitudes). An unpleasant taste in the boiled water might be masked by a pinch of salt. Particulate matter should be removed by filtering or straining, for instance, through clean panty hose.

Bismuth subsalicylate has been used with some success for the prophylaxis of travellers' diarrhea. However, high doses are necessary, which are inconvenient, expensive, and expose the traveller to unnecessary risk of adverse effects. Prophylactic use of 60 mL of bismuth subsalicylate 4 times daily is reported to provide a 65% protection rate.

Loperamide should not be used prophylactically to prevent travellers' diarrhea, since it will cause constipation. Prophylactic use of lactobacilli preparations is ineffective. In view of the generally mild, self-limited nature of travellers' diarrhea, prophylactic use of anti-infective agents is not recommended.

Treatment

Travellers' diarrhea is usually self-limited and patients recover in 3 or 4 days without treatment. Fluid replacement is the most important feature in its management. In mild cases, this can be achieved with soft drinks, fruit juices, hot tea, or safe water

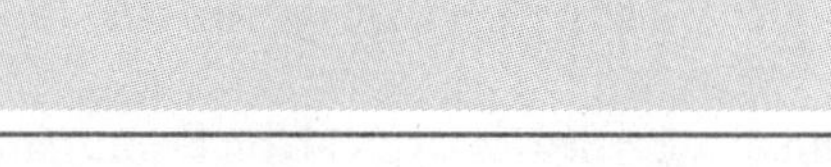

TABLE 11: Foods Associated with High and Low Risks of Travellers' Diarrhea

High-Risk Foods	Low-Risk Foods
Leafy green vegetables	Steam-cooked foods, served hot
Fresh cheese	Bread, tortillas
Buffet meats/food	Bottled water, beer, soft drinks
Milk from doubtful source	Fruits that can be peeled
Spiced sauces in open container	Fresh citrus fruits
Food from street vendors	Packaged butter and jam
Tap water, ice cubes	
Dessert	
Hamburger	

(boiled or bottled). Moderate diarrhea in adults should be treated with solutions containing a more favorable electrolyte content, such as *Gatorade* or sweetened mineral water. Patients with severe diarrhea are best treated with a commercial oral rehydration preparation. Rehydration preparations available in dose packets are smaller and easier to travel with than cans or bottles. It is essential the solution be reconstituted with clean water.

Loperamide provides symptomatic relief within a few hours. Antimotility agents should be avoided in patients with dysenteric symptoms or high fevers. These symptoms may signify *Shigella*, *Salmonella* or *Campylobacter* infection that can be prolonged or worsened by antimotility agents. These patients should be referred for formal diagnostic evaluation.

Bismuth subsalicylate (30 mL every 30 minutes for 8 doses) reduces the number of evacuations by 50%, although it does not reduce overall water loss. Other locally acting agents shown to be both safe and beneficial in reducing the symptoms of travellers' diarrhea (and other acute infectious diarrhea) are polycarbophil (twelve 500 mg tablets/day) and attapulgite (six 1,500 mg doses/day).

If necessary, the fever of travellers' diarrhea may be managed with acetaminophen.

Occasionally travellers' diarrhea develops into chronic or recurrent diarrhea. Patients with symptoms persisting after returning home should be seen by a physician.

ADVICE FOR THE PATIENT

Diarrhea

- Since the most important method of transmission of enterotoxic pathogens is by fecal-oral transmission, it is very important to always wash the hands with soap and water especially after using the toilet or changing a diaper.
- Try to drink 120 to 150 mL per hour of liquid while you are awake. Drinking frequent small amounts of fluid is better than large occasional drinks. Drinking a large volume at one time may cause vomiting, especially in children.
- If travelling to a developing country, heed the adage when considering whether food is safe to eat: Boil it, peel it, cook it or forget it.

PATIENT ASSESSMENT QUESTIONS

Q How long have you had the problem?

For adults, diarrhea lasting for more than 3 days is often more severe and may require specific therapy. A child under 3 years of age with diarrhea for more than 24 hours should be referred to a physician.

Q Is the diarrhea watery? Are the stools red or black?

Watery diarrhea is typical of noninflammatory diarrhea, which often is mild or moderately severe, and can safely be managed symptomatically. Bloody diarrhea suggests infection by an invasive pathogen, necessitating immediate referral to a physician.

Q What is the age of the individual?

Very young children and older individuals are at greatest risk of dehydration and attendant morbidity and mortality from acute diarrhea. Diarrhea in any infant under 4 months of age must be referred to a physician.

Q Is the patient experiencing excessive thirst, dry mouth, decreased urination and/or lightheadedness? If a child, is there a lack of tears? Are mucosal membranes dry? Is the skin loose or flaccid?

These are indicators of dehydration and may signify more severe illness.

Q Is there abdominal pain or fever?

Severe abdominal pain, especially in the lower left quadrant, or high fever (>38°C in infants under 2 months of age, >40°C in children under 2 years of age, >41°C in older children, or >40°C in adults) requires referral to a physician.

IRRITABLE BOWEL SYNDROME

ETIOLOGY

Irritable bowel syndrome (IBS) is defined as a functional bowel disorder in which abdominal pain is associated with defecation or a change in bowel habit, and with features of disordered defecation and distention. Since both the small and large bowels are involved, older terms such as spastic or irritable colon should no longer be used.

It is a chronic, benign disorder, often developing gradually in late adolescence or early adulthood. It occurs worldwide in 10 to 30% of the population, although probably fewer than half its sufferers seek medical care for it. Slightly more women than men suffer from IBS. While not a life-threatening condition, IBS profoundly affects those afflicted. It is disabling and one of the most common reasons for seeking health care. Work, leisure, travel and personal relationships all are affected.

The pathophysiology of IBS is poorly understood. It is an expression of intestinal hypersensitivity with no signs of anatomic or physiologic abnormality. This disordered motility is believed to be usually associated with life stress and emotional tension. Patients with IBS score higher for depression, anxiety and disordered thoughts than do control subjects in psychometric testing. Bowel spasms often are precipitated by emotional or stressful events. Nevertheless, the association of IBS with psychological disturbances may simply reflect co-morbidity rather than a cause and effect relationship.

Dietary factors probably play a role at least in a subset of patients. Abdominal pain may be provoked by "gassy" foods such as beans, milk, onions, cabbage and melons (Table 4). In some patients, ingestion of fat stimulates an exaggerated gastrocolic response resulting in smooth muscle spasms and postprandial pain. Alcohol, caffeine and sorbitol-containing gum are other common offending agents.

It was recently suggested that many cases of IBS may be due to abnormal resident gut flora. A study by Andrews and Borody showed that antibiotic pretreatment followed by bacterial replacement therapy with a mixed culture of 18 nontoxic bacteria typical of normal gut flora relieved symptoms in 76% of constipated IBS patients.

IBS symptoms may be exacerbated during menses, possibly accounting for the apparent female predominance among IBS patients. Progesterone and/or prostaglandins may be involved in the mediation of changes in bowel symptoms.

IBS was once considered to represent a spectrum of responses to a fibre-depleted diet. It is now known not to be as simple as that, but edible fibre is still an important component in its management.

SYMPTOMS

The clinical features of IBS are summarized in Table 12. Typically, patients with IBS experience intermittent episodes, characterized either by spastic constipation or by diarrhea, often alternating. There is severe, often disabling, abdominal crampy pain, usually but not always alleviated by passage of stool. Abdominal distention often accompanies the constipation and cramps and may be due to changes in bowel wall tone. Although IBS patients may believe this distention is due to excessive flatulence, the quantity and distribution of intestinal gas is normal. In most patients the passing of flatus usually relieves the symptoms, although this is not universal. The diarrhea usually is not associated with pain, although occasionally particularly severe cramps may be precipitated by an episode of diarrhea. In the constipation phase, the stools are hard pellets (rabbit-like) and may be coated with mucus. The diarrhea phase is marked by the frequent passage of small volumes of watery or pasty, unformed stools. The 24-hour stool volume is no greater than normal. Exacerbations and remissions are common throughout a personal history of many years with IBS.

Symptoms mimicking IBS may be due to lactose intolerance, food poisoning, laxative abuse, diverticular disease, amebiasis, or even colonic cancer. Thus, while IBS has a mortality rate of zero, patients must initially be referred to a physician for diagnosis, usually by exclusion of possible organic causes of the symptoms. This may necessitate a battery of tests by a gastroenterologist.

TREATMENT

IBS should be managed nonpharmacologically as far as possible. Edible fibre, accompanied by generous fluid intake, is the mainstay of a management regimen. These so-called bulk-forming agents exert a laxative effect in constipation-predominant IBS. By absorbing water, they also provide symptomatic relief of diarrhea. Over several months, fibre acts to reduce intraluminal rectosigmoid pressure, thereby relieving the cramp-like symptoms of IBS. Some patients benefit markedly from wheat bran while many report no effect. Usual practice is to start with 1 tablespoonful of bran 3 times daily with meals, adjusting the dose according to response. Colloidal fibre gels, such as psyllium, have a higher water-binding capacity than bran and may be more effective. In any case, fibre supplementation requires a long-term commitment and is unlikely to be more effective than placebo during the first month. A 6-month trial period is recommended for fibre therapy. The placebo response to any therapy of IBS symptoms ranges from 40 to 70%.

The naturally occurring fibres have few side effects, but they can cause increased flatulence and borborygmi (the sound of flatus in the intestines, sometimes jocularly called rumble-tum). Usually these side effects are transient, but certain patients cannot tolerate them, particularly from bran. Other patients find one or more forms of fibre unpalatable.

Calcium polycarbophil at a dosage of 6 g/day can benefit IBS patients with constipation or with alternating diarrhea and constipation; it has been suggested for patients complaining of significant bloating. Another alternative synthetic fibre is methylcellulose.

Other laxatives should be avoided as much as possible. Their use increases the risk of fluctuation in bowel function. Furthermore, IBS is a chronic syndrome, and chronic laxative use may be habituating. Should occasional use of a laxative be necessary, osmotic laxatives such as milk of magnesia are the drugs of choice. Long-term use of stimulant laxatives may permanently damage the myenteric plexus of the bowel.

Simethicone may be used safely in an effort to combat symptoms of flatulence in IBS. Like bran, it is at least a rational placebo agent. Alpha-galactosidase (*Beano*) has also been promoted for gas-related symptoms. However, elimination of offending dietary factors (lactose, fructose, sorbitol, etc.) is a better long-term approach.

Patients with diarrhea-predominant IBS may be treated with loperamide. This can be especially useful when a patient anticipates a diarrheal attack at the time of an important engagement. Regular use of this drug for longer than 2 days should not be

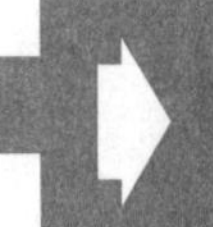

ADVICE FOR THE PATIENT

Irritable Bowel Syndrome

Lifestyle adjustments may help decrease the frequency of IBS episodes:

- Avoid commonly offending foods (caffeine, gas-producing foods, sorbitol-containing products);
- Eat smaller, more frequent meals;
- Follow a high fibre diet;
- Increase water intake.

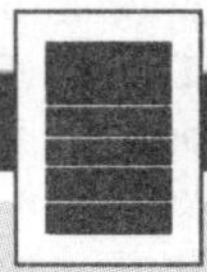

TABLE 12: Clinical Features of Irritable Bowel Syndrome

Definitive:

- Continuous or recurrent symptoms of:
  - abdominal pain (usually lower), may be severe
    - relieved by defecation and/or
    - associated with a change in frequency of stool and/or
    - associated with a change in consistency of stool
  - Irregular pattern of defecation at least 25% of the time (two or more of:)
    - altered stool frequency
    - altered stool form (hard/pellets or loose/watery)
    - altered stool passage (straining, urgency, or feeling of incomplete evacuation)
    - small stools (constipated or diarrheal)
    - passage of mucus
    - bloating or feeling of abdominal distention
  - Symptoms may be correlated with periods of stress

Suggestive:

- Age at onset less than 50 years
- Symptoms long-standing
- Symptoms not steadily progressive
- No nocturnal symptoms (awakening patient)

Exclusionary signs (excluding organic disease):

- Gradual onset of symptoms
- No abrupt change in a previously characteristic symptom pattern
- No rectal bleeding, negative occult blood test
- No rapid or unexplained weight loss
- No fever
- Normal blood count
- Normal sigmoidoscopy/colonoscopy
- Normal biochemical system

undertaken without the supervision of a physician.

Pain relief is best afforded by measures other than analgesics. Rest, local heat to the abdomen, and lukewarm tap water enemas are usually effective. Short-term use of acetaminophen is safe but is unlikely to provide significant relief.

Antispasmodic (anticholinergic) agents have been used extensively for the symptomatic management of IBS, but there is little evidence of their clinical value. These agents may have some utility in patients with pain as the predominant feature. Predictable postprandial pain might be alleviated by an antispasmodic drug taken before meals.

To better cope with their condition, sufferers of IBS need to be informed about its nature, its possible causes and management. The patient needs to be reassured periodically that the condition is not life-threatening. The sympathetic attention of a health professional is probably responsible for the significant placebo response observed in some studies. Patients may appreciate learning about the IBS Network, an independent organization that publishes a quarterly newsletter for IBS sufferers. Those interested should write to the Irritable Bowel Syndrome Network, Centre for Human Nutrition, Northern General Hospital, Sheffield, England or the International Foundation for Bowel Dysfunction, P.O. Box 17864, Milwaukee, WI (414) 964-1799.

PATIENT ASSESSMENT QUESTIONS

Q ***What is the usual pattern of your bowel movements? Has the frequency of your bowel movements or the consistency of your stools changed recently? Do you strain at stool? Have you experienced pain with the bowel fluctuations? Have you been examined recently by your physician?***

There is a wide range of frequency of bowel movements among healthy individuals. An abrupt change in bowel pattern may indicate an underlying bowel disease, including colonic cancer. However, a pattern of intermittent diarrhea and/or constipation, accompanied by crampy abdominal pain, is suggestive of IBS. The patient should initially be referred to a physician for a definitive diagnosis. Thereafter, the condition is appropriately managed with nonprescription measures.

Q ***Are your symptoms associated with particular times of the day, with environmental factors or stress, or with particular dietary factors?***

IBS often follows a pattern that may be associated with times of psychological stress or with ingesting certain foods. Awareness of this can help the patient cope with the condition.

NAUSEA AND VOMITING

ANATOMY AND PHYSIOLOGY

Nausea, a feeling of sickness in the stomach and/or the throat, is the sensation of impending vomiting. Vomiting, or emesis, is the forceful oral expulsion of stomach contents, usually preceded by spasmodic retching, whereas regurgitation refers to a more passive reflux of stomach contents into the esophagus and mouth. The vomiting manoeuvre is a protective reflex found in many species, presumably evolved for the expulsion of toxic substances ingested by the animal.

The vomiting centre (VC) located in the medulla oblongata is responsible for coordinating the abdominal and diaphragmatic contractions, together with gastric and esophageal relaxation that comprise the vomiting reflex. The VC responds to direct afferent input from sensory receptors in the stomach, and to indirect stimuli mediated by the chemoreceptor trigger zone (CTZ) on the surface of the medulla. Activation of the CTZ itself is believed to originate from the cerebral cortex (e.g., in response to unpleasant odors, sights or emotions), from the vestibular apparatus of the inner ear (disturbances of balance, such as motion sickness), and from xenobiotics such as drugs or toxins in the bloodstream. This latter function requires that the CTZ be located in a region of the brain not

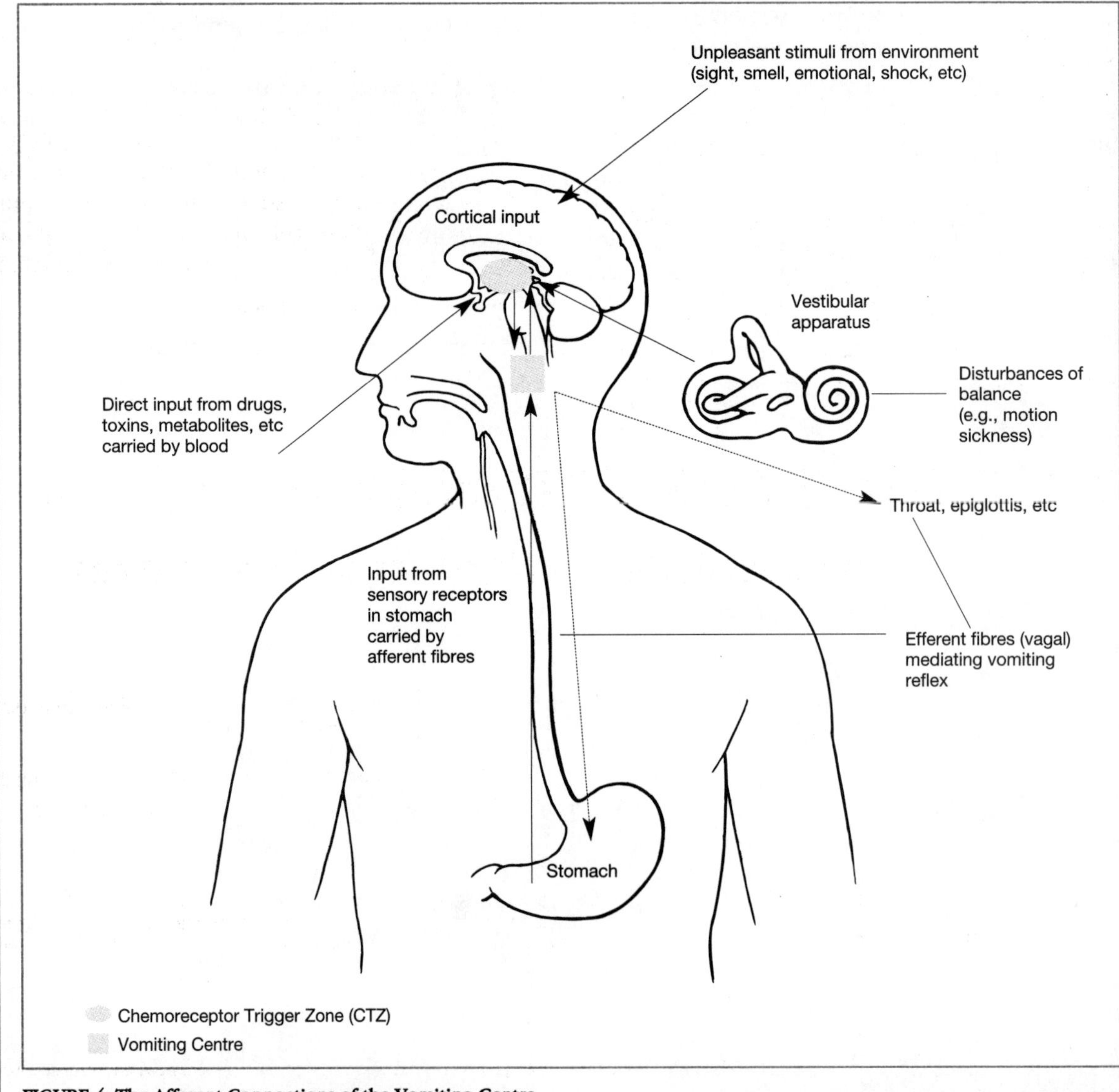

FIGURE 4: The Afferent Connections of the Vomiting Centre

protected by the blood-brain barrier. The anatomic structures involved in the vomiting reflex, showing the sites of action of antiemetic drugs, are illustrated in Figure 4.

ETIOLOGY

Motion Sickness

Motion sickness arises usually from overstimulation of the vestibular apparatus or semicircular canals of the inner ear, the mechanism responsible in vertebrates for maintaining equilibrium. Movement of the fluid in the semicircular canals is monitored by hair cell receptors, guiding the brain to make postural adjustments. Rotation of the head in two axes simultaneously, especially when the individual does not have control of the motion, may induce nausea and vomiting. Combined vestibular, visual and somatosensory inputs are integrated and compared with past sensory memories. A mismatch signal is believed to stimulate the VC via a histaminergic pathway. Cholinergic receptors are involved in the generation of signals for sensory conflict. The neural pathways mediating motion sickness are illustrated schematically in Figure 5.

In some individuals, simulation of such movement by watching a merry-go-round from close proximity or by watching a motion picture taken from a roller coaster can precipitate motion sickness. Here, visual input alone is sufficient to initiate the mismatch signal. Usually, after exposure to the same sort of motion for 1 or 2 days, an individual is able to develop tolerance to motion sickness (get one's sea legs), or acquire habituation to the provoking motion.

Morning Sickness

Nausea and vomiting occur commonly during the first trimester of pregnancy, usually beginning in the first 1 or 2 weeks, peaking at about 10 weeks, and almost always resolved by the fourth month.

ADVICE FOR THE PATIENT

Nausea and Vomiting

- Eat small meals throughout the day, so you are never too full or too hungry.
- Avoid rich fatty foods. Foods rich in carbohydrates will give you a sense of satiety without stomach upset. Try eating baked potato without butter or sour cream, white rice, and dry toast. Bland gelatin desserts (e.g., Jell-O) and nondiet ginger ale are generally well tolerated.
- Avoid nauseating smells.
- Avoid unnecessary use of drugs.

FIGURE 5

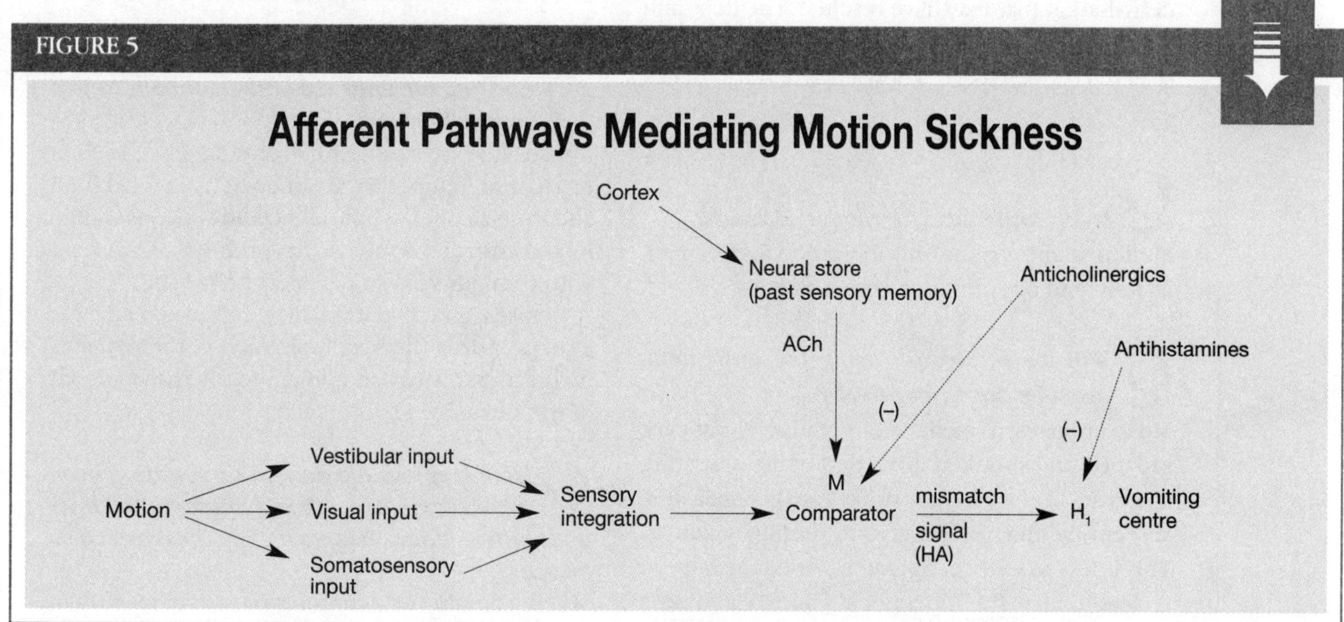

Adapted with permission from: Takeda N, Morita M, Hasegawa S, et al. Neuropharmacology of motion sickness and emesis. Acta Otolaryngol Suppl 1993;501:10–15.

Nausea and Vomiting

Some degree of morning sickness occurs in about 50% of all pregnant women. The cause of morning sickness is not completely understood, but seems to be related to elevated levels of chorionic gonadotropin, a hormone produced in the placenta.

Infectious

Nausea and vomiting often accompany diarrhea and fever secondary to enteric infections such as gastroenteritis and travellers' diarrhea. Vomiting is an early symptom of many infections; like diarrhea, the emesis represents the body's defence mechanism for ridding itself of the noxious agent.

Other

Many chemotherapeutic drugs stimulate the CTZ via serotonergic, and perhaps dopaminergic pathways. Opiates and certain other drugs, as well as many other toxic agents, also have emetic effects.

Vomiting not readily ascribed to an extrinsic stimulus or to pregnancy may be a sign of a respiratory, cardiovascular, gastrointestinal, renal, endocrinological, neurologic or psychiatric disorder.

TREATMENT

Nonpharmacological Treatment

Motion sickness can often be relieved or minimized by giving the person a stable visual earth reference. A passenger prone to car sickness usually obtains relief by sitting in the front seat and looking forward. Looking sideways or reading will provoke nausea. Alternatively, sitting in a semiprone position with the head braced at an upward angle minimizes the sensory conflict. Ship and airplane passengers who are prone to motion sickness should position themselves as near to the centre of the vehicle as possible, to minimize the extent of non-forward motion.

?

PATIENT ASSESSMENT QUESTIONS

Q *How old is the patient?*

True vomiting in an infant, as opposed to regurgitation, requires immediate referral to a physician for assessment and control, and for correction of dehydration that may have resulted. The dose and dosage form of a suitable agent can only be selected on the basis of knowledge of the patient's age.

Q *Is this antiemetic for motion sickness?*

Motion sickness is the only indication for self-medication with nonprescription antiemetics.

Q *Will the individual using the antiemetic agent be driving a vehicle?*

Most antinausea medications cause significant sedation and should not be used while operating a vehicle. In any case, car drivers are generally less susceptible than passengers to motion sickness. This is less so for boat operators, since the motion is less under the operator's control and less predictable.

Q *Is the nausea or vomiting due to pregnancy?*

Self-medication during pregnancy should be discouraged. Nonpharmacologic measures are often helpful. Severe persistent vomiting in pregnancy may signify additional complications requiring referral to a physician.

Q *Can you attribute the nausea or vomiting to some situation?*

Nausea may be caused by overindulgence in food or alcohol. Temporary abstinence from solid food and from alcohol, while maintaining adequate fluid intake, usually resolves the problem. Treatment with bismuth subsalicylate may be helpful.

Nausea and vomiting may represent adverse effects of drug therapy. Evaluation of the patient's medication history should guide the management of the situation.

Q *How long has the nausea or vomiting been a problem? Are other symptoms such as abdominal pain, headache or diarrhea also present?*

Severe vomiting or symptoms persisting more than 1 or 2 days require referral to a physician.

Excessive consumption of food or alcohol before or during travel should be avoided. At the same time, travel should not be taken on an empty stomach, when blood glucose levels are low, since this too can precipitate nausea.

Most cases of morning sickness can be managed by nonpharmacologic measures such as eating frequently throughout the day, limiting oneself to small meals of low fat, high carbohydrate foods. Plain baked potato, white rice, dry toast, gelatin dessert, and nondiet ginger ale are generally well tolerated. Strong or unpleasant odors should be avoided.

Acupuncture and acupressure have been found helpful against both motion sickness and morning sickness in up to 60% of subjects in studies where the placebo response was 30%. *Sea-Band* are one inch wide elasticized bands with a plastic button on the underside. They are worn high on both wrists, so the button exerts even pressure on the pericardial median that, according to the traditional tenets of acupuncture, controls the heart and breathing.

Pharmacological Treatment

The only indication for nonprescription drug treatment of nausea and vomiting is motion sickness. Antimotion sickness drugs are most effective if therapy is commenced before exposure to motion. Usually oral therapy should be commenced about 30 minutes before departure and repeated if necessary.

PHARMACEUTICAL AGENTS

ALGINIC ACID

Alginic acid compound products contain either alginic acid or sodium alginate, in combination with varying amounts of antacid, such as aluminum hydroxide or magaldrate. Mixed with saliva and then exposed to gastric acid, alginic acid forms a viscous foam that floats on the surface of the stomach contents. This serves as a mechanical barrier, reducing the frequency of gastroesophageal reflux. Suppression of reflux is effective only when the patient is sitting or standing. When reflux does occur, the foam has a demulcent and buffering effect, coating and protecting the esophageal mucosa from gastric acid.

Some of these products contain insufficient antacid to neutralize the gastric contents and should not be considered antacids. Because of the low dose, they also lack the side effects of antacids on bowel function. However, many combination products contain significant amounts of antacid and will have the characteristic side effects.

Alginic acid products are neither more, nor less, effective than gastric antacids in promoting healing of GER disease.

ALPHA-GALACTOSIDASE

This enzyme (*Beano*) hydrolyzes alpha-linked oligosaccharides of d-galactose (raffinose, stachyose and verbascose) into their component digestible monosaccharides and disaccharides. Thus, the oligosaccharides do not reach the colon where they would be broken down by bacterial flora to produce carbon dioxide and hydrogen, inducing flatulence. The enzyme is derived from *Aspergillus niger*, and persons sensitive to molds may react. Hypersensitivity reactions, though rare, have included gastric distress and dermatological reactions. Diabetics should be aware that use of this enzyme will render these sugars metabolically available.

ANTACIDS

Gastric antacids are bases with low solubility. Ideally, their action is limited to the lumen of the upper gastrointestinal tract. The agents used are aluminum hydroxide, calcium carbonate, magnesium hydroxide and magaldrate. The use of sodium bicarbonate as an antacid should be actively discouraged. Its action is rapid but short-lived. Worse, it may produce systemic alkalosis. Because of this and its high sodium content, it is contraindicated in people with impaired renal function, congestive heart failure or hypertension.

The selection of an antacid for occasional self-medication of dyspepsia should be based on palatability, convenience, cost and side effect profile. For GER, acid neutralization capacity (ANC) should also be considered.

Aluminum Hydroxide: Aluminum hydroxide is a slow-acting antacid with a relatively low ANC. Its principal advantage is its constipating effect, which may usefully counteract the cathartic action of magnesium hydroxide.

Aluminum-containing antacids are now believed to exert a cytoprotective action against various ulcerogenic and necrotizing agents by mechanisms independent of acid neutralization. Antacids apparently have advantages over the antisecretory agents in protecting the gastric mucosa against alcohol-induced necrosis and in preventing stress-induced ulcers in critically ill patients.

Aluminum hydroxide given immediately after meals and at bedtime can form a complex with phosphorus compounds in the gastrointestinal tract, preventing their absorption and leading to hypophosphatemia.

Aluminum is neurotoxic. Chronic heavy drinkers, who are likely to be frequent users of antacids, may have increased intestinal permeability to aluminum. A slowly progressive accumulation of aluminum in the brain has been hypothesized to be one of many factors in the development of alcoholic dementia. Aluminum is also suspected as a contributing factor in the development of Alzheimer's disease.

Calcium Carbonate: Calcium carbonate has a high ANC per g of salt. Significant amounts of calcium ion are absorbed, and the increased plasma calcium levels may stimulate gastrin secretion. This in turn stimulates more gastric acid secretion. The clinical consequences of this acid rebound effect have not been proven.

Magnesium Hydroxide: Magnesium hydroxide also has a high ANC. It is a relatively fast-acting antacid, a popular ingredient in gastric antacid products.

Magnesium hydroxide is also used as a saline laxative, and the most common side effect of its antacid use is diarrhea. This is best dealt with by combining its use with aluminum hydroxide.

Approximately 5% of the magnesium ion is absorbed systemically. Adults with normal renal function eliminate magnesium with no particular medical consequences. However, patients with impaired renal function may develop hypermagnesemia, leading to neurotoxicity. Early signs of hypermagnesemia include sedation and confusion, as well as muscle weakness, hypotension and electrocardiogram changes.

Magnesium/Aluminum Hydroxide Combinations: The most popular antacid products contain combinations of magnesium hydroxide and aluminum hydroxide, designed to balance the laxative effect of magnesium salts with the constipating effect of aluminum. Several products have equal concentrations of each, but others have more or less magnesium than aluminum. The product can be selected according to the particular needs of the user. The health professional should be aware that different products in a name product line may differ in the ratio of ion content. Product labels should be consulted to be sure of the composition of the product.

Magaldrate: Magaldrate is sometimes described as hydroxymagnesium aluminate, and has the approximate molecular composition $AlMg(OH)_7$ H_2O. Like magnesium hydroxide, the hydroxymagnesium moiety reacts rapidly with acid while the aluminate reacts more slowly. Magaldrate's buffering action does not peak as sharply as that of physical mixtures of magnesium and aluminum hydroxides, and it is sustained at a more or less constant level for over 1 hour in vitro.

Drug Interactions: Antacids interact with a variety of other drugs by several mechanisms, significantly altering the pharmacokinetics (rate or amount of absorption, or rate of renal excretion) of the second drug. Clinically significant interactions are summarized in Table 13.

Increasing gastric pH can decrease oral bioavailability of some drugs, although most antacid drug interactions involve the formation of insoluble salts or complexes with the polyvalent metal ions. Altering gastric pH obviously may alter the dissolution rate of enteric coated products.

High doses of antacids can affect urinary pH as well, increasing urinary excretion of acidic drugs and decreasing renal excretion of weak bases.

ANTICHOLINERGIC AGENTS

All anticholinergic (antispasmodic) agents should be avoided or used with caution by patients with gastroesophageal reflux disease, benign prostatic hyperplasia, narrow angle glaucoma or heart disease. Their most common side effects are dry mouth, dizziness and blurred vision. These agents are not recommended for use in children under 6 years of age.

Belladonna Alkaloids: Atropine sulfate, hyoscyamine sulfate and scopolamine hydrobromide are natural products with anticholinergic action. Theoretically they inhibit peristaltic motility of the bowel, but this action is seen only at doses that block cholinergic transmission at other sites as well, resulting in a high incidence of adverse side effects. Since diarrhea is primarily due to impaired absorption or excessive secretion, and is often characterized by decreased smooth muscle activity, the rationale for the use of antimotility agents is weak. Inclusion of these alkaloids with locally acting agents in some nonprescription antidiarrheal products is of questionable value. Their use as antispasmodics is also limited by adverse effects.

TABLE 13: Drug Interactions with Antacids

Drug	Nature of interaction	Corrective measure
Iron	Reduced absorption by up to 97%	Separate drugs by 2 hours
Salicylates	Reduced plasma salicylate by 30–70%	Avoid combination or adjust dosage
Thyroxine	Significantly reduced absorption	Adjust dose or discontinue antacid
Tetracycline	Reduced absorption by 50–90%	Separate drugs by 2 hours
Quinolones	Significantly reduced absorption	Separate drugs by 2 hours
Digoxin	Reduced absorption by 30%	Separate drugs by 2 hours
Nitrofurantoin	Reduced absorption by 20–50%	May need to adjust dosage
Penicillamine	Reduced absorption by 34%	Separate drugs by 2 hours

Dicyclomine: Dicyclomine, a nonprescription antispasmodic agent, is indicated for irritable bowel and spastic constipation. Once used for infantile colic, dicyclomine has been associated with apnea in infants and is no longer indicated for patients under 6 months of age.

Glycopyrrolate and Propantheline: These are synthetic anticholinergic agents, also indicated in adults for symptomatic treatment of irritable bowel. The efficacy of these quaternary ammonium agents has often been called into question. Like other anticholinergics, their therapeutic action is usually accompanied by side effects.

ANTIDIARRHEALS

Local-Acting Antidiarrheals

Attapulgite: Attapulgite is a hydrated magnesium aluminum silicate clay that is activated or dehydrated thermally for pharmaceutical use. It reputedly has adsorptive properties superior to kaolin, and has been demonstrated to be superior to placebo in restoring normal intestinal transit time in acute diarrhea in children. Nevertheless, because use of any antidiarrheal agent may mask fluid loss, attapulgite is contraindicated in infants under 2 years of age.

Bismuth Subsalicylate: Bismuth subsalicylate is popular, effective in reducing stool frequency and stool weights and improves stool consistency in travellers' diarrhea, although it has not been shown to reduce total fluid loss. Bismuth subsalicylate has the same effects in acute bacterial diarrhea in children when used as an adjunct to oral rehydration therapy. Internalization of bismuth by enteroinvasive bacteria is believed to interfere with the ability of the organisms to invade mucosal cells. Bismuth may also bind directly with bacterial enterotoxins.

In contrast, it plays no role in rotavirus elimination. Since this is the most common cause of acute childhood diarrhea, and in light of a possible association of salicylate with Reye's syndrome, routine use of bismuth subsalicylate in childhood diarrhea is not advised. As with other antidiarrheal agents, its use in infants under the age of 2 is contraindicated.

Excessive use of bismuth subsalicylate, especially by elderly patients who may have diminished renal function, can result in subacute salicylate toxicity (salicylism) manifested by lethargy, weakness, diminished hearing, vertigo and acidosis. Although ASA is the only salicylate strongly linked to Reye's syndrome or that irreversibly inhibits cyclooxygenase, salicylate absorption from bismuth subsalicylate also carries some risk for children and for patients with bleeding disorders.

Because bismuth is poorly absorbed from insoluble salts such as the subsalicylate, its toxicity is often overlooked. However, long-term daily ingestion of recommended doses of this product has led to CNS toxicity, characterized by progressive confusion and memory loss with possible delirium and seizures. Most patients recover gradually after discontinuing use of the drug. Patients with AIDS may be at particular risk from bismuth toxicity; a common opportunistic infection occurring with AIDS is cytomegalovirus, which causes colitis, perhaps enhancing bismuth absorption. Bismuth subsalicylate should be used for no longer than 6 or 8 weeks, followed by an 8-week bismuth-free interval.

Patients should be advised that bismuth subsalicylate will impart a transient and harmless black discoloration to the stool, due to the formation in the gut of bismuth sulfide. This discoloration does not interfere with tests for occult blood.

As a metal cation, bismuth has been considered likely to interact with drugs with chelating properties. However, in contrast to aluminum compounds, bismuth had no significant effect on the bioavailability of a single oral dose of ciprofloxacin in healthy volunteers. Salicylate can interact significantly with other drugs, and bismuth subsalicylate should not be used by patients taking anticoagulants, oral antidiabetic medications or medications for gout. *Pepto-Bismol* tablets contain calcium carbonate and should not be taken within 2 hours of ingesting tetracycline or quinolone antibiotics.

Kaolin/Pectin: Although kaolin, a natural clay, has long been thought to adsorb enteropathogens and toxins, more recent studies have shown it to be inefficient. It probably does weakly bind water. Pectin is a gel-forming carbohydrate. Combination products containing approximately 20% kaolin and 0.5 to 1% pectin have been popular home remedies for mild acute diarrhea. While safe, they have not been shown effective.

Lactobacillus Acidophilus: Dietary supplementation with lactobacilli after oral rehydration shortens the diarrheal phase of illness in young children with rotavirus infection, compared with oral rehydration alone. The lactobacilli enhance local immunoglobulin production. Prophylactic use of lactobacilli has given equivocal results in preventing iatrogenic diarrhea from amoxicillin. Perhaps more surprising is its apparent utility in diarrhea caused by other drugs such as sertraline. Unpasteurized yogurt, but not pasteurized yogurt, is probably as effective as pharmaceutical products containing live, lyophilized *Lactobacillus acidophilus*.

Antimotility Agents

Loperamide: Loperamide may be used for symptomatic relief of travellers' diarrhea and other cases of acute or infectious diarrhea in otherwise healthy adults. It reduces the number of unformed stools. Loperamide may also be used for symptomatic control of chronic diarrhea, but its long-term use should be undertaken only with a physician's supervision.

Loperamide exerts agonist actions at enteric mu-opiate receptors and antagonist actions at cholinergic receptors. It may also inhibit the local release of acetylcholine. In any event, virtually all of its antidiarrheal actions are antagonized by naloxone, an opiate antagonist. Loperamide affects both water transport and bowel motility, inhibiting fluid secretion, stimulating circular smooth muscle contraction and increasing internal anal sphincter tone. It reduces sensitivity of the recto-anal inhibitory reflex and improves rectal compliance in incontinent patients with diarrhea.

The recommended adult dosage for acute diarrhea is 4 mg (2 capsules or tablets) initially, followed by 2 mg after each unformed stool to a maximum of 16 mg per day. Loperamide is a safe, effective and long-acting bowel stopper for use in patients 12 years of age and over. Its use in children is not recommended except with the advice of a physician, and it is contraindicated in children under the age of 2. Its use in infants has led to lethargy, hallucinations, severe abdominal distention and paralytic ileus, ending in several infant deaths.

Unlike other opioids, loperamide is poorly absorbed from the gut and lacks analgesic or euphoric actions. Nevertheless, a case has been reported of physical dependence on loperamide in an adult who habitually ingested 320 mg daily during a 4-month period.

ANTIEMETICS

Dimenhydrinate: Dimenhydrinate is the 8-chlorotheophyllinate salt of diphenhydramine. Like diphenhydramine it possesses antihistaminic properties. Its antinausea properties may result from a combination of both its antihistaminic and anticholinergic actions. It is thought to block acetylcholine in the vomiting centre and chemoreceptor trigger zone. Its duration of action is about 6 hours.

Dimenhydrinate is marketed under various brand names and in a variety of dosage forms. Adult dosage forms include 50 mg tablets, 50 mg chewable tablets, 75 mg long-acting capsules (25 mg immediate release, 50 mg sustained release), and 50 or 100 mg rectal suppositories. Pediatric dosage forms are 15 mg film-coated tablets, 15 mg chewable tablets, 25 mg rectal suppositories and a liquid containing 15 mg per 5 mL. The fruit-flavored liquid also contains sorbitol and alcohol (4 to 6%). Dimenhydrinate is also available as injectable solutions for intravenous and intramuscular use. For recommended dosages see Table 14.

Dimenhydrinate is useful for mild to moderate motion sickness. For patients with severe nausea and vomiting, the oral route is impractical, and the drug may be used parenterally. Other drugs are generally more effective for severe symptoms.

Excessive sedation is a common problem of dimenhydrinate. It may also cause dizziness. Paradoxically, it sometimes causes excitement, especially in children, and nausea. Its anticholinergic action may cause dry mouth. It is contraindicated in patients with glaucoma, chronic lung disease and benign prostatic hyperplasia.

Large doses of antihistamines have been known to cause convulsions and eventually coma in young children, especially in the presence of dehydration. Doses in excess of 500 mg have produced hallucinations; doses of 700 and 800 mg are implicated in the deaths of two 2-year-old children.

In recent years dimenhydrinate has become a readily accessible and inexpensive drug of abuse. Teenagers have found it to have a mild euphoric effect and often use it in combination with alcohol or with other drugs. Many cases of dimenhydrinate overdose among teenagers have been reported across Canada, causing serious toxicity, and several provinces have legislated or encouraged the restriction of its accessibility. Dimenhydrinate products should be placed behind the counter and sold only by a pharmacist.

Diphenhydramine: While not marketed specifically as an antiemetic, diphenhydramine is also indicated for motion sickness. Like dimenhydrinate, this antihistamine possesses significant anticholinergic

TABLE 14: Recommended Dosages of Antiemetic Agents

Agent	Dosage
Dimenhydrinate	*Adults:* Oral: 50–100 mg every 4 hours PRN; or 150 mg (2 x 75 mg capsules) every 8 hours PRN Rectal: 50–100 mg every 6–8 hours PRN *Children:* 8–12 yrs of age: Oral: 25–50 mg every 6–8 hours PRN; max 150 mg/day Rectal: 25–50 mg every 6–8 hours PRN 6–8 yrs of age: Oral: 25–50 mg every 6–8 hours PRN; max 150 mg/day Rectal: 12.5–25 mg every 6–8 hours PRN 2–6 yrs of age: Oral: 15–25 mg every 6–8 hours PRN; max 75 mg/day <2 yrs of age: Only on the advice of a physician
Promethazine	*Adults:* 25 mg initially, followed by 10–25 mg every 4–6 hours PRN; max 100 mg/day *Children:* 2–12 yrs of age: 0.25–0.5 mg/kg every 4–6 hours
Scopolamine	*Adults:* 1 patch every 3 days

and sedative properties. Its use and side effects are similar to those of dimenhydrinate.

Diphenhydramine hydrochloride is available as 25 mg caplets and capsules, 50 mg capsules, an elixir containing 12.5 mg/5 mL in a 15% alcohol vehicle, and an alcohol-free children's fruit-flavored liquid containing 6.25 mg/5 mL. The children's liquid is sweetened with cyclamate and sorbitol.

Promethazine: Promethazine is another antihistamine whose antiemetic action has been considered to be mediated largely by inhibition of acetylcholine in the medullary centres. In higher dosage ranges it may have a longer duration of action (12 hours) than dimenhydrinate and is advocated for more severe motion sickness. It, too, frequently causes drowsiness. Dryness of the mouth is a common side effect. More rarely, blurred vision, dizziness and muscle weakness have been reported. Rarely, hyperexcitability and nightmares have occurred, especially in children. Allergic reactions and photosensitivity are also rare. Promethazine is contraindicated in patients who are hypersensitive to other phenothiazine drugs, and in patients with glaucoma. It is not recommended for infants under 2 years of age.

Promethazine is supplied as 10, 25 and 50 mg tablets and as a syrup containing 10 mg/5 mL. The syrup also contains sucrose (3.6 g/5 mL) and alcohol (3%). For recommended dosages see Table 14.

Scopolamine: One of the belladonna alkaloids related to atropine, scopolamine is an anticholinergic agent. Its antinausea action probably results primarily from inhibition of cholinergic transmission between the vestibular apparatus and the medullary centres. It may also act directly on the vomiting centre. It is effective in quelling severe motion sickness, but to be effective orally, scopolamine needs to be administered hourly.

Scopolamine is available without prescription as a skin patch. Each patch or disc contains 1.5 mg scopolamine and is designed to release 1 mg over 3 days. Maximum blood levels are reached in about 12 hours, and urinary excretion of scopolamine continues for up to 12 hours after removal of the patch.

Each disc is sealed in a separate pouch. It must be applied immediately after removal from the pouch. For optimal absorption, the disc is placed on a dry, hairless area on the back of the ear, the most permeable skin on the body. It should be applied 8 to 12 hours before the antiemetic effect is required. If protection is not needed for 3 days, the patch should be removed at the end of the journey. If therapy is needed for longer, the first disc should be removed after 72 hours and a second applied behind the other ear. The used discs should be disposed of securely out of reach of children and pets. The hands should be washed thoroughly after handling the discs, and the patient should refrain from fingering the attached disc to avoid contaminating the eyes with scopolamine. Should it come into direct contact with the eyes, it is likely to cause pupil dilation and blurred vision temporarily.

About 40% of users of transdermal scopolamine experience transient dryness of the mouth, and 12% report blurred vision; some of the latter probably due to inadvertent transfer to the eye by the fingers. Irritation of the eyelids occurs occasionally, as does local irritation at the site of application. Drowsiness also occurs occasionally. Reports of other CNS effects such as dizziness, impaired memory, confusion and hallucinations are rare. Urinary retention occurs rarely.

Withdrawal of scopolamine after several days use may lead to transient dizziness, nausea, vomiting, headache and disturbances of balance.

Scopolamine is contraindicated in patients with angle-closure glaucoma or a predisposition to glaucoma. Patients with a history of intraocular pressure pain or blurred vision must not use scopolamine without first having an ophthalmological examination to exclude glaucoma. Scopolamine should be used in pregnancy only if the anticipated benefit outweighs the potential risk to mother and fetus.

Pyridoxine: In doses of 25 or 50 mg, 2 or 3 times daily, pyridoxine (vitamin B_6) is effective against morning sickness. While the mechanism of its antinausea action is not known, it may affect the balance in the CNS between GABA, an inhibitory neurotransmitter, and glutamate, an excitatory transmitter. Pyridoxine is believed to be nonteratogenic.

Phosphorated Carbohydrate Solution: This is an oral solution containing glucose, fructose and sufficient phosphoric acid to produce a pH of 1.5 to 1.6. It is reputed to act locally on the wall of the hyperactive gastrointestinal tract, reducing smooth muscle contractions and relieving nausea. Data supporting its efficacy are lacking.

The usual adult dose is 15 to 30 mL at 15-minute intervals for a maximum of 5 doses. Because its effect depends on its osmotic action, the solution should not be diluted, and the patient should refrain from drinking other fluids within 15 minutes before or after taking a dose of phosphorated carbohydrate solution.

GRIPE WATER

Gripe water has not been shown effective in the management of colic. There is some concern about the alcohol content of some of these products.

HISTAMINE H_2-RECEPTOR ANTAGONISTS

Cimetidine[1]: Cimetidine has been in Canada as a prescription drug since 1977. It was the first of a group of drugs known as histamine H_2-receptor antagonists. These drugs inhibit the production of gastric acid by blocking the action of histamine on parietal cells in the stomach. All histamine H_2-receptor antagonists are equally effective in suppressing acid secretion, although they require different doses. These agents should not be used for more than 2 weeks without a physician's supervision. As in the case of antacids, these drugs may provide relief of symptoms of hyperacidity without necessarily healing the underlying cause. Persistent or recurrent symptoms should be investigated by a physician. Even as prescribed drugs, H_2-antagonists are less effective in healing GER disease than they are against PUD. Patients should be advised not to use histamine H_2-antagonists to relieve dyspeptic symptoms associated with NSAID use (including nonprescription use of ASA, ibuprofen and naproxen).

If approved for nonprescription use for heartburn and dyspepsia, cimetidine will be available as 100 mg tablets, with a recommended dose of 1 to 2 tablets up to 4 times a day, not exceeding 800 mg/day.

Cimetidine has been associated with a low incidence of mild and transient diarrhea, as well as skin rash and, occasionally, hives. Cimetidine is able to enter the central nervous system, sometimes leading to side effects such as headache and dizziness.

[1]Switch from prescription to nonprescription status expected in 1996.

High doses over a prolonged period may cause confusion, especially in elderly patients who may not be able to metabolize the drug as efficiently as younger adults. Excessive dosage of the drug can also have hormonal effects, causing breast growth in men and sexual dysfunction. These side effects are reversed on discontinuation of the drug.

It is important that patients using other medication seek the advice of a pharmacist or physician before taking cimetidine. Cimetidine can interfere with the metabolism of a number of other drugs, resulting in the equivalent of an overdose of the other drug. It can increase blood alcohol levels.

Famotidine[1]: Nonprescription famotidine would be marketed as 10 mg tablets, with a maximum daily dose of 2 tablets.

Like cimetidine, famotidine enters the central nervous system and may cause headache, dizziness and anxiety. Except for low incidences of transient diarrhea or constipation, it is not known to cause other side effects. Famotidine has not been shown to interact with other drugs or with alcohol.

Ranitidine[1]: Although ranitidine is believed not to enter the central nervous system, its side effect profile is very similar to those of the other histamine H_2-receptor antagonists, including mild diarrhea, skin rash and hives. It does not inhibit the hepatic metabolism of other drugs, although it does inhibit gastric alcohol dehydrogenase, and thus can increase blood alcohol levels.

LACTASE

Lactase is a normal constituent of the small intestine. Its deficiency is probably hereditary, with highest prevalence in non-Caucasians. This enzyme cleaves the unabsorbable lactose into its constituent monosaccharides, glucose and galactose, which can then be absorbed. Pharmaceutical products containing lactase derived from yeasts are available in liquid and in tablet form. The liquid is intended to be added to milk prior to use. Five drops will hydrolyze approximately 70% of the lactose in 1 L of milk at refrigerator temperature in 24 hours or 2 hours at 30°C. The tablets are to be ingested immediately prior to eating food containing lactose. While dosage varies according to the individual and to the amount of lactose consumed, the usual dose is 3 tablets.

LAXATIVES

Laxatives are usually classified according to the nature of their action. They include bulk-forming agents or fibre products, osmotic laxatives, so-called stimulant or contact laxatives, lubricants, and stool-softeners or emollients. This classification is somewhat anachronistic, as it implies inaccurate descriptions of their mechanisms of action. However, the classification scheme is convenient for discussing some features.

Table 15 classifies the agents according to their onset of action.

Side Effects

The incidence of abdominal cramps after the use of sennosides and diphenylmethane laxatives is about 10%, three times more than after placebo. Dosage of sennosides is easier to adjust to avoid cramps and diarrhea than that of diphenolics. Saline laxatives may disturb the systemic electrolyte balance; in patients with impaired renal function, magnesium sulfate and even magnesium hydroxide can cause hypermagnesemia.

Toxicity

Laxatives in use today are well tolerated and safe drugs. Laxative abuse (taken in excessive doses) can lead to hypokalemia, metabolic alkalosis and renal tubular damage. However, regular use of doses sufficient to produce soft, formed stools has not been shown to cause any untoward effects.

Use of laxatives for chronic constipation for between 10 and over 60 years led to so-called cathartic colon in 27 documented cases. This syndrome was characterized by loss of haustration (circular muscle segmentation), dilated lumens of both the colon and terminal ileum, mucosal atrophy and other macroscopic and microscopic pathologies. It is now believed that cathartic colon was caused by the use of podophyllin. Several of the victims had also used aloe and/or calomel. While aloe is still found in some products, podophyllin and calomel laxatives are no longer available. All reported cases of cathartic colon occurred in patients who began their laxative use before 1960.

Long-term use of anthraquinones and, to a lesser extent, diphenylmethanes is known to produce melanosis coli, due to the presence of pigment-

[1]Switch from prescription to nonprescription status expected in 1996.

loaded macrophages in the submucosa. The laxatives damage the colonocytes, which migrate to the intercryptal space where they are phagocytized by macrophages. The pigment derived from anthraquinones is darker than that from the other drugs, and so the melanosis is more closely associated with senna and danthron. The pigmentation is reversible on discontinuation of laxative use and has no apparent pathophysiologic consequences. There is no statistical link between habitual laxative use and colorectal cancer.

The damage to the autonomic myenteric plexus of the colon alleged to be caused by anthraquinones is controversial. Nerve damage was observed in experimental animals given danthron in high doses for 4 months, but not in lower doses. Because it is absorbed from the small intestine, danthron may cause systemic toxicity. Chronic administration of clinically relevant doses of sennosides, both in patients and in animals, has not been shown to produce any morphological damage of the autonomic nervous system of the colon. On the other hand, abnormalities of the nerve plexus have been observed in constipated patients, with or without laxative use.

Dietary Fibre and Bulk-Forming Laxatives

Edible fibre, not digested before it reaches the colon, is unabsorbed. Natural fibre is partly depolymerized by colonic bacteria, forming small organic anions that contribute an osmotic effect, drawing water into the lumen of the colon. The principal mechanism of action of fibre, however, is absorption of several times its mass of water, swelling and increasing the bulk of the intestinal contents. The resulting mechanical distention stimulates a reflex peristalsis, while the absorbed water also softens the stools. These effects appear within 24 hours, but if fibre is used repeatedly, the full effect may be delayed for several days. Fibre is considered to con-

TABLE 15: Laxative and Cathartic Agents

Agent	Type	Adult Dosage
Onset of action: 1-3 days		
Bran	bulk	6-12 g/day
Methylcellulose	bulk	initially: 5-15 mL three times daily maint: 5-15 mL once daily
Polycarbophil	bulk	4-6 g/day
Psyllium hydrophilic mucilloid	bulk	3.5 g one to three times daily
Docusate calcium	stool softener	50-300 mg/day
Docusate sodium	stool softener	50-300 mg/day
Mineral oil	lubricant	15-45 mL/day
Lactulose	osmotic	15-30 mL/day
Onset of action: 6-12 hours		
Bisacodyl tablet	stimulant	5-10 mg/day
Phenolphthalein	stimulant	30-70 mg/day
Cascara sagrada	stimulant	dose varies with dosage form
Senna	stimulant	dose varies with dosage form
Onset of action: 15-60 minutes		
Bisacodyl suppository	stimulant	1-2 suppositories
Glycerin suppository	stimulant	1 suppository
Phosphate enema	osmotic	100 mL
Mineral oil enema	lubricant	100 mL
Bisacodyl microenema	stimulant	5-10 mL
Bowel evacuants		
Magnesium citrate	osmotic	15 g
Magnesium hydroxide	osmotic	1.2-3.6 g/day; or up to 50 mL of 8% solution
Magnesium sulfate	osmotic	5-10 g

tribute to the regulation of too fast or too slow gut transit times. Good sources of dietary fibre are bran, whole grains, fresh or dried fruit, and vegetables. The fibre content of selected foods is listed in Table 7.

Edible fibre commonly causes flatulence and abdominal distention. This is usually transient, caused by bacterial metabolism of the agent. It can be minimized by increasing fibre intake gradually, over a couple of weeks, thus allowing adjustment of the colonic flora. Should one source of fibre, bran for example, cause persistent flatulence, switching to or supplementing with a different type should relieve this. Excessive bran may interfere with mineral absorption.

Edible fibre has been shown to provide some protection against cancer of the colon. Different types of fibre are believed to exert different, synergistic, effects. Insoluble fibre adsorbs potential carcinogens in the gut, while the more fermentable soluble fibre produces higher levels of short chain fatty acids that are required for normal colonocyte proliferation and differentiation.

Pharmaceutical fibre, or bulk-forming laxatives, represent a concentrated form of nonstarch polysaccharides. It is useful for individuals who cannot take adequate dietary fibre. It is most useful in preventing constipation and helpful in mild constipation but rarely adequate in severe cases. It should not be used where there is fecal impaction or megacolon. Bulk-forming laxatives must be taken with adequate fluids to avoid esophageal and colonic obstruction, and fecal impaction.

Bran Products: Raw wheat bran contains more than 40% insoluble fibre; processed bran 25%. Wheat bran is widely considered to be the most effective, as well as the most cost-effective, dietary measure for preventing constipation. Recommended daily intake varies from 6 to 12 g, up to 30 g, in divided doses.

Methylcellulose: The recommended dose is 5 to 15 mL, 3 times a day initially, tapering later to 5 to 15 mL, once daily.

Polycarbophil Calcium: This is the calcium salt of a synthetic loosely cross-linked highly hydrophilic polycarboxylic acid resin. It is not absorbed and has no pharmacological action. Its hydrophilicity enables it to absorb many times its own mass of water by hydrogen bonding.

The recommended adult daily dose of polycarbophil calcium is 4 to 6 g (2 or 3 chewable 500 mg tablets, 4 times a day). For children over 6 years of age, the dose is 1 tablet, 3 or 4 times daily. Polycarbophil calcium in this dosage regimen is effective for management of both constipation and diarrhea. In both instances, concomitant intake of adequate water (at least 250 mL) is imperative.

Psyllium Hydrophilic Mucilloid: Psyllium, a product of plantago seed, consists largely of a mucilage that swells into a gelatinous mass when mixed with water. As with other pharmaceutical fibre products, it is not absorbed and has no systemic effects. Psyllium can cause serious allergic reactions in sensitized individuals when either ingested or inhaled. This is particularly hazardous in manufacturing plants where airborne psyllium dust may be present, but the fine dust can be aerosolized when dispensing or measuring individual doses.

While indicated as a bulk-forming laxative, psyllium has been shown to be more effective than either wheat bran or polycarbophil calcium in improving fecal consistency and viscosity in experimentally induced diarrhea in healthy volunteers.

The usual adult dose is 3.5 g, 1 to 3 times daily. Psyllium products are available in a number of dosage forms, including flavored or unflavored, plain or sugar-free, regular or effervescent powders, granules and fibre wafers. The plain powders are approximately 50% dextrose. The effervescent preparations have a high sodium content. *Fibrepur* powder is 100% psyllium hydrophilic mucilloid with no additives.

The usual method advocated for administration of psyllium powder is to suspend it in 240 mL of cool water or fruit juice, and drink it immediately before the mixture thickens or settles out. Some individuals may find it more convenient and palatable to sprinkle the powder on their breakfast cereal in place of sugar. In either case, the ingestion of an additional 240 mL of fluid is recommended.

Sterculia Gum: Sterculia or karaya gum is related to tragacanth. It is a hygroscopic bulking agent, available as granules, which are to be placed directly on the tongue and swallowed with plenty of fluid without chewing. Allergic skin reactions and asthma have been ascribed to sterculia.

Osmotic Laxatives

These are ions or small molecules that are poorly absorbed from the gut. Their presence increases the osmotic pressure in the lumen of the bowel, drawing water from the mucosa in an effort to dilute the osmotically active solution. These agents are helpful when stools are hard.

Saline Laxatives

Saline laxatives act within ½ to 3 hours. They are used primarily for acute evacuation of the bowel before diagnostic or surgical procedures, and after certain anthelmintics to eliminate parasites. Side effects of saline laxatives include fluid and electrolyte depletion. Their toxicities are due to the cationic components. Magnesium salts can cause CNS toxicity in patients with renal dysfunction, while sodium salts are toxic in patients with congestive heart failure.

Magnesium Salts: Magnesium ions are poorly absorbed from the gut. Magnesium ion is believed also to stimulate the release both of cholecystokinin, a hormonal stimulant of intestinal secretion, and of prostaglandins, modulators of intestinal motility. Thus the laxative effect of magnesium salts is thought to be mediated by a combination of osmotic and hormonal mechanisms.

The poorly soluble magnesium hydroxide may safely be used occasionally for simple constipation. The dose should be adjusted to produce a soft formed stool. Usual adult doses range from 1.2 to 3.6 g per day, or up to 50 mL of 8% hydrated magnesium hydroxide suspension.

Soluble salts, such as magnesium sulfate (*Epsom Salts*) and magnesium citrate, often produce abdominal distention and the sudden passing of a large liquid stool. These salts are partially absorbed, which can lead to dangerous CNS depression in renal insufficiency or with chronic use. Magnesium salts are contraindicated in infants under 2 years of age, and are not to be used orally in children under 6. The use of magnesium citrate is generally restricted to bowel cleansing before investigative or surgical procedures. The adult purgative dosage is 15 g, preceded by at least four, hourly intakes of 250 to 300 mL of clear fluid, and followed by 300 mL/hour for 3 more hours. The solution can be made more palatable by chilling beforehand. Laxative doses for constipation are one-quarter to one-half this evacuant dose.

PEG-Electrolyte Lavage Solutions: These preparations are intended primarily for whole bowel irrigation, preparatory to a diagnostic or surgical procedure. They may also be used under medical supervision to treat fecal impaction in the elderly or children. The polyethylene glycol together with iso-osmotic concentrations of electrolytes allows the administration of large volumes of the solutions unaccompanied by net absorption or secretion of ions or water. To maintain the proper osmolality, no additional flavorings or other ingredients may be added to the solution.

Up to 4 L of the solution is administered over 3 hours (240 mL every 10 minutes) to completely flush the bowels. Each portion of the solution is preferably drunk rapidly, "chugged" rather than sipped. Lavage is complete when the fecal discharge is clear.

When used for bowel cleansing, solid foods must be avoided for at least 3 hours prior to use and until after the diagnostic or surgical procedure.

Contraindications to the use of PEG-electrolyte lavage solutions include ileus, intestinal obstruction or perforation, and megacolon. Caution should be used in patients with ulcerative colitis. Use in children must be carefully supervised to avoid dehydration.

Nausea, abdominal fullness and bloating are reported by up to 50% of patients. Cramps, vomiting and anal irritation may also occur. Other medications taken orally within an hour of starting gastric lavage are likely to be flushed from the gastrointestinal tract before their absorption is complete.

Carbohydrate Derivatives

Lactulose: A disaccharide that is not hydrolyzed by pancreatic enzymes, lactulose is poorly absorbed from the small bowel. It is hydrolyzed by colonic bacteria, then oxidized to smaller anions that exert an osmotic effect similar to that of the saline laxatives. The expected onset of laxative action is 24 to 48 hours. Some patients cannot tolerate the sweet taste of lactulose. As with edible fibre, flatulence and abdominal distention are common, caused by bacterial metabolism of the agent, and can be minimized by introducing the therapy gradually. Lactulose (15 to 30 mL/day) is highly effective in severe constipation, including impaction, and may be used safely for prolonged therapy. However, because of its nutrient effect, lactulose disrupts intestinal flora, and its effectiveness may diminish with continued use.

Inulin: Solutions of inulin are useful for infant constipation.

Mannitol: Mannitol is used as a bowel evacuant by only about 5% of gastroenterologists in North America. It is used as a 1.5% (w/v) solution in doses of 6 to 17 mL/kg.

Stimulant Laxatives

The term stimulant laxative is used to characterize three groups of chemically and pharmacologically unrelated agents once believed to act by somehow stimulating smooth muscle contraction of the colon. They are now known to act primarily by modulation of fluid secretion by the colonic mucosa.

Anthraquinone Derivatives

Anthraquinone Glycosides

These natural products act as prodrugs. They are biologically inactive carrier forms that are not digested or absorbed in the small bowel. The sugar group is hydrolyzed by colonic bacteria, releasing the active anthraquinone aglycones to the colon. The glycosidic linkage can be of two types, the O-glycosides, which are almost completely hydrolyzed by colonic bacteria, and the somewhat more lipophilic C-glycosides, which are partially absorbed and less completely hydrolyzed in the colon. Absorption of the aglycone from the colon is minor (≈ 2%). Anthraquinones stimulate active secretion of chloride ions by epithelial cells in the colon and exert an indirect action via serotonin, prostaglandin and histamine neurohormonal pathways. No pathologic damage to the mucosa has been detected after chronic administration of therapeutic doses.

The onset of action of the anthraquinone glycosides is about 6 to 12 hours. The agents are ideally taken at bedtime, with an expectation of results after breakfast the following morning. The importance of allowing time for defecation after breakfast should be emphasized.

Senna (leaves, seed pods): Products containing standardized crystalline sennosides are the stimulant laxatives of choice. Products containing the crude drug are likely to cause griping.

The glycosides of senna are mainly the desirable O-glycosides. Standardized senna has been described as a physiological bowel motility regulator. Taken in appropriate doses, it may enhance the postprandial gastrocolic reflex rather than having a laxative action per se. Senna may have an advantage for chronic atonic constipation in the elderly. A senna/fibre combination has been found to be more effective and more economical than lactulose, producing a greater frequency of bowel movements, with better stool consistency and greater ease of evacuation.

In appropriate doses, standardized senna is well tolerated, with a low incidence of adverse effects. The nonsennoside components of senna products may discolor the urine and feces.

Cascara (bark): The glycosides of cascara sagrada have been standardized as casanthranol, which consists of both O- and C-glycosides. The product is less potent and perhaps has a less predictable action than standardized senna.

Rhubarb (root): The glycosides of rhubarb are so far unstandardized, and products are therefore more likely to be irritant, griping and generally undesirable.

Aloe: Extracts of aloe consist largely of C-glycosides as well as aglycones. They are irritant, griping and spasmogenic. Aloe has also been found to cause nephrotoxicity. Products containing aloe should be avoided.

Danthron: This is a synthetic anthraquinone. Lacking the sugar group, danthron is absorbed and extensively metabolized. Absorption is increased when the drug is combined with docusate. Some of the absorbed drug is glucuronidated and excreted in the bile; the glucuronide is hydrolyzed in the colon, releasing the active drug. The absorbed fraction rarely may lead to hepatotoxicity. Danthron has about 10% of the potency of standardized senna.

Triphenylmethane Derivatives

Bisacodyl and phenolphthalein both are absorbed extensively. Much of the dose (up to 20% of bisacodyl) is excreted in the urine. Phenolphthalein will color alkaline urine pink. Some of the absorbed drug, though, is glucuronidated in the liver and excreted in the bile. The glucuronide remains unchanged and unabsorbed in the small bowel but is hydrolyzed by bacteria in the colon, releasing the active drug. The laxative action of these drugs has been postulated to be due to induction of the synthesis of nitric oxide, a smooth muscle relaxant and mediator of electrolyte secretion. The triphenylmethanes have narrow therapeutic dosage ranges and commonly produce a watery stool. Both drugs appear in breast milk and can be expected to have a laxative effect in a nursing infant.

Bisacodyl: This drug is available as enteric coated tablets, rectal suppositories and as a microenema. Taken orally, its laxative action is seen in 6 to 12 hours. The rectal dosage forms produce a laxative action in a few minutes to an hour. The patient should be encouraged to retain the rectal dosage form for as long as possible to maximize its effectiveness. The suppositories may cause a burning sensation, and repeated use can lead to local inflammation.

Phenolphthalein: Phenolphthalein is marketed in a variety of oral dosage forms, such as tablets, chocolate wafers and chewing gum. Probably because of the way it has been promoted, phenolphthalein is widely used and abused. Its chronic abuse can lead to osteomalacia. More common adverse effects of phenolphthalein are allergic reactions, especially skin reactions including fixed-drug eruptions, Stevens-Johnson syndrome and lupus erythematosus.

Miscellaneous

Castor Oil: The active constituent of castor oil is ricinoleic acid, which initiates a secretory response in the gastrointestinal tract, acting primarily on the small intestine. Castor oil acts in 1 to 3 hours, producing a watery stool. It is intended only as a bowel evacuant and should not be used as a laxative.

Lubricant Laxatives

Mineral Oil: A mixture of saturated hydrocarbons, so-called heavy mineral oil (liquid petrolatum) (e.g., *Nujol*) coats the stool and bowel wall with a water-immiscible film. The fecal mass is softened and lubricated, making its passage easier, and colonic reabsorption of water is retarded. Taken in doses of 15 to 45 mL, it acts in 6 to 8 hours.

Mineral oil is absorbed to a limited extent but not metabolized or eliminated, so it accumulates in the lymph nodes, gastrointestinal mucosa, liver and spleen, causing a foreign body granulomatous reaction. Oral use of mineral oil can lead to a fatty liver. While more palatable in emulsified form, its absorption is enhanced by emulsifying agents. It crosses the placental barrier.

Ingestion of mineral oil around mealtime inhibits absorption of the fat-soluble vitamins A, D, E, K and of calcium and phosphorus. Daily use in pregnancy can produce significant hypovitaminosis K and hypoprothrombinemia within 2 weeks.

Oral administration of mineral oil carries with it a risk of aspiration, which could cause lipid pneumonia, especially if the patient lies down after taking it. Another disadvantage of mineral oil is the possibility of anal leakage, with sequelae such as anal itching and hemorrhoids. Finally, mineral oil use has been implicated statistically in intestinal cancer.

The oral use of mineral oil is best avoided altogether. In particular, it should not be given to elderly, bedridden, pregnant patients or to children under 6 years of age.

The use of mineral oil enemas is safe but messy.

Stool Softeners

Docusate Calcium and Docusate Sodium: Stool softeners exert a surfactant activity, enhancing the penetration of water into the feces. They should not be considered laxatives, and they are ineffective at alleviating constipation. They may help prevent constipation and are often recommended for cardiac patients and patients with hemorrhoids or other painful anorectal conditions. Their usefulness and safety alone or in combination with laxatives is debatable. Docusate is absorbed significantly. It is believed to enhance the hepatotoxicity of other drugs.

Combination Products

Some combinations of laxative agents acting by different mechanisms are marketed. Significant are stimulant laxatives with other agents. Standardized sennosides with docusate sodium is rational, if docusate is useful. It is indicated for cardiac patients in whom straining must be avoided, as well as for constipation in the presence of hemorrhoids or anal fissures. It is sometimes recommended for postpartum constipation as well, although it should be avoided by nursing mothers. Products combining danthron and docusate should be avoided for any patient. The docusate component is strongly suspected to enhance the absorption and hepatotoxicity of danthron.

The combination of psyllium with senna is rational for relief of acute constipation and obstipation and, in particular, for constipation in elderly patients who have diminished muscle tone and gastrocolic reflex.

Concomitant use of mineral oil and docusate should be avoided since the surfactant docusate will likely increase absorption of the oil.

Enemas

Enemas are indicated in acute constipation, especially in the presence of fecal impaction. They are also used for cleansing the bowel before rectal examination, pre- and post-operatively to relieve fecal or radiographic impaction, collecting stool samples during pregnancy, before and after delivery and radiography. Warm tap water or saline enemas are preferable to soaps, which are likely to irritate the colonic mucosa. Hypertonic phosphate enemas are most efficacious, but they too may be irritating. A properly administered enema will cleanse the distal colon within an hour.

Unskilled administration of an enema can lead to colonic perforation. Repeated use of phosphate enemas can cause electrolyte imbalance: the ions may be absorbed from the rectum, and other ions are lost in the ensuing evacuation. Tap water and soap enemas in the presence of megacolon can cause water intoxication. Medically unsupervised use of enemas in infants under 2 years of age is contraindicated.

Bisacodyl microenemas are an alternative to the suppositories for adults, delivering 10 mg of bisacodyl to the rectum. The 5 mL volume is too small to permit delivery to the colon.

Suppositories

Rectal suppositories are less effective than enemas but are more acceptable to most patients. They may be used for evacuating the distal colon but are ineffective if the stool is dry and hard.

Glycerin suppositories have an osmotic effect that dehydrates the rectal mucosa, producing local irritation and stimulating the peristaltic reflex. Evacuation occurs within 30 minutes of insertion. Glycerin suppositories are considered safe and may be used in pregnancy and even in infants, although administration to children under 6 is not recommended except on the advice of a physician.

ORAL REHYDRATION THERAPY SOLUTIONS

Infants with acute diarrhea should be rehydrated during a 4- to 6-hour period, optimally with a commercially available oral rehydration therapy solution. These products are properly constituted to provide fluid and electrolytes in concentrations optimal for absorption and physiological balance. Decarbonated soft drinks do not provide sufficient electrolytes, and cola drinks have an additional diuretic action due to their caffeine content. Homemade salt solutions carry the risk of causing sodium overload.

Pedialyte and *Lytren* both contain citrate that will help to correct acidosis, and glucose (dextrose) to provide the energy required for active absorption of the ions. *Gastrolyte* is supplied as single dose packets of crystals for reconstitution in water. This makes possible the use of a few doses when needed and storage of the unopened remainder for future occasions. Opened containers of these solutions may be stored in a refrigerator for up to 24 hours. *Gastrolyte* has the potential disadvantage of improper reconstitution by the parent, who should be carefully counselled on the importance of following the dilution directions on the label. There may be a temptation to underdilute the product to make it even better or stronger, and this may exacerbate osmotic diarrhea. Overdilution would lead to inadequate electrolyte absorption.

Rehydration of older children and adults suffering from acute diarrhea can be achieved safely by drinking noncaffeinated and nonalcoholic beverages. Children under the age of 3 who have had diarrhea for less than 24 hours and who do not exhibit signs of dehydration can also be managed this way, or by use of a homemade remedy of fruit juice containing honey or corn syrup and a pinch

TABLE 16: Home Treatment of Acute Diarrhea

Glass I	Glass II
240 mL fruit juice (source of K^+) 2.5 mL honey or corn syrup (glucose) 1 pinch salt (NaCl)	240 mL tap water (preferably boiled and cooled) 1.25 g baking soda ($NaHCO_3$)

Directions: One glass of each is prepared and taken alternately. Supplement with other fluids.*

*These dextrose-electrolyte solutions may also be obtained commercially.

Reprinted with permission from: Frail DM. Antidiarrheals. In: Carruthers-Czyzewski P, ed. Self-medication. Reference for Health Professionals. 4th ed. Ottawa: Canadian Pharmaceutical Association, 1992:323.

of salt (Table 16), alternating with a 0.5% solution of baking soda.

SIMETHICONE

Simethicone is a chemically and physiologically inert substance that is not absorbed from the gastrointestinal tract. It reduces the surface tension of small gas bubbles so they break or coalesce to produce free gas or bubbles large enough to be easily expelled from the stomach by belching. However, since symptoms of bloating and abdominal distention are not usually associated with excessive gas in the stomach, treatment of these symptoms with simethicone is often not successful.

The efficacy of simethicone remains a matter of controversy. Drops containing simethicone 40 mg/mL (0.5 to 1 mL) given before meals were shown to decrease the amplitude and frequency of colicky crying attacks. Other anecdotal reports suggest simethicone is no more effective than placebo. Perhaps the best advice is to give it before feeding a child subject to colic rather than after the child is already crying. There is general agreement that simethicone is harmless and causes no side effects.

RECOMMENDED READING

Dyspepsia

Ching CK, Lam SK. Antacids: indications and limitations. Drugs 1994;47:305-17.

Various authors. Gastroenterol Clin North Am 1993;22:43-57.

Various authors. J Physiol Pharmacol 1993; 44(3 Suppl 1).

Gastroesophageal Reflux

Garnett WR. The one-minute counselor: a pharmacist's guide to the treatment of GER disease. Amer Pharm 1993;NS33 (1): insert.

Various authors. Gastroenterol Clin North Am 1990;19.

Gastrointestinal Gas

Levitt MD. Excessive gas: patient perception vs. reality. Hosp Pract 1985;20(11):163.

Levitt MD. How to handle complaints of "too much gas". DrugTherapy 1987;17(10):76-79, 83-86.

Infantile Colic

Vesterfelt KL, Steinberg SK. The pharmacist's role in counselling new parents. Infant Care 1989; (May):14-18.

Constipation

Almond P. Constipation: a family-centred approach. Health Visit 1993;66:404-405.

Various authors. Pharmacology 1993;47 (suppl 1): 138-260.

van der Horst ML, Sykula JA, Lingley K. The constipation quandary. Can Nurse 1994;90(1):25-30

Diarrhea

Various authors. Gastroenterol Clin North Am 1993;22:483-707.

Irritable Bowel Syndrome

Dancey CP, Backhouse S. Towards a better understanding of patients with irritable bowel syndrome. J Adv Nurs 1993;18:1443-1450.

Pattee PL, Thompson WG. Drug treatment of the irritable bowel syndrome. Drugs 1992;44: 200-206.

Various authors. Gastroenterol Clin North Am 1991;20(2):235-390.

13

HEMORRHOIDAL PRODUCTS

PATRICIA CARRUTHERS-CZYZEWSKI

CONTENTS

Hemorrhoids 325
- Anatomy and Physiology
- Epidemiology
- Etiology
- Pathophysiology
- Symptoms
- Treatment

Other Anal Conditions 330
- Anal fissures
- Pruritus Ani

Pharmaceutical Agents 331
- Anesthetics—Local
- Anticholinergics
- Astringents
- Counterirritants
- Keratolytics
- Protectants
- Vasoconstrictors
- Other Agents

Recommended Reading 334

HEMORRHOIDS

Anorectal diseases, including hemorrhoids, are annoying, discomforting and potentially serious.

The word hemorrhoid is derived from the Greek haema, meaning blood, and rhoos, meaning flowing. Hemorrhoids are common and their treatment dates back nearly 4,000 years.

ANATOMY AND PHYSIOLOGY

In discussing anorectal diseases, three parts of the body are of concern: the perianal area, the anal canal and the lower portion of the rectum. The perianal area is the portion of the skin and buttocks immediately surrounding the anus. The anal canal connects the end of the digestive tract with the outside of the body.

Hemorrhoids or piles are thought to be normal features of the human anal canal, forming pads or cushions that bulge into the lumen. They have a mucosal lining, a stroma with smooth muscle and connective tissue and blood vessels and are attached to the internal sphincter musculature by small fibres. These hemorrhoidal vessels line the anal canal and may serve as a minor continence mechanism. Just before the lower portion of the rectum, the skin lining changes to mucous membrane, and this level is called the dentate line.

The anal canal is surrounded by two sphincters, which control defecation. The external sphincter, located at the bottom of the anal canal, is under voluntary control. The internal sphincter, a muscle under autonomic control at the top of the anal canal, allows the passage of feces into the anal canal. Resting tone is supplied largely by the internal sphincter. The external anal sphincter accounts for 15 to 27% of anal resting tone. The skin covering the anal canal acts as a barrier against absorption of substances into the body.

Blood to the anal canal is supplied by three rectal arteries, which drain into the portal circulation through the superior rectal veins. In the rectum and the anal canal, the veins run close to the arteries. Drainage occurs through two plexuses. The superior venous plexus lies above the pectinate line and is covered by the mucosa of the rectum and the upper anal canal. It drains into the portal system via the inferior mesenteric vein. The inferior venous plexus lies beneath the pectinate line underneath the anal skin and drains into the systemic circulation via the internal ileac veins. Since these two systems interconnect, the portal and systemic circulations are connected in the hemorrhoidal plexuses. Substances absorbed through the rectal mucous membrane may enter the systemic circulation without passing through the liver.

Hemorrhoids are often described as varicose veins in the anal canal. However, hemorrhoids are not veins at all. They do not look like varicose veins and the blood from them is bright red, not dark as that from veins. Hemorrhoids are displaced anal cushions. The cushions are normal structures that have a rich arterial supply leading directly into distensible venous spaces. They help seal the upper anal canal and contribute to continence.

There are usually three anal cushions: two right and one left but each may be further subdivided by vertical folds. Whatever their contribution to anal resting pressure, the anal cushions also act as a compliant and comfortable plug.

EPIDEMIOLOGY

Canadian prevalence can be estimated from U.S. statistics. A U.S. survey showed a prevalence of 4.4% in the general population. Its incidence may be overestimated because it is the most common anal problem described. Some estimates have indicated that, while patients complain of hemorrhoids, only 50% actually have hemorrhoids; the other problems include thrombosed hemorrhoids in approximately 18.5% of patients with anal complaints, fissures in 8% and miscellaneous problems in 23%.

Hemorrhoids are found primarily in populations consuming the diet of the western world, a diet high in white flour, sugar and fibre-depleted carbohydrate foods. However, fibre intake and the prevalence of hemorrhoids are not associated.

ETIOLOGY

The attachment of the pads or cushions to the wall of the anal canal is normally quite lax. With increasing age, the anchoring connective tissue fibres start to disintegrate, and the cushions loosen even more. The resulting congestion within the anal canal causes the cushions to hypertrophy and protrude further down. Thus, hemorrhoids are anal cushions that have been disrupted from their internal attachments.

The exact cause is unknown. Many factors may be associated with the development of hemorrhoids. Straining, usually as a result of constipation, is the main contributing factor. When the individual tries to pass small, firm stools, the intrarectal pressure rises, blocking the venous return from the anal canal and leading to more straining. The shearing action of the fecal mass passing over the area causes a loosening of the underlying connective tissue. Diarrhea, either acute or chronic, can also cause hemorrhoids, due to futile and protracted straining. Regular bowel movements help to prevent hemorrhoids.

The suggestion that the human upright position has led to the development of hemorrhoids is unlikely. Hemorrhoids are not a universal problem, but are mainly an affliction of the western world. The condition seldom occurs in the rural populations of Asia and Africa.

Heredity is not an important factor. The only connection between heredity and hemorrhoids is the similarity of diet and personal habits in members of the same family.

Hemorrhoids often develop during pregnancy, but pregnancy is not the cause. Pregnancy is believed to precipitate the onset of hemorrhoids in susceptible women. The woman who has hemorrhoids in the last few months of pregnancy may have become symptomatic due to increased abdominal pressure, allowing already existing piles to present themselves. Other possibilities are that during pregnancy there may be a softening of the elastic tissue that supports anal cushions or that the woman may be more constipated, especially if she takes an iron supplement. In any case, these hemorrhoids usually resolve after parturition.

Other possible causes of hemorrhoids include increased abdominal pressure due to the type of work, cardiac disease, obesity and physical exertion.

PATHOPHYSIOLOGY

Hemorrhoids may be classified symptomatically according to their degree of formation. First-degree hemorrhoids swell in the anal cushion due to straining. This swelling is seldom noticed by the sufferer, but can be observed by a physician during a rectal examination. First-degree hemorrhoids are usually painless.

During the second stage, a small part of the anal mucosa or cushion may protrude at the anus during defecation. After the bowel movement, the hemorrhoid spontaneously returns to its normal position.

Third-degree hemorrhoids remain in the prolapsed position after defecation, but may be replaced manually within the anus.

Fourth-degree hemorrhoids cannot be replaced after a bowel movement, and thus create a permanent bulge at the anus. This condition is quite painful, and it is usually at this stage that individuals should consult their physician.

SYMPTOMS

Bleeding, protrusion and pain are the major complaints of hemorrhoid sufferers. Other conditions that cause pain and may coincide with hemorrhoids are anal fissures, inflammation and blood clots. Blood clots occur when a vessel within the anal canal expands or bursts. This can occur anywhere along the anal canal or completely outside the anus within a permanently prolapsed pile. The cause is not known, but one possible explanation is that a prolapsed hemorrhoid was pinched by the external sphincter muscle of the anal canal, causing the rupturing of a blood vessel. If no other complications develop, the blood clot usually resolves spontaneously after about 1 week.

Bleeding is usually noticed as a bright red streak on toilet paper or on the surface of the stool. Blood may also spot the person's underclothing or drip after a bowel movement, especially when the individual is constipated. If the blood is dark in color or present in large amounts, other pathologies may be involved, and a physician should be consulted promptly.

For many patients, the first symptom is a painful mass present at the anus lasting several days to weeks and sometimes accompanied by the sudden relief of pain following rupture of the skin overlying the thrombus and bleeding.

Other symptoms include itching, swelling and burning. Swelling is probably the main cause of pruritus ani. Individuals often have fecal soiling of underwear. Prolapse often coincides with the beginning of a troublesome amount of discharge as a result of increased mucus production.

High Fibre Diet

- Unprocessed wheat bran has been recommended as the least expensive, least perishable dietary source of vegetable fibre. Vegetables and fruits vary in their ability to absorb moisture. Carrots have the greatest absorption capacity of the vegetables, about half that of bran. Other high absorption vegetables are brussels sprouts, eggplant, spring cabbage and corn. High-absorption fruits include apples, pears and oranges.

TREATMENT

Nonpharmacological Treatment

A liberal increase in fluids (8 to 10 glasses of water/day) is recommended to establish good bowel habits. Since constipation and straining are major causes of hemorrhoids, increasing the daily intake of fibre by consuming a bran-containing cereal may help to regulate bowel habits. Adding fibre to the diet (20 to 30 g/day) is usually adequate to relieve symptoms of piles in individuals with first- and second-degree hemorrhoids.

The second most important preventive measure is good toilet habits. The urge to defecate should not be postponed, or it will weaken. The largest daily meal should be eaten at the same time each day. A healthy meal usually takes 36 hours to digest. One should not remain on the toilet more than 1 to 2 minutes. Straining should be avoided. Any prolapsed hemorrhoids must be replaced with a moistened tissue. After each bowel movement, the anorectal area should be cleaned with soap and water and wiped with wet toilet tissue.

If these general measures do not relieve hemorrhoidal symptoms, the individual may be advised to use a sitz bath 3 to 4 times daily. A sitz bath consists of a tub of warm water (about 46°C) in which the individual sits for 15 minutes at a time. Plastic sitz baths may be fitted over the toilet seat rim for greater convenience.

Pharmacological Treatment

Treatment is directed toward relief of symptoms. Oral analgesics, such as acetaminophen, may provide relief of mild discomfort or pain. Also, stool softeners, like docusate sodium, can alleviate pain associated with constipation and straining with defecation.

A variety of hemorrhoidal products is available that claim to relieve pain and burning. These products may relieve the discomfort; however, the degree of relief attributable to a placebo effect has yet to be determined. Hemorrhoidal products are classified into groups based on the pharmacologic action of the ingredients. Available products contain local anesthetics, anti-inflammatory agents, protectants, counterirritants, astringents, vasoconstrictors, anticholinergics, wound-healing agents,

TABLE 1: Active Ingredients in Hemorrhoidal Products

Drug Component	Usual Concentrations Ointments/Creams	Suppositories
Anticholinergics		
Belladonna	0.45%	11.25 mg
Antiseptics		
Benzethonium chloride	0.1%	NA
Boric acid	NA	226.7 mg
Domiphen	0.05%	NA
Oxyquinoline	1.2%	NA
Astringents		
Hamamelis water	10-50%	NA
Zinc oxide	5-10%	225-250 mg
Counterirritants		
Menthol	0.5%	NA
Keratolytics		
Allantoin	0.1%	NA
Local anesthetics		
Amylocaine	1%	NA
Benzocaine*	1-4.5%	50 mg
Dibucaine	0.5-1%	2.5 mg
Pramoxine	1%	20 mg
Protectants		
Calamine		
Glycerin	10%	NA
Shark liver oil	3%	66 mg
White petrolatum		
Zinc oxide	5-10%	225-250 mg
Vasoconstrictors		
Ephedrine	0.1-0.31%	2.5 mg
Naphazoline	0.04%	NA
Wound-healing agents		
Balsam Peru	1%	22.6 mg
Shark liver oil	3%	66 mg
Yeast	1%	22 mg
Zinc sulfate	0.5%	10 mg
Other		
Horse chestnut	2.5%	NA

*Stick preparations contain 20%.
NA=not available
Developed from: Carruthers-Czyzewski P, ed. Compendium of Nonprescription Products. Ottawa: Canadian Pharmaceutical Association, 1995.

antiseptics and keratolytics. Table 1 provides a list of ingredients in commercial products. Available preparations provide only relief; none are curative.

The safest compounds are the protectants, vasoconstrictors and some astringents. If not used for prolonged periods of time, some of the local anesthetics are relatively safe and may relieve pain.

Many of the commercially available hemorrhoidal products contain combinations of two or more active ingredients. The combination of ingredients should be rational, safe and effective (e.g., avoid the combination of local anesthetic and counterirritant).

When diet alone is not sufficient to relieve constipation, a stool softener or a bulk-forming laxative may be added.

If drug treatment fails, the individual should be referred to a physician.

Other Treatments

Surgical hemorrhoidectomy is the most definitive treatment; less than 3% of individuals undergoing this procedure experience recurrence.

More than 80% of people respond to medical treatment, rubber banding or infrared coagulation, and these methods cause much less discomfort and entail much less time off work than does hemorrhoidectomy.

In rubber band ligation, two elastic bands are placed over the pedicle of the hemorrhoid. The aim is to cut off the blood supply and produce necrosis of the hemorrhoid and subsequent sloughing of the lesion. This procedure is indicated for internal hemorrhoids only, because any such procedure below the pectinate line would cause severe pain.

Infrared coagulation uses infrared as a source of heat. Infrared radiation is generated by a tungsten halogen lamp and mounted on an instrument that resembles a gun with a trigger. The tip of the instrument is placed just toward the head of the internal hemorrhoid and "fired" for 0.5 to 3 seconds. The sensation produced is heat at the time of application and a feeling of fullness following treatment.

ADVICE FOR THE PATIENT

Hemorrhoids

➤ To prevent and alleviate symptoms, it is important to establish good bowel habits:

- drink 8–10 glasses of water/day
- add fibre to your diet
- do not postpone the urge to defecate
- do not remain on the toilet for more than 1 to 2 minutes and avoid straining.

➤ A sitz bath may help to relieve symptoms. Sit in a tub of warm water for 15 minutes 3 to 4 times a day.

➤ Nonprescription hemorrhoidal products should be used after each bowel movement for maximum effect.

➤ Nonprescription hemorrhoidal products for external use should be applied sparingly. They should not be inserted into the rectum.

➤ Before any nonprescription hemorrhoidal product is applied, the anorectal area should be washed with mild soap and warm water, rinsed thoroughly and gently dried by patting or blotting with toilet tissue or a soft cloth.

➤ Products containing local anesthetics should be used only in the perianal region or the lower anal canal.

➤ If symptoms worsen or do not improve after 7 days, or if bleeding, protrusion or seepage occurs, see a physician as soon as possible.

PATIENT ASSESSMENT QUESTIONS

Q *What are your symptoms and how long have you experienced them?*
People with hemorrhoids often complain of pain and the appearance of bright red blood after a bowel movement. Diagnosed, uncomplicated hemorrhoids usually resolve quickly. When symptoms persist for more than 1 week, a physician should be consulted. If the blood is dark or present in large amounts, refer the individual immediately to a physician for a definitive diagnosis.

Q *Have you been straining at stool?*
Constipation precipitates the development of hemorrhoids. If the individual has been straining at stool, advise that bowel habits be regulated through a high-fibre diet, adequate fluid intake and good toilet habits.

Q *Have you recently been pregnant?*
Pregnancy, especially in the third trimester and at parturition, often precipitates hemorrhoids in previously well women. It is believed pregnancy only accentuates an existing problem. Hemorrhoids in these people usually resolve soon after parturition.

Q *Have you tried anything for this condition?*
Knowing what products have been tried in the past aids in selecting a more appropriate preparation. Also, it may alert the health professional to a more serious problem.

OTHER ANAL CONDITIONS

ANAL FISSURES

Fissure *in ano* is a crack or cut in the lining of the anal canal. Ulcer *in ano* is a fissure in its chronic stage. The lesion is usually associated with bleeding and intense pain at the time of defecation.

Most patients complain of hemorrhoids. Severe, indescribable pain and intense cutting, tearing and knife-like sensations lasting many hours are common symptoms. Bleeding is always bright red and the pain is associated with and immediately follows a bowel movement. Many patients are so fearful of having a bowel movement that they hold it and in so doing, exacerbate the situation by producing harder stools.

Diagnosis can only be confirmed by physical examination.

Acute fissures should be treated conservatively with bulking agents or stool softeners to promote a softer stool. Individuals should be encouraged to have a bowel movement as soon as the first signal comes. Local ointments and creams (e.g., anesthetics) may provide some relief. Sitz baths may also be helpful.

PRURITUS ANI

Itching of the anus is one of the most common complaints associated with this part of the human anatomy. Most people, however, complain of hemorrhoids. It is a common condition affecting up to 5% of the population, with men affected more commonly than women by a ratio of 4:1. It occurs in all age groups but is most common in the fourth, fifth and sixth decade of life.

In most cases, the condition has no demonstrable cause, whereas, in others, the etiologic factors could include diet, personal hygiene, various systemic disorders, gynecologic conditions, anatomic compromise, such as obesity, neoplasm, diarrhea, radiation, drugs, dermatologic conditions, infections and psychogenic factors. Generally, the condition is self-limited. For the most part, anxiety, stress and dietary factors are to blame. Among children, a common cause is pinworms.

Individuals complain of an irresistible urge to scratch the anus. Although the symptoms occur at any time, they are most common following a bowel movement, especially after liquid stools and most peculiarly at bedtime, just before falling asleep. Some may also experience intense itching during the night. At times, itching is so severe, it tends to "drive" the person crazy.

As for treatment, careful attention should be paid to the person's dietary habits. Individuals affected should be discouraged from using any topical anesthetic preparations as they may exacerbate the problem. The individual should be referred to a physician. Sitz baths may be suggested for symptomatic relief of itching until a doctor is consulted.

PHARMACEUTICAL AGENTS

ANESTHETICS—LOCAL

Some of the local anesthetics found in commercially available preparations include amylocaine, benzocaine, pramoxine and dibucaine.

Local anesthetics block nerve conduction in an effort to temporarily relieve itching, irritation and discomfort. Most local anesthetics are classified according to chemical structure into esters or amides.

Local anesthetics should not be used more than 5 to 7 days at a time because of the danger of masking more serious conditions, such as anal fissures, cryptitis, fistulas, abscesses, and benign or malignant tumors of the lower colon or rectum.

Local anesthetics may produce allergic reactions, both locally and systemically. Hypersensitivity reactions are more common with the ester type of anesthetic. There appears to be no cross-sensitivity between the amide and ester types. Pramoxine exhibits less cross-sensitivity because it does not have the usual amide or ester structure. Local reactions may cause burning and itching that are indistinguishable from symptoms of hemorrhoids. If symptoms return after cessation of therapy, a physician should be consulted.

The risk of adverse effects from the absorption of local anesthetics can be decreased by combining it with a vasoconstrictor, for example, ephedrine or naphazoline. As well as reducing toxicity, the vasoconstrictors increase the duration of action of the anesthetic by slowing down absorption into the hemorrhoidal tissue.

Local anesthetics should only be used in the perianal region or the lower anal canal.

Amylocaine is a local anesthetic of the ester type found in combination with other drugs for anorectal disease.

Benzocaine, an ester type local anesthetic, is found in aerosols, ointments, suppositories and sticks and may be applied up to 6 times daily. The most common adverse effect to topical benzocaine is sensitization (e.g., contact dermatitis).

Dibucaine base and dibucaine hydrochloride (also known as cinchocaine) is a local anesthetic of the amide type. The ointment may be administered each morning and evening and after each bowel movement. Additional ointment may be applied topically to anal tissues. No more than 30 g of ointment should be used by adults in any 24-hour period.

Pramoxine hydrochloride may be used externally as an ointment or a suppository twice daily (morning and evening) and after each bowel movement. Adverse effects are rare. Initial burning or stinging may occur following topical application. Pramoxine hydrochloride has a low index of sensitization, and cross-sensitization with other local anesthetics is unlikely.

ANTICHOLINERGICS

Anticholinergics act systemically to prevent or inhibit the action of acetylcholine.

Anticholinergic agents (e.g., belladonna) are claimed to act as counterirritants, but no evidence exists that they are effective as such in anorectal conditions.

Belladonna can be absorbed systemically to produce anticholinergic toxicity. Anticholinergics are not recommended for use in nonprescription hemorrhoidal preparations.

ASTRINGENTS

Astringents are used to relieve the irritation and burning sensation of hemorrhoids by protecting the underlying tissue.

By coagulating proteins in the fluid between epidermal cells, astringents form a superficial protective layer. Their action is almost entirely limited to cell surfaces and the interstitial spaces of the skin and mucous membranes.

Astringents are applied to the skin or mucous membranes. When appropriately used, astringents contribute to drying by reducing mucus and other secretions. This drying effect helps relieve local anorectal irritation and inflammation.

The most commonly used astringent is zinc oxide. Zinc sulfate also exhibits astringent properties. Zinc oxide or sulfate may be applied internally or externally up to 6 times daily after each bowel movement.

Witch hazel (hamamelis water) is recommended for external use only and is available commercially as pads or wipes. Its effectiveness is due primarily to its alcohol content. It is applied after each bowel movement and may be used up to 6 times daily. Hamamelis provides temporary relief of itching and burning. Hamamelis is incorporated in ointments. Hamamelis water is used as a cooling application in rectal pads.

Pharmaceutical Agents

COUNTERIRRITANTS

Counterirritants are used to relieve pain and itch by providing a sensation of coolness, which distracts from the sensation of pain.

The only counterirritant found in commercial hemorrhoidal preparations is menthol in concentrations of 0.5%.

Menthol has a cooling effect when applied in low concentrations (0.1 to 2%). At these concentrations, it selectively stimulates sensory nerve endings, causing a cooling sensation and analgesia.

Menthol should not be used intrarectally, as the rectal mucosa does not contain any sensory nerve endings. The main adverse effect of menthol is the potential for sensitivity reactions.

KERATOLYTICS

Keratolytics cause desquamation and debridement or sloughing of epidermal surface cells. By allowing cell turnover and loosening surface cells, keratolytics may help to expose underlying tissue to therapeutic agents.

Keratolytics appear to have some value in reducing hemorrhoidal itch, but their exact mechanism of action is unknown.

The keratolytic used externally in hemorrhoidal ointment preparations is allantoin (aluminum chlorhydroxyallantoinate). It may be applied up to 6 times daily.

PROTECTANTS

Protectant compounds provide a physical barrier to irritation by forming a protective layer over the mucous membranes lining the anorectal region, thereby preventing excessive water loss from the tissues. This is important because drying of the area can intensify any itching, burning or pain already present. Protection of the perianal area from irritants, such as fecal matter, leads to a reduction in irritation and concomitant itching.

Commonly recommended protectants are aluminum hydroxide gel, kaolin, cocoa butter, lanolin, mineral oil, glycerin and white petrolatum. Protectants recommended only when used in combination with other protectants are calamine, shark liver oil and zinc oxide. Many substances classified as protectants are also used as vehicles and bases.

The bismuth salts (bismuth subcarbonate, bismuth subnitrate, bismuth subgallate) that are found in some hemorrhoidal preparations are not recommended as protectants. Bismuth subnitrate is not considered safe because it may be absorbed, producing toxic symptoms (e.g., gastrointestinal disturbances, skin reactions, discoloration of mucous membranes, methemoglobinemia). The effectiveness of bismuth subcarbonate and subgallate as protectants in the anorectal area has not been established.

Protectants are quite safe, because, with the exception of bismuth compounds, they are seldom absorbed through intact or broken skin or through mucous membranes.

Ingredients of Hemorrhoidal Products

The ideal hemorrhoidal product would contain:

- a vasoconstrictor
- a local anesthetic
- a protectant or protectants making up at least 50% of the ingredients

VASOCONSTRICTORS

Vasoconstrictors are agents that are structurally related to epinephrine or norepinephrine. Vasoconstrictors stimulate alpha-adrenergic receptors in blood vessels, causing constriction of the arterioles.

Vasoconstrictors are used temporarily to reduce swelling of hemorrhoidal tissue by constricting blood vessels. Vasoconstrictors also relieve itching by producing a slight anesthetic effect. **Ephedrine** and **naphazoline** are found in nonprescription hemorrhoidal preparations. Locally applied vasoconstrictors are not effective in controlling bleeding. If rectal bleeding occurs, this may be a sign of a more serious disease, and a physician should be consulted.

While significant absorption is not very likely when vasoconstrictors are used externally on intact skin, there is a possibility of systemic absorption following application of the drug to abraded and irritated skin.

Unpleasant side effects can occur following absorption of vasoconstrictors. These include increased blood pressure, cardiac arrhythmia, central nervous system disturbances, and aggravation of symptoms of hyperthyroidism.

Ephedrine sulfate is readily absorbed through mucous membranes in the rectum. Applied topically, its onset of action ranges from a few seconds to 1 minute and its duration of action is 2 to 3 hours. It effectively relieves itching and swelling and is applied up to 4 times a day. Some topical hemorrhoidal products containing ephedrine sulfate may cause nervousness, tremor, sleeplessness, nausea and loss of appetite.

Naphazoline is found in some hemorrhoidal preparations in concentrations of 0.04%.

OTHER AGENTS

Anti-inflammatories

Topically applied hydrocortisone-containing products have the potential to reduce itching, inflammation and discomfort. The combination of hydrocortisone with other hemorrhoidal ingredients is not currently available as a nonprescription product. Hydrocortisone alone is not generally recommended and should only be used temporarily for minor external anal itching due to minor irritation or rash.

Antiseptics

An antiseptic's purpose is to inhibit microbial growth in the area where it is used.

The use of antiseptics, such as boric acid, benzethonium chloride, domiphen and oxyquinoline benzoate, in the anorectal region has been described as scientifically unsound. It is unlikely that antiseptics make much difference considering the large numbers of microorganisms normally present.

It is advisable to keep the perianal area clean with soap and water; antiseptics should be regarded only as possible adjuncts to good personal hygiene.

These agents are considered unsafe (e.g., boric acid may produce systemic toxicity during repeated use) and have not been clearly shown to alleviate hemorrhoidal symptoms.

Wound-healing Agents

Several ingredients in nonprescription hemorrhoidal products are claimed to be effective in promoting wound healing or tissue repair in anorectal disease. To date, there are no studies that have found that wound-healing agents relieve hemorrhoidal symptoms. However, these agents claim to accelerate tissue healing and thus relief of symptoms may accompany healing.

In particular, a substance found in *Preparation-H,* a live yeast cell derivative (LYCD), has been extensively tested in in vitro and in vivo wound healing models. LYCD has been shown to stimulate oxygen consumption, increase angiogenesis (development of the vessels), and promote collagen synthesis. It is the subject of considerable controversy. Some clinical trials support the manufacturer's claim but overall, there is insufficient evidence to confirm this.

Shark liver oil, a form of vitamin A, is another agent claimed to promote wound healing. The value of shark oil as hemorrhoidal wound healer remains equivocal; its value as a protectant in hemorrhoidal products is a bit less equivocal.

Balsam Peru has not been demonstrated effective as a wound healer.

Miscellaneous Agents

Horse chestnut (aesculus) is still found in some nonprescription hemorrhoidal preparations. The horse chestnut contains several active ingredients including esculoside and aescin, which is a mixture of saponins.

Delivery Forms

- Hemorrhoidal preparations are available in a variety of dosage forms: creams, ointments, suppositories, aerosols, cleansing pads and sticks. Ultimately, the choice of delivery form lies with the consumer or physician. Many people prefer suppositories, but these products are often not effective because they tend to slip into the rectum and melt, bypassing the anal canal where the medication is needed. Suppositories with a multiple aperture tip may overcome this problem, but the possibility of self-inflicted trauma exists.
- In general, creams and ointments are preferable to suppositories. They are easier to apply and usually contain the same or similar ingredients as suppositories. Aerosols may be simplest to use, but delivery tends to be erratic and thus ineffective.

RECOMMENDED READING

Bassford T. Treatment of common anorectal disorders. Am Fam Physician 1992;45:1787–94.

Hodes B. Hemorrhoidal products. In: Handbook of Nonprescription Drugs. Washington: American Pharmaceutical Association, 1992;469–78.

Loder PB, Kamm MA, Nicholls RJ, et al. Hemorrhoids: pathology, pathophysiology and aetiology. Br J Surg 1994;81:946–54.

Mazier WP. Hemorrhoids, fissures and pruritus ani. Surg Clin North Am 1994;74:1277–92.

Sause RB. Self-treatment of hemorrhoids. US Pharmacist 1995;20:32–36, 39–40.

14

HERBAL PRODUCTS

R. FRANK CHANDLER

CONTENTS

Introduction 335

Medicinal Herbs 338
- Plants Generally Regarded as Foods
- Flavors and Spices
- Medicinal Teas
- Common Herbal Medicines

Special Considerations 353
- Safety Concerns
- Poisonous Plants
- Pre- and Peri-Natal Issues
- Drug Interactions

Recommended Reading 360

INTRODUCTION

Man has depended on plants for shelter, clothing, food and medicine throughout history. Through trial and error he has learned which plants are safe to eat, which are poisonous and which are effective medicines.

The use of herbs as medicines appears to date back to Neanderthal times, some 60,000 years ago. Today, about 25% of all prescription drugs are based on herbs and in some developed countries herbal preparations are used extensively as alternatives or as complements to conventional medicine.

A lack of faith in conventional medicines, concern about their side effects and cost, hope for a cure of a chronic or terminal illness and the fallacious belief that medications prepared from herbs are not harmful to humans are cited as reasons for the dramatic revitalization of herbal medicine in North America in the past 2 decades.

Most American physicians, however, are unaware of the significant body of research published in botanical journals and in foreign medical journals on the healing benefits and adverse effects of herbal products.

Taxol, the active ingredient from the Pacific yew tree that is taken in the treatment of breast and ovarian cancer, has recently received widespread media attention; but it is only one of countless possibilities for deriving healing agents from botanical sources. Saw palmetto *(Serenoa repens)*, a palm tree native to Florida, has been found effective in 90% of patients with benign prostatic hyperplasia, while the most commonly prescribed conventional drug has been shown effective only 57% of the time. Scientific evidence supports the use of feverfew *(Tanacetum parthenium)* for migraine headache, licorice *(Glycyrrhiza glabra)* for ulcers, chaste tree berry *(Agnus castus)* for premenstrual syndrome (PMS), valerian *(Valeriana officinalis)* for its tranquilizing effects, milk thistle *(Silybum marinum)* for helping the liver detoxify environmental pollutants, hawthorn berry *(Crataegus oxyacantha)* for heart disease, bilberry *(Vaccinium myrtillis)* for capillary fragility, echinacea *(Echinacea angustifolia)* for prevention and mediation of colds and flu and for its ability to stimulate the immune system, and ginkgo, maidenhair tree, *(Ginkgo biloba)* for increasing vasodilation and peripheral capillary blood-flow, especially cerebral blood flow.

The numerous studies showing the clinical benefit of various herbs, their low cost and low level of side effects leave little doubt they are cost-effective in certain situations.

However, the possibility of adverse effects and interaction with conventional medicines makes a thorough history of herbal preparations used a necessary component of a drug history, especially in individuals with specific illnesses or who are pregnant.

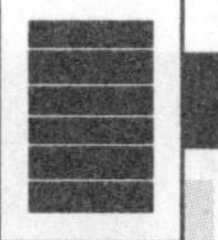

TABLE 1: Guidelines for Appropriate Use of Herbal Products

Buy herbal remedies from reliable and trusted sources.

Purchase an herbal remedy only if the package clearly states which herb(s) it contains.

Always ask for the exact directions for use.

Do not collect herbs in the wild, unless you are well able to distinguish poisonous and innocuous herbs from one another.

Store herbal remedies as you would allopathic medicines.

Do not use herbal remedies that you have kept for years.

Do not use herbal remedies for serious illnesses.

Stop using an herbal remedy if you start experiencing side effects.

Do not exceed the dose range stated in the directions for use.

To avoid possible chronic effects, do not use herbal remedies for prolonged periods.

If you are pregnant or breast-feeding and want to use an herbal remedy, do so only after consulting your physician or pharmacist.

Your physician or pharmacist must be informed if you are using an herbal remedy with conventional drug therapy.

Source: De Smet PAGM. Drugs used in nonorthodox medicine. In: Dukes MNG, Beeley L, eds. Side Effects of Drugs Annual 14. Amsterdam: Elsevier, 1990:429–51.

Allopathic Medicines

Some herbs or their products have become entrenched in current allopathic medicine and no viable alternatives exist. They play a major role not only in medicine but also in commerce. Between 1959 and 1980, drugs obtained from flowering plants and trees were present in about 25% of all prescriptions dispensed in the United States. This use represented an estimated $3 billion in sales in 1973 and $8 billion in 1980. Following are a few examples of familiar medicines in this category.

Foxglove (*Digitalis purpurea*): Used in domestic medicine in the United Kingdom as far back as the 10th century, it was introduced into medical practice by Dr. William Withering in 1775. He obtained knowledge of its value in dropsy (edema) from an old woman herbalist. Its mechanism of action in congestive heart failure and the nature of its active ingredients were determined later. Digoxin, the major constituent of *Digitalis lanata*, has largely replaced foxglove and its major constituent, digitoxin, in current medical practice.

Quinine: Still one of the most important antimalarial drugs, it was first isolated from cinchona bark (*Cinchona* species) in 1820. However, its value had been known to the Europeans since 1739, when a Peruvian Indian medicine man had cured a Jesuit missionary of malaria by administering a cinchona bark preparation. Several synthetic antimalarial drugs have been introduced to the market, but quinine is regaining importance in treating chloroquine resistant organisms.

Carbenoxolone: Before cimetidine, this was the only effective therapeutic agent available that stimulated the healing of gastric and duodenal ulcers. Carbenoxolone is derived from glycyrrhetinic acid, the major sapogenin of licorice (*Glycyrrhiza glabra*), a plant long used to alleviate gastric pain and oral ulcers.

Snakeroot (*Rauwolfia serpentina*): For centuries it was used in India to treat illnesses ranging from snakebite to insanity. Not until 1952 was the value of this plant and its alkaloids recognized. Reserpine was the first drug available to effectively control some forms of anxiety and psychosis, and is useful in essential hypertension. Rauwolfia and reserpine are still the basis of several preparations used for their antihypertensive and antipsychotic effects.

Tubocurarine, isolated from *Chondodendron tomentosum*: One of the major alkaloids of curare, a South American arrow poison, its skeletal muscle relaxant action (paralyzing effect on voluntary muscles) has been successfully transferred to the operating theatre. It allows for muscle relaxation without deep anesthesia.

Although beneficial, each of these drugs has its own list of adverse effects.

Alternative Health Care

- Alternative health care differs from conventional medicine in that it is concerned with the ongoing health of the entire person and is often referred to as "holistic medicine." Conventional medicine may take many factors into consideration, but most doctors do not dwell on nutrition or the psychological condition of the patient when prescribing a treatment. Alternative therapies tend to be more oriented to prevention and, when illness does occur, treating it with natural substances that enhance the body's inherent fighting ability.
- In January 1993, Dr. David M. Eisenberg and his colleagues at Harvard Medical School reported that more than one-third of Americans have turned to alternative therapies. A broad range of people use alternative medicines, the study found, with no significant differences by gender, insurance coverage, or size of community. They are most likely to be affluent, well educated, white baby boomers who live in the West. Overall, 34% of respondents used at least 1 of the 16 targeted alternative therapies during the 12 months preceding the survey. Only one-tenth saw a health care provider for treatment. Three per cent of Americans used herbal medicine during this period.
- A 1991 Canada Health Monitor survey of Canadians found that 20% had used an alternative health therapy, compared to 25% who used services provided by conventional medical practitioners. About 6% had sought advice from a health food store.
- Alternative therapies are most commonly used for chronic conditions such as back problems, anxiety, headaches, depression, arthritis, sprains and strains. They are also frequently used by patients with cancer, acquired immunodeficiency syndrome, chronic renal failure, and eating disorders. All too often this translates into the elderly patient with a chronic or terminal condition that conventional medicine has been able to do little for.
- It is sometimes argued that alternative therapies may delay the application of conventional medical treatments, leading to reduced health status and increased medical expenditures. However, no studies have shown this to be a problem.
- Increased consumer awareness of side effects and the unknown long-term effects of conventional pharmaceuticals will create a surge in the popularity of natural remedies, says the British consulting firm McAlpine, Thorpe and Warrier, even though the long-term adverse effects of herbal medications remain largely unknown.
- The American survey found that 72% of those reporting use of an alternative therapy did not tell their medical doctor.
- In the same year, Americans spent $13.7 billion on alternative treatments, $10.3 billion of this out of pocket. This figure is more than 80% of the $12.8 billion spent out of pocket annually for all hospitalizations in the United States and nearly 44% of the $23.5 billion spent on all physicians' services.
- Sales of herbal products are growing rapidly, although there are no figures available for the industry as a whole. About 220 companies produce herbal medicine in the United States, according to McAlpine, Thorpe and Warrier. They sense that the herbal remedy market is growing faster than conventional nonprescription medicines, with overall industry growth estimated at between 12 to 15% a year. Europeans spend $500 million to $600 million (U.S.) annually on natural remedies and food supplements. It is estimated that the U.S. herbal industry had a retail value of up to $1.5 billion in 1994. In 1993, ginseng and garlic alone saw a 46% increase in sales to $82 million. The size of the Canadian herbal market has been estimated at $4 million to $5 million for 1994.

MEDICINAL HERBS

PLANTS GENERALLY REGARDED AS FOODS

Some plants are generally regarded as safe to consume as foods. Few would challenge the safety of asparagus, lettuce, broccoli, cucumber, carrots, peas, kidney beans, apricots and potatoes. However, in spite of their general safety, the last 3 can cause severe toxicity. Fatalities caused by apricots and potatoes have been recorded. The toxins (lectins) in kidney beans (*Phaseolus vulgaris*), which cause severe stomach upset, are destroyed by boiling. The kernels of apricots (*Prunus armeniaca*), contain hydrogen cyanide and can be fatal if consumed in sufficient quantity. Potato (*Solanum tuberosum*) sprouts, fruit, vines and green tubers contain the poisonous alkaloid solanine that may cause stomach upset, vomiting, headaches and death. Only the tuber, free of green portions, should be consumed.

A number of herbs known primarily as foods may also be used for medicinal purposes.

Parsley (*Petroselinum crispum*): The leaves have been used for centuries as a garnish and nutrient, the seeds as a carminative and the root as a diuretic. The plant has been used to treat arthritis, and with its oil, as an emmenagogue (to promote menstrual flow). Adverse effects from ingesting the oil have included headache, giddiness, loss of balance, convulsions and renal damage. The oil comprises about 0.1% of the root, about 5% of the seeds and contains at least two biologically active compounds, apiol and myristicin. Apiol is an antipyretic and, like myristicin, a uterine stimulant. Apiol was once available in capsules for use as an abortifacient. The Russians have an apiol product used to stimulate uterine contractions during labor. These constituents are likely responsible for the observed diuretic effect of parsley. Because these compounds may stimulate the uterine muscles, the seeds, juice and oil of parsley should not be administered to pregnant women. Oil of apiol is a prescription drug in Canada.

Cassava (*Manihot esculenta* or *Manihot utilissima*): A small shrub native to Brazil, it is widely cultivated throughout the tropics. The rhizomes are used in many parts of the world as a starchy food similar to potatoes or rice. Cassava has also been employed as a medicinal herb, primarily for dermatological ailments and as a counterirritant.

Traditional methods of preparation as a food consist of carefully washing and cooking the rhizomes to remove the hydrogen cyanide present throughout cassava. The skin of sweet cassava (*Manihot dulcis*) and possibly the flesh may also contain hydrogen cyanide; it must be peeled before eating. The hydrogen cyanide is present as the water-soluble glucoside linamarin.

Commercially, the fleshy rhizomes of cassava and sweet cassava are washed, sliced and pulped. The pulp is placed in a strainer and the starch washed out by a powerful stream of water. The starch is allowed to settle, then removed and dried. Known as Brazilian-, Bahai-, Rio-, or Para-arrowroot or manioc starch, it may be used as a nutrient, a thickening agent or in preparing tapioca.

The hydrogen cyanide in cassava has been the cause of both acute and chronic toxicity, the latter especially in some African populations where cassava is consumed regularly.

Pokeroot, poke, pokeberry or pokeweed (*Phytolacca americana*): Long a favorite spring potherb in the southern United States, the young leaves and shoots are boiled, usually twice, and eaten as greens, like spinach. Occasionally, a few young leaves are added to salads to provide tang. Commercial preparations are also available. As an herbal remedy, pokeroot has been promoted primarily as an emetic, cathartic and remedy for chronic rheumatism. Overdoses have sometimes been fatal.

Pokeroot is a common weed of southeastern Canada and the eastern United States, growing to a height of 2 metres. The white flowers develop into juicy, dark purple berries. All parts of the pokeroot are toxic, the highest concentration in the rootstalks, less in the mature leaves and stems, and least in the berries. Leaves collected in the spring before acquiring a red color are edible if boiled for 5 minutes, rinsed and reboiled. Similarly, the berries are edible when cooked. Poisoning often results when pokeroot is collected in error for parsnips, Jerusalem artichoke or horseradish.

Ingestion of the poisonous parts of pokeroot causes severe stomach cramping, nausea with persistent diarrhea and vomiting, slow and difficult breathing, weakness, spasms, hypotension, severe convulsions and death. Several investigations have reported deaths in children following the ingestion of uncooked berries or pokeberry juice. The toxic principle is thought to be the triterpoid saponin, phytolaccigenin, of undetermined structure.

Poke presents a much more insidious risk to health than acute poisoning. It contains a proteinaceous mitogen that may produce blood abnormalities when absorbed. The United States Food and Drug Administration (FDA) classifies this herb as one of undefined safety, adding: ". . . contains an acidic steroid saponin. Emetic action is slow but of long duration. Narcotic effects have been observed."

The Herb Trade Association (a former consumer education organization) issued a policy statement declaring pokeroot must not be sold as a herbal beverage or food. It further recommended all packages containing pokeroot carry an appropriate statement warning of the product's toxicity and its potential danger when taken internally. However, one author states, "With or without a warning label, pokeroot is definitely not recommended for either internal or external use by human beings."

FLAVORS AND SPICES

Most flavors and spices used as medicines are also employed in low amounts for their familiar flavor or the zest they add to foods; some are used to flavor medicines. In higher doses, most exhibit a medicinal action. Most flavors are volatile oils, which as a group, are noted for their carminative and stomachic activities. As a food they are subject to standards for preparation and adulteration found in Part B of the Canadian Food and Drugs Regulations. Used as herbal remedies, they do not always comply with these regulations. Other herbs (e.g., hibiscus and passion flower) are not subject to these controls.

Aniseed, or anise, is the dried fruit of *Pimpinella anisum*. The fruit (seeds) contains 1 to 3% volatile oil (anise oil). Anethole (80 to 90%) is the primary ingredient. Anise oil is also obtained from the Chinese star anise (*Illicium verum*). This oil also contains 80 to 90% anethole, but, unlike *Pimpinella anisum*, contains traces of safrole, a known carcinogen. The safety of anethole has been questioned, but it was concluded that it does "not seem to be potent enough or persistent enough to be of serious practical concern at this time." The FDA lists both herbs as safe. The Food and Drugs Regulations state that *Pimpinella anisum* is the spice, and both *Pimpinella anisum* and Chinese star anise may be used in obtaining anise oil.

Apart from its extensive use as a licorice flavor in foods, beverages, drugs, cosmetics and confectionaries, anise oil is a well established folk remedy for treating flatulence, colic, dyspepsia and hard, dry coughs. The carminative and expectorant activities of the oil have been established, and it is the active ingredient in a number of proprietary cough remedies. It is also present in a number of stimulant laxative preparations to diminish griping (cramping of the bowels). The oil should be used with caution; as little as 1 mL can result in nausea, vomiting, pulmonary edema and seizures.

Although anise exhibits many biological activities, it is used primarily as a condiment and flavor. Anise may cause sensitization in some individuals, but it is normally safe and effective when employed in the traditional manner.

Fenugreek (*Trigonella foenum graecum*), the dried, ripe seeds of a small southern European herb, is one of the oldest medicinal plants and one of the most versatile seed spices. It is used as a spice and flavor, especially in imitation maple syrup and curry.

Fenugreek seeds contain a hydrophilic mucilage that has a soothing effect on the skin and mucous membranes, accounting for its external use in various ointments and poultices. Internally, the mucilage has a soothing effect on the gastrointestinal tract and may be of benefit in coughs and minor mouth and stomach disorders. Fenugreek also displays a laxative action due to the indigestible nature of the mucilage, but its reported hypoglycemic activity is equivocal. The plant appears to produce no serious toxic effects.

Its content of sapogenins, particularly diosgenin, makes fenugreek seed a potential future source of sapogenins for the manufacture of steroid hormones. Because it is an annual herb, the time required for planting-to-harvesting is much shorter than that for *Dioscorea* species, the current source of diosgenin, and fenugreek may eventually prove to have a distinct advantage.

Oregano, according to the Canadian Food and Drugs Regulations, the spice is the dried leaves of *Origanum vulgare* or other *Origanum* species.

However, oregano is known to be derived from several genera of plants, mainly from two families, Labiatae and Verbenaceae. The two most commonly encountered genera are *Origanum* and *Lippia*. Over two dozen species yield leaves or flowering tops that have the flavor recognized as oregano. The most commonly used are *Origanum vulgare*, *Lippia graveolens* and *Lippia palmeri*, the latter two referred to as Mexican oregano.

The botanical distinction between oregano and marjoram is not well defined. Carvacrol is the main constituent of the volatile oils of oregano, marjoram, thyme and summer savory.

Oregano is not a significant medicinal herb. The literature lists it as useful in toothache, oral inflammations, rheumatism and nervous headaches. It is also recommended as a carminative, a diaphoretic, a tonic and an emmenagogue. Because of its fragrance, it was also used as a strewing herb.

Noting that oregano has been used as an emmenagogue, the Expert Advisory Committee on Herbs and Botanical Preparations of Health Canada suggested oregano be labelled to indicate its contraindication in pregnancy. However, even allowing liberal usage in cooking, it is inconceivable that anyone might ingest enough oregano (one-quarter of the average kitchen spice bottle) in one meal to induce toxicity. Of greater concern is the purchase of the oil of oregano, thyme and marjoram, as toxic doses could then be easily consumed.

Oil of wintergreen (*Gaultheria procumbens*) is used as a flavoring agent in candies, chewing gum, soft drinks (e.g., root beer) and dental preparations. The leaves and berries, which persist throughout the winter, have been used by the Indians for survival food. The berries have been used in pies and the leaves to make an herbal tea. Both are used as a condiment and a refreshing nibble, especially on a hot day in the woods.

All parts of the plant yield oil of wintergreen, which contains about 95% methyl salicylate. It is primarily a counterirritant, analgesic and antipyretic but is also used as a carminative, antiseptic, anti-inflammatory, diuretic, stimulant and has many other uses. Small doses stimulate the stomach, but large doses cause vomiting.

Toxicity is unlikely to occur from ingesting the plant. However, as little as 10 mL of the oil (representing about 1 kg of the leaves) can be fatal to a child.

Hops (*Humulus lupulus*) are used primarily for flavoring and preserving beer. Since the Middle Ages, when it was observed that hop pickers tired easily, this herb has been reputed to have sedative and hypnotic effects. The active ingredients are thought to be the bitter, acidic compounds humulone and lupulone, but their action is erratic owing to their instability in light and air. Different varieties of hops seem to vary considerably in their sedative effects. Despite lack of scientific proof for the central nervous system depressant effects, the herb and its extracts are widely used in herbal sedative preparations. Hops are generally regarded as safe although they have been known to cause contact dermatitis.

MEDICINAL TEAS

Many herbs are consumed as teas, whether for beverage or medicinal purposes. To use the volatile oils or delicate plant parts such as the flowers and soft leaves, the herbs are steeped for 10 to 20 minutes in water that has been brought to a boil, usually in a tightly covered container. To extract the essences from coarser leaves, stems, barks and roots, the herbs are simmered uncovered until the volume of water decreases by about half through evaporation. The beverage teas are made using 1 to 5 g of herb per 500 mL of water; medicinal teas are usually made using about 30 g of herb. Thus, medicinal teas range from about 6 to 60 times stronger than beverage teas. If fresh herbs are used, the quantity of plant material is doubled. The usual dose of medicinal teas is one-half to 1 cup (125 to 250 mL) taken 3 times daily.

Consumption of more than 3 cups a day of any herbal beverage, including regular tea and coffee, is considered by some to be immoderate. Herbs used in herbal beverages cover a full range of safety, from those offering only flavoring and coloring to those that are quite toxic, including chronic toxicity.

Hibiscus: The red flowers of hibiscus (*Hibiscus sabdariffa*) are popular ingredients in jams, jellies, sauces, acidic beverages and teas. Hibiscus contains various pigments plus relatively large amounts of citric acid (12 to 17%), hibiscic acid (23%), the lactone of hydroxycitric acid and lesser amounts of malic, tartaric and other acids. The pigments impart a red color to the preparation. The acids are responsible for the tart, refreshing taste of various hibiscus beverages. In medicinal preparations they probably account for the mild laxative and diuretic effects attributed to the plant. Other medicinal claims for this plant need to be verified. Hibiscus is free from known side effects.

Chamomile: Two plants, closely related botanically, chemically and pharmacologically, have long enjoyed popularity as beverages and folk remedies for digestive disorders, cramps and various skin conditions. They are known as German or wild chamomile (*Matricaria chamomilla*) and Roman or garden chamomile (*Anthemis nobilis*). The active ingredients are found in the volatile oil, which is particularly abundant in the mature flower heads.

Although numerous claims are made for chamomile, most are without adequate support. Scientific evidence substantiates three medical claims. In common with many other aromatic plants, chamomile possesses carminative activity and therefore aids digestion. The terpenes, chamazulen and alpha-bisabolol, are major components of the volatile oil and primarily responsible for anti-inflammatory activity in various afflictions of the skin and mucous membranes. The terpenes and other constituents exhibit smooth muscle spasmolytic activity, useful in treating various cramps, especially menstrual cramps. The flavonoids (e.g., apigenin, luteolin and quercetin) and coumadins (e.g., scopoletin-7-beta-glucoside) enhance this activity. The therapeutic value of chamomile does not rest on a single constituent, but on a complex mixture of chemically different compounds.

Since much of the value of this plant lies in its volatile oil, it is unfortunate that even a strong tea contains only about 10 to 15% of the volatile oil originally present in the plant material.

Because these "drugs" include the flower heads, and therefore pollen, tea made from them may cause contact dermatitis or other hypersensitivity reactions in allergic individuals. The contact dermatitis is thought to be due to the alpha-methylene-gamma-lactone group of the sesquiterpene lactones present. Although these reactions are not common, individuals allergic to ragweed, asters, chrysanthemums or other members of the compositae family should be cautious about using chamomile. In nonallergic individuals, no serious undesirable effects have been reported with moderate use of chamomile; it is generally regarded as safe.

Gordolobos: Another popular herbal tea, formerly regarded as safe, it is now known to be a serious chronic poison and responsible for a number of deaths. The hepatotoxicity of the pyrrolizidine alkaloids found in Gordolobos tea has been widely publicized. The tea is used extensively in the southwest, daily by some, for many common ailments, such as sore throats. The symptoms may occur rapidly, especially in young people, but more commonly take decades to appear. Symptoms may progress even after withdrawal of the herb. At least in part, the use of this tea accounts for the high death rate from cirrhosis in Arizona, which consistently runs up to 25% above the national average, even when corrected for deaths known to be due to alcoholism.

Gordolobos is not a consistent preparation, but commonly contains plants rich in pyrrolizidine alkaloids, such as *Senecio longilobus*. The tea is derived from plants grown throughout southwestern and western United States. Some, or close relatives, are found in the northern United States and parts of Canada. The teas are widely available through commercial distribution. Various species of the *Crotalaria* are also responsible for much of the liver disease in Jamaica, where the plant is used as a bush tea.

COMMON HERBAL MEDICINES

The list of herbs used as traditional drugs is virtually endless. A few examples demonstrate how some of these are, or have been, useful medicines. Other examples touch on the problems encountered and questions about herbal medicines that need to be answered. A summary of some data on a number of popular herbs is presented in Table 2.

Valerian (*Valeriana officinalis*) is a popular plant used as a sedative/hypnotic, especially in parts of Europe. It is a common constituent in herbal preparations intended for tranquillization or sedation. A group of constituents known as the valepotriates has been shown to have definite central nervous system depressant effects in humans and is marketed as a sedative in Germany. Other constituents augment this activity. The depressant activity is not synergistic with alcohol, and the incidence of undesirable side effects is less than with diazepam. The valepotriates exhibit cytotoxic and antitumor activities. The valepotriate content of valerian can vary widely, depending mainly on preparation and storage conditions. No toxicities for valerian or the valepotriates have been reported in humans and no adverse effects attributed in controlled clinical trials. Although there is little evidence that the valepotriates are effective cytotoxic agents in vivo, there is a concern about the safety of valerian preparations, particularly following long-term use.

Overall, valerian appears to be a safe and effective drug. Stabilization and standardization of the constituents should produce products of considerable importance to the layman and medical practitioners.

Feverfew (*Tanacetum parthenium*, synonym *Chrysanthemun parthenium*) has traditionally been used as an antipyretic, an antispasmodic, an emmenagogue, a carminative and an anthelmintic. More recently it has become popular in Europe as a prophylactic treatment for headaches. Relief for menstrual pain, asthma and arthritis has been claimed for its extracts.

The chemistry of feverfew is poorly defined. The plant is rich in sesquiterpene lactones, principally parthenolide, cited as its active and toxic ingredients. Members of this class of compounds have spasmolytic activity. An aqueous solution dramatically suppresses prostaglandin synthesis. The mechanism of action is not known but appears to differ from that of the salicylates. Feverfew extracts are also potent inhibitors of serotonin release from platelets and polymorphonuclear leukocyte granules, providing a possible connection between the claimed benefits of feverfew in migraines and arthritis.

Several clinical studies have clearly established the beneficial effects of feverfew as prophylaxis against migraines, decreasing both the incidence and severity of symptoms. The abrupt withdrawal of feverfew in one study led to incapacitating headaches in some people. Most subjects experienced anxiety, poor sleep and muscle and joint stiffness. This effect has been referred to as "post-feverfew syndrome."

Side effects are noted by about 20% of feverfew users, the most troublesome (11%) being mouth ulcerations. Other side effects include widespread inflammation of the oral mucosa and tongue, often with swelling of the lips and loss of taste. Dermatitis and increased heart rate were reported by some users.

The herb has been used to promote menstruation and should be regarded as an abortifacient.

Feverfew, with its established benefits and relatively low incidence of adverse effects, represents a solid prospect for effective prophylactic therapy for migraine headaches. At the very least, studies with this herb should help clarify the nature of migraines.

Coltsfoot (*Tussilago farfara*) is one of several plants recently identified as potentially hazardous when consumed chronically. *Tussilago* is derived from the Latin *tussis*, meaning cough, and the plant has a long history of use as an antitussive. Either the leaves or the flower heads are used. The active ingredient is a mucilage that acts as a demulcent and expectorant.

Although coltsfoot is effective for the purposes claimed, the leaves and flowers contain pyrrolizidine alkaloids. Some of these alkaloids are hepatotoxic and carcinogenic. Senkirkine is present in young flowers and senecionine is found with it in the leaves. Both are known hepatotoxins and carcinogens.

No cases of confirmed coltsfoot poisoning have been reported, which is not surprising as the pyrrolizidine alkaloids are chronic, cumulative poisons. The argument that the plant has buffers or neutralizers to prevent the toxic effects is not supported by one study with rats. Two-thirds of those receiving greater than 4% coltsfoot in their diet developed hemangioendotheliosarcoma of the liver. That coltsfoot can no longer be considered safe therapy is reinforced by the recent death from hepatotoxicity of an infant whose mother consumed an herbal tea throughout her pregnancy that contained coltsfoot. This raises the question of long-term safety of many herbal preparations.

Comfrey (*Symphytum officinale*) is one of the most common herbs sold in North America. Modern herbalists have widely promoted the leaves or roots as poultices for wounds, burns, sprains, swellings and bruises. Comfrey, it has been claimed, heals gastric ulcers and hemorrhoids and suppresses bronchial congestion and inflammation.

The healing properties of comfrey are probably due to its content of allantoin, an agent that promotes cell proliferation. Ointments containing comfrey have been found to have anti-inflammatory activity, which appears to be related to allantoin, rosmarinic acid or a hydrocolloid polysaccharide. The roots are 0.6 to 0.8% allantoin and 4 to 6.5% tannins, the leaves 1.3% allantoin and 8 to 9% tannins. Both roots and leaves have large amounts of mucilage.

Despite its common use, the long-term ingestion of comfrey may pose a health hazard. Like Gordolobos tea and coltsfoot, comfrey contains several pyrrolizidine alkaloids known to be hepatotoxic and carcinogenic. The type and amount of alkaloids present vary with plant part and species of *Symphytum*. Echimidine is the most toxic of the alkaloids found in *Symphytum*, but does not appear in *Symphytum officinale*. The roots and leaves of this plant are hepatotoxic and carcinogenic (liver and urinary bladder) in rats fed in concentrations as low as 0.5 to 8% of their diet, respectively. Numerous human toxicities also appear in the literature.

Pyrrolizidine alkaloids are recognized as compounds of toxicological significance. A detailed report of human pyrrolizidine toxicity described an outbreak of hepatic disease among Afghani villagers who ate wheat contaminated with *Heliotropium* seeds, which contain hepatotoxic alkaloids. Within 2 years, 23% of the 7,200 inhabitants observed had severe liver impairment.

Oral ingestion of pyrrolizidine-containing plants, such as comfrey, poses the greatest risk; the alkaloids are converted to pyrrole-like derivatives, which are responsible for the toxicity. Additionally, the alkaloids of comfrey applied to the skin of rats were detected in the urine, and lactating rats in the experiment excreted pyrrolizidine alkaloids into breast milk.

The Henry Doubleday Research Association (growers and marketers of comfrey in the United Kingdom) stated publicly that until further research clarifies the long-term health hazard of comfrey ingestion, "no human being or animal should eat, drink, or take comfrey in any form." Due to the lack of scientific evidence of a therapeutic effect, the consumption of comfrey and its teas cannot be recommended until its safety and efficacy have been demonstrated.

TABLE 2: Commonly Available Herbs Used for Beverages and Medicines[a]

Name	Part Used	Major Uses	Ingredients[b]	Side Effects[c]	Efficacy[d, g]	Safety[e, h]	Comments
Aloe *Aloe barbadensis*	fresh juice	wound healing, burns	gel (mucilage)		+	+, 3	loses its healing activity if dried; aloe gel prudent to avoid in pregnancy
	dried latex	cathartic	anthraquinones	diarrhea, cramping	+	+, 3	habitual use may cause excessive irritation to the colon; aloe latex contraindicated in pregnancy
Aletris, Unicorn root *Aletris farinosa*	roots and rhizomes	female discomforts, estrogenic activity	diosgenin, gentrogenin	vertigo	e	s	contraindicated in pregnancy
Althaea, marshmallow *Althaea officinalis*	root	demulcent for topical wounds, sore throat, stomach ailments	mucilage, asparagine	–	e	s	found to have spasmolytic and anti-inflammatory activities
Ammi *Ammi majus, A. visnaga*	aerial parts	vasodilator (asthma and angina) increases HDL	coumarins, psoralens (khellin)	ophthalmic changes, photo-sensitization, dermatitis, nausea, vomiting	e	n	cromolyn sodium based on components of *A. visnaga;* contraindicated in pregnancy
Angelica *Angelica archangelica*	root, fruit, leaves	diuretic, carminative emmenagogue, flavor, etc.	volatile oil	–	–	–, 2	contraindicated in pregnancy
Anise (Star anise) *Pimpinella anisum (Illicium verum)*	fuit (seed)	carminative, cough, dyspepsia, flavor	volatile oil (anethole)	oil may cause nausea, vomiting, seizures and pulmonary edema	NA	NA, 2 (NA, 1)	licorice flavor
Arnica *Arnica montana*	flower heads	anti-inflammatory, analgesic	unidentified	ingestion can cause severe gastrointestinal and CNS disturbances and can result in death	+	+, 1	plant should not be ingested
Aspidium, male fern *Dryopteris filix-mas*	rhizomes	vermifuge	oleoresin filicin, filmarone	headache, dyspnea, vertigo, diarrhea, muscular weakness, coma, blindness	e	n	contraindicated in pregnancy
Australian	see: Tea tree						
Autumn crocus *Colchicum autumnale*	corm and extract	gout, rheumatism, etc.	colchicine	thirst, nausea, vomiting, diarrhea, renal impairment, agranulocytosis, etc.	e	n	being investigated for management of chronic inflammatory hepatic diseases; contraindicated in pregnancy

TABLE 2: Commonly Available Herbs Used for Beverages and Medicines[a] *(cont'd)*

Name	Part Used	Major Uses	Ingredients[b]	Side Effects[c]	Efficacy[d, g]	Safety[e, h]	Comments
Barberry, Oregon grape *Berberis vulgaris, Mahonia aquifolium*	root and stem bark	antibacterial, many others	berberine, isoquinoline alkaloids	stupor, daze, diarrhea, nephritis	e	n	effective in bacterial-induced diarrheal conditions
Bearberry	see: Uva ursi						
Betel nut *Areca catechu*	nut	stimulant	arecoline, etc.	leukoplakia, squamous cell carcinoma of mouth, affects respiration and heart rate, tetanic convulsions, death	e	n	the "quid" consists of the sliced areca nut, and slaked lime wrapped in betel leaves *(Piper betel);* contraindicated in pregnancy
Betony *Stachys officinalis,* syn.=*Betonica officinalis*	aerial parts	astringent to treat diarrhea, headache	15% tannins, flavonoids	high doses may cause gastro-intestinal irritation	e	i	flavonoids may be hypotensive; contraindicated in pregnancy
Black cohosh *Cimicifuga racemosa*	rhizomes and roots	antirheumatic, uterine stimulant, etc.	actein, cimicifugin	nausea and vomiting	-	±, 1	may potentiate hypotensive drugs; contraindicated in pregnancy
Bloodroot *Sanguinaria canadensis*	root and rhizome	dental antibacterial	sanguinarine, etc.	nausea, vomiting, CNS depression, hypotension	e	s/n	toxic if ingested; considered safe as an anti-plaque agent in oral rinses and toothpastes
Blue cohosh *Caulophyllum thalictroides*	rhizomes	emmenagogue, uterine stimulant	methylcytisine, caulosaponin and caulo-phyllosaponin glycosides	mucous membrane irritant, seeds are GIT irritants	i	n	contraindicated in pregnancy; roasted seeds are a coffee substitute
Boldo *Peumus boldus*	leaves	diuretic, "hepatic tonic", laxative	boldine and other alkaloids	CNS stimulation, paralysis, death	e	i/n	clinically significant diuresis; contraindicated in pregnancy
Boneset *Eupatorium perfoliatum*	aerial parts	antipyretic	eupatorin, tremetrol, sesquiterpene lactones	severe diarrhea, hypoglycemia, weakness	i	n	contains pyrrolizidine alkaloids; contraindicated in pregnancy
Borage *Borago officinalis*	leaves and tops	diuretic, astringent (diarrhea)	tannins, mucilage	-	- to ±	±, 3	contains traces of pyrrolizidine alkaloids; prudent to avoid during pregnancy
Broom *Cytisus scoparius*	flowering tops	diuretic, cathartic, emetic, sedative	sparteine, hydroxytyramine	-	+	-, 1	mind-altering properties when smoked; contraindicated in pregnancy

TABLE 2: Commonly Available Herbs Used for Beverages and Medicines[a] *(cont'd)*

Name	Part Used	Major Uses	Ingredients[b]	Side Effects[c]	Efficacy[d, g]	Safety[e, h]	Comments
Buchu *Barosma* spp.	leaves	urinary antiseptic, diuretic	diosphenol	–	± to +	+, 2	prudent to avoid during pregnancy
Burdock *Arctium* spp.	roots	skin disorders, diuretic	polyphenolic acids	–	–	+, 2	
Calamus *Acorus calamus*	rhizomes	digestive aid, cough, flavor	volatile oil	–	±	– or +, 1	some varieties contain the carcinogen, beta-asarone; prudent to avoid during pregnancy
Calendula, marigold *Calendula officinalis*	florets	anti-inflammatory, wound healing, antipyretic	calendulin, triterpenes	allergic reactions	i	i	
Capsicum *Capsicum* spp.	fruit	counterirritant, digestive aid	capsaicin	burning sensation, rarely blisters	+	+, 2	affects nerve endings but not capillaries
Catnip *Nepeta cataria*	leaves and tops	carminative, sedative, etc.	volatile oil (nepetalactone)	oil may cause CNS toxicity	±	+, 3	possible psychotropic when smoked
Cayenne	see: Capsicum						
Chamomile *Matricaria chamomilla, Anthemis nobilis*	flower heads	carminative, anti-inflammatory, antispasmodic	volatile oil, (chamazulene, alpha-bisabolol)	contact dermatitis	+	+, 3	
Chaparral *Larrea tridentata*	leaves and twigs	diuretic, antiseptic, anticancer	nordihydro-guaiaretic acid	lesions in the mesenteric lymph nodes and kidneys	–	–, 2	prudent to avoid during pregnancy
Chaste tree *Vitex agnus-castus*	fruit	various effects on female reproductory system	volatile oil, iridoids, flavonoids	minor GI upset, itching	e	s	used in Germany to treat PMS, potentially useful in managing abnormal menstrual cycles, hyperprolactemia and increasing milk production in lactating women
Coltsfoot *Tussilago farfara*	leaves and/or flower heads	antitussive, demulcent	mucilage	–	+	–, 2	low levels of pyrrolizidine alkaloids; prudent to avoid during pregnancy
Comfrey *Symphytum officinale*	roots and leaves	wound healing agent	allantoin, mucilage, tannin	hepatotoxic, carcinogenic	+	–, 2	contains high levels of pyrrolizidine alkaloids; Canadian laws recently amended to permit only the leaves of *S. officinale* eligible for DINs; prudent to avoid during pregnancy
Cucurbita pumpkin, squash *Cucurbita* spp.	seed	vermifuge, prostate disorders	cucurbitin	none reported	e	s	effective vermifuge

TABLE 2: Commonly Available Herbs Used for Beverages and Medicines[a] *(cont'd)*

Name	Part Used	Major Uses	Ingredients[b]	Side Effects[c]	Efficacy[d, g]	Safety[e, h]	Comments
Dandelion *Taraxacum officinale*	roots and leaves	diuretic, laxative, digestive aid	inulin, bitter resins	-	±	+, 3	leaves weaker in action
Devil's claw *Harpagophytum procumbens*	tubers	antirheumatic, anti-inflammatory	harpagoside	-	-	+, 2	activity is still controversial; contraindicated in pregnancy
Dioscorea *Dioscorea* spp.	tubers	none	diosgenin	-	NA	NA, 1	source of most steroid drugs
Echinacea, cone flower *Echinacea* spp.	flower	immunostimulant, wound healing, anti-inflammatory	polysaccharides, isobutylamides, alkamides	none reported	e	s	
Ephedra, Ma Huang *Ephedra* spp.	aerial parts	CNS stimulant	ephedrine, pseudoephedrine	nervousness, headache, insomnia, palpitations, skin flushing, vomiting	e	s	most N.A. species are devoid of alkaloids and are used to produce nonstimulating teas; contraindicated in pregnancy, and heart disorders, hypertension
Fennel *Foeniculum vulgare*	fruit (seeds)	carminative, coughs, digestive	volatile oil (anethole)	oil may cause nausea, vomiting, seizures and pulmonary edema	+	+, 3	
Fenugreek *Trigonella foenum graecum*	seeds	demulcent, laxative, digestive aid, flavor	mucilage	-	±	+, 2	also contains diosgenin and others
Feverfew *Tanacetum parthenium*, syn.=*Chrysanthemum parthenium*	leaves	migraine prevention, carminative, antipyretic, emmenagogue	parthenolide	oral ulcers	+	+, 3	contraindicated in pregnancy
Garlic *Allium sativum*	bulbs	hypertension, atherosclerosis	allicin	contact dermatitis	+	+, NA	
		antibacterial, diuretic, antihyperlipemic, antitumor, etc.			+		
Gentian *Gentiana lutea*	rhizomes and roots	appetite stimulant, digestive aid	gentiopicrin and amarogentin	nausea and vomiting	+	+, 2	
Ginger *Zingiber officinale*	rhizomes	motion sickness prevention, carminative	volatile oil, resin	-	+	+, NA	

TABLE 2: Commonly Available Herbs Used for Beverages and Medicines[a] *(cont'd)*

Name	Part Used	Major Uses	Ingredients[b]	Side Effects[c]	Efficacy[d, g]	Safety[e, h]	Comments
Ginkgo, maidenhair tree *Ginkgo biloba*	leaves	asthma, circulation disorders, dilation of arteries, capillaries and veins, inhibits platelet aggregation; antioxidant	ginkgolides, flavones	mild GI effects, headache, severe allergic reactions with fruit pulp	e	s	pulp and seed are toxic, appears to increase otic and cerebral circulation
Ginseng *Panax* spp.	roots	tonic, adaptogen (anti-stress)	triterpene glycosides	"corticosteroid poisoning"	±	±, 3	
Goldenseal *Hydrastis canadensis*	rhizomes and roots	dyspepsia, stop post-partum bleeding	hydrastine, berberine	dangerous in high doses	± to +	+, 1	contraindicated in pregnancy
Gotu Kola *Centella asiatica*	leaves (seeds, roots)	wound healing, anti-inflammatory, cicatrising agent	madecassol, asiatic acid, asiaticoside	few, contact dermatitis	e	s	*Madecassol* don't confuse with *Cola nitida*, a caffeine-containing stimulant, sedative in small animals
Guarana, Zoom *Paullinia cupana, P. sorbilis*	seed paste	stimulant, diuretic, fasting agent	caffeine	as for caffeine	e	s	3–5% caffeine by dry weight, (coffee contains 1–2%); contraindicated in pregnancy
Gymnema *Gymnema sylvestre*	leaves (stems)	hypoglycemic activity	gymnemic acid	as for hypoglycemia	e	s	appears to act similarly to the sulfonylureas
Hawthorn *Crataegus oxyacantha*	fruit, leaves, flowers	vasodilation, hypotensive	flavonoids and triterpene glycosides	-	+	+, 1	may enhance digitalis toxicity
Hibiscus *Hibiscus sabdariffa*	flowers	diuretic, laxative, coloring agent	citric and hibiscic acid, pigments	-	± to +	+, 3	
Hops *Humulus lupulus*	fruit (strobiles)	sedative flavoring and preserving beer	polyphenolics	dermatitis	+ to + +	+, 2	occasionally smoked to obtain a mild euphoria
Horse chestnuts *Aesculus hippocastanum*	seeds, bark, leaves	vasoconstriction, anti-inflammatory, anti-exudative	esculin, escin saponins, etc.	toxic, muscle twitching, weakness, vomiting, diarrhea, depression, paralysis	e	n/i	safe topically for hemorrhoids, *Proctosedyl*
Horsetail *Equisetum* spp.	aerial parts	diuretic, astringent, antihemorrhagic	saponin, flavones, alkaloids	-	- to ±	+, 1	prudent to avoid during pregnancy; contains thiaminase

TABLE 2: Commonly Available Herbs Used for Beverages and Medicines[a] *(cont'd)*

Name	Part Used	Major Uses	Ingredients[b]	Side Effects[c]	Efficacy[d, g]	Safety[e, h]	Comments
Hydrangea *Hydrangea arborescens, Hydrangea paniculata*	rhizomes and roots, leaves	diuretic, lithotriptic mild euphoric	flavonoids, resins, mucilage, phenolic and cyanogenic glycosides	vertigo in large doses, vomiting, nausea	– +	±, 2 –, 2	leaves are smoked; narrow margin between pleasure and toxicity
Juniper *Juniperus communis*	fruit (berries)	diuretic, antiseptic, carminative, flavor	volatile oil, resin, flavonoids	kidney irritation, contact dermatitis	+	±, 1	the berries and oil are contraindicated in pregnancy and kidney disease; related species should not be used.
Licorice *Glycyrrhiza glabra*	rhizomes and roots	expectorant, demulcent, flavor, etc.	glycyrrhizin	sodium retention, hypokalemia, "pseudo-aldosteronism"	+	±, 1	may be used in Herpes infections
Life root *Senecio aureus*	entire plant	emmenagogue	pyrrolizidine alkaloids	hepatotoxic	±	–, 1	contraindicated in pregnancy
Linden flowers *Tilia* spp.	flowers	diaphoretic, beverage	flavonoids, volatile oil	–	+	+, 2	contraindicated in heart disease
Lobelia *Lobelia inflata*	leaves and tops	nauseant, expectorant, psychotropic antiasthmatic	lobeline	vomiting, paralysis, convulsions	+ + NA	±, 1 –, 1 NA	nicotine-like action; death can result; prudent to avoid during pregnancy
Mate, Paraguay or Jesuit's tea, Yerba mate *Ilex paraguariensis*	leaves	stimulant, diuretic	caffeine, etc.	as for caffeine, may increase risk of esophageal cancer (dose-dependent)	e	s/i	used as a coffee substitute, similar caffeine levels; contraindicated in pregnancy
Mistletoe *Phoradendron tomentosum* *Viscum album*	leaves leaves	hypertensive, smooth muscle stimulant; hypertensive, antispasmodic	phoratoxins, tyramine; viscotoxins	gastric irritation, bradycardia, hemagglutination	± ±	–, 1 –, 1	cytotoxicity of lectins being studied for anticancer activity; contraindicated in presence of MAO inhibitor; prudent to avoid during pregnancy
Mormon tea *Ephedra nevadensis*	stems	diuretic, astringent (diarrhea), tonic	tannin, volatile oil	constipation	+ –	±[f], 1 ±[f], 1	N. Am. *Ephedra* devoid of alkaloids
Neem *Azadirachta indica*	all parts	panacea, insecticidal, hypoglycemic	fixed oil, azadirachtin, etc.	safe for adults, 5-30 mL of oil in infants caused Reye's syndrome-like symptoms, death from hepato-encephalopathy	e	s/i	seeds are poisonous in large doses; contraindicated in pregnancy

TABLE 2: Commonly Available Herbs Used for Beverages and Medicines[a] *(cont'd)*

Name	Part Used	Major Uses	Ingredients[b]	Side Effects[c]	Efficacy[d, g]	Safety[e, h]	Comments
Nettle *Urtica dioica*	aerial parts	diuretic, astringent	unidentified	local irritation to the stinging hairs	+	+, 3	
		antiasthmatic, antirheumatic			–	+, 3	
Parsley *Petroselinum crispum*	leaves and stems,	digestive aid; diuretic	volatile oil (apiol and myristicin), furanocoumarins	nausea, vomiting, dizziness, swollen liver, polyneuritis, phototoxicity	±	+, 2	roots and oil are contraindicated in pregnancy
	fruit (seeds), root	digestive aid, diuretic, emmenagogue			+	± to +, 2	
Passion flower *Passiflora incarnata*	flowering and fruiting tops	sedative, antispasmodic	alkaloids, flavonoids, maltol	hypotension	± to +	+, 2	
Pau d'Arco *Tabebuia* spp.	bark	anticancer, antimicrobial	naphthaquinones (lapachol)	nausea, vomiting, anemia, hemorrhage	–	±, 1	therapeutic index is low
Pennyroyal *Hedeoma pulegioides*	leaves, oil	carminative, diaphoretic	volatile oil (pulegone)	nausea, vomiting, diarrhea, CNS depression, kidney irritant	±	±, 2	contraindicated in pregnancy
Mentha pulegium		emmenagogue, abortifacient	volatile oil (pulegone)		+ to ±	–, 2	
Pokeroot *Phytolacca americana*	roots, leaves	antirheumatic, laxative, inflammatory conditions of the upper respiratory tract, anticancer	phytolaccigein, mitogens	severe cramping, vomiting, weakness, hypotension, spasms, death	–	–, 0	should not be consumed
Red clover *Trifolium pratense*	flowers	expectorant, anticancer	phenolic glycosides	–	–	+, 3	
St. John's Wort *Hypericum perforatum*	leaves and tops	tranquilizer, anti-inflammatory	volatile oil, tannins, hypericin	photosensitizer	+	+, 1	
Sarsaparilla *Smilax* spp.	roots	diuretic, flavor	volatile oil sapogenins	none recorded	+	+, 2	
Sassafras *Sassafras albidum*	root bark	antirheumatic, tonic, diuretic, diaphoretic	volatile oil (safrole)	hepatotoxic, carcinogenic	–	–, 2	Sassafras and safrole are listed as food adulterants in Food and Drugs Regulations B.01.046; contraindicated in pregnancy
		flavor	safrole		+	–, NA	
Saw palmetto, sabal, cabbage palm *Serenoa repens*	berry	benign prostatic hypertrophy	phytosterols	no significant side effects reported, headache	e	s/i	contraindicated in pregnancy, children, and those with hormone-dependent illnesses

TABLE 2: Commonly Available Herbs Used for Beverages and Medicines[a] *(cont'd)*

Name	Part Used	Major Uses	Ingredients[b]	Side Effects[c]	Efficacy[d, g]	Safety[e, h]	Comments
Senega *Polygala senega*	roots	expectorant, emetic, diaphoretic	saponins	nausea, vomiting, diarrhea	+	+, NA	low therapeutic index; prudent to avoid during pregnancy
Senna *Cassia acutifolia* *Cassia augustifolia*	leaflets, pods	cathartic	anthraquinones (sennosides)	griping	+	+, 1	habitual use may cause excessive irritation to the colon; prudent to avoid during pregnancy
Shavegrass *Equisetum hyemale*	aerial parts	diuretic, hemostatic, astringent	tannin, alkaloids (nicotine, equisetine)	lassitude, diarrhea	NA	NA, 1	confusion exists regarding safety; prudent to avoid during pregnancy
Skullcap *Scutellaria lateriflora*	aerial parts	sedative, antispasmodic	volatile oil, flavonoids	–	–	+, 2	considered to be essentially inactive
Slippery elm *Ulmus rubra*	inner bark	demulcent, urinary tract inflammations, throat irritations, topically for cold sores and boils	mucilage, phytosterols	contact dermatitis	e	s	contraindicated in pregnancy; efficacy in urinary tract is unconfirmed
Snakeroot	see: Senega						
Taheebo	see: Pau d'Arco						
Tansy *Tanacetum vulgare*	leaves and flowers	anthelmintic, emmenagogue, tonic	volatile oil (thujone)	nausea, vomiting, convulsions, death	±	– to ±, 2	contraindicated in pregnancy; oil is quite toxic
Tea tree *Melaleuca alternifolia*	leaf oil	topical antiseptic, vaginal infections	volatile oil, terpinen-4-ol	topical and vaginal irritation	e	i	safer and more effective products are available
Tubocurarine *Chondodendron tomentosum*	bark and stems	skeletal muscle relaxant	alkaloids	hypotension, cardiovascular collapse, respiratory failure	NA	NA, NA	a constituent of curare
Unicorn root	see: Aletris						
Uva ursi *Arctostaphylos uva-ursi*	leaves	diuretic, astringent, urinary antiseptic	arbutin (prodrug of hydroquinolone), ursolic acid, isoquercetin	mild CNS depression	+	+, 2	urine is often green
Valerian *Valerianna officinalis*	rhizomes and roots	tranquilizer	valepotriates	–	+	+, 2	disagreeable odor; commercial products available in Europe
Wintergreen *Gaultheria procumbens*	leaves and stems	counterirritant, analgesic, flavor	volatile oil (methyl salicylate)	oil is toxic (salicylism)	NA	NA, 1	

TABLE 2: Commonly Available Herbs Used for Beverages and Medicines[a] *(cont'd)*

Name	Part Used	Major Uses	Ingredients[b]	Side Effects[c]	Efficacy[d, g]	Safety[e, h]	Comments
Woodruff, sweet *Galium odoratum*	aerial parts	sedative, antispasmodic, anti-inflammatory, diuretic, diaphoretic	coumarin, asperuloside		i	s	used primarily as a flavor and fragrance
Wormwood *Artemisia absinthium*	leaves and tops	anthelmintic, flavor, tonic, mind-altering effects	volatile oil (thujone), sesquiterpene lactones (absinthin)	absinthism (trembling, convulsions, dementia, death)	+	–, 1	contraindicated in pregnancy; thujone is thought to be the toxic ingredient; it is nearly water-insoluble (teas), therefore teas may not be as toxic as alcoholic extracts
Yellow dock *Rumex crispus*	rhizomes and roots	astringent, laxative	tannins, anthraquinones	diarrhea, nausea, polyuria	+	+[f], 1	prudent to avoid during pregnancy
Yerba Santa *Eriodictyon californicum*	leaves	expectorant, liniments for bruises and rheumatism	volatile oil, eriodictyol, eriodictyonine	none reported	i	s	
Yucca *Yucca spp.*	fruit, leaves	arthritis, migraines, hypertension	saponins	nontoxic orally	i	i	

a This table does not comment on the desirability or feasibility of using any of the herbal remedies listed, even those indicated as being apparently efficacious and probably safe. Appropriate references should be consulted for detailed explanations of the many complex factors regarding the use of these drugs which could not be included in this brief summary.

b This column indicates the major ingredient(s) or class(es) of compounds identified. This may not be the active ingredient as often these have not been identified.

c This column lists the symptoms most commonly seen following doses generally considered to be excessive.

d Efficacy as scored by Tyler; +=effective; ±=efficacy inconclusive; –=ineffective; NA=not listed.

e Safety, in normal individuals when used appropriately, as scored in the first column by Tyler: +=safe; ±=safety inconclusive; –=not safe and in the second column by Duke: 0=very dangerous, Duke wouldn't drink a cup of it; 1=more dangerous than coffee, Duke wouldn't be afraid to drink 1 cup containing 10 g of herb steeped; 2=as dangerous as coffee, Duke wouldn't be afraid to drink. 2 cups a day; 3=Duke considers it safer than coffee and wouldn't hesitate, for health reasons, to drink 3 cups a day; NA=not listed.

f All tannin-rich drugs may have carcinogenic potential in long-term usage.

g Efficacy as interpreted from *The Lawrence Review of Natural Products* (up to December 1994), St. Louis, MO: Facts and Comparisons. Efficacy in normal individuals when used appropriately: "e"=efficacious, "i"=efficacy inconclusive, "n"=not efficacious.

h Safety as interpreted from *The Lawrence Review of Natural Products* (up to December 1994), St. Louis, MO: Facts and Comparisons. Safety in normal individuals when used appropriately: "s"=considered safe, "i"=safety is inconclusive or unknown, "n"=not safe/toxic.

SPECIAL CONSIDERATIONS

SAFETY CONCERNS

Herbal medicines are now widely available and widely used, but regulations to ensure quality products and their safe and effective use are largely nonexistent or ineffective. The consumer still cannot be absolutely sure the package actually contains what the label says or implies. Table 3 lists information that should appear on every label. The literature contains many examples of poor quality herbal preparations, with the characteristic constituents present only in negligible amounts or absent altogether.

The undeclared ingredients in herbal remedies can lead to unforeseen reactions. Intentional adulteration of herbal preparations with toxic components or allopathic medications continues: heavy metals, atropine-like alkaloids, cocaine, synthetic corticosteroids and/or nonsteroidal anti-inflammatory drugs, estrogen-like substances and other drugs have all been found in herbal preparations. Deaths from products containing some of these contaminants have been recorded.

Herbal products in a number of developed countries are not controlled by their drug regulations and can escape premarketing surveillance of their toxic potential; they can be marketed as dietary supplements. In Canada, the Health Protection Branch can grant a Drug Identification Number (DIN) to a herbal drug based on folklore and the anecdotal evidence or insist that it go through a premarket assessment for efficacy, labelling and quality. Though no DIN has been applied for, herbal substances sold as food or diet supplements can be clearly intended by the manufacturer to be used as drugs. Consumers use them to treat various ailments, frequently not knowing the proper method of preparation, the proper dose, the proper duration, or if the herb has any adverse effects or might be contraindicated in their particular case. It is even more complicated as the part of the plant used is often significant. Numerous patients may be exposed to unnecessary risk before the results of independent risk-assessments are available.

Uninformed individuals often believe that "natural" is a guarantee of harmlessness and exhibit little hesitation in consuming doses of herbal remedies larger than tradition provides. They do not consider herbal remedies to be drugs and rarely consider the possibility of adverse interactions when simultaneously taking nonprescription or prescription medications. Some herbal preparations are contraindicated for subpopulations with certain diseases or medical conditions, (e.g., the use of *Ephedra* species (Ma Huang) in hypertension).

Acute toxic response to most herbal products is uncommon (demonstrated by lengthy folk histories), but not unknown. There have been several deaths reported from ingesting Chinese herbs for pain relief that contain aconite. Acute toxic reactions to an herbal product, e.g., dermatological reactions, are quite likely to be recognized by herbal healers and the consumer. However, they are unlikely to recognize the subtle, chronic effects of some compounds: pyrrolizidine alkaloids, safrole, aristolochic acids, hydrogen cyanide, or other toxic compounds associated with the long-term use of some herbs. We know very little about the chronic toxicity of most herbs. Toxicities, including deaths, continue to be reported; interactions with other drugs have been documented.

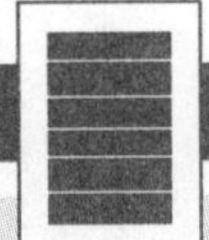

TABLE 3: What Every Label Should Have
Original supplier's certification that material is what is claimed.
List of ingredients showing amount of each and source by botanical name.
Part of plant used and whether it is an extract or powder.
The traditional use(s) and how it should be prepared.
Clear instructions for uses.
Any adverse effects that might occur.
Any persons who should not take this product.

Special Considerations

POISONOUS PLANTS

A poison is any substance that, in relatively small amounts, produces injury to the body by its chemical action. Most of us can probably relate an incident or story about a plant or plant product involved in an untoward event. Many poisons are highly active substances, and since ancient times have served the purposes of murder and suicide. In suitable doses they may also be important as medicines. Other pharmacologically less active substances may make a plant poisonous because they are present in high concentration or they accumulate in the body with chronic use. Often, the only difference between medicinal and poisonous plants is the dose. The poisonous nature of a plant (the presence and concentration of its active constituents) can be and often is subject to the plant part, the degree of maturity of the plant and environmental conditions.

Some plants are generally regarded as poisonous rather than medicinal. The following are examples, although most also have medicinal applications: rosary pea (jequirity bean, *Abrus precatorius*), water hemlock (*Cicuta maculata*), poison hemlock (*Conium maculatum*), bittersweet (*Solanum dulcamara*), deadly nightshade (*Atropa belladonna*), lily of the valley (*Convallaria majalis*), daffodil (*Narcissus nux-vomica*), mistletoe (*Viscum album*).

PRE- AND PERI-NATAL ISSUES

It is well recognized that drugs taken during pregnancy can produce devastating effects on fetal development. Dysmorphic teratology is considered the major risk, but behavioral teratology is an additional concern. Behavioral effects are less obvious, not as easily recognized as dysmorphic effects. The effects of caffeine, tobacco, alcohol and many illicit and licit drugs are well documented. However, the effects of herbal remedies on fetal and neonatal development are just starting to be realized.

The deleterious outcome in animals and some reports of in utero toxicities to humans clearly demonstrate that herbs are not always harmless to the unborn. Yet pregnant women frequently use herbal beverages during pregnancy as substitutes for caffeine-containing beverages or for medicinal purposes. Additionally, herbs (including some potentially dangerous ones) are sometimes employed in the practice of midwifery.

A recent report documents the hazards associated with two commonly used herbs. A Swiss woman consumed an herbal tea, purchased from her pharmacy, daily throughout her pregnancy. Her infant died 11 days after birth from severe jaundice, massive hepatomegaly and ascites. The tea has been found to contain coltsfoot (coughwort, *Tussilago farfara),* and butterbur (*Petasites officinalis*), both members of the compositae family and known to contain hepatotoxic pyrrolizidine alkaloids. The mother incurred no clinically apparent harm.

Severe, even lethal, cases of **liver damage** in small children occur sporadically throughout the world associated with the use of herbs that contain pyrrolizidine alkaloids. Veno-occlusive disease of the liver once was common in children in Jamaica, where a "bush tea" (*Crotalaria fulva*) that contained pyrrolizidine alkaloids was in common use. More recently, two incidences of veno-occlusive liver disease were diagnosed in infants treated at home with an extract of *Senecio longilobus*, which is known for its pyrrolizidine alkaloid content. One of the infants died, the other developed cirrhosis of the liver. Other plants used as herbal remedies that contain pyrrolizidine alkaloids and, therefore, should be avoided in pregnancy and infants, if not altogether, are alkanet (*Alkanna tinctoria),* hound's-tongue (*Cynoglossum officinale*), butterbur (*Petasites* species), ragwort (*Senecio jacobaea),* groundsel (*Senecio vulgaris),* comfrey (*Symphytum* species), and other species of *Senecio*, *Crotolaria*, *Echium*, *Eupatorium,* and *Heliotropium*.

Before a patient consumes an herbal beverage or herbal remedy, the risk-benefit ratio must be considered. Females are generally advised against ingesting medications while pregnant. This is particularly true of medications that may induce uterine contractions and possibly lead to spontaneous abortion. Herbal drugs in this category are those used as stimulant laxatives, diuretics, and emmenagogues (drugs that induce menstrual flow, abortifacients). Plants containing known toxins and their close relatives should also be avoided during pregnancy, if not at all times.

Herbal **laxatives** include aloe (*Aloe* species), bryony (*Bryonia* species), senna (*Cassia* species), colocynth (*Citrullus colocynthis*), scammony (*Convolvulus scammonia*), croton oil (*Croton* species), gamboge gum resin (*Garcinia* species), jalap (kaladanna, *Ipomoea* species), podophyllum (mayapple, *Podophyllum pelatum*), cascara

(*Rhamnus purshiana*), rhubarb (*Rheum officinale*), castor oil (*Ricinus communis*), and dock (*Rumex* species). Other laxatives, such as the bulk and lubricating agents, should be used cautiously.

Plants used as **diuretics** include calamus (*Acorus calamus*), quack grass (*Agropyron* species), dogbane (*Apocynum cannabinum*), bearberry (uva ursi, *Arctostaphylos uva-ursi*), buchu (*Barosma betulina*), birch (betula, *Betula alba*), blue cohosh (*Caulophyllum thalictroides*), false unicorn root (*Chamaelirium leuteum*), chicory (*Cichorium intybus*), black cohosh (*Cimicifuga racemosa*), broom (*Cytisus scoparius*), shavegrass (horsetail, *Equisetum* species), fumitory (*Fumaria officinalis*), licorice (*Glycyrrhiza glabra*), juniper (*Juniperus communis*), squaw vine (*Mitchella repens*), parsley (*Petroselinum crispum*), boldo (*Peumus boldus*), elder (*Sambucus nigra*), saw palmetto (*Serenoa repens*), ragwort and groundsel (*Senecio* species), and nettle (*Urtica dioica*).

Herbs used as an **emmenagogue** include alder (*Alnus incana* and other *Alnus* species), wild ginger (*Asarum canadense*), blue cohosh (*Caulophyllum thalictroides*), false unicorn root (*Chamaelirium leuteum*), black cohosh (*Cimicifuga racemosa*), wallflower (*Cheiranthus cheiri*), blessed thistle (*Cnicus benedicta*), saffron crocus (*Crocus sativus*), fleabane (*Erigeron canadensis*), euphorbia (*Euphorbia* species), lavender (*Lavandula latifolia*), lionsear (*Leonotis leonurus*), pennyroyal (*Mentha pulegium*), squaw vine (*Mitchella repens*), and rue (*Ruta graveolens*).

Other herbs that have **mutagenic or teratogenic** properties (in addition to coffee, alcohol, some licit and illicit drugs) include: rosary pea (jequirity bean, *Abrus precatorius*), colchicine (*Colchicum autumnale*), podophyllum (mayapple, *Podophyllum pelatum*), *Senecio* and other pyrrolizidine alkaloid-containing species as described above.

A popular prenatal formula used by some American mid-wives contains false unicorn root (*Chamaelirium leuteum*), black cohosh (*Cimicifuga racemosa*), blessed thistle (*Cnicus benedicta*), pennyroyal (*Mentha pulegium*), squaw vine (*Mitchella repens*), red raspberry leaf (*Rubus idaeus*), and skullcap (*Scutellaria lateriflora*). "This formula is taken 5 to 6 weeks prior to the birthing date. It is an aid in giving elasticity to the pelvic and vaginal area and strengthening the reproductive system." The author states that most of these herbs can be taken singly, but for pregnant women, ". . . a much safer and reliable action will be accomplished by using these herbs combined together . . . ." Maybe so, but in light of the above, the risks are even less if the formula is not consumed!

DRUG INTERACTIONS

The World Health Organization estimates that 80% of the earth's population relies on traditional medicines as a part of their health care, with herbs as the most common therapy. This figure does not simply represent significant use of herbs in Third World nations but also in numerous industrialized countries. An estimated 30% of medical doctors in France and 80% in Germany use herbal medicines as a regular part of their practice. Less than 1% of American doctors prescribe any herbal remedies.

Most consumers believe that being natural is a guarantee of safety, and they have no concerns about taking prescribed conventional medicine in conjunction with herbal remedies. Many ethnic populations have their own traditional medicine practices, which they frequently combine with conventional medical care. Generally, little is known about the consequences of such combinations, although the clinical reports of interactions that infrequently appear in the medical and pharmaceutical press suggest that many more interactions may occur than are identified, and are not reported in the literature.

There is an alarming lack of scientific data about the possibility of drug interactions between herbal remedies and allopathic medicines. It is complicated at present by lack of knowledge about what many of the herbs and herbal medicines contain. Herbal products have the potential to enhance the activity of allopathic medications when their bioactivities are of a similar nature, or if they block elimination pathways. They may reduce the absorption of allopathic medicines due to the presence of tannin or phytates, or they may enhance their metabolism. When original reports of reactions and interactions are carefully screened, it becomes obvious many of the cases where herbal products have been associated with actual human poisoning were not in fact caused by the herbs alleged to be in the product. The poisoning was caused by substitution or contamination of the declared ingredients, intentionally or by accident, with a more toxic botanical, a poisonous metal, or a potent nonherbal drug substance.

Special Considerations

The sparse reports of drug interactions between herbal products and western medicines neither confirms their safety in use nor suggests that the incidence of such interactions is low. The simple fact is that most interactions of this type will not be recognized as such by the self-treated patient, will not be reported to an orthodox medical practitioner and therefore, will not appear in medical or pharmaceutical literature.

Herbal products are in some circumstances a mixture of herbs or mixtures with other ingredients of nonherbal origin (e.g., arsenic or lead) or undeclared western drugs (e.g., prednisolone, nonsteroidal anti-inflammatory/antirheumatic agents and paracetamol) as found recently by Karunanithy and Sumita in traditional Chinese antirheumatic medicines. Readers are also referred to the comprehensive reviews by De Smet on adulteration and contamination of oriental herbal products with toxic metals, synthetic drug substances and drugs used in nonorthodox medicine.

A recent article by D'Arcy reviews the proven and potential interactions of herbal remedies with conventional medicine. A classification of herbal products has been provided, designed specifically to identify herbal products that have actions, or that are reputed to have actions, in certain areas of therapeutics where an interaction with conventional medicines could be relevant. Some of the interactions indicated in this review, although based on a firm pharmacological basis, are speculative.

Herbal preparations containing **cardiac glycosides** that may potentiate the action of digitalis medications and produce digitalis toxicity include: false hellebore (adonis, pheasant's eye, *Adonis vernalis*), lily of the valley (*Convallaria majalis*), broom (*Cytisus scoparius*), yellow foxglove (*Digitalis lanata*), purple foxglove (*Digitalis purpurea*), Kyushin (Chinese medicine), white squill (*Urginea maritima*), and strophanthin (*Strophanthus kombé*). Herbal preparations reputed to contain diuretic agents and digitalis glycosides may enhance potassium loss and, consequently, potentiate the effect and toxicity of cardiac glycosides. The Chinese medicine, kyushin, has the dried venom of the Chinese toad *(Bufo bufo gargarizans)* as one of its ingredients. Due to their chemical similarity to digoxin, the constituents of the *Bufo* venom can cross-react with digoxin antibodies and give the false impression of high plasma digoxin levels in clinical laboratory assays. In these situations it is advisable to counsel the patient to stop self-treatment.

The following list of herbs is reputed to have **diuretic** action and may induce hypotensive episodes or make hypertension difficult to control: calamus (*Acorus calamus*), false hellebore (adonis, pheasant's eye, *Adonis vernalis*), agrimony (*Agrimonia eupatoria*), couch grass (quack grass, *Agropyron repens*), lady's mantle (parsley piert, *Alchemilia arvensis*), water plantain (*Alisma plantago*), pellitory (*Anacyclus pyrethrum*), dogbane (*Apocynum cannabinum*), bearberry (uva ursi, *Arctostaphylos uva-ursi*), buchu (*Barosma betulina*), birch (betula, *Betula alba*), shepherd's purse (*Capsella bursa-pastoris*), bluc cohosh (*Caulophyllum thalictroides*), false unicorn root (*Chamaelirium leuteum*), celandine (*Chelidonium majus*), chicory (*Cichorium intybus*), prince's pine (ground holly, pipsissewa, *Chimaphila umbellata*), curare (pareira brava root, *Chondodendron tomentosum*), black cohosh (*Cimicifuga racemosa*), stone root (*Collinsonia canadensis*), broom (*Cytisus scoparius*), wild carrot (*Daucus carota*), shavegrass (horsetail, *Equisetum* species), fumitory (*Fumaria officinalis*), cleavers (goosegrass, (*Galium aparine*), licorice (*Glycyrrhiza glabra*), rupture wort (*Herniaria glabra)*, hydrangea (*Hydrangea aborescens*), St. John's Wort (*Hypericum perforatum*), juniper (*Juniperus communis*), tamarack (larch, *Larix americans*), squaw vine (*Mitchella repens*), wood sorrel (*Oxalis acetosella*), parsley (*Petroselinum crispum*), boldo (*Peumus boldus*), elder (*Sambucus nigra*), sassafras (*Sassafras albidum*), ragwort and groundsel (*Senecio* species), saw palmetto (*Serenoa repens*), dandelion (*Taraxacum officinale*), nettle (*Urtica dioica*), and pansy (heartsease, *Viola tricolor)*. Again the prudent advice to the patient is to stop self-treatment.

Herbs reported to have a **sedative** action may potentiate the activity of alcohol, antihistamines and hypnotics: aconite (monkshood, wolfsbane, *Aconitum napellus*), celandine (*Chelidonium majus*), hemlock (*Conium maculatum*), common hop (*Humulus lupulus*), wild lettuce (*Lactuca virosa*), opium poppy (*Papaver somniferum*), passion flower (*Passiflora incarnata*), scopolia (*Scopolia carniolica atropoides*), skullcap (*Scutellaria lateriflora*), valerian (*Valerianna officinalis*); tropane alkaloid-containing plants, e.g., deadly nightshade (*Atropa belladonna* and other *Atropa* species), thorn apple (jimsonweed, *Datura stramonium* and other *Datura* species), henbane (*Hyoscyamus niger*) and mandrake (*Mandragora officinarum*). Tropane alkaloids found in solanaceous plants (*Atropa* species, *Datura* species, *Hyoscyamus* species, and *Mandragora officinarum*) are powerful anticholinergic agents and can elicit peripheral symptoms (e.g., blurred vision, dry mouth) as well as central effects (e.g., drowsiness, delirium); they can potentiate the effects of synthetic drugs with similar pharmacological activities (e.g., antidepressants, antihistaminics, antispasmodics).

Two reports have suggested, but not proved, an interaction between **ginseng** products and the antidepressant phenelzine. The therapeutic action did not appear to be altered, but the patients reported insomnia, headache, tremulousness, irritability and vague visual hallucinations as side effects. Yohimbine (*Pausinystalia yohimbe*, synonym *Corynanthe johimbe*), has also been shown to increase blood pressure in the presence of tricyclic antidepressants. Although these reports are little more than anecdotal, they suggest possible interactions. It would be wise, therefore, to advise patients being treated with any antidepressant not to take herbal remedies containing ginseng or yohimbine.

Herbs reputed to **lower blood pressure** may potentiate antihypertensive agents and induce hypotensive episodes or make hypertension difficult to control. The following are examples of such herbs: English hawthorn (*Crataegus oxyacantha*), rauwolfia (chotachand, *Rauwolfia serpentina*), hellebore (green hellebore, *Veratrum viride*), mistletoe (*Viscum album*) and yohimbine (*Pausinystalia yohimbe*, syn = *Corynanthe johimbe*).

Herbs reputed to **raise blood pressure**, such as licorice (*Glycyrrhiza glabra),* may also interact with antihypertensive agents and make hypertension difficult to control.

Licorice (root or extract) has **mineralocorticoid effects** due to the saponin glycoside, glycyrrhizin, which results in sodium and water retention and development of edema and hypertension. The control of hypertension may be difficult. Licorice is found in foods, confectioneries, beverages and some medications; however, the confectionery forms, beverages, chewing tobacco and some alternative medications are potentially hazardous.

The prudent advice in these situations is to have the patient stop or avoid these self-treatments.

Any substance containing large amounts of **vitamin K** will, if taken in sufficient amounts, antagonize the effect of anticoagulants. Horse chestnut (*Aesculus hippocastanum*), broccoli and other green leafy vegetables (especially species of *Brassica*) containing vitamin K in sufficient amounts to create problems when ingested in large amounts. Three cases have been reported of warfarin antagonism caused by excessive broccoli ingestion (230 to 450 g of broccoli daily). Once broccoli was eliminated from the diet, prothrombin times returned to those desired. Problems have also been encountered with patients taking herbal tea, especially those prepared from plants that contain coumarins, e.g., sweet vernal grass (*Anthoxanthum odoratum*), tonka bean (*Dipteryx odorata* and other species), sweet woodruff (*Galium odoratum*), sweet-scented bedstraw (*Galium triflorum*), and sweet clover (melilot, *Melilotus officinalis* and other species).

Glycemic control could be upset if diabetic patients, especially those on insulin or oral hypoglycemics, who take traditional medications containing **antidiabetic agents,** such as Damsissa (*Amni visnaga*), akee (*Blighia sapida*), Gymnema (*Gymnema sylvestre*), bitter gourd (*karela, Momordica charantia*). These herbs may affect blood sugar levels and interfere with the control of diabetes mellitus in patients on conventional antidiabetic therapy. A bulk-forming fibrous slimming aid, glucomannan, has been reported to reduce the plasma levels of glibenclamide, presumably by reducing its absorption. Concomitant dosage with antidiabetic agents and fibrous slimming aids could upset glycemic control, and diabetic patients should seek medical advice before starting any slimming course.

Guar gum, a bulk-forming fibre sometimes used as an antidiabetic aid and as a slimming preparation, comes from the endosperm of the seeds of the cluster bean (*Cyamopsis tetragonoloba*). In humans it has been shown to decrease both the peak concentration of phenoxymethylpenicillin and its area under the serum curve by about 25% when taken with the antibiotic; it similarly reduces the absorption of digoxin. It has also been repeatedly associated with esophageal obstruction. Guar gum may well reduce the absorption of other orthodox medicines and so it should not be used in combination with them.

Nephropathy has been associated with the ingestion of Chinese slimming products claiming to contain *Magnolia officinalis* and *Stephania tetrandra*. Due to the similarity of the symptoms and pathological findings, e.g., interstitial fibrosis, vascular lesions, urothelial atypia and transitional cell carcinoma, it is believed these products were

Special Considerations

contaminated with *Aristolochia fangchi*, a plant known to be nephrotoxic and thought to be the toxic agent in Balkan endemic nephropathy. Renal transplantations were required in some patients.

Starch-blocker is the generic name for a group of products manufactured from legumes such as the red kidney bean (*Phaseolus vulgaris*). It is alleged these products prevent the hydrolysis of starch, causing it to pass through the gut unchanged thereby facilitating dieting and weight loss. Doubts have been cast on its efficacy.

It is believed that **gynecomastia** and/or **galactorrhea** may be caused by rauwolfia alkaloids (*Rauwolfia serpentina)*, or ginseng, *(Panax schinseng* and other *Panax* species) and siberian ginseng (*Eleutherococcus* species), especially in combination with other drugs known to have these side effects, e.g., calcium channel blockers (diltiazem, nifedipine, verapamil), digitalis glycosides, ethionamide, griseofulvin, methyldopa, phenothiazines, spironolactone. The production of gynecomastia and galactorrhea by rauwolfia alkaloids was first reported in 1954, the site of action being at the hypothalamus level.

Although ginseng is reported to contain small quantities of estrone, estradiol and estriol, contrary to early reports, **estrogenic side effects** have not been conclusively associated with its use. In fact, it has been proven that the most discussed case of neonatal hirsutism, presumed to have been caused by ginseng, was caused by Chinese silk vine (*Periploca sepium*), a common commercial substitute of siberian ginseng, *Eleutherococcus senticosus*. Even the infamous ginseng abuse syndrome has been discounted. It appears that the most serious side effects attributed to ginseng are likely due to contaminants and adulterants. Awareness of this interaction and avoidance of unnecessary medication is all that can be advised.

Cassia bark, *Cinnamomum arommaticum,* (2 g in 100 mL) has been reported to reduce the in vitro dissolution from gelatin capsules of tetracycline hydrochloride and methacycline hydrochloride to approximately 20% of that seen in water. As a dose of 1 to 2 g of cinnamon is not uncommon, care should be taken not to use tetracycline and related substances with cinnamon at that dose level.

Visual hallucinations were reported to occur in 17.5% of 115 patients treated with propranolol for hypertension. Combining hallucinogenic herbs with these conventional drugs can be expected to increase the risk of hallucinations. Herbs in this category include: marijuana (cannabis, *Cannabis sativa*), periwinkle (*Catharanthus roseus*), cinnamon (*Cinnamomum camphora* and other species), yohimbine (*Corynanthe johimbe*), thorn apple (*Datura stramonium*), Californian poppy (*Eschscholzia californica*), common hop (*Humulus lupulus*), hydrangea (*Hydrangea paniculata*), lobelia (*Lobelia inflata*), mandrake (*Mandragora officinarum*), nutmeg (*Myristica fragrans*), passion flower (*Passiflora incarnata*), kava (kava-kava, *Piper methysticum*), and magic mushrooms (liberty cap, *Psilocybe semilanceata*). Some herbal substances act on indoles in the CNS to produce symptoms that can mimic acute toxicity and schizophrenic states. The effect is potentiated by alcohol, and there is obviously a serious risk of interaction with other psychoactive drugs that may be taken concomitantly.

Ephedrine, *Ephedra* species, Ma Huang, is found in diet supplements, fitness management products and "pep pills." There is a high incidence of adverse reactions to this **sympathomimetic** agent in persons with heart disease, thyroid disease, hypertension, diabetes, glaucoma or prostatic hypertrophy. Ephedrine can also cause a hypertensive crisis in patients taking monoamine oxidase inhibitors.

Plantago seeds, e.g., ispaghula (*Plantago ovata*) and psyllium (*P. psyllium or P. indica),* are widely used as bulk laxatives. A recent case report has raised the possibility that such agents may inhibit the intestinal absorption of lithium. Patients on lithium therapy should not use this bulk laxative.

Kelp, (bladderwrack, tang, *Fucus vesiculosus*) is the general name for dried seaweed (often of various species). It has been used in the treatment of obesity, but its high content of potassium iodide may evoke hypersensitivity reactions, hyper- or hypothyroidism, or extrathyroidal reactions such as skin eruptions. Theoretically, it could interfere with the activity of thyroid hormones and antithyroid drugs.

Germander, *Teucrium chamaedrys,* is used as an adjuvant in the symptomatic treatment of mild diarrhea, for topical use of the oral cavity for buccal hygiene and in dyspepsia, anorexia, chronic bronchitis, gout and rheumatoid arthritis. In 1992, the French health authorities suspended the marketing licence of herbal preparations containing *Teucrium chamaedrys*, after the use of such preparations had been associated with 26 cases of **acute hepatitis**, one resulting in death. Studies are in progress to determine whether contamination by pesticides or fungi may be implicated in the hepatitis and to determine whether the hepatitis is of toxicological or immunoallergic origin. There is a possibility there might be additive hepatotoxicity if taken together with other potentially hepatotoxic agents, including conventional medicines and herbal teas, especially those prepared from comfrey and other plants containing pyrrolizidine alkaloids. Use of products containing germander should be discouraged, at least until the origin of the toxicity is substantiated.

Ink cap, *Coprinus atramentarius,* contains bis(diethylthiocarbamoyl) disulfide, which is disulfiram, the active component of *Antabuse*. It reacts with small amounts of ingested alcohol to give a typical, unpleasant syndrome of systemic reactions (hypotension, nausea, vomiting, sweating, facial flushing, throbbing headache, tachycardia, accelerated and deepened respiration and giddiness). Fatalities have been reported. Health food consumers should be warned of this interaction since *Coprinus* is a component of some of these foods. Interaction between medicines containing small amounts of alcohol and health foods containing *Coprinus* could present a problem.

A number of studies have demonstrated that the leaves, the oil and the major active principle, eucalyptol, of eucalyptus, *Eucalyptus globulus, E. fruticetorum, E. smithii* and other species, can induce **microsomal enzyme activity** in both in vitro and in vivo tests. While there have not been any recorded interactions between eucalyptus and other drugs at the clinical level, a number of animal studies have indicated possible areas of concern: any therapy that may be affected by altering the pharmacokinetic profile of a drug, such as insomnia, asthma, and diabetes.

PATIENT ASSESSMENT QUESTIONS

?

Q Are you aware your herbal medicine may cause adverse effects?

The same side effects that occur with prescription and nonprescription medicines can also occur with herbal remedies, as they represent nearly every class of pharmacologic agents.

Q Are you taking any herbal beverages or medicines concurrently with any other medication?

Interactions between herbal remedies and prescription or nonprescription medicines may be expected to occur as readily as those between the latter two classes. Potentiation of prescription or nonprescription medications by herbal remedies is likely to be the most common type of interaction.

Q Are you aware there is no legislated guarantee of the quality of any herbal medicine, even those generally regarded as safe and effective.

Identification, adulteration and quality control are the three major problems. Herbs should be traded only by their Latin names, as common names often refer to more than one plant, especially in different geographic areas. Herbs have been deliberately adulterated for economy (supplier provides cheaper herb, charges for more expensive one) or for the "benefit" of the consumer (adulterant is often a potent chemical that provides an effect quickly). Without employing adequate analytical or animal assays, neither the purveyor nor the purchaser knows the strength of the preparation supplied.

Q In spite of its long-standing use, are you aware that the ingestion of comfrey is associated with chronic toxicity?

Comfrey (*Symphytum officinale*) has been shown to contain sizeable quantities of pyrrolizidine alkaloids known to be hepatotoxic and carcinogenic. Animal studies have confirmed the toxicity, and human toxicities have recently been reported. Other species of *Symphytum*, often sold as comfrey, are known to contain even more toxic alkaloids. The major problem here is that the toxicities are usually chronic, sometimes taking 30 to 40 years to become obvious.

Q Are you fully aware of the potential hazards of this herb when it is used as an emmenagogue?

An emmenagogue is an agent that induces menstrual flow. An abortion may result if a pregnant woman uses a preparation of this nature. Emmenagogues are commonly used to induce abortions, but the hazards are considerable, as many emmenagogues do not always produce complete abortion.

Q Do you know how to prepare this herb as a medicinal tea?

Medicinal teas are usually prepared by simmering about 30 g of herb in about 500 mL of water. When the volume has been reduced to about one-half, the tea is filtered from the extracted herb. Medicinal teas are usually 6 to 60 times stronger than beverage teas.

RECOMMENDED READING

Blumenthal M, ed. Herbalgram. Austin, Texas: The American Botanical Council and The Herb Research Foundation.

Bradley PR, ed. British Herbal Compendium. Bournemouth, U.K.: British Herbal Medicine Association, 1992.

Chandler RF. Herbal medicine. In: Carruthers-Czyzewski P. ed. Self-Medication, Reference for Health Professionals. 4th ed. Ottawa: Canadian Pharmaceutical Association, 1992: 493-511.

Der Marderosian A, Liberti L. Natural Product Medicine. Philadelphia: George F Stickley, 1988.

De Smet PAGM, Keller K, Hansel R, et al. Adverse Effects of Herbal Drugs. Vol. 1. Berlin: Springer-Verlag, 1992.

De Smet PAGM, Keller K, Hansel R, et al. Adverse Effects of Herbal Drugs. Vol. 2. Berlin: Springer-Verlag, 1993.

Foster S. Herbal Renaissance. Salt Lake City: Gibbs Smith, 1993:6-14.

Lampe KF, McCann MA. AMA Handbook of Poisonous and Injurious Plants. Chicago: American Medical Association, 1985.

Leung AY. Encyclopedia of Common Natural Ingredients Used in Food, Drugs, and Cosmetics. Toronto: John Wiley & Sons, 1980.

Mills SY. The Essential Book of Herbal Medicine. Toronto: Penguin Books, 1991.

Olin BR, ed. The Lawrence Review of Natural Products. St. Louis, Missouri: Facts and Comparisons.

Stelling K, ed. Canadian Journal of Herbalism. Toronto: The Ontario Herbalists' Association.

Dobelis IN, ed. Magic and Medicine of Plants. Montreal: Reader's Digest, 1986.

Tierra M. The Way of Herbs. New York: Pocket Books, 1990.

Tyler VE. The Honest Herbal. 3rd ed. New York: Pharmaceutical Products Press, 1993.

15

HOMEOPATHIC PRODUCTS

HEATHER BOON / MICHAEL SMITH / LINDA MUZZIN

CONTENTS

Introduction 361
- History
- Current Use of Homeopathy
- What is Homeopathy?
- Law of Similars
- Infinitesimal Doses

Homeopathic Remedies 364
- Choosing a Remedy
- Scientific Verification

Homeopathic Medicine 368
- Alternatives to Classical Homeopathy
- Homeopathic Standards
- Homeopathic Medicine in Pharmacies

Recommended Reading 373

INTRODUCTION

Homeopathy is a therapeutic approach currently gaining popularity in Canada. Based on the theory that "like cures like," the practice of homeopathy was founded in the late 18th century by Dr. Samuel Hahnemann. Although homeopathic practitioners are not licensed in Canada, an increasing number of physicians, dentists, veterinarians and naturopathic practitioners across Canada are educated in and qualified to practice homeopathic medicine. Homeopathic products are especially visible in Quebec pharmacies, and interest is growing in the rest of the country.

Unless you are trained in homeopathic medicine you may find many of the concepts unfamiliar. This chapter explains the basic principles so you can provide general advice to consumers. A discussion of the history and basic principles is followed by an examination of the scientific evidence that supports the claims of homeopathic medicine, a table of some common remedies and patient counselling tips. As a health professional, if you are interested in providing a homeopathic service to your clientele, a formal course is recommended. Many homeopathic organizations listed in the Resource List provide seminars or correspondence courses for health professionals.

HISTORY

Homeopathy was born in the late 18th century, a time when mainstream medicine relied on drugs and procedures that today would be considered primitive, dangerous and ineffective. Venesection (bloodletting) was popular and sanitation not yet common practice. Samuel Hahnemann (1755-1843), a German physician, coined the term *homeopathy*, which is derived from the Greek, *homos* meaning similar, and *pathos* meaning suffering. Hahnemann proposed that a substance that causes symptoms in a healthy individual can be used at diluted levels to cure an ill person with similar symptoms. The American Institute of Homeopathy, founded in 1844, was the first national medical association in the United States. By the turn of the century, 20 to 25% of all physicians in American urban areas identified themselves as homeopaths, supporting 22 homeopathic medical schools and more than 100 homeopathic hospitals.

Hahnemann's principles posed a philosophical,

clinical and economic threat to orthodox medicine. The American Medical Association (AMA) was formed in 1846, partially in response to the growth of homeopathy. After 1900, homeopathic medicine declined in North America for a variety of reasons: (i) strong opposition from the AMA; (ii) advances in modern medicine; (iii) the cultural effects of the Industrial Revolution; and (iv) divisions among homeopaths. Acceptance began to grow again in the 1970s. The most popular explanation for this rebirth has been the public's eroding trust in allopathic or conventional western medicine.

CURRENT USE OF HOMEOPATHY

The resurgence of homeopathy has been documented around the world. A recent survey published in the *British Medical Journal* indicates that 42% of British physicians refer patients to homeopathic physicians. A second study published in the *London Times* reported that 48% of physicians in Britain were referring patients for homeopathic treatment.

Homeopathy is enjoying similar success in France. A recent study showed that approximately 25% of the French public have tried or are presently using homeopathic medicines, and more than 20,000 French pharmacies sell homeopathic medicines. According to the same study, courses in homeopathy leading to a degree are offered in 6 medical schools and approximately 11,000 French doctors use homeopathic medicines in their practices. Homeopathy is taught in all pharmacy schools and in 4 veterinary schools. All German medical schools teach compulsory courses in homeopathy.

Homeopathy is even more widespread in Asia, especially India, Pakistan, and Sri Lanka. There are currently more than 120 homeopathic medical schools in India. Nineteen of the colleges are maintained by the state and most are affiliated with universities. In Brazil, pharmacists are required to complete a course in homeopathic pharmacology to graduate, and several conventional medical schools offer courses in homeopathy.

The renaissance of interest in homeopathy in North America is consistent with world trends. According to the *Washington Post* the number of American physicians who specialize in homeopathy doubled from 500 in 1980 to just over 1,000 in 1982. In Canada, homeopathic medicine is not regulated; however, an estimated 500 to 1,000 health care practitioners offer homeopathic services to the public.

WHAT IS HOMEOPATHY?

Homeopathy is a therapeutic approach that applies the Law of Similars and uses medical substances at infinitesimal doses. The Law of Similars in essence means there is a similarity between the toxic potential of a substance and its therapeutic action. Allopathic practitioners rely on a pathological classification of disease and attempt to suppress the symptoms or correct the underlying pathology directly. In contrast, homeopaths interpret disease symptoms as representative of weakness in the natural defense mechanisms of the body and attempt to stimulate these mechanisms to allow the body to heal itself. In classical homeopathy, where the patient's individuality is stressed, it is important to identify the remedy with the best fit to the patient's symptoms.

LAW OF SIMILARS

Homeopathy is based on three principles:

1. A biological substance can cause symptoms in a healthy individual that are **characteristic of the substance** used.
2. Anyone suffering from a disease will exhibit specific symptoms that are **characteristic of the disease**.
3. Homeopathic **therapy is individualized** to treat specific symptoms. The remedies act to stimulate the body's defences.

The Law of Similars is the cornerstone of all homeopathic treatment. According to homeopathic theory, every plant, animal or mineral substance will cause a unique pattern of symptoms in a healthy individual if ingested. Homeopaths believe that every individual presents with a unique pattern of symptoms when they fall ill. They attempt to match a person's pattern of symptoms (symptom picture) with the remedy whose pattern of symptoms, when given in large doses to healthy volunteers, most closely resembles it—"like cures like." A substance that causes symptoms when taken by a person in good health will be of medicinal value to a person who shows those symptoms in ill health. For example, raw onions cause many people to develop symptoms of watery eyes and runny nose. If an individual presented with a cold that was typified by watery eyes and runny nose, a homeopath might prescribe a homeopathic remedy derived from onions (Allium cepa).

Conventional or allopathic medicine sometimes uses this principle as well. For example, small doses of disease-causing agents are given to immunize patients against diseases. Methylphenidate (an amphetamine-like drug that causes a hyperactive state in adults) is used to treat hyperactive children; digitalis (which causes arrhythmias in larger doses) is prescribed in small amounts to treat some heart conditions.

To individualize therapy, classical homeopaths prescribe a single remedy that closely matches each individual's specific symptoms. Each ill person presents with a unique group of symptoms, and there will be only one homeopathic remedy that exactly matches the patient's symptom picture. Classical homeopaths undertake years of training to learn this skill.

Current homeopathy has expanded to include a wide range of products and prescribing practices. Many manufacturers are now marketing combination products that are disease-specific instead of patient-specific. Combination products contain 3 to 8 low potency (3X to 12X or 3C to 7C) homeopathic remedies often prescribed by homeopaths for individuals with specific diseases such as the common cold. This type of homeopathy is popular in Europe and becoming increasingly common in North America. Classical homeopaths maintain that the grouping of remedies will change their individual properties, but little research has been done comparing the effectiveness of combination and single-entity remedies.

INFINITESIMAL DOSES

The most controversial principle is the use of minimum dose. Hahnemann began using small doses as an alternative to the harsh doses of the allopathic medicines of the early 19th century, which often caused severe side effects. Specifically, homeopathic remedies derived from plant, animal and mineral substances, are reduced to an "infinitesimal dose" through a pharmaceutical process known as "potentization." This involves the successive dilutions of the original substance with alcohol (70 to 87%) and the succussion (vigorous shaking) of the mixture after each dilution. The more dilutions (and succussions) a product undergoes, the more potent it is said to be. More potent (e.g., more dilute) remedies act longer, heal at deeper levels, and require fewer doses. For many homeopathic practitioners, the level of dilution corresponds to the symptom picture: low potency for local symptoms, medium for more specific symptoms and high for psychological symptoms.

The controversy arises because many of the homeopathic remedies are diluted to a concentration smaller than Avogadro's number (6×10^{-23}, the number of molecules in one mole). Thus, laws of probability would predict that none of the molecules of the original substance will be left in the remedy if it is diluted beyond this point. Traditional science maintains that a substance with no molecules of the active ingredient cannot have a pharmacologic effect; homeopathic theorists, practitioners and researchers disagree.

HOMEOPATHIC REMEDIES

All homeopathic remedies are derived from plant, animal or mineral sources. First a base substance, or Mother Tincture (M.T. or Ø) is prepared by macerating the original substance, if it is soluble, in 99 parts of a hydroalcoholic mixture. If the substance is not soluble, it is triturated in 99 parts of lactose, and diluted with lactose until the resultant mixture is soluble in a hydroalcoholic solution (usually 3C), at which point the dilution will continue in liquid form. The manufacturer of the mother tincture follows strict quality controls set out in either French, German, or American pharmacopoeias. The Mother Tincture then goes through successive dilutions on a scale of 1:10 (the decimal scale) or 1:100 (the Centesimal scale) (Table 1). Usually the Mother Tincture is clearly differentiated from the medications that are subsequent dilutions; however, in some cases it may be considered to be the equivalent of 1X.

As shown in Figure 1, there are two types of Centesimal series dilutions that are distinguished by the manufacturing process. For the Hahnemannian Centesimal series (CH), one part of the Mother Tincture is placed in 99 parts of diluent and succussed (shaken) vigorously producing 1CH. One part of this is then placed in 99 parts of diluent and succussed vigorously to produce 2CH. This dilutional process may be continued up to 200CH.

In Canada, most remedies over 30C are Korsakovian dilutions, each series requiring only one glass vial, (which makes this both a more efficient and more cost-effective manufacturing process). A vial is filled with 99 parts of the Mother Tincture, and then the contents of the vial are

FIGURE 1: Centesimal Dilutions

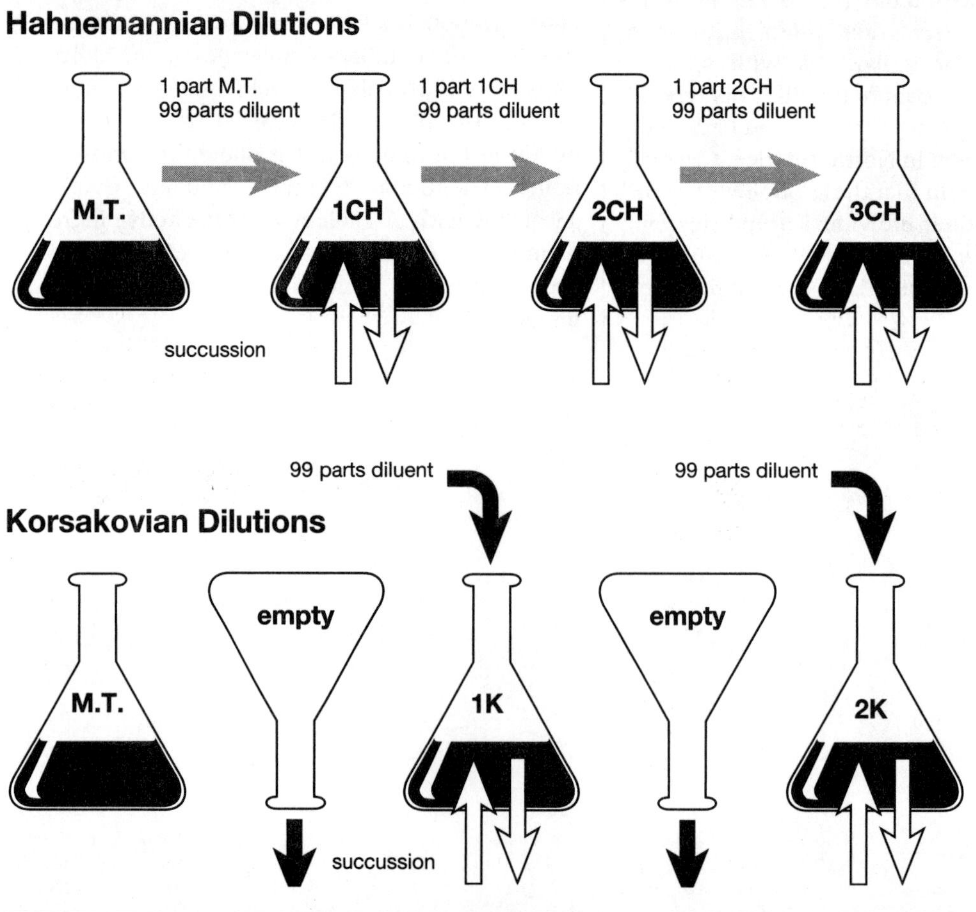

discarded. It is assumed that 1 part of the Mother Tincture will remain on the glass walls of the tube to which 99 parts of the diluent will be added. This is vigorously successed to produce a 1K solution that is then discarded and once more 99 parts of diluent are added to the vial, which is successed vigorously to produce 2K. This dilutional process may be continued to produce infinitely dilute remedies.

Although the CH and the K dilutional scales are mathematically identical, the resultant medications are not considered by some homeopathic practitioners to be interchangeable. Also, it cannot be assumed that C designates CH. Generally companies use the dilution designation of their country of origin, which is usually the Korsakovian method in the United States, Eastern Europe and India. In Canada and Central Europe the Hahnemannian method is more common for potencies under 30C but higher potencies are Korsakovian. However, the European Community has recently accepted the Korsakovian as their standard, which may result in some future changes.

Once the medication has reached its final dilution stage it is transferred to one of the dosage forms. Granules and pellets are saccharose and lactose cores that are impregnated with the potentized medication. The medication may also be transferred to a cream base, a syrup base or an alcoholic tincture.

Today most homeopathic dilutions are done in laminar flow hoods to prevent contamination because pollutants in the air are found in higher concentrations than many of the active ingredients in the remedies. Generally remedies of less than 15CH are considered low potencies and those of 30CH or higher are considered high potencies. The most common dilutions or potencies used today are 6CH to 30CH.

See Table 2 for a comparison of the different dosage forms available.

CHOOSING A REMEDY

Homeopathic practitioners rely on two types of reference texts, or their computerized equivalents: the Materia Medica, which lists all remedies and their symptom pictures; and the Repertory, which lists all symptoms and their associated remedies. There are several different Materia Medica and Repertories available; however, those most commonly consulted are those authored by William Boericke, T.F. Allen and J.T. Kent. All these references are derived from "provings," most of which were conducted over 200 years ago. Subsequent clinical research and experience have provided verification and modification of this original data. However, the concept of the "proving" is still an essential component of homeopathic medicine.

"Provings" must be done for every substance that is a homeopathic remedy. Healthy volunteers ingest the raw or potentized substance and record every symptom they feel. Homeopathic symptoms are much more inclusive than traditional allopathic symptoms, and include all mental, emotional and physical changes while taking the substance. These are recorded over the several weeks or months that the volunteers take the substance. Then the information from all the participants is combined to form the substance's "symptom picture."

The defining symptoms are those reported by all the volunteers, and the most useful symptoms are the unique ones for a particular substance. For example, if everyone had a fever, then this is a defining symptom, but because so many sub-

TABLE 1: Homeopathic Potencies

Dilution Ratio	Decimal Series	Centesimal Series
1/10 or 10^{-1}	1X	—
1/100 or 10^{-2}	2X	1C
1/1000 or 10^{-3}	3X	—
1/10 000 or 10^{-4}	4X	2C
10^{-12}	12X	6C
10^{-24}	24X	12C
10^{-60}	60X	30C

N.B. The Decimal Scale may also be represented by the letters D or DH. Similarly, the Centesimal Scale may also be represented by the letters CH or K. However, it is important to remember that although CH and K are mathematically equivalent, they are not considered clinically equivalent by many homeopathic practitioners and thus should not be interchanged.

Homeopathic Remedies

TABLE 2: Homeopathic Dosage Forms

Formulation	Excipients	Dosing	Route of Administration	Comments
Granules	Saccharose Lactose	Once daily	Usually sublingual	Single dose vials containing 200 granules Medium or high potencies Usually short-term use
Pellets	Saccharose Lactose	Multiple Daily dosing	Usually sublingual	10X or higher potencies 1 dose=3–5 pellets
Drops	30% alcohol	Varies	Oral	Low potencies One dose=15–20 drops
Tablets	Lactose	Varies	Varies	Disease-specific combinations Low potencies Frequent dosing

stances can cause a fever, it does not distinguish this remedy from all other remedies and thus is not considered a good symptom. However, symptoms such as: sensation of crawling ants over the surface of the head (Picric acid); moved to tears at the sound of bells (Antimonium crudum); time passing too swiftly (Cocculus); or symptoms worse at 2 a.m. (Kali bichromicum), are more useful because they are very distinctive.

The job of the homeopath is to try to match the patient's symptoms exactly to a remedy picture. Consider the case where 2 patients suffering from intercostal herpes zoster consult a homeopath. Patient A has an eruption and suffers from itching and burning pain that is relieved by cold compresses. The symptom picture is very similar to that of a healthy person who has been stung by a bee. Thus, the homeopathic remedy prescribed is bee venom in infinitesimal dilution. Patient B also has an eruption and burning pain, but her pain is worse at night and relieved by hot compresses. Her symptoms are different and thus she is prescribed potentized Arsenious anhydride although allopaths would say she is in the same disease state. In classical homeopathy, the choice of remedy is based on the complete symptom picture and the unusual or distinct symptoms give the best clues to which remedy to use.

SCIENTIFIC VERIFICATION

Basic Science

One of the first significant dilution studies done by scientists investigating the efficacy of homeopathy entitled "Effect on Mouse Peritoneal Macrophages of Orally Administered Very High Dilutions of Silica", was published in the *European Journal of Pharmacology* in June 1987. The study compared equivalent dilutions of silica and saline. It concluded that although the results could not be explained by present scientific knowledge, 19X (10^{-19}) silica was more active than 11X (10^{-11}) silica and that 19X (10^{-19}) saline was inactive.

In June 1988, the British journal, *Nature* reported a second dilution study entitled "Human Basophil Degranulation Triggered By Very Dilute Antiserum Against IgE." This study was undertaken in 6 different laboratories in 4 countries, including Dr. Bruce Pomeranz at the University of Toronto. The article was accompanied by an editorial, When to Believe the Unbelievable, which stated:

> *what the article shows is that it is possible to dilute an aqueous solution of an antibody virtually indefinitely without the solution losing its biological activity. Or rather, there is a surprising rhythmic fluctuation in the activity of the solution. At some dilutions, the activity falls off; on further dilution it is restored.*

The researchers ran blinded, double-coded experiments with controls and dilutions from 10^{-2} to 10^{-37} with agitation in a vortex. Their results showed that:

1. Agitation played a pivotal role in the activity of the highly dilute substances. They compared solutions that were pipetted up and down 10

times with solutions that had been vortexed for 10 seconds. The degranulation patterns of the 10^{-2} and 10^{-3} dilutions were superimposable, but although the two processes resulted in identical dilutions, no degranulation occurred at dilutions higher than 10^{-3} for the solutions that had been pipetted. Ten seconds of vortexing appeared to be the minimum time required to support the degranulation at higher dilutions, but increasing the vortexing to 30 or 60 seconds did not increase the high dilution activity. Thus, as homeopaths assert, the transmission of activity at high dilutions appears to depend on vigorous agitation.

2. Solutions diluted with water, ethanol or propanol all supported the phenomenon at high dilutions; however, dilutions with dimethyl sulfoxide did not. Increasing the proportion of water in dimethyl sulfoxide resulted in the reappearance of the activity at high dilutions. This suggests a dependence on polar diluents. Homeopaths have always diluted their remedies in polar solvents—usually water and alcohol combinations.
3. The activity of all highly diluted solutions was suppressed by heating, freeze-thawing and ultrasonication. It is of interest that all highly diluted solutions ceased to be active between 70 and 80°C. This suggests a common mechanism that operates at high dilutions and is independent of the nature of the starting molecule.

These startling findings led to an investigation of the study by a group including John Maddox, the editor of *Nature*; James "the amazing" Randi, whom *Time* calls "the scourge of clairvoyants, faith healers and spoon benders"; and Walter Stewart, a freelance fraud sleuth at the United States National Institutes of Health. Their report concluded that:

1. The phenomena are not reproducible.
2. The data lacked errors of the magnitude that would be expected and that are unavoidable.
3. Systematic errors, including observer bias, were not eliminated.
4. The climate of the laboratory was inimical to an objective evaluation of the exceptional data.

Dr. Jacques Benveniste, a pharmacologist at the French National Institute of Health and Medical Research, one of the original researchers, criticized the conclusions of the investigating group: "All in all, the judgment is based on 1 dilution tested on 2 bloods in awful technical and psychological conditions." The controversy continues.

Clinical Trials

The *British Medical Journal* published a criteria-based meta-analysis entitled "Clinical Trials of Homeopathy" in February 1991. The objective of this study was to establish whether there is evidence of the efficacy of homeopathy from controlled trials in humans. The researchers assessed the methodological quality of 107 controlled trials in 96 published reports, scoring the trials using a list of predefined criteria for good methodology. The outcome of each trial was then interpreted in relation to its quality. The results showed that most trials seemed to be of very low quality, but there were many exceptions. Regardless of the quality of the trial or the variety of homeopathy used, the investigators noted a positive trend in the results. Altogether, 81 of 105 trials indicated positive results for the homeopathic product. The researchers concluded that although their results were positive, there was not sufficient evidence to draw definite conclusions about the clinical efficacy of homeopathy; most of the trials were of low methodological quality; and the role of publication bias is unknown. However, the investigators argued that there appears to be a legitimate case for further evaluation of homeopathy by means of well-performed clinical trials.

HOMEOPATHIC MEDICINE

ALTERNATIVES TO CLASSICAL HOMEOPATHY

Homotoxicology

Homotoxicology is a specific discipline of complex homeopathy founded by Hans Heinrich Reckeweg. It is based on a theoretical model that describes 6 phases of disease that are defined by tissue type. Homeopathic remedies (up to 30X) are used in an attempt to stimulate the natural defense mechanisms of the body. Homotoxicology is widely practised in Europe, especially in Germany. In Canada, homotoxicology products are available as the Dr. Reckeweg or Heel product lines.

Tissue Salts

This biochemical system was developed by W.H. Schuessler in the 19th Century. It is based on the premise that there are 12 essential cell salts (biochemical or tissue salts) that allow the body to function properly. This theory is based on pathological theory rather than homeopathic provings; however, these salts have been incorporated into homeopathic practice. They are normally supplied in a 6X dilution.

The 12 tissue salts are:

- Silicean
- Natrum muriaticum
- Ferrum phosphoricum
- Kalium muriaticum
- Natrum phosphoricum
- Calcarea phosphorica
- Kali phosphoricum
- Calcarea fluorica
- Natrum sulfuricum
- Magnesia phosphorica
- Calcarea sulfurica
- Kalium sulfuricum

HOMEOPATHIC STANDARDS

The practice of homeopathic medicine is currently unregulated in Canada. However, naturopathic practitioners (NDs) who are regulated in British Columbia, Saskatchewan, Manitoba and Ontario study homeopathy as part of their naturopathic training. The Ontario Homeopathic Association (OHA), which represents a group of unlicensed homeopaths, is presently completing a Request for Regulation. If the Ontario government accepts this request, Ontario will become the first Canadian province to regulate homeopathic medicine.

The quality of homeopathic remedies is regulated through the Food and Drugs Act and Regulations, and most have been issued Drug Identification Numbers (DINs) by the Health Protection Branch. The Drug Directorate Guidelines entitled "Homeopathic Preparations: Application For Drug Identification Number" (Catalogue # H-42-2/21-1990) are available from the Canada Communications Group Publishing, Ottawa, ON, K1A 0S9. Health Canada may also be contacted for the Homeopathic Preparations Information Letter HPB No. 775, 1990. There is no Canadian pharmacopoeia, so manufacturers must abide by the requirements of the Pharmacopée française (PhF), the German Homeopathic Pharmacopoeia, or the Homeopathic Pharmacopoeia of the United States (HPUS). The HPUS can be contacted at P.O. Box 40360, Washington, D.C., 20016.

Definitions

Gemmotherapy: use of glycerin macerate diluted in 1D to drain toxins from specific organs or acting as anti-inflammatory agents.

Isopathy or Isotherapy: use of potentized substances obtained from the patient or his environment.

Lithotherapy: use of metals and minerals in 8D for drainage purposes.

Oligotherapy: use of very small quantities (mcg) called catalytic dosages of trace elements (oligoelements) normally found in the body to restore equilibrium.

Nosode: a potentized homeopathic remedy prepared from a diseased tissue or a product of disease.

Sarcode: an aspect of organotherapy in which a glandular or tissue extract is made into a homeopathic preparation.

HOMEOPATHIC MEDICINE IN PHARMACIES

Homeopathic products have been available for many years in Quebec, which represents the largest retail market; however, they are being produced and distributed by an increasing number of companies across Canada. Both single-entity remedies and combination disease-specific products are becoming widely available to patients in a variety of settings. Although some homeopathic products are available in health food stores, many manufacturers will only allow their products to be sold in pharmacies and practitioner's clinics. All homeopathic products are currently available without a prescription. Table 3 lists some of the common single homeopathic agents currently available in Canada.

TABLE 3: Common Acute Homeopathic Single-Entity Remedies

Remedy	Brief Symptom Picture	Common Uses
Aconitum napellus	Fearful and restless Sudden fever with hot dry skin Great thirst Tingling sensation of extremities	Fever Early stages of otitis Sore throat and U.T.I.
Allium cepa	Bland lacrimation Burning nasal discharge Sneezing Feel better outside Worse in warm room Symptoms move from left to right side	Allergic rhinitis Coryza Ear ache
Apis mellifica	Burning, smarting, stinging pain Redness and swelling Better with cold applications or drink (worse with heat) Little or no thirst	Sore throat Insect bites Conjunctivitis
Arnica montana	Bruised feeling Bed feels hard Want to be left alone	Trauma/injury
Arsenicum album	Fearful and restless Worse 1 a.m. to 2 a.m. Better if sip warm drinks Diarrhea and vomiting	Traveller's diarrhea Food poisoning
Belladonna	Acute, throbbing pain Flushed face Skin red and dry Dilated pupils High fever/severe pain Worse with touch, motion, sun, noise Unresponsive to environment	Sunburn Sunstroke Otitis media
Chamomilla Vulgaris	Capricious/demanding Inconsolable Very thirsty Intense pain	Teething pains

TABLE 3: Common Acute Homeopathic Single-Entity Remedies *(cont'd)*

Remedy	Brief Symptom Picture	Common Uses
Colubrina	Irritability, quick tempered Chilly Worse in dry/cold weather Sensitive to drafts Intolerant to many foods Crave stimulants (e.g., coffee, alcohol, tobacco)	Hangovers Indigestion Heartburn Work stress Indigestion
Euphrasia	Bland nasal discharge Excoriating lacrimation Bursting headaches Intolerance to bright lights	Eye conditions Hayfever
Gelsemium Sempervirens	Droopy eyelids, drowsiness No thirst Fearful, sense of inadequacy Chills up and down spine Diarrhea Occipital headache	Stage fright Influenza Dysmenorrhea
Ledum palustre	Puncture wound Bruising, puffy skin Better with cold application Worse at night Angry and impatient	Insect bites Puncture wounds
Pulsatilla	Seek consolation, weepy Depressed, clingy Better in fresh air Worse in evening Yellow/bland discharge Thirstless, with dry mouth	Otitis media Upper respiratory infection Eye conditions

General Principles for Self-treatment with Homeopathic Medicines

Homeopathic self-treatment should be limited to minor, acute, self-limiting illnesses. Chronic or more severe illness may be treated by a homeopathic practitioner, or may require attention from a medical doctor. Do not interrupt or change medical treatment without first consulting the medical doctor who prescribed the treatment. Homeopathic medication may be taken concurrently with any other medical treatment and if it significantly improves the condition, the medical doctor may adjust treatment accordingly. Homeopathic medicine is not toxic to anyone when diluted to at least 4 CH.

Adults, seniors and children over 8 years of age may take the same dose of homeopathic pellets and granules. Three to 5 pellets are usually allowed to melt in the mouth 3 times daily. Granules are prescribed as a whole unit-dose tube for every dose. Children under 8 years of age may be given 3 pellets per dose. The pellets may be dissolved in water for administration to children under 2 years of age. Drops are traditionally taken, 15 to 20 drops at a time in a small amount of water 3 times daily. Children under 12 years of age, nursing or pregnant women, diabetics or those sensitive to alcohol should not be given drops because they are prepared in a 30% alcohol solution.

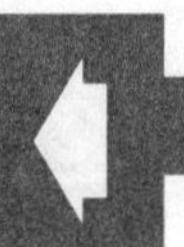

Most homeopathic companies manufacture nonprescription products that are designed specifically for self-treatment purposes. These are usually presented as blister-packed tablets that contain a combination of the most common homeopathic medications for common illnesses. It is recommended that one begin self-treatment with these products and as one's knowledge of homeopathy grows it is possible to move to single entity products (generics). Several good self-care books listed in the Recommended Reading section provide an introduction to the more common of these products.

Guidelines for Proper Care of Homeopathic Remedies

- Do not expose to intense light including sunlight, high temperatures, or strong odors.
- Remedies should be kept in their original containers.
- Do not contaminate the bottle cap when pouring doses, and replace the cap tightly.
- If you are unsure whether the remedy has been contaminated, replace it.

Homeopathic Medications That Should Never Be Used in Self-Treatment

- Bothrops
- Cactus
- Hepar sulfur
- Lachesis
- Lycopodium
- Mercurius corrosivus
- Mercurius cyanatus
- Naja
- Phosphorus
- Psorinum
- Sambucus
- Sulfur
- Thuya
- Tuberculinum
- Vipera

Always consult a homeopathic practitioner before using any of the above medications.

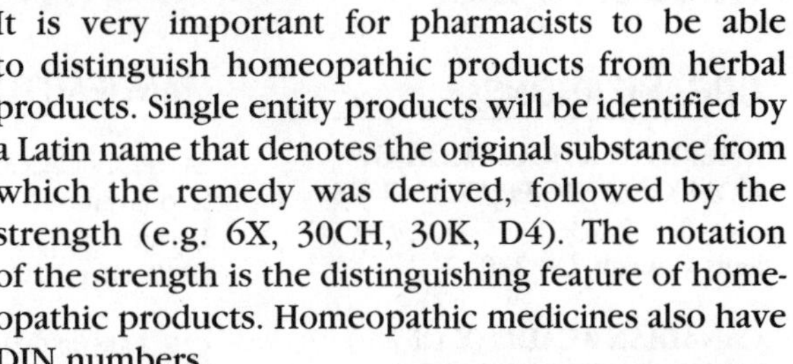

COUNSELLING TIPS

Homeopathy

It is very important for pharmacists to be able to distinguish homeopathic products from herbal products. Single entity products will be identified by a Latin name that denotes the original substance from which the remedy was derived, followed by the strength (e.g. 6X, 30CH, 30K, D4). The notation of the strength is the distinguishing feature of homeopathic products. Homeopathic medicines also have DIN numbers.

Generally there are no side effects when taking homeopathic products, although some higher potencies (more dilute products) can cause an initial aggravation in the symptoms known as a healing crisis. For this reason, self-treatment with homeopathic medicines should be restricted to remedies of 30CH or less. In some cases, if a poorly indicated remedy is repeated very frequently, the patient may also experience "proving" symptoms. These symptoms are seldom dangerous and normally disappear after the remedy is stopped.

There are generally no drug interactions between homeopathic products and other drugs; however, it is important to check the potency of the homeopathic product because there is the potential for possible drug interactions with remedies of low potency (not very dilute). The higher the potency, the less likely the possibility of drug/remedy interactions.

Most homeopathic dosage forms are dissolved in the mouth. Some, such as syrups, are ingested, and it is usually recommended they be taken on an empty stomach. Most homeopathic vials have special lids that enable the patient to pour their dose into the lid and then directly into their mouths. Remedies in an alcohol base are usually taken in some water, and granules or pellets may be diluted in water when given to babies.

There is some evidence that certain substances and procedures can counteract homeopathic remedies, which allows the symptoms to return. Substances containing caffeine and camphor should be avoided during homeopathic treatment and for 48 hours after the last dose. Volatile substances, such as mint, menthol or oil of eucalyptus, should be avoided, including cough drops, mouthwashes and flavored toothpastes. These substances do not always counteract homeopathic remedies so patients should be instructed to continue with their prescribed dosing regimen unless the symptoms that were previously getting better suddenly worsen after exposure to one of the above. If worsening occurs, it may be necessary to repeat the dose that has been counteracted.

Homeopathic Medicine

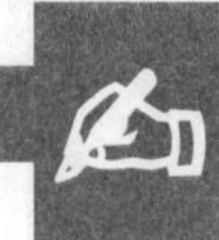

Resource List

ORGANIZATIONS

AMERICAN ASSOCIATION OF HOMEOPATHIC PHARMACISTS
P.O. Box 2273
Falls Church, CA 22042

CANADIAN ACADEMY OF HOMEOPATHIC MEDICINE
111 Simcoe Street North, Unit #2
Oshawa, ON L1G 4S4
(905) 433-8666

THE BRITISH INSTITUTE OF HOMEOPATHY (CANADA)
Ste 1205,
86 Gloucester St.
Toronto, ON M4Y 2S2
(416) 921-7887
Fax: (416) 921-5765

CEDH CANADA
Centre d'études et de documentation homéopathiques
814 Guimond
Longueuil, QC J4G 1T5
(514) 422-9921
Fax: (514) 442-3077

INTERNATIONAL ACADEMY OF HOMEOPATHY
3255 Yonge Street
Toronto, ON M4N 2L5

NUPATH (National United Professional Association of Trained Homeopaths)
P.O. Box 2766, Yorkdale
Toronto, ON M6A 3B8

ONTARIO HOMEOPATHIC ASSOCIATION
P.O. Box 852, Station P
Toronto, ON M5S 2Z2
(416) 488-9685

RHM (Regroupement pour l'homéopathie médicale)
828 Abbés Primeau
Boucherville, QC J3U 3T8
(514) 449-7533

MANUFACTURERS & DISTRIBUTORS

BOIRON CANADA INC.
816 Guimond
Longueuil, QC J4G 1T5
(800) 361-1010

C.E. JAMIESON & CO. LTD.
(distributor of BOERICKE & TAFEL (B&T) products)
4025 Rhodes Drive
Windsor, ON N8W 5B5
(800) 265-5053

DOLISOS CANADA INC
1400 Hocquart
St. Bruno, QC J3V 6E1
(514) 441-2121
(800) 668-7543

DR. RECKEWEG CANADA
518 Meloche Avenue
Dorval, QC H9P 2T2
(514) 631-0006
(800) 361-6663

HOMEOCAN
1900 rue Ste Catherine est
Bureau 400
Montreal, QC H2K 2H5
(514) 525-6303

HOMEO VIA
(distributor of DOLISOS products)
P.O. Box 56603
8601 Warden Avenue
Markham, ON L3R 0M6
(905) 513-0619
(800) 668-7543

SEROYAL CANADA INC
(distributor of UNDA and GENESTRA products)
44 East Beaver Creek Road, Unit 17
Richmond Hill, ON L4B 1G8
(905) 764-6355
(800) 2635861

STANDARD HOMEOPATHIC CANADA
(distributor of HYLANDS products)
317 Knowlton Road, Box 116
Knowlton, QC J0E 1V0
(514) 242-1256
(800) 363-8933

THORNE RESEARCH DISTRIBUTING LTD
(distributor of BIOPATH products)
111-20530 Langley Bypass
Langley, BC V3A 6K8
(604) 530-3639

RECOMMENDED READING

Introductory and Self-Care Books

Cummings S, Ullman D. Everybody's Guide to Homeopathic Medicines. Los Angeles: Jeremy Tarcher, 1991.

Lockie A. Family Guide to Homeopathy. Toronto: Penguin Books, 1989.

Panos M, Hemlich J. Homeopathic Medicine at Home. New York: G.P. Putnam's Sons, 1980.

Picard P, et al. The Canadian Guide to Homeopathic Self-Medication. Montreal : Les Éditions de la Chenelière, 1995.

Ullman D. Discovering Homeopathy: Medicine for the 21st Century. Berkeley, CA: North Atlantic Books, 1991.

Vithoulkas G. Homeopathy: Medicine for the New Man. New York: Arco, 1979.

Philosophy, Methodology and Research

Coulter HL. Homeopathic Science and Modern Medicine: The Physics of Healing With Microdoses. Berkeley, CA: North Atlantic Books, 1981.

Hahnemann S. Organon of Medicine. Los Angeles: J.P. Tarcher, 1982. Reprint.

Jouanny J, et al. Homeopathic Therapeutics. Lyon: Boiron, 1994.

Vithoulkas G. The Science of Homeopathy. New York: Grove, 1979.

Materia Medicas and Repertories

Allen HC. Keynotes and Characteristic of the Materia Medica. New Delhi: B. Jain. Reprint.

Boericke W. Pocket Manual of Materia Medica with Repertory. Santa Rosa: Boericke and Tafel. Reprint.

Kent JT. Lectures on Homeopathic Materia Medica. Berkeley, CA: North Atlantic Books, 1979.

Kent JT. Repertory of Homeopathic Materia Medica. New Delhi: B. Jain. Reprint.

Schroyens F. Synthesis Repitorium Homeopathic Synthetic. London: Homeopathic Book Publishers, 1993.

History of Homeopathy

Coutler HL. Divided Legacy: A History of the Schism in Medical Thought (3 volumes). Berkeley, CA: North Atlantic Books, 1975, 1977, 1981. Of special interest is Volume III: Divided Legacy: The Conflict Between Homeopathy and the American Medical Association.

Grossinger R. Planet Medicine: From Stone-Age Shamanism to Post-Industrial Medicine. Berkeley, CA: North Atlantic Books, 1987.

Handley R. A Homeopathic Love Story. Berkeley, CA: North Atlantic Books, 1990.

Nichols P. Homeopathy and the Medical Profession. Beckenham, England: Croom Helm, 1988.

16

MEDICAL DEVICES

MARIE BERRY

CONTENTS

Introduction 375

Aids for Daily Living 377
- Bathroom Safety
- Ambulation

Incontinence 382
- Urinary Incontinence
- Fecal Incontinence
- Incontinence Products

Ostomy 388
- Appliances and Equipment

Home Diagnostics 397
- Blood Pressure Monitors
- Pregnancy Testing and Ovulation Prediction Kits
- Cholesterol Home Tests
- Fecal Occult Blood Home Tests
- Peak Flow Meters
- Ear and Throat Examination Kits
- Diabetes Home Tests

Respiratory Aids 406
- Humidifiers and Vaporizers

Home Intravenous Programs 407

Recommended Reading 409

INTRODUCTION

This chapter is intended as an overview of medical devices, touching on aids for daily living, incontinence products, ostomy care and appliances, home diagnostics and home intravenous programs. More information can be obtained from the various references and resource groups cited.

Medical devices are a key to the home health care market, which is estimated at $30 million in Canada. It has grown from the traditional durable medical equipment to include first aid, wound care, sports medicine, incontinence, palliative care and diagnostic aids.

Home health care is an alternative or adjunct to government-funded programs such as community health centres, local hospitals and veterans' affairs organizations. Improved technology permits early diagnosis and self-treatment.

As government funding decreases, hospital beds are no longer used.[1] Less expensive alternatives include early discharge of patients for home recovery and/or day surgery.

By the year 2005, it is expected that 32% of the Canadian population will be over 80 years of age. More people will be requiring medical devices in their homes to carry on their day-to-day living.

The public benefits not only in money saved, but in reducing, if not eliminating, disability. Orthopedic patients, e.g., those with hip replacements or fractures, may be more mobile. Brain damaged patients, e.g., stroke or accident victims who have suffered hemiplegia, are able to cope with everyday life. Rheumatoid arthritis, amyotrophic lateral sclerosis (ALS), and multiple sclerosis (MS) patients cope better with their diseases. And amputees are not institutionalized. The caregivers, as well, find their tasks much less onerous.

The various provincial departments of health are responsible for many of these areas and organizations such as the Victorian Order of Nurses provide support for the patient at home. Some examples of medical devices are found in Table 1.

TABLE 1: Some Examples of Medical Devices

Category	Example
Durable medical equipment	Bathroom/toilet and mobility aids such as commodes, shower chairs, walkers, wheelchairs
Self-care equipment	Diagnostic items such as blood glucose monitors, cholesterol test kits, pregnancy test kits; blood pressure monitors; massagers; hot/cold therapy
Patient comfort aids	Pressure therapy; pillows; cushions; surgical stockings; back, neck and limb braces
Respiratory aids	Asthma nebulizers, peak flow meters, allergy sprays, vaporizers, humidifiers
Wound care products	Generalized first aid products, surgical bandages, specialized dressings
Incontinence aids	Undergarments, protectors, sheaths, drainage bags, bed wetting alarm systems
Surgical sundries	Personal hygiene products, ear plugs, gloves, medicine measures, manicure accessories
Sports and orthopedic products	Belts, braces, supports
Home intravenous products	Accessories

AIDS FOR DAILY LIVING

Aids for daily living (ADLs) range from ambulation aids such as wheelchairs and canes to adaptive clothing and handle grips for cutlery. They make day-to-day life easier for both patient and caregivers and may enable an individual to avoid institutionalization.

Occupational therapists teach people, using repetition and practice, to relearn skills, to perform tasks in a new way, or to use equipment to perform a task. They often recommend ADLs that simplify daily activities. The emphasis is on simplifying the task, planning ahead, organizing the task, sitting and resting when possible and regularly, and using correct body mechanics (Table 2).

BATHROOM SAFETY

About one-half of the falls in the home occur in the bathroom, and of those, two-thirds involve getting into or out of the bathtub. Bath oils and bubble bath make tubs slippery. Showers are an alternative, but some people have difficulty standing in a shower. Something as simple as a bath mat with suction cups will reduce the risk of falls. Bathtub and shower grab bars along with tub rails make a bathroom safer. Proper installation by a carpenter or qualified person is needed because rails and grab bars should be screwed into studs. Hand held or portable showers are another alternative.

For people confined to a bed or wheelchair, shampoo trays make hair washing possible. Inflatable vinyl tubs that fit over a bed come with a hand held shower and hose to allow bathing in bed.

Bath boards sit across the bathtub and usually have hand grips. They are ideal to hold soap and sponges within easy reach, and to steady stepping out of the bathtub. Bath seats are set right in the tub or across the tub to allow sitting down while bathing. Some have back rests, and all have suction cups to avoid movement.

Shower seats are similar to bath seats. Suction cup legs to stabilize, adjustable seat heights, back support, nonslip covering, and easy to clean surfaces are desirable.

Bathtub transfers, when most falls occur, are the cause of the greatest anxiety in debilitated individuals. Needing someone to assist in a bathtub transfer is also a sign of lost independence and privacy. Transfer benches straddle the bathtub with two seating areas, one inside the tub and the other outside. The individual sits on the outside seat much like they would a chair. While seated they can move their legs one at a time over the bathtub edge and into the tub, then pull themselves over to the portion of the seat positioned above the bath water.

Transfer benches are adjustable. A couple of trial runs without bath water and with the patient

TABLE 2: Some Examples of ADLs

Dishes	Partitioned, lip or higher edge, suction cup fixed on base, heated, food guards
Cups	Easy to hold handles, detachable handles, attached straws and/or spouts, nose cut outs, weighted bases, insulated, holders to stabilize
Utensils	Plastic coated spoons, weighted handles, easy to hold grips, swivel utensils, extension handles, specialized handles for odd angles, foam tubing to increase grip, putty to create a customized grip
Kitchen	Electric and manual knives and peelers with easy to hold handles, cutting boards with nails to hold food for cutting, cutting boards with corner guards, easy to use and hold can and jar openers
Home accessories	Door knob and tap turners and grippers; easy grip scissors; long reach sponge mops, dusters and vacuums; reading lights and magnifiers; book holders; reachers
Personal care	Extension combs and brushes, handle grippers for toothbrushes, zipper pulls, elastic shoe laces, sock and panty hose aids, button hooks
Communications	Games, stickers and communication boards; pen grips; computer accessories
Recreation	Playing card holders and shufflers, knitting needle holders and mobile bridges for pool cues

clothed are usually necessary to adjust the bench to the correct height. The sitting surfaces must be slippery enough that the transfer is easy, but not so slippery that one could slip off the surface, especially if it is wet.

Transfer benches should be easy to clean and, if not permanent, light and easy to position. Suction cups are used to anchor the bench to both the bathtub and the floor. Most have side grab bars and back rests. They also should be adjustable so a person can enter the tub from either the right or the left. Tubs with doors present problems for both bath boards and transfer benches; an appropriate model must be found or the tub doors removed.

Wash mitts, wash sponges, some with a pocket for a bar of soap, long handled scrubbing brushes and sponges, along with tap turners make bathing easier.

Raised toilet seats ease sitting down and getting up and transfers from a wheelchair to the toilet seat. Most raised toilet seats add 10 cm (4 inches) to the toilet height, although some adjust up to 16.25 cm (6½ inches). All raised toilet seats are attached directly to the toilet bowl, and some can be attached permanently by means of clips.

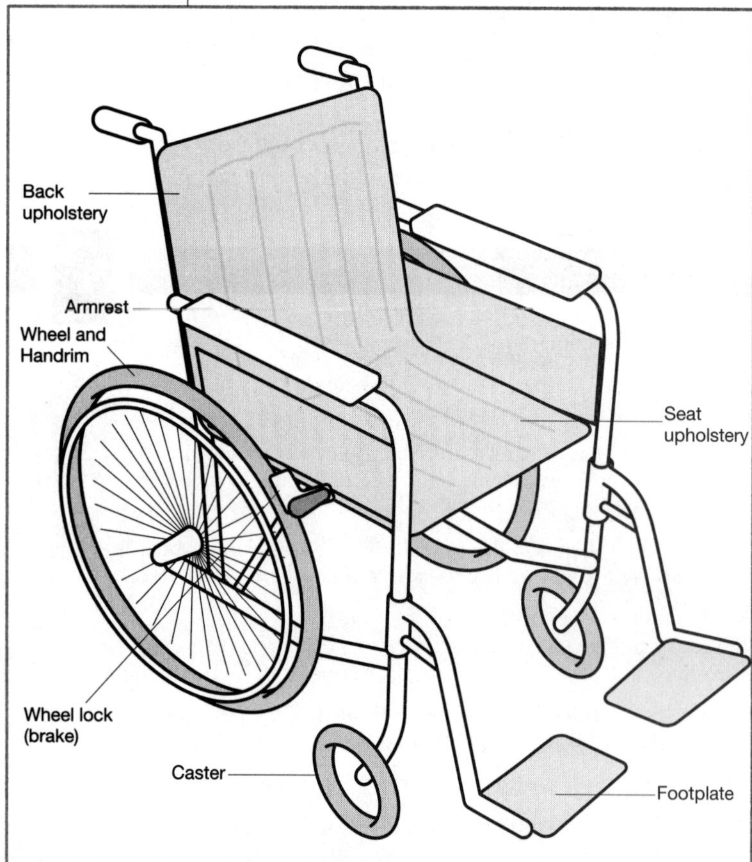

FIGURE 1: Wheelchair

Portable raised toilet seats are preferred when travelling. Some raised toilet seats have cut out areas that accommodate various lower extremity disabilities where the normal flexed sitting position is prevented, e.g., a hip joint that will not bend. Some raised toilet seats have armrests and safety rails. A safety bar can be attached to the wall next to the toilet; a trial run will help with the appropriate placement of the safety bar.

The toilet tissue dispenser should be within easy reach. Toilet tissue aids enable those without manual dexterity to use toilet tissue.

Splash guards can be attached to any toilet, raised seat or not. Attaching a raised toilet seat to a toilet means that the toilet lid is always up and a plush or fuzzy toilet seat cover cannot be used.

AMBULATION

Wheelchairs

Wheelchairs should provide comfortable and functional mobility. The user's daily routine must be considered before making a choice and many features can be customized to meet specific needs (Figure 1).

The method of propulsion of the wheelchair may be independent or assisted by another person. Independent propulsion is not only propelling by hand, but also electrically by hand, mouth, leg, or foot movements.

Positioning in a wheelchair needs to be balanced with adequate support. The buttocks should bear equal weight, and there should be adequate back support. Ideally, the shoulder should align with the elbows, with the arms resting at right angles. The knees and ankles should be at right angles as well. More severely disabled people may not be able to achieve the ideal, and adaptation may be needed.

The wheelchair seating dimensions should match the body dimensions. A too large or too small chair will not function well for the patient. The seat and back should not sag. The dimensions of an empty chair are not the same as the shape and dimension of a chair with the user sitting in it. And, if a seat cushion is used, the dimensions change again.

If the chair is to be used indoors, its size and ability to manoeuvre and the architectural features of the building or room in which use is anticipated must be considered. Measuring doorways and checking the turning axis are required. It must fit through doorways, both at home and work.

Wheelchairs used outdoors should be able to negotiate uneven ground, slopes, and curbs. This is the major limitation of wheelchairs. Designed to function on man-made surfaces, they perform poorly in the park or on the beach.

Wheelchairs used for leisure activities may require high performance features and should be easy to transport. Certain sports, e.g., basketball and track, require specialized wheelchairs that are light and strong. Appearance and styling may be important.

When transporting, close access to a car seat is required for transferring. Lightweight chairs with detachable or pivoting arm and foot rests, make transfers and transportation easy. See Table 3 for common wheelchair features.

Different manufacturers use different terms to describe the same features. Checking with the manufacturer will help to clarify the terms and descriptions. The Canadian Standards Association has several wheelchair standards, e.g., nomenclature, terms, definitions; determination of overall dimensions, mass and turning space; determination of brake effectiveness (Tables 4, 5 and 6).

Canes and Walkers

Canes and walkers reduce instability and give confidence and mobility. Wooden canes and walkers are less expensive, but heavy. Aluminum canes and walkers are light and more easily manoeuvred.

Canes and walkers should be measured to ensure a correct fit. The distance from the top of a cane's handle to its tip should equal the distance from the wrist crease to the ground, measured with the individual standing erect and wearing every day shoes. If the cane is too short, the user will lean forward, if too long, lean backward. Adjustable and telescopic canes help in finding the correct fit.

ADVICE FOR THE PATIENT

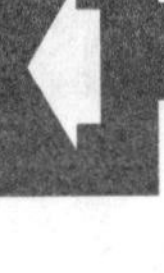

Where to Find a Wheelchair

- Renting a wheelchair is an option if it is required for a short period or a trial run of a specific model is desired, and the service is available in your area.
- Local chapters of resource groups such as the Canadian Paraplegic Association Inc. and the Canadian Rehabilitation Council for the Disabled may be aware of what is available. The Red Cross Society and the Victorian Order of Nurses may provide information, and service clubs sometimes supply wheelchairs to individuals. Public Health Departments and Home Care may also be able to arrange wheelchair rental.
- The yellow pages of the local telephone book will list retail outlets that sell wheelchairs; some will rent them. Sometimes arrangements can be made for a rent-to-buy purchase. Because wheelchair outlets are not licensed, comparison shopping is recommended before purchasing. The staff of retail wheelchair stores usually has some training in fitting them, and these stores may offer discounts to members of certain resource groups.
- Wheelchairs are expensive; if purchasing is a necessity, provincial health coverage, private health insurance plans, and even benevolent organizations may offset some of the cost.

TABLE 3: Common Wheelchair Features

Frame style—outdoor or amputee	Foot rests—fixed, pivoting or swing away, removable, elevated
Frame construction—regular or light weight	Wheels—spoked, composite, quick release axle
Seat height—standard or hemiplegic height	Casters—width
Arm rests—fixed, removable, pivoting, full length, desk length, adjustable, wrap around	Tires—pneumatic, semi-pneumatic, solid
Drive—regular, one handed, electrical	Upholstery and frame color
Back rest—height, reclining, sectional	

TABLE 4: Wheelchair Characteristics

Seat width	Ease of folding
Seat height	Type of release mechanism available
Overall width, chair folded and unfolded	Maneuverability or minimum turning radius
Weight (manufacturers usually quote weight without any foot rests)	Adjustability
Ease of propulsion	Quality of upholstery

TABLE 5: Considerations When Purchasing a Wheelchair

The individual's self-image, personality, preferences

The activities the wheelchair will be used for (e.g., home, work, leisure, school, community activities, outdoors)

The environment or terrain where the wheelchair will be used (outdoors or indoors). It is much less expensive to order a wheelchair to suit the environment than to do extensive renovations. An individual may need different wheelchairs for different environments

The type of transfers performed by the individual

The practicality of transporting the wheelchair

The individual's seating and postural needs

The individual's physical status (e.g., range of motion, endurance, sitting). If the individual's status is likely to change with time, the wheelchair should meet future as well as current needs

The individual's cognitive and perceptual status

The maintenance needs of the chair and the individual's ability or willingness to meet them

The individual's dimensions and weight. Allowances must be made for growing children

The expected lifetime of the wheelchair

The cost and availability of funding

TABLE 6: Wheelchair Accessories

Cushions—to accommodate urinals, to reduce pressure sores, (e.g., sheep skin, head cushions and supports)

Harnesses for support and safety

Trays—elevated, with cup holder

Pushing gloves and cuffs

Bag to carry personal items or for shopping

Stump boards

Hoods and umbrellas to protect from rain

Transfer boards

Portable ramps

Walkers are measured in the same manner, and most are adjustable.

A cane handle should afford an easy, yet firm grip. A swan's neck handle is easier for balancing, and many handles have molded grips. Metal and wood cane tips or walker feet tend to slip, requiring soft rubber tips, which are replaceable. For canes there is a flip back ice gripping tip that can be used in winter to provide extra stability. Quad bases add balance to canes. Canes are most comfortably held in the dominant hand, but holding the cane in the contralateral hand will provide greater balance. With a compromised joint, canes should be used on the opposite side to that joint.

Walkers may have wheels on 2 to 4 of the legs, and they may be permanent or removable. Some walkers have wheels that can be attached to the two front legs, the two back legs, or all four legs; others have wheels that can be locked in place. Because of the increased risk of accidents associated with the greater mobility of four-wheeled walkers, these brakes or wheels should be easily locked and the individual using these walkers familiar with the safety features. Walker accessories include tote bags and attached seats. A folding walker will ease transportation.

Crutches

Crutches require greater upper body strength and may not be suitable for all individuals. They offer more support in those conditions involving the lower limbs. Two basic types are available: underarm or axillary crutches are used temporarily, e.g., for a broken bone in the ankle; forearm crutches are meant for long-term use.

Axillary crutches should fit comfortably under the arm while standing erect. Various lengths are available to accommodate youths as well as adults; most are adjustable in both length and placement of handgrips. Metal crutches are lightweight, but wooden crutches are more economical. Axillary crutches can be rented for short-term use.

Compression Stockings

Elastic compression stockings decrease superficial venous pressure, increase the upward flow in unoccluded deep and superficial veins and raise local interstitial pressure. Compression of the leg also relieves some discomfort by preventing some edema. Compression stockings are designed to give gradual support with most pressure exerted at the ankle, less at the calf and the least at the thigh. Stockings can vary in their compression and range from 12 mm Hg compression at the ankle to 60 mm Hg.

A correct fit requires accurate measurements of the unedematous leg first thing in the morning. To assure good compression, the stockings should be washed and dried according to the manufacturer's instructions and replaced about every 2 to 3 months. They are intended to be removed at night and put on in the morning before beginning to walk. Manual dexterity is needed to put the stockings on.

Antiembolism stockings are worn by the nonambulatory to prevent venous emboli secondary to inactivity. They provide less support and are not suitable for ambulatory patients.

PATIENT ASSESSMENT QUESTIONS

?

Q *Why are you seeking an ADL? Has it been recommended?*

The ADL recommended depends on how long it will be used, e.g., crutches for a broken leg would be short term and adjustable axillary crutches would be suitable, but fitted forearm crutches suit paraplegia.

Q *What are your measurements?*

ADLs must fit correctly, and accurate measurements are necessary for a proper fit. Having a tape measure available will enable a check of these measurements, which must be done of the correct area under the right conditions, e.g., first thing in the morning for compression stockings. Attention must be paid to the unit of measure and if conversion is necessary, e.g., inches into centimetres, it must be checked.

Q *Do you have assistance at home? Has a home assessment been done?*

Many ADLs are expensive and used by more than one person in the home, e.g., bath-tub benches. A home evaluation by an occupational therapist (some provincial health departments do them) can identify barriers and indicate economical solutions before expensive purchases are made.

Q *What is your lifestyle?*

The ADL must suit the client's lifestyle, e.g., a wheelchair for an athlete or a wheelchair suitable for use at work in the narrow hallways of an office. If the client lives with others, the ADL should not cause problems in the home, e.g., a permanent raised toilet seat would not be suitable for a client living with a family in a one-bathroom home.

INCONTINENCE

Incontinence is the inability to control defecation or urination. Loss of bladder and/or bowel control is a medical problem but has psychological and social implications.

Seventy-five per cent of those who experience urinary incontinence are women, and half are under 60 years of age. It is important that urinary incontinence, as well as fecal incontinence, is not viewed as merely a sign of aging, but as a symptom of an underlying condition that must be treated.

URINARY INCONTINENCE

Urinary incontinence is identified as either transient or chronic. The causes of transient urinary incontinence include functional problems, the use of medication, acute urinary tract infections and fecal impaction. Chronic urinary incontinence is related to a malfunction of the urinary tract itself (Table 7). See Figure 2 for bladder and urinary anatomy.

Micturition

Three muscles and their accompanying nervous system controls are responsible for micturition:

- the detrusor smooth muscle of the bladder;
- the smooth muscle of the proximal urethral sphincter;
- the striated muscle of the external urethral sphincter.

The detrusor muscle is primarily innervated by the parasympathetic nervous system. Stimulation of the beta-adrenergic receptors located in the body of and fundus of the detrusor muscle contributes to bladder relaxation and promotes filling of the bladder. This smooth muscle expands to accommodate increased volumes of urine in response to stretch receptors found in the bladder submucosa.

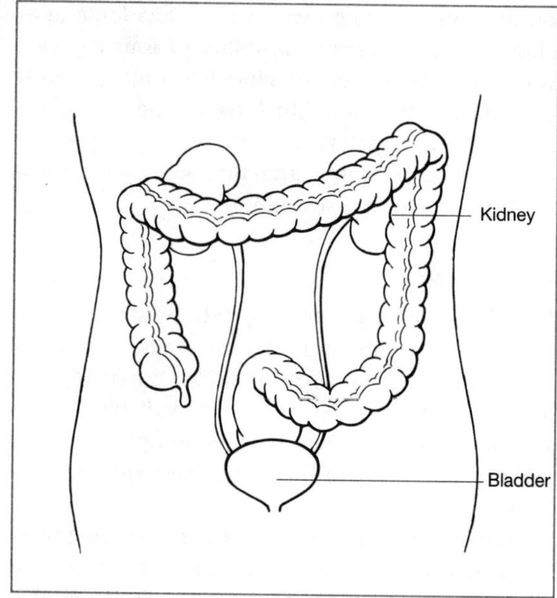

FIGURE 2: Kidney and Bladder

The alpha adrenergic innervation of the smooth muscle of the urethra responds to norepinephrine, to constrict the urethra and close the bladder. Estrogen may play a role opening an unobstructed internal urethral sphincter. In postmenopausal women, lack of estrogen induces atrophic changes in vaginal and urethral mucosa. Local urethral inflammation, usually a result of decreased estrogen (or infection) can also contribute to laxity of the sphincter and development of stress incontinence. Estrogens may have a role in maintaining the integrity of the internal sphincter in women: one of the ways gonadotropic hormones influence the urinary tract is by modifying the reponses to adrenergic stimulation.

TABLE 7: Types of Urinary Incontinence

Transient	Chronic
Functional incontinence	Urge incontinence or detrusor instability
Medication caused incontinence	Overflow incontinence
Acute urinary tract infection caused incontinence	Stress incontinence
Incontinence secondary to fecal impaction	Psychogenic incontinence
	Mixed incontinence

The striated muscles of the external urethra are under voluntary control. Acetylcholine stimulates these muscles to close the sphincter and bladder outlet, reinforcing the internal sphincter.

As the bladder progressively fills with urine, the tension in the bladder wall increases until a threshold is reached. A nervous reflex called the micturition reflex is elicited. It greatly increases the pressure in the bladder and simultaneously causes a conscious desire to urinate. The detrusor muscle contracts emptying the bladder of urine. The micturition reflex also initiates the appropriate signals from the nervous system to relax both the internal and external sphincters allowing for the passage of the urine.

The micturition reflex is a completely automatic spinal cord reflex, but it can be inhibited or facilitated by centres in the brain. The hypothalamus and the upper pons, both found in the brain stem, contain facilitory centres, while the higher centres keep the micturition reflex inhibited. When the time arrives to urinate, the cortical centres facilitate the micturition reflexes and inhibit the external urethral sphincter. Delay of micturition for short periods via voluntary contraction of the external sphincter is possible.

For predisposing factors to urinary incontinence see Table 8.

Transient Incontinence

Functional incontinence is the inability to get to the toilet. It is most common in institutional settings. Inaccessible call lights, restraints, side rails, patient immobility, communication problems, debility, and even cold air or tight undergarments all contribute. Some medications, e.g., hypnotics, sedatives, and diuretics may aggravate functional incontinence by making a trip to the toilet even more difficult.

The treatment of functional incontinence is aimed at making toileting more accessible. Increased toileting frequency, moving the individual closer to the toilet, or installing a bedside commode increases accessibility. Restricting fluids, especially those with diuretic activity, such as tea and coffee, and especially in the evening, may eliminate overnight accidents.

Medication alone may cause incontinence. The classic example is diuretics. Sedatives and hypnotics can cause nocturnal incontinence. Anticholinergics may cause inhibition of the detrusor contraction and are implicated in urinary retention and overflow. Numerous drugs, e.g., antidepressants, antihistamines, antipsychotics and some antispasmodics have anticholinergic side effects, especially urinary retention, and may contribute to incontinence (Table 9).

Acute urinary tract infections can result in urinary incontinence, which can lead to urinary tract infections. Severe cystitis causes frequency, urgency, and incontinence, which treatment of the infection may eliminate.

Painful urination can complicate both a urinary tract infection and urinary incontinence. The individual prefers to hold in the urine rather than experience pain at voiding. Frequent voiding flushes the infection from the urinary tract and prevents incontinence. The urinary analgesic, phenazopyridine, acts on the urinary tract mucosa to relieve the burning, urgency, and frequency.

In immobilized elderly patients, fecal impaction can cause urinary incontinence, thought to be due to local irritation and a change in the urethrovesical angle. Breaking up the fecal impaction is required, either digitally or with an enema. Prevention—increased fibre and fluid intake, regular bowel habits and exercise—is preferred.

Chronic Urinary Incontinence

Detrusor instability or urge incontinence, overflow incontinence and stress incontinence are the three most common forms of chronic urinary

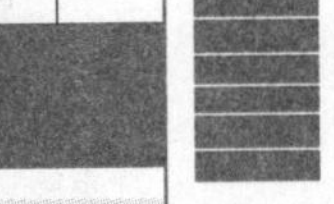

TABLE 8: Predisposing Factors to Urinary Incontinence

Age
Decreased bladder capacity
Inability to postpone voiding
Decrease in urethral or bladder compliance
Decreased urinary flow rate
Increase in post voiding residual volume
Increase in detrusor contractions
Decreased kidney ability to concentrate urine
Involuntary—increase in prostate volume
In Women
Menopause leading to atrophic vaginitis, urethritis, and weakening of periurethral tissues
Physical Factors
Genitourinary surgery, lack of post partum exercise
In Men
Benign prostatic hypertrophy leading to urinary retention and decreased urinary flow rate

TABLE 9: Drugs That May Contribute to Urinary Incontinence

Drug	Example(s)	Effect
Alcohol		Increased volume and frequency, decreased attention to bladder cues; impaired mobility
Alpha agonists	phenylpropanolamine, pseudoephedrine	Urinary retention (in patients with prostatic hypertrophy)
Alpha blockers	prazosin, terazosin	Decreased urethral closure pressure
Anticholinergics	propantheline, trihexyphenidyl	Urinary retention, overflow incontinence, fecal impaction
Antidepressants	imipramine, amitriptyline	See anticholinergic effect Decreased attention to micturition control
Antihistamines	diphenhydramine	See anticholinergic and sedative effect
Antipsychotics	chlorpromazine	See antidepressant effect Urinary retention is rare, most often occurring in patients with prostatic hypertrophy Decreased attention to micturition control
Antispasmodics	cyclobenzaprine	See anticholinergic effect
Anxiolytics	diazepam, alprazolam	Decreased attention to bladder cues Long acting benzodiazepines may accumulate in elderly patients causing confusion
Beta agonists	salbutamol	Urinary retention
Beta blockers	propranolol	Urinary retention
Calcium channel blockers	verapamil, nifedipine	Urinary retention
Diuretics	furosemide, hydrochlorothiazide	Increased volume and frequency
Skeletal muscle relaxants	baclofen, dantrolene	Urethral relaxation (weakness of the external sphincter) and sedation
Narcotic analgesics	codeine	Sedation and fecal impaction
Sedatives/Hypnotics	temazepam, triazolam	Sedation and urinary retention
Sympatholytics	reserpine, methyldopa	Urethral relaxation

incontinence. In fact, 65% of urinary incontinence in elderly individuals 65 years of age or older involves detrusor instability.

The detrusor muscle provides the propulsive force for emptying the bladder. It is located above the bladder and innervated by the parasympathetic autonomic system. Any physical condition or drug able to interfere with the detrusor muscle directly or indirectly will cause incontinence. A spastic or uninhibited bladder results in uncontrolled contractions and bladder emptying.

Nervous system conditions such as dementia, stroke, multiple sclerosis, Parkinson's disease and Alzheimer's disease worsen detrusor control. Small bladder volume, which can be natural or caused by bladder stones or tumors, makes the incontinence more pronounced. Aging means that the detrusor muscle does not function as it once did. Vaginitis is able to worsen this type of incontinence and can be corrected with topical or systemic estrogen replacement.

Overflow incontinence occurs when the pressure in the bladder is greater than the pressure in the urethra. Individuals "wet" themselves without knowing. Men with benign prostatic hypertrophy and partial bladder outlet obstruction experience overflow incontinence. By 80 years of age virtually all men have benign prostatic hypertrophy; the mean age for developing the condition is 65 years of age. Treatment of the prostate condition with either surgery or medication will improve overflow incontinence.

Individuals with large neuropathic bladders, such as diabetics, are also prone to overflow incontinence. Anticholinergic drugs can cause urinary retention and secondary urinary overflow. No matter what the cause, frequent toileting will improve overflow incontinence.

Stress incontinence is most common in postmenopausal women. There is urinary leakage on physical exertion such as coughing, sneezing, climbing stairs, or even turning over in bed. It is attributed to a weakening of the bladder neck either due to weakening of the pelvic floor musculature and supportive tissues surrounding the bladder outlet and urethra, or to damaged innervation of the smooth muscle of the bladder neck and proximal urethra. Pubococcygeal muscles support lower abdominal organs and rapid weight gain, pregnancy or lower abdominal surgery may result in poor muscle tone. The sphincter muscles clamp down and close off the urethra and rectum; there are several of these muscles around the vagina. All of these muscles lose tone with pregnancy, surgery and age. Estrogen deficiency, urethra and vaginal atrophy and pelvic floor weakening all may contribute to stress incontinence.

In postmenopausal women, estrogen replacement either topically or systemically will reduce stress incontinence. Exercise to strengthen the pelvic floor is useful. Walking, running, yoga, and aquacise all strengthen the pelvic floor. Kegel exercises are specific for the muscles of the pelvic floor. Kegel exercises are also recommended for men suffering from urge incontinence after prostatectomy. However, for maximum effectiveness they must be performed faithfully.

With Kegel exercises, the individual is taught to identify the muscles of the external sphincter by stopping the flow of urine during micturition. The muscles are drawn up slowly and held for a count of 10, then relaxed for a count of 10. This exercise is performed sitting on the toilet (applies to men and women) at each urination. Colloquially, the manoeuvre is known as the "faucet". The exercise should be repeated 30 to 80 times a day for up to 6 weeks, both during voiding and away from the toilet when the individual first feels the urge to void.

To strengthen the posterior muscles, the muscles of the anus are squeezed slowly and held for a count of 10, then relaxed for a count of 10. Again, these exercises should be repeated 30 to 80 times daily, or alternatively, 10 times in a row, 3 to 8 times daily. These Kegel exercises can be performed throughout the day in any location—working at a desk, doing dishes, stuck in traffic—and are known colloquially as the "wave."

Biofeedback to relax the muscles of the bladder, scheduled toileting to establish a fixed routine, and/or bladder retraining to increase the interval between voiding, are used along with the pelvic floor exercises to treat stress incontinence.

Specialized cones, known as vaginal cones are inserted and held in the vagina for 15 minutes to strengthen the pelvic floor muscles.

Stress incontinence is sometimes treated with tricyclic antidepressants or alpha adrenergic agonists to stimulate the nerves of the urinary sphincter. Phenylpropanolamine and pseudoephedrine are two alpha adrenergic agonists used as single ingredient therapy that are available as decongestants. Dosage regimens and duration of therapy vary along with the success of these agents.

Severe depression and/or psychosis sometimes involves incontinence as an attention getting device. The underlying condition needs to be treated.

Enuresis

Enuresis or bed wetting is involuntary micturition during sleep in an individual who usually has voluntary control. It is a parasomnia more common in children and usually occurs 3 to 4 hours after bedtime. Parasomnia is a state in which there is no response to stimuli, verbal or mental, except that of a reflex nature, thus the urge to urinate is not recognized, the individual does not wake up and wets the bed.

Urinary tract disease, e.g., infection, carcinoma and insulin dependent diabetes mellitus can cause enuresis. The majority of incidents are sleep related problems. The child is too sound asleep to feel the urge to go to the toilet. Sometimes restriction of fluids and taking the child to the bathroom when the parents go to bed, improves the condition.

In infants the sacral spinal reflex arc alone controls urination, but as the nervous system matures, the higher brain control develops over the spinal reflex and establishes control over urination and defecation. By about 2½ to 3 years of age, 90% of children have established bladder control. The remaining 10% are normal children who have a delayed maturation or a familial tendency.

Lack of bladder control beyond the age of 3 should be investigated. However, children with organic disease will be incontinent during the day as well as the night.

Bedwetting alarms and behavior modification programs train the individual to arouse themselves either when they begin to urinate or when they feel the urge to do so. Besides potential electrical shocks associated with some alarms, the cost may be a deterrent. Catheterization is an option, but requires training in technique.

FECAL INCONTINENCE

Continual dribbling of fecal matter through the anus is prevented by tonic constriction of the internal and external anal sphincters. The internal anal sphincter is a circular mass of smooth muscle that lies immediately inside the anus. The external anal sphincter is striated voluntary muscles controlled by the somatic nervous system.

The defecation reflex is responsible for defecation. When feces enter the rectum, extension of the rectal wall sends signals to the descending colon and sigmoid causing peristalsis. When the peristaltic wave reaches the internal anal sphincter, this sphincter is relaxed and if the external anal sphincter is also relaxed, defecation occurs.

The defecation reflex on its own is weak, but is reinforced through parasympathetic signals sent to and by the sacral segments of the spinal column. The signals entering the spinal column are responsible for other effects such as taking a deep breath, closure of the glottis, and contraction of the abdominal muscles.

The normal individual prevents defecation until a socially acceptable time by the voluntary contraction of the external anal sphincter. Taking a deep breath and contracting the abdominal muscles elicits new defecation reflexes. These new defecation reflexes along with the voluntary relaxation of the external anal sphincter combine to enable evacuation of the bowel. Unfortunately, defecation reflexes produced in this way are never as strong as those that arise naturally and for this reason individuals who routinely inhibit their natural reflexes are more prone to constipation.

Newborn babies and individuals with spinal cord damage have no voluntary control over their external anal sphincter. The defecation reflex causes automatic emptying of the lower bowel and fecal incontinence.

Anal sphincter impairment, either internal or external, can lead to fecal incontinence. Anorectal surgery, e.g., fistulotomy, hemorrhoidectomy; neurological disorders; and obstetric tears and episiotomy can all impair the integrity of either anal sphincter.

Diarrhea due to any cause can cause short term fecal incontinence, e.g., viral infections, bacterial infections such as *Escherichia coli*, shigella, cholera, salmonella, protozoal infections, ulcerative colitis, and Crohn's disease. Fecal impaction can contribute and complicate fecal incontinence.

Psychogenic fecal incontinence is an attention getting device. Fecal incontinence can accompany dementia and/or Alzheimer's disease and results from an individual's inability to voluntarily control the external anal sphincter.

INCONTINENCE PRODUCTS

Undergarments, diapers, bedside commodes, disposable pants for ambulatory individuals and disposable bed pads for institutionalized people are used to assist incontinent individuals. It is estimated that although widely available and widely advertised, 80% of ambulatory incontinent people do not use these products. Embarrassment purchasing the product and the cost are the two most often cited reasons.

The undergarments are available as fitted briefs, pull-on undergarments with folded or elasticized legs, and pads or shields. The fitted briefs must be sized, and a measurement of the user following the manufacturer's instructions is necessary. The fitted briefs are available with elasticized legs for greater comfort and security. Some undergarments have drop fronts and side fastenings for ease of wearing. All incontinence products are available in a variety of absorbencies.

Incontinence undergarments have three layers. The layers absorb urine, keep the skin dry, and contain fecal material. A waterproof polythene backing protects clothing. Cellulose fluff and/or sodium polyacrylate acts as an absorbent. The top lining is layers of hydrophobic material that keeps moisture away from the wearer's skin. The undergarments are not one-way systems, so as soon as the absorbent layer(s) are saturated moisture will flow back to the skin.

Most undergarments and pads are made for adults. Fitted briefs are worn like clothing, and sometimes instead of underwear. Undergarments have tabs on the side that enable the product to be adjusted to the user's size. They are intended to be worn under underwear. The absorbent pads are suitable for moderate to mild incontinence, especially stress urinary incontinence, and some are marketed specifically to women. These absorbent pads are preferred over menstrual pads for urinary incontinence, because menstrual pads are not designed to absorb urine.

When choosing an incontinence undergarment, consideration must be given to the individual's manual dexterity, daytime versus nighttime only use, the volume of urine or feces, the bulkiness, the fit (possibility of adjusting product to fit hip and waist), and whether fecal incontinence is part of the condition.

Knitted reusable briefs with a front opening for a disposable pad are available. These briefs are not suitable if fecal incontinence is a problem or if urinary incontinence is frequent and/or large in volume.

Body worn urinals, both male and female, are available, however the female versions are rarely used because of their high failure rate.

Condom drainage, also known as external catheters, is an option for men. These systems are penile sheaths of latex with reinforced tips and a drainage outlet. They are not suitable for men who have a retracted penis, are confused and may pull off the condom, or are unable to apply the condom. Problems include allergies to latex; condoms that are too tight resulting in edema, ischemia, and necrosis; pressure sores; pooled urine causing dermatitis; and "blow outs" with sudden voiding of large amounts of urine. The condoms should be removed daily and the area washed with soap and water, then dried well.

A condom drainage system should be drained into a drainage bag or clamped shut to prevent dribbling. If drainage bags are used, they should have nonreturn valves to prevent infection. The drainage bags ideally are emptied and cleaned daily if they are reusable, otherwise disposable drainage bags are more convenient. Drainage bags can be attached to catheters as well.

Internal catheters are used when other methods for managing urinary incontinence fail. Catheter diameter is measured in French gauge or Charriere size, (e.g., 1Fr or Ch = 0.33 mm = the external diameter of the catheter shaft). The catheter selected should be the smallest capable of giving adequate drainage while providing maximum comfort for the patient. Catheters most commonly range in size from 8 Fr to 14 Fr and most catheters are silicone coated for easy insertion. Shorter catheters, 21 cm versus the standard 40 to 45 cm length are available for female patients.

Problems with internal catheters include leakage, blockage, infection, rejection and psychological difficulties. Choosing the correct size, careful monitoring and appropriate antibiotic use will eliminate most problems; however, lack of psychological acceptance of catheterization may complicate problems that do occur.

PATIENT ASSESSMENT QUESTIONS

Q *When do you notice the incontinence?*

Identifying the type of incontinence can help in the recommending of a product. If the client wets himself/herself and doesn't realize it, it may be overflow incontinence. If the client wets himself/herself on exertion, e.g. sneeze, it may be stress incontinence. If the client feels the urge to wet himself/herself, it may be urge incontinence.

Q *Do you have any disease conditions or take any medications?*

Conditions such as vaginitis, prostatitis or diabetes can exacerbate or cause incontinence; treating the underlying condition may alleviate it. Medications and their timing, e.g., diuretics at bedtime, can produce incontinence as a side effect. A change in medication or dose may correct the problem.

Q *What is the frequency and severity of your incontinence? What is your lifestyle?*

Recommending an incontinence pad or brief depends on the frequency and volume of fluid. Although suitable for infrequent or small volume, lifestyle may make a pad impractical: frequent changing may not be possible at work; nighttime incontinence may require a brief, while a pad is adequate during the day.

Q *Is fecal incontinence an aspect of your problem?*

Because some products are not designed for fecal incontinence, which may increase the frequency of changing, the choice of product is paramount.

Q *What is the condition of your skin?*

Incontinence can cause skin irritation and proper care must be emphasized when counselling.

OSTOMY

An ostomy is an artificial opening made surgically in the body. The name is derived from the Greek word stoma, meaning mouth. A colostomy involves the colon, ileostomy the ileum or small intestine, and urostomy the urinary tract.

Half a million North Americans have ostomies and over 100,000 ostomy operations are performed each year in the United States and Canada. No particular age or ethnic group has more ostomies, but, in general, more women than men have ostomies. The older the adult the more likely the ostomy surgery will be a colostomy because of cancer or obstruction related to disease. Inflammatory bowel disease (IBD) is a common reason for an ileostomy. IBD occurs more commonly in whites than blacks or Asians with an increased incidence in Jews compared to non-Jews, and its peak occurrence is between ages 15 and 35. Urostomies are common in infants and older individuals. Illustrations of the common colostomies, ileostomies and urostomies are presented in Figures 3 and 4.

Cancer is one of the most common reasons for ostomy surgery. The location of the cancer will determine the type of ostomy. Cancer is the leading cause of urostomies in adults.

Inflammatory bowel disease, which includes chronic ulcerative colitis and Crohn's disease, may necessitate ostomy surgery to control the disease, and to remove damaged scar tissue. Events such as abdominal stabbing or automobile accidents resulting in puncture wounds may result in ostomies that may be temporary until the abdominal injuries have healed.

Ostomy surgery can be the result of a familial history of polyps that increases the risk for cancer or the development of polyps in young children. In spina bifida, peristalsis may be weak or ineffective and/or the micturition reflex inoperative, both of which necessitate ostomy surgery. Birth defects such as neonatal necrotizing enterocolitis and imperforate anus usually require ostomy surgery, which can be temporary.

Two-thirds of all ostomies are colostomies. Usually older individuals, men and women equally, have colostomies. In a colostomy, part of the large intestine is disconnected or removed, and depending on the location of the colostomy, it is referred to as ascending, transverse, descending, sigmoid, loop or double barrel. Descending and sigmoid colostomies are the most common.

In most cases the colostomy is permanent and the rectum and anus are removed. Loop and double barrel colostomies are temporary in that they give the lower bowel time to heal and once healed the colostomy is reversed. In a double barrel colostomy the colon is severed and both ends are brought to the surface as stomas. In a loop colostomy the colon is not cut completely through, but rather sliced along one side with both edges brought to the surface as one stoma.

About 20 to 25% of ostomies are ileostomies. The entire large intestine including the rectum and anus is removed and the end of the ileum is brought through the abdominal wall to form the stoma. Sometimes an ileostomy is temporary allowing the large intestine below to heal. Once healed the intestine is reconnected.

Urostomies account for about 10 to 15% of ostomy surgery with one-quarter of them occurring in young children. Birth defects are the most common reason for childhood urostomies; for adults, it is spinal cord injury and cancer. A urostomy diverts urine away from a diseased or damaged bladder, urethra, or ureters. Sometimes the conduit is part of the small intestine (an ileal conduit) and sometimes part of the colon (a colonic conduit). Another, less common type of urostomy is the ureterostomy in which the ureters themselves are used.

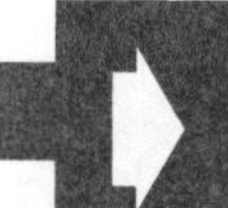

ADVICE FOR THE PATIENT

Enterostomal Therapy Nurses

- Enterostomal therapy nurses or ET nurses are specialized stoma care nurses. Their expertise is in ostomy and wound care, and they have postsecondary education in these fields. ET nurses may be involved in ostomy clinics, patient home visits, and hospital based pre- and postsurgical programs.
- Public Health Departments, provincial Home Health Care, hospitals that perform ostomy operations and organizations such as the Victorian Order of Nurses usually employ ET nurses. Manufacturers and retailers of ostomy appliances also may employ these specialist nurses.
- There is a national association of ET nurses: Canadian Association of Enterostomal Therapy Nurses, c/o Canadian Nurses Association, 50 The Driveway, Ottawa, ON K2P 1E2.

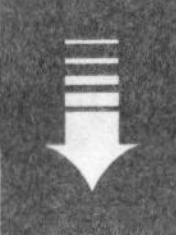

FIGURE 3: Colostomies

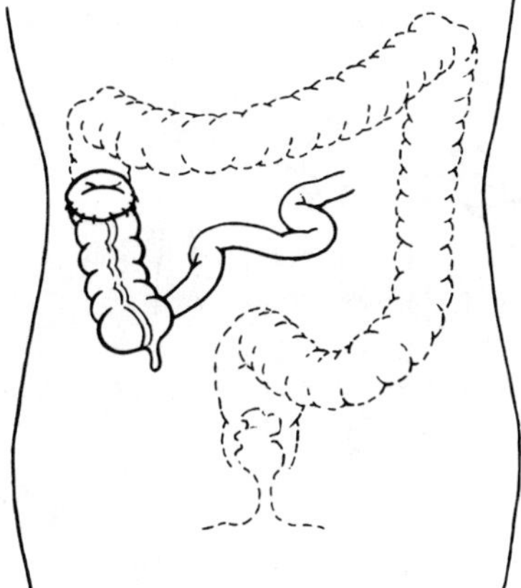

Ascending Colostomy

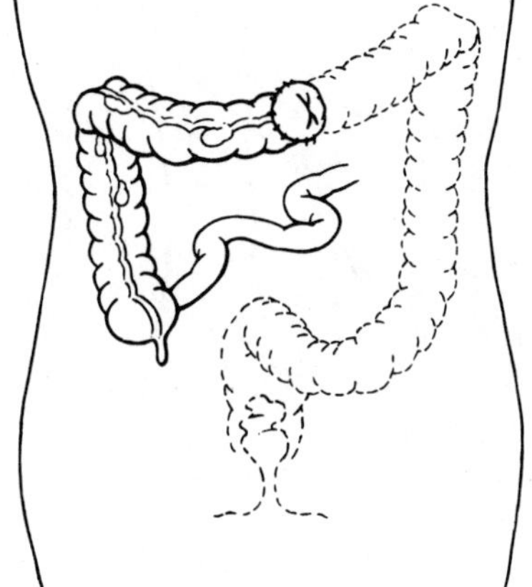

Transverse Colostomy

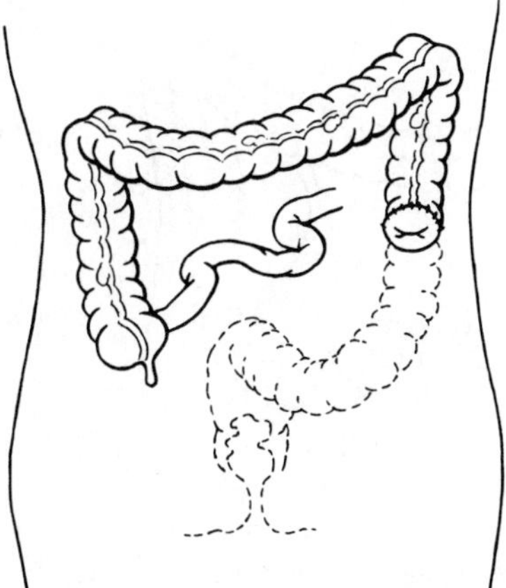

Descending Colostomy

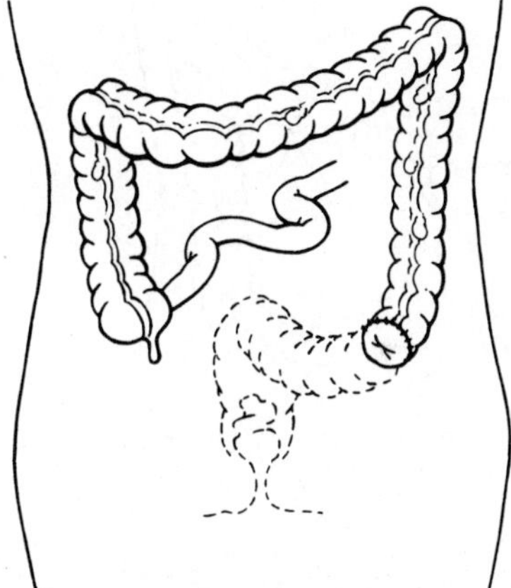

Sigmoid Colostomy

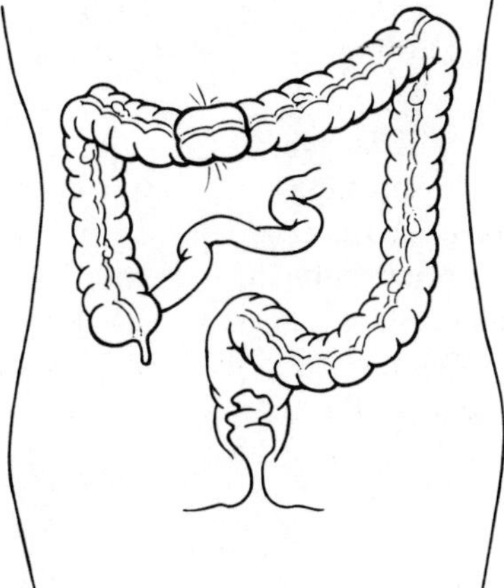

Loop Colostomy

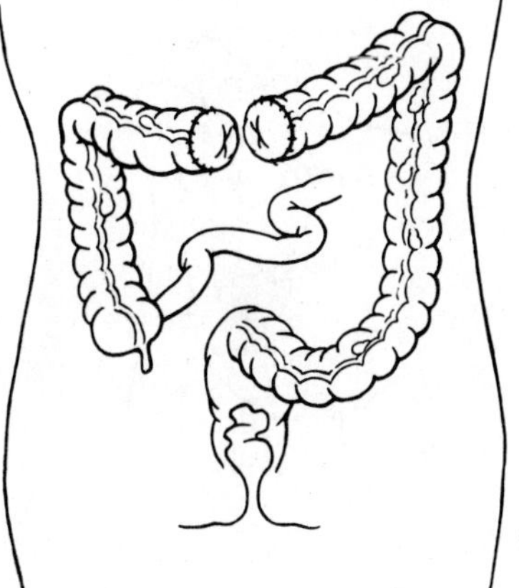

Double-barrel Colostomy

FIGURE 4: Ileostomies and Urostomies

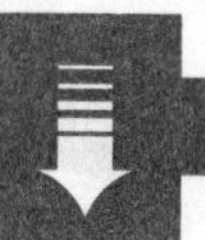

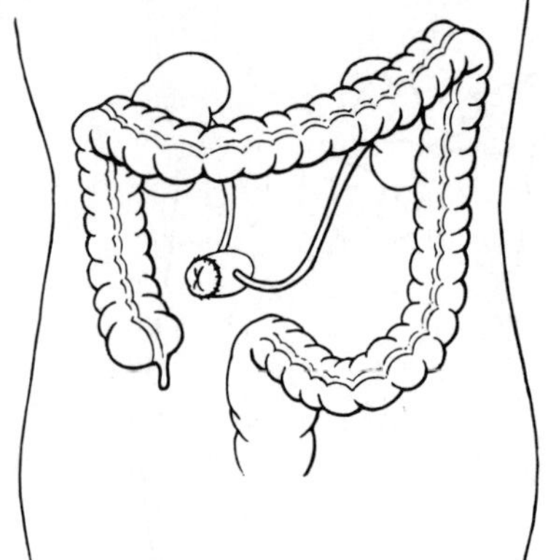

Ileal Conduit

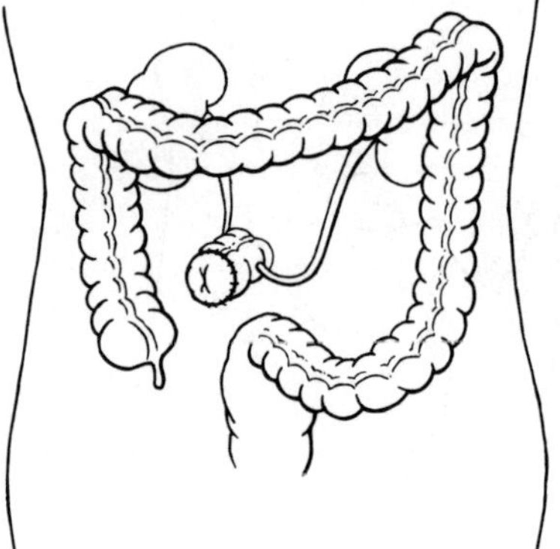

Colonic Conduit

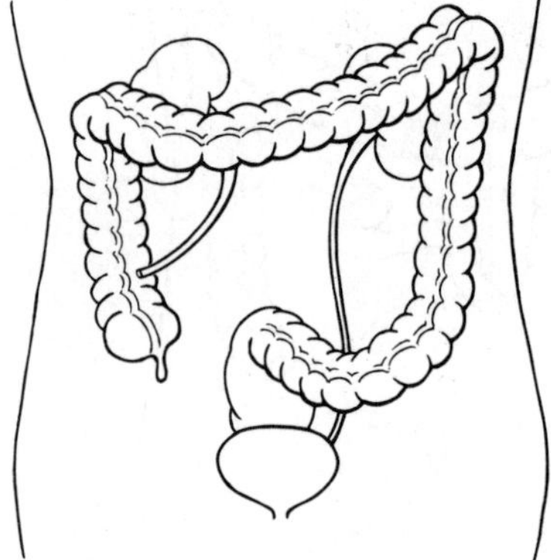

Unilateral Ureterostomy

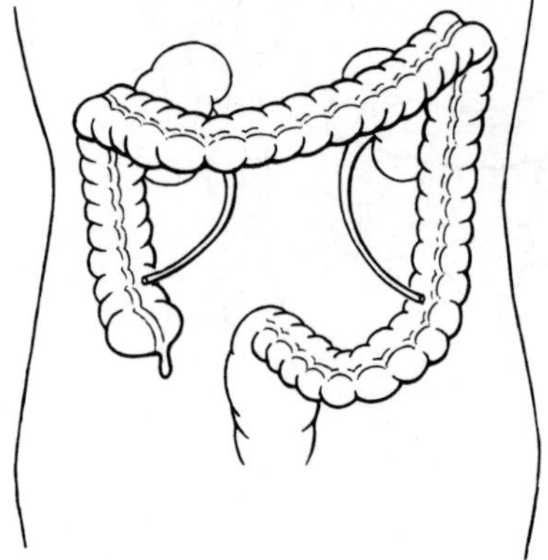

Bilateral Ureterostomy

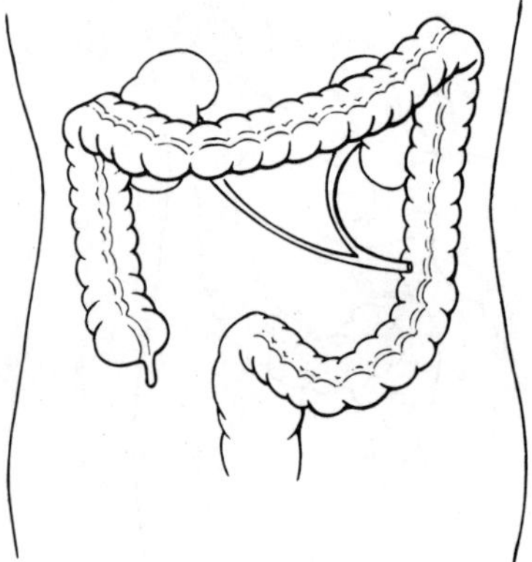

Transureteroureterostomy

The pelvic pouch procedure is a two-stage surgical procedure that involves a temporary ostomy (Figure 5). It is used to treat ulcerative colitis and familial polyposis, and in effect cures the disease while not requiring a permanent ostomy. In the first stage, the diseased colon is removed and a pouch constructed from the ileum. A temporary ostomy is constructed. After 3 to 4 months, the pouch has healed, and the gastrointestinal tract reconnected, closing the ostomy. A fully functioning, although shorter, bowel results. The pelvic pouch procedure can be differentiated by the shape of the reservoir created: S-shaped, J-shaped or side-to-side.

APPLIANCES AND EQUIPMENT

An appliance or pouch is used to collect waste at the stoma. Not all colostomies require appliances, however. Because urine always remains in liquid form, being discharged continuously, urostomy surgery always requires an appliance.

Irrigation

Irrigation is an option for some individuals with colostomies. It is less expensive than wearing appliances and affords some fecal outflow control. In irrigation, squirting water through the stoma into the intestine stimulates peristaltic movements, which forces waste out. It is usually performed in the bathroom with an irrigation bag that is much like an enema bag.

Approximately a quart of lukewarm water passes through a tube, through the stoma and into the intestine. An irrigation sleeve fits over the stoma and about 5 minutes after all the water has flowed into the bowel and the tube has been removed from the stoma, waste will begin to flow

FIGURE 5: The Pelvic Pouch Procedure

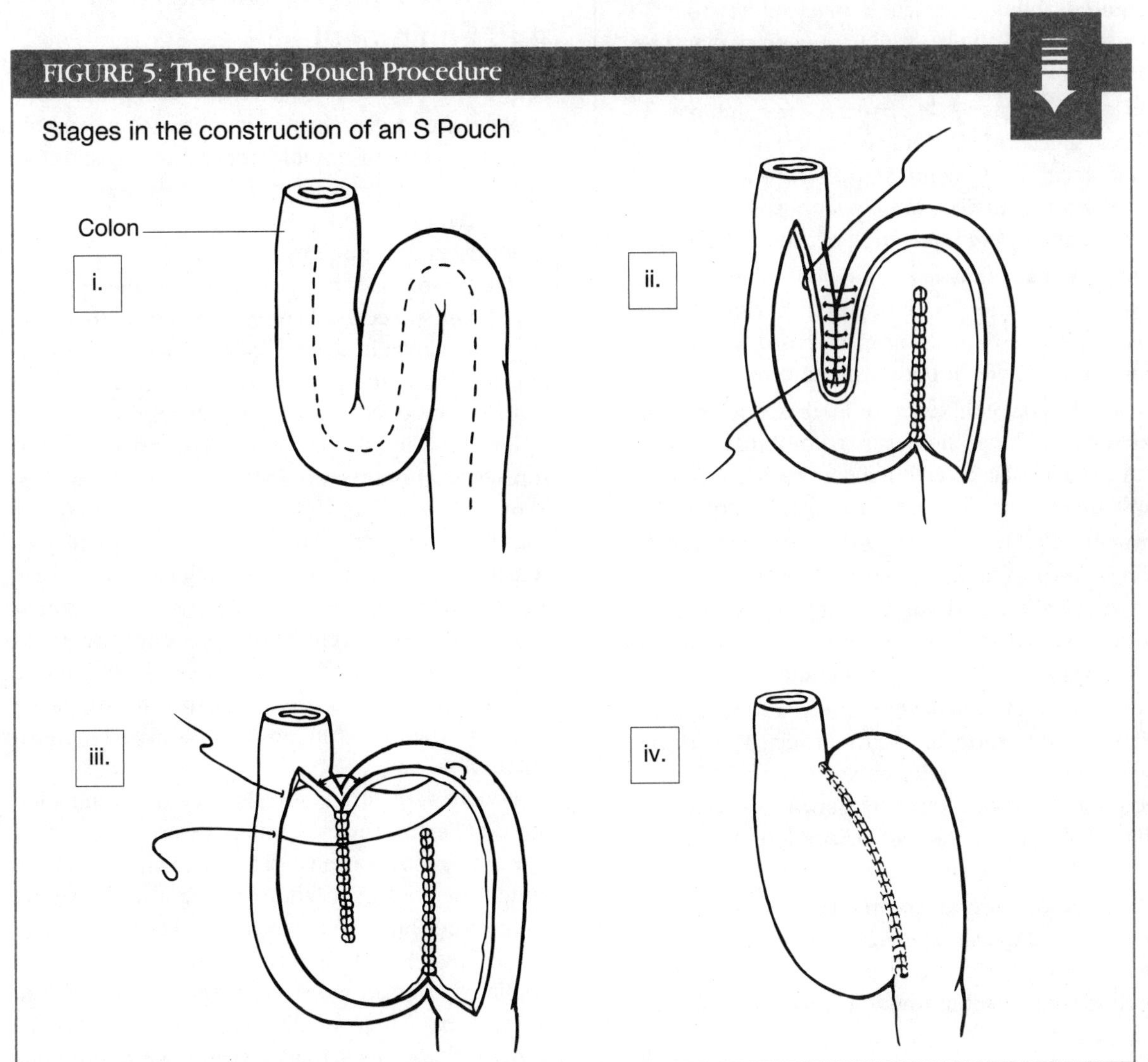

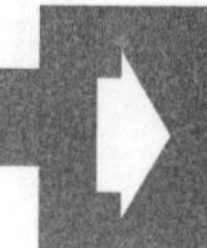

ADVICE FOR THE PATIENT

Skin Care for the Ostomy Patient

- Skin barriers are used to protect the skin adjacent to the stoma from discharge and include pastes, powders, and sprays. Skin barriers also provide varying degrees of adhesiveness improving the fit and security of an appliance.
- Some skin barriers are available as wafers that layer the combination of protectant and adhesive ingredients between a polyethylene film and a paper backing. These wafers must be cut to fit the stoma and appliance. Wafers are sometimes affixed directly to the face plate of an appliance surrounding the flange and no cutting is needed.
- Desirable characteristics of a skin protectant product are: nonirritating; nonstinging; alcohol free; low allergenic potential; bacterial/fungal growth inhibiting ability; premoistened; no wetting required; ability to remain in place; ability to "breathe"; and ability to fill in uneven skin and be leak proof.
- Most protectants or skin barriers are combinations of polysaccharides, cellulose, gums such as karaya gum, gelatin and pectin. *Stomahesive* and *Hollihesive* contain gelatin, pectin, sodium carboxymethylcellulose and polyisobutylene.
- Karaya gum is rarely used alone but in combination with other agents. Urine breaks down karaya gum making it an unwise choice for urostomies, and the gum melts readily at body temperature.
- Gelatin has been linked with increased growth of bacteria and fungi; however, in combination with other agents this growth may not be seen. Topical nystatin powder is used for fungal overgrowth.
- Protectant pastes, e.g., *Premium* and *Stomahesive*, can be used to fill in skin surface irregularities to prevent leakage and skin irritation. These pastes should be applied to the appliance not the skin and allowed to dry for at least 10 minutes.
- Solvents and cleansers help remove effluent and clean the skin surrounding the stoma. They should be used sparingly on the skin and not contain potential irritants such as perfumes. Alcohol due to its drying nature should be avoided. Wipes are used to remove adhesive.
- Specialized creams and ointments are available for peristomal skin care and are labelled as such. These products are nonirritating and do not interfere with appliance adhesion while providing moisture and protection.

out of the stoma in spurts. The spurts pass through the irrigation sleeve and fall into the toilet bowl. After the first 10 to 20 minutes the majority of the waste has been eliminated and the bottom of the irrigation sleeve can be clipped so daily activities can continue.

Irrigation is popular in the United States, because it is more economical and Americans for the most part pay for their own ostomy supplies. Many North American homes, as well, have two or more bathrooms, one of which can be occupied for the 30 to 45 minutes required for irrigation.

Other times, a stoma cap or even a pad is all that is required to cover the stoma. Irrigation is performed regularly, ranging from every 24 hours to every fourth day. A convenient time may be after the largest meal of the day, because of the stimulated peristalsis.

Characteristics of Appliances and Equipment

An ideal appliance is lightweight, leak-proof, spill-proof and odor-free. Appliances are either reusable (permanent) or disposable (temporary). Disposable are more costly because they are thrown away after 3 to 7 days of use, but reusable must be cleaned routinely and thoroughly.

There are, as well, one- and two-piece appliances. One-piece appliances attach directly to the skin using an adhesive or sealant. Two-piece appliances have a face plate that is self-adhesive. The pouch is attached to the face plate and is ideal for individuals in whom excessive removal and replacement of their appliances irritates their skin. Manual dexterity and good eyesight are required to use two-piece appliances. The face plate can remain in place for up to a week. Because both one- and two-piece appliances usually can be emptied from the bottom, even the one-piece appliance can remain in place for up to a week. However, routine emptying is required—usually when the appliance is about one-third full. Some systems have interchangeable pouches.

Pouches are either closed-ended or open-ended for drainage. Urinary appliances are most often open-ended with a valve to allow drainage. Closed-ended pouches are used most often by colostomy patients because the waste material is more solid.

A flange is the opening in the face plate or appliance. Flanges are sized depending on the size of the stoma. There are different shapes and sizes of flanges themselves that accommodate different body contours and locations of stomas. Sizes for children, both face plates and appliances, enable accurate and comfortable fitting. Obesity may be a problem in fitting and maintaining an appliance.

Skin barriers prevent irritation, and are essential with urostomies and ileostomies because the effluent can cause skin damage. Some adhesives have added skin barriers. Other skin barriers are powders, sprays, or pastes. It is a good idea to test a skin barrier before using it. Applying the product to an inconspicuous area of skin for 48 hours is usually sufficient to determine if there is any sensitivity.

To avoid damage to the skin the appliance should be peeled off carefully and the skin around the stoma washed gently with warm water and mild soap. Any hair on the abdomen should be clipped, not shaved, as shaving damages the epidermis. The appliance should not be too tight as edema, ischemia, and fistula formation may result. All the adhesive areas should be in contact with the skin and the skin folds smoothed out.

The most common problem is sore skin, the result of too frequent removal of the pouch by an anxious individual. The skin around the stoma becomes damaged: red, swollen, burning, itchy. The average for changing an appliance is about every three days but varies from person to person.

Ill fitted or badly applied appliances leak around the seal. Alcohol should not be used to clean the skin, as it can cause more damage. Warm water and mild soap are preferred, and the soap must be completely washed off.

The adhesive is the most common cause of allergies, but the pouch material may cause skin reactions. A patch test prior to use will avoid most allergies, but if a skin reaction does occur, a switch to another brand of adhesive or pouch will usually resolve the problem.

Appliance covers prevent rustling and skin irritation due to rubbing. Some ostomy patients tape down their appliances, and others wear ostomy belts that hold their appliances in place. Ostomy belts are most often used by urostomy patients to reduce the strain on the adhesive from the weight of the urine in the pouch.

The appliance must suit the type of stoma, be leak-proof, odor-proof and an adequate size. Pouches of different lengths and capacities are available to contain the varying amounts of waste material. Selection of a drainable or nondrainable pouch will depend on the site of the stoma, the consistency of motions, and whether the task of drainage and cleaning the pouch is acceptable to the individual. Clear, opaque or decorated pouches are available, and the choice depends upon the individual's eyesight and preference.

Problems

Flatus filters containing a layer of charcoal are incorporated into some appliances. Deodorants are available for inclusion in pouches. Skin irritation may be caused by contact with the pouch itself, and a bag cover may be needed. A number of preparations are available for the prevention and treatment of damaged skin, but greasy preparations will prevent appliance adhesion. For proper adhesion the skin must be dry before the appliance is applied, and for urostomy patients this may be a problem in that urine drains continually.

Crystalline phosphate deposits may build up on urostomies and cut into the mucosa. Vinegar dabbed on the stoma when the appliance is cleaned will dissolve these crystals. A few drops of vinegar in the appliance will reduce the smell of stale urine, as well.

When bleeding of the stoma occurs, it is usually due to aggressive cleaning. Proper cleaning technique is required — gentle yet thorough. If bleeding persists, it may be an indication that the original disease has recurred, or alternatively, a new condition is developing, e.g., an infection or an ulcer.

Fistula formation appears as leakage around the base of the stoma and causes skin erosion. Surgical

ADVICE FOR THE PATIENT

Foods with Implications for Stoma Patients

- *Bulk-forming foods:* celery, Chinese foods, foods with seeds or kernels, nuts, coleslaw, dried fruits, coconut, wild rice, popcorn, meats in casings, whole vegetables, whole grains.
- *Diarrhea-causing foods:* green beans, broccoli, spinach, raw fruit, highly seasoned food, beer (other alcoholic beverages are not common offenders)
- *Odor-forming foods:* fish, eggs, asparagus, onions, garlic, some spices, peas, beans, cabbage, broccoli, turnips
- *Gas-forming foods:* string beans, dried beans, mushrooms, beer, carbonated drinks, cucumbers, onions, brussels sprouts, peas, spinach, corn, cabbage, broccoli, radishes, cauliflower, yeast, dairy products

PATIENT ASSESSMENT QUESTIONS

Q What is the type, size and shape of your stoma? Have there been any changes in it?

The type, size and shape of the stoma determines the type, size and shape of the ostomy appliance the client uses. Changes in the stoma, e.g., bleeding, retraction, fistula formation, may indicate an underlying condition that should be treated or may indicate overly aggressive cleaning.

Q How long do your appliances last?

Use of disposable or reusable appliances depends on how long the client wears one. Reusable appliances last longer but require more care.

Q What is your lifestyle?

Activities and diet affect the choice of appliance and accessories for it. A client who swims regularly needs a different appliance from one who works at a desk.

Q Do you have other medical conditions?

Medical conditions may make the attachment of the appliance to the stoma difficult, e.g., Parkinson patients.

Q What is the condition of your skin?

Skin irritation can be a problem for clients with ostomies, and proper care must be emphasized when counselling.

refashioning of the stoma is sometimes required. Retraction or prolapse of the stoma always requires surgery. It is usually due either to faulty fashioning of the stoma to begin with, or major changes in the individual's weight.

Unless there are any medical contraindications, individuals should be advised to eat a normal, varied diet, making their own adjustments to omit foods that change the consistency of the feces, or cause odor or gas. Those most often cited are brans, fish, onions, carbonated beverages and beer.

Individuals with colostomies are prone to constipation; fluid, fibre and exercise are recommended to avoid this problem. Those with ileostomies should exercise caution with foods containing large amounts of cellulose that may cause blockage.

Anyone with an ileostomy lacks a normal reserve capacity for absorption of water, sodium and potassium, and should be advised to take extra fluid and electrolytes after exercise and in hot weather. Specialized fluid and electrolyte replacement drinks used by athletes, e.g., *Gatorade*, are ideal. Some individuals need routine potassium supplementation, and particular attention should be paid to plasma potassium levels if a diuretic is used.

Diet is the most common source of constipation, diarrhea, and odor problems. Identifying what food is causing the problem and changing the diet usually solves these problems. Modern pouches are odor free, provided they are changed regularly, emptied as needed, cleaned properly, have no flaws or pinholes, and have a reliable seal. Emptying a pouch will often be accompanied by odor, but there are several deodorants that help control this. They are placed into the pouch after each emptying.

Individuals with an ileostomy will notice that high fibre foods remain undigested, sometimes causing stomal blockage. Corn, celery, mushrooms, peas, Chinese vegetables, pineapple, oranges, grapefruit, raisins, prunes, popcorn, nuts, coconut, shrimp, and relish should be introduced into the diet one at a time. Eating them in small quantities, chewing well and drinking fluids along with them will help avoid problems.

Ostomy wearers should be assured they can wear their ordinary clothing and that if the pouch is changed and emptied as necessary it will not be visible. If a woman wants, she can continue to wear control top panty hose, but an elastic girdle may need adapting with an opening to prevent pressure on the stoma and pouch.

An ostomy does not interfere with exercise, sport, work or sexual activity. There are specialized stomal caps and pouches intended for wear when swimming. A smaller sized pouch or even emptying the regular sized pouch, along with bathing suits of patterned fabric or boxer trunks for men, may help an ostomy patient feel more comfortable on the beach.

Bathing and showering is possible with or without the appliance in place. Soap and water will not injure a stoma, but bath oils and some soaps may leave a greasy film that can prevent the appliance from adhering. If a long soak in the bath tub is contemplated and the stoma will be below the water line, a cap can be used to prevent water from seeping into the stoma and the bowel. A wearer wishing to attach a night drainage system to their appliance will require a free standing holder or one that slides between the box spring and mattress.

When travelling, individuals with ostomies should always carry their supplies in their hand luggage. Manufacturers will provide travellers with addresses for supplies at their destination. A summary of problems and coping techniques is provided in Tables 10 and 11.

TABLE 10: Coping With Ostomy Problems

Problem	Symptom	Coping Technique
Leakage	Most often seen with urostomies and ileostomies	Proper fit, clean and change pouch, proper adhesive
Odor	Odor from waste material and from gas	Diet, clean appliance, change appliance. Chlorophyll copper complex and activated charcoal are the most common ingredients in commercial internal odor products. A vinegar rinse of the appliance is sometimes used. External deodorizers include zinc ricinoleate, chlorine, quaternary ammonium compounds and phosphoric acid. Most appliances now include odor control.
Gas	Some appliances have safety valves with charcoal filters—the gas is released and the charcoal absorbs odors	Diet, use an antacid, eat yogurt, eat slowly and chew food well, avoid drinking with a straw, avoid chewing gum, limit intake of gas producing foods, especially prior to social occasions
Bleeding	Foul odor, signs of pus	Check cleaning technique, if other symptoms appear or bleeding has ocurred for a prolonged period of time, seek medical attention
Infection	Chills, fever, fatigue, foul odor, pus, dark colored urine	Drink plenty of liquids to avoid urinary infections if urostomy, clean appliance properly, seek medical attention if symptoms do not abate
Constipation		Diet, increased bulk and fluid, exercise
Obstruction or food blockage	Cramping, abdominal pain, vomiting, stoma swelling, watery foul smelling waste material	Chew food properly, increase fluid intake, remove pouch if stoma is swollen, mild exercise such as walking
Fluid electrolyte problems:		
1. Fluid loss	Dry mouth, increased thirst, dry skin, decreased urine output, fatigue, stomach cramps, shortness of breath	Increase fluids (any kind), fluid intake should be 2 to 3 L daily
2. Sodium loss	Stomach cramps, loss of appetite, fatigue, cold sensation in arms and legs, feeling faint	Increase foods and fluids high in sodium, (e.g., *Gatorade,* broth, tomato juice, cottage cheese, potato chips)
3. Potassium loss	Muscle weakness, fatigue, shortness of breath, decreased sensation in arms and legs, bloating	Increase foods and fluids high in potassium, (e.g., *Gatorade*, bananas, orange juice, tomatoes, fish)
Hernias		Avoid heavy lifting or improper lifting, additional surgery may be needed
Abscesses or fistulae		Proper stoma care, surgery
Kidney stones	Ileostomy and urostomy have increased risk for kidney stones	Increased fluid intake, kidney stones will pass through an urostomy as they would through an intact urinary tract
Stricturing	A narrowing that most often occurs in urostomies	Surgery

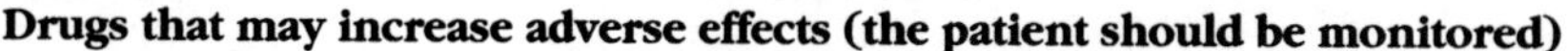

TABLE 11: Medication Concerns

Drugs with no additional adverse effects:	
Alcohol	
Salicylates	
Drugs that may increase adverse effects (the patient should be monitored)	
Antibiotics	Broad spectrum antibiotics may alter the normal flora of the intestinal tract resulting in diarrhea or fungal infections of the skin surrounding the stoma
Antimotility drugs	May cause constipation or diarrhea in colostomy and some ileostomy patients
Antidiarrheals	May cause constipation in colostomy patients
Antacids	Aluminum containing antacids can cause constipation in colostomy patients, calcium containing antacids can cause calcium stone formation in urostomy and ileostomy patients, magnesium containing antacids can cause diarrhea in ileostomy patients
Corticosteroids	Immunosuppression
Diuretics	May cause excess fluid loss and dehydration, fluid and electrolyte balances of ileostomy patients should be monitored
Laxatives	May result in perforation for colostomy patients, stool softeners are preferred for colostomy patients, enemas should be avoided by ileostomy and colostomy patients
Opiates	May cause constipation in colostomy patients
Salt substitutes	May produce hyponatremia in ileostomy patients
Stool softener	May result in diarrhea for ileostomy patients
Sulfa drugs	Crystallization in the kidney may be more prominent in patients having difficulty with fluid and electrolyte balance, urostomy patients are especially at risk, sulfa drugs should be accompanied with fluid intake
Drugs that may be ineffective because they are poorly absorbed	
Antibiotics	
Vitamins	Especially vitamin B_{12}
Drug formulations that may be problematic	
Enteric coated or timed release	Pass through the intestinal tract without being absorbed, liquids and chewable tablets are preferred
Drugs that discolor the feces	For example, iron (black); bismuth preparations (greenish-black); salicylates, especially ASA (pink to red or black); senna (yellow); antacids, aluminum containing (whitish or speckled)

HOME DIAGNOSTICS

The thermometer is an example of a home diagnostic device. It enables an individual at home to diagnose a possible health problem, e.g., a fever.

Home diagnostic devices are used for early diagnosis, to determine if a therapy is effective and to monitor a medical condition. Besides the thermometer, home diagnostic devices include blood and urine glucose tests and monitors, blood pressure monitors, pregnancy and ovulation tests, cholesterol tests and monitors, fecal occult blood tests, peak flow meters, ear examination kits, and throat examination kits. Thermometers are discussed in the *Pain and Fever Products* chapter.

Many medical devices require the user to observe color change or see a numerical display, and many require manual dexterity, e.g., the positioning of a blood pressure cuff. Displays with large, visible numbers, devices with easy to read colors and tests with simple steps are available and should be recommended for users with visual or manual dexterity limitations.

BLOOD PRESSURE MONITORS

Home blood pressure monitoring enables an individual to evaluate a new drug or treatment, to chart their course, which may act as motivation for compliance, and avoid unexplained elevations associated with visits to physicians' offices commonly known as "white coat" hypertension. Home blood pressure monitoring should never be considered self-diagnosis of hypertension. If blood pressure is elevated, medical advice should be sought.

Blood pressure is taken with a sphygmomanometer, Greek for "pulse, pressure meter." A sphygmomanometer has a cuff, stethoscope and meter connected to a column of mercury. Sometimes the stethoscope is attached to the cuff itself. The mercury-containing sphygmomanometer is the most accurate. It is important to use a properly fitted cuff for the size of the patient's arm.

The cuff becomes a tourniquet cutting off blood flow, then loosened by releasing air. To measure blood pressure, an individual listens with the stethoscope in the crook of the elbow for sounds, called Korotkoff sounds, in the brachial artery, the arm's main artery. Korotkoff sounds are rhythmic beatings as the blood flows through the artery to the lower arm. While the cuff is inflated there is no flow or no sounds, but once flow resumes the sounds resume.

The arm being tested should be at heart level when testing. The pressure in the mercury column is read when the first Korotkoff sound is heard; this represents the systolic pressure or the pressure the heart exerts as it pumps. As the cuff continues to deflate, the Korotkoff sounds become fainter, until they disappear. The pressure is measured at the point where the sounds disappear; this becomes the diastolic pressure or the pressure when the heart is at rest.

Aneroid blood pressure cuffs use the air pressure from the cuff to move a needle on a circular gauge instead of forcing mercury up a column. The same listening for Korotkoff sounds is required, although the stethoscope is sometimes attached directly to the cuff.

Although sphygmomanometers, both mercury and aneroid models, are available for home use, they do require coordination and experience. Usually the gauge is held in the left hand with the cuff on the left arm, if the individual is right handed. Problems arise when the cuff is not positioned properly and there is inexperience in recognizing Korotkoff sounds.

Electronic Models

Electronic models are ideal for home use because they require less coordination than the sphygmomanometers, and there is no listening for Korotkoff sounds. Electronic models measure pressure by analyzing changes in pressure of the cuff rather than detecting sounds by a stethoscope. The pressure in the inflated cuff changes as blood moves through expanding and contracting blood vessels.

Some models use a single microphone or sensor that must be positioned accurately over the brachial artery. Other models have cuffs that are fully pressure sensitive or oscillometric. Most have a liquid crystal diode display, which means reading the blood pressure numbers is easy. Pulse readings are often provided along with the blood pressure readings.

Accuracy can be a problem with electronic models. If the reading is consistently too high or too low, it may still be used to evaluate trends, but if the model reads too high one time and too low the next, the readings have no value. Once purchased, electronic models should be compared for accuracy against a sphygmomanometer, either mercury or aneroid, and the comparison should be done by a health care professional experienced in using the sphygmomanometer.

The proper technique for using blood pressure monitors is important and should be checked from time to time to ensure no bad habits have developed. The blood pressure reading should be taken under the same circumstances (e.g., same arm, same person) and at approximately the same time each day. Blood pressure changes with daily cycles and is typically the lowest during sleep. Public speaking can produce a 10 mm Hg rise in blood pressure; strenuous exercise a 60 to 70 mm Hg rise; sex up to 100 mm Hg rise for men and 80 mm Hg rise for women; and a competitive video game 20 mm Hg rise. Cigarettes, caffeine and strenuous exercise should be avoided for about an hour before the blood pressure measurement is taken.

It is recommended that 2 or 3 readings be taken at one time, resting several minutes between each reading. The reading can be compared and averaged. Keeping a log of the blood pressure readings will reflect what is normal for an individual and what effect various activities or medications have on the reading.

Finger Units

Finger units measure blood pressure from an artery in the index finger. Blood pressure measuring devices found in shopping malls employ finger units. These devices are not usually as accurate as either the electronic models or sphygmomanometers. One study showed fluctuations over a range of 22 mm Hg for the systolic reading, and 18 mm Hg for the diastolic reading.

People with impaired peripheral circulation are not able to obtain accurate reading from finger units. When measuring, the unit must be held exactly at heart level.

PREGNANCY TESTING AND OVULATION PREDICTION KITS

Ovulation occurs about mid cycle, that is day 14 of a 28-day cycle. It is triggered by a sudden release of luteinizing hormone (LH) from the pituitary gland known as the LH surge, which causes the mature follicle to rupture and release an ovum. The detection of the LH surge, which occurs about 24 to 36 hours prior to ovulation, is the basis of ovulation prediction kits.

If the ovum is fertilized and implanted in the endometrial wall, human chorionic gonadotropin (HCG) is produced by the placenta. HCG is detectable in the urine about 9 days after fertilization and implantation. At this time the woman will not have missed a period because it is not normally due for another 5 days. In healthy women, HCG is a specific marker for pregnancy, because it is only produced by the placenta.

HCG is a glycoprotein produced by the trophoblastic cells of the placenta and maintains the corpus luteum. It replaces LH. HCG can be detected in the serum as early as 6 to 8 days after fertilization, which is about the time of implantation. In the urine HCG reaches between 80 to 100 IU/L by the time of the expected period. Its highest concentration is between 9 a.m. and noon. It doubles in concentration about every 2 days to a maximum in 60 to 70 days, then it decreases to a lower level for the rest of the pregnancy. The half life of HCG is about 5.6 hours, and following termination of the pregnancy it returns to a baseline within 10 days. The detection of urine HCG is the basis of home pregnancy testing kits.

In choosing ovulation prediction kits and pregnancy testing kits, a woman should pay attention to the ease of the test (fewer steps are easier), speed in obtaining results, the inclusion of a control in the test, the accuracy of the test, ease of interpretation of results and cost.

Pregnancy Testing Kits

Prior to the advent of a biological assay for HCG, pregnancy tests were done by injecting a woman's urine into a female rat. After 5 days the rat was sacrificed. HCG causes swelling of the corpus luteum and the uterus; if the rat's uterus was heavy the woman was most likely pregnant.

In the 1960's immunoassay technology meant that an antibody could be synthesized that would combine with HCG to produce a precipitant or to change a colored substrate. There are three generations of pregnancy testing kits that reflect the improvement in technology.

FIRST GENERATION

First generation pregnancy testing kits used polyclonal antibodies that recognized multiple binding sites on HCG. Unfortunately these antibodies also reacted with other substances such as LH and follicle stimulating hormone (FSH). They required care in looking for the characteristic ring at the bottom of a test tube.

Because of their susceptibility to technical errors, they are no longer marketed.

SECOND GENERATION

Second generation pregnancy testing kits employ monoclonal antibody technology. Most pregnancy testing kits are second and third generation.

The anti-HCG antibody is bound to a solid surface such as a stick, bead, or filter paper. If HCG is present in the urine, it forms a complex with the antibody to produce a change in color of a chromogen reactive enzyme. The HCG actually becomes sandwiched between two antibodies, one attached to the test surface and the other attached to the color producing enzyme.

Second generation tests can detect HCG as early as the first day of a missed menstrual period and take a shorter time, 1 to 30 minutes, to perform. And, because these tests employ monoclonal technology, they are more specific for HCG.

THIRD GENERATION

The technology is even more refined in third generation pregnancy testing kits. An antibeta subunit, HCG monoclonal antibody, is linked to a color substrate. If present, HCG in the urine binds to this antibody, and the resulting complex binds to a second monoclonal antibody bound to a solid

COUNSELLING TIPS

Pregnancy Testing Kits

Pregnancy testing kits are usually sealed to prevent tampering so the consumer sees only the information on the outside of the package. More information about the various products may be required to make a decision on a suitable kit. These hints may help educate the consumer:

- Be more informative. Sit down and go over the directions with the consumer, making sure they know the directions. Know what color a positive result is and what color a negative result is. If the consumer does not have time to discuss the testing kit, make sure they know there are full instructions in the package and usually a toll-free number for problems.
- Be able to compare the various tests based on accuracy, efficiency, cost and whether they include a control or not.
- Provide information on which kits have the fewest steps to get the quickest result. The testing kits that use the stick technology are the easiest to use.
- Know how soon after a missed period a consumer can use a pregnancy testing kit. Women with irregular periods may have difficulty identifying the missed period day.
- Know if the consumer can use the test at any time of day and whether it has to be the first morning urine. Third generation technology means that pregnancy testing kits can be used at any time during the day as long as there is a large enough volume of urine with a sufficient concentration of HCG.
- Medications and alcohol do not affect test results with third generation technology. The hormone HCG can affect results, but if present, it is usually the result of a medical condition.
- Although the accuracy of third generation tests is high, if the client has a negative test and does not start her period or has a positive test and does start her period, she should seek medical attention.
- Place the testing kits in a more private area; next to the feminine care products and/or condoms may be a high traffic area. The consumer needs time and privacy to compare and examine the various kits available.
- Make sure that out of date kits are not available. Pregnancy testing kits contain test solution that does expire and, if expired, can give erroneous results.
- Encourage the consumer to perform the test in a well lit room, and if the client has trouble seeing or seeing specific colors, encourage them to have someone else available to read the results.

surface. The second monoclonal antibody is the alpha subunit and elicits the color change. Ease of use and accuracy are advantages of the third generation tests.

False positive and false negative results are possible regardless of which generation of test is used. Human error is most often the cause; however, the easier a test is to use, the less likely are human errors.

Several second generation and most third generation tests have controls built into them, to eliminate this human error. If the control test does not work, the test is classified as "no result". Examples of human errors leading to false results include: soap residue in the urine sample; warm or hot water rinses of the test surface; the use of wax paper cup to collect the urine sample; and exposure of the test reagents to extremes of heat or cold (freezing or above 30°C). With the urine stream tests, many of these sources of error have been eliminated.

Testing too early or too late—after the 60 to 70 days—can lead to false results, as can testing after a missed or incomplete abortion. Ectopic production of HCG by nontrophoblastic tumors will produce a false positive test result. Any exogenous HCG may produce a positive test result, e.g., HCG given for infertility problems. Some postmenopausal women normally have low levels of circulating HCG, which has the potential to produce a positive test result, but most tests are not sufficiently sensitive to detect these low levels in the urine. The hormone LH also has the potential to cross react with the test; however, most tests have compensated for this.

Drugs have the potential to interfere with the earlier generations of pregnancy tests, as do blood or protein in the urine and cloudy, pink, red, or strong urine odor. Third generation technology has virtually eliminated these concerns; however, corticosteroids in large doses can sometimes interfere with test results.

Pregnancy testing kits afford early detection in privacy, and early detection of pregnancy enables avoidance of harmful chemicals, x-rays, drugs, e.g., retinoic acid analogs, misoprostol, and elective surgery. Prenatal care can begin earlier. A positive result should be the impetus for a woman to seek medical care; a negative result with symptoms suggestive of pregnancy should also be confirmed. The tests are easy to use, readily available and about 96 to 99% accurate. They offer speed, convenience, confidentiality, and are economical.

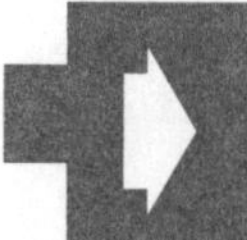

COUNSELLING TIPS

Ovulation Prediction Kits

- Home diagnostic kits give an approximate time of ovulation and an indication of when a woman may be more fertile. They do not indicate when a woman is not fertile and cannot be used as a method of contraception.
- Each ovulation prediction kit has a chart or graph that the client can compare to her cycle to choose the correct day to start the test.

Ovulation Prediction Kits

Ovulation prediction tests identify the LH surge, meaning a woman will know when she is most likely to ovulate and can plan her sexual activity to increase the chances of conception.

Monoclonal antibodies are used. One antibody is bound to a test surface and another to an enzyme. If LH is present, it becomes sandwiched between the two antibodies and produces a color change on the test surface. With no LH in the urine, the second antibody bound to the enzyme is washed away, and no color change occurs. The color intensity depends on the amount of LH present.

Most ovulation tests are mixtures of polyclonal and monoclonal antibodies. The polyclonal antibodies may bind with either the alpha or beta subunit of LH or even the entire molecule. The monoclonal antibodies are usually specific for the beta subunit, which is a more accurate identifier of LH.

More recently, tests are beta subunit specific antibodies bound to colored latex particles. The second monoclonal antibody is bound to the test surface. With LH, the two are sandwiched together producing a color change on the test surface. Without LH, the antibody bound to the colored latex particle is washed away.

Usually test kits contain 5 tests that require 3 to 60 minutes. Using the average length of her cycle, a woman uses a chart to determine the day of her cycle she should begin testing. Some test results are compared to a base line color chart, some to the previous test, and others to a control window. These tests are considered to be up to 98.3% accurate if performed properly.

Urine is collected at the same time each day, and while some tests are to be done on the first urine in the morning, others can be performed anytime during the day, as long as there is a sufficient volume to ensure an effective concentration of LH. As with pregnancy tests, human error accounts for the majority of false readings. The inclusion of test controls and the comparison of the results to the previous days' results reduce the chances of false results.

CHOLESTEROL HOME TESTS

Elevated cholesterol levels increase the risk for coronary heart disease. Screening of high risk individuals and therapy with diet or medication to lower cholesterol levels reduces mortality and morbidity.

Cholesterol home tests enable screening. These tests use an optical reader to determine total cholesterol in a blood sample. A drop of blood is placed on a test strip. Most test strips do not require wiping but use a capillary action to move the blood sample to the optical reader.

The test strip is impregnated with a reagent that reacts with cholesterol in the blood sample to produce a color change. The optical reader uses light absorption to determine the degree of color change, and thus the cholesterol content of the sample. The results are expressed digitally in millimoles (mmol) on a liquid crystal diode display.

The cholesterol blood test results take 3 to 15 minutes and represent total cholesterol. The results are considered to be 95% or greater in accuracy. A record is usually kept to observe trends in an individual's cholesterol levels over time and under various conditions.

Cholesterol home tests do not distinguish between low density lipoproteins (LDLs), high density lipoproteins (HDLs) and triglycerides. To obtain a breakdown of the cholesterol fractions, a laboratory procedure is required. The technology is being improved, however, so that eventually a fractioning of the various components may be possible, and even perhaps a noninvasive test, that is, a bloodless test.

There are, as well, pads or strips that will test for cholesterol levels. A drop of blood is placed on the test area, which changes color. The color is compared to a chart that indicates the range the cholesterol level is in. These tests are not very accurate, in that many factors, from touching the strip to air humidity, can alter the results.

FECAL OCCULT BLOOD HOME TESTS

(Extracted from: Heschuk SA. Diagnostic aids. In: Carruthers-Czyzewski P, ed. Self-Medication Reference for Health Professionals. 4th ed. Ottawa: Canadian Pharmaceutical Association, 1992.)

Detection of occult (hidden) blood in the stool is useful in detecting disease of the gastrointestinal tract. Ingestion of certain foods or drugs (salicylates, steroids, indomethacin, iron, colchicine and reserpine) is associated with increased gastrointestinal blood loss. Pathologic conditions such as bleeding gums, peptic ulcers, dysentery, ulcerative colitis, hemorrhoids, and fissures or colorectal cancer can cause occult blood in the feces. Cancerous lesions within the colon may bleed even before they are well developed; stool testing for occult blood may help provide early diagnosis. Colorectal cancer is one of the most prevalent cancers in the western world; the mortality rate is as high as 60% (Table 12).

A dark red to black tarry appearance in the stool indicates a loss of 0.5 to 0.75 mL of blood from the upper gastrointestinal tract. Chemical testing is required to prevent confusing bloody stool with coloring from diet or drugs.

In the 1960s, the guaiac test for occult blood in the stool was introduced. A positive reaction for hemoglobin is a result of its pseudoperoxidase activity. Guaiac undergoes phenolic oxidation in the presence of hemoglobin in the stool and hydrogen peroxide in the test reagent, turning the stool sample blue.

For tests using the guaiac reaction, false positive results can be caused by several substances (Table 13). A negative test for occult blood does not necessarily rule out cancer. Some cancerous lesions do not bleed; others bleed infrequently. Roughage encourages early, small cancerous lesions to bleed and increases the accuracy of the test. Since lesions bleed intermittently, more than one stool specimen must be tested. Testing of 3 consecutive stools is recommended. If the test is intended to detect blood from colorectal cancer, the individual should not begin the procedure if actively bleeding from a known source, e.g., nosebleed, hemorrhoids, rectal fissures, diarrhea, menstruation, diverticulitis, gastrointestinal ulcers or proctitis.

A person who obtains a positive result for a fecal occult blood test is advised to consult a physician for proper diagnosis.

TABLE 12: Risk Factors for Colorectal Cancer

Risk Factors
Age 40 or over
Ulcerative colitis (lasting more than 7 years)
Prior adenoma of colon
Family history of polyposis syndrome
Female genital cancer
Prior cured colorectal cancer

Source: Gossell TA. Fecal occult blood testing products. US Pharmacist 1986;11(4):40–51.

TABLE 13: Occult Fecal Blood Test Interference

False Positive	False Negative
Foods with peroxidase activity: turnips, horseradish, parsnips, cauliflower, broccoli, cantaloupe, artichokes, mushrooms (for tests using guaiac reaction)	Failure to ingest high residue diet
Red meat or rare meat	Ascorbic acid (>250 mg daily)
Drugs: iron, salicylates, NSAIDs, steroids, reserpine and colchicine	Lesions not bleeding at time of test
Pathological: bleeding gums, nosebleed, peptic ulcers, dysentery, ulcerative colitis, hemorrhoids, fissures, diverticulitis or proctitis	Noncompliance with test procedure
Menstruation	Test kit outdated or deteriorated
Toilet bowl cleaners (for tests developed in toilet bowl)	

Source: Home Health Care. Winnipeg: Canadian Council on Continuing Education in Pharmacy, 1988;VIII(4).

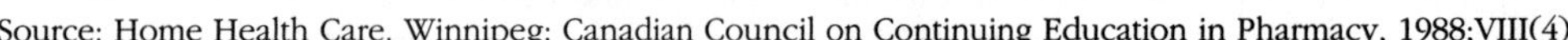

Until the cause for colorectal cancer is discovered, early detection and treatment probably offer the best hope for improving the outcome of this disease. Health Canada's Task Force on the Periodic Health Examination has recommended periodic testing of all Canadians over the age of 45 years. This recommendation is under review. Currently, insufficient data exist to indicate that screening for colorectal cancer by fecal occult blood testing reduces mortality from the disease. Controlled clinical trials are now underway, but more time is needed for assessment of survival benefit, risk possibilities and economic feasibility. These trials involve initial screening by fecal occult blood testing and the study of positive occult blood reactions by barium enema, endoscopy or both.

The success of a screening program depends largely on the acceptability of the test to the patients. The collection and handling of a stool sample may inhibit compliance. Newer tests, e.g., *Coloscreen Self-Test*, do not require collection of a stool sample. A test pad is simply dropped into the toilet after a stool has been passed and if there is occult blood present an indicator patch will change color. In 1990, Pye et al compared the *Coloscreen Self-Test* with a conventional slide test (*Haemoccult*). Compliance was higher with the test that did not require collection of a stool sample, but it was much less sensitive in detecting colonic and rectal cancers. As a result, Pye et al did not recommend *Coloscreen Self-Test* as suitable for screening asymptomatic patients. Uchida et al have developed a new monoclonal antibody test for fecal occult blood utilizing enzyme-linked immunosorbent (ELISA) of human hemoglobin with much greater specificity for human hemoglobin than previous tests. If and when these tests become available to the home care market, they should improve the rate of detection of colon cancer and eliminate the necessity for dietary and therapeutic restrictions.

PEAK FLOW METERS

Peak flow meters help prevent and predict exacerbations in chronic obstructive pulmonary problems such as asthma. They enable home monitoring of a patient's lung function and a titration of their medication in response to their lung function.

Peak flow meters measure the peak expiratory flow (PEF) or the amount of air that can be forced out of the lungs after the lungs are fully inflated. It is a mouthpiece with a gauge, an indicator and scale. There are usually two sizes to accommodate children and adults.

The individual inhales as deeply as possible, places the meter in their mouth, and blows out as hard and fast as possible. The final position of the indicator on the scale is the PEF reflecting litres per minute. Three tests are done with the highest of the three being the reading that is recorded. Children as young as 4 are able to do this test.

Daily measurements at 12-hour intervals are recommended, e.g., 7 a.m. and 7 p.m. A log or graph is kept (many meters come with a graph). If inhaled steroids or beta agonists are used either before or after the test, a note is made.

It is the accumulated data that is important. There are charts for adults and children based on height, weight and sex, to which the test results can be compared. A better approach is comparison with the individual's personal best.

A zoning system makes the test reading relevant for the patient. One frequently used is based on traffic lights. A result in the green zone correlates to 80 to 100% of the individual's personal best; yellow zone to 50 to 80%; and red zone below 50%. In the yellow zone, medication may have to be re-evaluated, and in the red zone a bronchodilator is immediately required. If readings appear in the red zone twice in 48 hours, medical attention should be sought.

Problems that can cause false readings include: the wrong size of mouthpiece; the indicator not at the bottom of the scale before the test is begun; fingers blocking some part of the mouthpiece opening; and atmospheric pressure effects.

EAR AND THROAT EXAMINATION KITS

Earaches and sore throats account for approximately one-quarter of walk-in clinic visits. Earaches may be a symptom of childhood otitis media or even earwax impaction, and sore throats are a concern if a "strep" infection is suspected, especially for individuals with rheumatic fever.

Early detection of ear and throat problems enables early and appropriate treatment. *Dr. Dedo's Family Throat Examination and Ear Examination Kits* enable such early detection. Both are home versions of throat and ear lights used by health care professionals, and both come with fully illustrated guide books.

DIABETES HOME TESTS

Monitoring a diabetic's glucose levels can increase compliance, give them better control of their condition and promote referral for medical attention when appropriate. Long-term complications such as vision loss can be reduced. Both urine and blood testing are possible, but blood testing is more accurate. Visual testing and monitoring with a meter are options in blood glucose testing; the latter is less influenced by human error.

Urine glucose testing measures the percentage of glucose present in the urine. The volume of the test sample, the concentration of the urine, diet and drugs, e.g., high doses of vitamin C, can all affect the results.

Blood glucose testing is a direct sampling of the blood glucose and enables the tailoring of insulin, diet and/or medication to the individual. The diabetic can participate in the control of the condition and may become more knowledgeable. Visual blood glucose tests compare the test color to a chart of colors; blood glucose monitors display the reading numerically.

Two types of technology are used in blood glucose monitors. Reflectance or optical meters measure the amount of color, that is, the light that is reflected from the test strip. A drop of blood is applied to the reagent pad on the strip; the blood glucose reacts with enzymes and sensitive dyes. The color change is quantified by the meter: the darker the color change, the higher the glucose concentration. Dirt and blood on the optical window can cause false readings, and these meters must be cleaned regularly.

Electrochemical or amperometric meters measure the amount of energy generated by a chemical reaction that occurs with an application of a drop of blood. The blood glucose reacts with enzymes and produces an electrical current. The current is directly proportional to the glucose concentration. Dirt and blood do not usually affect the result in these meters.

Human error accounts for the majority of false readings: failure to calibrate the meter when using a new box of test strips, failure to clean the optical window, failure to change batteries, use of too much blood, use of too little blood, use of the wrong strips. Blood glucose meters usually will not provide a result if there are errors. An error message will be displayed, and some meters will indicate the type of error. Some test strips are designed so that a capillary action moves the blood to the test site, eliminating errors involving the size of the blood sample.

Proper meter usage includes understanding the test procedure, sampling technique and reading the test results. Those using blood glucose meters must be familiar with maintenance, systems check procedure and battery replacement. A record should be maintained to observe trends.

PATIENT ASSESSMENT QUESTIONS

?

***Q** Have you been diagnosed with hypertension? Do you take medication to control hypertension?*

A client with hypertension may be using a blood pressure monitor to observe trends in their blood pressure or to monitor the effects of medication; however, it must be stressed that a normal reading does not mean they are cured.

***Q** Will your lifestyle facilitate using a blood pressure monitor?*

Blood pressure should be taken at about the same time each day and under the same conditions. The readings should be taken regularly to observe trends and the machine checked for accuracy routinely.

***Q** Do you have regular periods?*

A client who does not have regular periods may have difficulty determining the day of her missed period and could test too early or too late with pregnancy testing kits.

***Q** Do you have to perform the pregnancy test first thing in the morning?*

With third generation technology, the client can usually test anytime during the day as long as there is sufficient volume of urine with a sufficient concentration of HCG. The package directions will spell out the ideal timing.

***Q** Have you been diagnosed with elevated cholesterol? Are you taking medication or using a diet to control cholesterol levels?*

Cholesterol home tests do not differentiate among the types of cholesterol, and an elevated reading may not be an accurate depiction of the client's lipid profile.

***Q** Do you have a condition or take any medications that may interfere with a fecal occult blood test?*

Any condition or drug that causes occult blood loss may produce a false positive result.

***Q** Which system of measurement do you use for your peak flow meter?*

There are several systems of measurement, e.g., red, green and yellow lights or zones, and the client should use one system consistently.

***Q** Do you have a condition or potential for a condition that requires an ear or throat examination kit?*

Ear and throat examination kits facilitate early detection of conditions such as otitis media, but the client should be warned that the kits do not replace and should not delay medical attention.

***Q** Have you been diagnosed with diabetes? Are you taking medication or using diet to control it?*

Home monitoring ensures better control of the condition but must be done routinely and accurately. Comparing the results with those of a health care professional or a diabetes clinic will provide the client with an indication of their condition's status and alert them to developing trends.

***Q** Do you use urine or blood testing? If blood testing, is it performed visually or by a monitor?*

The procedure for urine and blood testing differs and varies according to product. The correct strip must be used for each monitor.

RESPIRATORY AIDS

HUMIDIFIERS AND VAPORIZERS

Vaporizers use heat to disperse moisture in the air and, because they are hot, increase the temperature of the space they are used in and can cause burns. Humidifiers require no heat. They increase humidity by physically dispersing water droplets in the air.

Distilled water prevents some mineral build-up in humidifiers, but vaporizers require some degree of mineral in the water to boil and disperse water vapor. Regular cleaning is essential for both to prevent infection and allergic reactions. Medication should not be added to humidifiers and only placed in a medication cup (not the water reservoir) of a vaporizer.

Ambulatory respiratory and hospice patients may require oxygen therapy and with available technology, e.g., face mask, nasal cannula, oxygen concentrators, tracheal or endotracheal tube, this therapy is more portable. Oxygenated water and ozone therapy are touted as beneficial. Both, however, are expensive with no supporting evidence of effectiveness.

HOME INTRAVENOUS PROGRAMS

Patients with chronic illness and serious infections may require long hospitalizations away from family, friends and work; however, they may be well enough to function daily if they have the required medication. Home intravenous programs have grown to meet this need.

Home intravenous programs are the fastest growing segment of the home health care market. Several factors are responsible: more reliable means, e.g., better catheters, home infusion pumps; increased patient awareness and involvement; cost savings; and home health support from health care professionals.

The home intravenous business was worth $2.6 billion in 1990 in the United States, and every year it is estimated that it grows by about one-third. Sixty per cent of home intravenous programs involve antibiotics, nutrition, or chemotherapy. Other drugs, hydration and fluid replacement account for the balance. Included in home intravenous programs are analgesic pumps.

To succeed with a home intravenous program, a patient and their family must feel comfortable with the technology and technique required. There must be cognitive function with no psychosis or drug addiction problems (Table 14).

Most home intravenous users have a catheter at one site to which tubing and a prepared intravenous drug are attached. The drug infusion takes place over a period of time. The catheter is usually a long term in-dwelling intravenous catheter, e.g., Broviac, Hickman, Groshong. They require a heparin lock and are usually rotated to retain venous patency.

Subcutaneous infusion pumps are implanted devices used to infuse medication, blood products, fluids or nutrition. They are completely under the skin and appear as a raised area. There is a port with a self-sealing silicone rubber septum through which a Huber needle is inserted. The medication enters the body through tubing attached to the Huber needle.

Analgesic pumps are portable external pumps that administer analgesics through tubing into a small needle placed in the subcutaneous skin. The pump controls the flow of medication and is usually programmed to provide a set dose per time period. The pump can also be used manually with the patient giving themselves a dose of analgesic, but then the pump is programmed to provide no more than a maximum quantity per time period. The pump is hung outside the tub when showering or bathing, and placed under the pillow or hung on a hook when sleeping. Humidity, heat, and freezing should be avoided.

TABLE 14: Criteria for Home Intravenous Programs

Positive	Negative
Medical stability	Substance abuse
Manageable infection/disease	Impaired vision
Compliance	Home without running water, electricity, refrigeration
Educability	
Venous access	

TABLE 15: Examples of Conditions Treated in Home Intravenous Programs

Antibiotics	Infective endocarditis, septic arthritis, cystic fibrosis, osteomyelitis
Chemotherapy	Breast cancer, Hodgkin's disease, leukemia, testicular cancer
Nutrition	Short bowel syndrome, inflammatory bowel disease, chronic intractable diarrhea, chronic idiopathic intestinal obstruction syndrome
Analgesia	Secondary to cancer

PATIENT ASSESSMENT QUESTIONS

Q *Do you have a condition that can be controlled by a home IV program?*

Clients with chronic illness or serious infections may be well enough to function but require a medication that can only be given intravenously. Client comfort and cost savings are the benefits.

Q *Do you have the qualities that make a desirable candidate for a home IV program?*

Clients who are medically stable, compliant, motivated, educable, and who have accessible veins, good vision and a treatable condition are ideal candidates. The client's home should have refrigeration and running water.

Nutrition may be either enteral or parenteral. Enteral nutrition is directly infused into the intestine where it is absorbed into the circulation. Parenteral nutrition bypasses the gastrointestinal tract completely and is infused into the circulation. With total parenteral nutrition (TPN) there may be a loss of gastrointestinal function.

Phlebitis, infiltration and infection at the catheter site are the most common problems. Air embolus, dislodged catheters, migrating ports, catheter leaks, and occlusion can also occur. The prepared intravenous solutions must be stored carefully, most often in the refrigerator, and sometimes even in the freezer. Pharmacies venturing into home intravenous programs will require a sterile working environment and a laminar flow hood for preparation of solutions.

For examples of conditions treated in home intravenous programs see Table 15.

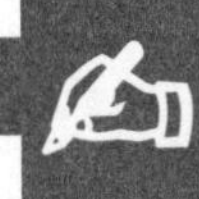

Resource List

The Amyotrophic Lateral Sclerosis Society
Suite B101
90 Adelaide St. East
Toronto, ON M5C 2R4

The Arthritis Society
Suite 901
250 Bloor St. East
Toronto, ON M4W 3P2

The Canadian Head Injury Coalition
29 Pearce Ave.
Winnipeg, MN R2V 2K3

Canadian Paraplegic Association Inc.
Suite 320
1101 Prince of Wales Dr.
Ottawa, ON K2C 3W7

Canadian Rehabilitation Council for the Disabled
Suite 801
45 Shephard Ave. East
Toronto, ON M2N 5W9

The Canadian Standards Association (CSA)
178 Rexdale Blvd.
Rexdale, ON M9W 1R3
Tel: (416) 747-4000

The Multiple Sclerosis Society of Canada
1000 - 250 Bloor St. East
Toronto, ON M4W 3P9

Victorian Order of Nurses (VON) Canada
5 Blackburn Ave.
Ottawa, ON K1N 8A2

Incontinence

The Simon Foundation of Canada
P.O. Box 264, Station E
Toronto, ON M6H 4E2
Tel: 1-800-265-9575

Ostomy

The Canadian Association for Enterostomal Therapy
311 - 167 Lombard Ave.
Winnipeg, MN R3B 0T6

The Canadian Cancer Society
200 - 10 Alcorn Ave.
Toronto, ON M4V 3B1
or the local branch

Crohn's and Colitis Foundation of Canada
Suite 301
21 St. Clair Ave. East
Toronto, ON M4T 1L9
Tel: 1-800-387-1479

The International Association for Enterostomal Therapy Inc.
P.O. Box 254
New Bedford
Pennsylvania, USA 161400

The International Ostomy Association
E701-500 Eau Claire Ave. S.W.
Calgary, AB T2P 3R8

United Ostomy Association
5 Hamilton Ave.
Hamilton, ON L8V 2S3

RECOMMENDED READING

Aids for Daily Living

Finlayson M, Havixbeck K. A post-discharge study on the use of assistive devices. Can J Occup Ther 1992;59(4):201-07.

Pedretti MS, Zoltan B. Occupational therapy practice skills for physical dysfunction. 3rd ed. Toronto: CV Mosby Company, 1990.

Trombly CA, ed. Occupational therapy for physical dysfunction. 3rd ed. Baltimore: Williams & Wilkins, 1987.

Incontinence

Horner ES. Urinary incontinence. US Pharmacist 1993;18(4):65-80.

Mandelstam D. Incontinence and its Management. Dover: Croom Helm, 1986.

Urinary incontinence in adults: Clinical practice guideline. Rockville, MD: Agency for Health Care Policy and Research, 1992. AHCPR 92-0038.

Ostomy

Brandt LJ, Steiner-Grossman P, eds. Treating IBD. New York: Raven Press, 1989.

Broadwell DC, Jackson BS. Principles of Ostomy Care. St Louis: CV Mosby Company, 1982.

Hampton BG, Bryant RA. Ostomies and continent diversions. Nursing Management 1992.

Phillips RH. Coping with an ostomy. Wayne: Avery Publishing Group Inc., 1986.

Home Diagnostics

Clark NM. Asthma self-management education. Chest 1989;95(5):1110-13.

Evans CE, Logan AG. The Canadian consensus on hypertension management. Montreal: Canadian Hypertension Society, 1990:1-12.

Fletcher M. Electronic blood pressure monitors. Canadian Consumer 1987;17(2):21-24.

Hunter KA, Bryant BG. Educating parents and children about asthma. US Pharmacist 1993; 18(11):84-96.

Home Intravenous Programs

Anon. Five therapies account for 60% of home infusion. US Pharmacist 1993;18(4):16.

17

MEN'S HEALTH CARE PRODUCTS

DENIS BÉLANGER

CONTENTS

Jock Itch 411
Etiology
Signs and Symptoms
Treatment

Contraception 416
Types of Condoms
Contraceptive Effectiveness
Condom Failure
Allergic Reactions
Advances in Male Contraception

Premature Ejaculation 419
Assessment
Treatment

Pharmaceutical Agents 421

Recommended Reading 423

JOCK ITCH

Jock itch, also known as tinea cruris or ringworm of the groin, is frequently found in obese men in the summertime. Tinea pedis is often present at the same time. While perspiration that occurs with exercise is probably the most common factor, heat, friction and maceration may also predispose to this infection.

ETIOLOGY

The dermatophytes *Trichophyton rubrum (T. rubrum)* and *Epidermophyton floccosum (E. floccosum)* are molds that can invade the stratum corneum of the skin or other keratinized tissues derived from epidermides such as hair and nails. They may cause infections at most skin sites, although the feet, groin, scalp, and nails are most commonly affected. Dermatophytes produce keratinases that allow them to penetrate keratin. They also produce elastase, which has been proposed as a factor in the development of inflammatory responses.

T. rubrum is the most common cause of tinea cruris in temperate climates. Once rare in the eastern hemisphere, the infection has spread rapidly during the past 40 years, largely through contact with infected desquamated skin scales. This usually occurs in bathing areas or shower rooms where large numbers of individuals share common facilities (e.g., athletic centres, military camps, factories). Transfer is through arthrospores, vegetative cells with thickened cell walls shed from the primary host with skin scales. These dermatophyte arthrospores can survive for considerable periods outside the host; direct contact between the infected individual and another is not necessary for transmission. The transfer itself is poorly understood, but skin invasion appears to follow adherence of fungal cells to keratinocytes.

SIGNS AND SYMPTOMS

The infection starts with scaling and irritation of the groin. The rash usually involves the anterior aspects of the thighs. The leading edge extending into the thighs is prominent and may contain follicular papules and pustules. The infection may also spread to the anal cleft. The rash is symmetrical and often has a butterfly appearance with clearly defined, raised borders. There is a tendency for central clearing, and the scrotum is seldom involved. Tinea cruris may also affect women, particularly in

TABLE 1: Differential Diagnosis of Tinea Cruris

Condition	Appearance of Rash	Diagnostic Tests
Tinea Cruris	Usually involves anterior aspect of the thighs Leading edge if prominent and may contain follicular papules and pustules Infection may spread to anal cleft Rash is symmetrical, has raised borders, butterfly appearance Often find central clearing Scrotum is seldom involved	Potassium hydroxide test[a] is positive
Candidiasis	Bright, intensely erythematous eruption with poorly defined borders Appearance of satellite papules and pustules Scrotum is often affected	Potassium hydroxide test is positive
Intertrigo	Not as erythematous as candidiasis Not as sharply demarcated as tinea cruris	Potassium hydroxide test is negative
Erythrasma	Velvety appearance with fine scales Leading edge is less prominent than in tinea cruris	
Psoriasis	Vivid red and uniformly scaling rash Usually at least 1 other site with typical psoriatic plaques Erythematous, sharply circumscribed, covered by loosely adherent silvery scales	Fluoresces coral-pink under Wood's light

[a]The potassium hydroxide test is used to confirm the presence of fungal infection.

the tropics, where the infection is often less well delineated and spreads in a band around the waist area.

People complaining of jock itch may present with symptoms of pruritus, which may be intense, and discomfort due to the inflamed intertriginous tissues rubbing together. Many eruptions, however, may be asymptomatic.

Other causes of groin rash include candidiasis, intertrigo, psoriasis, seborrheic dermatitis, and erythrasma, all of which can be misdiagnosed as tinea cruris. A guide to differential diagnosis is provided in Table 1.

TREATMENT

Nonpharmacological Treatment

Advise patients with tinea cruris to keep the affected area as dry as possible by thorough drying and applying fragrance-free talcum powder after showering or bathing. Also advise the individual to wear loose fitting undergarments.

Patients can be reinfected or infect others through dermal shedding. Strict personal hygiene is necessary during active infections. All skin in the vicinity of the lesion should be treated. The infected individual should use a personal washcloth, towel and grooming aids. Clothing, bedding and personal items should be carefully laundered in hot water or dry cleaned.

Pharmacological Treatment

The ideal drug for treating jock itch should have several properties:

- a broad spectrum of action against all dermatophytes;
- the ability to penetrate the keratin layer to effectively reach the dermatophytes;

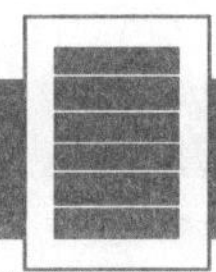

TABLE 2: Topical Nonprescription Antifungal Drug Products Not Generally Recognized as Safe and Effective

Alcloxa	Nystatin
Alum, potassium	Oxyquinolines (benzoxiquine, oxyquinoline, oxyquinoline sulfate)
Aluminum sulfate	Parabens (methylparaben, propylparaben)
Amyltricresols, secondary	Phenolates (phenol, phenolate sodium)
Basic fuchsin	Phenyl salicylate
Benzethonium chloride	Propionic acid
Benzoic acid	Resorcinol
Borates (boric acid, sodium borate)	Salicylic acid
Camphor	Sodium propionate
Candicidin	Sulfur
Caprylates (sodium caprylate, zinc caprylate)	Tannic acid
Chlorothymol	Thymol
Coal tar	Tolindate
Dichlorophen	Triacetin
Menthol	Zinc propionate

Reprinted from: Federal Register 1992, 57:38568.

- fungicidal, rather than fungistatic activity;
- safety when used according to instructions.

The nonprescription topical antifungal products that come close to meeting these criteria have one of the following agents: clioquinol, clotrimazole, miconazole nitrate, tolnaftate, and undecylenic acid and its salts. All have been shown effective in eradicating *T. rubrum* and *E. floccosum*, although studies demonstrate mycological cure rates ranging from 40 to 96%. Clotrimazole, miconazole and tolnaftate appear to have the higher cure rates.

A number of other agents have been shown safe, but their effectiveness remains to be proven (Table 2).

Studies of clotrimazole 1% cream or solution and miconazole 2% cream used twice daily for 2 to 6 weeks have shown mycological cure rates ranging from 85 to 96%, with the cream formulation producing slightly better results. Tolnaftate and undecylenic acid and its salts have had cure rates reported similar to and less than those achieved with clotrimazole. The U.S. Food and Drug Administration (FDA), in its review of nonprescription medicines, found cure rates for undecylenic acid and its salts to be only about 50%.

Improvement rates of 68% and cure rates of 45% have been reported in patients treated with a flumethasone pivalate/clioquinol cream twice daily for 28 days. No adverse reactions were reported.

Regardless of what agent is used, it may require several days of treatment to experience symptomatic relief and 2 to 4 weeks or longer to cure the infection. During this period, the medication must be used exactly as directed. Application should continue for several days to 2 weeks after all signs and symptoms have subsided.

Nonprescription antifungal products are safe when used correctly. Prolonged use on a macerated groin can lead to absorption and possible adverse effects. An individual with a chronic disease (such as diabetes) should be referred to a physician.

An antifungal product may provide symptomatic relief of infection without actually eradicating the dermatophytes. If the disorder persists, even though symptoms are lessened, an alternate product may be indicated. If symptoms are not relieved within several weeks of therapy, patients should be referred to a physician. Treatment failure may be due to bacterial infection or more serious pathology. Excessive oozing of vesicular eruptions or foul odor suggest a bacterial infection.

TABLE 3: Selecting a Suitable Dosage Form for Tinea Cruris

Vehicle	Advantages	Disadvantages
Solutions	Usually the most effective way to deliver antifungal drugs to their site of action	May not be as suitable for jock itch because of poor substantivity at the site
Ointments and creams	Hold the active ingredient at the site longer Preferred for chronic treatment Ointments adhere well to dry skin	Ointments may not cling as well to moist, oozing or sweating skin Ointments should not be used on macerated or fissured areas because they are occlusive
Powders	Not efficient for delivery of high concentrations of drug	Absorbent action may be beneficial because dermatophytes thrive poorly in a dry environment
Aerosols	Evaporate quickly, leaving the drug in contact with the skin which is then solubilized by skin moisture Evaporation also imparts antipruritic action to help relieve itching	

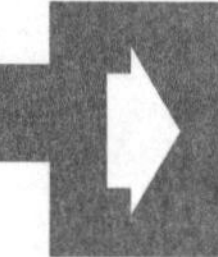

ADVICE FOR THE PATIENT

Jock Itch

- Be sure to follow directions for use on the label of this product. Do not miss doses. If you do, apply the dose as soon as you think about it.
- Cleanse the skin with soap and water and dry thoroughly before applying a nonprescription antifungal product.
- If using a cream or ointment, apply the smallest quantity to cover the area and rub it in well.
- If using an aerosol, shake the canister well. Hold the spray 15 to 25 cm from the affected area and spray evenly. Do not inhale the powder or vapor or use the product near an open flame.
- This product is for external use only. Do not use it near the eyes, nose or mouth. Wash your hands thoroughly after applying it.
- If irritation occurs, or if there is no improvement within 2 weeks, discontinue use and consult your doctor.
- Unless otherwise directed by a doctor, continue this medication after the infection is healed for the time shown on the label.
- Wear clean, loose fitting undergarments made of cotton or other absorbent material.
- During active infection, use your own washcloth, towel and grooming aids.

Selecting the Best Dosage Forms

Selection of the appropriate dosage form of a nonprescription antifungal product should be individualized to the patient. The medication must gain access to the fungal colony to exert action. The vehicle must be acceptable to the consumer to maximize compliance (Table 3).

Patients with pre-existing dermal sensitivities to topical drug application may be more prone to local irritation from repeated drug use. Irritation that persists or worsens while using a nonprescription antifungal product is cause for the individual to consult a physician.

Occasionally, severe pruritus with intensive scratching will damage the skin, increasing the chance for developing a secondary bacterial infection. Patients should be counselled not to apply an ointment based topical antibacterial product. Ointments may occlude the area and perpetuate the dermatophytic infection. A cream-based product would be appropriate. A physician should be consulted if infection persists.

?

PATIENT ASSESSMENT QUESTIONS

***Q** Have you been diagnosed with jock itch in the past?*

If the individual has had a previous medical diagnosis, they will be familiar with the symptoms.

***Q** Can you describe the physical appearance of the rash?*

The appearance of the rash will help in ruling out other possible conditions. In tinea cruris the rash is often symmetrical with raised borders and a butterfly appearance. In candidiasis and intertrigo the borders are less defined; in erythrasma it is a velvety patch; and in psoriasis it is the typical silvery scalely patch.

***Q** Are there any pustules or papules? If yes, where are they located?*

This will help you to rule out candidiasis. In tinea cruris there may be papules or pustules along the edges of the rash. In candidiasis, there are often satellite papules and pustules.

***Q** Is the penis or scrotum involved?*

The penis and scrotum are rarely involved in a tinea cruris infection.

***Q** Is the rash moist or oozing, or is the skin macerated or fissured?*

It is important to determine this prior to recommending a particular product formulation. An ointment, in this case, would not be appropriate. Ointments do not cling well to wet, moist areas, and they may occlude the macerated skin.

***Q** Is there a foul odor from the rash?*

A foul odor suggests the presence of a bacterial rather than a fungal infection. Nonprescription therapy is not effective for bacterial infections; therefore, you should see your physician.

***Q** Have you used a product for jock itch before? If yes, did it work for you? Did you experience any adverse effects to the product?*

This will be helpful in recommending a suitable product. Compliance will likely be enhanced if it was previously effective for the individual.

***Q** Do you have diabetes or suffer from any other chronic disease?*

Anyone with a chronic disease should be referred to their physician.

CONTRACEPTION

The history of condoms goes back to medieval times when sheaths of linen or animal intestine were used. Today, the condom is a sheath of latex or processed lamb cecum that fits over the erect penis. It provides a receptacle that prevents semen from reaching the vagina and cervix.

The use of condoms as a component of "safe sex" is widely publicized and encouraged to prevent the transmission of sexually transmitted diseases (STDs), including the human immunodeficiency virus (HIV).

TYPES OF CONDOMS

There are 2 major types available:

Lamb cecum condoms are not noted for elasticity and may slip off the penis during intercourse or withdrawal. It is claimed they provide better transmission of body heat and therefore greater sensitivity. Magnification of natural membrane condoms shows a surface riddled with pores of differing diameters that can allow the transmission of STDs. They are also more expensive.

Latex condoms are more elastic and more likely to remain in place during intercourse and withdrawal. Electron microscopy examination of a latex condom surface reveals no breaks or pores and they are considered impenetrable to STDs, including HIV. Latex condoms are also available in a number of variations: reservoir end, lubricated (wet or dry), lubricated with spermicide (nonoxynol-9), thin latex, extra strength, tapered, contoured, ribbed, studded, textured internal surface, colored and flavored. Most are produced in a regular size; however, small and larger sizes are also available.

In vitro studies have shown that nonoxynol-9 has bactericidal and virucidal action against many STD pathogens including herpes simplex viruses I and II and HIV. Latex condoms used with a spermicidal lubricant containing nonoxynol-9 may give added safety.

One manufacturer labels its condoms as made from sheerlon (a patented process to make latex stronger and silkier), claiming they are stronger and thinner than regular condoms.

CONTRACEPTIVE EFFECTIVENESS

Theoretically, condoms should be completely effective in preventing conception. In the real world, however, condoms are not so effective. The *USPDI* gives condoms a failure rate of 2 to 14%, while *Facts and Comparisons* gives them a failure rate of 3 to 36%. The broad range may result from study design, patient demographics, and socioeconomic status. Failures are attributed to breakage, improper use or inconsistent use.

The failure rate of condoms used in combination with a contraceptive foam is from less than 1 to 3%. This combination is the most effective nonprescription method available. Reported pregnancies per 100 women per year for other forms of contraceptives are:

combination pill—less than 1 to 2;
intrauterine device—less than 1 to 6;
mini-pill—3 to 6;
diaphragm with spermicidal foam or gel —3 to 18;
spermicide alone—3 to 21;
sponge with spermicide—3 to 28;
cervical cap with spermicide—5 to 18;
periodic abstinence (rhythm)—2 to 20.

CONDOM FAILURE

Most condom failures are thought to be due to incorrect use: after mucosal contact has already occurred, or only during certain types of sexual acts, or with oil-based lubricants that weaken the latex. The other leading cause of condom failure is user attitudes that lead to inconsistent use: reduction in physical sensations, uncomfortable feeling (inadequate lubrication), interruption in sexual activity, perception that sexual activity must be less vigorous, fear of sending a message that either the user or partner is unclean.

Quality control of condoms is very high. The main problem is that testing a specific condom renders it unfit for sale. Samples from each lot are tested but the condoms that actually reach the market are not. Nevertheless, the incidence of condom rupture or breakage is low (approximately 1%). Advantages and disadvantages of condoms are presented in Table 4.

ALLERGIC REACTIONS

Patients allergic to lanolin, wool or other sheep products may complain of itching or redness when using lamb cecum condoms.

Latex condoms may also cause this problem. It is estimated that up to 10% of the population is allergic to latex. Repeated exposure to certain proteins in the latex is thought to be the cause of allergies.

The connection between condom use and allergic contact dermatitis is easily missed. The allergy is an acquired immune reaction that may not develop for years after the initial exposure. Once an allergy develops, the allergic reaction itself may not appear for 72 hours following exposure. The most common symptom for both men and women is genital inflammation with redness, itching and burning. In more severe cases, intraepidermal edema leads to the formation of vesicles. Once the vesicles rupture, the skin weeps, oozes and crusts.

The recommended approach for women dealing with this problem is a lambskin condom worn over

TABLE 4: Advantages and Disadvantages of Condoms

Advantages	Disadvantages
Peace of mind	Interrupts lovemaking
Ease of use	Reduced sensation
Low incidence of side effects	Prompt withdrawal required
Convenience	Aware of its presence
Prolongs sex (less stimulation)	Less vigorous sex because condom may slip
Arousing to put on	Breaks
Easily obtainable	Difficult to put on
Lowers the risk of STDs in both men and women (latex)	Embarrassing
Inexpensive	Friction
Good for people who engage in sexual acts infrequently	Does not stay on
Used without medical supervision	Difficult to dispose of
	Messy to use

PATIENT ASSESSMENT QUESTIONS

Some people choose a nonprescription contraceptive method because they do not wish to talk to a health care professional. However, if the opportunity arises, the following questions may help the health professional advise the consumer about condom selection.

Q *Have you used condoms before? If yes, which brand(s)?*

If the individual has used condoms before, he will be familiar with this line of products.

Q *How do you use a condom correctly?*

This question will help assess the patient's knowledge and identify any missing information, which the health care professional can then fill in.

Q *What do you like or dislike about the condoms you have used? What does your partner like or dislike about the condoms you have used?*

This will help identify problems (e.g., lack of sensitivity, size, allergic reaction) the patient is having with the certain product he has chosen and will guide the health care professional in selecting a more appropriate condom.

Q *What problems have you or your partner had when using condoms?*

This will help identify any problems related to the improper use of a condom (e.g., breakage caused by lack of lubricant, condom slips off because it is not unrolled completely to the base of the penis).

Q *Are you using a condom as a contraceptive or as protection from a sexually transmitted disease?*

Patients concerned with sexually transmitted diseases should use a latex condom. Patients who require condoms as a form of contraceptive could use either latex or lamb cecum condoms along with a spermicide (if the condom does not already contain one).

Q *What variety of condoms are you aware of?*

Make certain the patient understands the difference between lamb cecum and latex condoms (e.g., elasticity, transmission of STDs, sensitivity). This will help identify which type of condom is best suited for the patient.

a latex condom; if the man is allergic, a lambskin condom can be worn under the latex condom. Sheerlon condoms are derived from latex and can also cause a reaction in a latex allergic individual. An alternative is "Femidom or Reality", a female condom manufactured from polyurethane.

Allergic reactions may also be caused by lubricants or spermicides; condoms free of these chemicals can be used. If the irritation persists, a physician should be consulted as the symptoms could be caused by an STD, not an allergy.

ADVANCES IN MALE CONTRACEPTION

Using a new polyurethane material, a British company, London International Group, has developed the first plastic condom for men, claimed to not cause allergic reactions. Duron has double the strength of latex so the condom can be thinner, which will improve sensitivity for its users. Clinical trials are now being conducted in the United States.

A German company, Neue Technologien, has invented a new form of male contraceptive, an implant that electrocutes sperm before they leave the man's body. The small capsule implanted into both seminal ducts has a galvanized element that produces a weak electrical current that destroys the sperm when they flow through. The galvanic effect of seminal fluid running between the 2 metals in the capsule apparently generates around 0.1 micro-amps, enough to render the sperm infertile. The manufacturer hopes to market the device within 2 years.

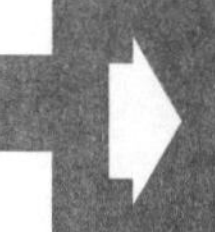

ADVICE FOR THE PATIENT

Condoms

- Store condoms in a cool, dry place. Do not use if they are sticky, discolored, brittle, or damaged.
- Examine the condom for an expiration date; if past this date, discard and use another.
- Open the condom package carefully to avoid damaging the condom with fingernails.
- Use condoms during every act that involves contact with the penis. Place the condom on the penis after it is fully erect and before any vaginal, oral or anal contact. Leakage from the penis prior to ejaculation can cause HIV transmission and pregnancy. Unprotected contact with female body fluids can also carry HIV to the male.
- Identify which side of the rolled-up condom is the outside and which is the inside. This is important because a male applying the wrong end to the penis at first, then reversing to the correct sides will allow some fluid to accidentally reach the partner.
- If the condom does not contain a spermicidal lubricant, the male may place a small amount of spermicide inside the tip.
- If uncircumcised, pull the foreskin back before placing the condom on the penis.
- Ensure adequate lubrication on the exterior surface of the condom prior to penetration.
- Unroll the condom completely to the base of the penis. If the product does not have a receptacle end, leave about 1.25 cm of empty space at the end (to catch semen, prevent leakage and reduce breakage), squeezing all air out of this space.
- Added spermicide and/or lubricant on the outside of the condom increases efficiency.
- Safe lubricants include water-soluble products (e.g., *K-Y jelly*) and spermicidal jelly or foam. Never use vaseline, mineral or vegetable oil, cooking oils, shortening, butter or margarine, baby oil, hand or body lotions, or oil-based cosmetics such as cold cream. All of these can damage the condom and result in breakage.
- Should the condom break during use, stop and withdraw immediately. An immediate application of spermicide might help prevent pregnancy and HIV infection.
- Immediately after ejaculation, the male must hold the condom at the base of the penis to prevent spillage and withdraw while the penis is still erect.
- Condoms must not be re-used. Dispose of the condom in a sanitary receptacle.

PREMATURE EJACULATION

Premature ejaculation is the most prevalent male sexual dysfunction. Studies that attempt to establish incidence and prevalence are difficult to equate because their definitions differ, but the disorder is common, with prevalence estimates ranging between 22 and 38%.

Historically, sexual dysfunctions of all kinds were regarded as a byproduct of severe psychopathology. Recently, however, they have been viewed as problems amenable to treatment, and effective interventions have begun to emerge.

Premature ejaculation has been defined in terms of varying duration of intravaginal contact, number of thrusts prior to ejaculation, number of partner-achieved orgasms, or the ratio of intercourse frequency to partner satisfaction. Masters and Johnson defined premature ejaculation as the man's inability to inhibit ejaculation long enough for his partner to reach orgasm 50% of the time. The revised 3rd edition of the Diagnostic and Statistical Manual of Mental Disorders (DSM-III-R) defines premature ejaculation as "persistent or recurrent ejaculation with minimal sexual stimulation before, upon, or shortly after penetration and before the person wishes it."

There is no reliable documentation identifying the cause or causes of premature ejaculation, although theories abound, physiological to psychological. One theory views it as the consequence of hypersensitivity in the glans penis, resulting in excessive stimulation of the spinal cord section that elicits ejaculation. A review by Shapiro of 1,130 cases, however, concluded that physiological explanations accounted for fewer than 4%. The psychoanalytic theory attributes it to generalized anxiety, passive-aggressive disorder, castration anxiety or unconscious negative feelings towards women.

A few biological approaches have been presented. One behavioral approach links the role of anxiety in decreased ejaculatory latency. Since anxiety and ejaculation are sympathetically mediated responses, it was speculated that sympathetic arousal related to anxiety could accelerate ejaculation. More recent knowledge, however, indicates that ejaculation appears to be mediated by both sympathetic and parasympathetic innervation, the sympathetic nervous system governing emission of semen into the posterior urethra and the parasympathetic nervous system responsible for the delivery of ejaculate.

Another behavioral explanation for premature ejaculation identifies the role of learning and conditioning in the etiology of the disorder. Situations such as sex with a prostitute or sex in situations where discovery might be imminent (e.g., a car or home when parental return may be imminent) condition the male to pair rapid ejaculation with sexual intercourse. Masturbation practices have also been suggested in the etiology of premature ejaculation. When masturbation is hurried out of anxiety, fear of discovery, or guilt, a speedy response may follow.

ASSESSMENT

The assessment of premature ejaculation should be multidimensional to reach a sound treatment decision and include self-reporting, behavioral, physiological and medical evaluations. Patients should be referred to their physician for the proper diagnosis. Organic factors are implicated in a relatively small proportion of cases. They include trauma to the sympathetic nervous system, prostatic hypertrophy, prostatitis, urethritis, alcoholism, diabetes, arteriosclerosis, cardiovascular disease, venous leakage and polyneuritis. Premature ejaculation has been described following withdrawal from antipsychotics and narcotics. It has also been associated with the use of desipramine and with alcohol-related peripheral neuropathy. Evaluation of premature ejaculation always inquires into genitourinary symptoms, symptoms of generalized or localized neurological disease, previous abdominal or pelvic trauma, and the use of prescription and nonprescription drugs.

TREATMENT

Nonpharmacological Treatment

The treatment of choice today is the "pause-squeeze" technique elaborated by Masters and Johnson, a modification of the original "pause" technique by Semans. Although this continues to be the recommended treatment, the reasons for its effectiveness are still not understood. The squeeze is reported to eliminate the ejaculatory urge.

To use this technique, the partner puts her thumb on the frenulum of the penis, with her 1st and 2nd fingers just above and before the coronal ridge. A firm grasping pressure is applied for

4 seconds and then released. The pressure, applied front-to-back, is proportional to the degree of erection present: a firm squeeze with an erect penis; a moderate squeeze when the penis is more flaccid. The squeeze may lead to a temporary 10 to 25% decrease in the erection. Masters and Johnson initially reported an overall failure rate of only 2.7%. Others, however, have not been able to replicate these results; overall improvement rates have ranged from 43 to 65%. Most data is based on uncontrolled case reports or program description, making success rates difficult to compare. The squeeze technique is less effective when self-applied.

The "pause-squeeze" technique is part of an elaborate treatment regimen. Initially used during mutual masturbation, after several days of practice the process is transferred to coitus. Later, a basilar squeeze technique may be taught, where the partner applies the squeeze technique to the base of the penis, so intercourse is not disrupted by repeated dismounting.

Pharmacological Treatment

A variety of pharmacological agents have been reported to delay or block an ejaculatory response. These include topical anesthetics, neuroleptics, antidepressants, alpha blockers, beta blockers, anxiolytics, and intracavernous injections of smooth muscle relaxants. Of these, only topical anesthetics are available to patients without a prescription.

A 1% dibucaine ointment showed improvement in ejaculatory latency. The authors stated that if sexual intercourse was undertaken at the height of anesthesia (e.g., 2 to 3 hours after application) the males were able to prolong the act for whatever period of time, usually 10 to 30 minutes, necessary for their partners to reach climax. The dibucaine neither prevented orgasm nor diminished its intensity. There was no anesthetic effect on the vaginal mucosa of the partner, since before intercourse, the penis was washed free of all remaining ointment and dried. Limitations identified were reduced sexual sensation and the need to plan sexual relations in advance and apply the ointment 2 to 3 hours prior to the act. Although commercially available in Canada, dibucaine ointment is not marketed as approved for use as a premature ejaculation retardant.

One clinical trial studied the effects of a 3% benzocaine cream in delaying climax in 13 men who complained of premature ejaculation. The 13 cases presented as follows: In 11 cases, orgasm occurred before the penis was inserted into the vagina; in 1 case it took place immediately on intromission, and in another case about 1 minute later. Approximately 2 g of the cream were massaged over the glans of the penis. After 5 minutes, the excess cream was wiped off and then the volunteer proceeded to coitus. The degree of anesthesia produced by the application was complete in 10 cases and partial in 3, with an average duration of 25.2 minutes. The average interval between intromission of the penis into the vagina and the orgasm was lengthened to 1.6 minutes (range 0.5 to 5 minutes). There were no untoward effects in any case. The local anesthetic did not affect the female partner's sensation in any way.

Another study involved 9 volunteers, 18 to 42 years old, who did not claim to have a premature ejaculatory problem. The subjects massaged a small amount (2 g by weight) of benzocaine 3% cream over the glans penis, waited 5 minutes, wiped off any excess and proceeded with intercourse once daily for 3 days in 5 cases and once daily for 30 days in 4 cases. The average duration of topical anesthesia on the mucous membranes with the 3% cream was 19.4 minutes. The average delay in orgasm with the 3% cream was 2.8 minutes. No adverse effects were reported.

The effectiveness of a 7.5% benzocaine ointment and placebo were compared on 120 men with premature ejaculation problems during intercourse. Results showed 90% of the men benefited, maintaining average (at least 2 minutes) control over their ejaculatory reflex when using the benzocaine compared to 7% with the placebo. Seventy-two per cent benefited substantially (3 minutes or more) from using the benzocaine. Seventy-two and a half per cent of the female partners achieved climax when the benzocaine ointment was used compared to only 2.5% with placebo.

Pharmacological treatment may be worth a trial in patients who fail to benefit from or who reject psychological approaches.

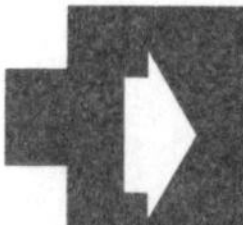

ADVICE FOR THE PATIENT

Premature Ejaculation

- Apply gel liberally to the head and shaft of the penis.
- Apply 5 to 10 minutes before intercourse.
- Wipe off any excess gel before commencing intercourse.
- After intercourse, wipe off any remaining benzocaine to minimize the risk of an allergic reaction.
- Do not continue if irritation occurs.

PHARMACEUTICAL AGENTS

Benzocaine: A local anesthetic of the ester type, it acts by blocking nerve conduction first in the autonomic, then in sensory and finally motor nerve fibres. Nerve conduction appears to be blocked by a decrease in the permeability of the nerve cell membrane to sodium ions.

Applied topically, benzocaine is relatively nontoxic; however, sensitization may occur. When used as a male genital desensitizer, benzocaine generally does not adversely affect orgasm in female sexual partners and does not appear to anesthetize the clitoris or vagina. If a rash or irritation develops during use, the drug should be discontinued and a physician consulted. Benzocaine should not be used in individuals with known hypersensitivity to the drug or other ester-type local anesthetics. It should be used with caution if the sexual partner is sensitive to local anesthetics, sunscreens, sulfa medications or hair dyes.

Benzocaine is available as a 7.5% gel for use as a male genital desensitizer applied to the head and shaft of the penis 5 to 10 minutes before intercourse. After intercourse, patients should wash off any remaining gel to minimize the chance of an allergic reaction.

Clioquinol: A halogenated 8-hydroxyquinidine-derivative topical antifungal (formerly, iodochlorhydroxyquin), clioquinol's precise mechanism is unknown. It inhibited the growth of various mycotic organisms such as *Microsporum*, *Trichophyton*, and *Candida albicans* and gram-positive cocci such as *Staphylococci or Enterococci* in in vitro studies. Also amebicidal, it was previously used orally to treat intestinal amebiasis. The oral use was barred worldwide due to reports of neurotoxicity. Clioquinol exerts a bacteriostatic rather than a bactericidal action.

Applied topically, only 2 to 3% of the dose is absorbed systemically. Under occlusive dressing, however, up to 40% of the dose can be absorbed. Generally, topical application is well tolerated. Local irritation, rash and sensitivity reactions have been reported occasionally; if any occur, the drug should be discontinued and a physician consulted. Cross-sensitivity with hydroxyquinoline and quinoline derivatives (e.g., antimalarials) and, occasionally, iodides can occur. Clioquinol can stain the skin and fabric; discoloration of the hair and nails has been reported rarely. Percutaneously absorbed clioquinol, which contains iodine, may interfere with certain thyroid function tests, and the manufacturer recommends that at least 1 month elapse between discontinuance of topical therapy with the drug and these tests. Use of clioquinol in children is not recommended, and use in those younger than 2 years of age is contraindicated.

Clioquinol is available as a 3% cream or ointment, applied topically 2 to 4 times daily after cleansing the affected area with soap and water and drying thoroughly. Treatment should be continued for 2 weeks; if there is no improvement, the drug should be discontinued and a physician consulted.

Clotrimazole and Miconazole Nitrate: Synthetic, imidazole-derived antifungal agents, these drugs interact with the fungal cell wall and inhibit the enzymatic conversion of lanosterol to ergosterol, which is required for cell membrane formation in actively growing organisms. With altered permeability, the cell membrane is unable to function as a selective barrier, and potassium and other cellular constituents are lost. Imidazole antifungals also inhibit fungi's ability to synthesize triglycerides and phospholipids. They inhibit oxidative and peroxidative enzyme activity, and toxic amounts of hydrogen peroxide accumulate intracellularly.

Both agents inhibit many fungi, including yeasts and dermatophytes. They are also active against some gram-positive bacteria. Only very small amounts of clotrimazole appear to be absorbed systemically following topical application. There are no reports indicating that miconazole is absorbed following application to intact skin.

Irritation and burning have occasionally followed cutaneous application of miconazole and clotrimazole creams. To avoid maceration in intertriginous areas, the creams should be used sparingly. If sensitization occurs, the drug should be discontinued.

Clotrimazole is available as a 1% cream and topical solution. Miconazole nitrate is available as a 2% topical cream. They should be applied sparingly and rubbed gently into the cleansed, affected area and surrounding skin in the morning and evening. Clinical improvement and relief of pruritus usually occur within 1 week. Tinea cruris is usually treated for 2 weeks; if results are inadequate, the drug should be discontinued and a physician consulted.

Pharmaceutical Agents

Povidone-Iodine: Effective against a broad assortment of bacteria, yeast and fungi. Povidone-iodine 10% has significant antifungal activity for treatment of jock itch but has not been studied for this indication. Elemental iodine is released from the physical complex at a rate equivalent to tincture of iodine in activity.

Povidone-iodine, available as a 10% ointment and solution, is safe for self-use and well tolerated.

Tolnaftate: Tolnaftate is fungistatic and fungicidal to *T. rubrum*, *T. tonsurans*, *T. mentagrophytes*, *T. schoenleinii*, *Microsporum canis*, *M. gypseum*, *M. audouinii* and *E. floccosum*, but does not act against bacteria or yeast. It is believed to distort the hyphae (the filaments that comprise the body [mycelium] of the fungi) and stunt mycelial growth in susceptible fungi.

Adverse effects include mild dermatitis, erythema, irritation and itching. If irritation or hypersensitivity occurs, or if the patient's skin disease does not improve within 10 days, the tolnaftate should be discontinued and a physician consulted.

Tolnaftate is available as a 1% solution, cream, powder, aerosol and 0.072% aerosol liquid applied topically twice daily to the affected areas, which have been washed and dried. The powder is used alone for the treatment of mild infections or as an adjunct to the cream or solution when drying of the lesion is desired. Pruritus, burning, and soreness may be relieved within 24 to 72 hours, but treatment continued for at least 2 or 3 weeks (2 weeks after the disappearance of all symptoms to prevent recurrence of infection).

Undecylenic Acid, Zinc Undecylenate: Fungistatic, fungicidal and a weak antibacterial, it is fungistatic against a wide variety of pathogenic fungi.

Undecylenic acid can be used on its own; but more often is combined with its zinc salt, which reportedly provides astringent action that helps reduce inflammation. It is available alone in a 10% solution or in combination with zinc undecylenate as a powder, medicated spray and cream. These preparations are usually nonirritating, but some individuals experience a transient, mild, stinging sensation if they are applied to excoriated areas.

Applied topically twice daily after cleansing the affected area, the cream should be used at night and, with ambulatory patients, the powder during the day. When a drying effect is desirable, the powder may be used alone. Treatment should be continued for 2 weeks.

RECOMMENDED READING

Anon. Condoms for prevention of sexually transmitted diseases. MMWR 1988;37(9):133-37.

Arndt KA. Fungal infections. In: Manual of Dermatologic Therapeutics. Toronto: Little, Brown, and Co., 1986.

Lookingbill DP, Marks JG. Scaling papules, plaques and patches. In: Principles of Dermatology. Toronto: Saunders, 1986.

Mandell GL, Douglas R, Bennett JE. Dermatophytosis and other superficial mycosis. In: Principles and Practice of Infectious Diseases. New York: Churchill Livingstone, 1990.

Masters WH, Johnson VE. Human Sexual Inadequacy. Boston: Little, Brown, and Co., 1970.

18

NUTRITION PRODUCTS

Nadeem Bhanji / Shirley Heschuk

CONTENTS

General Principles of Nutrition 425
- Normal Nutrition and Canada's Food Guide to Healthy Eating
- Basic Nutrients
- Nutritional Assessment

Principles of Infant Nutrition 455
- Breast-Feeding
- Infant Formulas

Principles of Weight Control 463
- Symptoms of Obesity
- Treatment Principles
- Eating Disorders: Anorexia Nervosa and Bulimia Nervosa

Special Nutrition Requirements 471
- Nutrition Requirements for Specific Health and Disease States
- Nutrition for Older Individuals
- Nutrition for the Athlete

Pharmaceutical Agents 479
- Vitamin Products
- Selected Minerals
- Enteral Products
- Infant Formulas
- Appetite Suppressants and Diet Aids
- Alternative Sweeteners
- Salt Substitutes
- Pharmaceutical Agents for the Athlete

Recommended Reading 487

GENERAL PRINCIPLES OF NUTRITION

This chapter deals with nutrition and its relevance to everyday practice.

The phrase You Are What You Eat emphasizes the vital and diverse roles nutrition plays in our lives. An adequate and balanced diet is central to growth and maintenance as well as good health. Through the processes of digestion and absorption, nutrients found in foods are incorporated into body structures and energy is produced via the various metabolic pathways.

Carbohydrate, fat, protein, vitamins, water, and some minerals found in foods are considered essential nutrients. They are required to sustain life and must be obtained from exogenous sources. During metabolism, the energy-yielding nutrients (fat, carbohydrate and protein) are catabolized to provide energy that can be used by the body; in contrast, water, vitamins and minerals do not supply energy, though they are actively involved in the processes of metabolism.

NORMAL NUTRITION AND CANADA'S FOOD GUIDE TO HEALTHY EATING

A nutritious and balanced diet provides variety, adequate nutrients and maximum protection against chronic disease. Health Canada, through its Scientific Committee on Nutrition, has addressed the need for an adequate diet for the Canadian population by establishing a recommended nutrient intake (RNI) for most nutrients. The RNIs, based on epidemiological and experimental data, have been designed to meet the needs of the majority of the healthy population and are intended to be a basis for planning a healthy diet. Specific RNIs are available according to age, sex, physiological status (e.g., pregnancy) and biological variations (Tables 1 and 2).

RNIs have been established for essential vitamins and minerals or micronutrients. Macronutrients, such as carbohydrate, fat and protein, are best expressed as a percentage of total calories consumed per day. Average amounts recommended are found in Table 3.

Despite their usefulness, the RNIs are not practical or convenient for the average Canadian. Guidelines have therefore been established by Health Canada's Scientific Review Committee recommending levels of essential nutrients that minimize the risk of chronic diseases. These recommendations are intended for healthy individuals over 2 years of age (Table 3).

More recently, in 1992, Canada's Food Guide to Healthy Eating (see pages 428–29) was developed

TABLE 1: RNI[a] of Vitamins Expressed as Daily Rates

					Fat-Soluble Vitamins			Water-Soluble Vitamins					
Age	Sex	Energy kcal	Weight kg	Protein g	Vitamin A RE[b]	Vitamin D µg	Vitamin E mg	Vitamin C mg	Folate µg	Thiamine mg	Riboflavin mg	Niacin NE[c]	Vitamin B_{12} µg
Months													
0-4	Both	600	6	12[d]	400	10	3	20	25	0.3	0.3	4	0.3
5-12	Both	900	9	12	400	10	3	20	40	0.4	0.5	7	0.4
Years													
1	Both	1100	11	13	400	10	3	20	40	0.5	0.6	8	0.5
2-3	Both	1300	14	16	400	5	4	20	50	0.6	0.7	9	0.6
4-6	Both	1800	18	19	500	5	5	25	70	0.7	0.9	13	0.8
7-9	M	2200	25	26	700	2.5	7	25	90	0.9	1.1	16	1
	F	1900	25	26	700	2.5	6	25	90	0.8	1	14	1
10-12	M	2500	34	34	800	2.5	8	25	120	1	1.3	18	1
	F	2200	36	36	800	2.5	7	25	130	0.9	1.1	16	1
13-15	M	2800	50	49	900	2.5	9	30[e]	175	1.1	1.4	20	1
	F	2200	48	46	800	2.5	7	30[e]	170	0.9	1.1	16	1
16-18	M	3200	62	58	1000	2.5	10	40[e]	220	1.3	1.6	23	1
	F	2100	53	47	800	2.5	7	30[e]	190	0.8	1.1	15	1
19-24	M	3000	71	61	1000	2.5	10	40[e]	220	1.2	1.5	22	1
	F	2100	58	50	800	2.5	7	30[e]	180	0.8	1.1	15	1
25-49	M	2700	74	64	1000	2.5	9	40[e]	230	1.1	1.4	19	1
	F	1900	59	51	800	2.5	6	30[e]	185	0.8[f]	1[f]	14[f]	1
50-74	M	2300	73	63	1000	5	7	40[e]	230	0.9	1.2	16	1
	F	1800	63	54	800	5	6	30[e]	195	0.8[f]	1	14[f]	1
75+	M	2000	69	59	1000	5	6	40[e]	215	0.8	1	14	1
	F	1700	64	55	800	5	5	30[e]	200	0.8[f]	1	14[f]	1
Pregnancy (additional)													
1st Trimester				5	0	2.5	2	0	200	0.1	0.1	1	0.2
2nd Trimester				15	0	2.5	2	10	200	0.1	0.3	2	0.2
3rd Trimester				24	0	2.5	2	10	200	0.1	0.3	2	0.2
Lactation (additional)				22	400	2.5	3	25	100	0.2	0.4	3	0.2

Adapted with permission from: Nutrition recommendations—the report of the scientific review committee. Ottawa: Health and Welfare Canada, 1990. With permission of the Minister of Supply and Services Canada, 1995.

a Recommended Nutrient Intake (RNI) is expressed on a daily basis, but should be regarded as the average recommended intake over a period of time, such as a week.

b Retinol Equivalents. 1 RE = 1 µg or 3.33 IU retinol. 1 RE = 6 µg or 10 IU beta-carotene.

c Niacin Equivalents. 1 NE = 1 mg niacin or 60 mg tryptophan. About 3% of ingested tryptophan is oxidized to niacin.

d Protein is assumed to be from breast milk and must be adjusted for infant formula.

e Smokers should increase vitamin C intake by 50%.

f Level below which intake should not fall.

to address current nutrition issues and recognize changes in Canadian eating patterns. This food guide essentially addresses the nutritional needs of the majority of Canadians 4 years of age and older.

Health care providers often encounter problems of undernutrition and overnutrition in their clients. Malnutrition due to primary deficiency (e.g., inadequate nutrients in the diet) is considered rare in western industrialized nations; however, secondary deficiencies are frequently encountered in patients with disease states that lead to malabsorption or increased destruction of nutrients normally present in the diet (e.g., cystic fibrosis, gluten allergy, etc.). Overnutrition is frequently encountered in practice

TABLE 2: RNI[a] of Minerals Expressed as Daily Rates

Age	Sex	Energy kcal	Weight kg	Protein g	Minerals: Calcium mg	Phosphorus mg	Magnesium mg	Iron mg	Iodine µg	Zinc mg
Months										
0-4	Both	600	6	12[b]	250[c]	150	20	0.3[d]	30	2[d]
5-12	Both	900	9	12	400	200	32	7	40	3
Years										
1	Both	1100	11	13	500	300	40	6	55	4
2-3	Both	1300	14	16	550	350	50	6	65	4
4-6	Both	1800	18	19	600	400	65	8	85	5
7-9	M	2200	25	26	700	500	100	8	110	7
	F	1900	25	26	700	500	100	8	95	7
10-12	M	2500	34	34	900	700	130	8	125	9
	F	2200	36	36	1100	800	135	8	110	9
13-15	M	2800	50	49	1100	900	185	10	160	12
	F	2200	48	46	1000	850	180	13	160	9
16-18	M	3200	62	58	900	1000	230	10	160	12
	F	2100	53	47	700	850	200	12	160	9
19-24	M	3000	71	61	800	1000	240	9	160	12
	F	2100	58	50	700	850	200	13	160	9
25-49	M	2700	74	64	800	1000	250	9	160	12
	F	1900	59	51	700	850	200	13	160	9
50-74	M	2300	73	63	800	1000	250	9	160	12
	F	1800	63	54	800	850	210	8	160	9
75+	M	2000	69	59	800	1000	230	9	160	12
	F	1700	64	55	800	850	210	8	160	9
Pregnancy (additional)										
1st Trimester				5	500	200	15	0	25	6
2nd Trimester				15	500	200	45	5	25	6
3rd Trimester				24	500	200	45	10	25	6
Lactation (additional)				22	500	200	65	0	50	6

Adapted with permission from: Nutrition recommendations—the report of the scientific review committee. Ottawa: Health and Welfare Canada, 1990. With permission of the Minister of Supply and Services Canada, 1995.

a Recommended Nutrient Intake (RNI) is expressed on a daily basis, but should be regarded as the average recommended intake over a period of time, such as a week.

b Protein is assumed to be from breast milk and must be adjusted for infant formula.

c Infant formula with high phosphorus should contain 375 mg calcium.

d Breast milk is assumed to be the source of the mineral.

Health Canada | Santé Canada

CANADA'S
Food Guide
TO HEALTHY EATING
FOR PEOPLE FOUR YEARS AND OVER
Enjoy a variety of foods from each group every day.
Choose lower-fat foods more often.
YOGOURT 2.2%
0.1%
SKIM MILK CHEESE
EVAP MILK
POWDER
2%
SKIM
TOFU

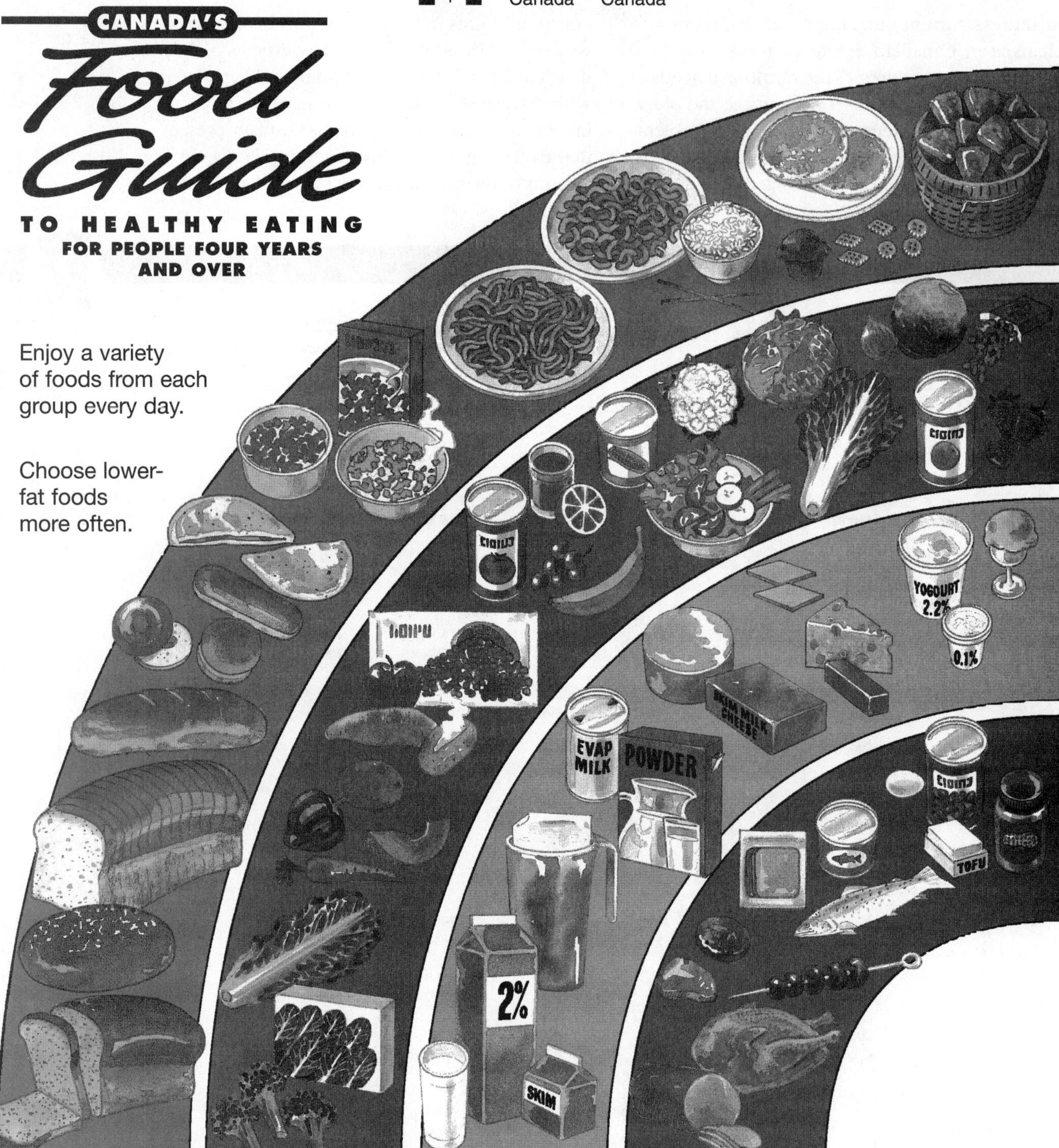

Grain Products
Choose whole grain and enriched products more often.

Vegetables and Fruit
Choose dark green and orange vegetables and orange fruit more often.

Milk Products
Choose lower-fat milk products more often.

Meat and Alternatives
Choose leaner meats, poultry and fish, as well as dried peas, beans and lentils more often.

Canada

CANADA'S
Food Guide
TO HEALTHY EATING
FOR PEOPLE FOUR YEARS AND OVER

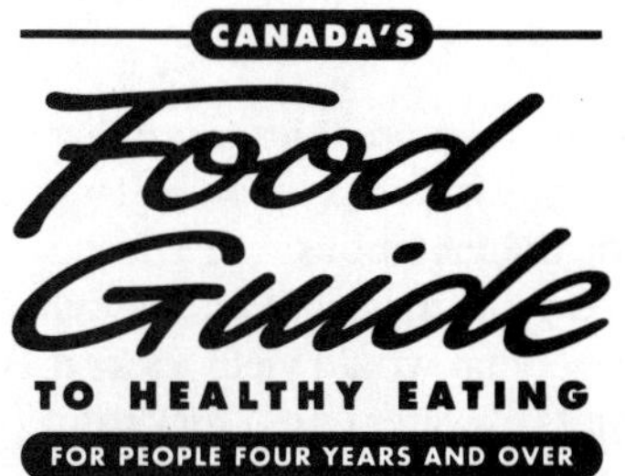

Different People Need Different Amounts of Food

The amount of food you need every day from the 4 food groups and other foods depends on your age, body size, activity level, whether you are male or female and if you are pregnant or breast-feeding. That's why the Food Guide gives a lower and higher number of servings for each food group. For example, young children can choose the lower number of servings, while male teenagers can go to the higher number. Most other people can choose servings somewhere in between.

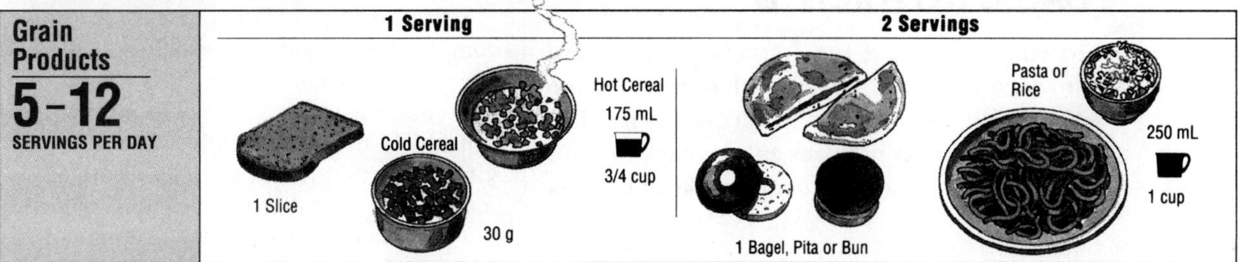

Vegetables & Fruit
5–10
SERVINGS PER DAY
1 Serving
1 Medium Size Vegetable or Fruit
Fresh, Frozen or Canned Vegetables or Fruit
125 mL
1/2 cup
Salad
250 mL
1 cup
Juice
125 mL
1/2 cup

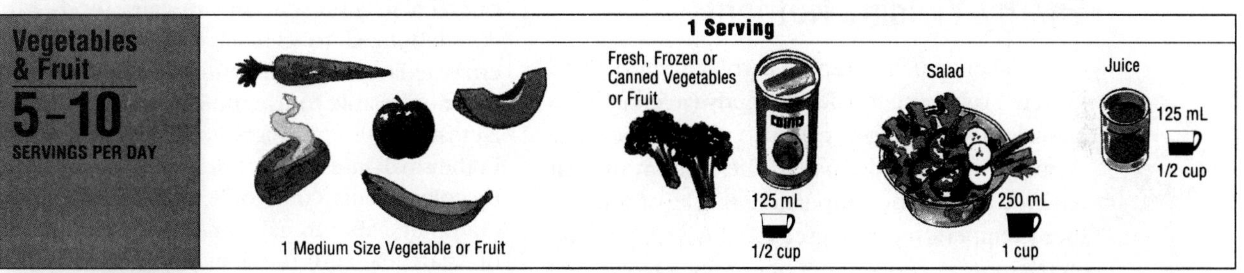

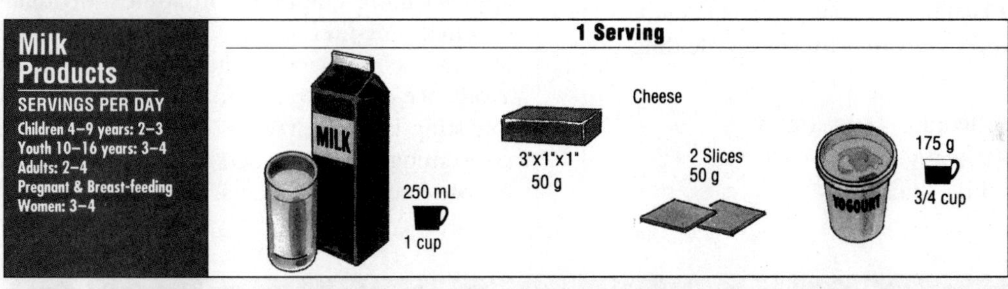

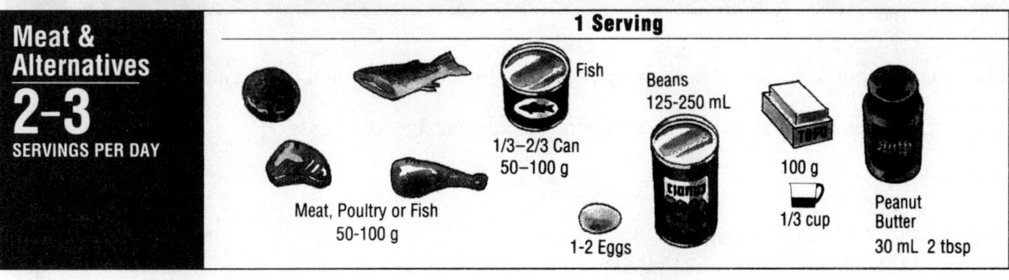

Other Foods

Taste and enjoyment can also come from other foods and beverages that are not part of the 4 food groups. Some of these foods are higher in fat or Calories, so use these foods in moderation.

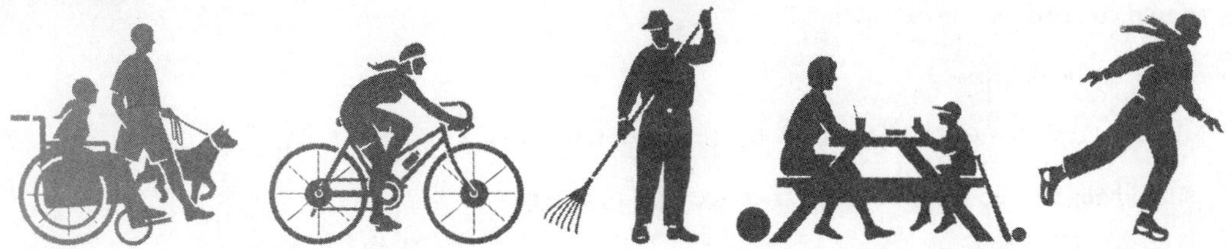

*Enjoy eating well, being active and feeling good about yourself. That's VITALIT*É

ISBN 0-662-19648-1

and is considered harmful. Increased consumption of fat and sucrose have conclusively been demonstrated to lead to atherosclerosis and dental caries, respectively.

BASIC NUTRIENTS

To effectively assist the consumer, health care providers should be familiar with nutrients in the diet and their normal physiological roles. The following section provides an overview of both energy-yielding and non-energy-yielding nutrients found in foods.

Energy-Yielding Nutrients

The oxidative metabolism of carbohydrate, fat and protein provide energy for the body (referred to as kilocalories or simply, calories). One kilocalorie (kcal) of energy is defined as the amount of heat required to raise the temperature of 1 kg of water at room temperature 1 degree Celsius (1°C). In the metric system, this amount of energy is expressed in joules, 1 kcal being equal to 4.184 kilojoules. The energy values provided by energy-yielding nutrients are as follows:

- carbohydrate—4 kcal/g;
- fat—9 kcal/g;
- protein—4 kcal/g.

The metabolism of fat provides more than twice the energy of carbohydrate or protein. To put this into perspective: the metabolism of 1 teaspoon of sugar (5 g) would yield 20 kcal of energy, while the metabolism of 5 g of fat would yield 45 kcal. Foods with large amounts of water (e.g., chicken) provide a lower calorie value by weight.

Carbohydrate occurs in nature in simple and complex forms. Simple sugars (also called mono- and disaccharides) are readily absorbed from the gastrointestinal tract into the bloodstream, and are considered the most rapidly available exogenous sources of energy. Monosaccharides (e.g., glucose and fructose) and disaccharides (e.g., sucrose, maltose and lactose) are the most abundant sugars found in foods. Sucrose is found in many foods, but lactose is present only in dairy foods. Lactose is catabolized to glucose and galactose by the enzyme lactase. An individual deficient in lactase will not be able to use the calories available from lactose in dairy products, it will remain undigested in the small intestine. Fermentation of lactose sugar by colonic flora commonly results in symptoms of cramp-like abdominal pains, bloating, acute onset of diarrhea and flatulence. Lactase deficiency appears more commonly in adult individuals of Oriental, Mediterranean and African descent. Management of lactose intolerance may include avoidance of all lactose-containing dairy products, ingesting lactase enzyme (e.g., *Lactaid*) prior to consuming dairy products, or consuming treated lactose-free dairy products.

TABLE 3: 1990 Nutrition Recommendations for Canadians
1. Energy consumption should be consistent to maintain body weight (e.g., calorie intake should equal calorie usage).
2. Diet should contain essential nutrients as specified in the Recommended Nutrient Intakes (RNIs).
3. Energy intake should be consumed as: <30% fats (33 g/1,000 kcal or 39 g/5,000 kJ); <10% saturated fats (11 g/1,000 kcal or 13 g/5,000 kJ); >55% carbohydrates (138 g per 1,000 kcal or 165 g per 5,000 kJ)
4. Protein intake should comprise 10 to 15% of the diet.
5. Salt consumption should be decreased.
6. Less than 5% of the total energy should be from alcohol (e.g., not more than 2 drinks per day).
7. Caffeine intake should not exceed 4 cups of regular coffee or tea per day.
8. Fluoridated water is recommended (1 mg/L).

Developed from: Nutrition recommendations—the report of the scientific review committee. Ottawa: Health and Welfare Canada, 1990.

Unlike simple sugars, complex carbohydrates (e.g., starch, dextrin and inulin) are digested in the gastrointestinal tract more slowly, making them ideal for individuals requiring a sustained release of energy (e.g., diabetics or individuals on a weight loss or control program). Since complex carbohydrates (e.g., whole grain products) often contain insoluble fibre, these foods may have a lower calorie content than simple sugars on a per gram basis.

Fat occurs in various structural forms (simple lipids such as fatty acids; compound lipids such as phospholipids; and derived lipids such as cholesterol and steroids or ketone bodies). Triglycerides (composed of glycerol and fatty acids) are the most abundant form of lipids in nature. Mammals use these compounds for energy storage, primarily as subcutaneous fat deposits and in skeletal muscle. Generally speaking, fatty acids do not occur singly in nature, they are used to form triglycerides and phospholipids.

Fatty acids occur in three forms: saturated, monounsaturated and polyunsaturated. Monounsaturated fatty acids contain one double bond, and polyunsaturated fatty acids contain two or more double bonds. They generally occur as oils at room temperature (e.g., olive oil or vegetable oil). Saturated fats (e.g., palmitic acid) have no double bonds, which results in solid fats such as butter and lard. Dietary fat (especially saturated fat) has been implicated in the etiology of cardiovascular disease. Cholesterol, which has also been linked to heart disease, occurs only in animal foods, generally major sources of saturated fats. Reduction of saturated fats is the most effective dietary means of lowering serum cholesterol. Olive and canola oils, which are made from monounsaturated fatty acids, are recommended as healthier alternatives to saturated fats.

Much has been said and written about cholesterol, which is synthesized by the body for production of bile acids and steroid hormones. However, its vital function is overshadowed by concerns with its role in atherosclerotic heart disease. Cholesterol is found in foods of animal origin, most notably full-fat dairy products, egg yolk, beef, pork, mutton, poultry and some seafood. Dietary ingestion of cholesterol can only partially suppress endogenous synthesis of cholesterol: up to 60% of normal synthesis cannot be suppressed. Limiting consumption of cholesterol-containing foods may only be part of the answer for individuals with severe hypercholesterolemias. Reduction of total dietary fat (especially saturated) plays a more significant role.

Finally, while most fatty acids can be synthesized *de novo*, certain polyunsaturated fatty acids (linoleic and linolenic acids) are required for normal physiologic functions (e.g., eicosanoid production), yet cannot be synthesized endogenously. They are obtained from dietary sources and are termed essential fatty acids. Present recommendations suggest that essential fatty acids should make up at least 3% of total energy intake. Total fat intake should be limited to no greater than 30% of total energy intake, with less than 10% of this being saturated fats. The 1990 Nutrition Recommendations do not specify cholesterol reduction, it is accepted that saturated fat limitation will also lead to cholesterol reduction in the majority of the population. (Cholesterol reduction is recommended for patients on lipid-lowering diets with underlying cardiovascular disorders.)

Protein is a complex molecule composed of amino acids. In the body, proteins occur as independent structures (e.g., antibodies) as well as in combination with other substances (e.g., mucoproteins or lipoproteins). Protein has to be broken down into constituent amino acids prior to absorption; once absorbed, these molecules are used primarily for the production of new body protein. They may also be used for energy when other sources have been depleted. Excess protein, typical of the North American diet, is either used for energy or converted to triglycerides with the nitrogen excreted as urea.

Proteins vary in their ability to maintain body functions, the quality judged on digestibility and relative content of essential amino acids. (Essential amino acids cannot be generated in vivo and must be derived from diet if the organism is to remain well.) In general, proteins from animals, fish, and fowl are easily assimilated and have a good balance of essential and nonessential amino acids. They are considered proteins of high biologic quality. With the exception of soybeans, vegetables are not considered of high biologic quality. However, a mixture of vegetable proteins from different sources (e.g., tubers, grains, seeds, nuts and legumes), each with a relative but different deficit of essential amino acids can make a complete or ideal protein mix.

Non-energy-yielding Nutrients

Water makes up 50 to 70% of total body weight (as an individual ages this percentage declines). The minimal daily requirement for water is highly variable and dependent on obligatory water losses such as urinary output, perspiration, water exhaled as vapor and loss via feces. Disease states and acute injuries may increase water loss. Daily water intake should meet or exceed expected water losses (approximately 2,500 mL, or 10 cups for an adult). Some free water is consumed through foods and beverages; however, additional intake as a beverage is highly recommended to facilitate normal function of the kidney and the gastrointestinal tract.

Fibre is an umbrella term that encompasses a heterogeneous group of substrates found in plants resistant to hydrolysis by human digestive enzymes. In addition to increasing fecal bulk and the frequency of bowel movements, it is agreed that fibre can alter nutrient digestion and absorption from the small intestine. Research indicates that dietary fibre may be essential in the prevention and treatment of many diseases. The benefits of fibre are summarized in Table 4.

Generally, increasing dietary fibre is recommended for most Canadians. An intake of 25 to 30 g of fibre per day can be easily achieved by following the guidelines outlined in Canada's Food Guide to Healthy Eating. Individuals should be counselled to gradually increase dietary fibre due to potential side effects such as bloating and flatulence. Some disease states (e.g., gastroparesis occurring secondary to diabetes mellitus or inflammatory bowel disease) may require a low-residue diet to prevent complications (e.g., bezoar formation) and to promote mucosal healing in inflammatory bowel disease.

Micronutrients: Vitamins and Minerals: Tables 5 and 6 summarize the key features of the lipid- and water-soluble vitamins. Table 7 provides an overview of key minerals required for normal body functions. These tables are not comprehensive but do provide an outline of key features of micronutrients.

NUTRITIONAL ASSESSMENT

As mentioned previously, Canada's Food Guide to Healthy Eating forms a sound basis for assisting clients to make positive changes in their dietary habits. A nutritional assessment is done to evaluate an individual's health from a nutritional perspective. In-depth assessments are most often done by dietitians or nutritionists, but screening based on nutritional and medical histories and physical observations can be done by other health care providers. A thorough nutritional assessment has several components: clinical and physical findings as well as an assessment of the individual's dietary habits.

Table 8 lists some physical findings in health and disease states that correlate with nutrient deficiencies. Clinical findings need to be correlated with biochemical (laboratory) tests prior to making therapeutic nutritional interventions. Some disease states and social conditions that require further referral are listed in Table 9.

A relatively simple yet useful assessment tool is the body mass index (BMI). This measurement, derived from the individual's height and weight, is useful for estimating the risk associated with overnutrition (see the section on weight control). A guide for determining the BMI for adults and the

TABLE 4: Benefits of Fibre*

Effects	Soluble Fibre†	Insoluble Fibre‡
Delay gastric emptying	√	×
Increase fecal bulk and frequency of bowel movements	√	√
Regulate colonic transit time	√	√
Slow glucose absorption from small intestine and reduce postprandial blood glucose levels during clinical tests	√	×
Lower total serum cholesterol and low-density lipoprotein cholesterol during clinical tests	√	×

* On the basis of physiochemical properties, fibre may be divided into soluble and insoluble fibre.
† Soluble fibre occurs as pectin (bananas, oranges and apples), gum (oatmeal and legumes), and mucilage (seeds, seaweed and psyllium).
‡ Insoluble fibre occurs as cellulose (wheat bran, orange peels and apples), lignin (cereal grains and potatoes), and hemicellulose (wheat bran and whole wheat).

associated degree of obesity for the individual is presented in Table 10. The BMI should not be used for individuals less than 20 years of age.

A major limitation of the BMI is the inability to distinguish the pattern of fat deposition—a parameter with better correlation to risk of chronic illnesses. The waist-to-hip ratio (WHR) (described in greater detail in the section on weight control) appears to be a more crucial indicator of risk associated with obesity.

No nutritional assessment is complete without an assessment of the client's dietary habits. Clients may be asked to retrospectively list the foods consumed over the past several days (usually 3 to 7 days). However, there is a potential for recall bias with this approach. Alternatively, clients may be asked to keep a food diary that would list all foods consumed over a 3- to 7-day period. This method, while being more accurate, is also subject to individual biases (e.g., modification of the diet from the normal pattern during weekends or on holidays). The Patient Assessment Questions outline some suggested approaches to nutritional assessment.

COUNSELLING TIPS

Vitamins and Minerals

Health care providers are often asked about the need for vitamin supplementation; consumers may request information on the benefits and uses. Parents with growing children often request information regarding a multivitamin supplement for their "finicky eaters." The lay person is bombarded with often-conflicting information from scientific journals and the media on the so-called antioxidant epidemiological trials.

- The need for a well-balanced diet from a variety of food groups should be emphasized to maximize the variety of nutrients from dietary sources. In general, a balanced and adequate diet composed of a variety of foods should provide all the necessary vitamins and minerals. Canada's Food Guide to Healthy Eating is an excellent basis for evaluating dietary habits and recommending changes. Free copies are available from Health Canada, municipal health units and provincial health ministries.
- Despite the positive results generated by several antioxidant trials, no firm conclusions can be made regarding universal micronutrient supplementation. On-going trials need to be completed before pharmacological supplementation with vitamins C, E and β-carotene can be routinely recommended.
- Consumers not convinced their diets are adequate, who want to supplement them with vitamins and minerals (e.g., a multivitamin product) may benefit from information on their potential risks and benefits as well as on appropriate doses to take. Warn those who wish to take individual vitamin and/or mineral supplements of the risk of megadosing and imbalancing other vitamins/minerals.
- In general, water-soluble vitamins (B and C) are relatively safe. The concern is that high levels can lead to obligatory diuresis of excess vitamins with concomitant dehydration. In addition, consumers should be counselled not to abruptly discontinue prolonged therapy with megadoses of vitamin C as rebound scurvy may occur.
- Fat soluble vitamins (A and D in particular) should not be routinely recommended unless for a specific therapeutic purpose. Vitamin E may be consumed safely in larger doses (Table 5). Vitamin K is sold by prescription only.
- Controversial areas regarding supplementation include: the appropriate doses of antioxidants in the diet; whether supplementation through dietary sources may be superior to ingesting pharmaceuticals (presumably because the latter may not include beneficial substances found only in foods); and the long-term benefits and hazards of supplementation.
- Where warranted, instructions regarding the proper storage and administration, signs and symptoms of toxicity, length of therapy, and other factors should be discussed with the client.

Alcohol

➤ Alcohol may be present in the diet as 5% by volume of beer, 12% of wine or 40% of spirits. One gram of alcohol provides 6.983 kcal compared to 4 kcal provided by protein or carbohydrate.

➤ Metabolically, alcohol is handled differently in the body, with increased consumption of oxygen and increased production of heat. Biochemically, chronic alcohol use may also diminish the use of vitamins and interfere with the absorption of amino acids.

➤ Chronic consumption of alcohol is linked to hypertension, liver disorders and central nervous system dysfunction. Positive correlations have also been noted with oral, laryngeal, esophageal and possibly, breast cancers.

➤ Alcohol consumption may have two possible effects on pharmacotherapy: acute ingestion of alcohol with drugs metabolized in the liver can lead to a competition for mixed function oxidases, which can prolong drug response or delay it if the agent is a prodrug; chronic consumption of alcohol (over several weeks) can lead to rapid induction of hepatic enzymes, which is characterized by a quicker onset and diminished response to drug therapy.

➤ In pregnancy, alcohol does not demonstrate any benefits, and chronic consumption leads to fetal alcohol syndrome (characterized by growth- and mental-retardation).

➤ The "French Paradox" is a phenomenon attributed to the people of France who consume wine without demonstrating a concomitant increased risk of cardiovascular disease. This is likely due to elevation of HDL lipids in the body. Alcohol also increases serum triglyceride levels and is discouraged in patients with any degree of hypertriglyceridemia.

➤ In view of the adverse effects of alcohol on blood pressure and the possibility it can replace foods that supply essential nutrients, adults who consume alcohol should limit their intake to less than 5% of total energy intake or 2 drinks per day, whichever is less.

➤ Diabetic individuals should regard alcohol as fat calories (1 alcoholic beverage = 2 fat exchanges), even though alcohol is primarily carbohydrate. Alcohol can be safely consumed by diabetics with caution: alcohol should never be consumed on an empty stomach, due to possible hypoglycemia; heavy alcohol consumption can lead to dangerous hypoglycemic episodes when taken concomitantly with insulin or hypoglycemic agents; and, hypoglycemic episodes can often mimic intoxication (e.g., fruity odor of breath due to ketone body production in insulin-dependent diabetics, "spaced out" feeling).

TABLE 5: Principal Micronutrients: Fat-soluble Vitamins

VITAMIN A

Function

Photoreceptor mechanism of retina; night vision; reproductive function; integrity of epithelial lining of eyes, skin, mouth, gastrointestinal and genitourinary tracts; lysosome stability (resistance to infection); glycoprotein (mucus) synthesis.

Principal Food Sources	Signs of Deficiency	RNI*	Signs of Toxicity
Preformed vitamin: fish, liver oils, liver, egg yolk, butter, cream, vitamin A-fortified milk and margarine. *Provitamin carotenoids:* dark green leafy vegetables, yellow fruits, sweet potato, tomato, carrots.	Dermatitis; nyctalopia; keratomalacia; xerophthalmia; morbidity and mortality in children.	800–1,000 RE/day **Therapeutic Dose†** 10,000–30,000 RE **Toxic Dose** >10,000 RE/day chronically	*Acute:* headache, irritability, desquamation, cheilitis, nausea and vomiting. *Chronic:* increased cerebrospinal pressure, dry scaly skin, bone thickening, hypercalcemia, pruritus, changes in nails and hair.

Comments

Three natural forms of vitamin A exist: *retinol* for reproductive function; *retinal* for vision; and *retinoic* acid for growth and differentiation.

1 µg retinol equivalent (RE) = 1 µg retinol
= 6 µg β-carotene
= 12 µg other provitamin carotenoids
= 3.3 international units (IU) retinol
= 9.9 IU β-carotene

Due to nonequivalent IU values for retinol and β-carotene, RE values are preferred as they are less likely to cause confusion.

Carotenoids (e.g., β-carotene, lycophene, and lutein) are yellow to red pigments that are widely distributed in plants. Not all carotenoids are converted to vitamin A in the body, and those commonly found in human diets (e.g., β-carotene and lycophene) can serve as singlet oxygen quenchers and as antioxidants, a role not shared by retinol.

Large amounts of carotenoids can be ingested safely over a long time. Only 20–30% of a given dose of β-carotene is absorbed (being very bile-salt dependent), and 50–60% is metabolized; in contrast, 90% of preformed vitamin A is absorbed (in the presence of adequate fat), and is stored in the liver, adipose tissue, kidneys and lungs.

β-carotene (along with vitamins C and E) may reduce cancer risk due to antioxidant activity. (Large scale trials are currently underway to substantiate these claims.)

Isotretinoin and cis-tretinoic acid are vitamin A analogues approved for use in acne treatment. Etretinate is indicated in the treatment of severe dermatological disorders.

Vitamin A deficiency can occur due to malnutrition (a common cause of blindness in the developing nations) or secondarily, due to malabsorptive states and chronic liver disease. Other causes of secondary vitamin A deficiency states include: celiac disease, sprue, chronic pancreatitis, and cystic fibrosis. Therapeutic management in deficiency states requires the use of active vitamin A orally or by intramuscular injections.

In addition to the treatment of deficiency states, vitamin A may reduce mortality in patients with severe measles.
Note: Vaccination is still the first line of defense.

β-carotene and carotenoids should not be used for management of deficiency states.

Signs of toxicity may occur with acute or chronic ingestion (doses in excess of 10 times the RNI over a period of months or years) of vitamin A. Hypercarotenosis results from prolonged ingestion of large amounts of carotenoids in green and yellow leafy vegetables, or carrots (often as carrot juice by food faddists), citrus fruits or tomatoes. Yellow discoloration of the skin is especially prominent in nasolabial folds, forehead, axilla and groin, and on the palms and soles. The condition is benign and usually reverses upon discontinuation of the food or supplement.

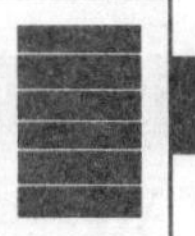

TABLE 5: Principal Micronutrients: Fat-soluble Vitamins (*cont'd*)

VITAMIN D

Function

Calcium and phosphorus absorption; resorption; mineralization and collagen maturation of bone; tubular resorption of phosphorus.

Principal Food Sources	Signs of Deficiency	RNI*	Signs of Toxicity
Ultraviolet radiation of skin is the major source; fortified milk is the main dietary source; fish liver oils, butter, egg yolk, liver.	Rickets (tetany sometimes associated), osteomalacia, hypophosphatemia, hypocalcemia, muscle weakness, secondary hyperparathyroidism. Deficiency common with long-term anticonvulsant therapy.	2.5 µg (100 IU)/day **Therapeutic Dose†** 10–40 µg (40–160 IU) **Toxic Dose** >25 µg/day (1,000 IU/day)	Hypercalcemia (anorexia, vomiting, diarrhea, polyuria, and mental changes), proteinuria, constipation, renal failure, metastatic calcification (kidneys and lungs), metallic taste.

Comments

1 µg = 40 IU vitamin D_3

D_2 (calciferol, ergocalciferol) and D_3 (cholecalciferol) occur naturally and are equipotent.

Major source of vitamin D in normal ambulatory adult is exposure to sunlight. Vitamin D production by the skin is related to latitude, and the further away from equator the lower the proportion of the year during which vitamin D can be synthesized.

90% of dietary vitamin D is absorbed from the small intestine and is converted by the liver and kidneys to the active metabolite (1,25-dihydroxycholecalciferol or calcitriol).

Calcitriol is indicated in chronic renal failure for management of hypocalcemia.

Breast-fed infants under 6 months of age, where sunlight exposure is low, require supplementation because maternal milk contains only small amounts of vitamin D, and because there is an increased demand for calcium for the growing skeleton. Generally speaking, vitamin D requirements are higher in infants, children, the elderly and in women who are pregnant or breastfeeding (Tables 1 and 2).

Theoretically chronic use of sunscreens, especially in the elderly population, may lead to vitamin D deficiency. This has not been evaluated in clinical trials. Patients may be advised to maintain sunscreen-free intervals (e.g., 10 minutes) on a routine basis. Alternatively, supplementation may be recommended (200–400 IU/day).

Calcipotriol (vitamin D analogue) may be useful in the management of psoriasis.

Large doses of vitamin D may have a role in the treatment of tuberculosis (possible immune strengthening effect), though it is generally not recommended.

TABLE 5: Principal Micronutrients: Fat-soluble Vitamins (*cont'd*)

VITAMIN E

Function

Intracellular antioxidant, scavenger of free radicals in biologic membranes.

Principal Food Sources	Signs of Deficiency	RNI*	Signs of Toxicity
Vegetable oil, wheat germ, leafy vegetables, egg yolk, margarine, legumes.	RBC hemolysis, neurologic damage (ataxia, muscle weakness, nystagmus, loss of touch), creatinuria, ceroid deposition in muscle.	6–9 mg (9–13 IU)/day **Therapeutic Dose†** 30–100 mg/day (44.7–149 IU/day) **Toxic Dose** Unknown	Little evidence of harmful effects with large doses; mainly gastrointestinal symptoms (nausea, flatulence, or diarrhea), potentiation of effects of oral anticoagulants.

Comments

d-α-tocopherol is the natural (and active) form of vitamin E (1 mg is equivalent to 1.49 USP units); dl-α-tocopherol is the synthetic form of vitamin E (1 mg being equivalent to 1 USP units). However, products labelled in USP units deliver equivalent amounts of vitamin E.

Absorption is 20–40% from the gastrointestinal tract, dependent on fat intake. It is decreased with hepatic failure and fat malabsorption states.

Possible role as an antioxidant in the prevention of cancer and/or cardiovascular diseases.

Unapproved uses: epilepsy, muscle cramps, Parkinson's disease, tardive dyskinesia, benign breast cancer. In epilepsy, vitamin E may have a role as an adjunct to antiepileptic drug therapy. In Parkinson's disease, vitamin E was not found to delay the progression of the disease.

Potentiation of anticoagulant effect may occur at doses >800 mg (1,200 IU/day).

Epidemiological studies have shown statistically significant inverse association between plasma vitamin E concentrations and mortality from heart disease and certain cancers. This has led to suggestions that dietary requirement for health, rather than avoidance of chronic deficiency, should be increased. Clinical trials utilizing 400 IU/day are currently underway in patients with pre-existing heart disease.

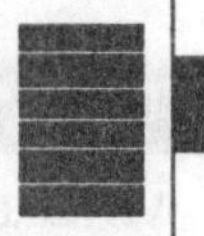

TABLE 5: Principal Micronutrients: Fat-soluble Vitamins (*cont'd*)

VITAMIN K

Function

Formation of coagulation factors II (prothrombin), VII, IX and X; plasma proteins C and S; and for normal blood coagulation.

Principal Food Sources	Signs of Deficiency	RNI*	Signs of Toxicity
Leafy vegetables, pork, liver, vegetable oils, intestinal flora (after newborn period).	Bleeding secondary to deficient clotting factors due to lipid malabsorption states; liver disease, use of extended-spectrum antibiotics (secondary to destruction of vitamin K-synthesizing intestinal bacteria or antagonism of vitamin K by N-methylthiotetrazole-containing second- and third-generation cephalosporins).	Not established for adults 2 mg orally or 1 mg intramuscular vitamin K_1 (neonates) **Therapeutic Dose†** 10 mg (warfarin overdose) **Toxic Dose** Nontoxic	Problems have not been encountered with high doses of vitamin K over extended periods of time; kernicterus has been observed with menadione in infants.

Comments

Phylloquinone (K_1) occurs in plants and menaquinone (K_2) is synthesized by intestinal flora; menadione (K_3) is a fat-soluble synthetic analogue.

Decreased amounts in hepatic failure, and with anticoagulation therapy.

Large amounts of dietary vitamin K (e.g., 250 mg of vitamin K in 8 oz of cauliflower, lettuce, spinach, or broccoli) may antagonize the hypothrombotic effect of oral anticoagulants.

Available only by prescription.

*RNIs are for adults 25–49 years old; complete RNIs for all age groups are presented in Table 1.

†Therapeutic doses are much larger than RNIs.

Note: Product monograph should be consulted when administering for specific indications.

Developed from: McCarter DN, Holbrook J. Vitamins and minerals. In: Herfindel ET, Gourley DR, Hart LL, editors. Clinical Pharmacy and Therapeutics. 5th ed. Baltimore: Williams and Wilkins, 1992:133–49.

McLaren DS, Loveridge N, Duthi G, et al. Fat-soluble vitamins. In: Garrow JS, James WPT, eds. Human Nutrition and Dietetics. 9th ed. Edinburgh: Churchill Livingstone, 1993:208–38.

Nutrition recommendations—the report of the scientific review committee. Ottawa: Health and Welfare Canada, 1990:82–92.

TABLE 6: Principal Micronutrients: Water-soluble Vitamins

VITAMIN B_1 (THIAMINE)

Function

Coenzyme in carbohydrate metabolism; normal growth; conduction of nerve impulses; acetylcholine synthesis.

Principal Food Sources	Signs of Deficiency	RNI*	Signs of Toxicity
Milk, pork, liver, nuts, whole grains, enriched flour and cereals.	Beriberi (peripheral neuritis ["pins and needles"], muscle wasting, edema, tachycardia, cardiomegaly, and pedal edema; loss of memory; depression). Wernicke's encephalomyelopathy (mental confusion, depression, nystagmus, ataxia, psychoses leading to coma).	0.8–1.1 mg/day **Therapeutic Dose†** 10–100 mg/day **Toxic Dose** >5 g/day for 4–5 weeks	Hypersensitivity, feelings of warmth, tingling, pruritus, pain, urticaria, weakness, sweating, nausea, restlessness, tightness of throat, angioedema, respiratory distress, cyanosis, pulmonary edema, GI bleeding, transient vasodilatation and hypotension, vascular collapse, and death have occurred occasionally, mainly following repeated IV administration. Neuromuscular and ganglionic blockade may occur with very large (5–10 g) parenteral doses.

Comments

Approved uses are as thiamine replacement (common in alcoholics), Wernicke's encephalopathy and coma. Thiamine does not appear to benefit Alzheimer's disease.

Unsubstantiated uses include: relief of anxiety, fatigue, irritability, tremors and depression, improved learning capacity and muscle tone maintenance.

Thiamine requirements are directly related to carbohydrate content of diet. Depletion occurs after 3 weeks of total absence of thiamine from diet.

Dialysis patients may require supplementation.

Thiamine may temporarily correct metabolic disorders associated with some genetic disorders including subacute necrotizing encephalomyelopathy (SNE, Leigh disease), maple syrup urine disease, and lactic acidosis associated with pyruvate carboxylase deficiency and hyperalaninemia.

VITAMIN B_2 (RIBOFLAVIN)

Function

Component of coenzymes FAD and FMN, which catalyze oxidative-reductive reactions in cells; required for building and maintaining body tissues.

Principal Food Sources	Signs of Deficiency	RNI*	Signs of Toxicity
Milk, cheese, eggs, meat (especially organ meats), liver, green leafy vegetables, enriched flour and grains.	Cheilosis, glossitis, seborrheic dermatitis, anemia, purplish tongue, burning and itching eyes, achlorhydria.	1–1.4 mg/day **Therapeutic Dose†** 10–30 mg **Toxic Dose** Nontoxic	No toxicity; large doses may cause yellow discoloration of urine.

Comments

Deficiency may appear in alcoholism and protein-calorie malnutrition (e.g., malabsorption states or elderly individuals).

Unapproved uses include: carpal tunnel syndrome and enhanced athletic performance. These claims have not been substantiated with double-blind, placebo-controlled studies.

Unsubstantiated uses: cataracts, skin, nail and hair ailments, stress relief, maintenance of adequate antibody and red blood cell production.

Patients on chronic tricyclic antidepressants or phenothiazines may require additional riboflavin due to impaired conversion of riboflavin to active coenzyme.

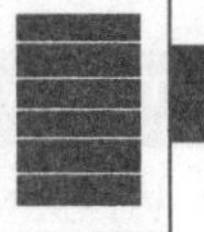

TABLE 6: Principal Micronutrients: Water-soluble Vitamins (*cont'd*)

NIACIN (NICOTINAMIDE, NICOTINIC ACID)

Function

Energy producing enzymes (NAD and NADP) involved in tissue respiration, fat synthesis, growth, healthy skin, protein metabolism.

Principal Food Sources	Signs of Deficiency	RNI*	Signs of Toxicity
Organ meats, fish, poultry, whole grains, corn, green vegetables, nutritional yeast, enriched flour and cereals.	Pellagra (dermatitis, diarrhea, dementia); erythematous eruptions, glossitis, insomnia, anorexia, abdominal pain and vertigo.	14–19 NE/day **Therapeutic Dose†** 300–500 mg (pellagra); 1.5–6 g, up to 9 g (antilipemia) **Toxic Dose** More common with long-term use of large doses	Cutaneous vasodilatation, pruritus, dizziness, nausea, gastrointestinal distress, hypotension, tachycardia, headache and blurred vision are common, nontoxic, reversible effects with larger doses of niacin. Long-term use may lead to rash, hyperpigmentation, dry skin, xerostomia, hyperuricemia (occasionally precipitating gout), peptic ulcer disease, amblyopia, visual disturbances, hyperglycemia, and glycosuria. Abnormal liver function tests (increases in serum bilirubin, AST, ALT and LDH), jaundice and chronic liver damage have occurred with niacin therapy.

Comments

Niacin (nicotinic acid) and nicotinamide (the amide derivative) are water soluble B-complex vitamins.

Tryptophan is converted to niacin in the body.

One niacin equivalent (NE) = 1 mg of niacin or 60 mg of tryptophan.

Niacin and nicotinamide are used to prevent niacin deficiency and to treat pellagra; however, only niacin possesses antilipidemic properties.

Fasting blood glucose, liver function tests, and uric acid levels should be monitored periodically with chronic niacin therapy. Extended-release products have been associated with greater incidence of liver damage.

Unapproved uses include: schizophrenia, Ménière's disease, stress situations, migraine, arthritis and to increase athletic performance. (Little or no scientific evidence is available for these claims.)

TABLE 6: Principal Micronutrients: Water-soluble Vitamins (*cont'd*)

VITAMIN B_6 (PYRIDOXINE)

Function

Transamination and transformation of amino acids, metabolism of tryptophan to serotonin, conversion of linoleic acid to arachidonic acid; formation of sphingolipids for the myelin sheath; regulation of gamma-aminobutyric acid (GABA). Essential for immune function.

Principal Food Sources	Signs of Deficiency	RNI*	Signs of Toxicity
Chicken, beef, pork, calves' liver, ham, fish, nuts, bread and whole grain cereals.	*Rare:* seborrheic-like skin dermatitis, stomatitis, peripheral neuropathy, anemia.	1.1–1.8 mg/day (suggested) **Therapeutic Dose†** 10–600 mg/day **Toxic Dose** Chronic (2 months to several years) ingestion of doses of 500 mg up to 2 g/day.	Sensory neuropathy (impaired sense of position and vibration, as well as progressive ataxia), paresthesia, nausea, somnolence, increased serum AST and decreased serum folic acid.

Comments

Deficiency states common in alcoholics, and in chronic drug therapy with hydralazine, isoniazid, pyrazinamide, phenelzine, cycloserine, penicillamine and estrogen (e.g., oral contraceptives).

Daily doses of 200 mg over a 4-week period have reportedly decreased serum phenobarbital and phenytoin levels.

Doses of 5 mg or greater antagonize the effect of levodopa; levodopa-carbidopa combination not affected by vitamin B_6.

May be used in the correction of deficiency states (2.5 to 200 mg/day); metabolic disorders (primary hyperoxaluria, primary homocystinuria, primary cystathioninuria, xanthurenic aciduria) (100–500 mg/day); sideroblastic anemia (200–600 mg/day); and drug-induced deficiency states (100–300 mg/day).

Unapproved uses include: premenstrual syndrome, carpal tunnel syndrome, and in improving athletic and mental performance. Studies show some benefit for the first two conditions. (Patients taking high doses should be monitored for toxicity.)

PANTOTHENIC ACID

Function

As a constituent of coenzyme A, metabolism of carbohydrates, gluconeogenesis, synthesis and degradation of fatty acids, synthesis of sterols, and steroid hormones, synthesis of porphyrins.

Principal Food Sources	Signs of Deficiency	RNI	Signs of Toxicity
Yeast, organ meats, poultry, fish, cereals, walnuts, fruits, vegetables, milk.	Rare, unless there is severe, multiple B-complex deficits.	Insufficient data to formulate RNIs **Therapeutic Dose†** 15 mg; 10–20 g/day **Toxic Dose** Nontoxic	Essentially nontoxic.

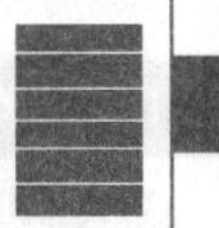

TABLE 6: Principal Micronutrients: Water-soluble Vitamins (*cont'd*)

VITAMIN C (ASCORBIC ACID)

Function

Collagen synthesis (poor wound healing and stress due to injury and infection); adrenaline synthesis in the adrenal gland; conversion of folic acid to folinic acid; synthesis and normal functioning of white blood cells; absorption of iron.

Principal Food Sources	Signs of Deficiency	RNI*	Signs of Toxicity
Citrus fruits, tomatoes, potatoes, leafy vegetables, melons.	Defects in collagen synthesis (poor wound healing, aching joints, weakened cartilage, and capillary walls); generalized fatigue, loss of appetite, low resistance to infection; scurvy (bleeding gums, loosening teeth, petechial hemorrhages, decreased wound healing).	30–40 mg/day **Therapeutic Dose†** 10–500 mg/day (scurvy); 4–12 g (other uses—see below) **Toxic Dose** Usually nontoxic; dose-related adverse effects.	Diarrhea and gastrointestinal distress with dosages of 1 g daily or greater. Hyperoxaluria occurs in about 5% of individuals. Ascorbic acid may cause acidification of urine, occasionally leading to precipitation of urate, cystine, or oxalate stones, or drugs in the urinary tract. Gout; lowered serum cholesterol; increased absorption of iron (hemochromatosis); interference with oral anticoagulants.

Comments

Concurrent administration with ASA may lead to decreased elimination of ASA and increased excretion of ascorbic acid.

Ascorbic acid may decrease the anticoagulant effect of warfarin; however, this interaction is of uncertain clinical significance.

Large doses may be useful in the treatment of pressure sores. Large doses (e.g., 1 g twice daily) may be beneficial in the prevention of diabetic neuropathy and cataract formation (possibly due to effects of vitamin C on sorbitol production).
Note: Urine based glucose tests may yield false positive or negative results (depending on the test) with increased vitamin C supplementation.

Cigarette smokers should increase vitamin C intake by 50% above RNI.

4–12 g/day of ascorbic acid has been used as a urinary acidifying agent; however, because of questionable efficacy, urinary pH should be confirmed with pH paper.

Studies that have evaluated vitamin C in cold prevention are nonconclusive (unsubstantiated by randomized, well-controlled, double-blind clinical studies).

TABLE 6: Principal Micronutrients: Water-soluble Vitamins (*cont'd*)

BIOTIN

Function

Porphyrin synthesis, carbohydrate metabolism, fat metabolism; normal growth and maintenance of nervous system tissue, skin, hair and blood cells.

Principal Food Sources	Signs of Deficiency	RNI	Signs of Toxicity
Liver, egg yolk, synthesized by intestinal flora.	Megaloblastic anemia.	None established **Therapeutic Dose†** 150–300 µg **Toxic Dose** Nontoxic	Essentially nontoxic.

Comments

Deficiency may occur during pregnancy.

FOLIC ACID (FOLACIN)

Function

Maturation of red blood cells; required for nucleic acid synthesis; formation and functioning of nervous system.

Principal Food Sources	Signs of Deficiency	RNI*	Signs of Toxicity
Liver, green leafy vegetables, nuts, asparagus, banana, strawberries	Megaloblastic anemia, glossitis and other gastrointestinal symptoms; possible neural tube defects (anencephaly and spina bifida) in offspring of folate-deficient expectant women.	185–230 µg/day **Therapeutic Dose†** 1 mg **Toxic Dose** >15 mg/day	No toxicity reported with doses up to 15 mg. Adverse GI effects such as anorexia, nausea, abdominal distention, flatulence, and bad taste. Adverse CNS effects such as altered sleep patterns, impaired concentration, irritability, overactivity, excitement, mental depression, confusion and altered judgment have been reported rarely in patients taking 15 mg of folic acid daily for 1 month. Vitamin B_{12} concentrations may be decreased with prolonged folic acid therapy.

Comments

Approved uses: anticonvulsant-induced folate deficiency, folate supplementation during pregnancy, during oral contraceptive usage, and for the treatment of megaloblastic anemia. Note: Large doses may lead to seizures in epileptics controlled by phenytoin (folate blocks uptake of phenytoin into neuronal cells).

Folate supplementation during pregnancy is recommended to reduce the likelihood of neural tube defects in the newborn. Supplementation should begin prior to pregnancy and be maintained throughout the first trimester of pregnancy. It is during the first 4 weeks of pregnancy that neural tube formation and closure occur. (Serum folate levels drop in the third trimester, due to plasma volume expansion—this is considered physiological and does not require supplementation.)

A minimum of 0.4 mg of folic acid is recommended for women planning to be pregnant; higher doses (4 mg) are recommended in women with a child with neural tube defect (under medical supervision).

While folic acid corrects vitamin B_{12}-induced megaloblastic anemia, it does not treat neurological disturbances associated with vitamin B_{12} deficiency. Therefore, the underlying cause of anemia should be evaluated prior to treatment.

Systemic folic acid does not treat phenytoin-induced gingival hyperplasia. Topical folate requires evaluation.

Unsubstantiated claims include: increased appetite, increased antibody formation, and healthy hair growth.

TABLE 6: Principal Micronutrients: Water-soluble Vitamins (*cont'd*)

COBALAMIN (VITAMIN B_{12})

Function

DNA synthesis; red blood cell formation.

Principal Food Sources	Signs of Deficiency	RNI*	Signs of Toxicity
Liver, meat, milk, eggs, cheese, yogurt, shellfish (fruits and vegetables are deficient in this vitamin).	Pernicious anemia, peripheral neuropathy, macrocytic anemia.	1 µg/day **Therapeutic Dose†** 100 µg/month **Toxic Dose** Nontoxic	Essentially nontoxic

Comments

Only approved use is for the correction of vitamin B_{12} deficiency (pernicious anemia).

Unapproved uses include: chronic fatigue syndrome, sleep-waking rhythm disturbances, placebo effect and increasing athletic performance. (A double-blind, placebo-controlled study found no difference between placebo and vitamin B_{12}-folate treatment for CFS.)

Patients on chronic (>2 years) H_2-antagonist therapy or proton pump inhibitors may require supplementation due to decreased gastric acid cleavage of cobalamin from food sources.

* RNIs are for adults 25–49 years old; complete RNIs for all age groups are listed in Table 1.

† Therapeutic doses are much larger than RNIs.

Note: Product monograph should be consulted when administering for specific indications.

Developed from: Halsted CH. Water-soluble vitamins. In: Garrow JS, James WPT, eds. Human Nutrition and Dietetics. 9th ed. Edinburgh: Churchill Livingstone, 1993:239–63.

Vitamins. In: McEvoy GK, ed. AHFS Drug Information 95. Bethesda: American Society of Health-System Pharmacists, 1995:2515–46.

Nutrition recommendations—the report of the scientific review committee. Ottawa: Health and Welfare Canada, 1990:99–131.

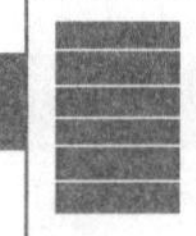

TABLE 7: Principal Micronutrients: Minerals

CALCIUM See Pharmaceutical Agents for discussion of calcium and osteoporosis.

Function	Principal Food Sources	RNI*	Signs of Deficiency
Normal integrity of muscular and nervous systems, for normal cardiac function, for activation of thrombin, and is a major component of bone.	Primarily from dairy products, though plant sources (e.g., broccoli, kale, spinach) do provide additional calcium.	700–800 mg/day	Tetany (acute); osteoporosis or osteomalacia (adults) and rickets (children) (chronic)

Comments

Interaction between parathyroid hormone, vitamin D and calcium is responsible for maintaining normal serum levels.

Absorption from small intestine is approximately 30%; may be increased to 50% during growth periods, pregnancy and lactation (in otherwise healthy individuals).

Chronic ingestion of 1–2 g of calcium per day is unlikely to cause problems.

Signs of calcium toxicity include: hypercalcemia, metastatic calcification, weakness, renal failure, psychosis.

Calcium from oyster shell is calcium carbonate which has the highest bioavailability amongst calcium salts. Bone meal and dolomite products may pose a risk due to possible contamination with lead.

CHLORIDE

Function	Principal Food Sources	RNI	Signs of Deficiency
Fluid-electrolyte balance, acid-base balance, gastric acidity.	Ubiquitous with sodium and potassium.	Not established	Chloride ion deficiency alone is rare.

Comments

Losses primarily due to gastrointestinal disorders, diarrhea, vomiting, and during tube drainage.

CHROMIUM

Function	Principal Food Sources	RNI	Signs of Deficiency
Favors normal glucose tolerance.	Meat, whole grains, nuts, legumes and brewer's yeast.	Not established	Impaired glucose clearance, peripheral neuropathy.

Comments

Required for normal glucose utilization.

Role in management of diabetes remains controversial.

Required for carbohydrate and lipid metabolism (though supplementation has not been proven in weight control or in improving athletic performance).

Lowers serum cholesterol and LDL and increases HDL.

COBALT

Function	Principal Food Sources	RNI	Signs of Deficiency
Integral component of B_{12}		Not Established	Pernicious anemia

Comments

Excessive amounts may lead to polycythemia

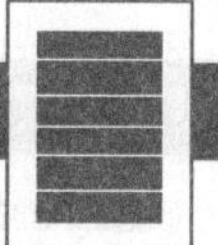

TABLE 7: Principal Micronutrients: Minerals (*cont'd*)

COPPER

Function	Principal Food Sources	RNI	Signs of Deficiency
Synthesis of melanin, collagen, hemoglobin, and connective tissue.	Liver, shellfish, nuts, high-protein cereals, dried fruits, meats.	Not established	Decreased red blood cell production and poor wound healing.

Comments

30% absorbed from diet.

Inversely related to zinc.

Essential for proper iron utilization (erythropoiesis), antioxidant protection and catecholamine synthesis.

Menkes' (kinky-hair) syndrome; absorption disorder.

Toxicity: Wilson's disease (a neurologic and hepatic disorder).

FLUORIDE

See Oral Health Care Products for fluoridation recommendations.

Function	Principal Food Sources	RNI	Signs of Deficiency
Contributes to structure of teeth and soft tissues.	Occurs primarily in water supply (naturally or added).	Not established	Dental caries.

Comments

Other use: osteoporosis (results equivocal).

Toxicity: fluorosis, mottled enamel.

IODINE

Function	Principal Food Sources	RNI	Signs of Deficiency
Synthesis of thyroid hormones, thyroxine and triiodothyronine.	Iodized table salt.	160 µg/day	Cretinism, goiter, myxedema.

Comments

Essential for homeostasis, growth, reproduction, cellular metabolism.

IRON

See Pharmaceutical Agents for toxicity from acute and chronic ingestion.

Function	Principal Food Sources	RNI	Signs of Deficiency
Oxygen carrier to all tissues, and functions in the respiratory chain.	Meats (animal); vegetables (green leafy vegetables) generally have lower bioavailability. (May be increased by consuming with orange juice or other citrus fruits.)	8–9 mg/day	Anemia (tiredness, pallor, nail changes). Severe cases may progress to heart failure. (Most common deficiency in the western world.)

Comments

Iron deficiency common in infants, children, adolescents, women of childbearing age, frequent blood donors, and chronic ASA users.

Dietary absorption is highly variable, ranging from 2 to 35% depending on the source and presence of acid environment.

Meat may increase iron absorption by stimulating gastric acid production. Iron from plant sources is poorly absorbed; ascorbic acid, meat, fish, or poultry may increase the bioavailability of iron from plant sources.

TABLE 7: Principal Micronutrients: Minerals (*cont'd*)

MAGNESIUM

Function	Principal Food Sources	RNI*	Signs of Deficiency
Nerve cell function, enzyme activator, synthesis of skeleton.	Cereals, fruits, vegetables and dairy products.	210–250 mg/day	Occurs in alcoholics, diabetics and malabsorption syndromes. Symptoms: tremor, spasm, irritability, lack of coordination, convulsions.

Comments

Uses in therapy: anticonvulsant, electrolyte replenisher, uterine relaxant (IV magnesium sulfate); oral supplementation, laxative, antacid (PO magnesium).

Depletion may occur secondary to mineralocorticoids, hypophosphatemia and alcohol ingestion.

Hypermagnesemia is rare except in renal impairment; excessive amounts may cause diarrhea.

MANGANESE

Function	Principal Food Sources	RNI	Signs of Deficiency
Cofactor for enzyme systems involved in bone formation, required for formation of mucopolysaccharides.	Fruits, grain products.	Not established	Not observed in humans.

Comments

May substitute for magnesium in some reactions.

MOLYBDENUM

Function	Principal Food Sources	RNI	Signs of Deficiency
Cofactor for xanthine oxidase.	Ubiquitous in all foods.	Not established	Not observed in humans.

PHOSPHORUS

Function	Principal Food Sources	RNI*	Signs of Deficiency
Skeletal synthesis, components of vitamins and essential for coenzyme formation, contributes to structure of teeth and soft tissue.	Found in all foods, especially those with large amounts of protein.	850–1,000 mg/day	Occurs secondary to excessive alcohol consumption or nonabsorbable antacids; prolonged vomiting, liver disease, hyperparathyroidism.

Comments

70% absorbed from jejunum, and maintained by renal resorption.

Dibasic calcium phosphate is used orally.

Hyperphosphatemia is associated with chronic renal disease, hypoparathyroidism, tetany.

TABLE 7: Principal Micronutrients: Minerals (*cont'd*)

POTASSIUM

Function	Principal Food Sources	RNI	Signs of Deficiency
Required for fluid electrolyte balance, acid-base balance, muscle activity, carbohydrate metabolism, protein synthesis.	Whole grain cereals, meats (all types), fish, dairy products, nuts, fruits, and vegetables.	Not established	Leads to painful, sore, weak muscles.

Comments

Major intracellular cation.

Losses occur in gastrointestinal disorders and diarrhea, used in the treatment of diabetic ketoacidosis.

Essential for fluid balance, along with sodium.

Potassium monitoring is essential with the use of potassium-depleting agents (e.g., diuretics, corticosteroids).

SELENIUM

Function	Principal Food Sources	RNI	Signs of Deficiency
Works with vitamin E as a cell membrane antioxidant.	Cereals (dependent on soil content), meat, dairy and poultry products.	Not established	Thigh tenderness, deficiency secondary to TPN or malnutrition.

Comments

Plays a role in prevention of cancer, along with vitamins C and E and β-carotene, in areas with low dietary selenium content.

Marginal deficiency where soil content is low.

SODIUM

Function	Principal Food Sources	RNI	Signs of Deficiency
Required for fluid balance, acid-base balance, cell permeability, normal muscle irritability.	Dietary salt (natural and prepared foods).	Not established	Gastrointestinal losses secondary to diarrhea: weakness, mental confusion, nausea, lethargy, and muscle cramping.

Comments

Major cation of extracellular fluid; serum concentration under control of aldosterone.

Depletion may lead to fluid imbalance, blood pressure changes, changes in membrane permeability, and altered neuromuscular function.

SULFUR

Function	Principal Food Sources	RNI
Skin and cartilage structure; important for coenzyme formation.	Cabbage, cauliflower and other cruciferous vegetables.	Not established

TABLE 7: Principal Micronutrients: Minerals (*cont'd*)

ZINC

Function	Principal Food Sources	RNI	Signs of Deficiency
Growth and maintenance of healthy skin; DNA and RNA synthesis; male sex organs functioning: uptake of insulin by adipocytes, normal olfactory system.	Meat, fish, poultry, dairy products, egg yolk.	9–12 mg/day	Loss of taste or smell, dermatitis, macular degeneration, poor wound healing. Increased losses during surgery, with diabetes, fever, alcohol consumption, and during therapy with corticosteroids, estrogen and thiazide diuretics.

Comments

Zinc therapy may be beneficial in facilitating wound healing (220 mg two to three times daily).

Acute toxicity: anorexia, lethargy, dizziness, and diarrhea.

Moderate doses (150 mg twice daily) have been shown to increase LDL/HDL ratio and to impair cell-mediated immunity.

High doses over prolonged time intervals (e.g. 150 mg/day) may result in copper deficiency.

*RNIs are for adults 25–49 years old; complete RNIS for all age groups are listed in Table 1.

Developed from: Nutrition recommendations—the report of the scientific review committee. Ottawa: Health and Welfare Canada, 1990:132–78. Garrow JS, James WPT, eds. Human Nutrition and Dietetics. 9th ed. Edinburgh: Churchill Livingstone, 1993:146–263.

General Principles of Nutrition

TABLE 8: Clinical Findings That May Reflect Nutrient Deficiencies

Body Area	Signs of Good Nutritional Status	Signs of Poor Nutritional Status	Nutrient(s) Implicated
General appearance	Alert, responsive	Listless, apathetic, cachexic	Energy or vitamin deficiency
General vitality	Endurance, energetic, sleeps well, vigorous	Easily fatigued, no energy, falls asleep easily, looks tired, apathetic	Energy or vitamin deficiency
Hair	Shiny, lustrous, firm, not easily plucked, healthy scalp	Dull and dry, brittle, loss of color, easily plucked, thin and sparse	Protein-calorie malnutrition, zinc
Face	Uniform skin color, healthy appearance, not swollen	Dark skin over cheeks and under eyes, flaky skin, facial edema (moon face), pale skin color	Vitamin A, iron, folate, and/or vitamin B_{12}
Eyes	Bright, clear, moist, no sores at corners of eyelids, and membranes moist and healthy pink color, no prominent blood vessels	Pale eye membranes, dry eyes (xerophthalmia), Bitot's spots, increased vascularity, cornea soft (keratomalacia), small yellowish bumps (xanthelasma), dull or scarred appearance	Vitamin A, riboflavin, pyridoxine, iron, folate, and/or vitamin B_{12}
Lips	Good pink color, smooth, moist, not chapped or swollen	Swollen and puffy (cheilosis), angular lesions at corners of mouth or fissures or scars (stomatitis)	Niacin, riboflavin
Tongue	Deep red, surface papillae present	Smooth appearance, beefy red or magenta colored, swollen, papillae hypertrophy or atrophy	Iron, niacin, riboflavin, folate, and/or vitamin B_{12}
Teeth	Straight, no crowding, no cavities, no pain, bright, no discoloration, well-shaped gums	Cavities, mottled appearance (fluorosis), malpositioned or missing teeth	Fluoride
Gums	Firm, good pink color, no swelling or bleeding	Spongy, bleed easily, marginal redness, recessed, swollen and inflamed	Vitamin C
Glands	No enlargement of the thyroid, face not swollen	Enlargement of thyroid (goiter), enlargement of the parotid (swollen cheeks)	Protein, iodine
Skin	Smooth, good color, slightly moist, no sign of rashes, swelling or color irregularities	Rough, dry, flaky, swollen, pale, pigmented, lack of subcutaneous fat, fat deposits around joints (xanthomas), bruises, petechiae	Vitamin C, niacin, riboflavin, vitamin A, protein, thiamine, zinc, hypercholesterolemia
Nails	Firm, pink	Spoon shaped (koilonychia), brittle, pale, ridged	Iron, vitamin C, zinc
Skeleton	Good posture, no malformation	Poor posture, bending of ribs, bowed legs or knock-knees, prominent scapulae, chest deformity at diaphragm	Vitamin C or D, protein

TABLE 8: Clinical Findings That May Reflect Nutrient Deficiencies (*cont'd*)

Body Area	Signs of Good Nutritional Status	Signs of Poor Nutritional Status	Nutrient(s) Implicated
Muscles	Well developed, firm, good tone, some subcutaneous fat	Flaccid, poor tone, wasted, underdeveloped, difficulty walking	Protein-calorie malnutrition
Extremities	No tenderness	Weak and tender, presence of edema	Protein-calorie malnutrition
Abdomen	Flat	Swollen	Protein-calorie malnutrition
Nervous system	Normal reflexes, psychological stability	Diminished or loss of ankle and knee reflexes, psychomotor changes, mental confusion, depression, sensory loss, motor weakness, loss of sense of position, loss of vibration, burning and tingling of hands and feet (paresthesia)	Thiamine, vitamin B_{12}
Cardiovascular system	Normal heart rate, rhythm, no murmurs, normal blood pressure for age	Cardiomegaly, tachycardia, elevated blood pressure	
Gastrointestinal system	No palpable organs or masses, (liver edge may be palpable in children)	Hepatosplenomegaly	

Adapted from: Bowman A, Stern ML. Parameters in nutritional assessment. In: Bell L, ed. Manual of Nutritional Care. 4th ed. Vancouver: British Columbia Dietitians' & Nutritionists' Association, 1992:71–88.

TABLE 9: Risk Factors for Poor Nutritional Status

Medical History	Social/Economic History	Drug History	Diet History
Alcoholism	Eating alone	Antibiotics	Anorexia nervosa
Anorexia	Inadequate food budget	Antineoplastics	Bulimia
Cancer	Lack of food preparation facilities	Anticonvulsants	Frequently eating out
Cardiovascular disorder	Poor education	Antihypertensives	Inadequate food intake
Circulatory problems	Poor self-concept	Catabolic steroids	Intravenous fluids (other than total parenteral nutrition) for more than 10 days
Constipation	Transportation problems	Oral contraceptives	No intake for 10 or more days
Dental disorders		Vitamins and other nutrient supplements	Poor appetite
Diabetes			Restricted or fad diets
Drug addiction			
Dysphagia			
Fever			
Gastrointestinal disorder			
Heart disease			
Hormonal imbalance			
Hyperlipidemia			
Hypertension			
Renal disorders			
Liver disorders			
Lung disease			
Mental retardation			
Multigravida			
Nausea			
Neurologic disorders			
Overweight			
Pancreatic insufficiency			
Paralysis			
Physical disability			
Pregnancy			
Radiation therapy			
Recent major surgery			
Ulcers			
Underweight			

Adapted from: Whiteney EN, Hamilton EMN, Rolfes SR. Understanding Nutrition. 5th ed. St. Paul: West Publishing Co., 1990:E-3.

TABLE 10: Correlation Between Body Mass Index (BMI) and the Degree of Obesity*

$$BMI = \frac{Weight\ (kg)}{Height\ (m^2)}$$

	BMI	Implication
Underweight	<20	Underweight
Acceptable weight	20–25	Healthy
Overweight	26–27	Caution
Severe overweight	over 27	High risk
Morbid obese	over 29	Very high risk

*The BMI and the waist-to-hip ratio (waist circumference/hip circumference) are used together to evaluate health risk associated with obesity.

TABLE 11: Some Medications Implicated with Weight Gain/Loss

Weight Gain		Weight Loss*
Amitriptyline	Maprotiline	Amphetamine
Amoxapine	Mesoridazine	Antineoplastics (all)
Astemizole	Nifedipine	Benzphetamine
Beta-adrenergic blockers	Nortriptyline	Dextroamphetamine
Chlorpromazine	Perphenazine	Diethylpropion
Chlorprothixene	Phenelzine	Ethacrynic acid
Clomipramine	Prochlorperazine	Fenfluramine
Clozapine	Promethazine	Fluoxetine
Combination oral contraceptives	Protriptyline	Furosemide
Cyproheptadine	Risperidone	Loxapine
Desipramine	Thiopropazate	Mazindol
Doxepin	Thioridazine	Phenmetrazine
Felodipine	Thiothixene	Phentermine
Haloperidol	Trifluoperazine	Phenylpropanolamine
Imipramine	Trimipramine	Pimozide
Ketotifen		
Lithium		
Loxapine		

*Generally weight loss is of short-term duration with the majority of these agents.
Adapted with permission from: Elbe D. Reference Guide to Drug and Nutrient Interactions. In: Bell, L. Manual of Nutritional Care. Vancouver: British Columbia Dietitians' & Nutritionists' Association and B.C. Pharmacy Association, 1992:453–528.

In summary, with greater emphasis on disease prevention, it is only natural for consumers to question the adequacy of their diets. Clinicians are routinely bombarded with questions on the need for supplements. In the majority of the population, vitamin or mineral supplements are not recommended or required. Canada's Food Guide to Healthy Eating forms a rational basis for an adequate and varied diet. Populations at risk for nutrient deficiencies are best referred to physicians and dietitians for assessment and management. In the following sections, principles of nutrition management are discussed for select population groups.

?

PATIENT ASSESSMENT QUESTIONS

Nutrition Products

***Q** Describe or list what you eat on a typical day (breakfast, lunch, snack and supper).*

Open questions are a useful indicator of dietary habits and provide a reasonable assessment of them. Some individuals may forget snacks and beverages consumed and specific questions may be required. Alternatively, keeping a food diary (over a 3- to 7-day interval) may show typical eating habits. Canada's Food Guide to Healthy Eating is a useful tool when assessing clients' diets, illustrating examples from the four basic food groups. Serving sizes are described (2 tablespoons of peanut butter, a source of protein and fat, would be considered one serving from the meat and alternatives food group).

***Q** Why do you feel that you require a vitamin, mineral, or a nutritional supplement?*

Nutritional supplements are frequently purchased by consumers concerned that inadequate nutrients are supplied by their diet, or who have subjective complaints such as tiredness or inability to concentrate.

By being familiar with Canada's Food Guide to Healthy Eating and knowing which natural foods supply RNIs, health care providers should be able to recognize clients with potentially high risk food patterns, such as vegetarian diets or other diets with deficient intake of one or more of the broad food groups. Appropriate physician or dietitian referral may be required for certain deficiencies. Generally speaking, most Canadians' diets meet their RNIs. However, the elderly, pregnant women, strict vegetarians, dieters, patients on certain medications and alcoholics may require additional supplementation (specific nutrient deficiency states and populations at risk are outlined in Tables 5, 6 and 7). Finally, some individuals may have reduced appetites or busy work schedules that warrant nutritional supplements (e.g., meal replacement products).

Further questioning and assessment of the individual may reveal the need for vitamin or nutritional supplements.

***Q** Are you taking any prescription or nonprescription drugs at the present time? Which ones, and how frequently?*

In addition to potential drug-nutrient interactions, some pharmacological agents may suppress the individual's appetite (fluoxetine or systemic decongestants). Table 11 lists drugs that may lead to weight loss or weight gain; additionally, pathological states (e.g., viral gastroenteritis, acquired immunodeficiency syndrome) often lead to appetite suppression. The time a medication is ingested in relation to meals should also be considered when making therapeutic interventions.

***Q** Do you have any chronic medical conditions or a family history of medical problems?*

Certain disease states (e.g., diabetes mellitus or hypertension) are factors that may influence interventions made by health care providers. Some diabetics and hypertensive patients may inquire about antiobesity agents as part of a weight-loss program. Unless recommended by a physician or a dietitian, health professionals should refrain from recommending products containing adrenergic blockers, such as phenylpropanolamine, or local anesthetics, such as benzocaine. (See the Principles of Weight Control Section.)

***Q** Describe your lifestyle. For example, do you smoke, drink, or exercise?*

Lifestyle modification should play the biggest role in nutritional problems. Individuals who want to increase or decrease their body weight should be informed of the benefits of exercise in increasing lean body mass (muscle).

Chronic alcohol ingestion leads to deficiencies in thiamine and other B vitamins. These individuals should be counselled on the benefits of adequate nutrition and decreasing the consumption of alcohol. Chronic alcohol ingestion can lead to appetite suppression, possibly because of its calorigenic effect.

Much has been discussed about the health risks of smoking. Smokers are at a higher risk for the development of lung cancer, as well as for coronary artery disease. Unfortunately, concern over rebound weight gain is often a major deterrent for individuals contemplating smoking cessation. Weight gain of up to 10 pounds may occur in a matter of several weeks to months in those who stop smoking. Clients concerned about potential weight gain should be reminded that the gain is not necessarily permanent, and may be prevented by following a sensible diet along with exercise.

PRINCIPLES OF INFANT NUTRITION

BREAST-FEEDING

Benefits of Breast-feeding: The Nutrition Committee of the Canadian Paediatric Society recommends breast-feeding until the infant is at least 9 to 12 months of age.

Benefits to both mother and child include:

Nutritional: correct balance of protein, fat, lactose, vitamins and minerals; easy to digest.

Immunological: colostrum (milk secreted in the first 5 days postpartum) is a rich source of antibodies; immunity to specific antigens can be passed via the mother to the infant throughout lactation.

Psychological: promotes mother-infant bonding.

Physical: oxytocin release stimulates contraction of uterus back to normal state more quickly; some protection against breast cancer; contributes to mother's weight loss, jaw and tooth development of infant from sucking.

Economical: extra calories required to feed lactating mother are less expensive than commercial formulas.

Convenience: safe, fresh and optimal temperature.

Contraindications to Breast-feeding: There are few instances where breast-feeding is positively contraindicated. Where there is a definite contraindication, alternative therapy may be possible. Absolute contraindications include:

If the mother:

- has breast cancer;
- has HIV/AIDS;
- is abusing drugs or alcohol;
- is taking certain drugs.

If the infant has:

- galactosemia or inborn errors of metabolism;
- phenylketonuria;
- urea cycle disorder;
- homocystinuria;
- tyrosinemia.

Composition of Breast Milk: The composition of breast milk varies little from day to day and woman to woman. Some nutrients (e.g., fatty acids, vitamins A, E and some B vitamins) have been shown to be influenced by the mother's intake (Table 12).

Establishment of Breast-feeding: The supply of breast milk depends on the demand of the infant and increases with frequent feeding (every 2 to 3 hours - 8 to 12 feedings/24 hours). As the infant's stomach capacity and efficiency at nursing increases, the interval between feedings lengthens.

Breast-feeding is considered sufficient if the baby:

- has 6 to 8 wet diapers/day;
- has frequent loose stools;
- swallows frequently while at breast;
- is content between feedings;
- has weight gain of about 30 g (1 oz)/day.

If the infant is not thriving, breast-feeding may be supplemented with appropriate formula. While supplementing, to keep up the mother's milk supply, express milk with a breast pump. The expressed milk can be used immediately or stored for future use.

Storage of Breast Milk: Place expressed breast milk in sterilized jars and refrigerate for 24 to 48 hours. Milk can be frozen at -20°C for up to 6 months. To thaw, set in a pan of warm water. Never let the milk stand at room temperature. Thawed milk must be refrigerated and used within 24 hours. Never refreeze breast milk.

Nutritional Requirements of Infants

- Infants have greater nutritional requirements for their weight than adults. They need nutrients for maintenance, growth and development, while the adult's requirements are primarily for maintenance.
- Energy and protein requirements are calculated using RNIs and based on the child's age, sex and body weight.

	Energy	**Protein**
Birth	500 kcal/day	2 g/kg/day
1 year of age	1,100 kcal/day	1.2 g/kg/day
Adolescence	2,500 kcal/day	1.0 g/kg/day

- Milk, ideally breast milk, provides all the nourishment a baby requires for the first few months of life. At 6 months, solid foods are added to meet nutritional needs.

TABLE 12: Composition of Mature Human Milk (15 days-15 months Postpartum)							
Protein (g/100 mL)	**Carbohydrate (g/100 mL)**	**Energy (kcal/100 mL)**	**Minerals (mg/100 mL)**		**Renal Solute Load (mOsm/L)**	**Fat (g/100 mL)**	
1.05 ± 0.20	7.2 ± 0.25	72 ± 5	Sodium	18 ± 4	290 ± 5	3.9 ± 0.04	
Whey: Casein	(100% Lactose)	(6% protein	Potassium	52.3 ± 3.5		Monounsaturated	38%
80:20		34% CHO	Calcium	28 ± 2.6		Polyunsaturated	15%
		55% fat)	Phosphorus	14 ± 2.2		Saturated	42%
			Chloride	42 ± 6			
			Iron	0.03 ± 0.01			

*Human milk consists of 88% ± 1 water. Adapted from: Wyeth-Ayerst Canada Inc. Infant Formula Comparison Chart, 1994; and Composition of mature human milk. Pediatric Nutrition Handbook. 2nd ed. Elk Grove Village, Ill: American Academy of Pediatrics, 1993.

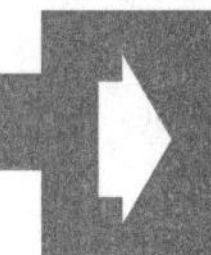

ADVICE FOR THE PATIENT

Breast-feeding

Breast-feeding is the best form of nourishment for young infants and the Nutrition Committee of the Canadian Paediatric Society recommends it until the infant is at least 9 to 12 months of age.

- A commercial formula should replace breast milk if weaning takes place before the infant is 6 months old.
- A totally breast-fed infant is rarely constipated; changes in frequency and consistency of stools can occur and are not considered a problem unless accompanied by other symptoms: vomiting, anorexia, frequent colic, failure to thrive, abdominal distress, etc.
- To express breast milk, either a hand expression technique or a breast pump may be used: refer to La Leche League or a public health nurse.
- Sore, cracked nipples should be checked by the physician or public health nurse for thrush (candida or yeast infection). If no infection is present, the best treatment is "hind-milk" expressed from the breast at the end of a feed and massaged into the nipple and areola area (it contains lysozyme, which is antibacterial). Any creams or ointments, if used, must be removed before breast-feeding the baby.
- Mastitis is any inflammation of the breast (e.g., plugged duct) and can be very painful. If an infection results, treatment with a systemic antibiotic is required. This should not cause disruption or termination of breast-feeding.

Vitamin/Mineral Supplementation of Breast-fed Infants: A summary table of vitamin and mineral supplement requirements for breast-fed infants can be found in Table 13.

Multivitamins should be given to breast-fed infants of mothers who are nutritionally at risk, e.g., poor dietary habits, marginal intake, low socioeconomic status.

INFANT FORMULAS

Commercial infant formulas are designed to simulate breast milk and provide the best alternative for the first 9 to 12 months. Three general uses for infant formulas are when:

- breast-feeding is contraindicated;
- breast-feeding is not chosen;
- supplementation is required (when mothers choose to omit a breast-feeding or mother's milk production is inadequate).

These products are available as powdered concentrates, liquid concentrates and ready-to-use liquids. Instructions for preparation should be strictly followed to avoid over or under dilution of nutrients and electrolytes. If formula is too dilute, the infant will not get enough nourishment; if too concentrated, it could cause hypernatremia, hyperkalemia and dehydration. The osmolarity or number of particles in 1 L of solution of infant formulas should be less than 400 mOsm/L. The osmolarity of infant formulas when diluted properly generally falls below this suggested limit (range of 150 to 380 mOsm/L). At the retail level, all infant formulas sold provide 284 kJ (68 kcal)/100 mL when prepared according to the manufacturer's label.

The Nutrition Committee of the Canadian Paediatric Society recommends that all formulas be fortified with iron (7 to 10 mg elemental iron/L). Low iron (1.5 mg elemental iron/L) formulas do exist to lessen the possibility of constipation and other feeding problems, though studies have shown that constipation is not a major problem and the only difference in iron-fortified formula users was a darker stool.

Types of Formulas

Cow's Milk Protein Formulas: These are the most commonly used commercial infant formulas. Unmodified cow's milk is casein dominant (whey: casein is 20:80) and high in total protein. The cow's milk based formulas are modified to resemble both the nutrient composition and digestibility of breast milk; they may be whey or casein dominant. Bovine whey and casein differ from human whey and casein. Although breast milk is whey predominant, bovine whey may be more allergenic. Beta-lactoglobulin, the most antigenic protein, is only present in trace amounts in human whey but is high in bovine whey. Since cow's milk is higher in total protein than breast milk, formulas have decreased protein levels, which have been heat treated to minimize allergenicity and maximize digestibility. The carbohydrate source is either all lactose, or a combination of lactose, corn syrup or cornstarch, although some formulations are now lactose-free. The fat of cow's milk formulas has also been altered and replaced with a more digestible form.

Recommended Use:

- routine feeding of most infants who are not breast-fed.

Soy Protein Formulas: These formulas contain methionine-fortified soy protein isolate (to enhance the biological value of the soy protein), vegetable oils and a carbohydrate source other than lactose. They are higher in protein (because of the decreased absorption of plant protein) and electrolytes than breast milk.

Recommended Use:

- intolerance to cow's milk protein. (Note: there may be cross-sensitivity between soy and cow's milk protein.);
- galactosemia;
- lactose intolerance (although a lactose-free cow's milk formula is available);
- infants of vegetarian families who avoid all animal protein.

Hydrolyzed Protein Formulas: The milk protein, either casein or whey, is hydrolyzed to peptides of

TABLE 13: Suggested Vitamin/Mineral Supplementation of Breast-Fed Infants

Vitamin	Dose	Comment
Vitamin B_1 (thiamine)	0.3 mg/day	If the mother is thiamine deficient
Vitamin B_{12}	0.3 µg/day	If mother is a strict vegetarian, supplement mother and infant
Vitamin D	400 IU/day starting at birth	Vitamin D content of human milk is low (22 IU/L) Especially important if deeply pigmented or little or no exposure to sunlight (rickets)
Vitamin K	Single dose at birth IM 0.5–1 mg or PO 1–2 mg	For prophylaxis against hemorrhagic disease of newborn Prevents or minimizes the postnatal decline of vitamin K dependent factors (II, VII, IX and X)
Minerals		
Iron	1 mg/kg/day at 6 months (if not given iron-fortified cereals)	Iron in breast milk has a high bioavailability so sufficient iron is provided for the first 6 months
Fluoride	Not recommended <3 years of age	Canadian Dental Association guidelines suggest supplementation only if >3 years and if fluoride in water supply is <0.3 ppm (mg/L)

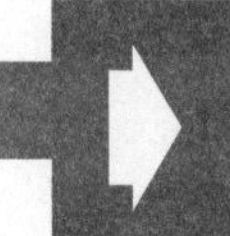

ADVICE FOR THE PATIENT

Nutrition for the Lactating Mother

- Prepare for nursing before birth by consuming approximately 2,050 to 2,850 kcal/day.
- Supplement meals on demand with nutritious snacks: milk, milk drinks, fruit, cheese, nuts and seeds, whole grain muffins, etc.
- Follow Canada's Food Guide to Healthy Eating (for breast-feeding). Consume a minimum daily quantity of: 3 to 4 servings of milk or equivalent; 2 to 3 servings of meat/fish/poultry; 5 to 12 servings of whole grain bread or cereal; 5 to 10 servings of fruit and vegetables.
- Caffeine consumption (coffee, tea, cola drinks) should be limited.
- Avoid alcoholic beverages or restrict use.
- Restrict nicotine use since it can reduce milk supply.
- Fluid intake should be at least 2 L/day.
- Use of a calcium supplement is recommended if unable to consume milk or intolerant to milk.
- Iron supplementation should be continued postpartum.
- Vitamin and mineral supplementation is not required if an adequate diet is maintained. Vegetarian lactating mothers require vitamin B_{12} and calcium (if no dairy products are consumed).

<1,200 molecular weight, which are small enough that they are incapable of eliciting an immunologic response in many infants. Casein hydrolysates have been on the market for about 40 years. The newer whey hydrolysates are not as extensively hydrolyzed and therefore have considerable antigenic potential.

Recommended Use:

- whey hydrolysate for managing milk protein or soy protein intolerance but not allergy;
- casein hydrolysate for infants with cow's milk protein intolerance and/or allergy;
- both are used for infants with severe feeding problems, e.g., cystic fibrosis where there are deficient intestinal enzymes.

Lactose-free Modified Cow's Milk Based Formulas: Formulations may consist of cow's milk or soy protein, and can be used temporarily or long-term, depending on the type of lactase deficiency.

Recommended Use:

- primary lactase deficiency;
- secondary lactase deficiency (e.g., postinfectious gastroenteritis, celiac disease, Crohn's disease, etc).

Fibre-containing Formulas: Recently, fibre-containing formulas have been shown to shorten the duration of diarrhea in infants and toddlers. The fibre, both soluble and insoluble, delays gastric emptying and increases fecal bulk. The protein is soy based. The infant must be rehydrated with an oral electrolyte solution for 1 to 2 days before starting the formula, which is taken for approximately 1 week, to minimize recurrence of the diarrhea. Following with a lactose-free formula temporarily may be indicated, then the infant returned to the original formula or breast milk.

Recommended Use:

- short-term feeding for infants and young children with loose, watery diarrhea.

Evaporated Milk: These formulas are not recommended for <6 months of age and >6 months is questionable. They do not meet requirements for essential fatty acids, folate, vitamin D or iron. They contain higher concentrations of electrolytes, protein, calcium and phosphorus than commercial infant formulas or breast milk. There is a greater chance for error in preparation.

Preparation:

- <6 months of age: 1:2 dilution of evaporated whole milk to water plus powdered dextrose or sucrose to yield 280 kJ/100 mL (67 kcal/100 mL), e.g., 30 mL evaporated whole milk; 60 mL water plus 5 mL of sucrose or powdered dextrose or sucrose (Dilute 1 can (1,155 mL) of evaporated whole milk with 2 cans (3,310 mL) of water and add 4 tablespoonsful of sugar.);
- >6 months of age: 1:1 dilution of evaporated whole milk to water plus powdered dextrose or sucrose to yield 280 kJ/100 mL (67 kcal/100 mL).

Formulas for Premature Infants: These formulas are used for premature infants until their weight reaches 1,800 to 2,000 g. Two categories exist—a hospitalization formula and a postdischarge formula, only the latter available retail. Both are concentrated forms of macro- and micronutrients that the neonate requires. The postdischarge formula may be used for up to 1 year in infants born prematurely. Hospital formulas may or may not contain iron. An iron formula is recommended; additional iron supplementation is not required unless anemia has been diagnosed. Additional vitamin/mineral supplementation is not required if the infant is receiving an appropriate premature formula.

Follow-up Formulas: These formulas are for infants >6 months of age and contain more iron, vitamin D and protein than other infant formulas. They offer little benefit to infants satisfied on breast milk or infant formula supplemented with solids. Some follow-up formulas are less costly, designed to minimize the early introduction of regular cow's milk.

Cow's Milk: Cow's milk is not recommended before 9 to 12 months of age; informed medical opinion tends toward 12 months because:

- iron from cow's milk is poorly absorbed;
- cow's milk decreases the absorption of other sources of iron, both dietary and medicinal;
- cow's milk may cause occult blood loss from the intestinal tract;
- cow's milk provides inadequate amounts of linoleic acid;
- cow's milk has a potentially high renal solute load.

If cow's milk is introduced before 12 months of age, it should be whole cow's milk rather than 2%, 1% or skim milk because the latter provide inadequate energy and linoleic acid, excessive protein and an unsuitably high potential renal solute load. Low-fat milk can be introduced at about 2 years of age.

Goat's Milk: Fresh goat's milk is not recommended; it is deficient in folate, vitamin D and C, and the fat is not easily digested. The three deficient vitamins have been added to evaporated goat's milk.

A management algorithm for infant nutrition for full-term infants is provided at Figure 1.

Vitamin and Mineral Supplementation for the Formula-fed Infant

Vitamins: Commercial infant formulas contain adequate amounts of vitamins, and no additional supplementation is required.

Iron: Infants on iron-fortified formulas that provide 7 to 13 mg iron/L do not require iron supplementation. At 6 months of age, the introduction of solids contributes additional iron that helps to maintain iron stores. The bioavailability of iron from fresh pasteurized cow's milk is poor (may be due to the high calcium and phosphorus and low ascorbic acid content). Therefore, fresh cow's milk is not recommended until 12 months of age, when the use of high-iron solids (iron-fortified cereals, strained meats and strained vegetables) and ascorbic acid-containing foods or fluids has been well established. If there are extenuating circumstances, e.g., socioeconomic population where cost is prohibitive, evaporated cow's milk may be used, since the protein is more digestible than regular cow's milk but strongly encourage doing so only under a physician's advice.

Fluoride: Supplementation is not recommended for children < 3 years of age regardless of fluoride content of water.

Introduction of Solids

The appropriate age for introduction of solid foods is 4 to 6 months. Single ingredient or first foods are introduced one at a time at intervals of several days to a week to identify intolerance. Rice cereal is usually well tolerated and is recommended as the first solid food. In the absence of any symptom of intolerance (skin rashes, diarrhea or wheezing), a second food such as oatmeal or barley cereal is presented. Note that *Milupa* cereals are not exclusively cereal as they also contain milk formula.

Guide to Introduction of Solids:

- 4 to 6 months of age: iron-enriched infant cereal.
- 6 to 9 months of age: (in the following order) pureed vegetables; pureed fruit and juices; pureed meat, fish, poultry; egg yolk; begin to vary texture with yogurt, cottage cheese, pureed well-cooked legumes, dried bread products (rusks).
- 9 to 12 months of age: mashed foods without sugar, butter, margarine, salt or other seasonings;

finger foods such as peeled fruit pieces, cooked vegetable pieces, dry toast, mild cheese; delay egg white until 12 months.

Water

Healthy infants usually require no supplemental water as the amount needed to replace water loss is available in human milk or infant formula. Additional water should be provided when the weather is hot, when fluid intake is low or extrarenal losses are increased, such as during an illness.

Weaning

Weaning should be done gradually over several months as more solid foods are added to the infant's diet. This can begin as early as 6 months of age but is more common at about 12 months of age, when the infant should be receiving some solid food. Once weaning is complete, 2 cups of milk a day should be consumed up to at least 5 years of age.

Vitamin and Mineral Supplementation After 12 Months of Age

No supplementation is required if the child's diet follows Canada's Food Guide to Healthy Eating and includes adequate sources of vitamin C and iron. If the child has an inadequate dietary intake (e.g., impoverished or fussy eater), a multivitamin preparation that supplies close to 100% RNI for each vitamin would help meet the requirements of proper growth. However, every effort should be made to correct poor dietary habits.

Children's multivitamin tablets are often not recommended for children less than 3 years of age because tablets cannot be properly chewed at this age. The vitamin drops are much more convenient. If the cost of the vitamin drops is a factor, the chewable children's multivitamin tablets may be broken and sprinkled onto food.

Common Concerns

It is quite common for toddlers to go through no-growth stages when their appetites are reduced. This is normal, and vitamin supplementation is not usually indicated.

Spitting is very common, usually resolves in 2 to 3 months without treatment and is not a concern for formula change.

Regurgitation may be due to gastroesophageal reflux but does not usually require a change in formula unless it persists.

Stool changes are usually not of concern unless the infant has chronic diarrhea (>2 weeks). If the stool has a high fluid content it may be a sign of carbohydrate intolerance or gastroenteritis (viral or bacterial); try a lactose- and sucrose-free formula, or a diarrhea formulation under a physician's advice. If the stool is large, bulky, pale or oily, it may be a sign of malabsorption; try a hydrolyzed protein, altered fat formula. The physician should be consulted regarding any formula change.

FIGURE 1

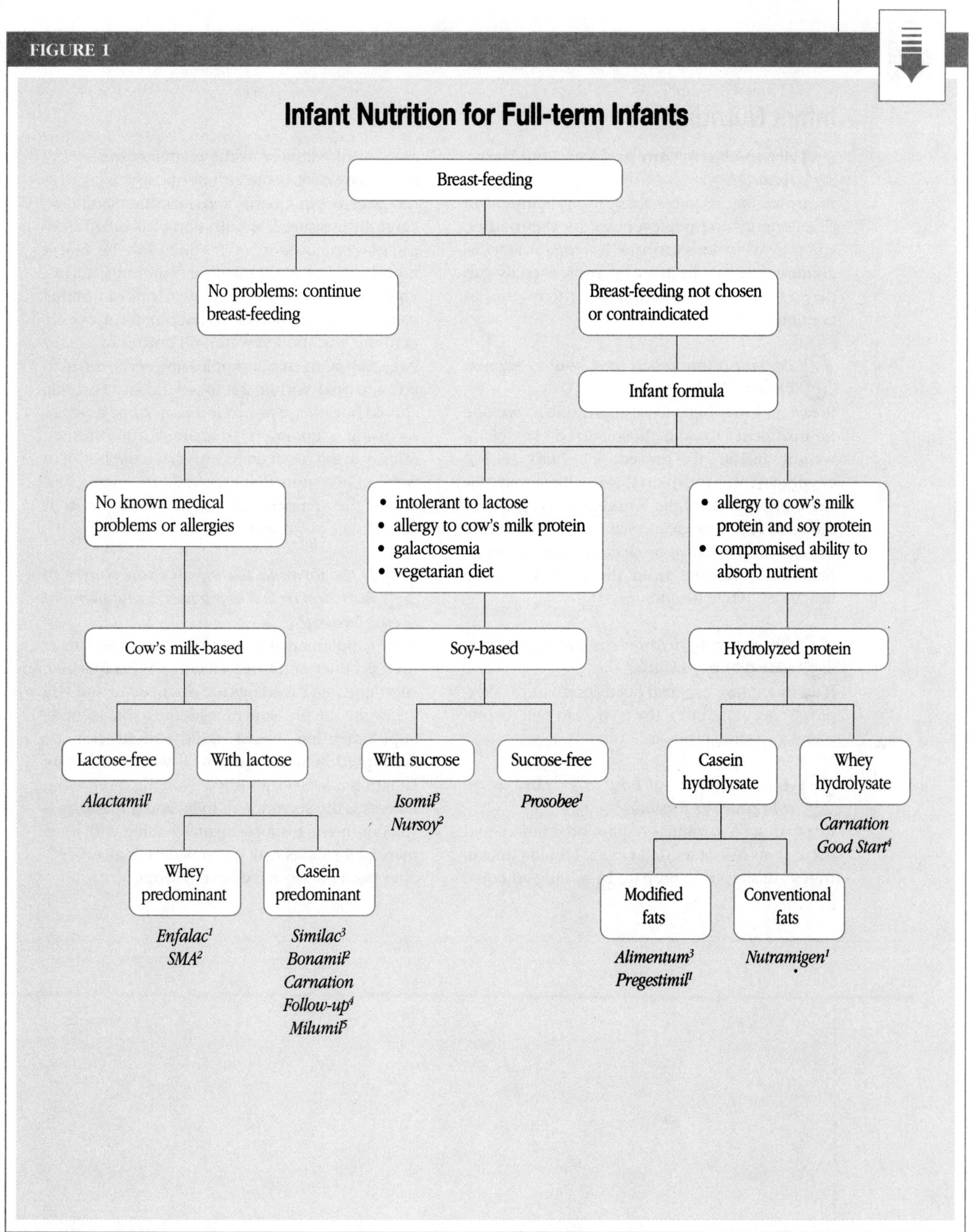

1–Mead Johnson 2–Wyeth-Ayerst Ltd. 3–Ross 4–Nestlé 5–Milupa (distributed by Wyeth-Ayerst Ltd.)

PATIENT ASSESSMENT QUESTIONS

Infant Nutrition

Q Are you having any problems with breast-feeding?

Breast-feeding requires a major commitment in time, energy and perseverance by the mother, and many situations can arise leading to early discontinuance. All health care professionals can play a major role in encouraging the mother to continue.

Q Do you know when and how to express breast milk?

Breast milk may need to be expressed: to provide nourishment to the hospitalized low-birth-weight infant; to prevent or help relieve engorgement; to help establish milk supply; for the convenience of the working mother. Breast milk can either be expressed by hand or with a breast pump (manual or electric). Further information is available from the local La Leche League or public health nurse.

Q Did your physician recommend a particular type of formula?

If an infant has a special need (premature, allergies, vegetarian, etc.), the physician will recommend a specific formula.

Q Are you aware of how to prepare, store and heat the formula?

Ready-to-serve formulas require no dilution, and there is no risk of mixing errors. Liquid concentrates are simple to prepare by adding an equal amount of water or as the manufacturer's label states. Powdered concentrates pose the greatest risk of errors in mixing, and quantities should be carefully measured. Sterilization of all infant feeding equipment is recommended for the first 4 months. Use water boiled for 5 minutes, and all equipment boiled for 5 minutes, tops of formula cans rinsed with boiling water; mix formula concentrate with boiled water, fill bottles or nurser bags, top with sterile nipples and seals, refrigerate and use within 24 to 48 hours. Formula should be either warmed in a pan of hot water or by using a commercial steam bottle warmer. Microwaving heats unevenly: shake the bottle to prevent hot spots that may scald the infant, and check the temperature on inside of wrist. It should feel warm, not hot.

Q Is the formula the infant's sole source of nutrition or is it being used to supplement breast-feeding?

Early supplemental feedings can decrease breast milk production. When lactation is established, supplementary feedings are not needed and will aggravate the problem of inadequate breast milk. Supplementing breast milk should not be attempted before the age of 8 weeks or before lactation is well established. Nursing more often increases the secretion of milk, and if the baby is still not thriving, supplemental feeding with commercial formulas may be considered, given only after both breasts have been offered.

PRINCIPLES OF WEIGHT CONTROL

SYMPTOMS OF OBESITY

Obesity is common in industrialized nations such as Canada. The results of the Canadian Health Promotion Survey (1988) indicate that 47.7% of Canadian women and 37.1% of Canadian men are obese according to the Body Mass Index (BMI). Studies found a greater prevalence of obesity in North American adults compared to similar populations in Europe and Australia. Nine to 15% of North Americans between the ages of 25 to 65 are likely to be severely overweight compared to 7% of age-matched counterparts living in Australia. Obesity and overweight are concerns for North American children as well. The prevalence of obesity appears to be increasing.

Obesity, simply defined, is characterized by accumulation of fat in the storage areas of the body that exceeds the amount required for normal body function. Various methods are used to quantify obesity.

An approach adapted in Canada since 1988 uses the BMI as a measure of obesity (see the section on Nutritional Assessment and Table 10). The Waist-to-Hip Ratio (WHR) is also an important determinant of the risks associated with obesity. Calculated by dividing the circumference of the waist by that of the buttocks/hips, a WHR of ≥0.95 for men and women indicates a greater risk for development of major illnesses such as diabetes and hypertension.

Despite its widespread prevalence, a single identifiable cause can only be found in a small proportion of individuals. Weight gain in excess of 1 kg per day invariably implies fluid retention and is frequently a sign of cardiovascular, renal or hepatic disorder. Drugs may also lead to fluid retention, either directly (e.g., glucocorticoids and related agents) or indirectly (drugs with high sodium content). Endocrinopathies such as insulinoma, Cushing's disease or thyroid dysfunction may also be implicated in weight gain. In the majority of cases, weight gain has no single identifiable cause, and may be considered as a group of heterogeneous disorders.

Obesity is associated with a number of metabolic abnormalities and complications for the individual. Relative insulin refractoriness (insulin burnout) is a significant metabolic complication in obesity: the individual consumes more calories for energy, resulting in a vicious cycle of weight gain. Severe obesity is often complicated by a number of serious coexisting disorders (Table 14). Central distribution of body fat (WHR ≥0.95 for men and women, "android" distribution) as well as "yo-yo dieting" (dieting that results in repeated cycles of weight loss and gain) appear to enhance the risk for developing coronary heart disease. Data suggest that moderately and severely obese individuals are at greater risk for morbidity and mortality.

The principal feature the obese client presents with is increased body weight with an obvious mass of fatty tissue. Some individuals may be overweight (e.g., athletes), but this increased muscle mass does not mean they are obese. Clients usually have cosmetic complaints (e.g., inability to wear certain types of clothes). Individuals with symptoms or complaints outlined in Table 15 should be referred to a physician for further diagnostic evaluation. They may require medical management for potentially serious illnesses such as congestive heart failure or sleep apnea.

TREATMENT PRINCIPLES

Those desiring to lose weight should be reminded that weight loss should be gradual, persistent and have several components for maximum success: social support; willingness to exercise; realistic expectations; and an attitude of self-acceptance. The treatment of obesity has to be multifactorial

TABLE 14: Conditions Associated with Obesity
Cerebrovascular disease
Congestive heart failure
Diabetes
Flat feet
Gallbladder disease
Hiatus hernia
Hyperlipidemia
Hypertension
Intertriginous dermatitis
Obstetric complications
Osteoarthritis
Respiratory distress syndrome
Varicose veins

Adapted with permission from: Tinks M, Garrison MW. Obesity and eating disorders. In: Herfindal ET, Gourley DR, Hart LL, eds. Clinical Pharmacy and Therapeutics. Baltimore: Williams & Wilkins, 1992:984–95.

and individualized; standard treatments quickly lead to noncompliance unless the program is tailored to the client's personality, lifestyle, and health status. Motivation and behavior modification along with reasonable goals and expectations are key elements. Crash diets and programs usually decrease weight initially (due to a fluid shift from glycogenolysis and proteolysis), but can quickly lead to rebound weight gain (yo-yo dieting) that in turn poses health risks to the client.

A comprehensive weight reduction program should incorporate diet management, exercise, counselling, and possibly pharmacologic and invasive treatments. Three critical and underlying factors for successful weight control are:

- calorie expenditure should exceed calorie intake (e.g., increasing activity);
- a permanent change in calorie intake must be continued to maintain a healthy weight; and
- a fixation on weight or the scale avoided as it can be discouraging.

Nonpharmacological Treatment

Calorie Restriction: A modest reduction in calorie intake by following Canada's Food Guide to Healthy Eating, decreasing fat intake and setting reasonable goals and expectations is the most palatable method of treatment. Based on the Harris-Benedict Equations[a], in theory, a 500 kcal/day deficit can be imposed to lead to a weekly weight loss of 0.5 kg. In reality, this degree of calorie restriction quickly leads to noncompliance and boredom in the client.

Canada's Food Guide to Healthy Eating is well suited to overweight individuals. It is easy to follow, represents relatively low energy intakes and ensures that nutrient recommendations are met with no added supplementation. It should be stressed to the client that dietary fat should not exceed 30% of the total energy intake as recommended in the guidelines (Table 16). Restriction of dietary fat is crucial to weight loss since the conversion of dietary fat, a concentrated form of energy, in the body occurs much more easily with lipids than carbohydrates. Several studies suggest benefits in using low-fat diets for weight reduction:

- Sheppard et al concluded that weight loss was more closely associated with the percentage of dietary fat rather than changes in total calorie intake;
- Prewitt and colleagues reported that increased weight loss occurred on a low-fat diet despite overall increased calorie intake;
- Kendall et al reported that weight can be lost by reducing dietary fat without any further restrictions of food intake.

Under no circumstances should clients undertake crash diets without medical supervision. The 200 to 500 kcal/day in a liquid meal provide a calorie deficit while aiming to preserve lean body mass. Advertised to consumers under such names as the "Last Chance Diet" or the "Cambridge Diet," they are potentially harmful. The "Last Chance Diet" resulted in dozens of cardiovascular fatalities due to negative nitrogen balance and subsequent protein tissue loss. These diets should be restricted to moderately-to-severely obese patients under close medical supervision, with special attention to cardiovascular monitoring. Diets below 1,800 kcal/day often lead to micronutrient deficiencies; a multivitamin and mineral supplement may be indicated.

Yo-yo dieting may also result, with continued on and off calorie restriction. During times of calorie reduction, the metabolism slows down, more efficiently using energy. When calorie intake increases, weight gain results. Over time, the body gets used to functioning on fewer calories, making weight loss difficult unless exercise is begun.

Exercise: The second component of weight reduction is physical activity. Regular aerobic exercise increases energy expenditure, favors the mobilization of adipose tissue and allows weight maintenance. Regular exercise increases the basal metabolic rate, which is normally diminished after prolonged calorie restriction. A regular exercise program undertaken at least 3 times a week over a

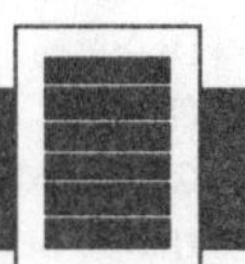

TABLE 15: Symptoms or Complaints that Require Further Evaluation

- Exertional or nocturnal dyspnea
- Persistent backache and low back pain
- Inflammation of weight-bearing joints
- Massive obesity
- Peculiar fat distribution
- Sudden or rapid weight gain
- Signs of depression or anxiety leading to repeated snacking

a The Harris-Benedict Equation is a formal method used to estimate caloric requirements for an individual:
men: resting energy expenditure (kcal/day) = 66 + (13.8 x weight in kg) + (5 x height in cm) - (6.8 x age in yrs).
women: resting energy expenditure (kcal/day) = 655 + (9.6 x weight in kg) + (1.8 x height in cm) - (4.7 x age in yrs).

30-minute interval should lead to an expenditure of at least 300 kcal (e.g., brisk walking, jogging or swimming). Aerobic exercise (e.g., walking) is the most effective for burning fat. The moderately-to-severely obese are often poor candidates for exercise, and any regimen should be preceded by a thorough medical evaluation.

Behavior Modification: Whether through group meetings or one-on-one counselling sessions, the primary goal of behavioral therapy is to modify eating behaviors. Therapy is targeted at levels:

Self-monitoring (e.g., daily food records or diary keeping) that identifies when and where foods are eaten throughout the day.

Modifying habits: Once aware of eating patterns and habits, the individual focuses on limiting the specific times and places food can be eaten. Other habits taught at this level include chewing food a specific number of times and taking sips between each bite.

Positive self-feedback: This stage reinforces the positive steps taken by the client toward weight reduction. Most studies demonstrate the effectiveness of behavioral modification in maintaining a prolonged period of weight loss compared to programs that do not include it.

Self-esteem: Examining the issues surrounding the need to eat when the stomach is full. Psychological counselling may be indicated.

Pharmacological Treatment

Appetite Suppressants: Drug therapy of obesity does not appear to provide greater benefits over previously mentioned therapies. The role of appetite suppressants appears to be fairly limited in the management of obesity and should not be routinely used for weight control. Early use of appetite suppressants in the management of obesity detracts the client from the importance of adhering to dietary and behavioral measures that are so critical to long-term success. Appetite suppressants should be reserved for the morbidly obese refractory to intervention by traditional methods alone. Any pharmacotherapy should be guided by a physician familiar with the uses (and misuses) of anorectic agents. Dieting products currently available directly to the consumer in Canada include benzocaine and bulking agents such as methylcellulose. These agents are not appetite suppressants per se; they have a locally acting effect on the gastrointestinal tract.

Information evaluating nonprescription anorectic agents is limited. Data suggest that benzocaine and methylcellulose may lead to limited weight loss over a 10-week period. However, no placebo-controlled trials exist to demonstrate the degree of weight loss that can be attributed to these agents alone. Products containing benzocaine should ideally be in a lozenge or chewing gum formulation to work at the site of action. Unfortunately, some appetite-suppressants are marketed as tablets, which bypass the site of action. In the United States, the Food and Drug Administration (FDA) has approved benzocaine as generally effective for short-term weight control. A dose of 3 to 15 mg (gum, lozenges or candy) taken prior to meals was generally safe and effective.

Phenylpropanolamine, it should be noted, is not approved by Health Canada for weight loss, but has been used by consumers attempting to lose weight. Problems include relapse (loss of efficacy occurring over weeks to months), and more importantly, a potential for toxicity (due to its narrow therapeutic index, with adverse effects on the central nervous and cardiovascular systems).

Phenylpropanolamine was approved for short-term weight control by the FDA in 1982. Doses of up to 37.5 mg (immediate-release products) and 75 mg (sustained-release products) have been approved as safe and effective for short-term weight control. Side effects such as nervousness, restlessness, insomnia, dizziness, perspiration, anxiety, headache, nausea and an excessive pressor response may occur when recommended doses are exceeded or when the drug is combined with other sympathomimetics (e.g., caffeine). Health care professionals should refrain from recommending phenylpropanolamine for weight control.

TABLE 16: Total Daily Fat Intake for Specific Kilocaloric Levels

Kilocaloric Levels	Grams of Fat Per Day
1200	27-33
1500	33-42
1800	40-50
2000	44-56
2200	40-61
2400	53-67

Note: Total fat intake restricted to 20-25% of total caloric intake. One portion of fries (25 pieces) contains more than 17 g of fat. 15 g of fat = 1 tablespoon fat (e.g., margarine, butter, oil, etc).

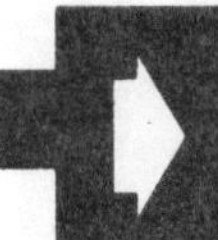

ADVICE FOR THE PATIENT

Behavioral Principles of Weight Loss

Stimulus Control

Shopping

Shop for food after eating.
Shop from a list.
Avoid ready-to-eat foods.
Don't carry more cash than needed for shopping.

Plans

Plan to limit food intake.
Substitute exercise for snacking.
Eat meals and snacks at scheduled times.
Don't accept food offered by others.

Activities

Store foods out of sight.
Eat all food in the same place.
Remove food from inappropriate storage areas in the house.
Keep serving dishes off the table.
Use smaller dishes and utensils.
Avoid being the food server.
Leave the table immediately after eating.
Don't save leftovers.

Holidays and parties

Drink fewer alcoholic beverages.
Plan eating habits before parties.
Eat a low-kilocalorie snack before parties.
Practice polite ways to decline food.
Don't get discouraged by an occasional setback.

Eating Behavior

Put the fork down between mouthfuls.
Chew thoroughly before swallowing.
Prepare foods one portion at a time.
Leave some food on the plate.
Pause in the middle of the meal.
Do nothing else while eating (e.g., read, watch television).

Reward

Solicit help from family and friends.
Help family and friends provide this help in the form of praise and material rewards.
Utilize self-monitoring records as a basis for rewards.
Plan specific rewards for specific behaviors (behavioral contracts).

Self-Monitoring

Keep a diet diary that includes:

Time and place of eating.
Type and amount of food.
Who is present/How you feel.

Nutrition Education

Use a diet diary to identify problem areas.
Make small changes that you can continue.
Learn nutritional values of foods.
Decrease fat intake; increase complex carbohydrates.

Physical Activity

Routine activity

Increase routine activity.
Increase use of stairs.
Keep a record of distance walked each day.

Exercise

Begin a very mild exercise program.
Keep a record of daily exercise.
Increase the exercise very gradually.

Cognitive Restructuring

Avoid setting unreasonable goals.
Think about progress, not shortcomings.
Avoid imperatives like *always* and *never*.
Counter negative thoughts with rational restatements.
Set weight goals.

Reprinted with permission from: Stunkard J, Berthold C. What is behavior therapy? A very short description of behavioral weight control. Am J Clin Nutr 1985;41:821–23.

Meal Replacement Products: Vitamins and minerals are present in some nonprescription weight-control products available as canned puddings and shakes as well as candy bars or wafers (e.g., *Ultra Slimfast*). The rationale behind these expensive products is meal substitution to reduce the total daily caloric intake. These products are not complete meal replacements, and the consumer is advised to have one regular meal a day or take vitamin or mineral supplements.

Most dieting aids state the nutrient composition. These products are low in sodium and provide moderate calorie reduction if followed as directed. Consumers not familiar with the label instructions can eat too many snacks or regular meals to compensate for the increased hunger.

Paradoxically, these aids may be useful for individuals desiring to gain weight. They can supplement Canada's Food Guide to Healthy Eating with the extra calories in these concentrated shakes or wafers.

EATING DISORDERS: ANOREXIA NERVOSA AND BULIMIA NERVOSA

By definition, anorexia nervosa is characterized by a refusal to maintain a minimally normal body weight for age and height: the individual exhibits an intense fear of gaining weight, though underweight; there is a grossly disturbed perception of their weight; the postmenarcheal female has amenorrhea for at least three consecutive months.

The principal features of bulimia nervosa include repeated episodes of binge eating followed by inappropriate compensatory behaviors, such as self-induced vomiting; misuse of laxatives, diuretics or other medications; fasting; excessive exercise.

An essential feature of both illnesses is a disturbance in perception of body shape and weight.

Eating disorders such as anorexia nervosa commonly appear in the teenage years and even with treatment, often persist into the lifetime of the affected individual. Anorexia nervosa appears to affect 1% of young North American women, usually between 12 to 15 years of age, predominantly in white middle and upper middle classes. Bulimia nervosa occurs in approximately 2 to 3% of young North American women, usually beginning in late adolescence or early adult life. Milder variants occur in approximately 5% of all women, and about 5% of all cases are found in men.

TABLE 17: Changes in Organ Systems in Anorexia Nervosa and Bulimia Nervosa

Organ System	Clinical Features
Dermatologic	Lanugo hair and thinning of scalp hair Dry skin Calluses on dorsum of hand (due to repeated use of hand for inducing vomiting reflex)
Gastrointestinal	Reduced gastric motility Parotid gland enlargement Esophageal tears Elevated serum amylase
Cardiovascular	Bradycardia and/or arrhythmias Hypotension
Renal/Electrolytes	Dehydration Edema, hypokalemia, hyponatremia
Metabolic	Decreased basal metabolic rate Hypercholesterolemia Hypercarotenemia
Endocrine	Amenorrhea
Musculature	Muscular wasting and weakness Osteoporosis
Dental	Dental caries (due to erosion by gastric juices)
Others	Decreased libido Cold intolerance and lack of energy Poor concentration, obsessive thoughts

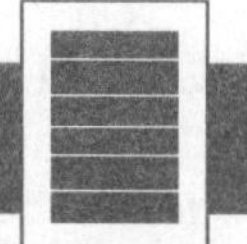

TABLE 18: Principles of Nutrition Intervention in Anorexia Nervosa

Increase kcal intake slowly, beginning with 800 to 1,200 kcal/day
Prescribe well-balanced diets, with some individual variations according to client preferences (e.g., vegetarian)
Give multiple vitamin-mineral supplements at RDA* levels
Enhance elimination with dietary fibre from grain sources
Reduce sensations of bloating with small, frequent feedings
In behavioral programs, link rewards to kcal intake, not weight gain
Use liquid supplements when the client cannot achieve desired intake with solid food
Reduce satiety sensations with cold or room-temperature foods and with finger foods (e.g., snacks)
Provide interactive nutrition counselling as an ongoing process
Reduce excessive caffeine intake
Provide parenteral nutritional support only in severe states of ill health, malnutrition, and wasting

*In Canada, to RNI levels.
Adapted with permission from: Rock CL, Yager J. Nutrition and eating disorders: A primer for clinicians. International Journal of Eating Disorders 6 (1987); 275, as cited in Nutrition and the M.D., July 1988. Reprinted with permission of John Wiley & Sons Inc., copyright 1987.

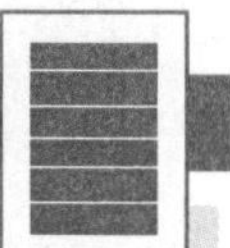

TABLE 19: Diet Recommendations for Bulimia

Avoid finger foods; plan meals with foods that require the use of utensils
Increase meal satiety by including warm foods, rather than cold or room-temperature foods
Include vegetables, salad, and/or fruit at a meal, to prolong the meal duration; choose whole-grain and high-fibre breads and cereals
Prescribe a well-balanced diet and meals, both to increase satiety and to increase the variety of foods eaten
Use foods that are naturally divided into portions, such as potatoes (rather than rice or pasta); 4- and 8-oz containers of yogurt, ice cream, or cottage cheese; precut steak or chicken parts; and frozen dinners and entrées
Include foods containing adequate amounts of complex carbohydrates (which promote meal satiety) and fat (which slow gastric emptying and further enhance the feeling of fullness)
Make sure meals and snacks are eaten sitting down
Plan meals and snacks, and keep a food diary by recording food prior to eating

Adapted from: Rock CL, Yager J. Nutrition and eating disorders: A primer for clinicians, International Journal of Eating Disorders 6 (1987); 277, as cited in Nutrition and the M.D., July 1988. Reprinted with permission of John Wiley & Sons Inc., copyright 1987.

Clinical features at presentation are often varied. The consequences of both illnesses relate to malnutrition induced by starvation, or to the physical effects of purging behaviors. A multitude of organ systems may be affected, especially in the later stages of the illness. Pathological changes are outlined in Table 17.

Treatment Principles

It is difficult to identify anorexics or bulimics without actively searching for the possibility of the illness; anorexics can conceal their illness by wearing loose-fitting, baggy clothing and may be reluctant to remove it for physical examinations. Community pharmacists may be the first health professionals to identify these individuals through their routine and repeated purchases of nonprescription laxatives and purging agents. Referral is the first step toward treatment.

Weight restoration forms the first treatment goal for the seriously underweight patient, and often results in improvement in obsessional thinking, mood and personality disturbances. The weight-gain target is determined by where the individual is healthy, with normal menstrual functioning. This goal is usually achieved at a BMI of 20 to 25. Seriously underweight individuals should be hospitalized and treated as inpatients; only highly motivated individuals with a good support network and few medical complications should be treated as outpatients. Bulimic patients are rarely ever treated as inpatients. Treatment strategies for both include nutritional therapy and/or nutrition counselling; individual or group therapy; family therapy; and pharmacotherapy with antiobsessive agents, antidepressants and appetite-promoting drugs (e.g., cyproheptadine). Table 18 outlines some general guidelines for the nutritional management of individuals with anorexia nervosa. Bulimic patients may benefit from dietary counselling advice outlined in Table 19.

PATIENT ASSESSMENT QUESTIONS

?

Q What is your age, height and weight?

Based on an individual's height and weight, it is easy to calculate the Body Mass Index (BMI) (Table 10). The BMI should only be used for individuals over the age of 20 years. Being overweight is not synonymous with being obese. A lean but heavily muscled person may be overweight according to the BMI, but not be obese.

Most individuals will present with physical complaints, e.g., chronic low back pain (secondary to truncal obesity) or dyspnea when lying down or bending down. Tables 14 and 15 outline conditions that are best managed under medical supervision. The waist-to-hip ratio (WHR) is a useful predictor of risk factors associated with obesity—a WHR $\geq$ 0.95 is more likely to lead to serious consequences.

Q How long have you had a weight problem?

Weight gain greater than 1 kg (2.2 lbs)/day implies fluid retention (e.g., due to cardiovascular, renal or hepatic disorders). Nonprescription drugs (e.g., ibuprofen) can lead to fairly rapid fluid retention in patients with underlying cardiovascular or renal problems.

A good rule of thumb is that clients who present with chronic weight problems (e.g., over a period of years) should not expect quick weight loss. This is an underlying principle of the healthy way to lose weight.

Q How many pounds overweight do you think you are?

Clients often have a distorted perception of how overweight they are. The BMI is a useful gauge of an individual's excess weight, but by no means should it form a sole parameter for assessing obesity. Other indices used in routine practice include the WHR and skinfold testing. (Both the BMI and WHR form a basis for an individual's healthy weight range.)

Q Are there certain times when you tend to eat excessively (e.g., when under stress or when anxious or tired)?

Habitual eating may be the hardest to change but can be one of the most important parameters in successful weight loss. There are behavioral changes that may be helpful to clients desiring to lose weight. It should be emphasized that the individual adapt one habit at a time, as a dramatic change can often lead to confusion and rapid dissatisfaction. It is important to know the time of day when most calories are consumed. Typically, most individuals will skip breakfast and/or lunch, then eat a large meal at supper. This form of eating results in more efficient storage of food as the body attempts to adjust to a fasting-feasting state. A rule of thumb advocated by weight loss experts is that 1/2 to 1/3 of total calorie intake should be consumed by suppertime.

Q Have you been on a diet? What were the dietary or behavior changes you made? Were you prescribed any supplements or diet products?

Numerous dieting aids are available to consumers in the form of powders, shakes, herbal products, etc. Unfortunately, diets often fail quickly because of various factors; they are often regimented and rapidly lead to boredom and noncompliance. They often promise a rapid weight loss (dehydration due to fluid losses) that is not sustainable over a long period of time. They do not attack the underlying problems that led to overeating in the first place (e.g., lack of physical activity or psychosocial problems). The best advice health professionals can give consumers is that weight loss does not have to come from shakes, mixes or powders; following Canada's Food Guide to Healthy Eating with an appropriate reduction in number of servings will lead to gradual and normal weight reduction. Just as important, physical activity (e.g., aerobic activity for at least 30 minutes 3 times a week) and behavioral changes should be part of a healthy plan to lose weight. It is a disservice to clients to prescribe or recommend dieting aids without confronting the underlying problem(s).

PATIENT ASSESSMENT QUESTIONS (*cont'd*)

***Q** Are you on any medication(s) at the present time? Have you been prescribed any medications for weight loss? Were you given a reasonable estimate of how much weight loss to expect?*

A number of agents can lead to gradual weight gain (e.g., prescription drugs such as tricyclic antidepressants, some beta-adrenergic blockers and other agents acting on the central nervous system; see Table 11 for a partial list). Nonprescription agents implicated in gradual weight gain include: astemizole, cyproheptadine and promethazine. Other agents may act indirectly, such as nicotine-resin gums, which are used in smoking cessation.

Prescription drugs should only be used for short-term management of weight loss due to undesirable adverse effects, e.g., elevating blood pressure, stimulant-like effects. Nonprescription products such as methylcellulose or benzocaine products have not been proven to lead to long-term weight loss. Low-calorie balanced foods may form an adjunctive component to weight loss, but should only be recommended by health professionals knowledgeable about possible nutrient deficiencies with these products.

A 500 kcal/day deficit can lead to a weekly weight loss of 0.5 kg (1 lb). However, such a dramatic calorie reduction (e.g., similar to skipping a meal daily), can quickly lead to boredom and craving. A modest daily reduction (along with a decrease in fat consumption) and an increase in physical activity should lead to a gradual and sustained weight loss.

***Q** Are you taking any prescription or nonprescription drugs at the present time? Which ones, and how frequently?*

In addition to potential for drug-nutrient interactions, some pharmacologic agents may suppress the individual's appetite (fluoxetine or systemic decongestants). Table 11 lists drugs that may lead to weight loss or gain. Pathological states, e.g., viral gastroenteritis, acquired immunodeficiency syndrome, often lead to appetite suppression as well. The time a medication is ingested in relation to meals should also be considered when making therapeutic interventions.

***Q** Do you have any chronic medical conditions or a family history of medical problems?*

Certain disease states (e.g., diabetes mellitus or hypertension) are factors that may influence interventions made by health care providers. Some diabetics and hypertensive patients may inquire about antiobesity agents as part of a weight-loss program. Unless recommended by a physician or a dietitian, health professionals should refrain from recommending products containing adrenergic blockers, such as phenylpropanolamine, or local anesthetics, such as benzocaine, found in dieting aids.

SPECIAL NUTRITION REQUIREMENTS

NUTRITION REQUIREMENTS FOR SPECIFIC HEALTH AND DISEASE STATES

Certain groups of people with concomitant conditions or illnesses are more likely to be deficient in nutrients or have specific nutritional requirements. They may need vitamin and/or mineral supplements. Generally, regardless of the individual's disease state, Canada's Food Guide to Healthy Eating forms a sound basis for making nutrient recommendations. For instance, the individual with hyperlipidemia will benefit from restricting total fat intake to no more than 30% of the total daily calorie intake (Table 3).

Table 20 outlines patient populations that may benefit from specific nutritional interventions.

NUTRITION FOR OLDER INDIVIDUALS

Older individuals have particular nutrient needs related to their process of aging accompanied by the increased prevalence of underlying chronic diseases. Physical, physiological and psychosocial factors all play a role.

Energy Requirements

Energy requirements decrease with age due to a normal decline in physical activity, a reduction in basal metabolic rates (approximately 20 to 25% reduction from the third to the seventh decade of life in men with a somewhat lesser decline in women) and a gradual reduction of muscle mass as the individual ages. To prevent unwanted weight gain or loss, energy balance is required. The following are approximate energy intakes as described in the Canadian RNIs (Table 1):

50 to 74 yrs:	males—2,300 kcal/day
	females—1,800 kcal/day
75+ yrs:	males—2,000 kcal/day
	females—1,700 kcal/day

Fat

All Canadian men and women, regardless of age, are advised to restrict the intake of total fat to 30% of total energy with no more than 10% of total energy from saturated fat. The reduction of dietary cholesterol is of less concern as there is no consensus that elevated plasma cholesterol in the elderly is associated with increased mortality from cardiovascular disease.

Protein

Requirements are estimated at 0.8 to 1.0 g/kg/day, the same as for the younger adult. Requirements may be increased in certain disease states (chronic lung disease, hypoalbuminemia infection, cancer, etc.). Protein deficiency causes a loss of lean body mass and subsequent hypoalbuminemia, which is important when protein-bound drugs are being taken (drug toxicity could result). Patients with impaired renal function should restrict protein intake to reduce renal damage.

Carbohydrate

Canada's Food Guide to Healthy Eating recommends increased complex carbohydrates. Dietary fibre plays an important role in increasing peristalsis thereby alleviating constipation.

Fluid

Older individuals are at risk of dehydration from their reduced thirst sensation, their usual low fluid intake (due sometimes to forgetfulness or concern with incontinence) and age-related disturbances in fluid balance. Daily fluid requirements are estimated at 30 mL/kg body weight. Overhydration, which may occur with acute illness or postoperatively, must be prevented as the elderly are prone to dilutional hyponatremia from reduced renal capacity to conserve sodium.

Vitamin and Mineral Supplementation

The RNIs for people over the age of 55 are the same as for younger adults with the following exceptions:

Vitamin A: Requirement decreases with age due to an increase in absorption from the gastrointestinal tract and a reduction in hepatic uptake.

Vitamin D: Requirement for both men and women over 50 years of age is increased to 200 IU/day as

Special Nutrition Requirements

TABLE 20: Nutritional Requirements for Specific Health and Disease States

Condition	Rationale or Nutritional Care	Specific Nutrition Needs
HIV positive/AIDS	Increased risk of malnutrition due to primary HIV infection and/or opportunistic infections Weight-loss may occur due to: — reduced appetite, gastrointestinal disturbance, or cachexia; — diarrhea, intestinal infection, drug use; — alterations in metabolism, e.g., secondary to fever	Nutritional support should be initiated when normal diet fails to meet nutritional requirements High protein, high energy diet may help maintain lean body mass Low-fat nutritional supplements are better tolerated than high-fat supplements Multivitamin and mineral supplements may be indicated Good nutritional status is recommended prior to progression to full-blown AIDS. Some studies suggest that micronutrient deficiencies (iron, zinc, folate, thiamine, niacin, riboflavin, vitamin E, ascorbic acid, and vitamin A) are inversely correlated to risk of progression to AIDS
Cancer	Cancer frequently leads to deterioration in nutritional status, either due to primary disease (e.g., neoplasms) or due to secondary effects of treatment (e.g., chemotherapy or surgical interventions)	Individuals with cancer may have hyper- or hypometabolic status; therefore, nutritional assessment should be individualized Oral route of feeding is preferred, but enteral or parenteral support may be required Multivitamin and mineral supplementation may be required in patients unable to tolerate food; megavitamin supplementation is controversial Nutritional supplements may be indicated in cachexia, anorexia or lactose intolerance Special problems such as esophagitis, xerostomia, thick saliva, dysgeusia should be treated as necessary
Diabetes mellitus	Target goal should be to maintain euglycemia without hyper- or hypoglycemic episodes Additionally, serum lipids should be maintained within physiologic range	Energy intake should be adequate to maintain a healthy body weight. Recommended protein intake for adults is 0.86 g/kg/day. Fat intake should not exceed 30% of total energy intake, and <10% should be as saturated fats. Carbohydrates should provide >55% of the energy, and should be preferably in the form of unrefined starch foods (e.g., whole grain cereals, breads, legumes and tubers) Artificial sweeteners are acceptable in moderation; nutritive sweeteners such as sorbitol, sucrose or fructose are acceptable in small quantities (less than 3 g/day)
Hyperlipidemia	Improving lipoprotein and lipid levels of individuals with dyslipoproteinemia reduces nutrition-related risk factor for coronary heart disease (CHD) Goal of lipid-lowering diet is: — total cholesterol <5.2 — LDL <3.4 — HDL >0.9 — triglycerides <2.2 Other risk factors should be reduced where possible (e.g., cessation of smoking) Extreme hypertriglyceridemia can also lead to pancreatitis	Reducing fat intake to ≤30% of the total energy intake facilitates reduction of total and saturated fat intake and cholesterol. While monounsaturated (10–15%) and polyunsaturated (≤10%) fats are recommended alternatives, their use should be within the range of total energy intake Sodium and caffeine intake may need to be reduced in the cardiac patient High fibre diet (especially soluble fibre—oat bran, beans) improves lipid profile Use of niacin for reducing elevated LDL cholesterol levels should be done under medical supervision Restrict alcohol (it can elevate triglyceride levels) Cholesterol intake should be <300 mg/day Canada's Food Guide to Healthy Eating is an excellent resource for the cardiac patient

TABLE 20: Nutritional Requirements for Specific Health and Disease States (*cont'd*)

Condition	Rationale or Nutritional Care	Specific Nutrition Needs
Hypertension	Avoid obesity, as insulin resistance and hyperinsulinemia are associated with hypertension	High fibre, and low fat, as for hyperlipidemia Low salt (<2 g/day) Low sugar Increase intake of calcium, magnesium and potassium Limit alcohol intake (<0.5–1 oz/day)
Congestive heart failure (CHF)	In CHF there is a loss of magnesium and a retention of sodium due to activation of renin-angiotensin-aldosterone system	Low salt (<2 g/day) Follow Canada's Food Guide to Healthy Eating to ensure the patient's nutritional status is maintained
Osteoporosis	Risk factors predisposing individuals for osteoporosis: — age — caucasian or oriental — females — small frame or lean — low bone mass — excessive alcohol use — smoking — lack of weight-bearing exercises — taking corticosteroids Sufficient calcium intake should be encouraged at an earlier age for minimizing bone loss later in life	The RNIs provide average recommended intake of calcium (Table 2) The National Institutes of Health Development Conference on Optimal Calcium Intake in the US recommends: — children and young adults (11–24 yrs of age) should ingest 1,200–1,500 mg/day of elemental calcium — women (25–50 yrs of age) should ingest 1,000 mg/day of elemental calcium to maintain positive balance — postmenopausal women (50–65 yrs of age) need 1,000–1,500 mg/day of elemental calcium; (>65 yrs) need 1,500 mg/day Dairy products remain the primary modality for calcium supplementation; however, mineral supplements may be an alternative in individuals unable to take dairy products Vitamin D (400 IU) and calcium (800 mg) recommended if osteoporosis already present
Pregnancy	Maternal nutrition is instrumental in determining the outcome of pregnancy Prepare for nursing before birth by consuming 2050–2850 kcal/day	In addition to adhering to Canada's Food Guide to Healthy Eating, the following recommendations may be made: — adequate fluid intake (6–8 cups/day) — prenatal supplementation with folate (0.4 mg/day) and iron (30–60 mg/day) (if pre gravid iron stores are low) — gradual weight gain during pregnancy — limit caffeine, alcohol and tobacco use
Alcoholics/ Drug abusers	Drug dependence can lead to micronutrient and macronutrient deficiencies in a variety of ways: — inadequate nutrition due to drug abuse and dependency — impaired absorption and conversion of nutrients due to pathophysiologic changes in the gastrointestinal system	Ideally, the individual should be treated for dependency, along with nutritional support Parenteral or oral B vitamins (especially thiamine) should be initiated Protein and carbohydrate deficiencies should be corrected as well
Anemias	Anemia has a variety of causes Correction of deficiency should not be undertaken without first evaluating the underlying cause of anemia. Several micronutrient deficiencies may lead to anemia: — iron deficiency — pyridoxine deficiency — folic acid deficiency — vitamin B_{12} deficiency	Treatment of anemias generally is as follows: — iron replacement: 100–200 mg/day of elemental iron — pyridoxine (sideroblastic) anemia: 50–200 mg/day — folic acid (megaloblastic) anemia: 50–100 µg/day — cobalamin (pernicious) anemia: 5–15 µg/day

Adapted with permission from: Whiteney EN, Hamilton EMN, Rolfes SR. Understanding Nutrition. 5th ed. St. Paul: West Publishing Co., 1990: E-3 and Bell L. ed. Manual of Nutritional Care. 4th ed. Vancouver: British Columbia Dietitians' & Nutritionists' Association, 1992.

compared to 100 IU/day for adults under 50. Vitamin D absorption is reduced with age due to pancreatic insufficiency and a reduction of bile acids, which are necessary for the absorption of fat-soluble vitamins. With age, skin loses its ability to convert the provitamin 7-dehydrocholesterol to the active form during exposure to sunshine and coupled with the reduced exposure to sunlight common in the elderly, the vitamin D deficiency is compounded. Optimal amounts of vitamin D improve calcium absorption, and this is important in slowing the progression of osteoporosis (a special concern for women).

B Vitamins: Individuals who abuse alcohol generally have thiamine and folic acid deficiencies. Achlorhydria may decrease Vitamin B_{12} absorption.

Iron: Postmenopausal women (>50 yrs) require less iron, 8 mg/day compared to 13 mg/day for women under 50. Achlorhydria, common in the elderly, interferes with iron and folate absorption. To prevent anemia, the diet should include iron-rich foods taken along with foods rich in vitamin C to increase absorption of iron.

Calcium: The RNI is 800 mg/kg (intakes of 1,000 and 1,500 mg/day have been shown necessary to maintain bone mass). Older individuals have decreased calcium absorption from the gastrointestinal tract and often, decreased vitamin D levels; dietary calcium supplements should be recommended where risk factors for metabolic bone disease are present.

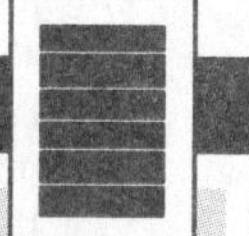

TABLE 21: Causes of Malnutrition in the Elderly

Causes
Loss of income—poverty
Social isolation
Diseases that reduce appetite, decrease absorption or utilization of nutrients or increase requirements for nutrients
Drugs that affect food intake, or the absorption, utilization or excretion of nutrients
Ignorance about good nutrition or food preparation
Dental problems
Depression or mental problems
Decreased physical ability to buy food or prepare a meal
Alcoholism

Reprinted with permission from: Roland DA. Nutrition in adulthood and the later years. In: Krause MV, Mahan LK, eds. Food, Nutrition and Diet Therapy. 7th ed. Philadelphia: WB Saunders, 1984:324.

Many seniors rely on multivitamin and mineral products for nutrition, but these alone cannot supply energy. There is rarely a need for extra-strength vitamins, and the best recommendation for supplementation would be a balanced multivitamin and mineral product containing calcium and iron.

Liquid Meals

If eating normal foods is difficult or impossible (e.g., due to dentition or swallowing difficulties), specially formulated liquid diets can provide a nutritionally complete substitute.

These products should be used as a supplement to meals rather than total meal replacement wherever possible to maintain quality of life. When used for prolonged periods of time, the taste may become boring and depress the appetite. To boost calories by diet alone refer to a registered dietitian or public health nutritionist.

Malnutrition

Some Canadian seniors are malnourished and this can have a deleterious effect on their health. When energy consumption is <1,800 kcal/day, it becomes difficult to meet the recommended nutritional requirements. Possible causes are outlined in Table 21.

Pharmacists, nurses, dietitians and other health professionals can play a role in observing declining health possibly due to poor eating habits and assisting the elderly by recommending appropriate products or community services such as Meals on Wheels, or referring to dietitians at the local public health unit or hospital.

NUTRITION FOR THE ATHLETE

For optimal health, the nutritional requirements for the athlete are the same as for any individual, e.g., adequate amounts, according to Canada's Food Guide to Healthy Eating, of the following nutrients: carbohydrate, fat, protein, vitamins, minerals and water. For peak performance, the athlete has a higher requirement for water and energy, which is provided most efficiently by carbohydrate, to a lesser extent by fat, and least efficiently by protein.

Energy Source

For optimal athletic performance, sufficient energy must be delivered to performing muscles. Adenosine triphosphate (ATP) is the energy-rich compound used by muscle cells. ATP is present in limited amounts and is continuously produced within the muscle cells through two processes: aerobic (requiring oxygen) and anaerobic (without oxygen). These two pathways work simultaneously. During the first few minutes of exercise, ATP is produced by the anaerobic breakdown of glucose to pyruvate and then to lactic acid, and this pathway provides most of the energy because oxygen-rich blood has not yet arrived in the muscles. Lactic acid accumulates and causes fatigue. When oxygen is available, lactic acid is cleared from the muscle into the blood, and pyruvate can enter the aerobic pathway. The anaerobic pathway produces two units of ATP per molecule of pyruvate, while the aerobic pathway is much more efficient producing 36 to 38 units of ATP. Training or conditioning increases the oxygen-use capacity of muscles and improves the athlete's ability to mobilize fat and spare glycogen, the storage form of body glucose.

The supply of glucose in muscles to produce ATP is limited (lasts for only about 10 seconds); therefore, glycogen and fat must be used to provide energy for activity to continue. During the first 20 minutes of moderate-intensity exercise, glycogen provides 60 to 70% of the fuel. The higher the carbohydrate content of the diet, the higher the muscle glycogen stores. For activity lasting longer than 20 minutes, fat is released to be used for energy with glycogen supplying 10 to 20% of the fuel. Protein is used as a source of energy only when fatty acids and/or glucose are in short supply.

Vitamins and Minerals

Supplementation in excess of the RNIs (Table 1) has no effect on athletic performance and does not prevent injury when a deficiency does not exist. There is no strong evidence to suggest that athletes have increased use, destruction or loss of vitamins associated with exercise that would necessitate supplementation.

Some of the claims that have been made (e.g., vitamin B complex) have not been shown to have an effect on muscular strength, endurance or recovery from exertion when a deficiency state does not exist. The evidence for vitamin C's ability to prevent injury and vitamin E's ability to increase aerobic capacity is not conclusive.

Is a daily multivitamin preparation beneficial to the athlete who has an unusual nutritional intake to avoid the development of a deficiency? Possibly. If the athlete has a well-balanced diet, vitamin supplementation has not been shown to enhance athletic performance.

Iron: Deficiency may result from poor dietary intakes, heavy sweating, gastrointestinal iron loss, hemolysis, hematuria and in females, menstrual losses. Those particularly at risk are endurance female and adolescent athletes. If the athlete has iron deficiency anemia, an iron supplement, or iron-rich food, is required. Excess iron is dangerous. In one study, men with high serum ferritin levels (>200 µg/mL) were more than twice as likely to suffer acute myocardial infarctions as their counterparts with lower ferritin levels when other risk factors were adjusted for.

Calcium: Calcium is important for strong healthy bones and muscle contraction; postmenopausal female athletes require 800 to 1,200 mg/day to prevent bone resorption. Other factors related to the development of osteoporosis include: estrogen level, alcohol and caffeine intake, vitamin D intake, family history and the amount and type of physical activity. Amenorrhea associated with low levels of body fat and high physical activity may hinder bone development and cause an increased risk of stress fractures. Consumption of 120% of the calcium RNI helps bones to develop properly and maintain density.

Diet for Optimal Performance

- 60 to 70% energy as carbohydrate (470 to 550 g): increase the number of food servings from the Grain Products Group and the Vegetables and Fruits Group.
- 25 to 30% energy as fat, no more than 10% of this as saturated fats.
- 15% protein (0.86 g/kg body weight)
  - — 1.0 g/kg during intense training,
  - — 1.2-1.5 g/kg during initial stage of training.

TABLE 22: Fluid Replacement Comparison Chart

Components	Recommended	Gatorade	Exceed	Homemade*	Coca Cola
CHO Source	Glucose Glucose polymer Sucrose Minimal fructose	Glucose Sucrose Glucose polymer	Glucose polymer Fructose	Sucrose Glucose Fructose	High fructose Sucrose
CHO concentration(%)	6-8	6	7.2	5.9	10.2
Sodium (mEq/L)	10-20	20	10	14	1.2
Potassium (mEq/L)	2.5-5	2.7	4.8	6.5	trace
Osmolality† (mOsm/L)	250-360	280-360	250	345	600-715

* Homemade solution: 2 L (66 oz) orange juice, 2 L (66 oz) water, 1 mL (1/4 tsp) salt.
† Osmolality refers to the concentration of the fluid.
Reprinted with permission from: Marriage B, Schnurr H. Sports Nutrition Resource Manual. Edmonton: Sports Medicine Council of Alberta, 1993:41.

Sodium: Adequate amounts of sodium are supplied by diet. Replacement may be necessary in extreme conditions, such as endurance events held in hot weather accompanied by a sodium-restricted diet.

Water: Water is required for all energy production in the body, for temperature control, for elimination of the by-products of cell metabolism and to prevent dehydration. See Table 22 for a comparison of fluid replacement options.

Carbohydrate Loading

This technique is used to maximize glycogen stores for endurance events (>90 minutes) or multiple event competitions.

The original carbohydrate-loading regimen involved depletion of glycogen by exhaustive exercising starting 7 days before competition followed by 3 days of a diet rich in fat and protein. The athlete then tapered the exercise and consumed a high-carbohydrate diet. Disadvantages of this procedure include: excessive weight gain due to water retention, gastrointestinal distress, loss of muscle tissue, etc. Recent studies indicate that maximal glycogen storage does not require prior glycogen depletion.

The recommendation now is that athletes follow a high-carbohydrate diet (55-65% carbohydrate, 350 g) throughout training and start tapering exercise 5 to 7 days prior to the event with complete rest 1 to 2 days before the event. During the 3 days prior to the event, the carbohydrate is increased to 70% of the energy or 525 to 550 g, whichever is greater. Sample menus can be obtained from the Sport Nutrition Advisory Committee of Canada.

Pregame Meal

The pregame meal should: prevent hunger during the competition; be quickly and easily digested to ensure the stomach and upper bowel are empty at the time of competition; provide an optimal state of hydration; provide about 500 kcal if taken 2 to 4 hours before the event (smaller meals are recommended if <2 hours); and have dilute forms of simple sugars (e.g., juice), it may cause diarrhea/bloating if not diluted.

High carbohydrate foods will provide the quickest and most efficient source of energy, and have neither the slow gastric-emptying problem of fats nor the dehydrating tendency of proteins. Commercial liquid meal replacements can satisfy all of the requirements for precompetition foods. They are high in carbohydrates and can contribute to both energy intake and hydration.

Fluid intake is important before and during the competition. Two to three glasses of fruit-flavored drinks or water should be consumed immediately pregame and hourly intakes of fluid or fruit juices scheduled during the competition.

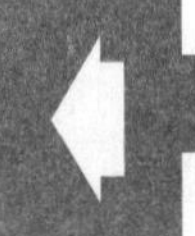

Postevent Meal

Muscle glycogen stores need to be replenished by consuming carbohydrate-rich foods and fluid and electrolyte losses replaced by consuming plenty of fluids with emphasis on fruit juices. Recent literature has indicated that including only a small amount of protein with the carbohydrate enhances glycogen repletion.

The Ideal Competing Weight

Ideal per cent body fat is an individual matter and varies according to the sport in which the person participates. Excess fat may hinder the basketball player or runner; however, the hockey player or wrestler may require extra cushioning or additional body size. The target per cent body fat for male athletes is 4 to 15% and for female athletes 12 to 25%. The amount of essential body fat is 3% for men and 12% for females. Insufficient body fat can decrease exercise performance, lower disease resistance, delay wound and injury repair and cause amenorrhea for the female athlete. Excess body fat can impair performance, cause heat exhaustion due to increased insulation and impair oxygen use during exercise.

Weight loss (fat loss) requires energy expenditure in excess of intake (approximately 3,500 calories for each pound of body fat). Weight loss accompanied by sufficient exercise and an adequate diet (no less than 2,000 kcal/day for an average male athlete) will cause loss of body fat. A weight loss >1 kg/week without exercise, relying on starvation, will result in a wasting of muscle tissue.

Weight gain (muscle gain) requires the athlete to take in more calories than they expend. From 500 to 1,000 kcal/day above that needed for weight maintenance, age and growth are recommended for weight gain. Specific training and conditioning programs (weight training) should accompany the high-calorie intake, if muscle and not fat is to be the major tissue component of added weight. Sufficient protein intake is recommended, but a dramatic increase is not warranted.

Protein Supplements

Athletic activity does not significantly increase the need for protein (RNI is 0.86 g/kg body weight/day). Endurance athletes or athletes in intense training may need slightly higher levels (1 to 1.5 g/kg body weight/day) due to muscle breakdown and a reduction in protein synthesis during such exercise. Only in the initial stages of training is additional protein required: 1.2 to 1.5 g/kg body weight/day. Growing young athletes may require 1.5 g/kg body weight because of increased needs for rapid growth. If they eat a varied and widely selected diet according to Canada's Food Guide to Healthy Eating, they will get all the protein they can use. Protein supplement powders on the market generally supply approximately 16 g protein/3 tbsp. If one consumes 3.5 oz light tuna in water,

ADVICE FOR THE ATHLETE

Nutrition

Optimum athletic performance can be attained with the following dietary recommendations:

- A high-carbohydrate diet promotes maximal energy storage for optimal performance: 60 to 70% of total energy for endurance athletes; 55 to 65% of total energy for recreational athletes. Increase the number of food servings from the Grain Products Group and the Vegetables and Fruit Group.
- A low-fat intake providing 25 to 30% of energy with no more than 10% of energy from saturated fats provides for optimal performance; choose lower-fat dairy products (skim, 1% milk, cheese with <20% milk fat, yogurt <2% milk fat) and lean cuts of meat (lean ground beef, sirloin and flank steaks). Bake or broil foods, rather than frying.
- Adequate (not excessive) protein is required to provide muscle maintenance and repair and production of antibodies to fight infection (0.86 g/kg body weight/day). This is easily met when 15% of the total energy is provided by protein in the diet.
- If a variety of foods are included in the diet, vitamin and mineral supplementation is not required.
- Adequate fluid levels are required to maintain proper hydration:
  600 mL—2 hours pregame
  250 to 500 mL—15 to 30 minutes pregame
  90 to 150 mL—every 15 minutes during
    exercise <3 hours: water is best;
    exercise >3 hours: dilute glucose and electrolyte solutions.

the amount of protein is 25 to 30 g. Vegetarian athletes are not at any additional risk for protein deficiency provided they consume a wide variety of protein choices.

Excess protein, especially animal protein, should be avoided because high quality animal foods (meat, whole milk, eggs, cheese) contain a lot of saturated fat. Excess protein intake is degraded and converted to energy or fat, and the nitrogen moiety is excreted in the urine.

Single amino-acid supplements and unbalanced protein supplements can interfere with the absorption of essential amino acids and lead to metabolic imbalance. Other detrimental effects include: increased work for the kidneys to excrete waste (urea) and increased fluid loss for elimination (dehydration). Dehydration leads to impaired exercise capacity, muscle cramping, and an inability to regulate body temperature, leading to heat stroke.

Protein supplements have not been shown to increase muscle size or to improve athletic performance. These products are also extremely expensive.

Nutritional Ergogenic Aids

Ergogenic refers to compounds or nutrients that enhance performance or improve exercise capacity. Many of the claims of the benefits of these compounds are unfounded and can be potentially dangerous, especially when used to replace a sound nutrition program. For additional information on ergogenic aids, refer to the Sports Medicine Products chapter.

PHARMACEUTICAL AGENTS

VITAMIN PRODUCTS

Folic Acid: In addition to its physiological roles in hemopoiesis and normal functioning of the nervous system, folic acid is important during embryogenesis. It is accepted that the presence of folate leads to closure of the neural tube during the embryonic period (generally the first 4 weeks post-fertilization). Therefore, women who are pregnant are encouraged to ensure adequate folate in their diets before (at least 6 weeks prior) and during the first trimester of pregnancy. Epidemiological studies have determined the incidence of neural tube defects (anencephaly and spina bifida) is inversely proportional to folate intake in the diet. Several organizations, including Health Canada, recommend women obtain at least 400 μg (0.4 mg)/day from dietary or supplementary sources prior to and during the first trimester of pregnancy. Higher doses (4 mg/day) are recommended in women with prior history of births with neural tube defects. Cross-Canada surveys indicate folate consumption is lowest in Atlantic Canada, and generally increases as one moves westward. At the present time, food fortification (e.g., cereals, wheat products) with folic acid is not undertaken due to concern with masking of vitamin B_{12}- deficiency by folate in anemic states. Prenatal vitamins (containing 0.8 to 1.0 mg of folic acid) should be recommended preferentially over regular vitamin formulas available in the market place.

Antioxidant Vitamins: Beta-carotene, vitamins C and E are the so-called antioxidant vitamins. They are believed to be beneficial to health because they help to protect the body from damage caused by free radicals (e.g., hydroxyl, superoxide, nitric oxide or unpaired oxygen atoms), or other highly reactive substances. Some clinical conditions in which oxygen free radicals have been postulated to cause damage include aging, atherosclerosis, bronchopulmonary dysplasia, hemochromatosis, cancer, cataractogenesis, emphysema, oxidant pollution, Parkinson's disease, radiation injury, rheumatoid arthritis, sickle cell anemia, skin injury from solar radiation and tissue damage due to cigarette smoking.

In vivo, a number of epidemiological trials have shown beneficial relationships between the antioxidant vitamins and the prevention or reduction of coronary heart disease and gastrointestinal cancers (vitamin E); lung cancer (vitamin C and beta-carotene); and esophageal cancer (antioxidant vitamins). While evidence suggests that vitamin E supplements (at doses of 400 IU/day) may protect against coronary heart disease, definitive recommendations await results from ongoing randomized trials of primary and secondary prevention. Patients interested in using antioxidant products, especially individuals with concomitant cardiovascular risk factors, should be encouraged to consult their physicians. Evidence for vitamin C and beta carotene is still under review. Under no circumstances should consumers view antioxidant products as a panacea for good health in lieu of appropriate lifestyle and dietary changes.

Clinicians should be cautious when recommending antioxidant vitamins. The importance of diet containing the recommended micronutrients should be emphasized to the consumer. Key questions regarding supplementation that remain to be addressed include: whether foods (in contrast to pharmaceutical products) provide the protective effects; the duration and dose of micronutrients needed; and at what stage of life should antioxidant therapy begin. When addressing consumers' questions, health care professionals should be knowledgeable about new developments in micronutrient supplementation. (Several review articles listed in the Recommended Reading section are a good place to begin.)

Multivitamin Preparations: Numerous combination products containing multiple vitamins and minerals are available to the Canadian consumer. The rationale behind a combination product is that vitamin deficiencies in the industrialized nations rarely occur for single nutrients. As a general rule, multivitamin preparations containing 2 to 5 times the recommended nutrient intakes are labelled "for therapeutic use only." Therapeutic vitamins should be used in deficiency states or in situations where absorption and usage of vitamins are reduced or requirements are increased. Single nutrient therapy for specific deficiency is preferable if specific deficiency can be documented by laboratory blood or urine tests and combined with clinical findings.

Supplemental vitamins are generally given to groups at risk for development of vitamin deficiency states. The following may be candidates for vitamin supplementation:

- Women with excessive menstrual bleeding may need to take iron supplements;
- Women who are pregnant have an increased requirement for all vitamins and minerals listed in the RNI (with the exception of vitamin A);
- During lactation, additional requirements (with the exception of iron) may necessitate supplementation;
- People with very low-calorie intakes (e.g., less than 1,800 kcal/day) frequently do not meet their needs for all nutrients;
- Some vegetarians may not receive adequate calcium, iron, zinc, and vitamin B_{12};
- Newborns, under medical supervision, are commonly given a single dose of vitamin K to prevent abnormal bleeding;
- Certain conditions and disease states (see section on Special Nutritional Requirements) have specific requirements that may include nutrient supplementation;
- Breast-fed infants may require vitamin D supplementation;
- Folic acid supplementation is given to expectant mothers to prevent nervous system complications in the offspring.

Stress Vitamins: Stress vitamins are not necessarily therapeutically superior to their regular counterparts, despite containing larger quantities of the B and C vitamins. They are marketed in the belief that, under physically stressful situations, energy requirements are higher than in nonstressful conditions. Although perceived to be superior to regular products, there is no difference from regular complete vitamin products.

Natural vs. Synthetic Products: Except for vitamin E, there is no significant difference between natural source and synthetic vitamins. A considerable body of scientific research now indicates that natural source vitamin E (e.g., d-alpha tocopherol or more properly designated RRR alpha tocopherol) is preferentially transported and retained by body tissues. Synthetic vitamin E is an equimolar mixture of 8 isomers of vitamin E, only one of which is equivalent to natural source vitamin E (RRR alpha tocopherol). Virtually 100% of all commercially available vitamins are synthetic in origin, with the exception of vitamin E and beta-carotene, which are available from both sources. The therapeutic efficacy of the two formulations is identical, and synthetic vitamins are usually less expensive and less likely to contain impurities than their natural counterparts.

Multiple Vitamins for Specific Populations: Pharmacy shelves are stocked with numerous brands of multiple vitamin products. Products with the same brand name are also marketed for different age and population groups (e.g., seniors, females, pregnancy, etc.). They contain varying amounts of vitamins and minerals reflecting the different RNIs for the different groups. It is generally felt that, with the exception of prenatal supplements, the adult multivitamin supplements are interchangeable for males, females and the elderly. This is because dietary intake over a prolonged period generally makes up for any nutrient deficiencies. In general, adult formulations should not be given to the pediatric population because of possible toxicity from iron or vitamin A. Some products may also contain undesirable ingredients such as alcohol (e.g., tonics marketed for the elderly).

SELECTED MINERALS

Calcium

Calcium is available in a variety of dosage forms. The calcium content of the various salts differs considerably, with calcium carbonate containing the greatest proportion of elemental calcium (40%) and calcium gluconate providing the least (9%) (Table 23). Calcium carbonate, the most frequently recommended form because of its high calcium content and low cost, requires an acidic medium for adequate absorption. Although 20% of the elderly are achlorhydric, recent data show that if calcium carbonate is administered with meals, adequate absorption will occur even in the presence of documented achlorhydria. Absorption of calcium involves mucosal uptake of the soluble calcium ion by an active transport mechanism. Vitamin D metabolites stimulate this transport system. In the absence of 1,25-dihydroxyvitamin D, less than 10% of dietary calcium may be absorbed. Supplementation of vitamin D intake to provide 600 to 800 IU/day has been shown to improve calcium balance. Other factors that may enhance calcium absorption include: estrogen, growth hormone and parathyroid hormone. (There is no conclusive evidence that magnesium, phosphate or caffeine enchance calcium absorption.) Factors that decrease calcium availability include: sodium and protein can increase urinary calcium excretion; glucocorticosteroids decrease calcium absorption

TABLE 23: Calcium Salts

Calcium Salt	Elemental Calcium	Comments
Calcium carbonate (40% calcium)	250 mg = 100 mg elemental calcium 300 mg = 120 mg elemental calcium 500 mg = 200 mg elemental calcium 600 mg = 240 mg elemental calcium	Available as tablets, syrup, or effervescent tablets To be taken in divided doses with meals to increase absorption and lessen GI irritation May cause bloating or flatulence Generally least expensive
Calcium lactate (13% calcium)	650 mg = 84 mg elemental calcium	May cause less GI irritation than calcium carbonate More expensive than calcium carbonate
Calcium gluconate (9% calcium)	650 mg = 60 mg elemental calcium	May cause less GI irritation than calcium carbonate Generally most expensive

Note: Excessive amounts of calcium (e.g., >2 g/day) should be taken under medical supervision, due to possible hypercalcemia, hypercalciuria and renal stone formation.

(therefore, arthritic patients on glucocorticosteroids may require calcium supplements).

Consumers may enquire about natural sources of calcium (e.g., dolomite or bone meal); these should not be recommended because they may be contaminated with impurities such as lead. Antacid preparations containing calcium carbonate (e.g., *Tums*) may be useful as an inexpensive and convenient calcium supplement, taken immediately following meals to maximize absorption and minimize adverse effects. The possibility of the milk-alkali syndrome is a theoretical concern.

Calcium (along with vitamin D) is important for maintaining bone density and preventing osteoporosis. Many Canadians (especially adolescents and women) without adequate calcium in their diets may develop osteoporosis later in life since maximal bone deposition occurs during adolescence and in the presence of estrogen. Calcium supplements may have a role for consumers who cannot tolerate or consume milk or dairy products.

Iron

Iron for the treatment of anemia is available in various salts and dosage forms. The choice of product depends on the elemental iron content, cost, and other ingredients. Ferrous salts are absorbed three times more readily than ferric salts. The ferrous sulfate and fumarate salts are the least expensive and provide a high content of elemental iron (Table 24).

Iron supplementation for the treatment of anemia is to correct the underlying cause and replace lost iron stores. To be effective, treatment should continue for 6 weeks up to 6 months. Since noncompliance can be a significant problem, patients should be reminded not to stop once they are subjectively improved.

Since iron can often cause constipation, some preparations contain stool softeners. In general, these combination products are more expensive, contain subtherapeutic doses of the stool softener and are not recommended. Sustained-release or enteric-coated products are often promoted as causing less gastrointestinal irritation than conventional dosage forms; however, they are more expensive and poorly absorbed as iron is transported beyond the duodenum and jejunum (sites of active iron absorption). Only patients unable to tolerate conventional iron preparations should take them. Iron products containing ascorbic acid are generally not recommended: although ascorbic acid enhances iron absorption by maintaining iron in the trivalent state (preferentially absorbed over the divalent form), doses of 500 to 1,000 mg of ascorbic acid only increase iron absorption by 10%. Clients may be counselled to take their iron tablets with a less-expensive glass of orange juice.

Oral iron salts should be taken on an empty stomach since food reduces absorption by 50%. Due to significant gastrointestinal irritation, iron preparations may be recommended with food, keeping in mind that absorption will be reduced significantly. Concurrent use of many drugs with iron supplements can influence iron absorption and should be avoided for at least 2 hours.

Adverse Effects: Nausea, abdominal pain and bloating, constipation or diarrhea, and vomiting are

TABLE 24: Iron Salts

Salt	Approximate Elemental Iron
Ferrous sulfate 300 mg	60 mg
Ferrous gluconate 300 mg	35 mg
Ferrous fumarate 200 mg	65 mg
Ferrous succinate 100 mg	60 mg

common; patients should be cautioned that iron preparations frequently turn stools dark. Individuals complaining of severe abdominal pain while taking iron therapy should be referred to their physician for evaluation. Liquid iron preparations can cause some staining of teeth, which is benign and temporary. To prevent staining, dilute the dose in water or juice and drink through a straw.

Toxicity: Iron toxicity is a significant problem with children since they are more subject to accidental poisoning than adults. Toxicity can occur with ingesting 30 to 60 mg of elemental iron per kg of body weight and appears in several stages. The acute stage (1 to 6 hours) is characterized by nausea, vomiting, abdominal distention, hypotension, tachycardia, or dehydration. Contacting the poison centre or emergency room at this stage should determine whether syrup of ipecac is indicated. If left untreated, the patient may develop shock, pulmonary edema, seizures or hyperthermia after 12 to 48 hours. Complications of poisoning include cirrhosis, brain damage and gastric stenosis.

ENTERAL PRODUCTS

Formulated Liquid Diet (FLD): As defined by Health Canada: "Sold or represented for sale as a nutritionally complete diet for oral or tube feeding of a person in whom a physical or physiological condition exits as a result of disease, disorder or injury."

These products are nutritionally complete and may be taken orally to supplement an inadequate diet or they can be used as a sole source of nutrition. The calorie content varies from 1 to 2 kcal/mL; protein from 0.4 to 0.7 g/mL; they may or may not contain fibre and generally are lactose-free. Hypercaloric formulas are ideal for those requiring extra calories in a smaller volume. Flavored versions are generally intended for oral use, as they may be hypertonic (>425 mOsm/kg), which may initially cause diarrhea in some tube-fed patients. Unflavored products are usually isotonic (300 to 475 mOsm/kg), and designed more for individuals being tube fed. Some patients with sensitivity to sweetness or flavor (e.g., chemotherapy patients) may prefer an unflavored product alone or mixed with a flavored one. These products are formulated for patients at nutritional risk: acutely ill patients (burns, pancreatitis, trauma, inflammatory bowel disease, prolonged vomiting/diarrhea, severe dysphagia); pre/postsurgical patients; cancer patients; dental/oral disorders; alcohol/drug abusers; eating disorder (e.g., anorexia nervosa/bulimic patients); AIDS patients; anorexia (e.g., rheumatoid arthritis, depression, nausea).

Meal Replacement Products: As defined by Health Canada: "Sold or advertised as a replacement for one or more daily meals and for use in a weight-reduction diet."

The nutrient distribution and vitamin/mineral content of these products is not nutritionally balanced and not designed for complete daily nutrition. Their calorie content is approximately 1 kcal/mL and protein is 0.5–0.6 g/mL. They are meant to be used to complement the diet, to replace a meal as a convenience or on a weight reduction diet and not to sustain a person for a long period of time. Healthy individuals who may require nutritional support include: pregnant women with nausea; lactating women; the elderly; weight control (gain or loss); athletes (to provide energy prior to and during activity, provide increased protein and energy for bulking); busy people who "eat on the run."

Formulated Liquid Diets may be more expensive than meal replacements because their nutritional content is superior. Health Canada does not permit advertising of FLDs to the general consumer so meal replacements tend to be more competitive in consumer sales and advertising.

Patients may have a taste preference for one product over another, as some are sweeter than others. Strong flavors/sweetness may cause nausea in some people. Taste fatigue may occur in those taking oral nutritional supplements for a prolonged period of time; some products are available in a pudding format or offer recipes for alternate methods of using the products.

Osmolality

Osmolality (mOsm/kg) and osmolarity (mOsm/L) are often used interchangeably. Isotonic formulas are about 300 mOsm/kg (the osmolality of normal body fluid) and are generally well tolerated.

INFANT FORMULAS

Cow's Milk Based Formulas: Recommended for full-term infants with no known medical problems or allergies. Many contain added whey protein to better simulate the ratio of whey and casein proteins in human milk. These products can be used as supplementation to or substitution for breast-feeding.

Modified Cow's Milk Based Formulas: The cow's milk protein has been partially broken down to decrease the antigen sites, which decreases the potential for intolerance or sensitivity.

Lactose-free Modified Cow's Milk Based Formula: Glucose polymers are substituted for lactose; these are recommended for lactose intolerance.

Soy Protein Formulas: All contain soy protein as the protein source and are lactose-free. The carbohydrate source is either corn syrup or sucrose. They were developed for use in infants allergic to cow's milk protein, but caution is warranted because of cross-sensitivity developing to soy protein. Soy protein formulas are recommended for use in infants with lactose intolerance, lactase deficiency, galactosemia and infants of vegetarian families, and with caution in infants with milk protein allergy.

Casein Hydrolysate Formulas: The casein protein is hydrolyzed or predigested and was developed for the infant sensitive to intact protein or unable to digest intact protein. They are lactose-free and recommended for infants with severe diarrhea or proven allergy to cow's milk protein. A disadvantage may be the unpleasant odor or bitter taste; however, most infants seem to tolerate these products well. These products are more expensive than routine formulas.

Fibre-containing Formulas contain soluble and insoluble fibre to delay gastric emptying and increase fecal bulk. The protein is soy based, and the carbohydrate is lactose-free. After oral rehydration with an electrolyte repletion product (24 to 48 hours), the formula may be used for 7 to 10 days, then a lactose-free formula may be indicated. Otherwise the infant may resume their regular formula.

Whey Hydrolysate Formulas: The casein portion of the protein is removed and the whey portion partially hydrolyzed to reduce antigenicity. The degree of hydrolysis is less than that with casein, and they do not have as unpleasant an odor or as bitter a taste. Recommended for infants with malabsorption problems, which may include food allergies, disaccharidase deficiency, idiopathic defects in digestion or absorption.

Formulated Liquid Diets

- Oral (flavored)
  - *Ensure/EnsurePlus/Ensure Fibre/Ensure High Protein/Ensure Pudding*
  - *Pediasure* (pediatric)
  - *Nutren Flavored* 1.0, 1.5, 2.0/ *Nutren Flavored with Fiber*
  - *Resource/Resource Plus*
  - *Isocal* (with or without fibre)
- Tube (unflavored)
  - *Osmolite HNR/Jevity*
  - *Pediasure* (pediatric)
  - *Nutren Unflavored* 1.0, 1.5/ *Nutren Unflavored with Fiber*
- Elemental
  - *Vital HN*
  - *Peptamen* (semi-elemental)
- Specialized
  - *Glucerna* (diabetes)
  - *Pulmocare* (CO_2 retention)
  - *Nepro* (hemodialysis)
  - *Suplena* (pre-dialysis)
  - *Advera* (AIDS)
  - *Sustacal* (high protein)

Meal Replacements

- *Essentials*
- *Boost*
- *Ultra Slim Fast*
- *Carnation Instant Breakfast*
- *Dynatrim*
- *Enervit*
- *Nutri Diet*

Preterm Infant Formulas: These formulas have a more concentrated nutrient content and are designed to meet the needs of small preterm infants. They use whey-predominant proteins, carbohydrate mixtures of lactose and glucose polymers and fat mixtures containing combinations of medium-chain and unsaturated long-chain triglycerides.

Follow-up Formulas: These formulas are for infants >6 months of age and contain more iron, vitamin D and protein than other infant formulas.

APPETITE SUPPRESSANTS AND DIET AIDS

For a summary of nonprescription weight-loss products in Canada see Table 25.

Also see the section on Formulated Liquid Diets (Enteral Products section).

ALTERNATIVE SWEETENERS

Alternative sweeteners are a substitute for sucrose without the calories. They are used in weight control and diabetic products and to help reduce dental caries. In diabetics, if used in larger amounts (>3 g), they may contribute to hyperglycemia unless counted as part of the carbohydrate allowance for the meal.

Saccharin is 300 times sweeter than sucrose and provides no calories. It is stable during food preparation and fully retains its sweetness. Its major disadvantages are a bitter after-taste and an association with a possible risk of bladder cancer, which has not been conclusively shown. In Canada, saccharin can be sold only in pharmacies. Saccharin products must state on the label that continued use may injure health and that it be used by pregnant women only on the advice of a physician.

Cyclamate is 30 times sweeter than sucrose. It acts synergistically with other sweeteners, is stable to heat and cold, and is used in drinks and table-top sweeteners. The major problem is an objectionable taste. There has been some controversy about carcinogenicity, but this has not been proven.

Aspartame is 200 times sweeter than sucrose. It is synthesized from the amino acids phenylalanine and aspartic acid. When exposed to heat or an alkaline pH, it decomposes into diketopiperazine, methanol and aspartylphenylalanine, all of which are nonsweet compounds, so it cannot be used in cooking. It works synergistically with other sweeteners and is used mainly as a low-calorie sweetener in carbonated soft drinks, diabetic and dietetic foods, chewing gums, fruit juices, gelatin jams and jellies and pharmaceuticals.

A safe level of aspartame intake has been determined to be 50 mg/kg body weight/day. At this level, toxicity is nonexistent. There have been reports of consumers complaining of adverse effects associated with aspartame consumption including: neurogenic and behavioral disorders, such as headaches, dizziness, insomnia and seizures; gastrointestinal effects, such as nausea, vomiting and diarrhea; rashes; menstrual irregularities. Some people may be more sensitive to aspartame. As one of the major metabolites of aspartame is phenylalanine, patients with phenylketonuria should avoid the use of aspartame because of an inability to tolerate phenylalanine. Most people have no problems tolerating aspartame consumption.

Acesulfame-K is 200 times sweeter than sucrose. It is rapidly absorbed, quickly excreted from the body unchanged and is nonmutagenic and noncarcinogenic. It is used as a sweetener in foods, beverages and pharmaceuticals.

Sucralose is 600 times sweeter than sucrose. It is produced from sucrose by substituting three atoms of chlorine for three of the hydroxyl groups in the sugar molecule. Sucralose is calorie free because the chlorine atoms strengthen the disaccharide molecule so it is not broken down during its passage through the body, absorbed only in limited amounts and excreted virtually unchanged. Sucralose is not toxic, does not accumulate in the body and is not carcinogenic. It is stable during food processing and storage and can be used in cooking. It is used in many foods, beverages, table-top sweeteners and as a sugar substitute in cooking.

Xylitol, Sorbitol and Mannitol: Xylitol is as sweet as sugar and has the same number of calories. Sorbitol is 60% as sweet as sugar and mannitol about 50% as sweet. Sorbitol and xylitol cause less tooth decay than sucrose and are used in chewing gums, jams, mints, candy and chocolates. These polyalcohol sweeteners, by an osmotic effect, can have a laxative effect if too much is consumed.

SALT SUBSTITUTES

These products are used in sodium-restricted diets for the management of hypertension and edema-

TABLE 25: Nonprescription Weight Loss Agents Available in Canada

Product	Mechanism of Action	Comments
Benzocaine	Local anesthetic to numb taste buds	Gum formulation may be better for constant snackers Limited data to demonstrate efficacy Safety data not available May also contain vitamins and other weight loss ingredients Available as gum, lozenge and tablets
Bulking agents or fibre (e.g., carboxymethylcellulose)	Delayed gastric emptying and absorption rate Creates a feeling of fullness and satiety	Clinical trials needed to evaluate efficacy Similar effect may be obtained by eating high-fibre vegetables and fruits
Phenylpropanolamine	Sympathomimetic activity with α and β stimulatory activity; temporary appetite reduction and possibly thermogenesis effect	Maximum daily dosage should not exceed 75 mg/day due to narrow therapeutic range Side effects: CNS stimulation and psychoses; high doses may lead to increased blood pressure in susceptible individuals. Drug interactions with irreversible monoamine oxidase inhibitors, tricyclic antidepressants, caffeine and antihypertensives Contraindicated in pregnancy, breast-feeding, diabetes, hypertension and hyperthyroidism Long-acting preparations are not advised if dietary indiscretion occurs at certain time of day
Meal replacement products	Rationale is to substitute for 1 or 2 meals, followed by a regular meal	Available as puddings, shakes, candy bars, powders and wafers Most products are supplemented with vitamins and minerals Provide a concentrated form of energy which is generally low in fat; thus may be useful as weight-promoting agents (in addition to regular meals) If products are recommended, appropriate counselling should include the importance of exercise and a balanced diet. Generally these products do not work over a long time period, unless behavioral changes are also undertaken

tous states associated with heart or liver failure. The principal source of sodium in the diet is salt added to food during its preparation and preservation, and at the table before eating. Each molecule of salt is approximately 40% sodium, and therefore 1 teaspoon of salt (5 g) contains about 2 g or 90 mEq of sodium. Mild sodium restriction usually means 2.4 to 4.5 g (100 to 200 mEq) of sodium used daily. Moderate sodium restriction usually means 1 to 2 g (45 to 90 mEq) of sodium daily. Severe sodium restriction usually means 0.5 to 1 g (20 to 45 mEq) daily but is generally not recommended as it is too severe for compliance.

A major problem of compliance with a low-salt diet is lack of palatability. Salt substitutes available contain potassium chloride, are rather bitter and not widely accepted. Hyperkalemia is a concern especially if the patient is on potassium-sparing diuretics and/or ACE inhibitors. A better approach is to add little or no salt at the table or in cooking, to avoid high-sodium convenience and fast-foods, to avoid foods that have salt added during processing and to encourage the generous use of spices that contain negligible (0.05–0.1%) amounts of salt. Eventually by cutting back on the amount of salt consumed, the taste buds adapt and less salt is desired.

PHARMACEUTICAL AGENTS FOR THE ATHLETE

Amino Acids: Promoted as stimulators of growth-hormone release to influence muscle growth, arginine and ornithine, in high doses, are the only amino acids that have any significant effect on growth-hormone release from the pituitary gland. Growth hormone stimulates protein synthesis, speeds up the breakdown of fat and decreases the quantity of carbohydrate used by the body. The release of growth hormone has been promoted to burn off fat and build muscles and is attractive to athletes. There are no long-term studies to support this contention. Growth hormone, in excess, causes gradual thickening of bones and overgrowth of soft tissue, resulting eventually in grotesque features. It may also result in symptoms of diabetes, hypothyroidism and arthritis.

Carnitine is a trimethyl amino acid derivative but is thought by the general public to be an amino acid. It is a popular product in health food stores, promoted to increase athletic performance by strengthening for endurance events. It is involved in the production of energy from fatty acids. Supplementation is not required as sufficient amounts are present in foods such as meat and dairy products and manufactured in the liver and kidneys, so it is not an essential amino acid.

Supplementation can be counterproductive. Most of the products available contain both the L form (active) and the D form (inactive). D-carnitine inhibits the transport of L-carnitine, which depletes tissue pools of L-carnitine. Use of the DL form can actually bring on symptoms of carnitine deficiency: muscle cramps and muscle weakness.

Protein Supplements: Gelatin is the usual base for protein supplements. It is derived from the collagen of animal bones but is one of the poorest quality proteins available. It contains glycinc, thc precursor of phosphocreatine, which has not been proven to improve athletic performance.

Sports Drinks: The ideal fluid replacement promotes rapid fluid absorption and does not cause gastrointestinal discomfort. Drinks containing 6 to 10% glucose or sucrose leave the stomach and are absorbed into the bloodstream from the intestine at a similar rate to that of plain water. Fructose solutions do not stimulate fluid absorption and may cause gastrointestinal distress. The sodium content of fluid replacement beverages is 10 to 20 mEq/L (230 to 460 mg/L), which is much lower than the sodium content of plasma (150 mEq/L) and therefore will not likely impair fluid absorption. See Table 22 for a fluid replacement comparison chart.

RECOMMENDED READING

Bell L, ed. Manual of Nutritional Care. 4th ed. Vancouver: British Columbia Dietitians' & Nutritionists' Association, 1992.

Gaziano JM. Antioxidant vitamins and coronary artery disease risk. Am J Med 1994;97(suppl 3A):18s–21s.

Hoffman RM. Antioxidants and the prevention of coronary heart disease. Arch Intern Med 1995; 155:241–46.

Johnson LE. The emerging role of vitamins as antioxidants. Arch Fam Med 1994;3:809–20.

Simon HB. Patient-directed, nonprescription approaches to cardiovascular disease. Arch Intern Med 1994;154:2283–96.

19

ORAL HEALTH CARE PRODUCTS

LINDA G. SUVEGES

CONTENTS

Oral Anatomy and Physiology	**489**
Dental Caries	**491**
Etiology and Pathophysiology	
Symptoms	
Treatment	
Prevention	
Periodontal Diseases	**496**
Etiology and Pathophysiology	
Symptoms	
Treatment	
Prevention	
Other Dental Problems	**499**
Dental Pain	
Dental Erosion	
Broken Teeth or Misfitting Restorations	
Teething Pain	
Cold Sores	**501**
Etiology and Pathophysiology	
Symptoms	
Treatment	
Canker Sores	**504**
Etiology	
Symptoms	
Treatment	
Candidiasis (Moniliasis)	**506**
Etiology	
Symptoms	
Treatment	
Other Causes of Oral Lesions	
Halitosis	**508**
Etiology	
Treatment	
Dry Mouth	**509**
Etiology	
Symptoms	
Treatment	
Product Information	**514**
Cold Sore and Canker Sore Products	
Dentifrices	
Denture Products	
Dry Mouth Products	
Fluoride	
Mouthwashes	
Plaque Disclosing Agents	
Plaque Removal Products	
Toothache Relievers	
Tooth Whiteners	
Summary	**528**
Recommended Reading	**529**

ORAL ANATOMY AND PHYSIOLOGY

The initial stages of food digestion are provided by mastication (chewing) and salivary secretion in the mouth. Various microorganisms make up the normal flora of the mouth; they create pathologic problems only when the host resistance is modified.

The inside of the mouth is covered by specialized epithelial tissue called the mucosa. In its normal healthy state, the mucosa is pinkish red. It protects the underlying muscles, nerves and vascular bed from food materials and bacterial contamination. The soft gum tissue surrounding the teeth is the gingiva. It is normally coral pink, because of its keratin content. The gingiva forms sharp, well-defined points, or papillae, between the teeth. To a large extent, the teeth are not protected by any tissue.

Anatomically, the tooth has two parts—the crown and the root (Figure 1). The crown is the part of the tooth normally completely exposed in the mouth and is responsible for mastication. The roots exist below the gingival line and are essential

Oral Anatomy and Physiology

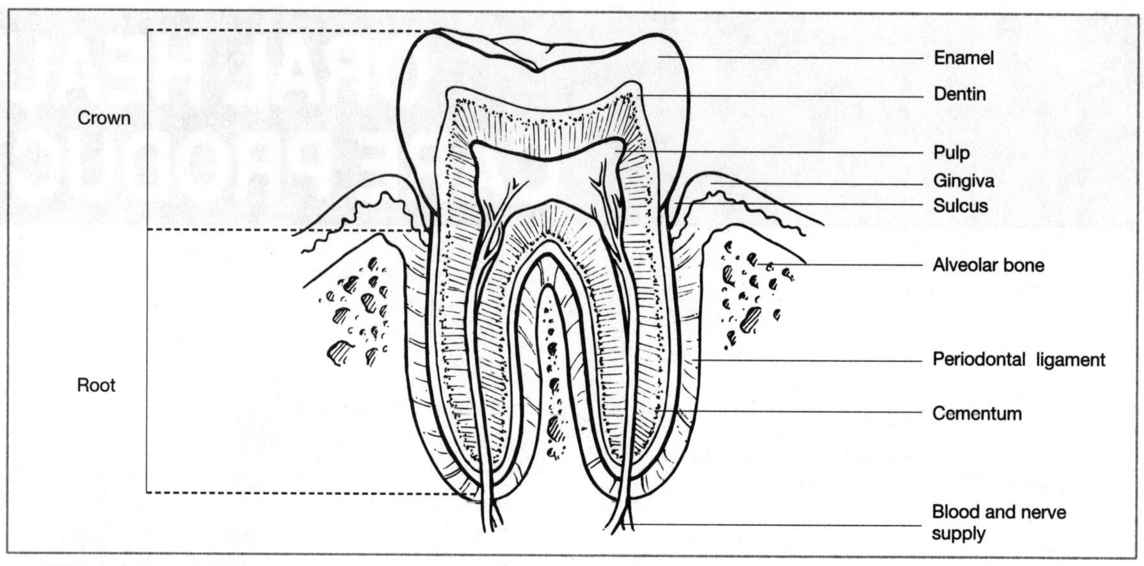

FIGURE 1: Anatomy of a Tooth

for support, attachment of the tooth to surrounding tissues and provide a pathway for innervation and blood supply for the tooth.

The **enamel** covers the crown of the tooth and protects the underlying structures of dentin and pulp. Enamel, the hardest and most densely calcified tissue in the body, is composed of crystals of a calcium phosphate compound known as hydroxyapatite. Unlike the enamel of certain animal teeth, human enamel cannot regenerate after injury or gradual loss. However, it is not an inert compound, as exchange and addition of ions can take place. This mechanism is the basis of the therapeutic application of fluoride ions, which replace hydroxy groups to form fluorapatite. This crystal is more stable, harder and more resistant to acid dissolution than hydroxyapatite. Characteristically, enamel is off-white in color, principally because of the underlying yellow dentin.

Dentin forms the bulk of the tooth. It is softer than enamel but is a calcified tissue similar to bone. It helps to protect the pulp and also distributes nutrients from the pulp. The **pulp** is a delicate, highly vascular material, continuous with the surrounding tissues through an opening at the apex of the root. Any stimulus, such as pressure, heat or cold, to the free nerve endings in either the pulp or the dentin causes pain.

A cervical margin marks the joining of the root and crown of the tooth. The channel formed between the tooth and gingiva is the sulcus. Entrapment here of bacteria and debris must be minimized to prevent dental disease.

The root of the tooth is covered with a calcified tissue called cementum. The tooth is attached in its socket in the alveolar bone by periodontal ligaments. During mastication, the tooth can move slightly because of the elasticity of these fibres but remains firmly in place in the dental arch. Collectively, the periodontium is made up of the cementum, periodontal ligament, alveolar bone and gingiva.

Calcification of the crowns of the teeth begins about the fourth month of gestation and continues until a child is 7 or 8 years of age. Various environmental influences, such as inadequate nutrition or the ingestion of toxic substances, may manifest after tooth eruption. The relationship between light-yellow to grey-brown pigmentation of dental enamel and the ingestion of tetracycline during tooth development is firmly established. The nature of the staining depends on the form, dosage and duration of tetracycline administration. The stains darken after tooth eruption. The use of tetracycline by pregnant women or children up to the age of 8 years is not recommended.

Other oral and extraoral tissues of the head and neck may be involved in certain pathological processes. The tongue is important in mastication, speech, taste and swallowing. Its upper surface is usually irregular and rough in appearance. Taste buds are located in or around various papillae or projections on the tongue. The salivary glands in the mouth secrete saliva. Saliva is an alkaline, slightly viscous, clear secretion with several components including enzymes, serum albumin, mucopolysaccharides, leukocytes and minerals. Normal salivary function is essential for good oral health.

DENTAL CARIES

ETIOLOGY AND PATHOPHYSIOLOGY

The oral health status of children in Canada and the United States appears to be generally better than that of children in other highly industrialized countries. However, dental caries or tooth decay remains the most prevalent disease among all age groups beyond infancy. Ninety-five per cent of the North American population experiences carious lesions, a frequency that has major economic and health implications. Unfortunately, the risk of dental caries is not evenly distributed over all groups. For example, by age 17, 84% of U.S. children have been affected by dental caries. However, members of high risk groups such as minorities, rural dwellers or those from less educated or poorer families are more affected: 25% of U.S. children have 75% of the dental caries.

In adults, dental caries tend to stabilize and remain dormant until root surface caries begin to develop because of exposure of cementum from gum recession or surgery.

Dental caries is the disease process involving the dissolution of tooth enamel, dentin and cementum, leading to the development of cavities. Formation of dental caries requires the presence and growth of cariogenic bacteria on the tooth surface. Caries susceptibility also depends on other factors, such as diet, saliva composition and flow, tooth placement and the physicochemical nature of the tooth surface. The influence of additional environmental factors, such as reduction in exposure to ultraviolet light, on caries susceptibility is currently being investigated.

When host resistance is modified, the normal flora of the mouth may create pathologic problems. Some of these microorganisms, especially *Streptococcus mutans* and lactobacilli, are cariogenic.

The pathophysiology of dental caries begins with the demineralization of tooth enamel by acid produced during fermentation of carbohydrates by the bacteria resident in dental plaque. Plaque is thought to start with formation of an acquired pellicle or protein coating that adheres to the clean tooth surface; saliva is a possible source. Bacteria and other components attach to the pellicle and tooth surface, forming a sticky mass called plaque. The high concentration of bacteria in plaque and its gel-like structure lead to acid accumulation at the tooth surface and a rapid fall in pH to a level at which demineralization can occur. Plaque prevents the washing and buffering effects of saliva from reaching the tooth surface, further enhancing caries production. Plaque also forms on dental restorations, appliances and dentures. Left unchecked, plaque thickens with food residues and proliferating bacteria. If not removed within 24 hours, plaque calcifies into calculus (tartar), which can only be removed by professional dental cleaning. Low accumulations of dental plaque are associated with significantly fewer dental caries, even in the adult population.

Not all enamel surfaces have the same potential for plaque formation and dental decay. Occlusal (top) surfaces of the molars and interproximal surfaces between the molars develop caries most often.

For caries to develop, a carbohydrate substrate must be present in the mouth. An individual's diet is thought to be an important determinant of susceptibility to dental decay, especially the form and frequency of sugar consumption.

Carbohydrate-containing foods differ in their cariogenic potential. Those with a high concentration of sucrose are strongly cariogenic because of rapid solubilization and fermentation to acids. The amount of sucrose ingested also influences the number of cariogenic bacteria able to colonize on tooth surfaces. When dietary intake of sucrose is limited, *Streptococcus mutans* colonizes only in small numbers. Because the average North American man, woman or child consumes over 1 kg of sucrose per week, dental caries remains a significant health problem. Much of this sugar is consumed in commercially prepared foods of all types.

Other sugars, such as fructose (in fruits and corn syrup) and lactose (in milk), are also cariogenic, but less so than sucrose. As well, starchy foods that adhere to the teeth may lead to dental caries because of prolonged availability for acid formation. The cariogenic potential of snack foods that contain fermentable carbohydrates and are also sticky, such as raisins and chewy granola bars, is greater than that of chocolate candy bars. However, high sugar concentrations also stimulate more rapid removal of carbohydrates from the tooth environment. Thus, breakfast cereal that is not sugar coated is actually retained in the mouth longer than sugar-coated cereal. The carbohydrate content of a particular food may therefore be a more important contributor to its cariogenic potential than has been generally believed. Some foods, such as milk, cocoa and peanuts, have cariostatic effects. Their presence in a food item may therefore also modify its cariogenic potential.

Although sucrose has long been implicated as a major factor in tooth decay, the relative cariogenicity of foods depends on variations in composition, solubility, retentiveness and ability to stimulate saliva flow. The cariogenic potential of foods also depends on the frequency and timing of eating those foods. Individuals who do not eat between meals have fewer decayed teeth than those who snack frequently.

After primary teeth erupt, some children who are bottle-fed for extended periods, especially while lying down, may also develop extensive caries of the upper incisors. This condition, "nursing bottle syndrome," can be largely prevented by avoiding the use of milk-containing or juice-containing bottles as pacifiers.

Children who require long-term therapy with a sugar-containing liquid medication are at increased risk of developing dental caries. Ingesting such medication should be followed by correct toothbrushing or at least by rinsing the mouth thoroughly with water.

Although the human preference for sweets appears innate, it can be modified greatly by environmental factors such as restricting sugar consumption from birth. Enamel decay is most common in young persons, reaching a peak between 11 and 18 years of age. Unfortunately, children and adolescents are in the group that finds sugary foods most attractive and may resist diet modification.

Some nutritive sugar substitutes, such as the hydrogenated sugars mannitol, sorbitol and xylitol, are less susceptible to rapid acid production by oral microorganisms, and therefore have lower cariogenic potential. These agents are used to sweeten a number of sugarless gums and candies. They satisfy cravings for sweet foods while reducing the opportunity for plaque formation and caries development. In addition, chewing sugarless gum after consuming sugary snacks may lessen the cariogenicity of such foods by stimulating saliva flow and delivering the saliva to interproximal areas of the teeth by mechanical action. Xylitol may also have some bacteriostatic properties that contribute to its cariostatic effects. The chewing of such gum for 10 minutes after consuming acidogenic foods is sufficient to return plaque pH to levels present before eating. Chewing xylitol-containing gum three times daily as part of a Canadian school-based dental program has also been shown to reduce the progression of dental decay over 24 months in children 8 to 9 years of age. Other noncariogenic, noncaloric, synthetic sweeteners include saccharin and cyclamates, but concerns exist for their safety in long-term use. Besides its noncariogenic properties, saccharin has been shown to inhibit bacterial growth and metabolism and to reduce plaque accumulation when used as a replacement for sucrose. Aspartame appears to be a safe and noncariogenic sweetener that also inhibits some bacterial growth and adherent plaque formation. It is about 200 times sweeter than sucrose.

SYMPTOMS

The demineralization of a tooth's enamel surface by acids produced by bacteria in dental plaque is chronic. Initially, a carious lesion exhibits no clinical symptoms and is difficult to detect without close examination with specific diagnostic instruments (Figure 2). Once the demineralization progresses through the enamel to the softer dentin, destruction is much more rapid and may produce a large cavity beneath only a small break in the enamel (Figure 3). At this point the individual may become aware of the lesion and complain of toothache. Any stimulus, such as heat, cold or percussion, to the affected tooth elicits pain. The quality of the pain—sharp, stabbing, dull or pulsating—indicates the proximity of the decay process

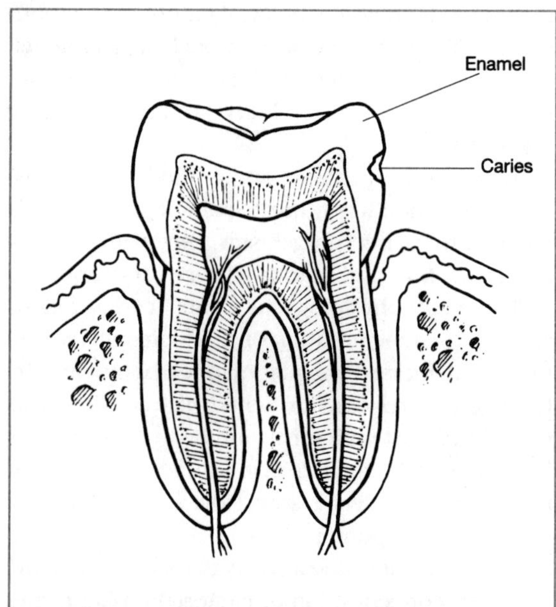

FIGURE 2: Enamel Caries

to the dental pulp. Progression of the carious damage to the pulp produces continuous, often excruciating, pain.

When a carious lesion is left untreated, infection of the pulp with bacteria elicits an inflammatory response, called pulpitis. Eventually, infection may spread to the periodontal ligament and bone (Figure 4). Such abscess formation can create a variety of signs and symptoms, including severe pain, edema and erythema of tissue around the tooth, or massive cellulitis and facial swelling. Some people may develop septicemia from untreated dental caries.

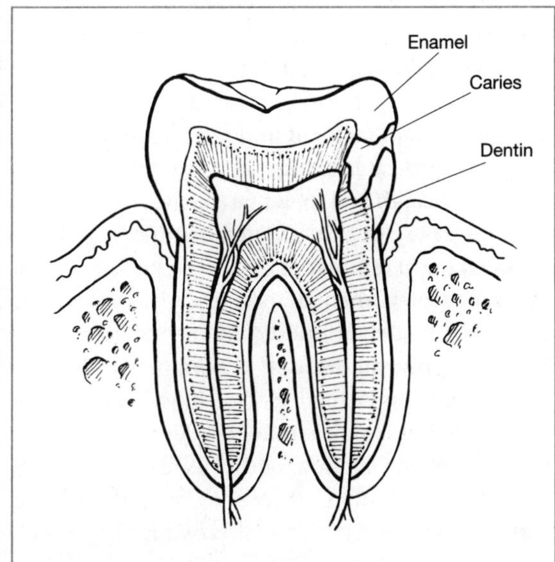

FIGURE 3: Dentinal Caries—Pulpitis

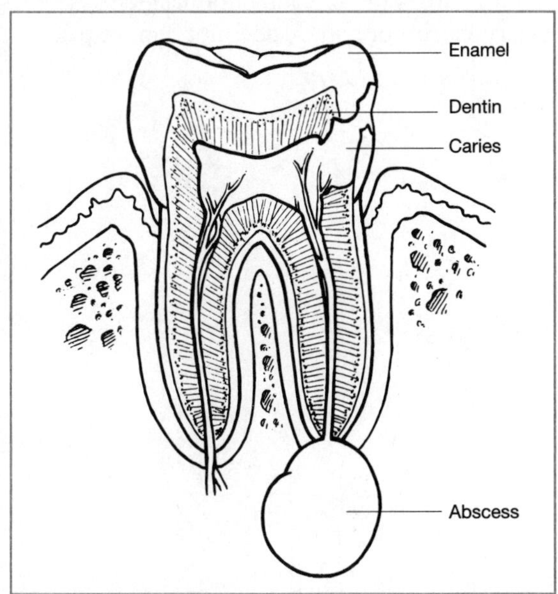

FIGURE 4: Advanced Caries with Pulp Necrosis and Abscess Formation

Other symptoms, such as bleeding and bad breath, more often relate to poor oral hygiene and periodontal disease than to dental caries.

TREATMENT

The untreated carious process, once initiated, cannot be reversed. It can be arrested by removing the external causes. Because the sequelae of dental decay are loss of enamel and bacterial infection of underlying tissue, the treatment of choice for very small lesions is remineralization of the tooth enamel. If this is unsuccessful, or if the lesion is larger, the infected hard tissue must be removed and the cavity filled with an inert material that restores the shape and function of the tooth. Such restorative treatment by a dentist is usually sufficient to relieve any associated pain. However, if the individual cannot receive such treatment immediately, nonprescription oral analgesics such as ASA, acetaminophen or ibuprofen may help. Adult doses of 650 to 1,000 mg of ASA or acetaminophen or 200 to 400 mg of ibuprofen are suggested. (See the Pain and Fever Products chapter for more detail.) In addition, an obtundent, such as benzocaine, applied to the cavity may help reduce the pain until dental treatment is received.

Because dental caries can eventually cause loss of tooth vitality and abscess formation, the health professional should encourage all people seeking nonprescription medication for toothache relief to see a dentist as soon as possible. They should also avoid any stimuli, such as sweet, hot or cold substances that may precipitate or aggravate pain.

PREVENTION

Most dental caries can be prevented. These factors must be present for dental caries to occur: a susceptible tooth; bacteria in dental plaque that can produce acids from carbohydrates; and fermentable carbohydrates in the diet. Measures to prevent caries focus on attempts to increase resistance of the teeth with fluorides and fissure sealants, to lower the number or cariogenicity of bacteria in contact with teeth by mechanical means or chemical agents, and to modify dietary patterns to reduce the amount and frequency of carbohydrate ingestion.

The prospects for reducing dental caries by altering the dietary habits of the public are not promising. Although the relationship between sugar and caries activity is accepted, significant

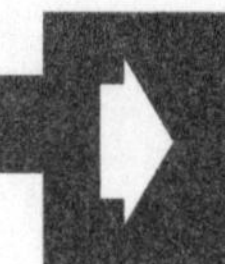

ADVICE FOR THE PATIENT

Prevention of Dental Caries

- Reduce the amount and frequency of eating sugar and processed foods.
  The bacteria in dental plaque produce acid when they metabolize sugar; it is important to consume foods that are low in sugars. Foods that stick to the teeth should also be minimized.
- Brush with a fluoride toothpaste and floss your teeth at least once or twice a day to remove dental plaque.
  Dental plaque contains bacteria that produce acid that in turn breaks down tooth enamel and leads to cavities. Regular removal of dental plaque is one of the best ways to prevent dental cavities (and gum disease). Fluoride helps to harden the tooth enamel and prevent its breakdown by acid.
- If you cannot brush after a meal, chewing sugar-free gum (e.g., *Trident*) for about 20 minutes will help to reduce dental caries.
  Chewing gum increases saliva flow and removes sugar and food from the tooth surface.
- Talk to your dentist about other fluoride treatments to help prevent dental caries.

reductions in sugar intake have not occurred. Perhaps the most practical recommendations a health professional can make are to suggest that sugary and starchy foods be restricted to meals, and the teeth be brushed promptly after all meals or snacks. If brushing is not possible, chewing a sugarless gum for 10 minutes after eating may help reduce the potential for caries development.

The use of fluoride in various forms continues to be the most effective way to prevent dental caries. Delivery methods include systemic ingestion of fluoridated water or fluoride tablets and topical application via various gels, varnishes, mouthrinses or dentifrices.

The method of fluoride therapy determines its effectiveness to a certain extent (Table 1). However, widespread availability of fluorides from various sources and the geographic mobility of society today has made it increasingly difficult to conduct additional research on the effectiveness of a single type of fluoride treatment. Perhaps the most important element in dental treatment is the frequent application of low concentrations of fluoride to the tooth and to dental plaque, such as with the regular use of a fluoridated dentifrice.

Mechanical removal of dental plaque is probably the most well known method of caries prevention. If dental plaque is periodically dispersed and the bacteria prevented from becoming sufficiently established, the incidence of periodontal disease as well as dental caries is reduced. Aids available for plaque removal include toothbrushes, dental floss, toothpicks and other devices. To clean the enamel surface completely, a mild abrasive is also usually necessary. Most dentifrices contain abrasives of varying properties. Chewing gum, rinsing the mouth with water or eating fibrous foods, such as celery, carrots or apples, does not remove plaque.

TABLE 1: Effectiveness of Various Methods of Administering Fluorides

Method	Concentration of Dose	Percentage Reduction in Dental Caries
Community water fluoridation	0.7–1.2 ppm	50–65
School water fluoridation	4.5 times optimum above	40
Dietary fluoride (F) supplements		
Home	Depends on age of child and F concentration in water	50–65
School only	2.2 mg NaF	30–35
Mouthrinses	0.05% NaF (daily) 0.20% NaF (weekly)	20–50
Dentifrices	0.40% SnF_2 0.76% MFP 0.22% NaF	20–30
Professionally applied applications	2.0% NaF 8.0% SnF_2 APF (1.2% F)	30–40

NaF = sodium fluoride
SnF_2 = stannous fluoride
MFP = monofluorophosphate
APF = acidulated phosphate fluoride
Adapted with permission from: Horowitz HS. The prevention of oral disease. Established methods of prevention. Br Dent J 1980;149:311–8.

PERIODONTAL DISEASES

Periodontal diseases afflict a significant portion of the adult population, although many causes are controllable and preventable. It has been commonly assumed that periodontal disease is the primary cause of tooth loss after age 35. However, recent studies indicate that caries, particularly in lower income individuals who have neglected their dental care, is a major reason for tooth extraction in adults. As the North American population ages and more people retain their teeth, the prevalence of periodontal diseases will remain high. Many people think that with increasing age, dentures are as inevitable as grey hair. However, natural dentition can be retained throughout a lifetime if there is proper and continuous attention to oral hygiene.

Periodontal diseases affect the supporting tissues of the tooth. They range from gingivitis to more severe conditions such as periodontitis. Although these conditions occur worldwide, the prevalence and severity of periodontal diseases are difficult to determine because of a lack of uniform descriptors or methods of measurement. It has been suggested that the periodontium of nearly every adult shows some deviation from normal. The incidence, extent and severity of periodontal disease increase with age because of the progressive nature of the condition and the cumulative effects of poor oral hygiene. Since the populations of industrialized countries like Canada and the United States are gradually aging and greater numbers of people are retaining much of their natural dentition, the incidence and prevalence of periodontal diseases may rise.

ETIOLOGY AND PATHOPHYSIOLOGY

Bacterial plaque is the single most important external etiologic agent in inflammation of the periodontium. As plaque accumulates on the tooth at the gingival margin, it produces an inflammatory reaction in the gingivae called gingivitis. The bacteria resident in dental plaque produce various metabolic compounds that are secreted into the gingival sulcus, activating host defense mechanisms. These metabolic products, rather than the microorganisms themselves, are thought to be responsible for the inflammatory changes in the periodontium. Further immunologic response within the gingivae enhances the destruction of the support tissue. As long as the bacterial plaque is left undisturbed, the inflammatory response continues. Eventually, alveolar bone may begin to break down, and the teeth become loose and fall out.

Although subgingival calculus does not initiate the inflammatory process, its presence can contribute to the chronicity and progression of periodontal disease. Calculus is porous enough to serve as a basis for further plaque growth. It also promotes retention of bacterial antigens and inflammatory mediators in the gingival area. Because calculus cannot be removed by normal toothbrushing, individuals must see a dentist regularly to have calculus removed from teeth.

Limited evidence suggests an association between smokeless tobacco use and gingival recession, but further research is needed on how this contributes to periodontal disease or dental caries.

The long-standing assumption that gingivitis inevitably progresses to destructive periodontitis has been challenged. Gingivitis is a poor predictor of periodontitis in people younger than 30 years of age. Some data suggest other host-related factors may be necessary to develop severe periodontitis.

SYMPTOMS

Healthy gingival tissue is coral pink, firm and adheres closely to the neck of the tooth. Periodontal disease begins as a marginal inflammation of the gums. The gingivae appear dark red and glossy and the interdental papillae become blunted and lose resiliency. At this stage the individual is usually unaware of the disease process, which may affect only part of the gingivae. When the disease involves most of the gum tissue, it is termed diffuse gingivitis.

As with dental caries, periodontal disease has a bacterial etiology and is usually a progressive or chronic disorder. Pain is not a feature until symptoms and tissue destruction are advanced. People most often complain about bleeding from the gums when they brush their teeth or chew hard foods. They may also complain about an offensive mouth odor.

The rate the disease intensifies depends on the individual's oral hygiene and oral habits. For example, mouth-breathing aggravates the symptoms around the anterior teeth due to a constant drying-wetting action. As the disease progresses to involve the rest of the periodontium, alveolar bone is resorbed and tooth attachment compromised. This stage of the disease is called periodontitis. Loss of gingival support and recession of tissue results in formation of pockets around the tooth, which may bleed or exude pus. The latter accounts for the outdated term pyorrhea used to describe periodontal disease. The individual may feel pain at this stage when drinking hot or cold fluids or when brushing the teeth because of stimulation of the now-exposed cementum.

Eventually, the teeth become loose and bacteria may invade the support tissue, causing an acute periodontal abscess or acute periodontitis to develop. The individual can usually pinpoint the site by symptoms of deep, throbbing or radiating pain. Prognosis for teeth with advanced bone loss, extreme mobility and recurrent abscess formation is poor. The usual treatment is extraction.

Although gingivitis is more often chronic in nature, acute forms of the condition do occur. One of these, acute necrotizing ulcerative gingivitis (ANUG), also termed Vincent's infection and trenchmouth, is characterized by extremely sensitive, bleeding gingival tissue. The interdental and marginal gingivae are covered with a necrotic, greyish pseudomembrane. When the necrotic tissue is removed with gauze, a painful, crater-like ulceration, which bleeds spontaneously or when touched, may be present. The individual may also complain of an offensive breath odor and a metallic taste as well as a wooden, dead or loose feeling in the teeth. Usually, fever and increased salivary secretion are associated with ANUG.

ANUG, seen most frequently in teenagers and young adults, seems to be associated with the presence of spirochete and fusiform organisms. Other predisposing factors may be anxiety and emotional stress, smoking, malnutrition and poor oral hygiene. Although it may resolve spontaneously, ANUG usually requires antibacterial therapy and a visit to the dental clinic to prevent septicemia or progressive destruction of the periodontium.

Acute gingivitis may also develop from the generally chronic course of periodontal disease as a result of physical irritation from such things as hard food particles, new or hard-bristled toothbrushes, toothpicks, hot foods or tobacco tars. The symptoms may vary from linear lacerations to eroded areas and vesicle formation.

Pregnancy gingivitis is an acute form of gingivitis usually confined to one or more sites on the gums. It is usually painless, but bleeding may occur. Inadequate oral hygiene is the primary cause of the condition, but the intensified tissue reaction is perhaps due to changes in hormone levels. Oral contraceptive use may also be associated with an increased incidence of gingivitis.

About 50% of people taking phenytoin develop a condition called gingival hyperplasia within 2 to 3 months of the start of therapy. The first sign of this condition is usually enlargement of the interdental papillae, particularly in the front of the mouth. Gingival tissue may eventually cover the teeth, interfere with mastication and be esthetically unacceptable. Development of gingival hyperplasia from phenytoin does not seem to be dose-related but is precipitated by poor oral hygiene. Surgery may be required to remove excess tissue even if the medication is discontinued.

Nifedipine and cyclosporine also cause gingival hyperplasia in certain people. About 27% of patients taking cyclosporine and about 20% of those on nifedipine will experience this side effect. When the two drugs are taken together, the proportion of patients experiencing gingival overgrowth may be as high as 48%. Although the condition appears to be caused by a direct stimulation of gingival fibroblasts, it can often be prevented by maintaining a high standard of oral hygiene, eliminating gingival irritation from such things as plaque. All people taking these drugs should be advised about effective and frequent toothbrushing and flossing techniques.

TREATMENT

The most effective method of treating periodontal disease in all stages is to remove bacterial plaque. In the early stages of gingivitis, the disease process can be completely reversed by thoroughly cleaning the teeth every day to remove plaque. As periodontal disease progresses, more concentrated and sustained oral hygiene measures must be undertaken to control the disease and to limit the amount of destruction to the support tissue.

To begin and maintain an adequate program of oral hygiene may require guidance from dental practitioners and pharmacists in using preventive aids. The use of toothbrushes and dental floss are completely outlined in the Product Information section. Advanced periodontal disease may require surgical intervention and, in certain cases, systemic antibacterial therapy.

Topical nonprescription medications are generally of little use in treating periodontal disease. Products containing oxygenating agents, such as sodium perborate, zinc peroxide, hydrogen peroxide and carbamide (urea) peroxide in concentrations of 1 to 30% have been promoted as adjunctive therapy. These products may be recommended by dentists for postoperative use or after other oral treatments. Any benefit derived from the use of oxygenating agents is thought to be due to loosening of adherent debris by the liberated oxygen. Long-term use of these agents may produce oral irritation or decalcification of teeth (due to the agents' acidity) and development of a black, hairy tongue. The use of sodium bicarbonate by individuals at home has not been shown to effectively treat periodontal disease. Because most studies on the use of sodium bicarbonate or hydrogen peroxide in periodontal therapy have also employed techniques such as root scaling and planing by the dental practitioner, the effectiveness of such adjunct therapy has been questioned.

Antibacterial mouthrinses may also be used to reduce plaque levels in individuals with periodontal disease, although they do not affect subgingival plaque found in periodontitis associated with deep pockets.

Recent experimental studies have demonstrated that oral administration of nonsteroidal anti-inflammatory drugs (NSAIDs), such as ibuprofen or flurbiprofen, may be useful adjuncts in the treatment of gingivitis and periodontal disease. Both agents have been shown to control gingival inflammation, especially during the early stages of gingivitis. Dental practitioners may advise patients to purchase nonprescription products, such as ibuprofen, as an adjunctive measure to reduce inflammation that may be contributing to oral pain.

PREVENTION

Because periodontal diseases are closely associated with accumulations of dental plaque, reducing or removing plaque from the teeth and gingiva is the best way to prevent them. Gingival stimulation may play a role, but removing plaque from both hard and soft tissues is essential to prevent gingival inflammation.

OTHER DENTAL PROBLEMS

DENTAL PAIN

Besides caries, dental pain may be caused by certain dental procedures, such as placing large restorations or fillings, or removing calculus. Both treatments may cause hypersensitive teeth.

Receding gingival tissue may expose the cementum or root of the tooth and create an area of hypersensitivity to certain stimuli. The major symptom of this condition is a short, sharp pain or shock elicited by cold food or beverages, cold air, sweet or sour substances, salt, touching the tooth surface with the fingernail or toothbrush, or, in some cases, closing the teeth together. The pain is usually transient and can sometimes be prevented by avoiding the stimuli or protecting the area with a desensitizing agent.

Individuals may also complain of a dull, mild, generalized pain in a number of maxillary teeth at the back of the dental arch. The cause of such pain is often infection in the maxillary sinuses (sinusitis). Sinusitis is most severe in the morning and is aggravated by bending over or going up and down stairs. It is less painful when lying down. The person may also describe symptoms, such as tenderness, sensitivity to cold fluids, and pain when the teeth are clenched together. Mild analgesics, such as ASA, acetaminophen or ibuprofen in recommended doses, may ease the discomfort of this type of dental pain, but complete relief requires medical assessment and proper antibiotic and decongestant therapy.

Another source of dental pain may be a tooth fracture, which may not be visually evident. The individual experiences a sudden, brief, unbearable, stabbing pain when chewing or when cold liquids contact the tooth. Avoiding such stimuli and promptly consulting a dentist are the only recommendations to give such people.

Vague tooth pain, especially in the early morning, may result from grinding the teeth together while sleeping or from an improperly contoured dental restoration. Nonprescription oral analgesics may help until the person can consult a dentist.

DENTAL EROSION

Although demineralization of tooth enamel is usually caused by acids produced by plaque-resident bacteria, teeth can be eroded by stomach acid when frequent vomiting occurs (e.g., in bulimia) or by acidic substances taken orally. Chewing large numbers of vitamin C tablets regularly may also lower saliva pH sufficiently to cause tooth erosion. People who take chewable products containing vitamin C should use such products judiciously and, if possible, brush the teeth after.

BROKEN TEETH OR MISFITTING RESTORATIONS

Broken teeth, besides being esthetically unappealing, can result in pulp exposure, pain, malocclusion and compromised mastication. Any break or chip in the natural dentition must be referred to a dentist for proper treatment. If a crown is chipped only slightly, restorative techniques may repair it. A large fracture may require root canal therapy or extraction. Occasionally a tooth that is knocked out, intact, from the dental arch can be reimplanted with prompt treatment. A dentist should be consulted immediately for appropriate instructions to ensure the greatest chance for possible reimplantation.

Lost or broken fillings and nonremovable prostheses, such as crowns and bridges, must also be evaluated and treated by a dental practitioner to prevent loss of normal function, discomfort and tooth breakdown.

Complete or partial dentures are removable prostheses used for partial correction of the loss of natural dentition. Dentures modify oral tissue and, later, the anatomy and physiology of the oral cavity. As well, they may have significant psychological effects. Wearing dentures satisfactorily requires the coordinated activity of the tongue and perioral musculature, as well as perseverance by the wearer and the clinician. To ensure maximal effectiveness, periodic professional attention is required. Although the time of useful service for a denture may be as low as 5 to 6 years, many denture wearers have had the same prostheses in place for much longer periods.

Ill-fitting or broken dentures can create several problems for the wearer, including accelerated bone loss with subsequent facial structure changes, ulceration, irritation, tumor growth and compromised oral function. Refitting, relining or repairing dentures to ensure proper functioning requires professional dental attention.

TEETHING PAIN

Normally, people are provided with two sets of teeth—primary or deciduous dentition, and permanent dentition. The deciduous teeth, commonly referred to as milk or baby teeth, begin to appear about 6 months after birth and are generally complete by the time the child is 24 to 30 months old. The first tooth to erupt is usually one of the mandibular or lower central incisors. This is followed by the fairly rapid and continuous eruption of the remaining primary teeth until the maxillary or upper second molars complete the dentition. There are 20 primary teeth, 10 in each arch. Generally, the first of the 32 permanent teeth to appear is the lower first molar, behind the primary second molar, at about 6 years of age. In some children the lower central incisors are the first permanent teeth to appear. Shedding a deciduous tooth is largely caused by root resorption stimulated by contact with the erupting permanent tooth beneath it. The permanent teeth are usually in place by age 13 except for the third molars (wisdom teeth), which usually erupt between 17 and 21 years of age.

The process of eruption of the deciduous teeth through the gingiva is referred to as teething. Although usually uneventful, teething may cause the gums to be swollen, irritated and painful. Some infants may also exhibit hypersalivation, irritability and sleep disturbances. They may also bite or chew on any available hard surface, including their hands or finger, toys or other objects in an apparent attempt to relieve the discomfort. When teething is accompanied by fever, nasal congestion or other symptoms, the child should be referred for medical assessment as these symptoms are more likely to be associated with an infection than with teething.

Older children and adults may also experience some pain as the rest of the molars erupt. This process may be associated with tenderness of the gum tissue, but patients who experience any significant amount of pain with molar eruptions should see a dentist for assessment.

Treatment

To relieve infant teething pain, parents may offer the child a frozen teething ring or a hard food such as a teething biscuit. Any object given to the child should be examined to make sure that it cannot be punctured or a small part bitten or broken off, which will cause choking. Parents may also apply a cold cloth or a small amount of a local anesthetic preparation to the gum tissue. An oral analgesic like acetaminophen may be given to relieve the pain and allow the child to sleep.

COLD SORES

The existence of disease caused by *Herpes Simplex* virus (HSV) has been known for at least 2,000 years. Despite identification of the virus in the 1940s and knowledge of its two varieties since 1960, developing effective treatment or preventive measures for herpes infections has been largely unsuccessful.

ETIOLOGY AND PATHOPHYSIOLOGY

Cold sores, or fever blisters, are usually caused by reactivation of latent *Herpes simplex* virus Type I (HSV-I), although HSV-II has been isolated from a few cases. Because the lesions commonly affect the lips or areas bordering the lips, cold sores are also known as recurrent herpes labialis (RHL). Although not as common, recurrent intraoral herpes (RIH) also occurs.

The peak incidence of primary infection with HSV-I is 6 to 36 months of age, but new cases appear in all age groups due to the contagious nature of the virus. An estimated 15% of adults will have the primary infection. The disease is thought to be transmitted by direct contact, usually with an individual suffering from recurrent herpes labialis. Virus excretion persists in all body secretions for 15 to 42 days after the onset of the primary herpes infection. In most cases of primary oral herpes, symptoms are subclinical or cannot be distinguished from other viral infections. The remainder experience an acute gingivostomatitis during the primary infection.

After the primary infection has healed, effective immunity develops in some people, but 20 to 45% have recurrent lesions. The virus apparently remains dormant in nerve cells until stimulated to reactivate. In North America, an estimated 7% of the general population have two or more bouts of herpes labialis annually. Recurrences may be precipitated by a number of factors, including fever, emotional stress, physical trauma, sunlight, systemic infections and menses (Table 2). People whose resistance is compromised may experience more severe lesions with slower healing.

SYMPTOMS

The onset of primary oral herpes infection is preceded by generalized systemic symptoms, including high fever, nausea, vomiting, headache and malaise for 1 to 2 days. Small vesicles that appear on the oral mucosa, tongue, lips or in the throat quickly rupture to form shallow round ulcers surrounded by inflammation. An important

TABLE 2: Features for Differential Diagnosis of Canker Sores and Cold Sores

	Primary Herpes	Recurrent Labial Herpes	Recurrent Aphthous Ulcers
Etiology	*Herpes simplex* virus	*Herpes simplex* virus	Unknown; possibly hypersensitivity or *Streptococcus sanguis*
Predisposing factors	None	Fever; stress; trauma; sunlight; infection	Heredity; food/drug allergy; trauma; stress; physiological factors
Prodrome	Slight fever; malaise; cervical lymphadenopathy	Burning; tingling sensation	Burning; tingling sensation
Lesions	Multiple vesicles; large superficial ulcers; diffuse erythema; yellow membrane; gingival inflammation	Small papules and vesicles; red centre; yellow crust; labial swelling	Small, multiple, erosive lesions; yellow or gray membrane; erythematous halo
Location	Labial mucosa; buccal mucosa; tongue; gingivae	Mucocutaneous junction of lips and adjacent skin	Buccal mucosa; labial mucosa; tongue, soft palate
Symptoms	Fever; intense oral pain; increased salivation; halitosis	Fever (only with other illnesses); lip pain; salivation unaffected; breath unaffected	Usually no fever; intense oral pain; localized hyperesthesia

diagnostic feature is acute marginal gingivitis. The person may also experience severe pain when the lesions are touched, increased saliva flow, malodorous breath and swollen neck glands. Table 2 outlines the features of primary and recurrent herpes. Primary herpes infection is usually a self-limiting condition and lasts 10 to 14 days. The lesions heal without scarring.

Recurrent herpes labialis (RHL) is often preceded for 24 to 48 hours by prodromal tingling, itching or burning of the lesion site (usually on or near the lips). A cluster of small vesicles then appears, ruptures and crusts over to form the typical cold sore or fever blister. The base of the lesion is reddened and edematous. A yellow crust on older lesions may indicate bacterial superinfection. Cold sores generally last from 3 to 10 days and are rarely accompanied by systemic symptoms. Patients who have frequent recurrences of RHL (such as an average of three recurrences within 6 months) may differ from the general population; those with frequent episodes may have multiple facial locations for their lesions.

The vesicles of RIH lesions break rapidly to form ulcers. These are typically 1 to 2 mm in diameter and cluster on the keratinized mucosa of the gingiva, palate or alveolar ridge.

TREATMENT

The treatment for acute herpetic gingivostomatitis is essentially symptomatic and supportive. Bed rest, adequate fluid maintenance and a soft diet supplemented by proteins are recommended. Oral analgesics such as ASA, acetaminophen or ibuprofen, in recommended doses, may be required to relieve pain and fever. Severe pain not controlled by nonprescription analgesics may require use of an opiate derivative, such as codeine. Because most primary herpes infections occur in children less than 6 years of age, sedation with diphenhydramine or prescribed agents may help.

Local therapy to ameliorate symptoms is also suggested. Cleansing mouthwashes with benzalkonium chloride 1:1,000, dilute hydrogen peroxide or a saline solution help clean and soothe involved mucous membranes. An appropriate saline solution can be prepared by dissolving 1/2 teaspoonful of table salt in 250 mL warm water.

Acute herpetic gingivostomatitis is one of the few conditions for which topical anesthetics are justified. Preparations containing benzocaine or lidocaine in vehicles that adhere to the oral mucosa, or that can be used as mouthrinses, are perhaps the most useful. The agents are applied as often as necessary to keep the individual comfortable, but should not be used long term due to the possibility, although rare, of hypersensitivity. Oral lesions may also be covered with an adherent protective paste, such as *Orabase* to relieve discomfort.

Recurrent herpes labialis is an annoying, cosmetically disfiguring and uncomfortable condition for which consumers often seek a health professional's advice. Unfortunately, no treatment reliably shortens healing time or lowers the recurrence rate of cutaneous herpes simplex infections. Ice applied within 24 hours of the prodrome may abort a cold sore, although controlled study of this preventive method has not been undertaken. Anecdotal reports show that cold sore vesicles may be resorbed and completely healed in 1 to 2 days if ice is applied continuously for 45 to 60 minutes to the prodromal area. To be effective, this treatment must be instituted as soon as possible after the prodromal tingling or burning is noticed.

When cold sore lesions are vesicular, cool compresses with tap water or Burow's solution applied for 10 minutes 3 to 4 times daily can be used. Bland emollients such as *AquaCare*, *Keri* products or white petrolatum are recommended to prevent drying lesions from cracking or fissuring. Secondary bacterial infections can be prevented by applying a topical nonprescription antibiotic ointment. The use of caustic agents, such as phenol or silver nitrate, are contraindicated in cold sore therapy. When an attack is precipitated by sunlight, nonprescription sunscreen products may be recommended to prevent cold sore development, although some individuals may still have a reactivation of HSV. Applying a topical corticosteroid to a cold sore for its anti-inflammatory action is controversial.

As outlined in Table 3, many topical agents have not proven clearly useful for herpes labialis. Well controlled, double-blind studies have not been published for several products, such as those containing propolis 2% and a combination of heparin with zinc sulfate.

TABLE 3 Treatments Ineffective or Not Proven Clearly Useful in Herpes Labialis

Ethyl ether	Alcohol
Chloroform	Lysine
Adenine arabinoside	Povidone-iodine
Vitamins C, E and B_{12}	Dye-light (photodynamic inactivation)
Lactobacillus	Silver sulfadiazine
Zinc	2-deoxy-D-glucose

CANKER SORES

Recurrent aphthous stomatitis (RAS) is a relatively common disease characterized by painful oral ulcers, often called canker sores. Although it is one of the most common conditions for which people seek treatment, the course of RAS is essentially unaltered by modern medical and dental therapy. At least 20% of the general population is affected, with women about twice as susceptible as men. RAS can occur at any age, but its incidence rises sharply after age 10. Susceptibility to RAS appears to be inherited, although the exact mode of genetic transfer has not yet been determined.

ETIOLOGY

Numerous etiologic factors for RAS have been suggested. These include hereditary predisposition, microbial agents, hypersensitivity, psychological factors, endocrine abnormalities, chemicals in food stuffs, trauma and foreign bodies. In particular, the pleomorphic, alpha-hemolytic *Streptococcus sanguis* may be partly responsible for canker sore development in predisposed individuals. These people seem to be hypersensitive to certain components of *Streptococcus sanguis,* although some reports do not substantiate this etiology. Most researchers have also implicated autoimmune mechanisms in the etiology of RAS. *Herpes simplex* virus has been ruled out as a causative factor.

Various endogenous precipitating factors have been associated with RAS (Table 2). Trauma from dental procedures, cheek-biting and hard foods commonly leads to canker sore development in susceptible people. Emotional stress and hormonal changes may also play a role for some individuals.

Deficiencies in cyanocobalamin, folic acid or iron have been reported for a small number of people. RAS may be associated with the presence of celiac disease. Consequently, dietary elimination of gluten has been suggested as a treatment. Certain other foods may precipitate or irritate canker sores, or may act as nutrients for oral streptococci. Smokers develop canker sores less frequently than do nonsmokers.

It has been suggested that RAS is caused by a complex interaction between host and environment. Apparently, a genetic component is required to establish susceptibility, but interaction with several environmental factors is essential for clinical expression.

SYMPTOMS

RAS is characterized by painful recurrent ulcerations of the oral mucosa. Ulcers are most often found on nonkeratinized tissues of the mouth, such as the buccal mucosa, lips, mucobuccal fold, tongue, floor of the mouth and soft palate. Aphthous lesions usually occur singly, although several areas of the mouth may be ulcerated simultaneously. Individuals may notice a prodromal burning or tingling sensation up to 24 hours before the ulcer appears. The lesion begins as a small macule that enlarges and progresses to a shallow ulceration 3 to 10 mm in diameter. The ulcer is round or ovoid with sharply delineated margins surrounded by an intense erythematous halo. A gray or yellowish membrane covers the ulcer crater. Canker sores are extremely painful and may make eating, talking, drinking or swallowing difficult. Lesions generally persist for 7 to 14 days and heal slowly from the margins without scarring.

TREATMENT

Nonpharmacological Treatment

Aphthous stomatitis therapy is aimed at controlling the pain, shortening the duration of lesions already present and aborting new lesions. Nondrug measures include rinsing the mouth with warm water, a saline solution (see the discussion of herpes labialis) or mouthwash as often as possible. Individuals should also avoid any known precipitating factors and irritating foods and remove any cause of trauma, such as ill-fitting dentures (Table 4).

Pharmacological Treatment

Topical anesthetics applied as often as needed are useful in relieving canker sore pain. These agents should be applied to small areas only or a disturbing "cotton-mouth" feeling and total loss of taste results.

Coating the ulcers with protectants, such as emollient mixtures or denture-adhesives, often alleviates pain. Protectants may be particularly helpful if applied before eating or retiring for the night. Chlorhexidine gluconate mouthwash 0.2% used 3 times daily may shorten the number of days with ulcers and reduce the discomfort of lesions. It is also effective when put on a gauze pad applied directly over the lesion.

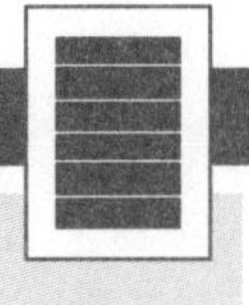

TABLE 4: Foods to Avoid During an Attack of Aphthous Stomatitis

Citrus fruits	Chocolate	Melons
Sour substances	Spices	Strawberries
Tomatoes	Vinegar	Walnuts

Patients who have frequent, large or numerous canker sores should be referred to a physician or dentist. Prescribed treatments for RAS include tetracycline compresses or mouthrinses, or topical corticosteroids in an emollient base (e.g., *Kenalog in Orabase*). Beclomethasone dipropionate aerosol spray has also been shown to reduce the severity and pain of RAS lesions. Levamisole, in immunostimulant doses, is effective for some people. People with vitamin or iron deficiencies may benefit from appropriate supplements.

Oxygenating agents, such as carbamide peroxide in 10% glycerol, oral zinc sulfate and lactobacillus preparations, are not useful in treating RAS.

CANDIDIASIS (MONILIASIS)

ETIOLOGY

Candida albicans is a true fungus that is part of the normal flora of the gastrointestinal tract and oral cavity in a large percentage of the population. The tongue serves as the primary oral reservoir for the fungus, which may then colonize other parts of the mouth.

Under certain circumstances, *Candida* can change from a commensal organism to a pathogen and cause a variety of mucocutaneous conditions. Associated predisposing factors include environment (warmth, moisture, maceration or occlusion); physiology (early infancy, pregnancy, old age or diabetes mellitus); compromised immune mechanisms (malignant diseases, immunosuppressive drugs, corticosteroids, cytotoxic drugs or radiation therapy); malnutrition and malabsorption (iron-deficiency anemia, pernicious anemia or alcoholism); drugs causing xerostomia (anticholinergics, antidepressants, antipsychotics, antihypertensives or antihistamines); and other changes in the host environment (antibiotic therapy, trauma or postoperative states).

SYMPTOMS

Acute oral candidiasis appears as acute pseudomembranous candidiasis or acute atrophic candidiasis. The most common form of candidal infection of the oral mucosa is the acute pseudomembranous type, often called thrush. It appears as white, milk-curd plaques attached to the mucosal surface. When the plaques are removed, erythematous, bleeding erosions are seen. Thrush is associated with some pain or soreness, but systemic symptoms are generally lacking or mild.

Acute atrophic candidiasis, sometimes referred to as antibiotic sore mouth, is thought to be similar to the form taken by thrush but without the white plaques. It is characterized by reddened painful mucosal areas in the oral cavity and commonly occurs with concomitant antibiotic therapy.

Two chronic candidal infections also exist—chronic hyperplastic candidiasis and chronic atrophic candidiasis. In chronic hyperplastic candidiasis (*Candida* leukoplakia), firm, well-attached and persistent white plaques are present on the inner cheeks, tongue, palate and lips. Individuals may complain of soreness, roughness or a white plaque that cannot be removed. This type of candidiasis may resist treatment.

Chronic atrophic candidiasis is also known as denture stomatitis or denture sore-mouth because it is commonly found in people wearing full or partial dentures. Symptoms include a diffuse inflammation of the denture-bearing area. Denture stomatitis generally can be distinguished from the trauma caused by ill-fitting dentures because the latter is localized to one spot. Individuals with chronic atrophic candidiasis may also experience soreness or a burning sensation.

An iron or vitamin B deficiency may also play a role in susceptibility to denture stomatitis, but colonization of the denture material appears necessary for it to develop. Failure to remove the denture at bedtime or to clean the denture worsens the condition. Angular cheilitis (inflammation at the corners of the mouth) is commonly associated with denture stomatitis. Cultures of these lesions frequently show *Candida albicans* or *Staphylococcus aureus* organisms.

TREATMENT

Treating oral candidal infection involves elimination, if possible, of such contributing factors as concurrent antibiotic or corticosteroid therapy, and the use of oral nystatin suspension. Clotrimazole or miconazole vaginal suppositories may also be dissolved in the mouth to treat thrush. Gentian violet 1 to 2% solution may also be used, although it is esthetically unappealing. Certain patients may also require therapy with oral antifungal agents; recently itraconazole and fluconazole have been used successfully in the treatment of oral candidiasis.

Because no nonprescription products are available to treat oral candidiasis, the health professional's role involves recognizing clinical symptoms and referring the individual to a dentist or physician. Pharmacists can also assist by providing advice on the proper use of antifungal agents. People with denture stomatitis should be reminded of the importance of regularly removing and cleaning dentures.

OTHER CAUSES OF ORAL LESIONS

Many other diseases and conditions also have oral manifestations, including bacterial infections, blood dyscrasias, dermatoses, allergies, metallic intoxication and neoplasms. As a general rule, any person exhibiting an oral ulcer that persist for 3 weeks or longer should see a dentist or physician.

People undergoing radiation treatment or drug therapy for cancer may experience various problems affecting the mouth. Problems include inflammation of the mucosa (mucositis), ulcerations and severe dental caries precipitated by loss of normal salivary function. These people may be treated with one of several protocols that take into account the individual's disease condition and treatments, as well as oral health status. Generally these treatments are prescribed by a dentist or physician. Health professionals can help the individual select appropriate dental care items.

HALITOSIS

ETIOLOGY

Bad breath or halitosis is an unpleasant problem caused by a mixture of the breath and malodorous compounds coming from the mouth, parts of the digestive tract or the respiratory tract. It can be a benign condition, easily treated, or the symptom of a serious disease.

Up to 85% of cases of bad breath are caused by disorders of the oral cavity. Halitosis is most frequently associated with poor oral hygiene, dental plaque or caries, gingivitis, stomatitis, periodontitis and oral carcinoma. Because there is no flow of saliva during sleep, putrefaction of saliva and debris in the mouth can lead to bad breath in the morning. Similarly, mouth-breathers may also experience bad breath. Other common causes of halitosis include various respiratory conditions, such as sinusitis, tonsillitis, rhinitis, tuberculosis and bronchiectasis. Gastrointestinal tract disorders above the gastroesophageal junction may also cause bad breath. In addition, the metabolism of certain foods and beverages, such as alcohol, garlic, onions and pastrami, produces volatile, malodorous compounds that are excreted through the lungs. The drug dimethylsulfoxide is also excreted in this manner, producing a breath odor similar to stale oysters. Other drugs can alter the senses of taste and smell and cause subjective halitosis. These drugs include lithium salts, penicillamine, griseofulvin and thiocarbamide.

TREATMENT

When not secondary to a specific disease, halitosis can usually be eliminated through good oral hygiene. This includes frequent brushing and flossing of the teeth and brushing of the tongue to remove bacterial plaque and food debris. Mouthwashes or other breath fresheners probably serve only to mask bad breath and to increase salivary flow. The American Council on Dental Therapeutics believes that nonprescription mouthwash rinses containing alcohol do not substantially contribute to oral health and may aggravate certain conditions because of alcohol content. If a marked breath odor persists after thoroughly cleaning the teeth, the individual should see a dentist to determine the cause.

DRY MOUTH

ETIOLOGY

Dry mouth or xerostomia is the subjective complaint of dryness of the mouth. Although a dry mouth is commonly thought due to disturbed salivary function, it may have multiple causes. Elderly people in particular complain of a dry mouth. Several studies have indicated that 20 to 49% of people older than 55 years may complain of a feeling of dryness in the mouth. The structure and function of the salivary glands do change with age, but xerostomia is unlikely to develop from the aging process alone. Four basic causes have been outlined for xerostomia: factors affecting the salivary centre (emotions, organic disease, and drugs, such as levodopa or morphine); factors affecting the autonomic nervous systems (encephalitis, brain tumors, cerebrovascular accidents and drugs); factors affecting salivary gland function (autoimmune disorders, such as Sjögren's syndrome, obstruction and infection, and irradiation); and factors affecting fluid or electrolyte balance (dehydration, edema, diabetes mellitus, cardiac failure, other systemic conditions and diuretics). The most frequent causes of dry mouth are drugs, autoimmune diseases and irradiation of the salivary glands.

SYMPTOMS

A complaint of dry mouth may be accompanied by a reduction in the amount of saliva produced or by a change in the properties of the saliva, although the condition also exists without any such measurable changes. People suffering from dry mouth may also complain of generalized burning or soreness in the mouth, ulceration, difficulty in swallowing or speaking, and poor denture retention. Taste acuity may decrease. A rapid progression of dental caries in dentate individuals may occur if effective oral hygiene is not practised. Cracks and fissures may appear at the corners of the mouth, and the tongue may be red and smooth. Bad breath and a sore throat commonly accompany xerostomia.

TREATMENT

Treating xerostomia effectively may be difficult and frustrating, but a multifaceted approach may be successful. Individuals should be thoroughly evaluated first to determine the causes of the condition, which may also give some insight into appropriate treatment. Although people often become tolerant to the xerostomic effects of drugs, a reduction in dosage or the use of an alternative therapy might be indicated and may solve the dry mouth problem.

In general, people with xerostomia should avoid dry and bulky foods, spicy or acidic foods, alcoholic or carbonated beverages, and tobacco. They should also sip water or thin soup throughout the day, unless medically contraindicated. They may also find that chewing dill pickles or sucking on ice chips relieves the dryness. Humidification of inspired air may provide benefit. Candy or chewing gum (preferably sugarless) may help by stimulating salivary production in people who have viable salivary glands. All these measures provide only temporary relief.

Salivary function may also be stimulated by various prescription medications or by a sialogogue, such as anetholtrithione, if the xerostomia is not related to an underlying condition, such as irradiation of the salivary glands. Citric acid and lemon oil have also been used successfully as salivary stimulants, but dentate individuals should be cautious in the chronic use of acidic solutions. Recently, saliva substitutes (artificial saliva) have proven useful in alleviating oral discomfort from a dry mouth.

FIGURE 5

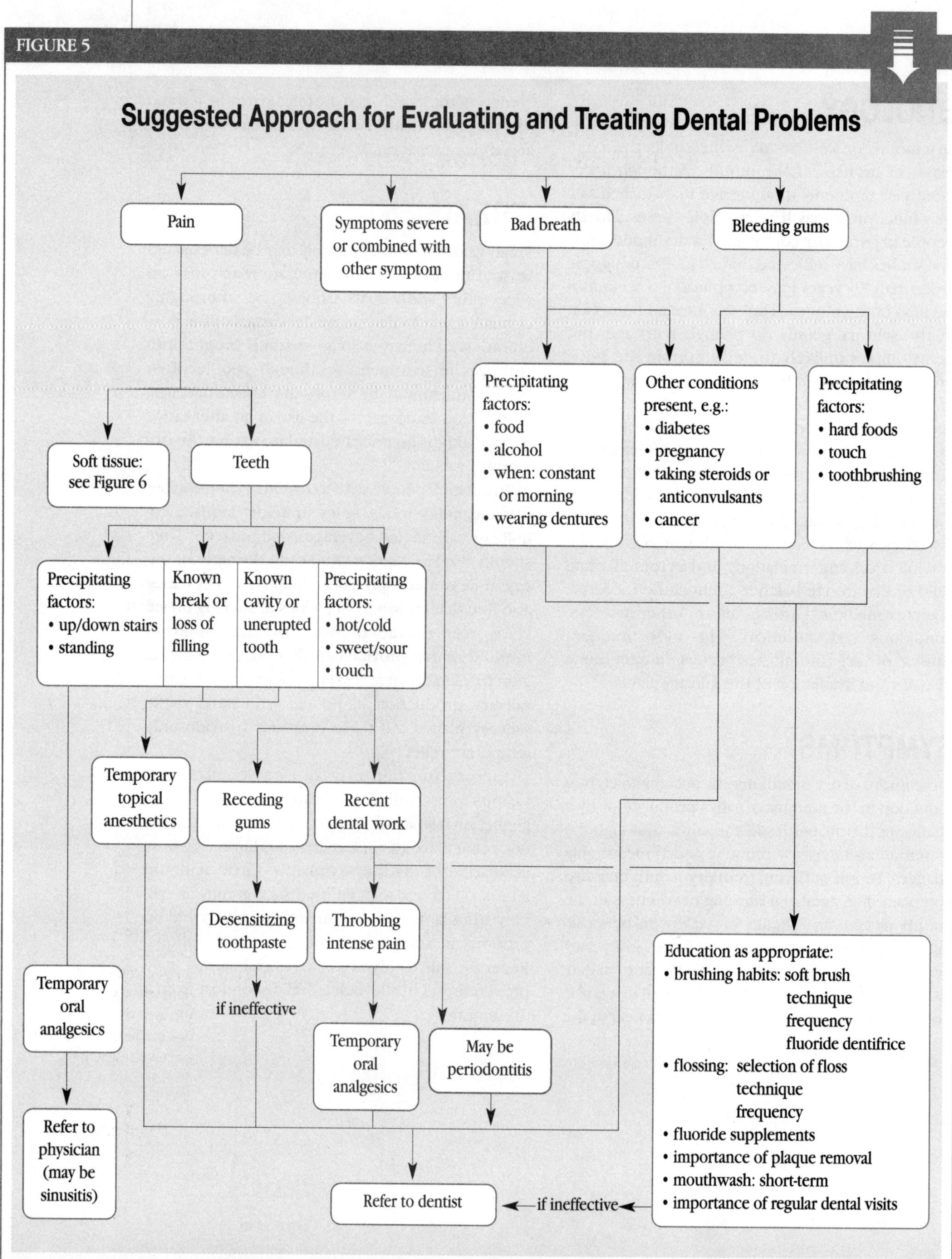
Suggested Approach for Evaluating and Treating Dental Problems
Pain
Symptoms severe or combined with other symptom
Bad breath
Bleeding gums
Precipitating factors:
• food
• alcohol
• when: constant or morning
• wearing dentures
Other conditions present, e.g.:
• diabetes
• pregnancy
• taking steroids or anticonvulsants
• cancer
Precipitating factors:
• hard foods
• touch
• toothbrushing
Soft tissue: see Figure 6
Teeth
Precipitating factors:
• up/down stairs
• standing
Known break or loss of filling
Known cavity or unerupted tooth
Precipitating factors:
• hot/cold
• sweet/sour
• touch
Temporary topical anesthetics
Receding gums
Recent dental work
Desensitizing toothpaste
Throbbing intense pain
if ineffective
Temporary oral analgesics
Temporary oral analgesics
May be periodontitis
Refer to physician (may be sinusitis)
Refer to dentist
if ineffective
Education as appropriate:
• brushing habits: soft brush
technique
frequency
fluoride dentifrice
• flossing: selection of floss
technique
frequency
• fluoride supplements
• importance of plaque removal
• mouthwash: short-term
• importance of regular dental visits

FIGURE 6

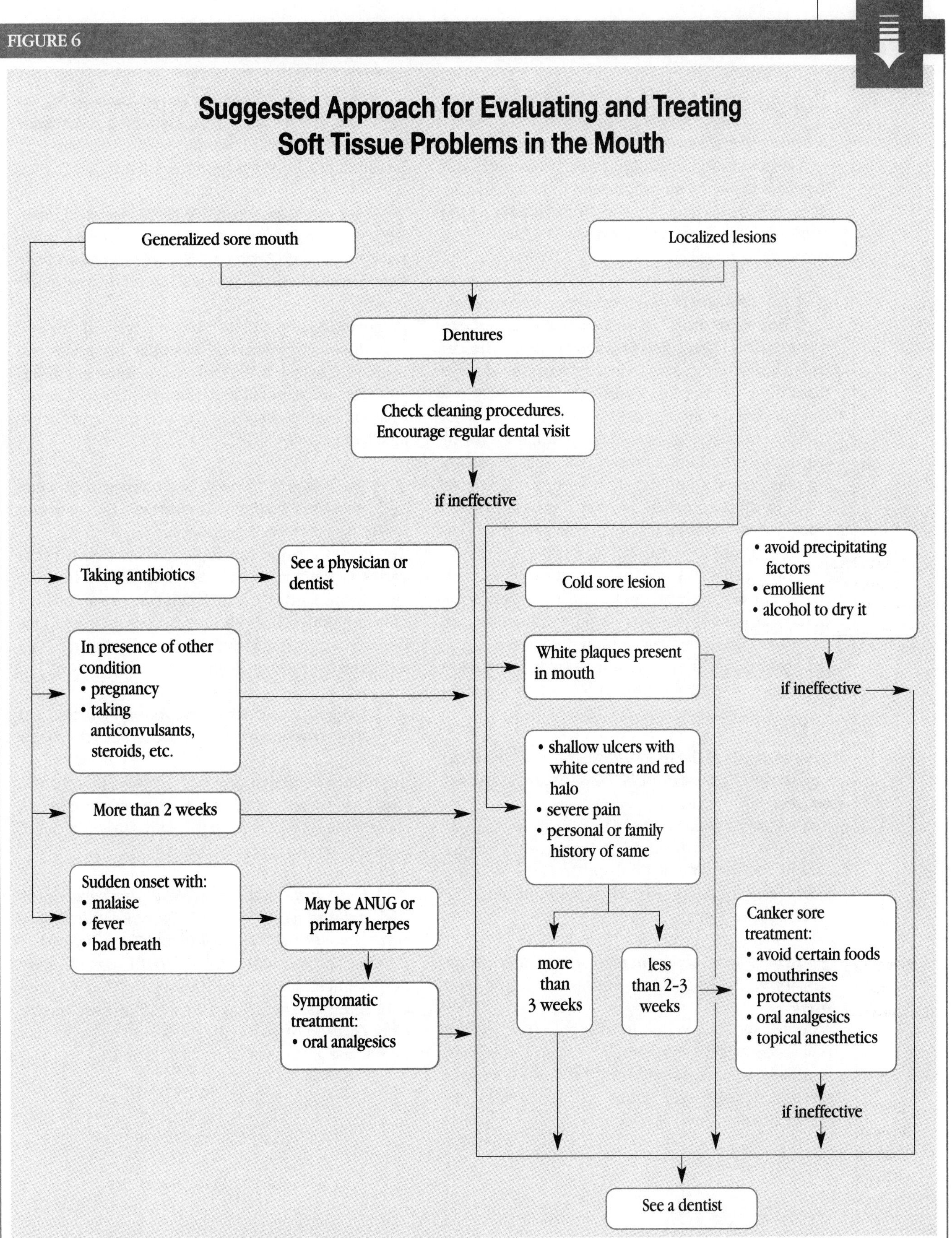
Suggested Approach for Evaluating and Treating Soft Tissue Problems in the Mouth
Generalized sore mouth
Localized lesions
Dentures
Check cleaning procedures. Encourage regular dental visit
if ineffective
Taking antibiotics
See a physician or dentist
In presence of other condition
• pregnancy
• taking anticonvulsants, steroids, etc.
More than 2 weeks
Sudden onset with:
• malaise
• fever
• bad breath
May be ANUG or primary herpes
Symptomatic treatment:
• oral analgesics
Cold sore lesion
• avoid precipitating factors
• emollient
• alcohol to dry it
if ineffective
White plaques present in mouth
• shallow ulcers with white centre and red halo
• severe pain
• personal or family history of same
more than 3 weeks
less than 2-3 weeks
Canker sore treatment:
• avoid certain foods
• mouthrinses
• protectants
• oral analgesics
• topical anesthetics
if ineffective
See a dentist

PATIENT ASSESSMENT QUESTIONS

***Q** How long have you had this dental problem? Did it begin suddenly or develop gradually? Is only one tooth involved?*
A history of vague, nondescript discomfort not localized to one tooth suggests periodontal disease. Acute gingivitis may develop from trauma to the gums, but, in general, periodontal disease is a chronic disorder.

***Q** How painful is it? Is the pain radiating, deep, intense or dull? Is it generalized or specific to one tooth? Is it triggered by hot or cold substances or by chewing? Is the pain lingering or does it resolve after removing the hot or cold drink?*
Dental pain precipitated by hot, cold or sweet substances suggests superficial dentinal caries or exposed cementum. Chronic pain that gradually becomes more intense and has deep, boring or radiating characteristics is associated with pulpitis from a deep carious lesion or the placement of extensive restorative material in one tooth. Nonprescription analgesics may provide temporary pain relief, but consumers should consult a dentist as quickly as possible for professional evaluation and treatment. Lingering pain is more indicative of pulpal abscess, and hence requires more immediate treatment. Acute pain that resolves when the stimulus is removed is more easily dealt with.

***Q** How old is the individual? Have all the teeth erupted in the mouth? What other symptoms are present?*
Infants may experience discomfort from teething as well as increased salivation and restlessness. Eruption of the permanent third molars—the wisdom teeth—may be associated with pain and possible swelling if an abscess forms.

***Q** Have you seen a dentist about this condition? When? What treatments have you tried?*
A dentist should be consulted for pain that may follow recent dental treatment. Nonprescription toothache remedies should only be used short term for any dental pain, as an emergency measure before obtaining dental treatment.

***Q** Is the pain altered by lying down, going up and down stairs, or by clenching your teeth?*
Symptoms such as these suggest the problem may be nondental in origin (e.g, sinusitis).

***Q** Are any teeth loose? Do the gums bleed when you brush your teeth? Do you have a continuous foul breath problem? How do you clean your teeth? How often? Do you use dental floss or toothpicks?*
Removing bacterial plaque by proper toothbrushing and flossing methods is essential for good oral hygiene. If plaque is allowed to accumulate, gingivitis and halitosis are possible. The improper use of dental floss or toothpicks may also precipitate an acute attack of gingivitis.

***Q** Do you use fluoride supplements? Is your drinking water fluoridated? Do you use toothpaste containing fluoride?*
The need for fluoride supplementation to prevent caries is determined by the amount of fluoride already ingested. Too much fluoride causes enamel mottling. Individuals should discuss their need for fluoride supplements with a dentist prior to taking any extra fluoride products.

***Q** Do you wear dentures? Are they loose? Do they cause sore spots? How do you clean them?*
Improperly-fitted dentures may create oral problems, such as sores, difficulty in chewing and destruction of supporting bone. Denture stomatitis may develop if dentures are inadequately cleaned.

***Q** How long have you had the sore in or around your mouth? Describe the lesion. Have you ever had a similar condition before?*
Harmless canker sores last up to 14 days. Primary herpes infections generally last from 10 to 14 days; cold sores last from 3 to 10 days. However, mouth ulcers caused by blood dyscrasias or an oral cancer persist and grow over a period of months.

?

PATIENT ASSESSMENT QUESTIONS (*cont'd*)

Q *Do you have any other symptoms such as fever, increased salivation, bad breath or flu-like symptoms?*
A young child with such symptoms may be experiencing a primary herpes infection. Bad breath, bleeding gums, fever and malaise, and cervical lymphadenopathy may indicate the presence of acute necrotizing gingivitis.

Q *Do you suffer from any chronic medical illness, such as diabetes mellitus, rheumatoid arthritis, heart disease, or epilepsy?*
Many diseases have periodontal manifestations, especially those of endocrine imbalances, blood dyscrasias, dermatoses and allergies. Some conditions, such as angina pectoris, have referred pain to the teeth. Sjögren's syndrome is commonly associated with rheumatoid arthritis, particularly in females, and presents as a chronic dry mouth condition.

Q *Are you allergic to any foods or medications? What are they?*
Certain foods may precipitate recurrent aphthous stomatitis. Topical anesthetics, such as benzocaine, may produce localized allergic reactions in the mouth. Drugs may also produce oral lesions as manifestations of an allergic response.

Q *What medications are you taking?*
Certain drugs may produce blood dyscrasias or allergic reactions that manifest as oral lesions. Drugs can also cause a dry mouth. Anticonvulsants such as phenytoin, and some other agents, may cause gingival hyperplasia.

PRODUCT INFORMATION

Both the Canadian Dental Association (CDA) and the Council on Dental Therapeutics of the American Dental Association (ADA) evaluate and recommend certain treatments for oral conditions. Products that meet established criteria may be eligible to carry a seal of recognition of either of these associations. In addition, several of the United States Food And Drug Administration (FDA) advisory review panels looking at nonprescription products have evaluated drugs used in oral health. These panels include dentifrice and dental care drug products, miscellaneous external drug products and oral cavity drug products. Publications from these panels are referred to where their recommendations are appropriate.

In Canada, the Bureau of Nonprescription Drugs of Health Canada has revised criteria for drug and cosmetic claims of plaque and tartar removal products. Claims that point to mechanical removal of plaque or tartar are now deemed cosmetic; those suggesting a chemical or antimicrobial effect are classified as drugs.

COLD SORE AND CANKER SORE PRODUCTS

Nonprescription products available to treat cold sores and canker sores are primarily intended to control pain and do not alter the course of either disease. They contain various protective, drying, counterirritant, anesthetic, antibiotic and antiseptic agents (Table 5). These products are marketed for sore mouth generally, or for canker or cold sores specifically. Many of these ingredients were evaluated by the FDA for the general treatment category of sore mouth. However, the FDA recommends that people with canker sores be treated by physicians or dentists. Because some people with an occasional canker sore or cold sore attempt to self-medicate, the following information may help pharmacists. Individuals with extensive lesions, frequent recurrences or ulcers lasting longer than 3 weeks should be referred for medical evaluation.

The most useful products to relieve canker sore discomfort are those containing a local anesthetic or a protective agent. Benzocaine is the most common anesthetic used. It is poorly absorbed and can be safely applied to ulcerated areas of the mucosa. Benzocaine provides local anesthesia for 5 to 10 minutes after application, although this effect may be prolonged with repeated use.

Lidocaine preparations are also available for use in the mouth. The FDA does not consider these preparations safe for nonprescription use.

Consumers should apply a local anesthetic only to the canker sore, or a "cotton-mouth" feeling occurs. If extensive areas of the oral cavity are anesthetized, individuals are unaware of such sensations as extreme heat. When eating or drinking hot food or beverages, they should be careful to prevent burning the oral mucosa and causing further discomfort. Prolonged use of local anesthetics may produce localized allergic reactions.

Demulcents, such as carboxymethylcellulose, benzoin or gums, are protective agents used to relieve irritation. These agents adhere to the mucosal surface and protect the lesion from friction. Consumers apply the product (such as *Orabase*) directly onto the lesion to create a smooth, slippery film. If the medication is rubbed in, it produces a granular, gritty sensation. These products may be applied as frequently as necessary to relieve discomfort.

An oxidizing agent such as hydrogen peroxide may be used as a cleansing agent for inflamed mucous membranes. When it touches the mucosa, oxygen is liberated and loosens debris. After dilution with an equal volume of water, a solution of 3% hydrogen peroxide is considered safe for use as a mouthrinse, gargle or topical application in the mouth. It can be used 3 to 4 times daily, but for no longer than 2 days unless recommended by a dentist. Since hydrogen peroxide is an irritant, prolonged unsupervised use can retard the healing of ulcerated mucosa.

Carbamide peroxide is another form of peroxide that is formulated in anhydrous glycerin. The glycerin increases the peroxide's stability and also helps the product adhere to the lesion. Concentrations of 10 to 15% can be used safely up to 4 times daily for 2 days. Sodium perborate and its modified forms also release oxygen, but these are considered ineffective and unsafe because of boric acid absorption and irritation to the mucosa.

Antibiotics available in canker sore products do not produce any beneficial effect. Topical tetracycline and cephalexin, which are effective against *Streptococcus mutans*, require a prescription by a physician or dentist. Antibiotics do not alter the

TABLE 5: Agents Found in Nonprescription Canker and Cold Sores Remedies

Agent	Purpose
Allantoin	Cleansing, debridement
Aluminum potassium sulfate	Astringent
Benzocaine	Anesthetic
Benzoin	Protective
Camphor	Counterirritant
Carbamide peroxide	Cleansing, debridement
Carboxymethylcellulose	Protective
Dequalinium chloride	Antiseptic
Ethanol	Antiseptic
Heparin sodium	Healing agent
Hydrogen peroxide	Cleansing, debridement
Iodochlorhydroxyquin	Anti-infective
Lidocaine	Anesthetic
Menthol	Counterirritant
Myrrh	Astringent
Para-aminobenzoic acid	Sunscreen
Polymyxin B	Anti-infective
Potassium chlorate	Astringent
Propolis	Antipruritic
Quinine bisulfate	Astringent
Sodium percarbonate	Oxidizing agent
Tannic acid	Astringent
Tyrothricin	Anti-infective
Zinc salicylate	Astringent
Zinc sulfate	Astringent

Adapted with permission from: Popovich NG, Popovich JG. What you should know about fever blisters and canker sores. US Pharmacist 1978;3(2):35–48.

course of recurrent herpes labialis. They may help prevent or treat a bacterial superinfection.

Antiseptics have limited use in treating RAS or herpes labialis. Agents such as benzalkonium chloride, dequalinium chloride or the phenolic compounds generally affect only a limited number of bacteria and have not been proven totally safe or effective. Ethanol (70%) denatures protein to destroy bacteria. Unfortunately, this concentration also irritates mucous membranes. Ethanol or other solvents, such as ethyl ether, applied to herpes labialis may dilute virus particles and dry the lesion. However, their therapeutic efficacy has not been substantiated in well-controlled studies.

Tannic acid and other astringents precipitate proteins when applied to the mouth, protecting the area from irritating substances. However, their effect is temporary.

Counterirritants, such as camphor, menthol and phenol, relieve discomfort by creating another sensation, such as irritation or warmth. However, they can increase irritation. They must be kept away from children, as camphor is toxic when ingested.

Silver nitrate sticks have been used in the past to cauterize canker sores. Although this procedure may relieve pain, it is not recommended because the ulcer itself may enlarge and heal slowly. The surrounding area of the gums and teeth may also be stained black.

A product containing propolis and flavonoids (*Probax*) has been marketed to treat cold sores, but published studies on its effectiveness are lacking. It is claimed to relieve the commonly associated itching and stinging. Another product containing heparin sodium and zinc sulfate (*Lipactin*) is also claimed to provide symptomatic relief from cold sores and may shorten the time required for the lesions to heal.

DENTIFRICES

Dentifrices are substances used with toothbrushes to clean teeth. Although toothbrushing alone is partly effective in controlling plaque buildup, dentifrices help remove stains, debris and dental plaque from tooth surfaces. Dentifrices have cosmetic functions (to improve the appearance of teeth and freshen breath), and they also provide therapeutic benefits, such as preventing dental caries and periodontal diseases because of plaque removal. In addition, therapeutic dentifrices may convey specific drug substances such as fluoride to the tooth.

Dentifrices are available in three forms: paste, gel and powder. Toothpastes are by far the most popular. Most dentifrice formulations contain the same types or classes of ingredients. These formulations include abrasives (cleaning and polishing agents), foaming agents and flavoring mixtures. Pastes also contain water, humectants and thickening agents or binders. Some products may also incorporate low levels of preservatives, and therapeutic dentifrices contain a drug substance.

Abrasives are the largest component of dentifrices and are responsible for physically removing plaque and debris. An ideal abrasive provides a maximum cleaning action with minimum abrasion of tooth surfaces. In addition, the abrasive agent must be physically compatible with the other dentifrice ingredients. If used correctly, dentifrice abrasives should not damage dental enamel appreciably. However, exposed cementum and dentin can be damaged by routine use of dentifrices and toothbrushes, particularly if an individual brushes the teeth aggressively.

Abrasives are pharmacologically inactive and insoluble compounds, such as silicates and calcium or phosphate salts, that vary greatly in abrasiveness. Individuals vary in the degree of abrasiveness required to keep their teeth free from stains. Some are able to keep their teeth stain-free by using only water and a toothbrush; others can achieve a similar effect using sodium bicarbonate as the dentifrice. Although low in abrasivity, sodium bicarbonate (baking soda) dentifrices do not appear to remove plaque as well as dentifrices containing silicates or other such salts and have shown no measurable therapeutic advantage in reducing plaque or gingivitis when compared to available commercial dentifrices. A low-abrasive toothpaste containing beads of poly(methyl)methacrylate as the abrasive was as effective as conventional toothpastes in removing plaque from teeth. However, brown staining of the teeth was worse with the low abrasivity product.

Most dentifrices sold in Canada and the United States are similar in abrasivity. None of these products appreciably abrade enamel. With normal use, they do not greatly affect dentin or cementum. In general, consumers may use any of these commercially available dentifrices safely, unless advised otherwise by their dentists. Dentifrices promoted to whiten and brighten the teeth may contain harsher abrasives and probably should not be used regularly by most consumers.

Generally speaking, dentifrice powders are more abrasive than pastes. Gel dentifrices are similar to pastes but are clear because the refractive indices of the abrasive and humectant systems have been carefully matched. Manufacturers of gel dentifrices claim that use of these products cause children to brush longer and more thoroughly. This claim was not substantiated in a study that examined toothbrushing times and patterns after initial use and after 1 month of use of either a gel or paste in matched groups of children aged 10 to 16 years.

Humectants are incorporated into toothpastes and gels to prevent loss of water and subsequent hardening of the product. Thickening agents or binders stabilize dentifrice formulations. Foaming agents in dentifrices are usually synthetic detergents; most consumers prefer to use a product with adequate foaming capabilities. Various flavoring systems are also used to appeal to dentifrice users. Most products use saccharin or sorbitol as their sweetening agent.

Fluoride Dentifrices

Certain dentifrices that contain stannous fluoride or sodium monofluorophosphate (MFP) have been accepted by the CDA and the ADA as providing a significant decrease in caries incidence compared to similar nonfluoride products. Formulation modifications have also produced sodium fluoride dentifrices that provide readily available fluoride ions to the tooth surface. Acceptable products bear the Seal of Recognition of the CDA.

The FDA approved the ingredients outlined in Table 6 as safe and effective for caries prevention. Although the safety of fluoride dental products has been questioned, the FDA stated on the basis of available evidence that toxicities do not occur with normal usage. It has been suggested that dental fluorosis is unlikely except in areas where water supplies contain excess fluoride (greater than 2 ppm), but some authors have challenged this contention. Although the quantity of dentifrice used and the proportion ingested varies, average brushing by an adult produces little systemic ingestion of fluoride. Concern has been expressed for young children who might swallow excessive amounts of toothpaste. The FDA and CDA have recommended that fluoride dentifrices be labelled for use by adults and children over 2 years of age, and that children

TABLE 6: Dosages of Approved Fluoride Ingredients

	In Dentifrice	In Rinse
Acidulated phosphate		0.02%
Sodium fluoride	0.22%	0.05% daily 0.2% weekly
Sodium monofluorophosphate	0.76%	
Stannous fluoride	0.40%	0.1%

Adapted from: Federal Register (U.S.) 1980;45:20666.

aged 2 to 6 use these products under parental supervision. Recent reports have also called for the development of dentifrices for children that would contain less fluoride.

Ad libitum toothbrushing with a recognized fluoride dentifrice reduces the incidence of dental caries up to 35%. Because most people prefer to use a dentifrice while brushing their teeth, health professionals should encourage regular use of a fluoride dentifrice by both children and adults. This recommendation holds true even in areas where drinking water is fluoridated. The use of fluoride dentifrices and mouthrinses provides added cariostatic benefits in such communities, although the cost-benefit ratio for school-based rinsing programs in fluoridated communities has been questioned. Fluoride dentifrice use has also been shown to reduce the incidence of caries, including root surface caries, in adults older than 54 years of age.

Desensitizing Agents

Dentifrices containing fluoride may reduce hypersensitivity by strengthening the tooth surface or remineralizing tiny flaws in the enamel. The FDA rates fluoride dentifrices safe but not proven effective for this purpose. These agents are currently under review by the FDA.

Dentifrices containing potassium nitrate 5%, strontium chloride 10% and sodium citrate have been accepted by the ADA for treatment of dentinal hypersensitivity. Products containing sodium citrate are not available in Canada. The council has also accepted *Sensodyne-F*, which contains a combination of potassium nitrate 5% and sodium MFP 0.76%, for use as a "desensitizing decay preventive dentifrice."

Tartar Control Dentifrices

Soluble pyrophosphates are crystal-growth inhibitors that interrupt the transformation of amorphous calcium phosphate into dental calculus. Use of a dentifrice containing these compounds has been shown to reduce the build-up of calculus or tartar on teeth above the gumline that were made calculus-free by professional dental cleaning. A sodium fluoride dentifrice containing a combination of soluble pyrophosphates was used *ad libitum* in an adult population for 6 months after dental prophylaxis. Compared to a control group using only a sodium fluoride dentifrice without the pyrophosphates, the test group showed a 32% reduction in newly formed calculus. In addition, the test group had fewer sites affected by calculus. Additional studies have supported these results. One study comparing anticalculus toothpastes did not find any difference in calculus prevention between brands.

The CDA does not yet recognize any toothpaste for tartar control alone. Both *Crest* and *Colgate Tartar Control* toothpastes are recognized for their anticaries activity.

Other Dentifrices

A dentifrice containing sanguinaria and zinc chloride has been evaluated for its effectiveness in preventing plaque formation and gingivitis. Although not effective when used alone, a combination of this toothpaste and a sanguinarine mouthrinse has reduced the amount of plaque and gingival inflammation in adult and orthodontic patients.

Dentifrices containing triclosan with zinc citrate or a copolymer of polyvinylmethyl ether maleic acid have also been effective in reducing plaque and gingivitis when used regularly in both short-term and long-term studies. A chlorhexidine dentifrice also has been shown to reduce plaque and gingivitis but its side effect of dental staining precludes widespread use without further product development.

DENTURE PRODUCTS

Denture Cleansers

Denture cleansing removes denture plaque, stain and debris. Regular removal of plaque and extrinsic materials from dentures helps control or prevent oral malodor and conditions such as denture stomatitis the same way toothbrushing and flossing prevent dental caries, periodontal disease and halitosis in dentate individuals. The suggested methods of cleaning acrylic resin dentures include mechanical and abrasive action and immersion in chemical solutions.

A common method for cleaning dentures is brushing with tap water and soap or pastes. This technique removes stain and plaque effectively when used meticulously. In general, a soft toothbrush or a specialized denture brush and low-abrasive denture cleaning powder or paste should be used instead of toothpaste. Denture-wearers should not use scouring powders to clean dentures.

The ADA has found no form of denture cleaning device or product superior to cleaning with a brush. Ultrasonic agitation devices may increase a disinfectant's effectiveness, but data conflict on their effectiveness in removing denture stains and plaque.

Chemical denture cleansers are dissolved in water and the denture immersed in the resulting solution for a period of time. Alkaline peroxide products (e.g., *Efferdent* and *Polident*) are the most commonly used chemical cleansers. They provide alkaline solutions of hydrogen peroxide that release oxygen and exert the cleaning action. They seem most effective on new plaque and stains when the denture is soaked overnight or for several hours. They are effective in the 15 minute time period recommended by manufacturers. A denture brush may be used after soaking to ensure thorough denture cleaning. Alkaline peroxide solutions are safe for denture cleaning, but routine use may cause bleaching of the acrylic resin material.

When two methods of denture cleaning (*Dentu-Creme* and *Efferdent*) were compared, an *Efferdent* soak reduced plaque bacteria levels significantly more than *Dentu-Creme* alone. Although a combination of the cream and soak did not produce additional reductions in microflora, regular use of such a combination regimen is recommended to effectively remove plaque, bacteria and debris from dentures.

Alkaline hypochlorite and dilute acid solutions are also available to remove stains and plaque on dentures. Overnight soaking is recommended when using these solutions. They should be used only weekly or biweekly as either solution can corrode metal denture parts. These products remove stains better than do alkaline peroxide solutions. Consumers should not use strong hypochlorite solutions, such as bleach, to clean dentures, because of possible damage to the denture material. Hot water or hot soaking solutions also should be avoided to prevent distortion of the dentures.

Some denture cleansers contain enzymes such as protease or mutanase. These enzymes break down the proteins and polysaccharides in plaque on the dentures. Use of such products has been shown to significantly reduce denture plaque when compared to placebo or Steradent solutions.

All dentures should be thoroughly rinsed before reinsertion into the mouth, and all cleaning products kept out of the reach of children.

Adhesives, Reliners, Cushions and Repair Kits

Even the best-fitting dentures result in chronic bone resorption from the dental arch. If a denture becomes loose or poorly retained, the individual should see a dentist for re-evaluation to ensure proper denture fit. Although denture adhesives may improve denture retention in some people, the chronic use of such products may lead to further pathological changes in the tissues under the denture.

Denture adhesives are available in powders and pastes based on ingredients such as methylcellulose, karaya gum, carboxymethylcellulose and gelatin.

Denture reliners and cushions damage the denture and the wearer if used for extended periods. Any person considering purchasing a denture reliner or cushion should see a dentist as soon as possible. The use of denture repair kits should be discouraged except in emergencies. Dentures can be properly fitted and repaired only by trained professionals.

DRY MOUTH PRODUCTS

Several approaches can be taken to relieve xerostomia: sialogogues or cholinergics may be employed to stimulate salivary flow if salivary gland function remains; a palliative mouthrinse may be used to relieve dryness; or a saliva replacement may be employed.

Mouthrinses that moisten and lubricate the mouth are effective only for short periods of time. Most examples of such mouthrinses contain water or a humectant glycerin-water mixture. Substances such as citric acid or lemon oil may be added to such mouthrinses or used alone as gustatory stimulants of salivary function. However, prolonged use of acidic substances should be avoided in dentate individuals due to their demineralizing effect on tooth enamel.

Cholinergic drugs, such as bethanechol or urecholine, act on the central nervous system to increase salivary flow; anetholtrithione acts directly on the salivary glands. Cholinergic drugs may be associated with significant systemic effects that may limit their usefulness in treating xerostomia. Anetholtrithione is generally well tolerated and may be prescribed by medical or dental practitioners for some people.

Artificial saliva describes preparations whose chemical and physical properties resemble those of natural saliva. An ideal artificial saliva should be long lasting, inhibit colonization by cariogenic bacteria, provide lubrication and coat and protect oral tissues. Such products relieve the feeling of mouth dryness longer than mouthrinses and have proven benefit for soft tissue care.

A thickening agent, such as methylcellulose or mucin, is the primary ingredient in artificial saliva. It gives the product viscosity and provides sustained activity. Mucin appears to be the better lubricant, acting much like natural saliva. Ingredients such as glycerin, sorbitol and lemon oil increase palatability because of their humectant and flavoring ability.

Although sorbitol does not promote tooth decay in people with normal salivary function, oral cariogenic microorganisms can also ferment sorbitol and enhance caries formation in people who constantly use artificial saliva. The ADA therefore recommends a professionally applied topical fluoride treatment for dentate individuals using artificial saliva.

All saliva substitutes currently available have similar viscosity, pH and ion content. However, *Moi-Stir* has the highest sodium content, which may be a consideration for people on sodium-restricted diets who wish to use the preparation frequently.

Xerolube is the only product that contains fluoride ion. Limited in vitro data indicate fluoride, along with the calcium and phosphate present in artificial saliva, promotes remineralization of tooth enamel. No clinical evidence exists that artificial saliva reduces caries. Fluoride rinses specifically designed to prevent caries are probably more effective for this purpose.

Artificial saliva products are used to relieve soft tissue discomfort whenever mouth dryness persists. Consumers should be encouraged to use them as often as needed to keep the mouth moist. They are particularly effective in relieving nocturnal xerostomia.

Artificial saliva may be recommended to any person experiencing a dry mouth, providing treatable causes (e.g., neoplasms) have been ruled out by a physician or dentist. Dentate individuals experiencing xerostomia should be reminded also of the importance of toothbrushing and flossing, and the need for regular visits to a dentist. Denture-wearers with dry mouth should clean their dentures frequently and see a dentist regularly.

A toothpaste developed to fight xerostomia contains enzymes and other agents found in saliva (*Biotene*). It is said to produce antibacterial levels of hypothiocyanate and hydrogen peroxide during brushing. However, clinical trials on its effectiveness have not been published.

FLUORIDE

The fluoride ion exerts its anticaries effects through several mechanisms. When it first touches the enamel surface, the fluoride ion combines to form calcium fluoride. It serves as a reservoir of fluoride ions in plaque, releasing fluoride ions during caries challenge at low pH. From this reservoir, fluoride ions slowly replace hydroxyl groups in hydroxyapatite to form fluorapatite. The latter is a denser, less soluble and more stable crystal that has a greater resistance to acid. Fluoride ions are also antibacterial in high concentrations, particularly to *Streptococcus mutans*, and also remineralize early or incipient caries.

Over the past 50 years, much controversy has developed around the idea of community water fluoridation. A large body of research has found fluoride to be a safe and effective method of preventing the major health problem of dental caries. Careful analysis of epidemiologic data from fluoridated and nonfluoridated communities have consistently concluded that fluoride does not increase mortality due to heart disease, cancer or other specific diseases. No congenital malformations are associated with ingesting fluoridated water during pregnancy.

Recently, the widespread availability of fluoride ions in the environment and the increased use of fluoride-containing oral health products has led to concern regarding the risk of excessive exposure to fluoride. Over-exposure to fluoride ion can lead to both dental and skeletal fluorosis, especially in young children who drink optimally fluoridated water and use other fluoride-containing products. Suggestions on controlling these risks include changes in optimal fluoride concentrations of water, the development of dentifrices with lower fluoride levels, especially for children, and educational programs targeted toward the appropriate use of such products.

Oral Fluoride Supplements

In Canada, 46% of the population is served by optimally fluoridated water. People living in areas where water supply is not fluoridated can reduce the incidence of dental caries by giving oral fluoride supplements to children at home or in school-based programs.

Although one study has shown that an almost caries-free dentition may occur in children whose mothers take 1 mg of fluoride daily during pregnancy, such supplementation is not routinely recommended for pregnant women. Instead, the Canadian Dental Association (CDA) recommends supplementation only for individuals who are at high risk of dental caries and where the estimate of average fluoride consumption from all sources indicates a need.

The optimal amount of fluoride necessary to reduce most dental decay, with the least amount of risk of dental fluorosis (discoloration of the enamel), is 0.7 to 1.2 mg/L (0.7 to 1.2 ppm). In areas where water is not fluoridated to this level, oral supplementation of fluoride according to the regimen in Table 7 is recommended by the CDA.

Fluoride supplements should be given under close professional supervision to ensure their correct, consistent use. Those prescribing fluoride supplements should consider the amount of fluoride consumed from all sources of drinking water, such as the home or a child-care facility, as well as the possible impact of water-filtration devices that may remove fluoride from drinking water.

The CDA recommends that chewable tablets or lozenges be used when fluoride supplementation is desired. Children should be instructed to dissolve or chew tablet dosage forms of sodium fluoride before swallowing, thus delivering fluoride to the teeth topically as well as systemically. For special care patients, the CDA recommends the use of fluoride drops that may be administered in fluids, except in milk, or directly onto a child's tongue. If the child is old enough, the fluoride drops should be swished around the mouth before swallowing. In addition, no food or beverages should be consumed for 30 minutes after taking the fluoride dosage.

Compounded sodium fluoride solutions should be dispensed in plastic containers, as aqueous preparations of fluoride slowly attack glass. Large quantities of fluoride should not be stored in the home. For safety reasons, no more than 264 mg of sodium fluoride (120 mg of fluoride) are dispensed at one time. Although most fatalities associated with fluoride toxicity have resulted from industrial exposure or accidental use of a fluoride compound in cooking, two fatal cases have been related to fluoride used for dental prophylaxis. Both fatalities were 3-year-old children; one died after swallowing

TABLE 7: Fluoride Supplement Dosages for Individuals or Groups at High Risk to Dental Caries Based on Fluoride Level in Water Supply

	Dosage of Daily Supplement	
Age of Child	**Fluoride in water supply <0.3 ppm (mg/L)**	**Fluoride in water supply ≥0.3 ppm (mg/L)**
<3 years	Not recommended	Not recommended
3, 4, 5 years	0.25 mg (0.5 mg if no regular use of fluoridated toothpaste)	Not recommended
6-13 years	1.0 mg	Not recommended

Source: Canadian Dental Association Policy on Fluoride Supplementation. Ottawa, 1996.

large amounts of material used in a professional prophylaxis treatment; the other child died after swallowing 200 sodium fluoride (1 mg) tablets.

Toxicity

Acute fluoride intoxication is associated with gastrointestinal symptoms, such as nausea, vomiting, diarrhea and abdominal pain. The more serious consequences of overdose include hypocalcemia and hyperkalemia, both of which may affect the cardiovascular system. The toxic and lethal doses of fluoride reported in the literature vary considerably. Mild gastrointestinal symptoms are usually associated with doses up to 5 mg/kg of body weight, and more serious systemic toxicity with any doses greater than that.

At levels less than 5 mg/kg, treatment for fluoride toxicity is calcium given orally to relieve gastrointestinal symptoms. Milk and ice cream are suitable as calcium sources. Any fluoride ingestion greater than 5 mg/kg requires induction of vomiting and treatment in an emergency facility.

Because of the widespread use of fluoride-containing products (in addition to possible ingestion of fluoridated water), mild dental fluorosis has been reported. Young children in particular must be supervised when using fluoride products to ensure their appropriate use, and a fluoride supplement should be taken only on the advice of a dentist.

MOUTHWASHES

A mouthwash is generally regarded as a medicated liquid used for cleaning the mouth or treating diseases of the oral mucosa. Such a description does not accurately define the contents of most products nor differentiate between cosmetic and therapeutic uses. General use of these products is undoubtedly for cosmetic purposes to relieve bad breath. However, a mouthwash may serve as a vehicle for a therapeutic or prophylactic ingredient, such as fluoride. Other terms that are used for mouthwashes are mouthrinses, oral antiseptics and gargles.

The most popular form of mouthwash is a liquid, although troches, lozenges, concentrates and sprays also exist. The basic ingredients in commercially available liquid mouthwashes are water, alcohol, flavoring oils and coloring materials. Other ingredients, such as humectants, astringents, emulsifiers, antimicrobial agents, sweeteners and therapeutic substances, may also be included.

Although water is the principal component of mouthwashes, ethanol is present in concentrations of 15 to 30% to enhance the solubility of other ingredients. A single container of mouthwash can supply an alcohol dose lethal to a small child. Consumers should be made aware that mouthwashes are not innocuous and should be stored out of the reach of children.

Claims that mouthwashes overcome mouth odors are viewed with skepticism. Consumers should be questioned first about the presence of any oral lesions or other symptoms accompanying the breath odor. In the absence of any other symptoms, proper toothbrushing and flossing techniques should be emphasized. A marked breath odor persisting after these measures should be investigated by a dentist to determine the underlying cause. Mouthwashes should not be relied on to mask odor.

The presence of antimicrobial agents in mouthrinse formulations is controversial. The most commonly used agents in this category are the quaternary ammonium compounds, such as cetylpyridinium chloride, benzethonium chloride and domiphen bromide, and phenolic substances, such as phenol, thymol, betanaphthol and hexylresorcinol.

The FDA and the ADA do not recognize mouthwashes as contributing substantially to the treatment of oral conditions when used unsupervised. Besides a lack of data on effectiveness, both groups expressed concern that use of such products might delay treatment of an underlying disease. Therapeutic use of mouthwashes should occur with appropriate evaluation and supervision by a dentist or physician.

In addition to a cosmetic breath-freshening function, some antiseptic mouthwashes have antiplaque activity. Specifically, mouth rinsing with chlorhexidine, stannous fluoride, cetylpyridinium chloride, volatile oils, benzethonium chloride or a combination of cetylpyridinium chloride with domiphen bromide may reduce dental plaque formation. Sanguinarine, an herbal extract, is also retained in the mouth and may have antiplaque activity, especially when a sanguinarine mouthrinse and dentifrice are used concurrently.

Volatile Oils: The mixture of volatile oils (eucalyptol, thymol, menthol and methyl salicylate) in *Listerine* has been used for over a century with little change in the basic formulation. The product has been evaluated recently for antiplaque action in several double-blind studies involving more than

700 people. Results from these studies vary, but generally indicate that the mouthwash helps reduce plaque by up to 50% depending on the study design protocol.

When used as a mouthrinse against pre-existing plaque deposits, twice daily rinses with *Listerine* produced no reductions in plaque when compared with a placebo. In short-term studies on plaque formation over 7 to 14 days, *Listerine* rinses 2 or 3 times daily as the only form of oral hygiene resulted in plaque scores significantly reduced compared to those found in placebo groups. Longer studies of 21 days in which the formation of plaque was evaluated after a dental prophylaxis, and when rinsing accompanied twice daily toothbrushing, showed plaque reductions of 38 to 43%. A nine-month trial of *Listerine* rinsing in conjunction with normal toothbrushing and flossing routines resulted in 50 to 60% less plaque, by wet weight, than the placebo rinse. Therefore, this agent appears capable of reducing plaque formation on a long-term basis. Its efficacy in combination with brushing is greater than that of a placebo rinse with brushing.

Listerine is also effective in helping to prevent gingivitis. Although a 21-day experimental gingivitis trial found no difference between *Listerine* and a placebo rinse when gingivitis development was evaluated, several studies have shown reductions of 28 to 36% in gingivitis scores after daily rinsing for 6 months or longer. *Listerine* is the first nonprescription mouthrinse to receive the Seal of Acceptance of the ADA Council on Dental Therapeutics as safe and effective in helping to prevent and reduce supragingival plaque and gingivitis. It is also recognized by the CDA. It is not yet known whether plaque inhibition by any chemical agent is of any long-term value in preventing periodontitis.

Further studies have indicated that *Listerine* is effective for gingivitis control used as a mouthrinse twice daily for 30 seconds. For plaque reduction, maximal results are seen with 60 seconds of use.

Quaternary ammonium compounds such as cetylpyridinium chloride, benzethonium chloride and domiphen bromide have shown excellent in vitro antimicrobial activity against plaque-resident bacteria. However, clinical trials of these compounds as antiplaque agents have produced variable results, perhaps because of their short retention time in the mouth. Although they rapidly adsorb to the tooth surface in a high concentration, they also release rapidly. Cetylpyridinium chloride rinses have significantly reduced plaque formation by an average of 30% in the absence of other oral hygiene measures. When used in addition to regular toothbrushing for 6 weeks, cetylpyridinium chloride rinsing reduced plaque wet weight by 25% and was also associated with reduced gingival inflammation when compared to placebo. Both cetylpyridinium chloride and a combination of cetylpyridinium chloride with domiphen bromide (e.g., *Scope*) have produced significant reductions of 15 to 20% in plaque accumulation, compared to rinsing with water, when used in conjunction with normal oral hygiene procedures over a 31-day period.

To prevent plaque formation to the same degree as that produced with twice-daily rinses with chlorhexidine, quaternary ammonium compounds need to be used 4 times daily.

Side effects with quaternary ammonium compounds include staining, ulcerations and discomfort. Long-term studies with *Listerine* generally show no soft tissue problems or extrinsic staining of the teeth or oral mucosa.

Sanguinarine is the chief constituent alkaloid found in sanguinaria extract. Studies of its activity as an antiplaque mouthrinse, used alone or in combination with a sanguinarine-zinc chloride dentifrice, indicate that it can reduce and prevent plaque formation and gingivitis. Although staining and taste alteration do not appear to be a problem with sanguinarine, the taste of the product has been subjectively rated as poor in one study.

Prebrushing Antiplaque Rinse: A combination product containing sodium lauryl sulfate, sodium borate and sodium salicylate (*PLAX*) has recently been extensively marketed as a prebrushing antiplaque rinse. However, initial reports of its efficacy in dissolving plaque by a detergent action have not been substantiated in further studies. Although using *PLAX* in combination with toothbrushing has been shown to remove plaque effectively, the amount of plaque removed has not been any greater than that removed with toothbrushing alone.

Recent reports have shown that a prebrushing rinse containing triclosan 0.03% and a copolymer (0.125%) was more effective than a placebo rinse in reducing plaque in both short-term (5 days) and long-term (6 months) studies. Because this product also apparently bears the name *PLAX*, at least in Great Britain, future reports on *PLAX* will have to be examined carefully to determine which product is being described.

Consumers who wish to use a mouthwash for plaque control should be advised to use it in addition to regular toothbrushing and flossing. It should not replace usual oral hygiene measures or visits to the dentist. A product containing cetylpyridinium chloride alone or in combination with domiphen bromide, or *Listerine* may help prevent plaque formation when used routinely 2 to 4 times daily along with mechanical plaque removal. Consumers should swish 30 mL of the product around the mouth for 30 to 60 seconds before expectorating. They should not rinse with water after this procedure, and should refrain from eating, drinking or smoking for at least 30 minutes after rinsing. The effectiveness of this rinsing is most significant if done immediately after brushing and/or flossing the teeth. The manufacturer of *PLAX* suggests it be used as a prebrushing rinse.

Products may receive the CDA Seal of Recognition if their ingredients are recognized as effective agents for the prevention of supragingival plaque accumulation and gingivitis.

Because of the widespread use of mouthwashes and a known link between frequent alcohol ingestion and oral cancer, several retrospective studies have attempted to determine if mouthwash use may also be involved in cancer development. When compared to control subjects, a small subgroup of women who had not been exposed to either smoking or alcohol use were shown to have a slightly higher risk of developing oral or pharyngeal cancer. However, these results have not been confirmed by other studies, and may be due to chance because of the small number of cases studied.

Fluoride Mouthrinses

Several mouthwashes containing fluoride and special fluoride rinses are available. The substances outlined in Table 6 have been approved as anticaries ingredients by the FDA; several may carry the Seal of Recognition of the CDA. Although these products appear particularly useful for people living in areas of nonfluoridated water, some cavity prevention benefits may be achieved even where water is fluoridated. Fluoridated mouthwashes for daily use currently available contain 0.05% sodium fluoride. The recommended procedure is to swish a mouthful through the teeth for 1 minute, once daily, and then expectorate. The individual should also be cautioned not to rinse the mouth after this procedure, nor to eat or drink anything for 30 minutes. Mouthrinses containing 0.2% sodium fluoride are also available for use once weekly.

In nonfluoridated areas, dentists may recommend certain fluoride rinses that must be diluted before use, or they may recommend others that are to be swallowed after rinsing. Consumers should be instructed in the appropriate use of the selected product.

PLAQUE DISCLOSING AGENTS

Disclosing agents make dental plaque visible. By staining plaque either at home or in the dentist's office, individuals can evaluate their oral hygiene techniques and identify areas needing improvement.

Disclosing agents are available as chewable tablets (*Red Cote*) or as a solution. These agents should be expectorated completely and the mouth rinsed with water, which also should be expectorated. Disclosing products commonly contain the dye FDC Red No. 3, which has the advantage of staining red to match soft tissues, and not markedly staining the teeth. However, plaque at the gingival margin may not be well differentiated. A combination of FDC Red No. 3 and FDC Green No. 3 or FDC Blue No. 1 is able to color differentiate between thick old plaque and thin plaque. All these dyes are considered safe when used at approved doses and expectorated. Disclosing agents are meant for occasional use as indicators and should not be used continuously (e.g., daily).

PLAQUE REMOVAL PRODUCTS

Toothbrushes

A wide variety of toothbrushes is commercially available. The selection of a toothbrush should take into account the individual's manual dexterity, oral anatomy and periodontal health. Prime functional properties of toothbrushes are flexibility, softness and diameter of the bristles, as well as the strength, rigidity and lightness of the handle.

For general adult use, multitufted brushes with soft, rounded nylon bristles are probably the best choice. The number of tufts per brush may vary. Brushes with 3 or 4 rows of 10 to 12 tufts or clusters of bristles are the most common. Four-row brushes tolerate increased pressure with flexing of the filaments; two or three row brushes, especially those with soft bristles, wear out the quickest.

Brushes with tufts arranged in a V-shape are no better at plaque removal than straight, multitufted brushes.

The use of hard-bristled brushes should be avoided. Hard brushes can damage the gingiva, causing the gums to bleed, or to recede, exposing the cementum; or cause hard tissue damage or tooth abrasion.

No official standard exists for use of the terms soft and hard in describing toothbrushes. Brands may vary in the bristle diameter and length that constitutes a soft brush. The experience of the user and dental practitioner may be the best guide for appropriate choice of a toothbrush for regular use.

Brushes with natural hog bristles are also available, but tend to be less durable. The bristles may loosen and become lodged in the gingiva and oral mucosa.

Handle shape varies among toothbrushes. Since there is no ideal handle shape, choice is a personal preference. Straight handles are the most common. Whatever shape is chosen, the handle should be long enough to fit comfortably into the hand. Dentists or dental hygienists may recommend brushes specially adapted for certain user characteristics, such as an angled handle to reach posterior dental areas or bristles of different lengths for orthodontic appliances.

Children should use a toothbrush with a small head and a thick handle for ease of manipulation. Adults who gag easily may also find a child's brush, or one with a smaller head, more useful than an ordinary toothbrush.

Worn toothbrushes do not remove plaque effectively. Toothbrushes should be replaced when they begin to show signs of matting or wear. This usually occurs after 3 months of daily use, but this time period may vary according to individual brushing technique and frequency of use. Most studies show that people do not replace toothbrushes as frequently as they should to achieve optimal plaque removal. Toothbrushes should be replaced 72 hours after starting an antibiotic regimen for strep throat.

The proper frequency and method of brushing for optimal oral health have not been well established. Suggestions for toothbrushing frequency range from 5 times daily to once every other day. Once-daily brushing should be a minimum recommendation because *Streptococcus mutans* requires at least 24 hours to organize on a clean tooth; however, about 60% of plaque may remain after daily brushing, lending support to more frequent and thorough brushing. The longer plaque remains undisturbed, the greater its pathogenic potential. Many dental practitioners recommend twice daily brushing to promote good oral health.

Thoroughness of brushing, without trauma, is more important than method of brushing. No one method of brushing has been proven superior to others in removing plaque. Individuals may need instructions in different brushing techniques to remove plaque completely. The scrub technique using short back-and-forth brush strokes is the most popular method of brushing and requires the least time. It may be the easiest method for children to learn and use, but may not remove plaque from the gingival sulcus and, when performed too vigorously, may cause abrasion of the tooth structure and gum recession. Although children should be encouraged to develop good preventive habits, such as toothbrushing at an early age, it is suggested an adult clean a child's teeth once daily to ensure complete and safe plaque removal until the child has mastered the technique.

A brushing method developed by Bass is currently the method most often recommended by dentists and dental hygienists. In the Bass method, the bristles of the brush are placed at a 45° angle to the tooth, covering about 6 mm of the gingiva above the crown of the tooth. The brush is then vibrated gently and swept away from the gingiva as

How to Select a Toothbrush

- For general adult use, choose a multitufted brush with soft, rounded nylon bristles, with the size of head that fits comfortably into your mouth. Children should use a toothbrush with a small head and a thick handle so they can manipulate it appropriately.
- Some toothbrushes have specially angled handles for individuals who have difficulty reaching the back of the mouth with a regular straight handled brush.
- Do not use a hard-bristled brush. It can cause gum and tooth damage and does not remove plaque any better than a soft-bristled brush.
- Replace your toothbrush when it begins showing signs of matting or wear, usually after 3 months of daily use.

it is lifted to the next tooth area. With this placement of the brush, the bristles actually displace the marginal gingiva and reach the base of the healthy sulcus (about 3 mm depth), thoroughly removing plaque. Consumers should also be instructed to brush the areas behind the back molars, the occlusal (top) tooth surfaces and perhaps the upper surface of the tongue to remove plaque.

Professional advice on recommended brushing times ranges from 3 to 7 minutes. Recent studies have shown that 90% of plaque is removed after 30 seconds of brushing a particular area, no matter what type of toothbrush is used. Although consumers significantly overestimate the time spent brushing their teeth, studies of actual brushing times show that, on average, people spend a total of 1 minute brushing their teeth. The use of a gel dentifrice fails to enhance toothbrushing time or thoroughness over that found with use of a conventional toothpaste. Although frequency and pattern of brushing affects children's plaque removal, duration of brushing produces the most significant effect on plaque removal. Smokers tend to have more plaque on their teeth, before and after brushing. This condition may be partly explained by their practice of brushing for shorter periods of time than nonsmokers, although other factors may also contribute to their poorer oral cleanliness.

Powered toothbrushes may benefit individuals with dexterity problems or those who brush longer because of the novelty of the item. However, most studies have shown that these brushes do not remove plaque any better than a manual toothbrush used correctly. A rotary electric toothbrush may remove plaque more effectively and prevent decalcification in adolescents undergoing orthodontic treatment with fixed appliances. Some studies have also shown that such toothbrushes may be more effective than manual brushing in patients with gingivitis or periodontal conditions, especially those previously noncompliant with oral hygiene procedures. Electric toothbrushes may be recommended for certain groups of patients who would benefit from their use.

How to Brush your Teeth

- Brush your teeth at least once a day. Dentists or dental hygienists may recommend a greater frequency—follow their advice.
- Whatever technique you use to brush your teeth, make sure that you do it thoroughly—you should brush each tooth area for about 30 seconds to remove most of the plaque.
- A popular method of brushing is to place the brush at a 45° angle to the tooth, covering about 0.5 cm (1/4") of gum. Then, gently vibrate the brush and sweep it away from the gum.

Water Irrigating Devices

The routine use of water irrigating devices is recommended only as an adjunctive measure for oral hygiene, as these devices do not remove subgingival plaque and may cause bacteremia in people with periodontitis.

Dental Floss

As the toothbrush has a limited efficacy for cleaning between the teeth, dental floss should also be used. Frequent interdental flossing reduces the incidence of proximal caries. Continued flossing for long periods increases the beneficial effect.

Dental floss is available from various manufacturers in waxed and unwaxed forms. Both types remove plaque effectively and improve oral health. No significant differences in physiological effects have been found in recent studies comparing waxed to unwaxed dental floss. On smooth, planed tooth surfaces, four types of dental floss (unwaxed, waxed, lightly waxed and Superfloss) removed plaque equally well. Lightly waxed floss was significantly better at removing plaque from rough unplaned surfaces than the other three products. In other studies, Superfloss, a 3-in-one product made up of unwaxed floss, a threader and a nylon brush, was not consistently superior to dental floss alone. Patients may prefer dental tape over floss because of ease of use.

Some people may prefer unwaxed floss because it is thinner and easier to manipulate. Most consumers in a recent study preferred waxed floss, presumably because it may pass between tight-fitting teeth more easily than unwaxed floss and without shredding. Lightly waxed floss may combine the benefits of both types. Flavored dental floss (e.g., mint) has also been shown to be preferable to plain waxed floss.

Flossing technique is important to remove plaque effectively. A length of floss is wound around the index finger of each hand and placed through the contact area of the teeth by gentle pressure with the thumbs. It is then guided into the gingival sulcus, flattened against the tooth surface and moved toward the crown of the tooth. The tooth surface above and below the gingival margin is cleaned before the floss is moved across the interproximal tissue to the adjacent tooth surface for similar cleaning. When the floss is removed from between the two teeth, the individual should check it and the gums for gingival bleeding, which indicates gingivitis and the need for more effective cleaning.

Children's teeth may be difficult to floss depending on the age of the child. Adults responsible for such a procedure may wish to floss only areas of the child's mouth where there is contact between adjacent teeth. They may also find knitting yarn or interproximal toothbrushes useful in removing plaque from surfaces where there are openings between teeth.

People with dexterity problems may find a floss holder easier to use. However, such flossing aids have not been shown to remove plaque any better that floss held between the fingers. Floss may also be passed interdentally by a floss threader in areas where contacts at the crowns of the teeth are too tight to prevent normal flossing techniques.

Other Interdental Cleaning Devices

Other interdental cleaning devices include interdental brushes, rubber points and toothpicks. Interdental brushes appear to clean interdental areas where the papillae are missing better than dental floss. Dental floss removes plaque much better than toothpicks for most people, although combinations of these cleaning techniques with toothbrushing does improve oral health. The rubber tips found on some toothbrushes are designed to massage the gingiva, which allegedly enhances blood flow into the area, increasing oxygen delivery and removal of waste products. However, these devices should be used only on the advice of a dentist. Above all, proper instruction and motivation of the individual are essential for effective oral hygiene.

Several chemical agents—chlorhexidine, quaternary ammonium compounds, volatile oils, enzymes and herbal extracts—have been used as antiplaque treatments. The most widely studied agent for this purpose is chlorhexidine, which reduces caries activity because of its antibacterial effect on cariogenic bacteria in plaque. Other agents, such as cetylpyridinium chloride and the combination of volatile oils in *Listerine*, also show antiplaque activity but have not been evaluated for caries prevention.

TOOTHACHE RELIEVERS

Most products marketed for relieving toothache contain eugenol or benzocaine.

Eugenol is the essential chemical constituent of clove oil and is principally responsible for its action. Eugenol acts as an antiseptic and in concentrations of 85 to 87% acts as an obtundent or analgesic. It is accepted by the Council for Dental Therapeutics for use by dentists, often as a zinc oxide paste formulation to cover exposed pulpal areas.

Because eugenol irritates, it must be applied carefully, only to the cavity in the tooth. It is so irritating that eugenol can actually destroy viable dental pulp. The FDA recommends eugenol be used only on irreparably damaged teeth (candidates for extraction or root canal therapy). People experiencing intermittent toothaches, indicating a viable and repairable tooth, should not use any nonprescription toothache product containing eugenol. Instead, they should make an emergency dental appointment, apply cold compresses or ice cubes, and take oral analgesics such as ASA, acetaminophen or ibuprofen, until the condition can be treated. If the pain is throbbing and relentless, the tooth is likely to be irreversibly damaged. When properly applied, eugenol preparations may bring some relief until dental attention is possible.

Benzocaine has been widely used for toothache relief since 1926. A recent clinical study confirmed the efficacy of 7.5% benzocaine in propylene glycol for the temporary relief of toothaches. When applied as directed to the tooth, its cavity and the surrounding gingival tissue, benzocaine is safe and noncaustic. However, it should be used only temporarily until dental service can be obtained. Benzocaine also provides effective relief of teething pain when rubbed on the gum tissue surrounding the erupting tooth. Only a small amount should be applied with a gauze pad or cotton-tipped applicator to prevent excessive numbness or swallowing of the product.

Other ingredients in combination products available for toothache relief include benzyl alcohol and phenolic compounds. None have been proven both safe and effective for this purpose. In addition, the alcohol present in some products may cause dehydration of the dentin. Products such as waxes, gums or cotton soaked with medication, are not recommended because their occlusive properties may prevent an abscess from draining.

TOOTH WHITENERS

Products containing oxidizing agents, such as hydrogen peroxide or carbamide peroxide, have recently been marketed as tooth whiteners. Most of these products are liquids or gels that are applied via a mouthguard tray, worn for several hours daily. Some others are toothpastes or consist of a multistep process (mouth-cleanser, gel and polishing cream). Some products are available by prescription from a dentist, while others are nonprescription products.

Although these products may be safe and effective, long-term safety data are not available. Concern has been expressed because of possible damage to oral soft tissues and the pulp of the teeth.

Recent decisions by the Bureau of Nonprescription Drugs of Health Canada mean that these products are now classified as cosmetics, when labelled solely for whitening or brightening the teeth. Labelling requirements include cautionary statements regarding seeing a dentist if irritation occurs and not using the product for a child under the age of 6 years, or for longer than 14 days unless on a dentist's advice. Patients are also to be cautioned not to allow gel products to contact the gums. In addition, manufacturers must ensure that products have a pH greater than 4 if they are to be sold as cosmetics.

The Canadian Dental Association believes that the public should only use these tooth whitening products after consultation with a dentist.

SUMMARY

Self-medication with nonprescription products is not generally recommended for most dental or oral problems. In most cases, diseases of the hard and soft tissues of the mouth require evaluation and treatment by a dentist. However, topical anesthetic preparations may provide temporary relief from toothache or teething symptoms, as well as from pain associated with canker sores or primary herpes infections. Protective agents also can be useful in relieving oral ulcer discomfort. Nonprescription mouthwashes may serve a cosmetic function but should not be used unsupervised to treat oral conditions.

On the other hand, products available to prevent dental diseases are numerous and varied. These include nonpharmaceutical items such as toothbrushes, dentifrices and dental floss, as well as fluoridated toothpastes and mouthrinses. Because all preventive techniques require cooperation and sustained effort on the part of the individual, the health professional may serve a valuable function by reviewing and reinforcing instructions for good oral hygiene.

RECOMMENDED READING

Adams RA, Mann WV. Oral hygiene techniques and home care. In: Stallard RE, ed. A Textbook of Preventive Dentistry. Philadelphia: WB Saunders, 1982:217–40.

American Dental Association Council on Dental Therapeutics. Accepted dental therapeutics. Chicago: American Dental Association, 1984.

Antoon JW, Miller RL. Aphthous ulcers: a review of the literature on etiology, pathogenesis, diagnosis, and treatment. J Am Dent Assoc 1980;101: 803–08.

Flynn AA. Counseling special population groups on oral health care needs. Am Pharm 1993;33: 33–39.

Flynn AA. Oral health products. In: Covington TR, ed. Handbook of Nonprescription Drugs. 10th ed. Washington, DC: American Pharmaceutical Association, 1993:401–31.

Gossel TA. Dry mouth and use of saliva substitutes. US Pharmacist 1986;11:22–28, 58.

Gossel TA. The role of fluorides in preventing cavities. US Pharmacist 1986;11:28–34.

Kanapka JA. Over-the-counter dentifrices in the treatment of tooth hypersensitivity. Dent Clin North Am 1990;34:545–60.

Mandel ID, Gaffar A. Calculus revisited. A review. J Clin Periodontol 1986;13:249–57.

Miller MA. Odontologic diseases. In: Lynch MA, ed. Burket's Oral Medicine. Toronto: JB Lippincott, 1977:283–301.

Popovich NG, Popovich JG. What you should know about fever blisters and canker sores. US Pharmacist 1978;3:35–48.

Pray WS. A coping strategy for oral ulcers. US Pharmacist 1993;18:37–41.

Pray WS. Dental hypersensitivity. US Pharmacist 1993;18:29–33.

Pray WS. Dry mouth syndrome: causes and treatment. US Pharmacist 1994;19:16–24.

Scully C, Porter SR. Recurrent aphthous stomatitis: current concepts of etiology, pathogenesis and management. J Oral Pathol Med 1989;18:21–27.

Serio FG, Siegel MA. Periodontal diseases: a review. Cutis 1991;47:55–62.

Tessier JF, Kulkarni GV. Bad breath: etiology, diagnosis and treatment. Oral Health 1991;(Oct): 19–24.

Volpe AR. Dentifrices and mouthrinses. In: Stallard RE, ed. A Textbook of Preventive Dentistry. Philadelphia: WB Saunders, 1982:170–216.

20

PAIN AND FEVER PRODUCTS

Yvonne M. Shevchuk / Alfred J. Rémillard

CONTENTS

Pain	**531**
Pain Transmission and Perception	
Headaches	
Arthritis	
Visceral Pain	
Dental Pain	
Musculoskeletal Pain	
Other Conditions	
Fever	**545**
Pathophysiology	
Differential Diagnosis	
Measurement of Body Temperature	
Fever in Specific Patient Groups	
Management of Fever	
Pharmaceutical Agents	**550**
Internal Analgesics	
External Analgesics	
Recommended Reading	**565**

PAIN

Pain remains a difficult term to define. In practice, the most useful definition is: "Pain is what the patient says hurts." It can be described as an unpleasant sensory and emotional experience associated with actual or potential tissue damage. Regardless of the definition, pain is always subjective, as only the person experiencing it can describe the pain and its intensity.

Pain can be classified into acute pain and chronic pain. Chronic pain is further divided into nonterminal pain, such as that associated with arthritis, and terminal pain, such as that associated with end-stage malignancy. The type of pain will dictate the type of treatment necessary.

Acute pain normally progresses from mild through moderate to severe, or vice versa, and is typically self-limiting. It serves to warn the individual that something is wrong, allowing appropriate protective actions. Acute pain is accompanied by the signs and symptoms of catecholamine release, e.g., increased blood pressure, tachycardia, sweating, increased gastric acidity and mydriasis.

Chronic pain is a more complex phenomenon that might be secondary to acute pain or be the primary event. By its nature, chronic pain no longer serves any purpose and eventually causes loss of sleep and appetite, anxiety and irritability, and begins to adversely affect social and sexual functions. A vicious cycle is entered, and the pain is no longer responsive to analgesic medication alone.

PAIN TRANSMISSION AND PERCEPTION

Neuroanatomy

The transmission of acute pain is the net result of complex neuronal mechanisms that detect, relay, interpret and respond to noxious or harmful stimuli.

As pain evolves from acute to chronic, different fibre pathways are used, and diverse areas of the brain become involved in pain perception and modulation.

Pain mechanisms are initiated with the nociceptors, which are free nerve endings serving as pain sensors in the skin, muscle, blood vessels and internal organs. They detect and respond to the various types of noxious stimuli, including thermal, mechanical (e.g., pinching) and chemical damage

Pain

to tissue. When the stimulus is sufficient to cause tissue damage, endogenous chemicals such as bradykinins, histamine, prostaglandins and substance P are released and the pain message is transmitted. Nociceptors function as transducers, converting energy into electrical signals that are then relayed to primary afferent (ascending to the brain) fibres.

Primary Afferent Fibres: The nervous system contains several types of primary afferents that are classified according to their diameters, degree of myelination (having a lipid layer or myelin sheath), type of stimulus needed for activation and anatomical location.

The A-beta afferent has the largest diameter of all fibres. It responds to light touch, pressure, vibration or electrical stimulation and is present primarily in nerves that innervate the skin. Normally this fibre does not transmit pain impulses. It may play a major role in the gate-control theory of pain modulation, discussed later in this section.

Two other primary afferents include the large diameter myelinated A delta fibre and the small diameter unmyelinated C-fibre axon. These fibres are present in the nerves of the skin, muscle and visceral structures or organs. The myelinated A delta fibre carries sharp, localized, and first pain sensations at high conduction velocities. The C-fibre conducts dull, diffuse pain (along with sympathetic impulses) at slower rates. Since the A-delta and C-afferents respond to intense stimuli to produce pain, they are known as primary afferent nociceptors or pain receptors.

Central Pathways for Pain: The afferent fibres that convey nociceptive information converge on the dorsal horn of the spinal cord (Figure 1). The dorsal horn contains the substantia gelatinosa, an important area involved in pain modulation. All pain fibres synapse in the substantia gelatinosa and release unique chemical transmitters, such as substance P, cholecystokinin and somatostatin. The transmitters then relay specific messages to secondary and tertiary neurons in the spinothalamic tract to the higher brain regions.

The large and fast A delta fibres are transmitted from the dorsal horn directly to the thalamus and then to the cortex, which is responsible for the conscious recognition of pain. This spinothalamic tract localizes and characterizes the intensity and quality of the painful stimulus in the body. Interruption of this pathway produces permanent deficits in pain and temperature discrimination.

The signals from the C fibres ascend mainly to the reticular formation (medulla), the periaqueductal gray (midbrain), the hypothalamus and the thalamus. From there, signals are directed by the thalamus to the cortex and the limbic system. The limbic system is responsible for the emotional components of pain, such as fear and anxiety, as well as other basic functions including temperature regulation. The reticular formation alerts the individual and sends messages to higher brain centres. Distractions at this arousal centre result in a decrease in intensity of pain. The hypothalamus, which receives information from the reticular formation, is responsible for autonomic responses to pain, such as sweating, nausea, increased heart rate.

Descending Pathways: The periaqueductal gray receives input from the higher brain centres to control the pain perception through descending neurons that terminate in the medulla. The medulla can facilitate or inhibit the noxious stimuli by activating a second series of descending neurons.

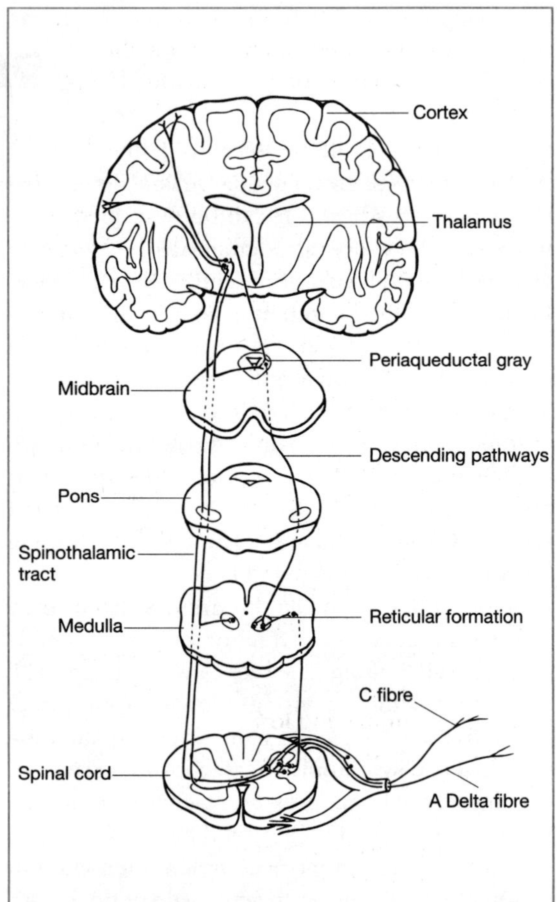

FIGURE 1: Pain Pathways

This transmission involves the endogenous opiates and enkephalins that interfere with neurons ending in the dorsal horn. The enkephalins are endogenous pentapeptides that act on the morphine receptors within the central nervous system (CNS). These peptides exert a presynaptic inhibition effect to reduce pain transmission by reducing the release of substance P, one of the chemical messengers for nociception. The descending pathway, as described, is an oversimplification of a very complex system. Similar inhibitory systems involving other sites in the brain and other neurochemicals are probably activated simultaneously.

Neurochemistry

The central processing of pain involves multiple neurotransmitter systems including monoamines, amino acids and neuropeptides. Much of their function remains unclear. Morphine-like peptides, such as enkephalins and endorphins, have been identified. With analgesic properties 20 to 30 times more potent than morphine, these peptides occupy opioid receptors and produce both presynaptic and postsynaptic inhibition of primary afferent transmission. Enkephalins are found within the limbic system as well as the pons, medulla, thalamus and dorsal horn.

Serotonin, which is widely distributed in the body, appears to be associated with enkephalin activity in the descending inhibitory system to exert postsynaptic control of nerve transmission and therefore suppress pain impulses. Norepinephrine, which is also found at various levels within the CNS, can enhance or antagonize opioid-mediated analgesia depending on where it is released in the brain.

Bradykinin and histamine activate pain fibres. Prostaglandins alone do not appear to stimulate the fibres, but their presence in inflammatory conditions seems to sensitize pain receptors to mechanical stimuli and low concentrations of chemical stimulants.

Substance P, an 11-amino acid peptide, serves a regulatory function both in peripheral afferent transmission of noxious stimuli and the descending nociceptive pathways to produce pain. It has been shown that depletion of substance P from the cord of experimental animals with capsaicin will cause analgesia.

Cholecystokinin, another peptide, is present in the same locale as substance P and also has pain modulating effects. Somatostatin is the major transmitter of pain located in unmyelinated sensory neurons, similar to substance P. Neurotensin elicits analgesia by inhibition of neuronal firing outside the opioid system.

It is not surprising that medications that alter or enhance these neurochemicals may have profound effects on pain modulation.

Gate-Control Theory

Many nonpharmacological modalities are effective in providing pain relief. In 1965, Melzack and Wall proposed the gate-control theory in an attempt to explain mechanisms by which noxious stimuli and cognitive factors can modulate pain transmission (Figure 2).

It is postulated that the substantia gelatinosa, located in the dorsal horn of the spinal cord, acts as a "gate" through which impulses reach the CNS. The gate can increase or decrease the flow of nerve impulses from peripheral fibres to pain centres in the central nervous system, including the reticular formation, thalamus, limbic system and cerebral cortex. The gate is thought to be controlled by the primary afferent fibres as well as descending pathways originating from higher brain function input.

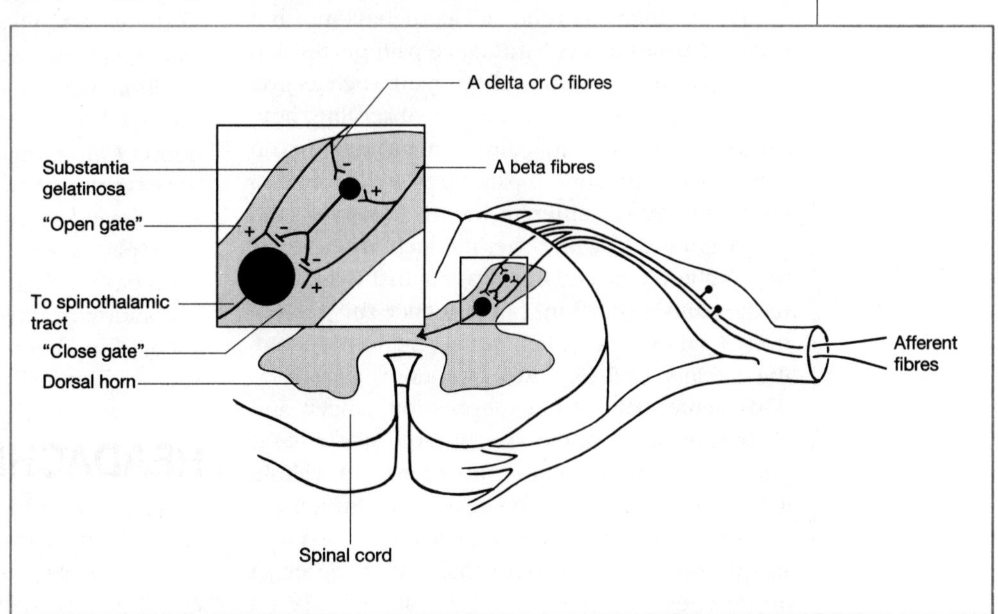

FIGURE 2: Gate Control Theory of Pain

The large A beta fibres carry touch, pressure and electrical stimuli. When stimulated, these fibres excite the substantia gelatinosa cells to close the gate and inhibit transmission of noxious stimuli or pain. The mechanism may involve the release of enkephalins in the dorsal horn. On the other hand, the A delta and C fibres, carrying cutaneous pain stimuli, inhibit the substantia gelatinosa, which opens the gate and facilitates pain transmission. The gate-control theory helps explain the mechanisms by which physical (e.g., back massage), thermal (e.g., counterirritants) or electrical stimulation (e.g., transcutaneous electrical nerve stimulation therapy - TENS) help relieve pain. These various forms of stimuli activate the larger, nonpain producing or non-nociceptor afferent A-beta fibre, which in turn inhibits the transmission of the smaller pain producing A delta and C fibres. A further example is how pain from a bump on the side of the head can be relieved by rubbing the injured area. There are other mechanisms in which non-pharmacological methods can produce pain relief. For example, acupuncture is thought to work by causing the release of endorphins.

Pain modulation can also occur at the cortical level. Treatment techniques, such as behavior modification, hypnosis, biofeedback and psychotherapy, have been shown effective in pain management.

Psychology of Pain

Pain is not simply a function of bodily damage. There are many psychological, behavioral and social variables that can influence pain perception and expression. Learning about pain, such as previous experience with pain or observing how someone responds to pain, can influence pain perception. Variations in pain threshold have been observed across different racial, religious and ethnic groups. Cognitive factors, such as a person's beliefs about pain and the meaning that is attached to the painful situation, can influence the perception of pain intensity. Emotional reactions, including anxiety and fear, are frequently associated with acute pain, while depression, anger and irritability are commonly observed in chronic pain. Other factors that influence pain threshold are coping style and strategies, family influences and social support. The influence of psychosocial factors on pain perception has led to different approaches in therapy aimed at modulating motivational and cognitive contributors to pain.

Psychological methods known to alleviate pain include:

- hypnotic suggestion techniques;
- techniques to diminish the frequency of pain-related behavior patterns;
- electromyography or other physiological indexes to teach patients to relax and develop an attitude that allows them to cope with pain;
- strategies to distract attention from or change the meaning of pain;
- psychotherapeutic or pharmacological techniques to relieve depression and anxiety.

Although these approaches alone may not abolish the pain completely, they may make some kinds of pain more bearable.

Inflammation

An inflammatory reaction is induced by damage to or irritation of tissue by various factors. These include microorganisms, chemical irritants, thermal and mechanical damage as well as immunological reactions. When injured, the cell releases biochemical mediators, such as histamine, serotonin and kinins, as well as arachidonic acid, which is biotransformed to thromboxane, prostacyclin, leukotriene and prostaglandin. Prostaglandins potentiate the effects of chemical mediators on the local pain receptors to increase pain and dilate blood vessels. This in turn increases blood flow causing heat and redness at the local site. The chemical mediators also increase the permeability of the vessels, allowing fluid to leak into the surrounding tissue, resulting in edema and swelling. In addition, white blood cells descend on the site of injury where they consume foreign particles and debris. Cells form a wall around the inflamed focus to prevent further spread of pathogens and toxins. Inflammation is characterized by swelling, redness, heat, pain and limited function. It is essentially a protective mechanism, cleansing the tissue and facilitating healing. However, on a chronic basis, such as in rheumatoid arthritis, it becomes the source of complication.

HEADACHES

An estimated 70 to 80% of the general population suffer from at least one headache per month. It is the most prevalent of all chronic pain conditions and the most frequent cause for missing work or school. The International Headache Society has classified headache syndromes into 13 major categories and 66 subcategories. This section will focus on the main recurrent syndromes, tension-type, migraine and cluster headaches, and the newly recognized medication-induced headache, a syndrome that health professionals can have a critical role in identifying, managing and preventing.

Health professionals should be alert to the many causes of acute headache pain that may signal a severe medical problem: leaking aneurysms, meningitis, increased intracranial pressure and tumors. It is rare that headache signifies ominous disease, however, if patients complain of the following symptoms, they should be advised to seek medical attention promptly:

- the worst headache ever for someone who seldom gets headaches;
- onset with exertion, never before experienced by the patient;
- decreased level of awareness and cognitive function not due to excessive use of analgesics;
- meningeal irritation (pain occurs when neck is flexed forward);
- abnormal physical exam, such as fever and worsening of pain while under observation.

Tension-Type Headaches

Tension-type is the new term for tension, muscle contraction, stress or ordinary headache. It is the most common recurrent headache syndrome, affecting nearly 50% of all patients who visit headache clinics, and up to 36% of the general population. It afflicts twice as many males as females and is more common in high stress jobs. Tension-type headache is characterized by a gradual progression of dull, nagging pain that is perceived to be deep and more frequently affects both sides of the entire head. There are no prodromal (warning) symptoms. Often the sufferer complains of a tight headband-like squeezing sensation. The pain tends to move from the neck to the forehead, usually worsening as the day progresses. During the attacks, sufferers often describe a stiffness of the neck and shoulders. The pathophysiology of tension-type headache is not well known. It has been suggested that muscle contraction of neck and scalp muscles produce ischemia and later pain.

Treatment

As with any headache, one must assess what has worked for the patient in the past. Nonprescription analgesics have been successful in the treatment of this condition. Most patients respond well to ASA or acetaminophen. Nonsteroidal anti-inflammatory drugs (NSAIDs) are also helpful but are generally used if there is a lack of response to ASA or acetaminophen. Ergot drugs are not effective for tension-type headaches and may actually worsen the pain.

Since psychological anxiety and tension play important roles in provoking attacks, management can be addressed by behavior modification, relaxation training and biofeedback as well as the elimination of tension-causing agents such as caffeine. Antianxiety agents may be required in certain patients who have difficulty self-inducing a more relaxed state, while antidepressants may be necessary if depression has been judged a significant cause of tension-type headache.

Migraine Headaches

Migraine headaches are considerably more debilitating than tension-type headaches, afflicting 20 to 25% of the general population, while 14% suffer from both migraine and tension-type headaches together. Twice as frequent in female compared to male adults, migraine affects both sexes equally in the prepuberty years. There is a genetic predisposition: 65 to 90% of the sufferers have a family history of migraine. The pain is described as intense and pulsating, and is usually associated with uncontrollable somatic complaints, including nausea, vomiting, diarrhea, photophobia (intolerance to light) and phonophobia (intolerance to noise). Although pain is unilateral in most cases, it may be bilateral as well as frontal, temporal or generalized. Pain may also be intensified by physical activity.

A distinctive feature of migraine is the presence of a prodrome (warning symptom) that appears one to several hours before the headache pain. Prodromal symptoms include rapid mood swings, changes in level of activity and inability to concentrate.

In some patients, triggering factors have been identified that may precipitate migraines. The more common factors are sleeping late, changes in weather conditions, fatigue/stress, menstruation, the use of oral contraceptives, diets high in tyramine such as cola, tea and coffee, alcohol and stimuli, such as bright, flashing lights.

Migraines are classified into two distinct forms depending on the presence or absence of an aura:

Migraine without aura, previously known as common migraine, accounts for 90% of migraine sufferers. The headache phase usually lasts from 4 to 72 hours, but rarely exceeds several days.

Migraine with aura is the new term for classic or complicated migraine. The aura precedes the pain by 15 to 60 minutes and consists of focal neurological symptoms. The most common element is some form of visual disturbance, such as photopsia (flashes of light), scintillating scotomata (blind spots with luminous borders) and loss of the visual field. Other aura symptoms may include tactile loss, weakness, aphasia (slurred speech), vertigo and paresthesia. The aura rarely continues into the headache phase, which usually lasts less than 6 hours.

Despite the different classifications, some patients may experience both types at different times.

Treatment

The initial management of a migraine should focus on identifying and eliminating trigger factors and implementing behavioral interventions to reduce frequency of attacks. For some, lying in a darkened room and avoiding disturbing light and sound may be all that is required. If interventions are unsuccessful or headaches frequently recur, drug therapy is indicated. The intense pain should be managed with ASA, acetaminophen or NSAIDs.

One of the primary reasons for treatment failure is too low a dose of analgesic. A good rule to remember is, medicate early with an adequate dose. Another reason for drug treatment failure is that patients are nauseated and gastrointestinal motility is greatly impaired. Pretreatment with an antiemetic prior to analgesic therapy is recommended. Since most nonprescription antiemetics have prominent anticholinergic effects, which can further decrease gastrointestinal motility, metoclopramide 10 mg orally, a prescription gastrointestinal motility modifier, is the treatment of choice.

If headache pain and associated symptoms cannot be controlled by simple analgesics, a prescription medication, such as ergotamine, butorphanol nasal spray or sumatriptan may be indicated. Only if all else fails should drug therapy with other narcotics be initiated.

Prophylactic therapy is indicated in patients whose headache occurs with intolerable frequency (e.g., greater than 2 to 3 per month), or who are not responding to or unable to tolerate the side effects of acute therapy. Patients must be taught to take the preventative medications on a continuous basis whether they feel an attack is impending or not. This regimen is often difficult to adhere to when the patient is headache-free. Recent studies have shown that patients taking low dose ASA for its antiplatelet properties have experienced a 20% reduction in migraine attacks. Since the treatment is effective at very low doses of 60 to 75 mg every other day, physicians may recommend it for patients who can tolerate it. Other prophylactic prescription medications include beta-blockers, calcium channel blockers, specifically flunarizine, methysergide, amitriptyline, selective serotonin reuptake inhibitors (e.g., fluoxetine) and pizotyline. Onset of action of prophylactic medications varies from 4 weeks to 3 months. Feverfew has gained attention as a prophylactic agent for migraine therapy. Refer to the *Herbal Products* chapter for more information.

Cluster Headaches

As the name implies, patients with this headache syndrome experience a rapid-fire succession of several headache clusters in a specific time frame. Cluster headaches are also known as migrainous neuralgia, histamine cephalgia and Horton's syndrome. The prevalence of cluster headaches in adults is estimated to be 0.4% of the general population. It affects males 4 to 5 times more often than females. There is no strong correlation between a family history of cluster headaches and the likelihood of affliction. Most patients experience their first attack between 20 and 30 years of age.

The pain of cluster headaches is reported to be the most intense of all recurrent headaches. Characterized by single-sided intense boring pain, often described as a red hot probe penetrating the skull, it may spread, radiating from the eye, temple, or forehead to the neck, ear or jaw. The pain lasts for 30 to 40 minutes and recurs up to 6 times per 24-hour period. Often the pain is associated with the following symptoms on the same side of the face: tearing, nasal congestion, sweating, decreased pupil size and drooping eyelid.

There are no prodromal symptoms in cluster headaches. They recur daily (or nightly) or even several times per day and may continue for a period of 6 to 10 weeks, may reappear once or twice a year, once every few years or once in a lifetime. Frequently the patient will awake from sleep with a cluster headache. About 10% of these patients may experience chronic attacks and become at high risk of self-inflicted trauma or suicide. The pathophysiology of cluster headache is not well understood. Since there is a male predisposition, hormonal contribution has been suggested. There is little evidence to support histamine as playing a major role.

Treatment

Although analgesics are a reasonable choice for most pain syndromes, they are not very useful in cluster headaches because of the short duration of the attack. A better approach is the application of hot or cold compresses to the affected area in conjunction with 10 minutes of vigorous exercise, as physical activity appears to shorten the pain episode. A third alternative is for the patient to inhale 100% oxygen at a rate of 7 L/minute for 10 minutes. Prescription therapies include ergotamine, sumatriptan, short-course prednisone, intranasal lidocaine, lithium, methysergide, calcium channel blockers and steroids.

Medication-Induced Headaches

Medication-induced headache (MIH), is also known as rebound or analgesic withdrawal headache. Nearly daily ingestion of medication partially relieves the headache in the short term; in the long term it increases frequency and sometimes severity. Since self-medication is frequent (90% in one survey), health professionals are in an ideal position to recognize MIH by monitoring the analgesic consumption of headache patients.

Several characteristics of MIH can be described, but in general the presence of daily or almost daily headache despite regular and increasing use of medication should alert the health professional to the possibility of this condition. Early morning headache is a hallmark of MIH; others may be awakened by a rebound headache 3 or 4 hours after falling asleep. Associated symptoms may include difficulty falling asleep or maintaining sleep, restlessness, forgetfulness, irritability, memory lapse and fatigue. MIH seems to be restricted to patients with a primary headache disorder; patients with other conditions, such as arthritis, taking large doses of analgesics do not develop MIH.

All medications used for the immediate relief of headache pain have been implicated in the etiology of MIH. Recent surveys have shown that many patients use two or more preparations and since each can contain three or more ingredients, the patient may actually be taking six to eight different drugs on a daily basis. Dihydroergotamine (DHE) as well as prophylactic migraine therapies, such as amitriptyline or beta-blockers, have not been implicated in MIH.

Patients in whom MIH is suspected should be encouraged to see their physician for medical assessment. Since patients are sensitive about the amount of medication they are taking, raising the possibility of MIH must be done tactfully. It is best to focus on the drug's efficacy rather than implying that the patient is at fault.

The successful treatment of MIH includes both psychological and pharmacological interventions. This begins by withdrawing the offending medication under a doctor's care. Unless patients were taking barbiturates, narcotics and possibly ergotamine, treatment can be initiated in an outpatient setting. Withdrawal symptoms and their duration will vary depending on which medication was taken, but the most common symptom is increased headache intensity beginning 24 to 48 hours after abrupt discontinuation of the analgesic.

During the difficult period of severe headache pain, the patient can be treated with either sumatriptan or DHE. Clonidine or the phenothiazines may be helpful for patients unable to tolerate other withdrawal symptoms, such as tremor, nausea or insomnia. After the initial withdrawal period, which can last 2 to 3 months, many patients' symptoms improve. They should then be fully educated on all medications with continued reinforcement of the need to avoid excessive doses of analgesics. For some, prophylactic medications may be required.

Patients should also be taught nondrug therapies for pain management. These include avoiding any precipitating factors, such as ingestion of alcohol; reducing normal daily stress that provokes headaches by taking 20-minute relaxation periods; avoiding activities that can put extra pressure on head and neck muscles, such as poor posture; placing cold compression ice packs on the back of the neck (others prefer moist heat or a hot pack); taking hot showers or baths, or even wrapping a tight cloth or towel around the head. Some patients may benefit from biofeedback, yoga meditation, massage and stress management programs. Regular follow-ups with health care professionals may be helpful for those at risk for a recurrence of MIH.

ARTHRITIS

Arthritis refers to a variety of disorders that cause pain or inflammation in various joints. An estimated 3.5 million Canadians have some form of arthritis. Although the incidence increases with age, it afflicts all patient groups: approximately 75,000 children have arthritic-related problems.

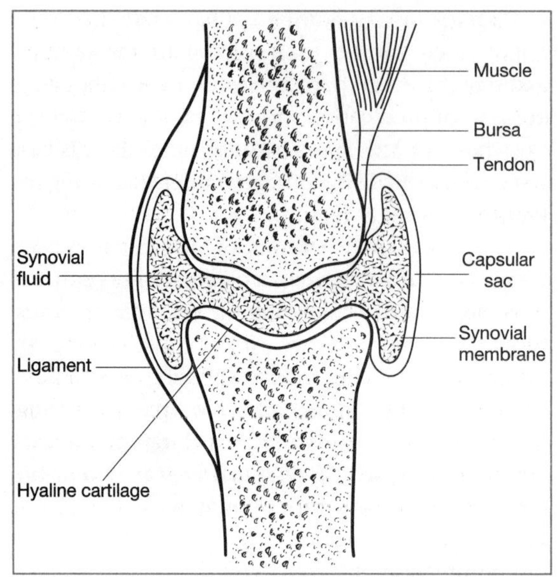

FIGURE 3: Knee Joint—Sagittal Section

Anatomy and Physiology

A joint is the junction of two bones held together by connective tissues; it provides flexibility and the ability to move. The human body contains three types of joints: fibrous, cartilaginous and synovial. The fibrous joints connect bony plates of the skull and allow little to no movement. Cartilaginous joints connect the spine and allow limited movement. Fibrocartilage connects each vertebrae along the full length of the spine and also helps to cushion joint components against body forces. The synovial joint, found in elbows, knees and hips (Figure 3), is more complex. The end of each joint is covered by hyaline cartilage to cushion the joint space from mechanical shock and friction. Bones are kept in position by fibrous connective tissue known as the capsular sac. This sac is lined with a thin layer of tissue called the synovial membrane, which secretes fluid. This fluid allows frictionless gliding and provides nutrition to the hyaline cartilage. Ligaments hold together the synovial joint and tendons attach bones to muscle. When muscles contract, the tendons pull the bones and create motion. Ligaments and tendons glide over articulating bone, the surfaces lubricated by sacs filled with synovial fluid called bursae.

Rheumatoid Arthritis (RA)

Rheumatoid arthritis is the most severe and painful form of arthritis, affecting 3% of the general population. It occurs in all age groups but peaks in the 4th to 5th decade. Although women are primarily affected by a ratio of 3:1, gender differences diminish in older age groups. Although the cause of rheumatoid arthritis is unknown, there appears to be a genetic predisposition. About 90% of patients possess a unique antibody known as the rheumatoid factor, which it is postulated, initiates an autoimmune reaction leading to destruction of tissue and bones.

The presentation of rheumatoid arthritis varies, but often starts as a generalized ache, fatigue, pain and joint stiffness, particularly in the morning or after periods of rest. Later, inflammation settles into specific joints, such as the knees or hands in a bilateral manner. These joints become tender, warm, swollen and painful with acute flare-ups. The painful joint limits motion and ultimately inhibits the patient's ability to function.

The pathophysiology of RA begins as synovitis. Pannus (the inflamed, proliferating synovial tissue characteristic of rheumatoid arthritis) spreads around the articular cartilage and grows over it; the excess synovial fluid produced causes swelling and pain in the joint. The pannus spreads from the synovial membrane, invades the joint and ultimately damages the underlying cartilage. (It contains lymphocytes, plasma cells and macrophages that produce factors that destroy bone protein and collagen.) The process continues with cartilage erosion, bone thinning and finally bone erosion. Eventually the ligaments, capsules and muscle of the joint become unstable and deformity appears first in the hands, knees, elbows, ankles, wrists and toes.

Treatment

The objectives of therapy are to reduce pain, maintain or improve joint function and quality of life, retard disease progression and minimize side effects. Nonpharmacological management includes physical and occupational therapy as well as patient and family education on the concepts of arthritis and its management. It is important that rheumatoid arthritic patients maintain a balance between resting and exercising joints. An early morning bath or shower can decrease morning stiffness. Active exercise should be performed twice daily for approximately 15 minutes and is most successful after heat application. Occupational therapists can help with the activities of daily living.

Nonsteroidal anti-inflammatory drugs remain the cornerstone of drug therapy for rheumatoid arthritis. Most patients with significant arthritis will be under the care of a physician. ASA is the initial treatment of choice in therapeutic dosages of 3.6 to 5.4 g/day. If there is no significant improvement or the patient cannot tolerate ASA because of adverse effects, other NSAIDs are used. In the elderly, shorter-acting drugs such as ibuprofen may be safer. If patients fail to respond to several trials of NSAIDs, disease modifying antirheumatic drugs (DMARDs) or systemic corticosteroids may be added.

Rheumatoid arthritis was previously managed using a pyramid approach. Therapy was initiated with the better tolerated drugs, such as NSAIDs; more toxic drugs were added when the disease progressed. This traditional approach has now been challenged. Evidence suggests that disease progression is rapid and that most erosion occurs within 2 years. If DMARDs do modify the disease, they should be started sooner. It has also been demonstrated that low doses of corticosteroids and several DMARDs are well tolerated while the NSAIDs have significant side effect profiles. For these reasons, low dose prednisone therapy (7.5 to 10 mg daily) and second line agents, starting with hydroxychloroquine, sulfasalazine, azathioprine and methotrexate followed by gold therapy, penicillamine and cyclophosphamide, may be initiated earlier in therapy. A short course of high dose pulse methylprednisolone (1,000 mg/d intravenously for 2 to 3 days) has proven effective for some severe cases of RA. Tenosynovectomy, tendon repair and joint replacement are surgical options for treatment of certain patients.

Although there have been suggestions that certain foods, through hypersensitivity reactions, may contribute to arthritis, the evidence is lacking. However, patients observing a strong relationship between a certain food and an exacerbation of arthritis should be advised to avoid the food. A lot has been said about the consumption of fish oil and its alleviation of arthritic symptoms. The omega-3 polyunsaturated acids found in cold water fish oil block the cyclo-oxygenase pathway and thus decrease the production of prostaglandins and leukotrienes. However, to achieve this pharmacological effect, 15 to 25 g of fish oil are required. At those doses, fish oil can prolong bleeding times and inhibit platelet function and should not be given concurrently with NSAIDs or ASA.

Osteoarthritis

Osteoarthritis is the most common arthritic condition, accounting for 30% of all musculoskeletal disorders. Almost everyone living long enough will have it to some degree. By age 50, more than 90% of individuals will have radiological evidence of this disorder although only one-third of affected joints will be symptomatic. A degenerative process that affects both sexes equally, it begins in the joint cartilage, causing pain and impaired joint motion. As the disease progresses, changes occur in the joint capsule, tendons, periarticular muscle and bone. Joint space narrows and proliferation of underlying bone leads to the formation of spurs that disturb normal joint alignment.

The primary symptom is stiffness and pain of varying intensity. Stiffness may last for 15 to 20 minutes, which is usually less than that experienced in rheumatoid arthritis and it is localized. The affected joints are those subjected to a lot of stress in vigorous or weight-bearing activities.

Treatment

The nonpharmacological and pharmacological management of osteoarthritis is similar to that of rheumatoid arthritis. In the early stages there is less evidence of inflammation; therefore, to avoid the adverse effects of NSAIDs, analgesics are usually employed. Acetaminophen 325 to 650 mg given 3 to 4 times daily, not to exceed 2.6 g/day, and administered regularly rather than as needed provides good relief. As the condition progresses and synovial inflammation becomes the source of pain, prescription therapy is warranted. Prescription agents include NSAIDs and intra-articular corticosteroid injections.

Gouty Arthritis

Gouty arthritis, simply referred to as gout, primarily targets men over the age of 40 and some postmenopausal women. This disorder has a tendency to be hereditary. Patients with gout have either impaired renal excretion of uric acid or overproduction of this metabolic product leading to hyperuricemia. When the blood is oversaturated, uric acid begins to crystallize and collect in the joints and kidneys. The first symptom of gout is usually a sudden attack of extreme pain and inflammation in one joint, most often the big toe. Early attacks, referred to as acute gouty arthritis, last a few days when properly treated. Chronic gouty arthritis, if left untreated, can result in permanent and severe damage to the joint or kidney.

Gout is first managed by resting the involved joint. Pain may be controlled with NSAIDs, such as ibuprofen 800 mg initially, then 400 mg every

6 hours with gradual tapering over 5 days. (Nonprescription strengths of ibuprofen are not effective.) Other NSAIDs are equally effective. Colchicine is also effective in relieving the pain of an acute attack at 0.6 mg every hour for 5 to 6 doses. However, since therapy must be initiated within 12 hours of onset and most cases do not present within this time, colchicine may have limited value. Also, at the necessary dose, nausea and diarrhea frequently occur. In more complicated cases, prednisone can be given at 20 to 40 mg/d for 3 days, then rapidly tapered. Probenecid, a uricosuric agent, or allopurinol should not be started in the acute gout phase because reduction of serum uric acid levels may be associated with prolongation of the attack.

Bursitis

Bursitis is inflammation of the bursae or closed sacs containing synovial fluid. Bursae are located in areas where tendons and muscles move over body prominences, such as the shoulder, elbow, hip, knee and foot.

The etiologies of bursitis include direct trauma to the bursa, chronic overuse or irritation as seen in tennis elbow or infection. Patients complain of localized pain with some radiation. Swelling and erythema may appear. Tenderness is commonly present.

Treatment

Rest is most important in the management of bursitis. If possible, the localized areas should be immobilized for 7 to 10 days and activities that aggravate the condition discontinued until symptoms have fully resolved. Ice compresses on the acutely inflamed area reduce swelling and provide relief from pain. Mild symptoms respond to ASA 650 mg orally, 4 times daily, while moderate symptoms require NSAID therapy such as ibuprofen 400 mg, 4 times daily. For severe symptoms, steroid injection (lidocaine/methylprednisolone) may be necessary. If, after appropriate management, or in the treatment of refractory cases, infection is suspected, the bursae may need to be aspirated, the aspirate cultured and antibiotic therapy instituted.

VISCERAL PAIN

Visceral pain originates in any large internal organ enclosed within the body cavity, especially the abdominal area. Nociceptors have been identified in all tissues and organs except the central nervous system. However, there are fewer nociceptors in the viscera than in the skin, and they may have a different activation profile. For example, cutting and burning mesentery, uterine cervix or other organs does not necessarily produce clinical pain, but traction, distention or ischemia will produce a type of pain. This pain is often diffuse and poorly localized and has a significant autonomic component. The visceral nociceptors have wide receptive fields, which prevents accurate localization of visceral sensation and may explain the phenomena of referred pain. This can complicate evaluation and diagnosis. For example, a patient cannot complain of pain in the pancreas itself, but of pain in the upper abdomen and back. Patients with any of several disease processes may present with similar pain complaints. Visceral pain, also known as deep pain, is particularly distressing because of its unrelenting and often progressive character. It is generally associated with a severe medical problem and should be referred to a physician.

DENTAL PAIN

Dental pain can occur for a variety of reasons. Tissue injury, such as formation of an abscess, surgical intervention, including teeth extraction, or simply a toothache are the most common. Patients with dental pain of unknown origin must be referred to a dentist as there are several medical conditions that may be responsible. These include sinus infection or inflammation, sickle cell anemia, lymphoma, angina, migraine and cluster headaches.

Treatment

Pain management in the dental patient is individualized to the quality of pain, its severity, cause and chronicity. Ibuprofen is a widely used analgesic for dental pain unless the patient has a platelet disorder or an active ulcer. Apart from its analgesic properties, ibuprofen reduces edema and fever, which may follow oral surgery. Acetaminophen is a good alternative when ibuprofen is contraindicated or not well tolerated. Since acetaminophen may not have clinically significant anti-inflammatory properties, its use in postoperative procedures is limited. ASA has now been largely replaced by ibuprofen unless cost is an issue.

Dental-related Pain

Besides the obvious odontological and periodontal diseases, there are common disorders that can be

associated with dental pain. Myofascial pain/dysfunction syndrome (MPD) is a psychophysiological disease where the muscles of mastication are in spasm. Common causes are chronic bruxism (grinding of teeth), muscular overextension (excessive opening of the bite) and muscular overcontraction (overclosure of the bite). Signs and symptoms of MPD are dull aching nonlocalized pain, joint tenderness, limited jaw motion and clicking sounds. Treatment includes a conscious effort to avoid clenching, a soft nonchewy diet, limitation of jaw movement, the use of moist heat and muscle massage. NSAIDs such as ibuprofen 400 to 600 mg, 3 to 4 times daily, may be useful as well as diazepam for its muscle relaxant effect.

Temporomandibular disorder (TMD), another common orofacial condition, is a dysfunction of the joint that connects the temporal to the mandible or lower jaw bones. It is marked by a clicking or grinding sensation in the joint, pain in or about the ears, tenderness and soreness of masticator muscle upon awakening. Pain is usually localized. The majority of affected patients have multifactorial problems, including psychological stress, joint disease, poor body mechanics and myofascial pain. Causes of TMD pain and dysfunction may be primarily of extra-articular origin, such as myofascial dystrophy, or intra-articular origins, such as arthritis or internal derangement of the joint. Treatment is similar to MPD with a soft diet and resting of the mandible. Local heat application can improve circulation. The already described analgesics are used for acute pain, and muscle relaxant drugs are used if muscle spasm is present. More severe cases may require injections of corticosteroids in the joint. Dental treatment includes insertion of a bite appliance that prevents the teeth from grinding.

ADVICE FOR THE PATIENT

External Analgesics

- The product is for external use only.
- Avoid contact with the eyes.
- Do not apply to wounds or damaged skin.
- Do not bandage tightly.
- Methyl salicylate products:
  - — avoid use when taking anticoagulants;
  - — avoid use if allergic to salicylates.
- All external analgesic products should be stored in a cool, dry, dark place. They must be stored out of reach of children, as ingestion may lead to severe toxicity.

For capsaicin, the following additional information should be provided:

- Application less than 3 times a day may not provide optimal pain relief and may cause the initial burning sensation to persist.
- With regular use, the transient burning sensation diminishes.
- Continued application for 3 to 4 weeks is necessary for optimal response.
- Discontinue use if condition worsens or does not improve after 28 days, and consult a physician.

MUSCULOSKELETAL PAIN

Musculoskeletal pain may result from chronic conditions, such as rheumatoid arthritis and osteoarthritis, or acute conditions, such as muscle soreness, strains, sprains and joint inflammation resulting from overexertion (e.g., on the job, housework, yardwork, etc.) and athletic activities. Typical musculoskeletal pain occurs with use of the affected muscle group or with weight bearing and is relieved by rest.

A **strain** is an injury to a muscle-tendon unit. Severity may be mild, with no loss of strength or motion, to severe with complete disruption of the muscle-tendon unit resulting in loss of function. A **sprain** refers to ligament injury. Since ligaments stabilize joints, joint instability may result. Severity ranges from mild (pain with no joint instability) to more severe with partial or complete disruption of the ligament. Acute injury to a joint through a direct hit or twisting motion can produce **traumatic arthritis** with swelling and joint effusion. **Fractures** and **dislocations** also cause musculoskeletal pain; obviously medical attention is required if either is suspected.

The acute management of strains, sprains, contusions and traumatic arthritis is generally with **RICE** therapy—**R**est, **I**ce, **C**ompression bandaging and **E**levation for at least 48 hours.

Other causes of skeletal pain include poor posture, prolonged, fixed or stressful conditions producing muscle strain, stiffness from cold, dampness, temperature changes and air currents.

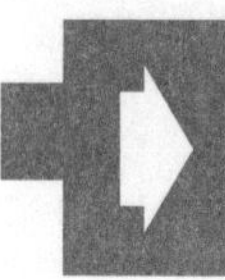

ADVICE FOR THE PATIENT

Pain

- If the pain lasts longer than 10 days in adults or 5 days in children, consult a physician.
- Acetaminophen, ASA or ibuprofen can be used short term to manage acute pain.
- ASA and ibuprofen are sometimes used under medical supervision long term for inflammation (e.g., in arthritis).
- For acute pain, effects will be noticed in 1 to 3 hours; however, when used for inflammation, full effects may not be seen for 3 to 4 weeks or longer.
- Application of heat or cold, bandaging, bracing or splinting is sometimes useful depending on the type of pain.
- Keep all medications out of the reach of children.
- If using this medication for headache, report daily or increasing numbers of headaches to your physician or pharmacist.

For acetaminophen

- Patients with a history of heavy drinking who continue to drink should consult their physician before using this product.

For ASA and ibuprofen

- Take this medication after meals, with food or antacids to reduce stomach upset unless you are using a product with a special coating (e.g., enteric coating).
- Take this medication with a full glass of water and avoid lying down for 15 to 30 minutes.
- Alcohol will increase the risk of stomach upset.
- Do not take if a vinegar smell is present (for ASA).
- Do not take this medication if you have peptic ulcers, bleeding ulcers, bleeding problems or are allergic to ASA or anti-inflammatory drugs.
- Consult a physician before taking this medication if you have congestive heart failure, liver disease, if you are pregnant, or if you are taking any of the following medications: warfarin, oral drugs for diabetes, steroids, drugs for gout, methotrexate, antihypertensives or furosemide.
- If you become pregnant while taking this medication, advise your physician as soon as possible.
- Do not administer to children with febrile illness.

For combination products containing codeine

- This medication may cause drowsiness, dizziness or lightheadedness. Do not drive or operate machinery that requires you to be alert until you know the effects of the medication.
- Do not take this medication on a regular basis unless advised by your physician.
- Codeine may be habit forming.
- This medication can cause constipation, especially during regular use. Add more fibre to your diet. Laxatives may be necessary. Check with your pharmacist or physician.
- This medication can cause dry mouth. Temporary relief can be obtained by using sugarless gum or candy or sucking on ice chips.

Treatment

The immediate pain following trauma is nociceptive pain, while delayed pain results from swelling, pressure and tissue damage with subsequent release of substances, such as prostaglandins and kinins. ASA and other oral NSAIDs or acetaminophen are regarded as the treatment of choice for most pain. However, in musculoskeletal pain, topical analgesics, which avoid the unwanted systemic side effects of internal analgesics, may provide the desired pain relief. Most medical references and sports medicine literature fail to mention topical analgesics altogether, perhaps because their efficacy is poor. If used, they are generally recommended after the 48-hour period of RICE therapy. It should be noted, however, that once tissues have been damaged, the natural process of repair must occur. There is little evidence currently that any method of treatment significantly reduces the time needed for this repair.

External analgesics are also purchased by consumers for chronic symptoms associated with osteoarthritis, rheumatoid arthritis, chronic tendinitis, bursitis or other chronic pain syndromes, such as postherpetic neuralgia. Consumers should again be reminded that topical analgesics do not alter the underlying disease process, but local treatment for short periods may provide temporary reduction or relief of pain.

OTHER CONDITIONS

There are numerous other causes of pain beyond the scope of discussion here. One chronic pain condition, postherpetic neuralgia, follows an acute reactivation of herpes zoster (shingles), particularly in immunocompromised or older individuals. Burning pain, aching or severe pruritus occurs in the dermatome(s) involved in acute infection. Response to systemic analgesics, tricyclic antidepressants and anticonvulsants is often disappointing; however, topical capsaicin may provide relief in some individuals.

PATIENT ASSESSMENT QUESTIONS

?

Pain

Q Do you have any other medical conditions?
It is important to identify medical conditions that could be causing or exacerbating the pain and that could be exacerbated by oral analgesic/antipyretic agents, e.g., ASA and peptic ulcer disease.

Q Are you taking any prescription or nonprescription medications?
Internal analgesic/antipyretics may interact with drugs in the patient's current medication regimen.

Q Are you allergic to any medications?
The answer to this question will guide the health professional's recommendations regarding choice of a product.

Q Can you describe in detail the pain you are experiencing? Are there any factors that precipitate the pain? Are there factors that alleviate the pain? Have you had this pain before?
The location, intensity and factors altering the pain all help the health professional determine the source of the pain. If the patient cannot localize the pain, it may be visceral in origin, and the patient should be directed to seek medical attention. A description of headache pain may help the health professional to classify it as a specific type (tension, migraine or cluster). An acute pain that the patient has never experienced before could indicate a significant medical problem.

Q What is the age of the patient?
ASA should generally be avoided in children, especially for the treatment of febrile illnesses presumed to be viral. Doses of analgesic/antipyretic agents are based on a child's age or weight. The elderly may be more predisposed to specific adverse effects.

Q How long has the pain been present?
Pain lasting longer than 10 days in adults and 5 days in children should be evaluated by a physician.

Q What has worked for the pain in the past?
This will help the health professional determine which agent to recommend.

PATIENT ASSESSMENT QUESTIONS *(cont'd)*

External Analgesics

Q What is the nature and location of the pain?
It is necessary to identify individuals who need referral to their physician. To self-treat, consumers should be able to specify the location of pain in a muscle, joint or bone. Pain that radiates to other areas should not be treated with external analgesics.

Q How long have you had the pain?
External analgesic products are used for short-term, self-limiting conditions, such as sprains or strains, or as temporary adjunctive treatment of chronic conditions, such as rheumatoid arthritis. If the pain has persisted for longer than 1 week, the consumer should be referred to a physician. Capsaicin, however, must be used for a minimum of 3 to 4 weeks for optimal pain relief.

Q Is the occurrence of pain associated with a particular event such as strenuous exercise, recent injury or particular work?
This information is used to assess the need for referral to a physician. If the condition is associated with broken or irritated skin, external analgesics should not be recommended. External analgesics may be recommended for muscle aches and pains associated with strenuous exercise or work.

Q Is the pain associated with a joint? Is the joint red, swollen or hot to touch? Is the pain worse in the morning, but lessens as the day progresses?
Rheumatoid and other types of arthritis should be diagnosed by a physician. Redness and swelling of a joint may be associated with many conditions, including septic arthritis, gout and rheumatoid arthritis. The characteristic pattern of improvement as the day progresses is suggestive of rheumatoid arthritis; worsening of pain and swelling might occur with an untreated infection. If infection of the joint or gout is a possibility, the person should be referred to a physician. If the individual has been diagnosed as having an arthritic condition, adjuvant therapy with external analgesics can be recommended for temporary relief of pain.

Q Do you have signs and symptoms of a flu-like illness?
Viral infections may be associated with muscle aches and pains as well as fever. Systemic analgesic/antipyretic products may be more appropriate than external analgesics in this situation.

Q What is the age of the individual?
Children may absorb topical products to a much greater extent than adults. External analgesics are not recommended for children less than 2 years of age.

Q Do you have any allergies?
Look specifically for ASA hypersensitivity. Systemic absorption of salicylates does occur, and agents containing methyl salicylate and triethanolamine salicylate should not be recommended to people with salicylate allergies.

Q Have you treated this condition before? What was tried and did it work?
The answers to these questions help the health professional choose products to recommend or to reinforce the appropriate use of specific products. The need to refer the person to a physician also may be ascertained.

FEVER

Almost all children have a fever at some time; adults also have fevers with certain disease processes. Fever is generally considered to be caused by infection; however, noninfectious causes include inflammatory diseases, neoplasms and immunologically mediated conditions, such as some drug fevers.

While the definition of fever varies, anything above the normal range for body temperature can be defined as fever. An individual's body temperature varies with the time of day (normal circadian variation): lowest at approximately 6 a.m. (anything above 37.2°C [98.9°F] orally would be a fever) and highest between 4 and 6 p.m. (37.7°C [99.9°F] orally is the upper limit of normal in adults). The mean amplitude of variability is 0.5°C (0.9°F). Outside the neonatal period, children generally have a higher temperature than adults; however, this is poorly documented. Basal core temperatures decrease toward the adult range by 1 year of age and continue to decrease until puberty. One study has suggested that the definition of fever in young children should be: >38.0°C rectally in infants less than 30 days of age, >38.1°C in 1-month-old infants and >38.2°C in 2-month-old infants.

Mild elevations in body temperature occur with exercise, ovulation, pregnancy, excessive clothing (overbundling of infants) and ingestion of hot foods or liquids.

Rectal temperatures are approximately 0.5°C higher and axillary temperatures approximately 0.5°C lower than oral temperatures. A high fever is usually defined as a temperature greater than 40.5°C (105°F). Neurological damage does not occur below a body temperature of 41.7°C (107°F).

PATHOPHYSIOLOGY

The thermoregulatory centre in the anterior hypothalamus normally controls core temperature within a narrow range by balancing heat production by tissues with heat dissipation. With fever, the thermoregulatory set point is elevated. Endothelial cells of the organum vasculosum laminae terminalis, located in the hypothalamus, release arachidonic acid metabolites when exposed to pyrogens in the circulation. Prostaglandin E_2, released by the hypothalamus, is thought to be the major substance producing an elevation of the thermoregulatory set point. With an elevated set point, there is vasoconstriction of peripheral blood vessels to conserve heat, shivering to increase heat production and behavioral changes such as seeking warmer environments and clothing. When the set point is reduced, e.g., by administering antipyretics or disappearance of pyrogens, there is vasodilation and sweating as well as behavioral changes such as removal of clothing.

There are both exogenous and endogenous sources of pyrogens—substances that cause fever. The most common exogenous sources are microorganisms, their products or toxins (e.g., lipopolysaccharide endotoxin of gram negative bacteria). Exogenous pyrogens induce formation and release of endogenous pyrogens. Endogenous pyrogens or pyrogenic cytokines are polypeptides produced by host cell macrophages, monocytes and other cells. The most common are interleukin 1β, interleukin 1α and tumor necrosis factor.

DIFFERENTIAL DIAGNOSIS

Fever should be differentiated from hyperthermia, which is an increase in core temperature without an increase in hypothalamic set point: body temperature is elevated above the set point as a result of insufficient heat dissipation. Hyperthermia occurs with exercise, in hot environments and with the use of drugs that inhibit perspiration. If hyperthermia is suspected, the patient should be referred to a physician; antipyretics are not useful.

MEASUREMENT OF BODY TEMPERATURE

There are five ways to measure temperature—oral, rectal, axillary, tympanic membrane and transcutaneous routes. Oral, rectal and axillary temperatures may be taken with a standard mercury in glass thermometer or an electronic thermometer with digital display.

Electronic thermometers are safer and easier to use because they are faster and easier to read. Generally, they require 30 seconds to 1 minute while adequate equilibration times up to 10 minutes are required for standard glass thermometers. Their major disadvantage is that they are significantly more expensive.

Fever

Problems associated with the use of standard thermometers are:

- insufficient time is allowed for equilibration when taking the temperature (3 to 4 minutes orally, 2 to 3 minutes rectally, and 4 to 10 minutes axillary);
- they are improperly read;
- the user fails to reset the thermometer;
- or it is incorrectly placed in the mouth.

The rectal route is preferred for newborns, in children less than 5 years old when an axillary temperature is not sufficient, and when the oral route is not suitable due to mouth breathing. It is contraindicated in premature infants, the immunocompromised and in the presence of rectal anomalies, recent anorectal surgery or severe hemorrhoids. A rare complication is perforation of the rectum.

In children, the thermometer and anus should be lubricated with petroleum jelly, the thermometer gently inserted into the rectum 2 to 3 cm with one hand, the buttocks closed against the thermometer with the other hand. This is best done by laying the infant or younger child across the parent's lap. The thermometer should be left in place for 2 to 3 minutes (standard thermometer). It is important to be gentle and reassuring when taking a rectal temperature because it can be very frightening and uncomfortable for children.

The oral route can be used in children over 5 years old and in adults. Younger children may bite the thermometer or have difficulty keeping it in the closed mouth for the required 3 to 4 minutes (standard thermometer). This may also be a problem for individuals who have difficulty understanding instructions, e.g., the mentally impaired or demented elderly. When nasal breathing is difficult due to viral upper respiratory tract infection, mouth breathing will cause spuriously low temperatures. Beverages, either hot or cold, and smoking should be avoided for at least 10 minutes prior to taking an oral temperature. The thermometer should be placed under the tongue or on either side of the mouth, held in place with the lips or fingers (not the teeth), the mouth closed.

Axillary temperatures have disadvantages. They take a long time to measure and are affected by a number of factors including hypotension, cutaneous vasodilation and prior cooling of the patient. Although most textbooks state that axillary temperatures are approximately 0.5°C lower than oral temperatures, good data are not available to correlate axillary with oral or rectal temperatures. The obvious advantages of axillary temperatures are that this route is very accessible, safe and much less frightening to children than rectal temperatures. The thermometer should be placed in the apex of the axilla, and the elbow held against the chest to stabilize the thermometer for 4 to 10 minutes (standard thermometer).

Tympanic membrane thermometers (TMT) measure infrared emissions from the tympanic membrane. Because the tympanic membrane and the hypothalamus share the same blood supply, these thermometers are considered to reflect core temperature measurements. The temperature is then converted by the thermometer to reflect oral or rectal temperatures, which may lead to some inaccuracy in the temperature reading. The aiming of the ear probe and proper placement in the ear canal are important for accurate measurements. Improper placement can result in a lower temperature reading from a lower outer ear canal wall temperature. The advantages of TMT include simplicity, speed and patient acceptance. Less than 2 seconds is needed to obtain a reading. Other advantages include lack of external influences such as hot beverage ingestion and no mucous membrane contact, therefore, minimal risk of disease transmission. Acute otitis media and nonobstructive cerumen do not appear to affect the accuracy of TMT. The prohibitive cost of TMT makes it impractical for most consumers.

The transcutaneous route uses a plastic strip that is placed on the forehead for 1 minute and indicates body temperature by changing color. The strip contains encapsulated thermophototropic esters of cholesterol (called liquid crystals) that change color in response to temperature changes. They are easier to read and require less time than a standard thermometer, but are less reliable because skin temperature is not a reliable indicator of core temperature. The strip incorporates a correction factor for this but assumes the factor is the same in all individuals. When studied in emergency departments, they were poor predictors of fever. Their accuracy is affected by ambient temperature (e.g., cold hands holding the strip and nearby heat sources such as a lamp). Because they can register afebrile temperatures in a truly febrile child, possibly delaying medical attention, their use is not recommended.

FEVER IN SPECIFIC PATIENT GROUPS

Children: Young children have an immature central nervous system thermoregulatory system, and in the first 2 months of life may have minimal or no fever during an infectious illness. Since neonates and infants are less able to mount a febrile response, when they do get febrile, it is more likely to indicate a major illness. After 3 months of age, the degree of fever more closely approximates that seen in older children.

Fever in children is usually due to bacterial or viral infection and, because children have had less previous exposure than adults to infectious agents, they are more susceptible upon initial contact, so fever is common. Reactions to vaccinations may also be a cause. Compared to adults, children are more sensitive to ambient temperature (due to a greater body surface area for heat exchange) and at higher risk for dehydration.

The biggest concern in children is febrile seizures, which occur in 2 to 5% of children 3 months to 5 years of age. Febrile seizures rarely result in neurological damage or a permanent seizure disorder; however, they concern and frighten parents. Many references state that the rate of temperature rise may be more important than the actual temperature reached, but there is no scientific evidence to support this theory. On the other hand, the height of the temperature is important. Febrile seizures are more common with temperatures over 40°C. A susceptible child, however, may have a seizure with only a moderate rise in temperature.

Antipyretics are universally recommended to prevent recurrences of febrile seizures, but studies have shown they may not be effective. Febrile seizures often occur at the onset of a febrile illness and may be the first sign of infection, making prevention with antipyretics difficult.

Health professionals often encounter febrile children who are teething. Although the literature is inconclusive or difficult to interpret, fever should not be attributed to eruption of teeth; other causes should be considered. However, a common treatment of teething pain is acetaminophen, which will treat a fever, if present, while managing the pain. Unfortunately, this may mask and delay treatment of potentially serious infections.

"Fever phobia" is common in parents of young children, who have many misconceptions about fever. They believe it can cause brain damage or that body temperature will continue to rise if treatment is withheld. These beliefs result in many unnecessary calls and visits to physicians. There are also studies suggesting that physician misconceptions about fever and aggressive management of children with fever (often only to console parents) may contribute to this phobia. Health professionals may not be providing parents with enough information about febrile illnesses. As a result, antipyretics are commonly used in children, perhaps when therapy is not warranted.

Older Individuals: In older individuals, axillary and oral temperatures are lower, but rectal temperatures are the same. Fever may be absent or blunted in older individuals with infection and so should not be relied on as an indicator of infection. The increase in oxygen consumption produced by fever may aggravate comorbid disease states in patients with congestive heart failure, coronary, pulmonary or cerebral insufficiency. Cognitive function may deteriorate and delirium may occur. Since older individuals appear to be more predisposed to gastritis and gastrointestinal ulceration from ASA and NSAIDs, acetaminophen is a safer alternative.

Pregnancy: Studies in humans suggest that exposure to fever and other heat sources during the first trimester of pregnancy is associated with increased risk of neural tube defects.

Acetaminophen crosses the placenta and is relatively safe for short-term use in pregnancy when therapeutic doses are used. ASA and NSAIDs can result in a number of problems. Since they inhibit prostaglandin synthesis, they may interfere with labor and cause premature closure of the ductus arteriosus. This can result in persistent pulmonary hypertension in the infant. Platelet aggregation is inhibited in the newborn if ASA is ingested by the mother within 7 days of delivery and salicylates displace bilirubin from protein binding sites. Increased bleeding has been reported in both mothers and infants if ASA is ingested close to the time of delivery.

Table 1 indicates individuals who may require treatment of fever.

MANAGEMENT OF FEVER

Mammals raise their body temperature in response to invasion by microorganisms, and studies suggest that fever enhances the ability to survive serious bacterial infections. At higher temperatures, the

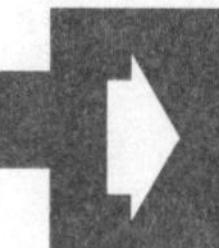

ADVICE FOR THE PATIENT

Fever

- Treat the child, not the fever. Fever itself is rarely dangerous.
- Use acetaminophen, not ASA, for fever in children.
- Medication can be given every 4 hours, if needed, but not more than 5 times a day.
- Do not wake a sleeping child to administer drugs for fever unless the child has had previous febrile seizures.
- Do not give fever medication for more than 3 days without consulting a doctor.
- Encourage fluids and remove excess clothing and bedding.
- Contact the doctor for: fever over 40.5°C, febrile children less than 2 months old, or if the child appears very ill, has a stiff neck, has a seizure, is confused or delirious or is crying inconsolably.
- Keep antipyretics and all other medication out of reach of children.

growth and virulence of some microorganisms is impaired. Therefore an argument can be made not to treat a fever. Other beneficial effects of fever include a greater phagocytic and bactericidal activity of neutrophils, increased antibody production and increased cytotoxic effects of lymphocytes. The use of antipyretics may impair the use of temperature as an important clinical tool for monitoring the progress of an infection or response to antibiotics. The most common consequences of fever are generally harmless: mild dehydration, febrile delirium, febrile seizures and discomfort.

Nonpharmacological Treatment

Sponging increases evaporation to promote heat loss. Tepid water sponging may be useful to reduce body temperature; however, it does not reset the hypothalamic set point; therefore, the body actually works harder to maintain the elevated temperature. If done, antipyretics should be administered 30 minutes beforehand to reduce the hypothalamic set point. Two studies did not show additional benefit from sponging after antipyretic administration, but it is a frequently recommended procedure in children with higher temperatures. The individual may feel quite uncomfortable, especially if cooler water is used. Shivering should not be induced when sponging because this will increase heat production. Many children find the procedure uncomfortable, and it is time consuming.

Tepid sponging should be done with water only. Isopropyl alcohol has resulted (rarely) in hypoglycemia, intoxication and coma from absorption through the skin or inhalation of fumes and should no longer be recommended. Sponging should be started approximately 30 minutes after administration of an antipyretic in children with a temperature >40°C. If the temperature is >41°C, the child has a seizure, or delirium is present, sponging can be started immediately after antipyretic administration. The child should be sitting in about 5 cm (2 inches) of water and the skin surface continuously bathed. Immersion in water is much less efficient. The water temperature should be lukewarm (29 to 32°C), but increased if shivering occurs. Generally sponging should be carried out for at least 20 minutes. The child's temperature will not usually fall below 38.3°C.

Particularly in infants, excess clothing and bedding should be removed to allow heat dissipation. It is important that fluid intake be increased to replace the increased insensible water loss in fever; dehydration can increase core temperature and reduce cutaneous blood flow. The ambient temperature should be maintained around 20 to 21°C to ensure efficient heat dissipation. Physical exertion should be avoided and physical activity reduced.

It should be stressed that treatment of fever should depend on the individual and their symptoms, and not solely the elevation of the temperature. Table 1 lists individuals who should be directed to seek medical attention.

Pharmacological Treatment

Acetaminophen, ASA and ibuprofen are currently recommended to reduce fever, but ibuprofen does not carry this indication for children under 12 years of age. These agents reduce body temperature in febrile patients by reducing the hypothalamic set point to normal. They do not lower normal body temperature. Antipyretics will suppress the constitutional symptoms of fever; in children this may reduce irritability and poor feeding. Intermittent administration of antipyretics may exaggerate swings in temperature, which may make the individual feel worse.

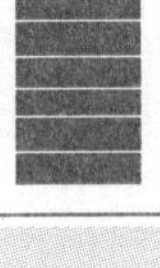

TABLE 1: Management of Fever

Referral to Physician	Individuals Requiring Treatment
Patients who recently received chemotherapy	Children with febrile seizures
Children less than 2 months of age	Pregnant women
Fever >40.5°C	Impaired cardiac, pulmonary or cerebral function
Fever associated with stiff neck or seizures	Temperature >41°C
Patient difficult to arouse, confused or delirious	
Child who appears very ill or with inconsolable crying	
Individuals with serious underlying disease	
Fever that persists >24 hours without obvious cause	
Fever that persists >72 hours	

There is no evidence that antipyretics are useful in low grade fever, only individuals listed in Table 1 require treatment. Acetaminophen is a safe and effective antipyretic with few contraindications, which can be used in any age group. ASA should be avoided in children less than 18 years old with a viral illness because of its association with Reye's syndrome in influenza and varicella. Since the cause of fever is unknown initially in many circumstances, generally ASA should be avoided in children. Ibuprofen, although effective, is considered a second-line agent. There is less experience with it than with acetaminophen or ASA; it can cause more adverse effects than acetaminophen, is more expensive, but less toxic in overdose. Based on their mechanism of action, antipyretics are not useful in hyperthermia.

In specific cases, fever may warrant treatment. Fever results in increased oxygen consumption and increased caloric and fluid requirements, which may be detrimental in pregnancy, in children or patients with cardiovascular or pulmonary conditions. Fever can produce discomfort, back pain, myalgias, arthralgias, anorexia, somnolence, chills, rigors and sweats. In children, febrile seizures are very frightening, especially to parents. Antipyretics are often recommended for those with previous febrile seizures.

When counselling on the management of fever, information should be provided on the appropriate dose of antipyretics for the age or weight of the child, instructions on how to take a temperature and instructions on sponging, if it has been recommended.

PATIENT ASSESSMENT QUESTIONS

?

Q ***Are you taking any prescription or nonprescription medications?***
Internal analgesic/antipyretics may interact with drugs in the patient's current medication regimen.

Q ***Are you allergic to any medications?***
The answer to this question will guide the health professional's recommendations regarding choice of a product.

Q ***Are there any symptoms accompanying the fever?***
Symptoms such as a stiff neck, a purulent wound or a specific rash can help the health professional determine whether a serious bacterial infection is present that requires medical attention.

Q ***How long has the fever been present?***
Fever lasting longer than 3 days without an apparent cause requires medical evaluation.

Q ***What is the age of the patient?***
ASA generally should be avoided in children, especially for the treatment of febrile illnesses presumed to be viral. Doses of analgesic/antipyretic agents are based on a child's age or weight. Older individuals may be more predisposed to specific adverse effects.

PHARMACEUTICAL AGENTS

INTERNAL ANALGESICS

Acetaminophen

Pharmacology and Pharmacokinetics: Acetaminophen works centrally in fever to restore the hypothalamic set point to normal, resulting in peripheral vasodilation. This is most likely from inhibition of prostaglandin synthesis in the preoptic anterior hypothalamic region. Its analgesic activity is poorly understood. Inhibition of prostaglandins in the central nervous system may result in analgesic effects. Acetaminophen may also have peripheral activity by blocking pain impulse generation or by inhibiting the synthesis or action of other substances responsible for sensitizing pain receptors.

At doses less than 1 g, acetaminophen does not have anti-inflammatory activity like ASA or NSAIDs. This may be partially explained by the observation that acetaminophen can block cyclo-oxygenase only in an environment low in peroxide such as the hypothalamus. Sites of inflammation, like the joints, generally have high concentrations of peroxides generated by leukocytes.

Oral absorption of acetaminophen is rapid and almost complete but may be reduced by a high carbohydrate meal. Absorption from suppositories is variable, both in rate and extent. Peak plasma concentrations occur in 30 to 60 minutes; the duration of effect is 3 to 4 hours, requiring frequent dosing for sustained effects. The elimination half-life is reported to be 1 to 4 hours (mean 2 h). This may be prolonged in neonates, older individuals, individuals with hepatic disease and with overdose. Acetaminophen is metabolized in the liver by conjugation with glucuronic acid (60%), sulfuric acid (35%) and cysteine (3%). Children have less capacity for glucuronidation. A small amount is metabolized to N-acetyl-p-benzoquinonimine, which is a highly reactive intermediate that normally reacts with sulfhydryl groups in glutathione. In overdose, when hepatic glutathione is depleted, this metabolite reacts with sulfhydryl groups in hepatic proteins resulting in hepatic necrosis. Renal tubular necrosis and hypoglycemia may also occur.

Acetaminophen is detected in breast milk of nursing mothers but has not been reported to cause adverse effects in infants.

Use, Effectiveness and Safety: Acetaminophen is useful for mild to moderate pain in conditions such as headache, myalgia, arthralgia, postpartum pain, postoperative pain and some malignancies, fever and the pain of osteoarthritis; it does not have anti-inflammatory activity at doses less than 1 g. Acetaminophen can be used in many situations when ASA should not or cannot be used, e.g., in hemophiliacs or individuals with thrombocytopenia, upper gastrointestinal disease, or on anticoagulants or uricosurics, or when there is intolerance or hypersensitivity to ASA.

It is the preferred antipyretic agent in pediatrics because of its relative freedom from adverse effects at therapeutic doses and ASA's association with Reye's syndrome. It is also available in liquid dosage forms, unlike ASA. On a mg per mg basis its efficacy as an analgesic and antipyretic are equivalent to ASA. Acetaminophen is available in a broad range of dosage forms including tablets, capsules, caplets, elixir, suspension, chewable tablets and suppositories.

Acetaminophen is a safe medication, except in overdose where hepatotoxicity is the major concern. In adults, single doses of 10 to 15 g can cause hepatotoxicity and 20 to 25 g are potentially fatal. Plasma acetaminophen concentrations 4 hours or longer after an overdose are valuable for predicting risk of hepatotoxicity in acute ingestions. It is important to ensure patients seek treatment following any suspected overdose, even if they are asymptomatic, because symptoms may be delayed for 24 hours or more. N-acetylcysteine is the antidote administered to prevent hepatotoxicity. A poison control centre should be consulted for information on management of acetaminophen overdose.

Precautions and Contraindications: Acetaminophen should be avoided in alcoholics because of increased risk of liver toxicity. Alcohol should be avoided in individuals taking high doses (>4 g/day) or those using acetaminophen for long periods of time (7 days or longer). Fasting may enhance hepatotoxicity at doses above those recommended (>4 g/day). Analgesic nephropathy has been reported with the use of large doses of analgesics for prolonged periods of time, primarily in individuals who use combinations of analgesics including acetaminophen.

Side Effects: See Table 2.

Dosage: For general dosing information see Tables 3 and 4.

TABLE 2: Internal Analgesic Side Effects

Agent	Immediate Medical Referral	Medical Referral	Medical Referral Not Required
Acetaminophen	*Uncommon* Allergic reactions, thrombocytopenia, neutropenia, pancytopenia	*Uncommon* Skin rash	
ASA	*Common* Signs and symptoms of overdose, GI hemorrhage (hematemesis, coffee ground emesis, bloody or black stools), hypersensitivity reactions *Uncommon* Hepatotoxicity, leukopenia, thrombocytopenia, agranulocytosis	*Common* Tinnitus or hearing loss (chronic ingestion), abdominal pain (GI ulceration), sodium and water retention, anemia, analgesic nephropathy, skin rash, regular daily use for headaches	*Common* Dyspepsia, heartburn, mild to moderate abdominal discomfort, nausea, vomiting, rectal irritation (suppositories)
Codeine	*Common* Respiratory depression *Uncommon* Anaphylaxis, histamine release (increased heart rate, decreased blood pressure, wheezing, face flushing), paralytic ileus, convulsion	*Common* CNS stimulation, allergic reaction, skin rash, confusion, constipation, changes in heart rate, antidiuretic effect, urinary retention *Uncommon* Depression	*Common* Drowsiness, blurred vision, dizziness, dry mouth, headache, nausea, vomiting, loss of appetite, nervousness *Uncommon* Biliary spasm, stomach cramps
Ibuprofen	*Common* Decreased renal function (glomerular filtration rate) *Uncommon* Gastric perforation/bleeding, anaphylaxis, renal toxicity, hemolytic anemia, thrombocytopenia, aplastic anemia, agranulocytosis	*Common* Epigastric pain, diarrhea, skin rash, fluid retention, anemia *Uncommon* GI ulcers, congestive heart failure, palpitations, hypertension, bleeding or crusty lips, bloody or cloudy urine, problems in urination, blurred vision or other ocular disturbance, hepatotoxicity	*Common* Mild to moderate abdominal discomfort or stomach cramps, decreased appetite, dizziness, drowsiness, headache, heartburn, indigestion, nausea *Uncommon* Bloating, appetite changes, sensitivity to sunlight

TABLE 3: Pediatric Dosing of Acetaminophen

Age	Weight	Dose
0–4 mo	2.5–5 kg	40 mg
4–12 mo	5–7.9 kg	80 mg
12–24 mo	8–10.5 kg	120 mg
2–3 yr	—	160 mg
4–5 yr	—	240 mg
6–8 yr	—	320 mg
9–10 yr	—	400 mg
11–12 yr	—	480 mg
over 12 yr	—	640 mg

ASA

Pharmacology and Pharmacokinetics: ASA is an antipyretic, anti-inflammatory and analgesic drug. It works by inhibiting prostaglandin synthesis through irreversible acetylation and inhibition of the enzyme cyclo-oxygenase, which catalyzes the conversion of arachidonic acid to prostaglandins and thromboxanes. In the central nervous system a decrease in brain concentrations of prostaglandin E_2 reduces the hypothalamic set point to reduce fever. In the periphery, prostaglandins are important mediators of inflammation hence the anti-inflammatory effect. Prostaglandins may act as pain mediators. ASA may also block pain impulse generation in the periphery through a central action in the hypothalamus.

ASA is generally rapidly absorbed; however, the rate is dependent on the dissolution characteristics of the dosage form. It is found in the plasma within 5 to 30 minutes and peaks within 1 hour. Fever reduction occurs within 1 hour and is maximal at 1 to 3 hours. Analgesia follows a similar time course; however, full anti-inflammatory effects with ASA may not occur for 3 to 4 weeks or more. Food will delay absorption but will not reduce the extent of absorption. Absorption from enteric coated preparations is delayed with the peak occurring at 6 to 8 hrs. Rectal absorption is slower, incomplete and unreliable, and doses are generally 25 to 50% higher.

ASA is hydrolyzed to salicylate in the gastrointestinal tract, liver and blood, and is considered the active moiety (although ASA has other activity as well, e.g., as an antiplatelet agent). At therapeutic doses it is 80 to 90% plasma protein bound. Salicylate is metabolized and excreted in the urine as salicyluric acid (75%), salicyl phenolic glucuronide (10%), salicyl acyl glucuronide (5%) and other minor metabolites. Excretion of free salicylate is variable depending on both the dose and urinary pH. Excretion is increased in alkaline urine.

The metabolic pathways to produce salicyluric acid and the phenolic glucuronide are saturable resulting in a longer half-life with higher or repeated doses. The half-life of ASA is 15 to 20 minutes. At low doses the half-life of salicylate is 2 to 3 hrs, 5 to 18 hrs at higher doses (such as anti-inflammatory doses of 3.6 to 5.4 g/d), and may be 20 hrs or longer with very high or toxic doses (>7 g/d). Elimination of ASA is reduced in dehydration or with reduced urinary output. This is of concern in an ill child where accumulation may lead to toxicity.

Salicylate clearance is reduced in newborns. The drug is present in the breast milk of nursing mothers.

Use, Effectiveness and Safety: ASA is useful for mild to moderate pain, fever and for inflammatory conditions such as rheumatoid arthritis. Headache, myalgia, arthralgia and neuralgia respond to ASA better than visceral pain. Moderate postoperative, postpartum, traumatic or dental pain may also respond. The drug can be used in dysmenorrhea; however, other NSAIDs may be more effective. It is also a useful adjunct in some cancer pain. In postoperative pain, 600 mg of ASA is equivalent to 60 mg of codeine or 50 mg of pentazocine. It is equivalent on a mg per mg basis to acetaminophen for antipyresis and analgesia.

As mentioned previously, it should not be used in pediatric patients to treat fever unless a viral cause, such as influenza or chickenpox, has been ruled out. In children receiving long-term ASA for treatment of inflammatory conditions, its use should be discontinued at the onset of a febrile illness until the cause of fever is determined. ASA is not available in a liquid dosage form making use in children less convenient.

ASA is available as regular tablets, chewable tablets, dispersible tablets, extended release tablets and enteric coated tablets and capsules. The enteric coated tablets are generally not considered useful for acute pain or fever management because of delayed absorption. This form, however, does produce less gastric irritation and is recommended in arthritic conditions requiring chronic therapy

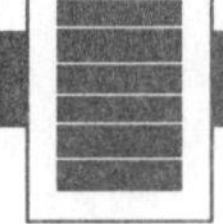

(e.g., rheumatoid arthritis and osteoarthritis). Combination products containing an alkali or buffer may be better tolerated (this has been disputed in some studies); however, if alkalinization of the urine occurs, the half-life may be reduced. ASA is also available as a rectal suppository and as chewing gum. Absorption from suppositories is slow, variable and depends on retention in the rectum.

Both acute ingestion and chronic administration can cause toxicity. Death can result in adults ingesting 10 to 30 g. Effects of overdose include acid-base disturbances (metabolic acidosis and respiratory alkalosis), hyperpyrexia, hyperventilation and respiratory failure, hyper- or hyponatremia, hypokalemia, hypo- or hyperglycemia, dehydration, nausea, vomiting, tinnitus, lethargy, disorientation, hallucinations, irritability, seizures and coma. A poison control centre should be consulted for management of overdose. Plasma concentrations of salicylate can be useful in predicting toxicity in acute ingestions.

Analgesic nephropathy has been associated with chronic use of analgesic mixtures containing ASA, although ASA alone may not be a risk factor.

Precautions, Contraindications and Drug Interactions: ASA's effects on prostaglandin production result in a number of precautions and contraindications to therapy. Ulceration and gastrointestinal (GI) hemorrhage result from direct toxic effects on GI mucosa as well as inhibition of synthesis of gastric prostaglandins I_2 and E_2 that provide a protective effect. Individuals with peptic ulcer disease or gastrointestinal hemorrhage should avoid ASA. The risk of GI bleeding is increased with concomitant alcohol ingestion. ASA should be taken with food.

Inhibition of platelet function results from inhibition of thromboxane A_2. Individuals with thrombocytopenia or bleeding disorders such as hemophilia should avoid ASA. At higher doses ASA has a hypoprothrombinemic effect through inhibition of hepatic synthesis of coagulation factors and should be avoided in individuals with pre-existing hypoprothrombinemia, vitamin K deficiency or hepatic damage. Individuals who rely on vasodilatory renal prostaglandins for renal function (congestive heart failure, hepatic cirrhosis with ascites, chronic renal failure and hypovolemia) may experience a reduction in glomerular filtration rate and renal blood flow and should use the drug cautiously.

Chronic high dose salicylate therapy has a number of effects in pregnancy. Prostaglandins have a

TABLE 4: Internal Analgesic Dosages

Acetaminophen Analgesic/Antipyretic	
Adults:	325–500 mg every 3 hours or 325–650 mg every 4 hours or 650 mg–1 g every 6 hours PRN while symptoms persist. For self-medication, recommend the physician be consulted if pain not relieved within 10 days in adults or 5 days in children, fever within 3 days or sore throat within 2 days.
Short-term:	up to 10 days not to exceed 4 g/day.
Long-term:	up to 2.6 g/day unless chronic treatment prescribed and monitored by physician.
Children:	10–15 mg/kg every 4–6 hours no more than 5 times daily (or 65 mg/kg/day)
Ibuprofen Analgesic (mild to moderate pain)/Antipyretic	
Adults:	200–400 mg every 4–6 hours PRN For self-medication do not exceed 1,200 mg/day
Children:	(2 to 11 years) 7.5 mg/kg up to 4 times per day Maximum 30 mg/kg/day
Codeine Analgesic	
Adults:	15–60 mg (usual 30 mg) every 3–6 hours PRN
Children:	500 mcg (0.5 mg)/kg up to 4 times daily (every 4–6 hours) or 15 mg/m^2 every 4–6 hours PRN
ASA Analgesic/Antipyretic	
Adults:	*Oral:* 325–500 mg every 3 hours or 325–650 mg every 4 hours or 650 mg–1 g every 6 hours PRN while symptoms persist. For self-medication, it is recommended that the total daily dose not exceed 4 g and that a physician be consulted if pain is not relieved within 10 days for adults or 5 days in children, fever within 3 days or sore throat within 2 days. Antirheumatic *(NSAID):* 3.6–5.4 g/day in divided doses. *Chewable Gum:* 454 g (2 pieces) every 4 hours PRN. Same precaution for pain and sore throat as above. (Note: not for fever). *Suppository:* Analgesic: 325–650 mg every 4 hours as symptoms persist. Same precaution as for oral ASA. Antirheumatic: same as oral doses.
Children:	10–15 mg/kg every 4 hours or 60–80 mg per year of age per dose no more than 5 times daily (see precautions above)

major role in initiation and progression of labor and delivery. Prolonged gestation, prolonged labor, complicated deliveries and increased risk of maternal and fetal hemorrhage have been reported. Chronic, high dose ASA should be avoided in pregnancy, particularly in the third trimester; occasional use for pain or fever is considered relatively safe, although teratogenic effects have been reported in animals.

ASA should also be avoided in those exhibiting hypersensitivity reactions to salicylates (including topical methyl salicylate) or other NSAIDs as cross-reactivity is reported. Cross reactivity also occurs to tartrazine (FD&C Yellow No. 5). Individuals with the triad of nasal polyps, asthma and allergies appear to be particularly susceptible. Signs and symptoms include vasomotor rhinitis, angioneurotic edema, generalized urticaria, laryngeal edema, bronchoconstriction and shock.

If possible, ASA should be discontinued 5 to 7 days prior to any surgical procedures to minimize blood loss and bleeding risk.

ASA is contraindicated in children less than 18 years of age with a viral illness because of its association with Reye's syndrome in children with chickenpox or influenza. A causal association has not been proven. Significant drug interactions are listed in Table 5.

TABLE 5: Significant Drug Interactions with ASA

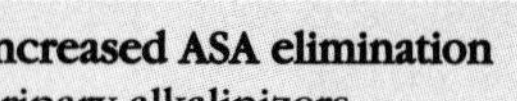

Interaction	Drugs
Increased ASA elimination	urinary alkalinizers
Displacement from plasma protein binding sites	warfarin sulfonylureas valproic acid
Impaired renal elimination	methotrexate (chemotherapy dose)
Reduced uricosuric effect	sulfinpyrazone probenecid
Additive toxicity	NSAIDs antiplatelet drugs alcohol warfarin corticosteroids

Note: Many other drug interactions are reported with ASA and have little clinical significance or are unsubstantiated. An appropriate drug interaction textbook should be consulted.

Side Effects: See Table 2.

Dosage: For general dosing information see Table 4. Administration in children should not exceed 5 times per day.

Salicylate Salts

Magnesium salicylate, sodium salicylate and combinations of choline and magnesium salicylates are available. They dissociate to salicylate in vivo and offer no significant advantages over ASA. In some studies, they were better tolerated with fewer GI effects, but the anti-inflammatory, antipyretic and analgesic effects are generally considered comparable to ASA. One major difference is that these preparations do not inhibit platelet function. The magnesium salt should be avoided in renal insufficiency, the sodium salt in congestive heart failure, hypertension and conditions exacerbated by excess sodium. All salicylates should be avoided in patients with ASA allergy.

Ibuprofen

Pharmacology and Pharmacokinetics: A propionic acid derivative, ibuprofen inhibits the activity of cyclo-oxygenase, the rate limiting enzyme converting arachidonic acid to prostaglandins and leukotrienes. Unlike ASA, this enzyme inhibition is reversible. This inhibition occurs both in the periphery and CNS. Recent evidence suggests that NSAIDs may affect the activity of other neuroactive substances that play a key role in processing nociceptor input within the dorsal horn.

Ibuprofen is rapidly and efficiently absorbed following oral administration with a bioavailability of 85%. Peak concentration occurs between 0.5 to 1.5 hours, and it is extensively plasma protein bound at 99%. Ibuprofen has a small volume of distribution of 0.14 L/kg. However, because it is a weak organic acid with low ionization constants (pKa), ibuprofen is highly concentrated in inflamed tissue, which has a low pH, and synovial fluid. Ibuprofen undergoes primarily hepatic metabolism with > 90% excreted in the urine as metabolites or conjugates. Dosage adjustment is not required in the presence of renal failure. The half-life is relatively short at 2 to 2.5 hours. Clinically, ibuprofen has an onset of 30 minutes and a 4 to 6 hour duration of action.

Use, Effectiveness and Safety: Although best recognized for its role in the treatment of inflammation and pain of arthritic conditions, ibuprofen can provide analgesia in other pain states such as postoperative oral surgical pain, postoperative pain, gout, dysmenorrhea, and soft tissue injury, as well as fever. Ibuprofen is also useful in the treatment of chronic pain of nonmalignant origin since it has low abuse potential, low CNS side effects and lacks apparent tolerance to effect. Clinical trials have shown that a daily dose of 1.2 to 1.8 g of ibuprofen is comparable in activity to a daily dose of 3.6 g of ASA.

Generally, ibuprofen is most useful in milder cases of inflammation and degenerative diseases. Since it exhibits a ceiling effect, maximum doses should not be exceeded. Because of its relatively short half-life, frequent dosing is necessary.

Although not indicated for children in Canada, it has been shown that as an antipyretic, 10 mg/kg of ibuprofen lowered temperature significantly more than acetaminophen 10 mg/kg in children. The maximum antipyretic effect of ibuprofen occurs in approximately 4 hours. As an antipyretic it has a longer duration of action, 8 hours as compared to 4 to 6 hours with ASA and acetaminophen. It appears to be well tolerated in children.

At doses recommended for self-medication, ibuprofen is considered a milder NSAID. Although it shares the same side effect profile of other nonsteroidal agents, including ASA, the severity of adverse effects appears less intense and frequent. In overdose, ibuprofen may be safer than acetaminophen and ASA.

The safety and efficacy of ibuprofen in children under the age of 12 years has not been established.

Nonprescription ibuprofen is available only in an oral formulation, as 200 mg capsules and tablets. The suspension is not available in Canada.

Precautions, Contraindications and Side Effects: Ibuprofen is not recommended during the second half of pregnancy. It may adversely affect the fetus by causing premature closure of the ductus arteriosus. It may also prolong labor and promote excess bleeding. Ibuprofen does not appear to be excreted in breast milk.

As a prostaglandin inhibitor, ibuprofen's most disturbing adverse effects are those associated with impaired physiologic activity of prostaglandins. This includes decreased protective mucus production and flow, increased acid secretion and impaired platelet aggregation, leading to peptic ulcer formation. Prevention of upper gastrointestinal bleeding is discussed at the end of this section. To prevent some of the GI upset, ibuprofen should be taken with food.

Drug Interactions: Studies with warfarin demonstrated no pharmacokinetic effect or hypoprothrombinemic changes; however, caution is required because of possible detrimental effects of ibuprofen on gastric mucosa and platelet function. Ibuprofen can impair the excretion of lithium and increase plasma levels by 15 to 30%. At greatest risk are older individuals. Concurrent administration should be avoided or the patient monitored carefully for lithium toxicity.

Renal clearance of methotrexate has been reduced by as much as 50% when administered with ibuprofen. This interaction is significant when methotrexate is used in oncological doses, and this combination should be avoided. Finally, NSAIDs have been reported to cause acute renal failure when combined with triamterene and can decrease the diuretic response of furosemide.

Contraindications: Ibuprofen should not be used in patients who have peptic ulcer or active inflammatory disease of the gastrointestinal tract. It should not be used in patients exhibiting hypersensitivity to the drug or in individuals with the syndrome of nasal polyps, bronchospastic reactivity and angioedema to ASA or other NSAIDs.

Side Effects: Approximately 10 to 15% of patients on ibuprofen must discontinue the medication because of adverse effects. See Table 2.

NSAID-Induced Gastropathy: Since NSAID therapy can cause upper gastrointestinal bleeding, several recommendations have been made to prevent this adverse effect. Replacing NSAIDs with acetaminophen is appropriate if only simple analgesia is required. Using the lowest effective dose may decrease the incidence and severity of gastropathy. Concurrent administration with antacids or the use of enteric coated NSAIDs have provided minimal success. Acute therapy does not warrant concurrent antiulcer treatment. If symptoms are present, control may be attempted first with antacids. If this approach is unsuccessful, prescription therapy, such as sucralfate, is warranted. Patients with a significant history of gastrointestinal bleeding warrant misoprostol therapy. Individuals with other risk factors (e.g., increasing age, disability, concurrent prednisone use) require careful consideration.

Dosage: For general dosing information see Table 4.

Caffeine

Caffeine is available in combination with mild analgesics such as acetaminophen and ASA. It is rapidly and completely absorbed from the gastrointestinal tract. After oral administration, peak plasma levels are reached in 30 to 60 minutes. Caffeine is extensively metabolized by the liver with only 1 to 5% excreted unchanged in the urine. Liver diseases such as cirrhosis and viral hepatitis can decrease the rate of the drug's metabolism. The rate of caffeine clearance appears not to be affected by age. Drug interactions leading to impaired caffeine elimination have been reported with oral contraceptives, cimetidine and disulfiram.

Although a few studies have shown that caffeine alone may have analgesic properties, e.g., 130 mg of caffeine but not 65 mg was better than placebo in the relief of nonmigrainous headache pain, the major role of caffeine is as an analgesic adjuvant. Earlier studies that failed to demonstrate the efficacy of caffeine were most likely due to poor study design, e.g., either patient samples were too small or the methods used were not sensitive enough to evaluate mild analgesic effects. Based on the current literature, it seems reasonable to conclude that the addition of at least 65 mg of caffeine to acetaminophen or ASA, results in more effective analgesia.

In a placebo controlled study, ASA with caffeine was found to be more effective than ASA alone. The combination product had a faster onset of action (15 vs 30 minutes) and delivered a higher level of analgesia (by a factor of 23 to 44%) as determined by pain assessment scales. These observations are consistent with pharmacokinetic data that caffeine can increase the rate and extent of absorption of ASA, perhaps by increasing gastric secretion and gastric mucosal microcirculation.

In a more recent report, 6 placebo-controlled clinical trials evaluated the efficacy of 130 mg of caffeine as an analgesic adjuvant combined with either acetaminophen (1,000 mg) or acetaminophen (500 mg) and ASA (500 mg) to either acetaminophen (1,000 mg) alone or placebo in patients that were suffering from tension headaches. Both combination products were significantly superior to either acetaminophen or placebo; however, the combination products also had more clinically significant adverse effects including stomach discomfort, nervousness and dizziness.

The mechanism by which caffeine exerts analgesic adjuvant effects is not yet clear. Other than its potential pharmacokinetic effects, caffeine's role in headache pain may be due to its vasoconstrictive effect on cerebral blood vessels. Caffeine may also antagonize the release of peripheral mediators of pain and inflammation. As well, caffeine is a psychomotor stimulant and can enhance mood. Changes in affect may alter the manner in which patients perceive or respond to pain.

The literature suggests that a minimum dose of caffeine as an analgesic adjuvant is 65 mg, a dose much higher than is present in many over-the-counter analgesic formulations. An appropriate single dose is 100 to 200 mg. Caffeine is tolerated by most patients if the dose does not exceed 200 mg in a 3-hour period or 600 mg in a 24-hour period. Obviously the dose necessary to ensure safety and tolerability is also dependent on the patient's dietary consumption of caffeine in such products such as coffee, tea, cola beverages and chocolate.

In the management of fever, caffeine as an adjuvant provides no advantage over ASA or acetaminophen alone.

Codeine

Although codeine is a narcotic agent, it is available without a prescription (in products containing 8 mg or less per dose) in several products containing acetaminophen or ASA and caffeine. It is important for the health professional to remember that the following discussion is specific for codeine alone. In nonprescription products, one must consider the additive effects of other medications contained in the formulation.

Pharmacology and Pharmacokinetics: Opioid analgesics bind with stereospecific receptors at many sites within the CNS to alter processes affecting both the perception and emotional response to pain. Opioid analgesics may alter the release of various neurotransmitters from afferent fibres sensitive to painful stimuli. At least two types of opioid receptors (mu and kappa) mediate pain. Codeine exerts weak agonist activity primarily at the mu receptors, which are widely distributed throughout the CNS, especially in the limbic system, thalamus, striatum and several laminae of the dorsal horn of the spinal cord.

Codeine is absorbed rapidly following oral administration. Peak plasma levels occur in about 1 to 2 hours, and the plasma half-life ranges from 2 to 4 hours. The bioavailability of codeine is greater than that of morphine after oral administration with an oral:parenteral ratio of 2:3. The onset of analgesic action is 30 to 45 minutes with a duration of 4 hours. As an antitussive, codeine can last up to 6 hours. Codeine is extensively metabolized in the liver. About 10% is demethylated to morphine, which may contribute to its analgesic effect. In the kidney, 5 to 15% is eliminated as unchanged codeine and 10% as unchanged or conjugated morphine. Codeine has low plasma protein binding while plasma concentration does not correlate with the brain concentration or relief of pain.

Use, Effectiveness and Safety: Codeine occurs naturally in opium and is structurally related to morphine. In doses of 30 to 60 mg, it is more effective than placebo in relieving mild to moderate pain. Doses of less than 30 mg are generally considered ineffective. Codeine was reported less effective than ASA in postpartum, uterine or dental pain, which might be explained by ASA's anti-inflammatory action. However controlled studies have shown that 30 mg of codeine added to 650 mg of ASA is superior to 650 mg of ASA alone. The combination of a weak narcotic and a non-narcotic having different mechanisms of action may produce an additive analgesic effect. Tolerance to the analgesic effects of codeine usually develops, requiring an increased dose to provide continued relief.

Codeine phosphate is available in nonprescription products as 8 mg per tablet, capsule or caplet in combination with either acetaminophen or ASA and caffeine.

Precautions, Contraindications and Drug Interactions: Dependence liability of codeine is somewhat less than that of morphine, and physical dependence occurs only rarely after oral analgesic use. Withdrawal signs and symptoms of codeine are less severe than those of morphine. Codeine should not be used by individuals known to abuse medications and alcohol.

Codeine is not recommended during pregnancy as it enters fetal circulation and can cause respiratory depression as well as physical dependence. Codeine is secreted in breast milk, although at analgesic doses, concentrations are low.

Children up to the age of 2 are more susceptible to respiratory depression. Children are also more likely to experience paradoxical excitation.

Codeine is contraindicated in patients with respiratory depression and diarrhea secondary to pseudomembranous colitis or poisoning. It should be used with caution in those with head injuries, pulmonary disease and cardiovascular disorders.

Concurrent therapy with medications known to have similar pharmacologic properties to codeine should be avoided as the combination can cause additive adverse effects. These include CNS depressants, anticholinergic agents and hypotensive drugs. Codeine can antagonize the effects of metoclopramide on gastrointestinal motility.

Side Effects: Constipation occurs more often with codeine than with other opioids, especially during chronic therapy. If codeine is to be used on a regular basis, a laxative is recommended. For a listing of side effects see Table 2.

Dosage: For general dosing information see Table 4.

EXTERNAL ANALGESICS

Allyl Isothiocyanate

Allyl isothiocyanate, also known as volatile mustard oil, is obtained from the seeds of black mustard plant or produced synthetically. Black mustard seed contains the glycoside sinigrin. When the seeds are crushed and exposed to moisture, hydrolysis by myrosin results in the formation of allyl isothiocyanate. White mustard contains sinalbin, which is chemically related to sinigrin and has similar action. Allyl isothiocyanate is an extreme irritant and may produce blistering and severe pain if in contact with the skin too long. In plasters and poultices (mustard plaster), formation of allyl isothiocyanate is slower and therefore less likely to cause blistering. To avoid skin damage, plasters and poultices containing mustard oil should not be left on the skin longer than 15 to 20 minutes. Local effects may last 24 to 48 hours.

Few studies have examined the clinical usefulness of allyl isothiocyanate. Volatile oil of mustard 3% in simple ointment is effective in relieving pain caused by intramuscular injection of hypertonic saline under experimental conditions. Allyl isothiocyanate produces severe irritation but only mild flushing of the skin.

If ingested, gastrointestinal irritation with vomiting results.

Allyl isothiocyanate is usually applied in a concentration of 0.5 to 5%, not more than 3 to 4 times daily in adults and children older than 2 years.

Camphor

Camphor has weak analgesic and rubefacient action and may have mild local anesthetic action. It produces numbness at the site of application. It has a hot bitter taste; ingestion of small amounts produces a feeling of warmth in the stomach. Flushing of the skin may be minimal unless massage is vigorous. Natural camphor is obtained from the camphor tree, but most commercial camphor is produced synthetically.

The major problem with this external analgesic is accidental ingestion. In its pure form, it is often mistaken for castor oil. As little as 5 mL can result in life threatening illness and may be fatal to a child. Ingestion causes gastrointestinal tract irritation with nausea and vomiting, which may lead to shock and severe dehydration. Central nervous system toxicity occurs (excitement, hallucinations, delirium, muscular excitability, tremors and tonic clonic seizures). Other signs and symptoms include urinary retention, albuminuria and transient changes in liver enzymes. In some provinces (e.g., British Columbia and New Brunswick) camphorated oil is restricted to No Public Access areas of the pharmacy in an attempt to decrease the number of poisonings by this agent.

At concentrations of 0.1 to 3%, camphor exhibits analgesic properties. When used as a counterirritant, 3 to 11% is effective and may be applied 3 to 4 times daily.

Capsicum Preparations

Capsicum preparations are counterirritants derived from cayenne pepper and include capsaicin, capsicum and capsicum oleoresin. Small concentrations of capsaicin have been used topically for many years for short-term management of arthralgias and arthritis. Capsicum products are generally available in concentrations of 0.025 to 0.25% capsaicin. Recently, capsaicin has undergone both open and placebo controlled trials for management of chronic pain syndromes, such as postherpetic neuralgia.

Application of capsicum causes erythema and a feeling of warmth. The irritant action is potent, and severe burning can occur on tender skin. With continued use, tachyphylaxis to the burning sensation occurs. Capsaicin does not cause blistering, presumably due to a lack of effect on blood vessels. In normal male volunteers, application of capsicum 0.1% cream did not increase forearm blood flow despite local erythema and a sensation of warmth or burning.

Capsaicin is probably the most extensively studied topical analgesic. It exerts its analgesic effect by causing release of substance P from peripheral sensory C nerve fibres, reduced synthesis and subsequent depletion of substance P from the neuron.

On initial application, capsaicin produces burning and hyperesthesia followed by desensitization to burning and pain. The burning diminishes with repeated use, presumably as a result of depletion of substance P. Application 3 to 4 times daily is recommended for maximal effect. Less frequent application prevents adequate depletion of substance P resulting in decreased efficacy and increased local side effects. One study suggested pretreatment with topical lidocaine 5% for the first 2 weeks to control burning at the site of application. Other adverse effects include stinging or erythema at the site of application, cough and respiratory irritation. Dried residue from the hands can irritate the eyes.

Capsaicin is indicated for temporary relief of postherpetic neuralgia, rheumatoid and osteoarthritis (0.025%), and diabetic neuropathy, postsurgical neuralgia and rheumatoid arthritis (0.075%). It has also been used in idiopathic trigeminal neuralgia, postmastectomy neuroma, reflex sympathetic dystrophy, vulvar vestibulitis, psoriasis, apocrine chromhidrosis and hemodialysis-related itching. It has been studied in management of cluster headaches.

Initial research was in patients with postherpetic neuralgia. The results of both open and placebo controlled trials have been reviewed elsewhere; however, in general, pain relief occurred in 60 to 78% of patients. Intolerable burning was the major reason for dropout of study patients. Pain relief requires a minimum of 14 to 28 days of treatment. Maximum response occurs after 4 to 6 weeks of continuous therapy; some patients require therapy indefinitely to prevent return of pain. Both 0.025 and 0.075% cream have been studied.

Double-blind randomized trials of capsaicin 0.025% in rheumatoid arthritis and osteoarthritis indicate pain reduction in approximately 70 to 79% of patients after 4 weeks of treatment; however, 49 to 60% of patients reported improvement with the vehicle. These differences are statistically significant. Topical capsaicin 0.075% was studied in rheumatoid arthritis and osteoarthritis of the hands. Tenderness and pain in the joints were reduced in patients with osteoarthritis but not rheumatoid arthritis when compared to placebo. Swelling, grip strength, duration of morning stiffness and function showed no change.

The length of treatment required to achieve the desired response and the frequency of application must be stressed to the patient. Noncompliance will result in decreased efficacy and increased local adverse effects. The patient should also be advised that burning on application decreases with time.

Esters of Nicotinic Acid

A number of esters of nicotinic acid have been used as counterirritants, including beta-butoxyethyl nicotinate, benzyl nicotinate, ethyl nicotinate, n-hexylester nicotinic acid and methyl nicotinate. Methyl nicotinate is the most commonly used. Application results in vasodilation causing redness and warmth.

Application of a 5% solution results in redness, tingling and heat in 5 to 10 minutes, lasting 0.5 to 1 hour. In some cases a full response is delayed 2 to 4 hours. This may not correlate with pain relief.

The mechanism of nicotinic acid esters is thought to be due to vasodilation, which does not occur in people with brachial plexus injury; intact nerves may be required. These effects were not correlated to pain relief.

Studies of efficacy are few. Tetrahydrofurfuryl nicotinic acid 5% produces flushing, warmth and prickling when applied to the skin of healthy, normal volunteers, but fails to reduce pain resulting from intramuscular injection of hypertonic saline. The nicotinic acid ester was compared to volatile oil of mustard ointment, which produced severe irritation and was effective in reducing pain. The authors concluded that counterirritation relieved pain by producing skin pain of adequate intensity, and that local vasodilation as evidenced by flushing was not important.

A liniment containing esters of salicylic acid, nicotinic acid and benzoic acid was evaluated in 147 people with degenerative or rheumatoid arthritis. The following results were reported: 83 people found the medicated liniment superior, 27 people found the placebo superior, 33 people found them equally effective, and 4 people derived no benefit from either preparation. The only adverse effect reported was mild skin irritation. This finding suggests an important placebo component to application and massage of a liniment. Many people in this study requested the liniment be added to their previous medication regimen.

Esters of nicotinic acid penetrate the skin well. Fainting, caused by a drop in blood pressure, has been reported in some people who applied the product over large areas of the body. This adverse effect is due to generalized vasodilation.

Methyl nicotinate is used as a counterirritant in concentrations of 0.25 to 1% applied 3 to 4 times daily.

Eucalyptus Oil

Eucalyptus oil is in many counterirritant products, but there is little or no documentation of its pharmacologic effects or activity as a counterirritant or topical analgesic. Eucalyptol is the most important constituent of eucalyptus oil. This agent is listed as a flavoring agent and expectorant and as having bacteriostatic properties, but not as a counterirritant. Like camphor and menthol, it produces a cooling sensation when applied topically. Ingestion of eucalyptus oil may result in signs and symptoms of toxicity, such as a burning sensation in the mouth and throat, nausea, vomiting, seizures, ataxia, delirium, coma and pulmonary complications from aspiration. However, a retrospective analysis of 41 cases of ingestion (<10 mL to >45 mL) in children reports 77% were asymptomatic, and symptomatic patients required only symptomatic treatment suggesting eucalyptus oil may be less toxic than once believed. The usual concentration in external analgesics is 0.5 to 3% eucalyptus oil.

Menthol

Menthol is derived from peppermint oil or produced synthetically. It is an irritant that has a cooling effect when applied in low concentrations (0.1 to 2%). At these concentrations it selectively stimulates sensory nerve endings, causing a cooling sensation and analgesia. When used for muscle aches in rubs and liniments, a higher concentration (1.25 to 16%) produces a prickly or burning sensation. Topical application in counterirritant concentrations produces a feeling of coolness followed by a sensation of warmth. It is applied to the affected area 3 to 4 times daily. It may cause sensitization in some people, although this adverse effect is uncommon.

Methyl Salicylate

Methyl salicylate is the most common counterirritant ingredient and is readily identified by its characteristic odor. It is also referred to as sweet birch oil, wintergreen oil, gaultheria oil, betula oil and teaberry oil. It may be obtained from the willow or produced synthetically.

Pharmacology and Pharmacokinetics: Methyl salicylate is absorbed through intact skin. Initially, it was thought to have the systemic effect of salicylates. Metabolites of salicylates can be detected in the urine after topical application. Only 12 to 20% of the salicylate applied to various areas of the body, with occlusive dressing, is absorbed into the systemic circulation after 10 hours of application. Estimated steady state salicylate plasma concentrations are much lower than levels required for control of rheumatoid arthritis. In some cases, plasma concentrations and antiplatelet effects are detected only in the arm to which the counterirritant is applied. Although some absorption of methyl salicylate does occur, evidence to suggest a central or systemic effect is lacking.

A combination of 15% methyl salicylate and 10% menthol produces a feeling of warmth within 30 seconds of application and subjective improvement of pain in most people. In rheumatoid arthritis and osteoarthritis, subjective data indicate this combination is more effective than placebo cream in reducing pain, improving dexterity and increasing range of motion in the joint.

Use, Effectiveness and Safety: Systemic toxicity due to absorption through the skin is uncommon. Toxic levels are achieved only if methyl salicylate has been applied to damaged skin or to large areas of skin with occlusive dressings. Local application of heat should not be used in conjunction with methyl salicylate. The use of a topical methyl salicylate and menthol preparation with a heating pad in a 62-year-old man produced severe, local skin and muscle necrosis, and renal damage resulting in prolonged hospitalization. These severe effects were attributed to increased percutaneous absorption of the drugs due to local heat application. Levels of salicylate adequate to potentiate the anticoagulant effects of warfarin have been reported in at least 12 cases. There are no prospective studies available examining the potential interaction; however, case reports indicate elevated prothrombin times, evidence of bleeding and detectable salicylate blood concentrations in people using topical methyl salicylate and warfarin concurrently. Patients should be instructed to avoid the combination, particularly if increased potential for methyl salicylate absorption exists (e.g., applications to damaged skin). Methyl salicylate should be used sparingly in children and avoided in people with burns or skin diseases.

Side Effects: Adverse reactions to topical salicylates are uncommon. Local reactions such as redness, itching and dermatitis can occur. The dermatitis may reappear following oral ingestion of salicylate. Considering the widespread use of salicylates, the incidence of topical sensitization is probably low. In a survey of 30,000 users, only 2 verified cases were identified. People with hypersensitivity reactions to ASA should use caution since the salicylate moiety is absorbed to some extent through the skin.

The most serious adverse effect is toxicity from oral ingestion, especially by children. The characteristic odor may appeal to small children, especially since some candies have this odor and taste. As little as 4 mL in a child and 6 mL in an adult can be fatal. Intoxication results in gastrointestinal, acid-base, metabolic and coagulation disturbances. The characteristic odor will be present on the breath, in urine and in vomitus. A poison control centre should be contacted for details regarding symptoms and management.

Methyl salicylate is used in concentrations ranging from 10 to 60% and may be applied to the affected area no more than 3 to 4 times daily.

Strong Ammonia Solution

Strong ammonia solution is a counterirritant that produces redness. For this use, it must be diluted to a concentration of 1 to 2.5% ammonia. Undiluted, the solution is caustic and vapors are extremely irritating to the respiratory tract and eyes. Ingestion results in severe pain, coughing, vomiting and esophageal or gastrointestinal tract strictures or perforation. Convulsions may also occur.

Ammonia is usually formulated as a liniment. It should be applied no more than 3 to 4 times daily.

Triethanolamine Salicylate

Triethanolamine salicylate (TEA), a salicylate ester, is a topical analgesic agent. Although some controversy exists in the literature, it is unlikely that sufficient quantities of ester are absorbed through the skin to provide systemic analgesia. Oral radiolabelled ASA compared to radiolabelled TEA 10% results in serum salicylate levels much lower with the topical preparation than with the oral salicylate; topical application resulted in synovial fluid concentrations of about 60% of the oral concentration at 1 and 2 hours. Equivalent pain relief was observed with both topical and oral preparations in 4 out of 6 people.

A double blind study of 40 people with rheumatic pain compared 10% topical TEA to oral salicylate. Improvement was determined jointly by the physician and the user. Relief of mild to moderate and moderate pain was equivalent with TEA and oral salicylate. TEA was more effective than oral salicylate for severe pain. The response of people with osteoarthritis to both agents was poor. There was a tendency for TEA to provide faster pain relief. A significantly greater number of people experienced adverse effects with oral therapy, and the number of people requiring discontinuation was much higher in the oral salicylate group.

The use of 10% TEA in 25 people with osteoarthritis for 1 week produced the following results: 8 people preferred TEA, 6 people preferred placebo and 11 people had no preference. The results may be questioned because many people had severe arthritis and received concurrent oral anti-inflammatory agents.

Side effects of TEA are similar to other salicylates, although reports of toxicity due to ingestion have not been reported. One case report attributes postoperative bleeding secondary to marked suppression of platelet activity to extensive use of TEA by the patient.

Triethanolamine salicylate is available as a 10 or 15% cream and is massaged into the area of soreness 2 to 3 times daily.

Turpentine Oil

Turpentine oil, used as a counterirritant and available as turpentine liniment or white liniment, is distilled and rectified from pine trees. No published trials have reported the efficacy of turpentine oil as a counterirritant for arthritic conditions or muscle soreness. When applied it produces redness and a sensation of burning; hives and blisters may occur. Turpentine oil may sensitize the skin and result in eczema-like conditions.

Vomiting may occur in some individuals due to absorption through the skin.

Toxicity can result from ingestion of turpentine oil. As little as 15 mL may be fatal in children. Severe gastroenteritis, irritation of the urinary tract and pre-existing inflammatory processes occur. Petechiae and thrombocytopenia have been reported. Individuals may exhibit central nervous system excitation and seizures or central nervous system depression.

The topical dose is a 6 to 50% concentration applied 3 to 4 times daily.

Pharmaceutical Agents

External Analgesics

- An external analgesic is a topically applied drug used to relieve pain. It may have analgesic properties resulting from depression of cutaneous sensory receptors (e.g., camphor and menthol) or counterirritant properties to stimulate cutaneous sensory receptors (e.g., methyl salicylate, allyl isothiocyanate and methyl nicotinate). In general, the desired effect of external analgesics is from local action rather than percutaneous absorption and systemic effects. However, methyl salicylate and TEA are rapidly and well absorbed percutaneously following topical application, but blood levels remain very low.

- Counterirritants are rubbed into the skin over a painful joint, tendon, ligament or muscle to relieve pain. They may be described as rubefacients, which cause redness; vesicants, which induce blistering; or pustulants, which cause more severe irritation and ulceration. These differences are quantitative rather than qualitative. Higher concentrations of rubefacients or application for prolonged periods produce blistering or severe irritation.

- Few scientific studies deal with the mechanism of action or effects of counterirritants. Although articles published in the 1940s and 1950s report the effects of counterirritants, there is a scarcity of current data. Possible mechanisms of action and the effects of counterirritants are discussed despite the lack of scientific evidence.

- Counterirritants act by producing a transient, mild, local inflammatory reaction at the site of application. Pain relief is desired at another site, usually the underlying structure such as a joint or muscle. The intensity of response depends on the irritant used, its concentration, the solvent in which it is dissolved and the period of contact with the skin.

- A phenomenon called the pain paradox can be described simply as one pain inhibiting another. The pain paradox theory assumes the brain can deal with only a limited amount of information at any specific time. When a new stimulus is presented to the central nervous system, the brain is unable to process information about the pre-existing pain. Application of counterirritants acts as a new stimulus and distracts the brain, making it less likely to concentrate attention on the original pain. Application of counterirritants stimulates pain or other sensory receptors resulting in closure of the gate (see gate control theory above).

- Counterirritants cause local vasodilation, which results in a feeling of warmth and increased comfort. The extent of vasodilation is unknown; it may occur only on the skin surface. It is unlikely the effects reach deeper structures such as muscle. Table 6 lists other potential but unproven effects of counterirritants.

- The placebo effects of counterirritants should not be overlooked. These products have a medicinal smell and quickly provide visual and tactile evidence of activity in the form of redness, warmth and a burning sensation. This physical evidence provides the user with a sense of satisfaction. Also, applying the counterirritant may require massage of the affected area, which may provide some relief. The placebo effect may be particularly important in chronic debilitating conditions such as rheumatoid arthritis, osteoarthritis and postherpetic neuralgia. Topical application of placebo ointments produces high placebo response in single blind and double blind trials. Placebo response is important for two reasons. First, people with conditions resulting in chronic pain are potential placebo respondents and often purchase external analgesic products. Second, placebo response should be considered when evaluating the effectiveness of external analgesics in treating various conditions. Studies of counterirritant efficacy may provide little valuable information if a placebo control group has not been included.

External Analgesics *(cont'd)*

➤ Although the mechanism of action of these agents is far from clear, the response to counterirritants has been studied and a number of interesting results noted. For example, the number of rubs used to apply a counterirritant ointment does not affect the magnitude of the erythema or the time to achieve it. Redness is not proportional to the concentration used. Mild pain is often permanently relieved by counterirritants, but more severe pain may not be relieved at all. If counterirritation is too great, summation of pain with increased discomfort results; if too weak, there is little effect on the pain. The most effective intensity of counterirritation is slightly less than that which produces discomfort on normal skin. The most effective site of application is directly over the painful stimulus.

➤ Most commercially available external analgesic products contain more than one active ingredient. Although marketed as combinations, individual active ingredients are discussed in the preceding section according to the classification in Table 7. All doses given are those recommended for adults and children over 2 years of age. No guidelines are available for the use of these products in children less than 2 years of age. Rarely is the use of counterirritants appropriate for this age group.

➤ External analgesics offer the advantage of avoiding the potential adverse effects of internal analgesic products. When used appropriately, they have little toxicity, but consumers should be warned that significant adverse effects may result from overzealous application. These products should not be applied to broken or damaged skin. Occlusive dressings should be avoided. Many of these agents can be toxic if accidentally ingested. External analgesics should be stored away from children. Because efficacy has not been proven and toxicity reported with most topical analgesics, use of these products in general is not encouraged. Capsaicin is the best studied topical analgesic.

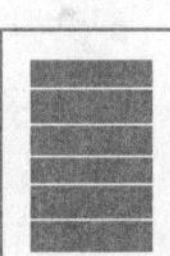

TABLE 6: Effects of Counterirritants

Effects
Local vasodilation
Dispersal of pain-producing substances secondary to vasodilation
Lower muscle action potential
Increase speed of nerve conduction
Increase muscle capacity to work
Placebo effect

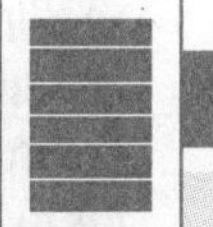

TABLE 7: Counterirritants

Irritants that produce cooling sensation	**Irritants that produce redness**
camphor	allyl isothiocyanate
menthol	strong ammonia solution
eucalyptus oil	methyl salicylate
Irritants that do not produce redness	turpentine oil
capsaicin	**Irritants that produce vasodilation**
capsicum	methyl nicotinate
capsicum oleoresin	

Source: Food Drug Cosmetic Reporter. Vol. 1 Drugs/Cosmetics. New monograph. Washington: Commerce Clearinghouse Inc., 1986:Sec:a)72,068.

Counterirritants: Clinical Considerations and Dosage Forms

- Nonprescription counterirritants are available in a number of dosage forms including liniments, gels, lotions and ointments. The massaging action of application may be an important component of efficacy. The desired effect is local rather than systemic. Ideally, absorption through the skin should be minimal, so the vehicle used in the product formulation is of some importance. Factors that influence absorption are skin condition (intactness), skin age (fetal and infant skin are more permeable than adult skin), regional skin site, skin hydration, drug concentration, solubility and molecular characteristics of the drug, and vehicle characteristics. The amount of rubbing and the period of time the medication is permitted to remain in contact with the skin also may have an effect.
- Liniments may be defined as solutions or mixtures of various substances in oil, alcoholic solutions of soap, or emulsions. They are applied to the affected area with friction or rubbing. The oil or soap base allows for ease of application and is preferred for massage. Alcoholic liniments are commonly used for rubefacient, counterirritant or astringent properties. They penetrate the skin better than the oily liniments. Liniments should not be applied to broken skin or bruised areas.
- Ointments are semisolid dosage forms for external application. They may be greasy (oleaginous) or water-soluble. Water-soluble ointments are easier to remove after application. Because ointments soften when applied to the skin, massage is easy to perform.
- Lotions are liquid suspensions or dispersions for external application. They require shaking before use to disperse the active ingredients. Gels are semisolid systems that are easy to apply and remove. Gels often provide a faster release of drug than ointments.
- Choosing a suitable dosage form depends on the individual. Some people prefer water-washable or greaseless preparations; others find the greasier, heavier preparations more soothing. Lanolin (wool fat) produces a number of allergic reactions, which should be considered when choosing a product.
- External analgesics should not be used for children younger than 2 years of age without first consulting a physician. No information is available about how long these preparations can remain on the skin. The Canadian Counterirritant Monograph states these products should be used no more than 3 to 4 times a day. If excessive burning, redness, irritation or a rash occurs, the product should be washed off immediately with soap and warm water or removed with olive oil. Overzealous application may lead to severe irritation and blistering, and consumers should be warned against excessive use. The use of heat in the form of heat lamps, heating pads and hot water bottles in combination with counterirritants may lead to severe burning and blistering or to systemic effects as a result of enhanced absorption. This combination should be used cautiously, if at all.
- No rationale exists for combining the use of more than one counterirritant product. If the condition worsens, fails to clear up or recurs within a few days of discontinuing the product, the individual should be referred to a physician. Seven days of use is a reasonable length of time for most products except capsaicin.

RECOMMENDED READING

Pain

Kubacka RT. Practical approaches to the management of migraine. Am Pharm 1994; NS34:34–73.

McBean Cochran B. Medication-induced headache: strategies for pharmacist identification and management. Halifax: BMC Health Associates, 1994.

Pray WS. Dental pain: refer your patient. US Pharmacist 1994;(Dec):22.

Fever

Bonadio WA. Defining fever and other aspects of body temperature in infants and children. Pediatr Ann 1993;22:467–73.

Schmidt BD. Fever phobia. Misconceptions of parents about fevers. Am J Dis Child 1980;134:176–81.

Schmitt BD. Fever in childhood. Pediatrics 1984; 74(suppl):929–36.

Styrt B, Sugarman B. Antipyresis and fever. Arch Intern Med 1990;150:1589–97.

Pharmaceutical Agents

Pain and Fever

Bhatt-Mehta V, Rosen D. Management of acute pain in children. Clin Pharm 1991;10:667–85.

Drwal-Klein LA, Phelps S. Antipyretic therapy in the febrile child. Clin Pharm 1992;11:1005–21.

Fye KH. Recent controversies in the treatment of rheumatoid disease. Hosp Formul 1990;25: 1220–32.

Kantor TG. Ibuprofen. Ann Intern Med 1979;91: 877–82.

Sawynok J, Yakish TL. Caffeine as an analgesic adjuvant: a review of pharmacology and mechanisms of action. Pharm Rev 1993;45:43–85.

Supernaw RB. Therapy of recurrent headache syndromes. US Pharmacist 1991;16:33–54.

Welch KMA. Drug therapy of migraine. N Engl J Med 1993;329:1476–83.

External Analgesics

Hoffman GS. Tendinitis and bursitis. Am Fam Physician 1981;23(6):103–10.

Lynn B. Capsaicin: actions on nociceptive C-fibres and therapeutic potential. Pain 1990;41:61–69.

Sherman M. Hot or cold: which treatment to recommend? Am Pharm 1980; NS20(8):46–49.

21

PERSONAL HYGIENE PRODUCTS

DEANNE P. WONG / STEPHANIE EDWARDS

CONTENTS

Introduction 567

Skin Hygiene 568
Soaps

Perspiration and Body Odor 571
Anatomy and Physiology
Prevention of Perspiration and Body Odor

Hair Care 574
Hair Anatomy and Physiology
General Hair Care
Shampoos
Surfactants
Conditioners

Pharmaceutical Agents 583
Antiperspirants
Deodorants

Recommended Reading 584

INTRODUCTION

Good personal hygiene is important both to individuals and the community in the prevention of disease transmission. The first requirement is cleanliness; equally important is the suppression of odor.

The healthy body participates in the cleansing process just as it protects itself against external disturbances. In the constant sloughing of the skin's uppermost horny cells, impurities that have migrated to the surface with the corneal cells are rubbed off by normal body activity. Bacterial flora on the skin assist in the degradation and removal of organic impurities. Old hair is shed and replaced by newly grown clean hair.

Humans have long used washing to help nature. It removes visible soil from skin, hair, and nails; dried perspiration or remnants of cosmetic preparations that make the skin and hair sticky; and prevents body odor. Water removes water-soluble soil, but a detergent, or soap is necessary to remove oil-soluble material. Keeping the body clean and odor free involves soaps, shampoos, conditioners, antiperspirants and deodorants.

SKIN HYGIENE

Most people should wash themselves twice a day (morning and evening) with soap and tepid, not hot, water. Soap should be on the skin for less than 5 minutes: extended bathing time is unnecessary for cleanliness. All traces of soap should be thoroughly rinsed and the skin dried gently. An emollient moisturizing lotion can then be used to combat dryness or a rough flaky appearance.

Dry or Sensitive Skin

When skin is excessively dry, washing less often and more quickly, using a minimal amount of soap will help. Tub baths may be limited to 1 or 2 per week. For daily cleansing, quick showers in warm water or sponge baths will clean areas that are dirty or odorous, such as underarms, genitals, feet, and hands. For people with dry to very dry, and/or sensitive skin, or who must remove heavy, oil based make-up, a cleansing cream will remove oil-soluble soil and deposit an emollient on the skin afterwards. Cleansing creams usually contain cetyl alcohol and/or spermaceti. Dry skin soaps may contain more fatty chemicals. Although these chemicals will provide a rich creamy feel, they may not lather as well as other soaps. Little benefit from these added moisturizers may be seen as only a small amount will remain on the skin after rinsing. Superfatted baby soaps instead of synthetic detergents may be preferred for patients with dry, sensitive, old, or eczematous skin.

Sensitive skin has a different meaning for the layman than for cosmetic scientists and dermatologists. To the lay person it means his or her skin has unwanted reactions to external factors such as personal care products. To the dermatologist it means irritant or contact dermatitis, urticaria, acnegenesis/comedogenesis caused by irritants or allergens in soap products (Table 1).

Fragrances or abrasives contained in some soaps may also irritate sensitive skin. Soaps labelled fragrance-free may contain small amounts of fragrance to mask the odor of the raw ingredients. Products marketed for sensitive skin are more likely not to contain a high concentration of fragrance or known irritants.

Oily or Problem Skin

For people with oily skin or acne, a degreasing cleanser containing alkyl sulfates may be appropriate. Superfatted or baby soaps are generally not suitable. Soaps targeted for oily skins may contain combinations of absorbent materials, such as clays or cosmetic oat flour, along with an astringent. Patients with acne already using either nonprescription or prescription drying agents should be advised to use a mild neutral pH soap once daily. Vigorous scrubbing of the skin does not improve acne.

Patients with impetigo, furuncles and infected cuts or abrasions should be referred to a physician for treatment with a prescription drug. Medicated soaps or surgical soaps may reduce skin flora but alone are not effective treatment for active skin infection or acne.

Children and the Elderly

In general, soaps have minimal contact time with the skin, and most children can tolerate any soap without adverse effects. For the routine care of babies, infants, and toddlers, a mild neutral pH soap may be preferred. Baby soaps are regular soaps with minimal additives.

Baby soaps usually do not contain antimicrobials, a large amount of fragrance, or abrasives. Bubble bath products may enliven bath-time for children, but they have been associated with genital

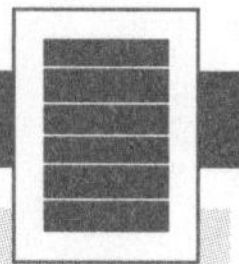

TABLE 1: Selected Ingredients with High Comedogenicity
Lanolin
Fatty acids and derivatives (e.g., isopropyl isostearate, myristate, isostearyl isostearate, myristyl myristate)
Alcohols, sugars and derivatives (e.g., laureth-4, oleth-3)
Oils (e.g., cocoa and coconut butter)
Xylene
Coal tar

and urinary tract irritation, especially in young girls. To minimize this, appropriate amounts should be mixed thoroughly with bath water.

The elderly may prefer bubble baths or foams as less physical effort is required than scrubbing with soap. Dry skin is usually a problem with the elderly; fewer baths and the use of moisturizers may help.

SOAPS

In chemical terms, soaps are the alkali metal salts of long-chain fatty acids. In the process of saponification, monocarboxylic fatty acids (lauric, myristic, palmitic, stearic, and oleic) derived from animal and vegetable sources react with lye (sodium or potassium hydroxide) to produce soap. Sodium hydroxide produces hard soaps; potassium hydroxide produces liquid or paste soaps.

The surface activity of soaps results from the soap molecule having a hydrophobic group and a hydrophilic group at opposite ends. In aqueous solution, oriented monolayers form at the surface, with the hydrophobic tails pointing outward to the air. In solution, soap molecules aggregate into micelles that are easily removed by water. Micelles are bundles of surfactant molecules, roughly spherical in shape, with the hydrophilic ends pointing outward. In hard water, soaps form a precipitate that reduces their activity. Synthetic detergents, which also possess surface activity but do not precipitate in hard water, have been a significant development. In synthetic soaps, sodium lauryl sulfate or a derivative is usually substituted for the natural fats and oils.

The use of soaps and synthetic detergents has been associated with skin dryness and aggravation of dermatologic conditions. Skin tightness normally precedes the development of flaking and scaling and may be the only sign of skin damage noted. A number of factors, including chemical structure, pH and cleansing ability have been implicated. Longer carbon chain length and heavier molecular weight soaps may be less irritating. Most irritation occurs with 12-carbon chain length compounds like sodium lauryl sulfate.

Ordinary soaps tend to be alkaline, with pH ranging from 9.5 to 10.5. Synthetic detergents are usually buffered to a pH of 7.5 or less. Normal skin

TABLE 2: Characteristics of Some Common Soaps

Soap/Synthetic Detergent	pH	Major Component	Comment
Alpha Keri	10.2	soap (superfatted)	neutral, transparent
Aveeno bar	5.4	sodium isethionate	
Camay	9-10	soap	
Caress	6.8-7.1		superfatted
Coast			deodorant
Cuticura	9.5	soap	
Dial	10	soap	deodorant
Dove	7.2	sodium-laurylisethionate, sodium soap	neutral
Fa	10.2	soap	
Irish Spring	9.4	soap	deodorant
Ivory	9.6	soap	floating
Jergens	regular	soap	
Johnson and Johnson Baby Soap	near normal		
Keri	10.2	soap (superfatted)	neutral
Lever 2000	10-11		deodorant
Lifebuoy	10-11	soap	deodorant
Lowila	6.9	lauryl sulfoacetate	neutral
Lux	10-11	soap	
Neutrogena	8.8	sodium and triethanolamine soaps	neutral, transparent
Palmolive Gold		soap	deodorant
Pears	9-10	sodium and triethanolamine soaps	transparent
Zest	9.4	sodium, potassium lauryl sulfate, magnesium and sodium soap	deodorant

pH ranges from 5 to 6. Washing the skin with soap causes a temporary increase in skin pH. Normal pH is rapidly restored by the buffering capacity of the skin surface. Data indicate pH in the range of 5.5 to 10 may have little or no influence on the irritation potential of soaps and detergent bars. Only prolonged contact with undiluted high or low pH compounds will irritate the skin. Fear of alkaline soaps may be largely unfounded and has been exaggerated in the past. Nevertheless, most dermatologists may recommend neutral pH soap. Too frequent washing may also be implicated in excessive removal of skin lipids and may cause dry, flaky skin. Soap manufacturers have added a variety of components to soaps to mitigate the inherent irritancy potential of their products and to appeal to a wider market. See Table 2 for characteristics of some common soaps.

Types of Soaps

Luxury soaps, which have a high percentage of perfumes (up to 5%) that may be irritating, are recommended for the body but not the face.

Deodorant soaps, which are often marbelized or striated, include antibacterial agents that inhibit odor producing bacteria, commonly triclocarban or triclosan.

Cream/moisturizing/superfatted soaps have a large percentage of refatting agents like extra fatty alcohols, lanolin, lecithin, vegetable oils, partial glycerides, and other lipophilic compounds.

Baby/hypoallergenic soaps may be superfatted and have low concentrations of perfumes or scents.

Skin protective soaps include refatting agents, and protein and milk components that reverse drying. They may also contain a variety of botanical materials.

Abrasive/scrub soaps contain abrasive additives for controlling skin blemishes or removing heavy dirt (quartz sand, almond bran, pumice, oatmeal, maize meal).

Floating soaps incorporate air into the formulation and have a specific gravity below 1 g/cm^3, enabling them to float in water.

Toilet soaps are 20 to 50% coconut oil and often the most basic personal care soap.

Transparent soaps contain glycerin, sugar, and ethanol, giving a clear, amber product (e.g., *Pears* and *Neutrogena)*.

Translucent soaps are similar to toilet soaps but contain polyhydric alcohols and special fatty acid blends, with no sucrose or ethanol, (e.g., *Body Shop* soaps). Chemically, transparent and translucent soaps are similar, but the consumer perceives the translucent soaps to be cleaner and more attractive.

Soapless/synthetic detergents are biologically degradable fatty alcohol sulfates or fatty acid isethionates used as surfactants and are combined with builders, refatting agents and other additives. They are soap like, powerful cleaners with a range of pH.

Medicated/surgical soaps may contain antibacterials, moisturizers and emollients and are usually liquids.

Liquid soaps are formulated with synthetic detergents or liquid soaps, or combinations.

Castile soaps, once made exclusively with olive oil, now may contain other vegetable oils and are rarely seen anymore.

PERSPIRATION AND BODY ODOR

ANATOMY AND PHYSIOLOGY

The secretory organs of perspiration found in the skin are the eccrine and apocrine glands. Each gland is a simple tubule with a coiled secretory segment deep in the dermis and a straight duct extending up to the skin's surface (Figure 1).

Two to 3 million eccrine sweat glands are distributed over all parts of the body surface. The eccrine glands play an important part in thermoregulation by secreting a hypotonic, practically clear, odorless fluid with a pH ranging from 4 to 6.8, to the skin surface. Dissipation of excess body heat occurs through evaporative cooling. The combined output of these glands may exceed 1.5 litres per hour.

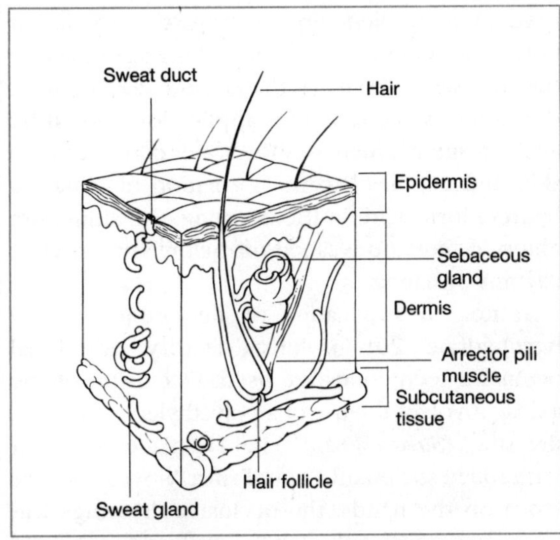

FIGURE 1: Hair Follicle

Apocrine sweat glands are localized to the axillary, inguinal, perianal areas, external auditory canals, and areolae of the breasts. They secrete viscid, milky, odorless material with a pH ranging from 6 to 7.5, a relatively high content of protein and carbohydrate waste materials, water and sodium chloride. The combination of eccrine sweat, sebaceous oils, normal skin debris, apocrine secretions at pH 6 to 7.5, and body heat provide ideal conditions for bacterial growth and the formation of odor.

Sweating is a normal body function caused by 3 major types of stimulation: mental or emotional, thermal and gustatory. Mental or emotional stress causes sweating mainly on the palms, soles or axillae. This is the most common form of sweating and is difficult to control due to the abundance of eccrine glands in these regions. Heat produces sweating mainly on the face, upper chest and back. Gustatory sweating occurs on the face following ingestion of spicy foods. Sweating may also be secondary to other conditions, such as infection, thyrotoxicosis, scleroderma, frostbite, trauma, alcohol withdrawal, or menopause.

Sweating may be general or localized to the palms, soles, axillae, intramammary regions, or groin. Excessive sweating, **hyperhidrosis**, either general or localized, usually occurs in otherwise healthy individuals. The skin in affected areas is often pink or bluish white. In severe cases, the skin, especially on the feet, may be macerated, fissured, and scaling. Axillary hyperhidrosis is socially embarrassing and causes wetness, staining, and rotting of clothing. Patients with excessive sweating of the hands are often reluctant to shake or hold hands and may become socially withdrawn. They are unable to grasp objects; papers become wet; ink runs; metals rust; and electric shock may occur. Excess sweating of the feet leads to foot odor, friction blisters, infection, and rotting of socks and shoes.

Body odor, **bromhidrosis**, is caused when degradation of apocrine secretions and cellular debris by bacteria and yeasts occurs. Two distinct types of body odor have been described. The weaker, sour odor is associated with the micrococcus bacteria and is especially common in women. The second, more prevalent in men, is acrid or pungent and brought about by lipophilic diptheroid bacteria and androsterol and androsterone (the decomposition products of the male sex hormone testosterone). Typical perspiration odor does not occur before puberty and the maturation of the apocrine glands. The presence of armpit hair has practically no effect on the amount or intensity of odor, although through sheer surface area, the hair may help the odor to spread.

PREVENTION OF PERSPIRATION AND BODY ODOR

Since no product can reduce apocrine secretions, most personal care products are designed to reduce the amount of eccrine sweating or to mask odor. The personal care products available are antiperspirants—nonprescription drugs that decrease perspiration, and deodorants—cosmetics that contain antibacterials and fragrance to retard odor formation. No one solution for excessive perspiration is suitable for everyone. Perspiration is not under voluntary control, and the degree to which an individual perspires is influenced by many factors.

Nonpharmacological Prevention

To prevent odor, removing perspiration with regular washing is paramount. Steps to control perspiration could include limiting physical activity; wearing loose, porous clothing; and lowering the humidity in the environment. Dress shields with waterproof linings help absorb perspiration to some degree, but primarily act as a barrier to the wetness.

For excessive sweating of the feet, patients should dry their feet carefully after bathing and apply an absorbent foot powder. Nonocclusive footwear such as leather shoes and cotton or wool socks should be worn. Rubber shoes and stretch socks made of synthetic materials should be avoided where possible.

Palmar and plantar hyperhidrosis may have a poorer response to topical antiperspirant therapy, and iontophoresis, a process where palms and soles are immersed in water through which an electric current is passed, may be tried. The induced current causes a nonspecific injury to the sweat duct that results in abnormal keratinization and keratin plugging of the sweat gland.

Pharmacological Prevention

Perspiration: The most effective and widely marketed agents for the control of perspiration are antiperspirants containing aluminum salts. Because of its high acidity and potential for irritation and damage to fabrics, aluminum chloride has been replaced in commercially available products by other salts such as aluminum chlorohydrate (aluminum chlorhydroxide), aluminum zirconium, and zirconium complexes.

Antiperspirants are marketed in a variety of forms: roll-ons, sticks or solids, aerosol sprays and creams. The effectiveness varies. In their testing, the United States Food and Drug Administration has shown that for average sweat reduction, as a class the lotions are the most effective and the aerosols least effective (Table 3).

The vehicles used in roll-ons are divided into 2 types: water based emulsions and dry (silicone based) suspensions. Dry suspensions offer a more comfortable application, eliminating the wetness and stickiness normally associated with water based roll-ons. Roll-on antiperspirant products containing aluminum zirconium tetrachlorohydrate offer the highest efficacy, with a sweat inhibition in the 40 to 60% range. Stick and solid forms also offer a dry application, and those containing aluminum zirconium tetrachlorohydrate provide efficacy in the 40 to 50% sweat inhibition range. Since zirconium compounds were found potentially toxic when inhaled, aerosol products use only aluminum chlorohydrate as the active ingredient. Aerosol formulations are delivered as a dry powder and can be shared by household members.

In situations where ordinary antiperspirants are ineffective, aluminum chloride hexahydrate 20% in anhydrous ethyl alcohol (e.g., *Drysol*®) may be used. It is applied directly from the applicator bottle, preferably at bedtime to take advantage of the relative inactivity of the eccrine gland during the night. Washing before application should be avoided since it increases the water content of the skin and may lead to the formation of irritating hydrochloric acid. In the morning, the aluminum chloride must be washed off before the onset of daytime sweating.

If normal application of aluminum chloride hexahydrate 20% is unsatisfactory, additional occlusive techniques are used. Occlusion of the axillae involves the use of a polyethylene occlusive dressings (*Saran Wrap*™) held in place overnight with rolled socks and a tight T-shirt. Vinyl gloves are worn on the hands, the occlusive dressings and socks on the feet. Although the occlusive technique is more effective, it is also more irritating. Whatever technique is used, the aluminum chloride hexahydrate should be applied nightly or on alternate nights until the desired degree of dryness is obtained. Thereafter, the agent should be applied as often as necessary. The manufacturer claims application once or twice a week can provide a continuing effect.

Nonaluminum-containing topical agents that have been tried include glutaraldehyde, formaldehyde and tannic acid (strong tea). Currently, no commercial products contain these agents, although pharmacists may be asked to compound a preparation. Of these, glutaraldehyde in concentrations ranging from 2 to 10%, is the most useful. Both the degree of effectiveness and the intensity of staining increase with the higher concentrations.

Methenamine 8% (e.g., *Dehydral®*) hydrolyzes on the skin to form formaldehyde and ammonia. The manufacturer of *Dehydral®* recommends that it be used only on the feet.

Body Odor: Deodorants act primarily by removing, killing, or inhibiting the growth of bacteria that decomposes sweat, and by masking unpleasant body odors with pleasant odors. Deodorants may contain antibacterial preparations, odor maskers, odor absorbers, and to a small extent, enzyme inhibitors or antioxidants as active ingredients.

Antiperspirant preparations also function as deodorants since their active ingredients are also capable of suppressing bacterial growth and bind ammonia and amines in the form of nonvolatile and consequently odorless salts. Accordingly, labels of many of these products display the dual description: antiperspirant/deodorant.

The most common antibacterial agents used are benzethonium chloride, triclosan and zinc phenolsulfonate. Only small concentrations (0.1 to 0.3%) are involved. Deodorants are usually sold as aerosols or sticks. Ethyl alcohol and propylene glycol present in these deodorant vehicle formulations also reduce the microbial flora immediately upon application.

Odor-masking fragrances, such as the essential oils, clove oil, menthol, and thyme oil, all have antibacterial properties. The body's own odor, along with the perfume, will form a composite odor, and individuals must discover their preferred scent in choosing a deodorant.

Deodorants are appropriately used after bathing or showering, and as needed in between. Scented sprays and pumps can be applied to the armpits as well as the adjoining chest, back and arm areas. One should not dress immediately after application, but wait until the solution evaporates and the active ingredients can be absorbed by the skin.

TABLE 3: Efficacy of Antiperspirant Dosage Forms

Dosage Form	Effectiveness
Aerosols	20-33%
Liquids	15-54%
Sticks	35-40%
Creams	35-47%
Roll-ons	14-70%
Lotions	38-62%

Reprinted from: Federal Register (U.S.) 1978, 43:46694.

HAIR CARE

The history of hair care is almost as old as the history of humans, as evidenced by combs and other hair-grooming materials found with the Cro-Magnon people. At different periods throughout history, hair care and styles have reflected fashion trends, power and wealth.

Although hair provides no vital function for humans, its psychological effect is immeasurable. Luxurious scalp hair is seen as desirable by both men and women; lack of scalp hair, although generally accepted in North American society, is still distressing to the male or female who experiences the loss. Men in particular often go to great lengths to encourage hair growth or have hair replacement treatments when they experience the first signs of balding.

Cleanliness is a relatively new cultural phenomenon. Its importance was emphasized with the discovery of the link between cleanliness and health. Today, cleanliness of hair and scalp are among the most important personal hygiene considerations.

HAIR ANATOMY AND PHYSIOLOGY

In the dermis layer of the skin, specialized cells develop into follicles, tubular invaginations that enclose hair. Follicles may vary in depth depending on the thickness and location of the skin. One or more oil glands are attached to each hair follicle. At the bottom of each follicle, papilla cells multiply and rearrange to form the hair bulb or root. The papilla is the only living part of hair. As the hair bulb grows, cells elongate, die and become the hair strand or shaft that eventually projects from the scalp. The hair shaft is pushed up the follicle to the surface of the scalp at a rate of about 8 to 12 mm per month (Figure 2).

The papilla, with its many blood vessels, is also a source of food and oxygen for fully grown hair. The health of hair is dependent on the circulation of blood in the papilla. Decreasing the blood supply or nutrition to the hair affects its appearance. This can occur with aging, heart disease, pregnancy or improper scalp care. Proper nutrition and scalp brushing or massage will make hair healthier and stronger.

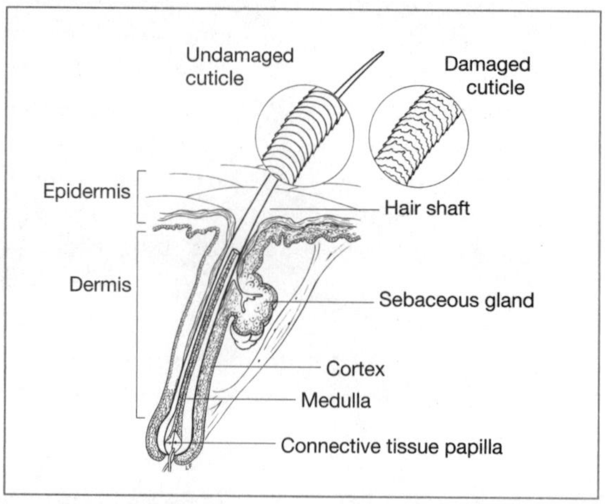

Hair Composition

Hair is composed primarily of the protein keratin; the main chemicals are carbon, oxygen, nitrogen, hydrogen, and sulfur. The chemical composition of hair varies with its color. Darker hair has more carbon and less oxygen, lighter hair the reverse. Hair cells group into three separate layers:

- **Cuticle**: The tough outer layer of transparent, overlapping, scale-like cells, pointing away from the scalp towards the hair ends, protects the inner structure of the hair. When these outer cells lie flat, the hair looks shiny and healthy. When hair is colored or permed, the chemicals raise these scales when they enter the hair cortex. Cuticle cells may become damaged or torn off, causing the hair to look dull and drab because light does not bounce evenly off this rough surface (Figure 2).
- **Cortex**: The middle layer is a fibrous substance formed by elongated cells. It gives strength and elasticity to the hair, and stores the pigment that gives hair its color.
- **Medulla:** The innermost layer, composed of round cells referred to as the pith or marrow of the hair shaft, may be absent in fine and very fine hair.

FIGURE 2: Hair Growth

Hair Growth

The hair follicle does not run straight out of the skin or scalp, but is set at an angle. The direction of hair as it grows out of the follicles determines each person's hair shape. Hair flowing in the same direction is known as the hair stream. Two such streams, sloping in opposite directions, form a natural parting of the hair. Hair may grow in a circular pattern, particularly at the crown, leaving a swirled effect; hair growing at an angle contrary to the rest of the hair is known as a cowlick.

Although hair growth is a continuous process, it is divided into 3 stages: growing or active (anagen), regressive (catagen) and resting (telogen). The anagen phase is the longest, usually lasting 2 to 8 years. Anagen follicles produce hair that is firmly fixed within the hair follicle. When the growth is complete, degeneration begins. The catagen stage, lasting a much shorter time, involves bulbar involution and destruction of the lower part of the follicle as cell growth slows and eventually ceases. During the telogen phase, about 100 days, the hair follicle is shortened, its base terminating in the vicinity of the sebaceous gland. Telogen or clubbed hair generally contains a thin shaft, transparent near the root and devoid of a medulla and keratogenous zone. The walls of the follicle firmly adhere to the stalk of the hair club until a new hair replaces the old hair in the follicle. Approximately 50 to 100 clubbed hairs are shed each day.

Factors such as sex, age, type of hair, heredity and health influence the duration of each of these cycles and therefore the duration of hair life. The duration of the growing cycle determines how long hair will grow if never cut. Although the exact life span of hair is not known, the average hair seems to grow for 2 to 6 years. During this time, the hair shaft can grow from 30 to 90 cm. In many people, hair grows only to a certain length, often shoulder length, and then seems to stop.

When a growing hair approaches the end of its life, a new hair begins to form in the follicle. This is a signal to the old hair that it must move out of the follicle. The departing hair, or club hair, falls out and the new hair moves up to take its place. If a hair is pulled out of the head before its natural time to depart, a new hair will not replace it, since no new hair will form in the follicle while a healthy shaft of hair is growing. However, if a club hair comes out prematurely, the new hair that is being formed will quickly replace it. In humans, the cycle of each follicle occurs independent of that of neighboring follicles. Thus human hair is constantly growing, falling out, and being replaced. In contrast, the hair growth cycles in animals are synchronized so all the hair falls out at once and is replaced by a new set of hair; this is the process of shedding.

The amount of hair a person has is determined genetically. No new follicles develop after birth. The average scalp contains from 80,000 to 150,000 hair follicles. In general, redheads have the least number of follicles, but red hair is thicker and coarser than other natural colors. Blondes have the most follicles and the hairs are thin and fine. Brunettes are somewhere in between, both in numbers of follicles and in thickness of hair.

Hair Types

Hair is usually categorized as oily, dry, treated, or a combination of these. Each hair type requires different care, different cleansing and conditioning products.

Oily hair: The tendency to oily hair is inherited; however, specific hair care practices can aggravate the condition. Excess oil-producing glands in the scalp are controlled by the ratio of estrogen and androgen hormones in the individual. During puberty, the ratio of these hormones can change. In some adolescents, this can lead to an increase in glandular oil production, resulting in oilier face and scalp. After puberty, the hormone balance may stabilize, leading to less oily skin and hair. In some people, the hormone balance remains unstable and oily hair becomes the norm.

Oily hair is very healthy hair and has a sheen that shows best after being freshly washed. This kind of hair is strong, often thick and can be processed without too much damage. Unfortunately, it can also lose its style very quickly, becoming stringy, greasy and limp. In some cases, it must be washed daily or even more often.

Recommended Care: If the oily hair problem is excessive beyond adolescence, a medical opinion should be sought to rule out possible endocrine problems such as polycystic ovaries or adrenal hyperactivity. Oily hair should be well brushed to maintain its sheen. A shampoo formulated to remove excess oil and dirt is recommended. The shampoo should contain fewer oils, waxes, and conditioners, and more and stronger detergents. Hair may be shampooed more frequently, daily if necessary. For very oily hair, 2 shampooings may be necessary. Shampoos that contain lemon juice/citric acid are especially good for use on oily hair; baby shampoos may not be very effective. Few conditioners are useful for oily hair as they contain too many substances such as oils, glycerin, wax, proteins, and balsam. The hair becomes limp, dull and oily very soon after shampooing.

Dry hair: Although dry hair can also be inherited, it is more often due to poor hair care, or lack of protection from sun, wind and other irritants.

Naturally dry hair is rare in young people. Individuals with dry hair usually have dry skin also. The dry hair is due to lack of water; the oil glands of the scalp do not produce enough oil to coat the hair and prevent water evaporation from each strand. In young people with naturally dry hair, the hair is frequently curly or wavy and a darker shade. It is often thick, healthy hair and normal care will keep it looking good.

Dry hair usually requires shampooing only once a week, unless conditions warrant it more frequently. Processing such as perming or coloring may cause even more drying of the hair; exceptional care must be taken during and after processing to prevent further water loss and hair damage.

Recommended Care: Dry hair should be cleansed gently with rich emollient shampoos that cleanse the hair and moisturize the strands. The cuticle is prone to developing little nicks and cuts on the surface, where the keratin fibres are shredded away by weathering or routine brushing and combing. Shampoos with protein, balsam and film-forming agents will help fill these cracks and keep the cuticle strong and firm, hair shiny and soft. Naturally dry hair is not weak like dry, processed hair. A conditioner that contains quaternary ammonium salts may be used; these soften the hair strands and make them smoother and more manageable. If ends are split, a creme rinse or conditioner with additional protein or balsam should be used. Alcohol-free gels and mousses are preferable styling agents to avoid increased dryness.

Baby Fine Hair: Fine, thin hair is the result of thin hair shafts, which may be half as thick as normal hair shafts. Blonde hair is the thinnest, red hair the thickest. Genetically determined, this hair quality cannot be altered except by products such as protein conditioners, hair dyes or permanents. Styling products such as mousses or gels are used to add body.

Treated Hair (permed, colored): Chemical processes/treatments such as coloring, waving, or straightening can cause normal hair to become very dry. The chemicals used are very alkaline, causing damage to the protein structure of the hair. They also leach water out of the hair, causing it to be brittle and dull.

Recommended Care: To restore natural moisture and increase protein, low pH shampoos rich in oil, proteins, and moisturizers should be used. The acidity of low pH shampoos shrinks the hair back to normal size and firms up the hair shaft. Hydrolysed protein, balsam, and other film-forming agents coat the surface of the hair, helping it retain a supply of water. Creme rinse conditioners are often too strong—they contain hair-softening chemicals (quaternary compounds) that can further weaken already fragile hair.

Split Ends

When the individual cell layers of the hair shaft separate, it is called split ends. The problem may be worse with long hair that is seldom cut. General good hair care helps minimize split ends. The best solution is to cut the hair off beyond the point of the splits, but several corrective hair products will temporarily repair or "fuse" the split ends, giving the hair a much healthier appearance. Some of these products retain their effectiveness through several hair washings.

Singeing the hair, an antiquated practice, can worsen the damage and actually promote split ends. Based on the erroneous belief that the hair has a hollow canal through which flows a nourishing, life-giving fluid, singeing was intended to seal the tip so the fluid could not escape.

Swimmer's Hair

Regular swimming, particularly in heavily chlorinated pools, can be very drying. Hair develops a dull appearance, tangles easily and often breaks.

Recommended Care: A mild shampoo formulated for dry, damaged hair should be used. Several products are marketed specifically for swimmer's hair. A short, simple hairstyle that requires minimal handling may be sensible.

Green Hair

Most often caused by increased concentrations of copper in tap water and swimming pools, green hair is most likely to affect blonde (natural or colored) and white hair. Less common causes include industrial exposure to cobalt, chromium and nickel, and the use of tar shampoos.

Copper absorption may occur more readily in hair physically damaged by curling irons, overbrushing, hot blow dryers, and sun exposure. Hair may be vulnerable if it has been chemically altered by bleaching, permanent waving or straightening, or exposed to alkaline shampoos.

Recommended Care: There are no simple remedies to remove green hair. Prevention is the best treatment.

Cradle Cap

The common name for seborrheic dermatitis in infants, cradle cap occurs in adults as a completely unrelated condition. In both instances, the pathogenesis is unknown.

Recommended Care: For treating most cases of cradle cap, a baby shampoo is usually all that is required. It should be applied to the scalp and left on until the scale is softened. After contact with the shampoo, gentle scrubbing will usually remove the scale. The scale may also be softened with olive oil before shampooing.

For persistent cases, medicated shampoos such as tar shampoos may be used. In adults, seborrheic dermatitis is treated with a medicated shampoo containing zinc compounds, salicylic acid or tar (see Dermatitis, Seborrhea, Dandruff and Dry Skin Products chapter).

GENERAL HAIR CARE

The goal of basic hair care is to minimize damage to the cuticle layer. After hair is washed and conditioned, it should be gently dried with a towel. Rubbing with a towel may rough up the cuticle surface or even break fragile hair shafts. After washing, hair should be combed using a wide-toothed comb, not a brush because wet hair is more delicate.

Brushing

An old myth suggested that brushing hair 100 strokes a day would make it grow faster and look better. Although hair brushing is essential, 20 strokes are probably as effective and less damaging than 100. Brushing too vigorously can irritate the scalp and damage the hair. Proper brushing improves the hair appearance by spreading oil along the shaft to add shine, while loosening and removing dust, grime, chemical residues, and dead cells. Brushing and combing stimulate blood circulation, ensuring adequate nutrition for growing hair.

Often debated is the type of brush to use for best results. Natural bristle brushes, many made with boar hairs, have naturally-rounded tips and soft, flexible bristles; they are recommended. In contrast, nylon brushes may have rough jagged edges and stiff bristles, and may cause hair breakage and scalp irritation. Better quality nylon brushes that have bristles with polished edges and rounded tips are often used for styling hair.

Brushes and combs should be washed frequently to remove all the debris transferred from the hair. Soak in warm water with a small amount of liquid shampoo for about 10 minutes. Hair and other debris may be removed by hand, or using the implements to clean each other. Rinse thoroughly and dry carefully with a towel.

Scalp Massage

If scalp circulation is poor, the capillaries at the root of the hair are no longer as effective at delivering oxygen and nutrients and getting rid of waste products. In extreme cases, hair cells grow very slowly, new hairs are no longer formed, and existing hairs may die. This can lead to thinning of the hair that may or may not be permanent.

As people grow older, the general body circulation slows, indirectly affecting scalp circulation. This is a major factor in the declining appearance of the hair as one ages.

To maintain healthy hair, scalp massage is often more beneficial than hair brushing as it stimulates the scalp circulation more quickly and is less likely to pull out or damage the hair. Although hairdressers and beauticians offer head massage service, it can be costly, particularly if one requires the service regularly. One of the best, and least expensive, ways to massage the scalp is with an electric scalp vibrator, until a tingling sensation is experienced. Begin at the scalp line on the front of the head, then go around the ears, over the top of the head, and finally, over the back of the head and neck.

Shampooing and Conditioning

The hair and scalp can accumulate many substances including natural oils and scales (normal or excessive sloughing of dead epidermal cells); hair styling products such as sprays, gels, and mousses; and dust, dirt and air pollution. The variety and quantity may vary depending on different biochemical, grooming and environmental factors. Hair that is soiled with these substances can look dull, feel oily and gritty to the touch, and may even give off an unpleasant odor.

When hair is in contact with water, it swells and becomes more fragile; therefore, shampooing should be done gently. Frequent shampooing will not cause hair loss, although excessive shampooing of very dry hair may cause hair breakage that could appear to be excessive loss. Hair may be washed as often as necessary to keep it looking healthy and the scalp feeling comfortable and clean. It is normal to lose 50 to 100 hairs per shampoo.

The hair care product line has evolved from shampoos only to creme rinses, hair conditioners and, more recently, combinations of shampoo and conditioner.

Although shampoos and conditioners are usually seen as very different products, with different uses, their formulations are surprisingly similar. The surfactant combinations in shampoos tend to be better cleaners, while those in conditioners, along with other ingredients, tend to make hair more manageable and healthy-looking. Individual choice is most likely based on visual appeal, fragrance, cost, peer recommendation, and the perceived benefits of a product from advertising.

Although choosing an appropriate shampoo from the available array can be very confusing, there are two major types: plain cleansing shampoos, often sold in hair salons or specialty hair care shops or conditioning shampoos. Many currently available products fall into the latter category. To choose a product based on ingredients is difficult because most shampoos sold in pharmacies and grocery stores do not list the ingredients, but there is often a 1-800 telephone number to call for information.

When an individual uses a shampoo, it is usually possible to tell after 1 or 2 shampooings whether the product is suitable. However, even when a shampoo is suitable in the beginning, it may seem to lose its effectiveness after being used a few times. This is most likely due to a buildup of conditioning ingredients on the hair shaft, which is not removed with subsequent shampooings. It is usually best to use more than one type of shampoo; a plain cleansing shampoo used every 2 or 3 times may remove some of the buildup, keeping the hair in better overall condition.

When choosing a shampoo, people should know their basic hair type—dry, normal, oily or processed—as well as any hair problems. There are shampoos for every possible hair type, problem and situation: split ends; dull, limp, thin, sun-dried, color-treated, permed, or damaged hair; hair that is shampooed daily, blow-dried frequently, or on which a large number of styling products have been used. In most cases they can be grouped into several large categories. Thus, shampoos for color-treated, permed, straightened, sun-damaged, and dry brittle hair all have similar formulations. Limp, fine or thin hair usually requires a shampoo with minimal oils and waxes, and additional protein and body-building agents. Since conditioning agents in shampoos (and conditioners) will give different results to different kinds of hair, several shampoos may have to be tried to obtain best results.

The first shampoos were soap-based, alkaline, hard on hair and not particularly good cleaning agents. The discovery of surfactants changed shampoos drastically, allowing better cleansing even in hard water. The early surfactants were efficient at cleaning, but were irritating, tended to dry out hair and scalp, and left hair in a flyaway state with a harsh feel. Gradually, products have changed, incorporating less irritating surfactants and many other chemicals to give optimal cleaning and conditioning.

The ideal shampoo is one that will safely and effectively remove the soil yet leave the hair and scalp in good condition. The shampoo must spread easily over the head and into the hair, should foam quickly and copiously in both soft and hard water and rinse out thoroughly. Neither hair nor scalp should feel tight or dry, and the hair should be left in a soft, lustrous, full-bodied and manageable state. Shampoos have become more sophisticated and are continuously being changed with the discovery of new and better chemicals and chemical combinations.

Safety and toxicity factors are also very important in accidental or intentional ingestion of haircare products. Reliable poison references indicate that accidental ingestion of nonmedicated liquid shampoos or conditioners has not resulted in significant toxicity, mild GI irritation being the worst symptom. Recommended treatment consists of giving the patient water to dilute the product, followed by observation. However, medicated shampoos, such as shampoos containing lindane, have been reported to cause clinically significant toxicity.

SHAMPOOS

The properties of a shampoo depend not only on its ingredients but on how much of each type it contains. While the average shampoo has 15 ingredients, many have up to 25. An individual can generally decide after 1 or 2 shampooings whether a product is satisfactory. The ingredients in a shampoo may or may not be listed on the label. When listed, they may either be in descending or ascending order according to amount; however, there is no standardized format. When the ingredients are not listed on the product, the manufacturer usually provides a toll-free number that the consumer can call for further information. Shampoos have many common ingredients, including:

- **Water** (usually purified or deionized)
- **Surfactants** (cleaning agents)
- **Other additives**:

  sequestering agents: prevent formation of insoluble calcium and magnesium soaps and prevent discoloration from iron contamination, e.g., disodium EDTA, citric acid (also used as a buffering agent to decrease pH—improves lustre and resilience of hair), tartaric acid

  foam stabilizers: do not contribute to the efficacy of the shampoo although the sudsing properties may enhance an individual's perception of the product, e.g., fatty acid alkanolamides

  foam builders: to control excessive foaming when a product is used on the hair, e.g., cocoamide EDTA, lauramide DEA (diethanolamine)

  preservatives: inhibit mold and bacterial growth in shampoos; must be chosen carefully for the following reasons: must be stable, properties must not be inhibited by surfactants, some (e.g., phenol) may give a brown discoloration to the shampoo, and some are irritant

  antioxidants and buffers: help prevent discoloration and the development of unpleasant odors in a shampoo (e.g., citric acid—decreases pH)

  coloring agents: no use other than to distinguish products; however, may contribute to product esthetics

  fragrances: no use other than to distinguish products

  conditioners: the agents used as separate conditioners are also used in shampoos, in amounts adjusted to reflect its intended use; no theoretical basis for influencing shampoo function and results (see Conditioners)

  opacifying agents/pearlescents: change the appearance of shampoo, but also soften (e.g., long-chain fatty alcohol sulfates or fatty acid esters)

  protein: many shampoos contain some protein (hydrolysed proteins, keratin, amino acids); hair has an affinity with protein, picking up a coating of protein from shampoo. The protein fills in the cracks in the cuticle caused by strong alkaline chemicals used in dyeing or perming, or damage from sun, wind or blow-drying; the layer of protein makes hair look thicker

  viscosity builders/thickeners: claimed to increase hair consistency and thickness; when combed into the hair, gives a thicker appearance and makes the hair fibres more rigid and adhere more to one another; removed with rinsing, however, as with most other shampoo ingredients, is of little value (e.g., natural gums such as tragacanth, karaya; hydroxymethyl- or carboxymethylcellulose; acrylic polymers, carbomer, salts such as sodium or ammonium chloride)

  pH balance: not an ingredient, rather the result of different additives; many shampoos may be alkaline, which makes the hair shaft swollen, flakey and weak; acidic or balanced shampoos can shrink the cuticle and make the hair shaft stronger or shinier

- **Miscellaneous ingredients** (natural ingredients, herbs, vitamins, sunscreens, etc): little or no scientific evidence to support the "beneficial" claims made by manufacturers; most special additives included to attract the attention of the consumer. Examples are:

  allantoin

  aloe: not thought to have an effect on the hair shaft

  balsam: a resin that stiffens the hair, adding volume and body

  beer/malt

  birch

  carrot oil: no value other than adds fragrance and color

  chamomile

  eggs

  geranium oil: no unique properties for conditioning; may cause allergic reactions

  henna

  herbs: some can brighten color, soften hair strands and soothe an irritated scalp; are potential allergens

  honey

  jojoba: claims for moisturizing properties without adding greasiness; expensive therefore the shampoo may contain a very small amount, which is rinsed off along with other shampoo ingredients *lemon/citric acid:* an excellent rinse for oily hair that will cut through the film left by oil and minerals to make the hair shiny and soft; even when shampoos claim to contain lemon, the amount is usually less than is required to be beneficial

milk: claimed valuable for its protein content; no studies available

panthenol (vitamin B_5): a cationic surfactant; listed in approximately 50% of products on sale in the United States; demonstrated essential for the strength and growth of hair; unlike most other vitamins, studies have shown that the hair does pick up panthenol and hold it inside the shaft

papaya

placenta extracts

silk: does not strengthen hair or fill in cracks in the surface of the shaft; acts like hundreds of tiny reflecting particles to make the hair appear shinier

sunscreens: the same ingredients used to block ultraviolet (UV) rays from the skin are added to shampoos, conditioners and other hair care products; wash out with the product, only effective in the leave-in conditioners; may protect the hair from the cross-linking and disintegration of the keratin fibres caused by UV rays, but cannot protect hair from the heat and dehydration of exposure to the sun

vitamin E: no benefit other than as a preservative/antioxidant

vitamins (A, D, E, B complex): for the most part, hair cannot absorb vitamins; with the exception of panthenol, have no effect on the appearance of hair

SURFACTANTS

Apart from water, surfactant compounds, both lipophilic and hydrophilic, are the second most common ingredient in shampoos. The hydrophilic polar group located at the end of a fatty chain renders the surfactant water soluble; any fatty material attracted to the hydrophilic end is easily washed away. Synthetic surfactants are classified according to the polar end in four categories:

- **Anionics** have excellent detergent, emulsifying and foaming properties, but are highly irritating and usually combined with other types of surfactants to counteract this. Examples are alkyl sulfates (sodium lauryl sulfate, ammonium lauryl sulfate, TEA lauryl sulfate), alkyl ether sulfates, etc.
- **Nonionics** have no polar end. With low foaming, good antistatic and antiseptic properties, they act as foam modifiers or stabilizers, and conditioners. They add body and lustre to hair while cleaning and make it more manageable. Most effective in the pH range 6.5 to 8.5, they are often used as counterirritants in products with sodium lauryl sulfate as the anionic surfactant. They are generally considered the mildest of all surfactants. Examples include aromatic amine oxides (dimethylalkylamine oxides), alkanolamides, polyethoxylated derivatives and polyhydroxy derivatives.
- **Amphoterics**, also called ampholytics, have both positive (cationic) and negative (anionic) charged groups. The cation portions are usually quaternary or amino nitrogens; the anion portions usually carboxylates, sulfates, or sulfonates. They have low foaming properties and are usually combined with anionics. Shampoos with this type of surfactant alone are difficult to

TABLE 4: Irritation Potential of Common Surfactants

Irritation Potential	Surfactant
High	Ammonium lauryl sulfate Sodium lauryl sulfate Dodecyl trimethyl ammonium bromide
Moderate	Sodium laureth sulfate—3EO Triethanolamine lauryl sulfate soap
Low	Sodium laureth sulfate—7EO Sodium cocoyl isethionate

thicken and difficult to opacify. The most commonly used amphoterics are either imidazoline or betaine derivatives. Imidazolines are highly compatible with anionic, nonionic, and cationic surfactants over a broad pH range. Examples include cocoamphoglycinate, cocoamphocarboxyglycinate, cocoamphopropionate and cocoamphocarboxypropionate. Betaine derivatives are effective foam boosters. Examples include coco- and laurylbetaines. Amine oxides are also useful amphoterics.

- **Cationics** are severe eye irritants, poor detergents, anionic foam depressants, and are incompatible with anionic surfactants. Therefore, although they add pronounced substantivity to hair and scalp, and good conditioning effects (improved combability while reducing fly-away), these surfactants have not been in popular use. Quaternary ammonium compounds are the best known cationic surfactants.

In spite of the apparent drawbacks of cationic surfactants, recent investigations have shown potential for various combination cationic-anionic systems in single-step shampooing and conditioning agents. The irritation potential of common surfactants can be found in Table 4.

Natural surfactants are primarily saponins found in various plants such as soap bark, soapwort, sarsaparilla, and ivy. They have good foaming properties, but their detergent properties are not good. They are often combined with synthetic surfactants to ensure good cleansing along with other desirable cosmetic qualities (nonirritating).

CONDITIONERS

Although conditioners cannot repair damaged hair or improve the quality of new hair growth, they can restore lustre, shine, manageability; ease of combing and detangling; and prevent static buildup. Most conditioners are in the pH range of 3.5 to 6, due to acids in their formulation and can restore the pH balance after an alkaline chemical treatment.

Similar to shampoo formulations, surfactants and water are the most important and abundant agents in conditioners. Many other agents used in shampoos are found in conditioners including moisturizers, humectants and emollients, viscosity builders, fragrance, color, and many natural ingredients. In most cases, these natural ingredients have

Types of Shampoos

Ordinary shampoos: These are common, designed to clean hair, provide combability and gloss without fluffiness and usually contain anionic surfactants.

Conditioning shampoos: The foaming and cleansing properties of shampoos were combined with the manageability of a conditioner for the convenience of consumers. In earlier formulations, there was sometimes an interaction between the shampoo and conditioning ingredients, forming insoluble complexes that did not clean as well as a cleansing shampoo or condition as well as a separate conditioner. However, improved technology allows products to combine the efficient cleaning of a quality shampoo and the conditioning one would expect from a separate conditioner.

Special care shampoos: Some shampoos are marketed for particular types of hair or particular conditions. Among them are moisturizing shampoos, medicated shampoos and shampoos for oily, dry, damaged, or treated hair, or for frequent use.

Mild or baby shampoos: In the 1950s, it was discovered that certain imidazoline-derived amphoteric surfactants were extremely mild, and later that adding an anionic surfactant could also reduce the irritation associated with shampoos. Any anti-irritant used in a shampoo should also contribute to its foaming, cleansing and conditioning abilities, or its market appeal. Surfactants are perfectly suited to this role since they are already used in shampoos and possess some of the properties required.

The use of an anionic surfactant with an amphoteric as the detoxifying agent has produced a very useful and popular product. At alkaline pH, which is normally how amphoterics are supplied, they are anionic and mild. However, in acidic conditions, which is normally how they are used, the molecule assumes a cationic character. The cationic form may be more irritant than the anionic or the neutral form. However, if combined with equimolar amounts of an alkyl or alkyl ether sulfate (anionic surfactants), the complex has very low irritating properties.

Dry shampoos: When people are unable to wash their hair with regular shampoos, either due to lack of water, illness, or disability, dry shampoos are very useful. They are primarily a combination of talc and an alkaline powder. After being brushed onto the hair, the dry shampoo is left on for a few minutes to absorb excess oil, then removed with minimal brushing so not to stimulate further oil production. There are some disadvantages: dirt and dandruff on scalp and hair cannot be completely removed; any shampoo left on the scalp may cause dermatitis; and hair may not feel as clean as with regular washing.

Types of Conditioners

Before commercial hair rinses and conditioners were available, vinegar and lemon juice (acid rinses) were used to remove the undesirable lime coating left on hair in hard-water areas. Lemon juice may still be added to conditioning products, although the amount added in most cases is not enough to be beneficial.

Instant conditioners are either designed to be left on the hair for a very short period (1 to 5 minutes) or left in the hair during styling. Conditioners improve wet combing, detangle wet hair and reduce static. They may be diluted or used in their original strength. The active ingredients are quaternary ammonium compounds. They usually contain humectants that absorb and hold moisture from the hair (e.g., sorbitol, ethylene glycol, butylene glycol, and propylene glycol). Cetyl alcohol and stearyl alcohol work as pearlizing agents and lubricants, and leave hair with a glossy finish. Lanolin and derivatives are often included in conditioning agents for fine hair because of their low molecular weight. Silicone oils such as simethicone are effective lubricants and emollients, but are easily removed with the next shampooing.

Deep conditioners are usually heavier, creamier formulations than instant conditioners, and have a longer application time (10 to 20 minutes). The main ingredients are quaternary ammonium compounds and natural oils such as lanolin, castor oil, apricot oils, etc., because of their ability to attach to hair strands (substantivity) and provide longer lasting protection.

Leave-in conditioners are designed to be left on the hair rather than rinsed off. Unlike the 2-in-1 shampoos (though popular, they leave the feeling the benefits are lost down the drain with the rinsing) these give customer satisfaction because the cuticle-coat product remains on the hair, contributing to improved appearance (shiny), feel (silky), and combability. These conditioners contain dimethicones and related materials. With leave-in conditioners, which are designed to be used on wet or dry hair, silicone buildup is not a problem because the basic cuticle coat formulations wash off easily during shampooing.

no benefit, other than enhancing buyers' perception of the product. Some of the useful agents are alkylolamides; fatty ingredients (fatty alcohols, fatty acids, fatty esters, lanolin, vegetable or mineral oil, etc); glycols (glycerin); silicones; nonionic surfactants (amine oxides); amphoteric surfactants; anionic-cationic complexes; cationic polymers, proteins (hydrolysed proteins, keratin, amino acids), and cationic surfactants (quaternary ammonium compounds).

Cationic surfactants remain the backbone of the formula because of their properties such as adding substantivity to hair, good emulsifiers, and good performance in an acid pH. In just over 10 years, conditioners have changed from cationic emulsions of cetearyl alcohol to the many forms now available. The recent trend has been away from fatty alcohols, oils and waxes and towards the use of silicones, proteins and other additives, particularly natural ingredients, with clear and leave-in conditioners replacing the greasy emulsions. Proteins in all forms are ideal for conditioners, since they also have natural substantive properties. Vegetable-based proteins have become more popular than animal-based proteins.

Many ingredients may be more useful in conditioners than in shampoos because they are less likely to be washed off.

PHARMACEUTICAL AGENTS

ANTIPERSPIRANTS

Aluminum and zirconium salts most likely act in the upper portion of the eccrine duct where an insoluble plug of amorphous material is formed. These plugs may physically inhibit sweat elaboration from an affected duct for up to 3 weeks following application of an aluminum salt. However, there are millions of ducts and they may not be predictably or uniformly plugged for that length of time.

Topical application is unlikely to result in substantial aluminum absorption.

Adverse effects of aluminum and zirconium salt antiperspirants are usually limited to irritation such as itching and burning. In severe cases, marked dermatitis and ulceration can develop. Rarely, contact sensitization occurs. Irritation normally subsides when the antiperspirant is discontinued. Topical hydrocortisone cream helps relieve irritation.

To be effective, aluminum chloride hexahydrate, and probably other aluminum salts, must remain on the skin for 6 to 8 hours. One should wait 24 to 48 hours after shaving before applying the medication. The skin, particularly in the axillae, must be dry before application, and sometimes it is helpful to blow-dry the axillae first.

Glutaraldehyde and **formaldehyde** are disinfectants. A glutaraldehyde 10% solution has been recommended for idiopathic hyperhidrosis of the feet, but its effectiveness remains questionable. Formaldehyde solution, in glycerol or alcohol may be used for sweating of the feet, but it is likely to cause sensitization reactions.

Methenamine is a synthetic antibacterial. Its antibacterial effect is dependent on the release of formaldehyde in an acid medium.

DEODORANTS

Deodorants commonly contain antibacterial agents, odor maskers and/or odor absorbers. The bacteriostatic effect of deodorants is to control the bacteria population and not eradicate and disrupt the balance of normal skin flora, thus enabling spread of pathological bacteria.

Benzethonium chloride is a quaternary ammonium disinfectant. It has bactericidal activity against gram-positive and some gram-negative organisms. Alcohols enhance the activity of quaternary ammonium compounds.

Phenolic compounds include triclosan and zinc phenolsulfonate. The phenolic compounds are compatible with soap and tend to last longer than other agents. **Triclosan** is a disinfectant that has bacteriostatic activity against gram-positive and most gram-negative organisms. Although rare, contact dermatitis has been reported with the use of triclosan. It is often found in deodorants and deodorant soaps. **Zinc phenolsulfonate** is often formulated in liquid products.

RECOMMENDED READING

Skin and Soaps

Greene DW. Cleanliness and the Health Revolution. Soap & Detergent Association (US), 1994.

Schoen LA, Lazar P. The Look You Like: Medical Answers to 400 Questions on Skin and Hair Care. New York: Marcel Dekker, 1990.

Hyperhidrosis and Antiperspirants

White JW. Treatment of primary hyperhidrosis. Mayo Clin Proc 1986;61:951-56.

Hair Care

Brauer EW. Your Skin and Hair: A Basic Guide to Care and Beauty. New York: Macmillan, 1969.

Cooper W. Hair: Sex, Society and Symbolism. New York: Stein and Day, 1971.

Forsch PJ. Principles of Cosmetics for the Dermatologist. St. Louis: CV Mosby, 1982.

Jellinek JS. Formulation and Function of Cosmetics. New York: Wiley Interscience, 1970.

Orfanos CE, Happle R, eds. Hair and Hair Diseases. New York: Springer-Verlag, 1990.

Schoen LA, Lazar P. The Look You Like: Medical Answers to 400 Questions on Skin and Hair Care. New York: Marcel Dekker, 1990.

Schoen LA, ed. The AMA Book of Skin and Hair Care. Philadelphia: Lippincott, 1976.

Zviak C, ed. The Science of Hair Care. New York: Marcel Dekker, 1986.

22

SLEEP AIDS AND STIMULANTS

Sandra Naidoo

CONTENTS

Introduction 585
Sleep Physiology 586
Sleep Architecture
Factors that Affect Sleep Patterns
Insomnia 589
Prevalence and Types of Insomnia
Sleep in Older Individuals
Caffeine-Induced Insomnia
Caffeinism
Management
Other Sleep Disorders 593
Narcolepsy
Sleep Apnea
Pharmaceutical Agents 595
Recommended Reading 596

INTRODUCTION

The recent widow, the ruminative worrier, the problem patient with chronic obstructive pulmonary disease, the melancholic depressive and the executive with jet lag all share the common problem of inability to sleep, but the cause and their therapeutic needs differ.

The drowsiness and chronic fatigue associated with sleeplessness can adversely affect the quality of life, impairing a person's ability to concentrate, cope with minor irritations and enjoy interpersonal relationships.

Each year traffic and industrial accidents attributable to daytime drowsiness result in thousands of injuries and deaths, and billions of dollars in damage. Many of these costs can be prevented or at least substantially reduced if those suffering from sleep problems are properly identified, supported and treated.

SLEEP PHYSIOLOGY

SLEEP ARCHITECTURE

Normal sleep consists of two phases: rapid eye movement sleep (REM) and nonrapid eye movement sleep (NREM) (Table 1). REM sleep is accompanied by a range of physiological functions such as muscle twitching, eye movement, blood pressure, respiratory and heart rate changes. This is also the phase in which most dreaming occurs. NREM sleep is characterized by a reduction in physiological activity: heart rate, blood pressure, respiratory rate and brain activity tend to decline. NREM is further subdivided into four stages, each characterized by specific electroencephalographic (EEG) patterns (Table 1).

We cycle back and forth through the four non-REM stages and REM sleep so that there are four or five different REM periods throughout the night, each successive one tending to be longer. The required amount of sleep is to some extent genetically determined, most individuals needing at least 8 hours, a few needing only 4, to function normally. The sleep pattern becomes more fragile with advancing age; in older individuals the number of nocturnal awakenings increases and REM sleep becomes more evenly distributed throughout the night.

A number of generalizations can be made about sleep in the normal young adult on a conventional sleep-wake schedule with no sleep complaints (see Figure 1 for a hypnogram of a normal young adult):

- Sleep is entered through NREM.
- NREM and REM sleep alternate approximately every 90 minutes.
- Slow wave sleep predominates in the first third of the night and is linked to the initiation of sleep. REM sleep predominates in the last third of the night and is linked to the circadian rhythm of body temperature.
- Wakefulness within sleep generally takes up less than 5% of the night's sleep.
- About 75% of sleep is NREM, 20 to 25% REM in four to six discrete episodes.

FACTORS THAT AFFECT SLEEP PATTERNS

Age: The cyclic alternation of NREM-REM sleep has a period of 50 to 60 minutes in a newborn versus 90 minutes in the adult. Slow wave sleep is maximal in young children and decreases markedly with age.

TABLE 1: The Stages of Sleep in Adults

NREM Sleep	Stage	Features	% Sleep time
Characterized by: Decreased respiration rate/body temperature/blood pressure Frequent body motions Dreams absent Divided into four stages NREM sleep is usually 75–80% of sleep time.	1	Transition between sleep and wakefulness Low voltage, mixed frequency EEG	2–5%
	2	Light sleep; subject easily awakened Sleep spindles, K complexes on EEG	45–55%
	3	Slow wave or delta sleep High voltage, slow delta waves on EEG	3–8%
	4	Slow wave, deepest sleep Nocturnal terrors and sleepwalking are associated with stage 4 sleep	10–15%
REM Sleep			
Characterized by: Fluctuations in blood pressure/respiratory rate/body temperatures Dream sleep REM sleep is usually 20–25% of sleep time, occurring in 4–6 discrete episodes.			

Circadian Rhythms: The circadian stage at which sleep occurs affects the distribution of sleep stages. REM sleep in particular occurs with a circadian distribution that peaks in the morning hours coincident with the trough in body temperature. If sleep is delayed until the peak of the REM phase of the circadian rhythm (e.g., the early morning), REM sleep will tend to predominate and even occur at the onset of sleep. This reversal of sleep pattern is often seen in normal persons who undergo a phase shift from shift work or jet travel across several time zones.

Temperature: Extremes in temperature in the sleeping environment tend to disrupt sleep. REM sleep is more sensitive to temperature-related disruption than NREM sleep.

Drug Ingestion: Drugs that are prescribed for medical or psychiatric disorders may contribute to disturbed sleep (Tables 2 and 3). Benzodiazepines tend to suppress slow wave sleep and have no consistent effect on REM sleep. Tricyclic antidepressants (TCAs) and monoamine oxidase inhibitors (MAOIs) suppress REM sleep. Withdrawal from drugs that selectively suppress a sleep stage tends to be associated with rebound of that sleep stage. Acute withdrawal from benzodiazepines increases slow wave sleep. Withdrawal of TCAs and MAOIs increases REM sleep. Acute presleep alcohol intake results in REM suppression early in the night often followed by REM rebound in the later part of night as the alcohol is metabolized. The sleep pattern of an alcoholic is often characterized by frequent awakenings and decreased slow wave and REM sleep. When an alcoholic withdraws from alcohol, REM sleep occurs more frequently in the sleep cycle and for longer periods of time causing a REM rebound effect with insomnia and daytime sleepiness. Nicotine tends to increase sleep latency (time taken to fall asleep), and the duration of sleep decreases with increased use. Sleep patterns revert to normal after withdrawal from nicotine.

Medical and Psychiatric: Sleep disorders as well as conditions that cause pain, anxiety or discomfort (cardiovascular, pulmonary and endocrine disorders, gastrointestinal disease) have an impact on the structure and distribution of sleep. Narcolepsy is characterized by abnormally short delay to REM sleep, marked by sleep onset REM episodes. It is thought the dissociation of components of REM

FIGURE 1

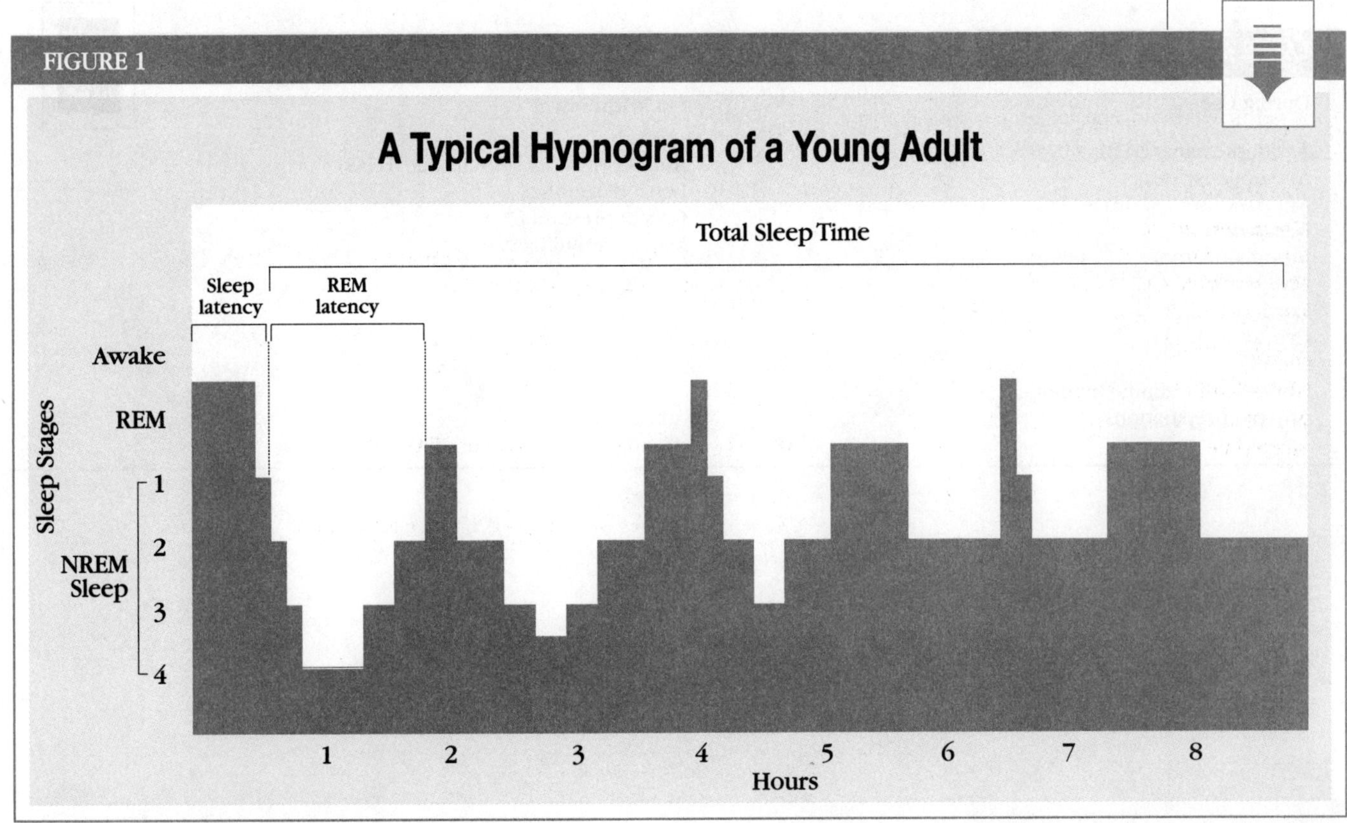

sleep into waking state results in hypnagogic (sleep inducing) hallucinations, sleep paralysis and cataplexy (see below). Sleep apnea may be associated with suppression of slow wave sleep or REM secondary to the sleep-related breathing problems. Suppression of slow wave sleep occurs more commonly in children with sleep apnea and REM suppression is more common in adult sleep apnea patients. Periodic movements during sleep, sleep apnea and chronic fibrositis may be associated with numerous arousals each night.

Psychosocial Factors: Difficulty initiating and maintaining sleep can be due to alterations in the patient's work status, finances and the loneliness caused by loss of a partner or friends. A change in residence due to extended visits with family, extended travel and hospitalization may be other causes.

TABLE 2: The Effect of Some Prescription Medications on Sleep Patterns

Medication	Effect on Sleep
Cimetidine Levodopa Methyldopa Phenytoin Theophylline Thyroid hormone	Delays the onset of sleep
Beta-blockers Quinidine-related agents Selegiline	Nightmares
Alcohol Nicotine, caffeine	Stimulant Frequent awakenings and disruption of sleep

TABLE 3: Prescription Medications That Can Disturb Sleep

During Use	On Withdrawal
Antidepressants (SSRIs) Anti-epilepsy drugs Antiparkinsonian drugs Beta-blockers Bronchodilators CNS stimulants Corticosteroids Cytotoxic drugs Diuretics Non-benzodiazepine hypnotics Thyroid preparations	Antidepressants (MAOIs and TCAs) Benzodiazepines CNS depressants Major tranquilizers

INSOMNIA

Insomnia can be defined broadly as the perception of insufficient or nonrestorative sleep despite an adequate opportunity to sleep. Jet lag, life-events, pain or underlying pathology (e.g., cancer) can cause insomnia (Table 4). It is a symptom rather than a disease, and the root cause must be fully explored.

PREVALENCE AND TYPES OF INSOMNIA

Most current studies rate the national incidence of insomnia in Canada and the United States at 30 to 35%. It affects both sexes, all ages, races and socioeconomic groups. It is more prevalent among women, older individuals, the divorced, widowed or separated, persons with chronic medical or psychiatric disorders, those with a history of alcohol or substance abuse, and those with multiple health problems. Basically, there are three broad categories of insomnia:

- Transient insomnia, which generally lasts only a few days, is often caused by jet lag or acute anxiety.
- Short-term insomnia, which typically lasts less than 3 weeks, is usually associated with self-limiting phenomena, such as grief, noise, or pain.
- Long-term or chronic insomnia, which lasts longer than 3 weeks, usually indicates some underlying pathology, e.g., major depression or rheumatoid arthritis.

SLEEP IN OLDER INDIVIDUALS

Contrary to popular belief, the requirement for sleep in adulthood does not decrease with age, but the circadian rhythm is affected, leading to decreased regulation of sleep. This may be caused by age-related changes in the brain, such as loss of neurons and a decrease in dendritic connections. Sleep therefore becomes redistributed over the 24-hour day. Older individuals spend more time in bed but less of that time asleep. With frequent daytime napping, total sleep time is often equal to that of younger people.

Older individuals most often complain of frequent awakenings, inability to return to sleep after these awakenings, early morning arousals, or a combination of these. Their insomnia is often a symptom of an underlying medical, psychiatric or pharmacological problem. They take many medications, prescribed and other, some of which may cause insomnia (Table 2). Alcohol, often used by these individuals as self-treatment for sleep, can cause frequent awakenings and disruption of sleep.

When an older individual complains of poor sleep, it is important to question them for possible causes. Pain from arthritis, duodenal ulcer and coronary artery disease may be sufficient to disrupt sleep on an ongoing basis. Neurological diseases, such as stroke and Parkinson's disease, may result in the patient being "cast" in an uncomfortable position leading to disturbed sleep.

TABLE 4: Causes of Insomnia

Pathology	*Medical conditions causing pain/discomfort:* rheumatoid arthritis, cancer, sleep apnea, hypothyroidism, chronic obstructive pulmonary disease, asthma, myoclonus, hypoglycemia, narcolepsy, Parkinson's disease, sclerosis, cardiovascular insufficiency and esophageal reflux. *Psychiatric disorders:* depression, schizophrenia, mania, dementia, obsessive compulsive disorder, anorexia nervosa and post traumatic stress disorder.
Substances	Caffeine, nicotine, alcohol, hypnotics, tranquilizers, prescription medications, substances of abuse
Circadian rhythm problems	Shift work, jet lag, delayed sleep phase syndrome, advanced sleep phase syndrome
Psychological factors	Stress, psychopathology, nightmares, inactivity, reinforcement for insomnia
Poor sleep environment	Noise, ambient temperature, light, sleeping surface, bedpartner
Poor sleep habits	Extended time in bed, naps and irregular schedule, bed as a cue for arousal

COUNSELLING TIPS

Insomnia in Older Individuals

- Provide information about the change in sleep patterns with age.
- Query the presence of psychiatric or medical causes of insomnia.
- Query drug-induced insomnia.
- Encourage good sleep hygiene:
  - Avoid the use of caffeine, nicotine or eating large meals before bedtime.
  - Delay onset of sleep time until after sleepiness occurs.
  - Exercise lightly every day.
  - Pursue special interests as well as quiet relaxing activities prior to bedtime.
  - Avoid daytime napping, but if needed, include in 24-hour sleep time.
- Provide reassurance.

Psychiatric causes include dementia that may lead to inversion of the sleep pattern: daytime sleep and nocturnal wakefulness. Nocturnal confusion and wandering may be seen as well. The sleep of Alzheimer's disease patients is marked by increased duration and frequency of awakenings as well as decreased slow wave and REM sleep. Depressed patients may have initial, middle or terminal insomnia, although early-morning awakening is the most common. Anxiety is generally associated with difficulty falling asleep.

CAFFEINE-INDUCED INSOMNIA

Caffeine is the most widely and regularly-used psychoactive substance in the world. Canadian statistics suggest that 80% of the population consumes coffee and that the daily per capita consumption is about 2 cups per day. More than a quarter of the adult population drinks 5 or more cups of coffee per day and 5% drinks at least 7 cups per day. Caffeine is present in many prescription and nonprescription medications and is used for the central nervous system stimulating effects, vascular headache relief or to enhance the effect of analgesics (Table 5).

Caffeine consumed 30 to 60 minutes before bedtime may cause delayed sleep onset, diminished sleep times, reduce the average depth of sleep, alter the normal patterns of sleep, increase early REM sleep (when most dreaming occurs), but may reduce late REM sleep. The number of awakenings also increases. These effects appear to be dose-dependent. More nondrinkers of coffee than habitual heavy drinkers of coffee report an increase in latency and a decrease in sleep quality after drinking coffee before bedtime. Caffeine clearance is significantly affected by concurrent drug use, smoking and pregnancy. Clearance is increased by smoking and decreased by pregnancy. Caffeine does not, however, reverse the effects of alcohol on the nervous system.

CAFFEINISM

Reported at doses of 1 g and greater (more than 10 cups of coffee), caffeinism is characterized by anxiety, irritability, agitation, hyperexcitability, tremulousness, dizziness, headache and muscle twitches. Tolerance to the effects of caffeine can

TABLE 5: Nonprescription Products Containing More Than 50 mg Caffeine

Products	Caffeine (mg) per dose/formulation
Alert	100 mg
Cafergot preparations	100 mg
Ergodryl preparations	100 mg
Excedrin preparations	65 mg
Gravergol capsules	100 mg
Instantine preparations	64.8 mg
Megral tablets	100 mg
Midol Multi-Symptom	60 mg
Norgesic Forte	60 mg
Wake-up tablets	100 mg
Wigraine tablets	100 mg

occur, but the overuse of caffeine-containing foods and beverages can result in insomnia.

Pregnant women should be counselled against the use of nonprescription products containing caffeine, and they should limit caffeine consumption. Children are very sensitive to the effects of caffeine. Their diets preferably should not include tea and coffee, and they should be encouraged to limit other caffeine-containing products like chocolate and colas (Table 6).

MANAGEMENT

Nonpharmacological Management

When the patient complains of insomnia it is important to question him/her for possible causes/contributing factors (see Patient Assessment Questions).

Before advising an individual on the proper use of nonprescription sleep-aid preparations, the Principles of Good Sleep Hygiene should be reinforced.

A number of nonpharmacological treatments have been found useful in insomnia, including progressive muscle relaxation, biofeedback techniques, bright light therapy, hypnosis and meditation. Insufficient data are available to offer clear guidelines for use.

Principles of Good Sleep Hygiene

- Establish a regular sleep-wake routine. Wind down activities before bedtime.
- Sleep and wake up at same time including weekends. Engage in regular, moderate exercise early in day.
- Reserve bedroom for sleep-related activities only. Do not read, watch TV or eat in bed.
- Improve sleep environment. Minimize noise and light. Avoid extremes in temperature.
- Avoid or minimize caffeine (tea, coffee, colas), alcohol, nicotine.
- Do not go to bed feeling hungry. Eat foods containing tryptophan such as milk or tuna before bedtime.

TABLE 6: Caffeine Content of Some Foods and Beverages

Product	Caffeine (mg)
Coffees (per 150 mL)	
Percolated	75–140
Instant	60-90
Decaffeinated	2-6
Filter drip	110-280
Teas (per 150 mL)	
Herbal	25–140
Regular	45–110
Iced	30-80
Soft Drinks/Colas (per 350 mL)	
Coca Cola	33
Ginger Ale	0
Mountain Dew	54
Pepsi Cola	38
Seven Up	0
Tab	32
Cocoa Products	
Cocoa (hot) 240 mL	50
Baking chocolate 30 g	25-35
Chocolate bar 30 g	3-6
Chocolate milk (225 mL)	27

Pharmacological Management

Both nonprescription and prescription sedative/hypnotics are available. Sedative/hypnotics should be used only when nonpharmacologic measures have failed, and other causes for insomnia have been ruled out. Nonprescription sedative/hypnotics are usually used to reduce the latency period. They should be used in conjunction with good sleep hygiene. There is consensus in the current literature that available sleep aids or nonprescription sedatives are of little value in treating insomnia. Patients who appear to warrant medical or psychiatric attention should be referred to a physician.

The Management of Insomnia

History

- Sleep hygiene
- Social habits—smoking, alcohol, caffeine consumption
- Sleep-wake pattern
- Medical/neurological diagnosis
- Psychiatric/behavior/mood disturbances
- Medication taken

Sequence of advice

- Sleep hygiene
- Referral to appropriate service for psychotherapy
- Psychotherapy goals:
  - Stress management
  - Improve emotional expression
  - Improve insight
  - Improve interpersonal relationships
  - Restructure lifestyle
- Specific measures under medical supervision:
  - Treatment of withdrawal states from drugs and alcohol
  - Treatment of medical and psychiatric causes of insomnia
- Pharmacological treatment as appropriate

Jet Lag

Symptoms of jet lag

- Daytime fatigue
- Inability to sleep at night in new time zone
- Difficulty concentrating
- Headaches
- Loss of appetite, upset stomach
- Irregular bowel movements
- Lightheadedness

Unproven but widely recommended treatments

- Increase hydration (air in plane is dry)
- Exercise—walking about during flight (especially relevant for pregnant and obese passengers)
- Short-acting hypnotic—triazolam in doses of 0.125 mg (preferably tried before flight to identify side effects and adjust doses—amnesia has been reported)
- Maintain social cues at destination—eat, sleep according to local time
- Exposure to bright light
- Dietary modification
  - timed caffeine intake—for overnight eastward flight avoid before and during flight, near arrival black coffee advances body clock
  - for westward flight avoid caffeine altogether
  - high carbohydrate diet (starch or sugars) on overnight eastward flight is thought to stimulate release of sleep-inducing neurotransmitters (serotonin) and on arrival a protein-rich breakfast (bacon and eggs) is thought to stimulate release of neurotransmitters to induce alertness
- Melatonin tablets (experimental—melatonin excretion from pineal gland normally increases at night and decreases during the day)

OTHER SLEEP DISORDERS

NARCOLEPSY

Excessive daytime sleepiness and cataplexy are the two most common symptoms of narcolepsy. Other symptoms include abnormal sleep, overwhelming episodes of sleep, hypnagogic hallucinations, disturbed nocturnal sleep and sleep paralysis. A chronic, genetically based disorder, narcolepsy is found in 1 in 5,000 to 10,000 in Europe and North America. Narcoleptic sleepiness differs from normal sleepiness in that it is not fully relieved by any amount of sleep.

Cataplexy is a muscular weakness usually brought on by excitement or emotion and is virtually unique to narcolepsy. It is frequently precipitated by laughter, other forms of emotion or athletic activities. Most typically the jaw sags, the head falls forward, arms drop to the sides and knees unlock.

Sleep paralysis can be defined as brief episodes of inability to move during the onset of sleep and on awakening.

Hypnagogic hallucinations are vivid dreamlike experiences that occur as the person is falling asleep. They may be visual, auditory or tactile.

Patients who complain of these typical symptoms of narcolepsy should be referred to a physician.

SLEEP APNEA

Defined as cessation of breathing for 10 seconds or more, it can occur 30 or more times during a 7-hour period of sleep. Daytime symptoms such as excessive sleepiness, impairment of intellectual performance, personality changes, psychiatric disturbances and morning headache may occur. Nocturnal symptoms include snoring, gasping, snorting sounds, excessive body movements, diaphoresis (excessive sweating) and enuresis. Systemic hypertension is a common consequence of sleep apnea. The hypoxia and carbon monoxide retention associated with nocturnal apneic episodes may contribute to the development of polycythemia (increase in total red cell mass of the blood) and the cardiovascular complications of pulmonary hypertension, cardiomegaly, right-sided heart failure and persistent cardiac arrhythmias.

The typical sleep apnea sufferer is an overweight, middle-aged man who snores heavily, has hypertension and is prone to daytime sleepiness. Referral to a physician is important because of the deleterious effects on the cardiovascular system and probable increased risk of death.

PATIENT ASSESSMENT QUESTIONS

Q What is your normal pattern of sleep? How long have you had this problem? How often does this occur? Occasionally? Regularly?
Transient insomnia is appropriate for self-medication with nonprescription sleep aids. Chronic insomnia may be due to an underlying pathology and requires referral to a physician.

Q What sort of sleep difficulties are you experiencing? Falling asleep? Staying asleep? Early morning awakening?
Nonprescription sleep aids are effective in decreasing the time it takes to fall asleep. They will not be effective for midsleep awakening or early morning awakening.

Q Have you been experiencing pain, worry, stress? Any work or family-related problems that could possibly relate to your sleep problems?
Some problems may cause secondary insomnia. If you are able to identify the reason for the insomnia, you should first try to eliminate it.

Q Do you suffer from any physical or emotional illness?
Certain medical conditions are often accompanied by insomnia. These include cardiovascular disorders, pulmonary disorders, gastrointestinal disease and endocrine disorders. Drugs prescribed for medical and psychiatric disorders may also contribute to disturbed sleep.

Q Do you drink cola beverages, coffee or tea? Are you taking any medications that contain caffeine?
Cola beverages, coffee, tea and certain medications may contain significant amounts of caffeine. Caffeine is a stimulant and can affect your sleep patterns, especially if consumed in large amounts. Caffeine-containing products should not be consumed for several hours before bedtime.

Q Has your bedpartner noticed that you are restless or snoring during sleep? Are you depressed, sleepy or irritable during the day?
Before trying a nonprescription sleep aid, you should consult your physician. A sleep aid may only aggravate the symptoms.

Q Does anyone else in your family have the same sleep problems?
The actual period of sleep required is to some extent genetically determined.

Q Is there anything that helps your problem? Exercise? Prescription or nonprescription sleeping pills?
The effectiveness of previous treatments may help you to determine an appropriate therapy.

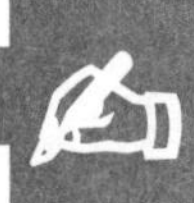

Resource List

Emotional support for persons with sleep disorders and their relatives can be provided by contacting the national office of Sleep-Wake Disorders Canada:

3089 Bathurst Street, Suite #304
Toronto, ON M6A 2A4
(416) 787-5374 Fax (416) 787-4431

or regional offices at:
Vancouver/Burnaby, BC (604) 433-8467;
Calgary, AB (403) 282-4623;
Edmonton, AB (403) 467-2411;
Montreal, PQ (French) (514) 486-1030;
(English) (514) 697-2041;
Saint John, NB (506) 633-4636.

PHARMACEUTICAL AGENTS

Nonprescription sedatives usually contain antihistamines as the active ingredient. These can sometimes cause significant delirium due to excessive sedation, especially in older individuals, who are often taking other sedating and anticholinergic drugs.

Diphenhydramine

Diphenhydramine is a potent antihistamine of the ethanolamine group with a high incidence of sedative and anticholinergic effects. Other side effects include dizziness, disturbed coordination and muscle weakness. Diphenhydramine should be administered with caution to patients with convulsive disorders. Diphenhydramine should be used with caution in narrow angle glaucoma, stenosing peptic ulcer, pyloroduodenal obstruction, bladder neck obstruction, prostatic hypertrophy and cardiovascular disease, because of the anticholinergic side effects. Also, concomitant use of medications that are highly anticholinergic, such as antidepressants, antipsychotics, benztropine or oxybutynin, may result in additive effects.

The CNS depressant effects of diphenhydramine are enhanced by other CNS depressants including barbiturates, antidepressants, antipsychotics, anxiolytics and alcohol.

Diphenhydramine should not be recommended as a sleep aid to pregnant women, or women who are likely to become pregnant. The drug's side effect, dizziness, could be a problem and there have been case reports of withdrawal in neonates: tremors and diarrhea. Diphenhydramine has been listed under Risk Category C in Drugs in Pregnancy and Lactation, Briggs et al. Risk category C is defined as: Either studies in animals have revealed adverse effects on the fetus (teratogenic or embryocidal or other) and there are no controlled studies in women, or studies in women and animals are not available. Drugs should only be given if the potential benefit justifies the potential risk to the fetus.

L-Tryptophan

L-Tryptophan is an essential amino acid that is ingested daily in amounts of 1 to 2 g in the normal diet. L-Tryptophan has been advocated as a "natural sedative/hypnotic" presumably relatively free of toxicity. It is converted in the body to serotonin, which is a sleep-inducing neurotransmitter. Foods rich in tryptophan include milk and tuna, hence the recommendation of a glass of warm milk and a tuna sandwich before bedtime as a sleep aid.

Stimulant Products

Nonprescription stimulant products contain caffeine as the active ingredient and are classified as stay-awake or stimulant products. A number of nonprescription analgesic products contain caffeine and are used by consumers to self-treat sleep problems (consult product labelling). The caffeine content of some foods and beverages commonly used can be found in Table 6. Users of these products should be advised of the effects of caffeinism: anxiety, irritability, agitation, hyperexcitability, tremulousness, dizziness, headache and muscle twitches.

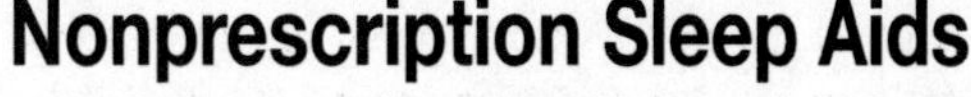

Nonprescription Sleep Aids

- Insomnia is generally a temporary, self-limiting condition, frequently caused by change in location, daily schedule or stress. In some cases it may be caused by a medical condition or drugs you are taking.
- Nonprescription sleep aids may cause drowsiness. Use caution when driving a car or operating machinery. Avoid concurrent use of alcohol and other drugs that can cause drowsiness.
- If you have persistent insomnia, contact your physician. It can be an indication of underlying disease.
- If you are pregnant or nursing, consult your physician.
- Use only for a short period of time. If you have chronic insomnia, consult your physician.

RECOMMENDED READING

Aldridge MS. Review: narcolepsy. N Engl J Med 1990;323:389-93.

Carskadon MA. Normal human sleep: an overview. In: Kryger MH, Roth T, Dement WC, eds. Principles and Practice of Sleep Medicine. Philadelphia: Saunders, 1994:16-25.

Filingim JM. Insomnia: diagnosis and treatment in general practice. Drug Ther 1992;3:77-93.

Gillin JC, Byerley WF. The diagnosis and management of insomnia. N Engl J Med 1990;322: 239-48.

Guilleminault C. Narcolepsy syndrome. In: Kryger MH, Roth T, Dement WC, eds. Principles and Practice of Sleep Medicine. Philadelphia: Saunders, 1994:549-61.

Leonard BE. Drug treatment of insomnia. In: Fundamentals of Psychopharmacology. Chichester: John Wiley and Sons, 1993:113-22.

Mendelson WB. Insomnia and related sleep disorders (review). Psychiatr Clin North Am 1993; 16(4):841-51.

Monane M. Insomnia in the elderly. J Clin Psychiatry 1992;53(6 suppl):23-28.

Raebel MA, Black J. The caffeine controversy. What are the facts? Hosp Pharm 1984;19:257-67.

Zorzitto ML. Sleep in the elderly. Mod Med Can 1983;38(1):77-82.

23

SMOKING CESSATION PRODUCTS

MELANIE RANTUCCI

CONTENTS

Introduction 597
- Epidemiology
- Harmful Components of Tobacco
- Health Risks
- Environmental Tobacco Smoke (ETS)
- Drug Interactions

The Smoking Habit 600
- Physical Addiction
- Psychological Addiction

Smoking Cessation 602
- Counselling
- Nonpharmacological Treatment
- Pharmacological Treatment

Pharmaceutical Agents 609

Recommended Reading 611

INTRODUCTION

Many gimmicks as well as legitimate programs and products have been used to help smokers quit, with variable success. Because they are highly regarded and trusted, the advice and guidance of a health professional can greatly enhance the chances of success in a smoking cessation program. Moreover, Canadians generally have contact with a doctor, nurse or pharmacist at least once a year.

A recent study found that 40% of smokers had tried to quit in the past year. Yet the general public is still largely uninformed about the damaging effects of smoking, the benefits of quitting, and how to go about it. Health professionals have the knowledge to explain the risks of smoking and provide information about how to quit and the products that can help.

EPIDEMIOLOGY

An estimated 5.4 million people in Canada smoke: 26% of Canadians over the age of 15 reported smoking daily in 1991. While the percentage of the population that smokes is declining (down from 41% in 1966), more young Canadians and more women are smoking. At present, men aged 20 to 44 are the largest group; in 1983 it was men aged 25 to 44. Although women aged 20 to 44 are almost as likely to smoke as men in this group (29 versus 32%), more women than men in the 15 to 19 age group now smoke (20 versus 12%). Statistics Canada predicts that smoking will be more prevalent among women than men within the next 5 years.

Education and employment status are related to the tendency to smoke. The unemployed and people with lower levels of education and low job status are more likely to smoke (Canadians with university education are half as likely to smoke as those with high school education or less).

HARMFUL COMPONENTS OF TOBACCO

There are more than 4,000 chemicals in tobacco smoke, many known to affect body functions. In the gaseous phase, the chemicals include aldehydes, alcohols, ammonia, carbon dioxide, carbon monoxide, creosols, cyanides, nitrogen oxides, volatile nitrosamines, volatile sulfur-containing compounds, volatile hydrocarbons and ketones. The particulate matter is comprised of water, nicotine and tar. The tar consists mainly of polycyclic aromatic hydrocarbons, including many documented carcinogens such as nonvolatile nitrosamines and benzapyrene. The tar also contains metallic ions and several radioactive compounds such as polonium 210.

The nicotine in tobacco smoke can affect the heart by increasing cardiac workload. The pharmacological actions of nicotine are complex: it affects a variety of neuroeffector junctions and has both stimulant and depressant mechanisms of action. For example, in small doses, nicotine stimulates autonomic ganglia, but in large doses it results in blockage of the ganglia. Effects on blood pressure and heart rate may also be stimulatory or depressive. In addition, effects may be seen on the central nervous system (respiratory depression), gastrointestinal tract (nausea, vomiting), and the exocrine glands (stimulation followed by inhibition of salivary and bronchial secretions). These vary according to the degree of tolerance to nicotine.

The carbon monoxide inhaled in tobacco smoke is also a significant contributor to heart disease.

HEALTH RISKS

Smoking is the single most common preventable cause of death and disability in Canada. A recent study linked tobacco to 1 in 5 deaths in Canada. Some of the more important health risks associated with smoking are listed below:

- Smoking accounts for about 30% of all cancer-related deaths. Cancer of the lung, pancreas, kidney, bladder, lip, oral cavity and pharynx, esophagus and larynx are all increased, 2 to 27 times for smokers compared with nonsmokers.
- Smokers have been found to have lower serum ascorbic acid than nonsmokers (25% lower in those smoking less than 20 cigarettes daily and 40% lower in those smoking more than 20 cigarettes daily) and need twice as much vitamin C.
- Smokers have 2 to 4 times higher risk of coronary artery disease, and a 1.5 higher risk of cerebral thrombosis.
- Oxidants in smoke particles and migration of inflammatory cells to the lung tissue lead to chronic obstructive lung disease from reduced ciliary function and an increase in mucus production by goblet cells.
- Smoking in pregnant women has been linked to lower birth weight infants (200 g on average) and a 25 to 50% increase in fetal and infant deaths.
- Smoking increases oral diseases such as leukoplakia (white patches on oral mucosa), smoker's palate, impaired gingival bleeding, periodontitis and ulcerative gingivitis.
- Delayed wound healing has been observed, possibly from cutaneous vasoconstriction, increased platelet adhesiveness and diminished proliferation of red blood cells, macrophages and fibroblasts.
- Chronic smokers have been found to have insulin resistance, with a recent study showing higher steady-state plasma glucose concentrations in smokers compared with nonsmokers in spite of similar steady-state plasma insulin concentrations.
- Smoking can cause wrinkles, bad breath, stained teeth and fingers.

Many of the physical effects of smoking are reversed when smokers quit (Table 1). There are immediate benefits to blood pressure, heart rate, and carbon monoxide and oxygen levels in the blood. Reductions in the risks of cancer and heart disease occur over 1, 5, 10 and even 15 years after quitting (after 15 years, the risk of dying is similar to that of a person who has never smoked).

ENVIRONMENTAL TOBACCO SMOKE (ETS)

ETS (or secondhand smoke) also puts the friends and family of smokers at risk. In 1989, 333 deaths in Canada were directly attributed to ETS. Effects include eye and throat irritation, coughing, rhinitis, headaches and various types of cancer, particularly lung cancer. ETS has been repeatedly linked to respiratory problems in infants and young children of parents who smoke. In addition, children with recurrent acute otitis media have been found to be twice as likely to come from homes where ETS is present.

DRUG INTERACTIONS

The various components of tobacco smoke may induce alterations in drug absorption, distribution, metabolism, excretion and effectiveness. The predominant action of tobacco smoke on drug action appears to be mediated through hepatic microsomal enzyme induction. Smokers may require larger doses or more frequent administration of many drugs such as theophylline, imipramine, estrogens, warfarin and certain analgesics to main-

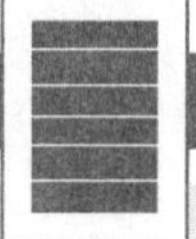

TABLE 1: Health Benefits of Quitting Smoking

Immediate Benefits	**Benefits After 5 Years of Quitting**
Within 20 minutes, blood pressure, heart rate and temperature of hands and feet become normal	Cancers of the oral cavity and esophagus risk drops 50%
After 8 hours, CO and oxygen levels in the blood return to normal	Risk of bladder cancer reduced by about 50%
Women who stop smoking before becoming pregnant have infants of the same birth weight as those born to someone who never smoked	Risk of stroke can return to the level of those who never smoked
	Benefits After 10 Years of Quitting
	Lung cancer risk drops 30–50%
Benefit After 1 Year of Quitting	**Benefits After 15 Years of Quitting**
Excess risk of coronary heart disease (CHD) reduced by half	Risk of CHD is similar to a person who has never smoked
	Risk of dying is similar to a person who has never smoked

Adapted with permission from: Butting out for life. A smoking cessation program for pharmacists. Laval, PQ: Merrell Dow Pharmaceuticals (Canada) Inc., 1993. The health benefits of smoking cessation: A report of the Surgeon General. Washington, DC: U.S. Department of Health and Human Services, Public Health Service, Center for Chronic Disease Prevention and Health Promotion, Office on Smoking and Health, 1990. DHHS publication no. (CDC) 90–8416.

tain therapeutic blood levels. Few studies have evaluated the effects of smoking on drug therapy, and the variability of the quantity and quality of smoke inhaled by individuals would make conclusions difficult to draw. Nevertheless, it has been suggested that smoking may:

- alter the integrity of the gastric mucosal barrier to peptic acid corrosion, or reduce alkaline pancreatic secretions, thereby interfering with the effect of H_2-antagonists and antacids;
- modify the efficacy of central nervous system drugs through lessened sedation;
- affect insulin absorption through reduced blood flow to the skin; and
- affect the efficacy of cardiovascular drugs and increase the risks of cardiovascular side effects of other drugs (e.g., increased risks for a smoker using oral contraceptives).

THE SMOKING HABIT

Tobacco dependency is defined as the inability to discontinue tobacco use despite awareness of medical consequences. This dependency involves physical, psychological and social factors.

PHYSICAL ADDICTION

Nicotine causes the physical addiction to smoking. The Surgeon General of the United States and the Health Protection Branch of Health Canada recognize smoking as a drug addiction.

As with other addictive substances, tolerance develops. There is a craving for continued use, a tendency to increase use, and profound physical and psychological symptoms elicited by withdrawal. Nicotine addiction is so strong that opiate addicts and alcoholics claim it is easier to do without these substances than cigarettes.

When smokers attempt to quit, they often feel the effects of nicotine withdrawal, including craving for nicotine, irritability, anxiety, difficulty concentrating, confusion, tremor and increased coughing (Table 2). Withdrawal symptoms generally begin 2 to 24 hours after the last cigarette and peak at 72 to 96 hours, although rebound withdrawal can occur several weeks after complete abstinence. The craving symptoms of withdrawal may continue for many years. There is a relationship between the severity of withdrawal symptoms and the level of nicotine intake, but it is weak and unreliable.

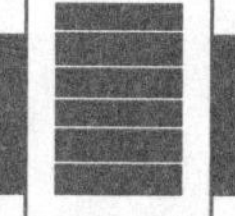

TABLE 2: Organic and Mental Effects of Nicotine Withdrawal
Severe urges to smoke or cravings for nicotine
Irritability, anxiety, restlessness, impatience
Difficulty concentrating
Difficulty sleeping or restlessness
Drowsiness
Increased hunger and eating
Gastrointestinal symptoms
Headaches
Light-headedness, dizziness, sweating and tremor

Adapted from: Hughes JR, Hatsukami D. Signs and Symptoms of tobacco withdrawal. Arch Gen Psych 1986;43:289–94.

PSYCHOLOGICAL ADDICTION

The psychological habit of smoking is a result of the repetitive nature of smoking. A behavioral conditioning results from the hand-to-mouth ritual with each cigarette. This behavior is repeated 250 times a day, or more than 90,000 times a year for a "pack-a-day" smoker, multiplied by the number of years of smoking. As well, the use of cigarettes in specific situations such as stress or emotional crisis adds to the psychological addiction.

The pleasure of smoking is also a positive reinforcement of the habit. Nicotine appears to produce euphoria or a "high" similar to that produced by some other addictive psychomotor stimulants. Within 7 seconds of puffing on a cigarette, nicotine is delivered directly to the brain. Smokers can self-regulate the positive effects of smoking by varying the rate of smoking, the depth of each inhalation and the amount of time they hold the smoke in the lungs. Once addicted, smokers continue to smoke to reduce the unpleasantness of withdrawal, as well as to alleviate the unpleasant moods produced by stressors.

Smoking is further reinforced by specific social situations: many smokers have a cigarette after a meal, while talking on the phone, or immediately on awakening. These acts occur repeatedly day after day. Friends and relatives may also smoke, making the habit more socially acceptable.

The weight gain associated with smoking cessation results from increased hunger and eating and is a reinforcement to continue smoking. An individual's "set point" body weight is suppressed by smoking (due to the acute metabolic effects of smoking). A subsequent weight gain (on average 1.8 kg) associated with smoking cessation is apparently a return to normal body weight rather than increased eating or hunger. This may be a psychological reinforcement to continue smoking in some people. One study of teen smokers found that both male and female smokers were more likely than nonsmokers to use diet pills, go on crash diets, use laxatives and make themselves vomit to keep weight off, suggesting that this age group may smoke because of weight-related concerns. However, another study of male and female adults in a quit-smoking program found that weight gain did not play a significant role in promoting initial smoking relapses.

The Smoking Habit

The physical and psychological addictions to smoking make the difficulty of quitting understandable. A recent study found that 40% of smokers had tried to quit in the previous year. Unfortunately, few smokers (20%, at most) succeed on their first or second attempt, and up to 60% may make 7 or more attempts. Relapse is very common after varying periods of abstinence up to 10 years, although most smokers are completely abstinent after 2 years.

Studies of the relationship between the demographic, behavioral, and health-related factors and smoking cessation indicate that the strongest predictors of smoking cessation are health related such as recent hospitalization and development of coronary heart disease. Diagnosis of cancer or changes in pulmonary function appear to have little effect.

Smoking cessation rates do not seem to differ by gender or age, although some studies have suggested that women may have a more difficult time quitting. Smoking cessation rates may be directly related to age when smoking was started and inversely related to the extent of daily cigarette use before attempting to quit.

SMOKING CESSATION

A recent analysis of 633 studies of smoking cessation concluded that on average, 6.4% of smokers could be expected to quit the habit without any intervention. Overall, for people using self-help methods (including nonprescription products) and various smoking cessation programs, the one-year success rate ranges from 8 to 25%. A combination of methods, particularly behavioral intervention with pharmacological therapy, appears to be the most successful.

COUNSELLING

Many smokers know the hazards of smoking but tend to dissociate themselves ("It happens to other people, not necessarily me."), so scare tactics will not work. Most smokers have tried unsuccessfully to quit before and need to know there is support available if they have a relapse. Smoking cessation counselling must therefore involve a number of specific approaches.

Preparing for Smoking Cessation Counselling

Smoking cessation counselling requires the health professional to be motivated and committed; have knowledge of the dynamics of quitting smoking and how to help the patient; and a practice environment consistent with smoking cessation.

A health professional simply discussing smoking cessation with patients can really make a difference. Studies show that a health professional offering to help patients stop smoking and providing encouragement through a 2- to 3-minute discussion can account for approximately 5 to 6% of the smokers who will have stopped smoking at the end of 1 year.

Opportunities for the health professional to discuss smoking cessation may arise from direct requests from the patient about ways to quit or about specific products for quitting; from concerns voiced by patients about their smoking habit; or as part of a medical history interview. Patients who are at greatest risk from smoking or environmental tobacco smoke because of their condition or because of the drug they are receiving can be identified as priorities for smoking cessation counselling. Some of these high-risk conditions are listed in Table 3.

In preparation, the health professional must become knowledgeable about the physical, psychological, and social factors of smoking and the dynamics of quitting to recognize areas to target during smoking cessation counselling. Knowledge of counselling techniques for each of the factors affecting smoking cessation is also needed.

The physical environment is important. No-smoking signs should be posted and a no-smoking policy enforced. Posters, displays and lapel buttons can further indicate commitment. Patient educational materials should be available and calendars used to help patients select a "stop date" to start their program.

Smoking Cessation Counselling Techniques

Current smoking cessation counselling programs use a strategy based on three simple steps: Ask, Advise, and Assist. There are three main factors involved in the smoking habit (physical, psychological and social), each needs to be addressed during each of these steps (Figure 1).

Ask the Patient

The first task is to identify the patient's risk due to a medical condition and smoking or environmental tobacco smoke (Table 3). Ask a high-risk patient whether he or she, or any family members smoke:

ASK: *"Your condition/your spouse's condition/your child's condition can be made worse by smoking or second-hand smoke. Do you or a family member smoke?"*

Secure a commitment from the patient to attempt to quit, and show a commitment to help. This is important in dealing with the psychological and social factors involved in the smoking habit.

ASK: *"I may be able to help you stop smoking. Would you be interested in stopping with my help?"*

Advise the Patient

Advice to the patient to quit smoking can have a considerable effect on the patient's decision to quit now or in the future. If the patient is not ready to quit smoking, still offer the advice.

FIGURE 1

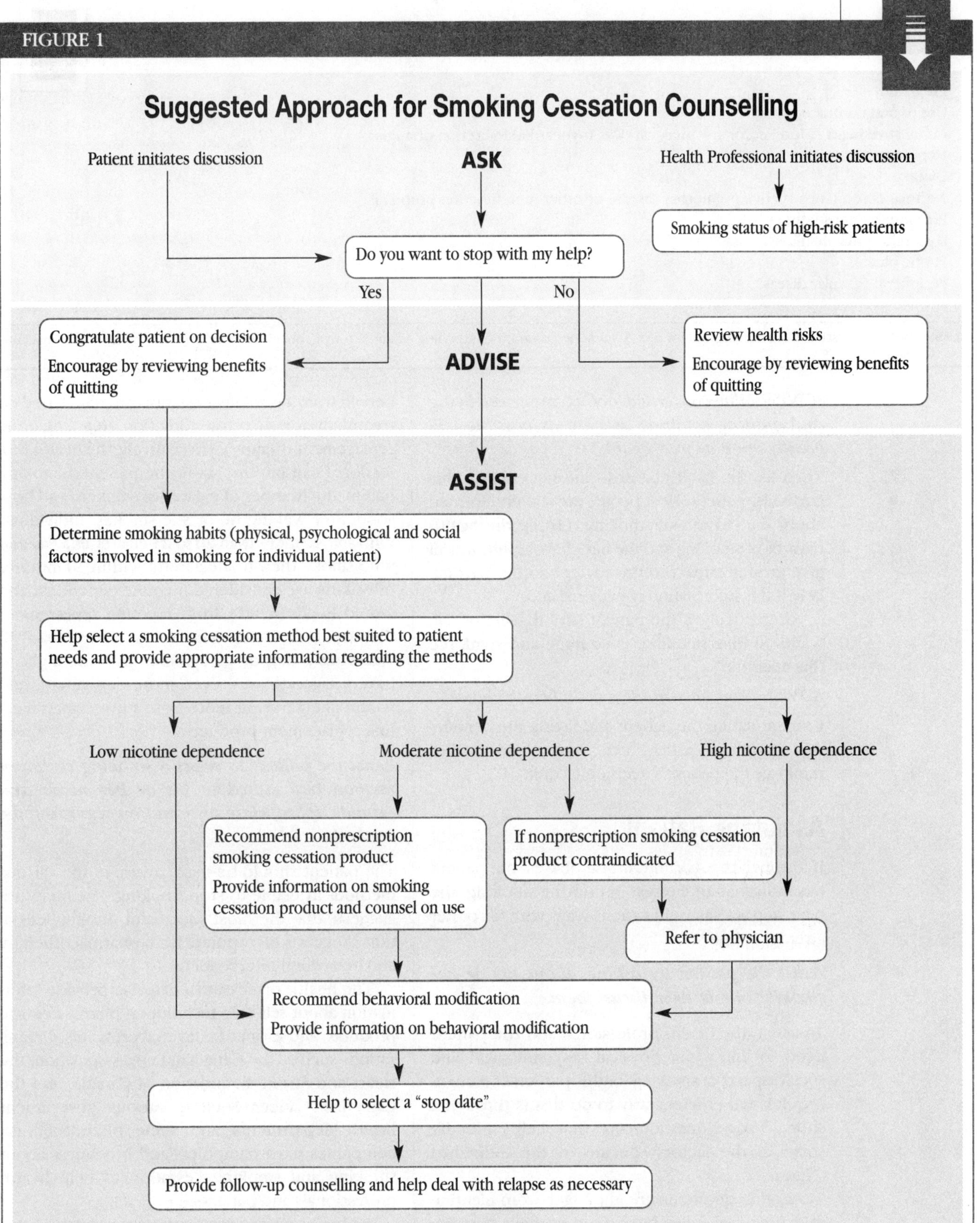

Adapted with permission from: Butting out for life. A smoking cessation counselling program for pharmacists. Laval, PQ: Merrell Dow Pharmaceuticals (Canada) Inc. 1993.

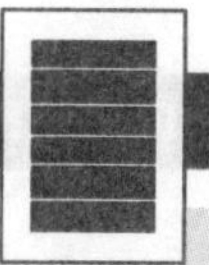

TABLE 3: Conditions Where Smoking Presents a High Risk for Patients

Pregnancy
Use of oral contraceptives
Congestive heart failure, coronary artery disease, myocardial infarction or angina
Hypertension
Diabetes
Asthma, chronic obstructive pulmonary disease or other lung function problems
Pre-surgery (anesthetics)
Hypercholesterolemia
Peptic ulcer
Peripheral vascular disease

Adapted with permission from: Butting out for life. A smoking cessation counselling program for pharmacists. Laval, PQ: Merrell Dow Pharmaceuticals (Canada) Inc., 1993.

ADVISE: *"I'm concerned about your well-being and quitting smoking as soon as possible will greatly improve your health."*

Then list the health hazards and benefits for this particular patient. Most people are still uninformed about the hazards of smoking. Listing the health hazards of smoking and the benefits of quitting will give greater impact to the advice to quit, particularly if this information is personalized.

Alternatively, if the patient says that he or she wants to quit smoking, encourage and reinforce this decision:

ADVISE: *"You have made a good health choice."*

Congratulating the patient and listing the benefits that particular patient can expect can further reinforce the patient's decision to quit.

Assist the Patient

If, through the *Ask* and *Advise* phases, the patient has indicated an interest in quitting smoking, the next step is to assist in various ways with his or her attempt to quit.

Assist the patient by asking about his or her smoking habits, then discuss them.

To assist, the health professional and the patient need to know the physical, psychological and social aspects of smoking for this particular patient. A quick and efficient way to do this is through a short, 1-page questionnaire that helps identify some of the factors specific to the individual (Figure 2).

Another questionnaire, the Fagerström nicotine tolerance scale, has been used to help patients determine the severity of their nicotine addiction. The score indicates whether a patient would benefit from a smoking cessation program based on treatment for nicotine addiction (e.g., nicotine replacement therapy). Alternatively, the health professional can inquire about the patient's smoking habits, the number of cigarettes smoked, and how soon after waking he or she smokes. Individuals who smoke more than 20 to 25 cigarettes a day and who smoke their first cigarette within 30 minutes of waking are considered nicotine dependent and would likely benefit from nicotine replacement therapy. Individuals who smoke more than 30 cigarettes a day, or who wake up in the night to have a cigarette, are even more dependent, and would likely benefit more from a prescribed nicotine replacement product.

Assist the patient to select a smoking cessation method best suited to his or her needs and provide appropriate information regarding the methods.

The patient should be made aware of the various methods available to stop smoking. The literature suggests that the most successful smoking cessation programs incorporate both pharmacotherapy and behavioral interventions.

The health professional can also provide information about self-help techniques, pharmaceutical products, and various behavioral programs. Organizations such as the Canadian Lung Association, the Heart and Stroke Foundation of Canada, and the Canadian Cancer Society, various government health departments and some pharmaceutical companies have pamphlets and brochures about smoking and smoking cessation to help health professionals and patients.

A physician's involvement is appropriate at this point if it appears the patient would benefit most from prescribed nicotine replacement therapy, or

FIGURE 2: The Why Test

The Why Test

Next to the following statements, mark the number that best describes your own experience.

1=Never 2=Rarely 3=Once in a while
4=Most of the time 5=Always

____ A. I smoke to keep myself from slowing down.

____ B. Handling a cigarette is part of the enjoyment of smoking it.

____ C. Smoking is pleasant and relaxing.

____ D. I light up a cigarette when I feel angry about something.

____ E. When I'm out of cigarettes, it's near-torture until I can get them.

____ F. I smoke automatically, without even being aware of it.

____ G. I smoke when other people around me are smoking.

____ H. I smoke to perk myself up.

____ I. Part of enjoying smoking is preparing to light up.

____ J. I get pleasure from smoking.

____ K. When I feel uncomfortable or upset, I light up a cigarette.

____ L. I'm very much aware of it when I'm not smoking a cigarette.

____ M. I often light up a cigarette while one is still burning in the ashtray.

____ N. I smoke cigarettes with friends when I'm having a good time.

____ O. When I smoke, part of my enjoyment is watching the smoke as I exhale it.

____ P. I want a cigarette most often when I am comfortable and relaxed.

____ Q. I smoke when I'm "blue" and want to take my mind off what's bothering me.

____ R. I get a real craving for a cigarette when I haven't had one in a while.

____ S. I've found a cigarette in my mouth and haven't remembered that it was there.

____ T. I always smoke when I'm out with friends at a party, bar, etc.

____ U. I smoke cigarettes to get a lift.

The Why Test Score Card

Write the number you put beside each letter in the Why Test beside the same letter below. For example, if you marked a "3" beside question "C" on the test, put a "3" beside the letter "C" below. Then, add up the numbers to get totals for each category.

"IT STIMULATES ME"

A___ H___ U___ Stimulation Total ______

With a high score here, you feel that smoking gives you energy, keeps you going. So, think about alternatives that give you energy, such as washing your face, brisk walking and jogging.

"I WANT SOMETHING IN MY HAND"

B___ I___ O___ Handling Total ______

There are a lot of things you can do with your hands without lighting up. Try doodling with a pencil, knitting or get a "dummy" cigarette you can play with.

"IT FEELS GOOD"

C___ J___ P___ Pleasure/Relaxation Total ______

A high score means that you get a lot of physical pleasure out of smoking. Various forms of exercise can be effective alternatives. People in this category may be helped by the use of nicotine replacement therapy if medically indicated.

"IT'S A CRUTCH"

D___ K___ Q___ Crutch/Tension Total ______

Finding cigarettes to be comforting in moments of stress can make stopping tough, but there are many better ways to deal with stress. Learn to use relaxation breathing or another technique for deep relaxation instead. People in this category may be helped by nicotine replacement therapy if medically indicated.

"I'M HOOKED"

E___ L___ R___ Craving/Addiction Total ______

In addition to having a psychological dependency to smoking, you may also be physically addicted to nicotine. It's a hard addiction to break, but it can be done. People in this category are the ones most likely to benefit from the use of nicotine replacement therapy if medically indicated.

"IT'S PART OF MY ROUTINE"

F___ M___ S___ Habit Total ______

If cigarettes are merely part of your routine, one key to success is being aware of every cigarette you smoke. Keeping a diary or writing down every cigarette on the inside of your cigarette pack is a good way to do it.

"I'M A SOCIAL SMOKER"

G___ N___ T___ Social Smoker Total ______

You smoke in social situations, when people around you are smoking and when you are offered cigarettes. It is important for you to remind others that you are a nonsmoker. You may want to change your social habits to avoid the "triggers" which may lead to smoking again.

Adapted with permission from: Butting out for life. A smoking cessation counselling program for pharmacists. Laval, PQ: Merrel Dow Pharmaceuticals (Canada) Inc., 1993.

if the patient's condition requires further evaluation before a nicotine replacement therapy can be recommended (e.g., cardiovascular disease, pregnancy).

Assist the patient to set a "stop date."

When the patient has decided on the behavioral and/or pharmacological methods to use in quitting smoking, the health professional can help set a "stop date." The best way to quit smoking is to stop smoking completely (also known as quitting "cold turkey"). To do this, the patient should select a specific day on the calendar. Ideally, it should be within 2 weeks of the decision to quit, and it is helpful if the patient is away from his smoking triggers (e.g., on vacation). The patient should avoid a time that might be associated with high stress, anger, frustration, anxiety, or depression. For example, a patient going for a job interview may be advised that the day of the interview might not be a good time to quit. It may be best to wait until after the first few weeks on a new job, when the level of stress is reduced.

Assist the patient with follow-up counselling, monitoring and encouragement, and help him or her deal with relapse.

Tell the patient you would like to stay in touch to follow his or her progress and discuss any questions or problems with their smoking cessation. This follow-up should be tailored to the patient's needs. Ask for a convenient time to call or meet after the first week of quitting. After the initial follow-up, determine through discussion with the patient how frequently further follow-up would be helpful. This could be weekly, then monthly, then 3-month intervals, continuing up to 20 to 24 months, when a patient can then be considered a "confirmed former smoker." In the follow-up discussions, reinforce the quitting decision by reminding the patient of the specific health benefits he or she can expect and help them recognize health benefits already occurring. Provide encouragement and offer suggestions for dealing with difficult social situations.

Since smoking may alter the effect of drugs in a number of ways (Table 4), it is important for the health professional to monitor ongoing drug therapy and suggest any necessary adjustments during the first few weeks of smoking withdrawal.

Make patients aware from the start it is likely they will have relapses. Research shows it often takes 7 or more attempts before a smoker quits entirely, with the highest number of relapses occurring within the first 3 months of smoking cessation. Encourage patients to keep in touch even if they have had a relapse. Tell them you can help them get started again. When patients suffer a relapse, help them identify what caused it and help them plan strategies to overcome the problems in the future.

TABLE 4: Potential Effects of Smoking Cessation on Other Medications

Drug	After Smoking Cessation	Significance
Acetaminophen	Increased blood levels	May need lower dose
Amobarbital	Slower elimination	May need lower dose
Benzodiazepines	Slower elimination	May need lower dose
Caffeine	Slower elimination	May experience more stimulation
Cimetidine	Enhanced drug action	May need lower dose
Estrogen supplements	Metabolized slower	Discuss with physician
Furosemide	Enhanced effect	Discuss with physician
Glutethimide	Reduced effect	May need higher dose
Heparin	Slower elimination	May need lower dose
Pentazocine	Slower excretion	May need lower dose
Phenothiazines	Enhanced effect	Discuss with physician
Phenylbutazone	Metabolized slower	May need lower dose
Propoxyphene	Greater effect	Discuss with physician
Propranolol	Greater effectiveness	Discuss with physician
Theophylline	Metabolized slower	May need lower dose
Tricyclic antidepressants	Slower elimination	May need lower dose
Vitamin C	Slower elimination	May require less

Adapted with permission from: Butting out for life. A smoking cessation counselling program for pharmacists. Laval, PQ: Merrell Dow Pharmaceuticals (Canada) Inc., 1993. Ferguson T. The Smoker's Book of Health. New York: Putnam, 1987.

NONPHARMACOLOGICAL TREATMENT

In addition to counselling, there are a number of nonpharmacological treatments available that involve behavioral intervention.

Acupuncture

Acupuncture involves needles or staple-like attachments placed under the skin on the surface of the nose or on the ear. Proponents claim it relieves physical withdrawal symptoms and stops hunger and "hand-to-mouth" urges. In a few poorly designed studies, quit rates have ranged from 8 to 40%, but there is no evidence the therapy relieves withdrawal symptoms. Acupuncture is attractive to smokers, since it is relatively quick and simple, and requires minimal effort by the smoker. It may be that a placebo effect helps the smoker handle the addictive component of smoking.

Hypnosis

Hypnosis is a deep, relaxed state of attention during which people are more responsive to suggestions. Hypnotherapy attempts to change patients' habits and attitudes to cigarettes. A review of this method by the National Institute of Health in the United States found contradictory results. One recent study found 23% of smokers treated with a single-session habit restructuring intervention involving self-hypnosis maintained abstinence for 2 years. The therapist's skill and experience are very important, as are the patient's susceptibility to hypnosis and desire to quit. The success of hypnosis can be improved with follow-up counselling and support, and by combining the therapy with other smoking cessation methods.

Laser Therapy

A laser beam is directed at certain key points of the body surface to relieve the physical craving for nicotine, apparently by triggering a release of endorphins. There is no scientific validation in the literature for reported success rates using this method of smoking cessation.

Group Support Programs

Many commercial and nonprofit programs are available. Most are listed under Smokers' Information & Treatment Centres in the yellow pages of the telephone book. *Countdown* is one provided by the Canadian Lung Association.

These programs usually involve behavior modification techniques such as relaxation training, stress management, cognitive restructuring, relapse prevention and the development of alternate adap-

ADVICE FOR THE PATIENT

Quitting Smoking

- Be aware of the various methods available to stop smoking. Smoking cessation programs that involve medication in combination with methods to change behavior are most successful.
- Pamphlets and brochures available from various sources have ideas on quitting.
- Smokers who consume more than 20 to 25 cigarettes, and who smoke their first cigarette within 30 minutes of waking, are considered nicotine dependent and would likely benefit from nicotine replacement therapy.
- Smokers who consume more than 30 cigarettes a day, or who wake up in the night to have a cigarette, are even more dependent, and would likely benefit more from a prescribed nicotine replacement product.
- A physician's involvement is necessary if medical conditions exist that require further evaluation before a nicotine replacement therapy can be recommended (e.g., heart disease, pregnancy).
- Follow the manufacturer's instructions carefully for use of the product.
- Select a specific day on the calendar as a "stop date." It should be fairly soon after the decision to quit (ideally within 2 weeks), and it would help to avoid smoking triggers.
- Be prepared to deal with smoking triggers, e.g., coffee breaks, tense situations.
- Be prepared for slight weight gain (2 kg on average). Consider modifying diet and exercise to limit weight gain as much as possible.
- Realize that relapse is not unusual, and if it occurs, try quitting again as soon as possible.

tive behaviors. Since no single method seems to work well for everyone, the best approach is to tailor the program to the individual. These programs have varying success. A recent report evaluating 42 clinics in the United States found an overall 1-year quit rate of 29% (ranging from 0 to 69%).

Computer Assisted Programs

A computer method (*Lifesign*) that helps wean smokers off cigarettes provides a type of behavioral modification, allowing smokers to program their own smoking behavior.

PHARMACOLOGICAL TREATMENT

Nicotine-containing products and products that seek to replace the tobacco in cigarettes with another material are the only nonprescription smoking cessation products for sale in Canada. Products that cause an unpleasant sensation when the individual smokes and products that simulate the tracheobronchial sensations elicited by smoking are no longer available. In the United States, all smoking cessation products except those containing nicotine have been ordered off the market because of the lack of data to substantiate claims.

In addition to these nonprescription products, nicotine replacement therapy is available in higher strengths by prescription only.

The effectiveness of nicotine replacement as a stop-smoking aid has been documented in many research papers, although success rates vary from 45% down to 6%. Comparisons have been made between the effectiveness of 2 mg and 4 mg nicotine resin complex and nicotine patches. In 1994, an analysis was made of 28 randomized trials of 2 mg nicotine resin complex, 6 trials of 4 mg nicotine resin complex and 6 trials of the nicotine transdermal patch, and their relative effectiveness in smoking cessation after 1 year. It was concluded that both nicotine resin complex and patch were effective aids to help nicotine dependent smokers. It was further found that for the most nicotine dependent smokers (as determined by Fagerström tolerance questionnaire), the 4 mg nicotine resin complex was most effective, enabling one third to quit. In less dependent smokers, the different preparations were comparable in efficacy. Overall, all types of nicotine replacement analysed helped 15% of smokers to give up smoking by 1 year.

Patients using behavioral intervention achieve higher quit rates than those using nicotine replacement alone. A study using 2 mg nicotine resin complex together with group counselling found abstinence rates for smokers of medium to low dependence of 73.3% after 6 weeks, 38.3% after 1 year and 28.3% after 2 years, compared with 41.5%, 22.6% and 9.4%, respectively, with placebo.

It appears reasonable that non-nicotine-dependent patients should be advised to attempt to quit without nicotine replacement. The health professional may recommend nicotine resin complex in 2 mg doses to those patients with moderate nicotine dependence or those with low dependence who have been unsuccessful on previous attempts to quit without nicotine replacement. Refer highly dependent patients to a physician for evaluation of a higher dose nicotine replacement product, such as a 4 mg dose of the resin complex or a nicotine patch. In addition, patients who are concerned about post-cessation weight gain may find that the use of nicotine replacement therapy slightly reduces this problem.

PHARMACEUTICAL AGENTS

Nicotine Resin Complex: Nicotine resin complex in a 2 mg dose is available as a nonprescription product.

As discussed above, the pharmacological actions of nicotine are complex, varying from stimulant to depressant effects on autonomic ganglia and the central nervous system. In nonsmokers, nicotine resin complex can cause an increase in blood pressure and heart rate and central nervous system stimulation, but these effects may not be detectable in smokers since the effects vary according to the degree of tolerance to nicotine. Nicotine also causes the release of catecholamines from the adrenal medulla, which is not decreased by tolerance.

The nicotine from the resin is absorbed through the buccal mucosa more slowly than from tobacco smoking. It does not produce the pleasure some people associate with cigarette smoking, but it can relieve the irritability, difficulty concentrating, and other symptoms associated with withdrawal. About 75% of the nicotine released by chewing is swallowed and metabolized first by the liver. The chewing pieces are buffered to pH 8.5 to enhance buccal absorption, and inhibit release of the nicotine in the acidic pH of the stomach, so that a significant amount would not be absorbed if the chewing piece were swallowed rather than chewed.

The nicotine released into the mouth through chewing over a 30-minute period results in a peak blood nicotine level of 5 ng/mL after 25 minutes; it stabilizes at 9 ng/mL following repeated chewing of a 2 mg piece every half hour. This is compared with a peak of 16 to 35 ng/mL reached within 5 minutes of smoking a cigarette with mild to moderate nicotine content.

Adverse effects from nicotine resin are generally minor and quite rare. Studies of prolonged use find little difference compared with placebo except for increased hiccups. Mouth or throat soreness, jaw ache and hiccups are the most frequently reported side effects. Some reports have also been made of gastrointestinal irritation, nausea, vomiting and aggravation of dyspepsia. Very rarely there have been reports of central nervous system effects (insomnia, dizziness or light-headedness, irritability and headache); cardiovascular effects (edema, flushing, hypertension, palpitations, tachyarrhythmias, tachycardia, chest pain); dermatological reactions (erythema, itching, rash, urticaria); respiratory symptoms (breathing difficulty, cough, hoarseness, sneezing, wheezing) and apparent severe allergic reactions.

The risk of these adverse effects can be reduced by giving the patient detailed instructions on proper use (Figure 3). In particular, the proper "chew and park" technique should be explained and the maximum frequency of 20 chewing pieces per day emphasized. If side effects do occur, the cause is likely improper use (often chewing too vigorously). Inquire about the method of use and review the instructions with the patient.

The resin may stick to full or partial dentures, dental caps or bridges, depending on their material, the amount of dryness of mouth and salivary

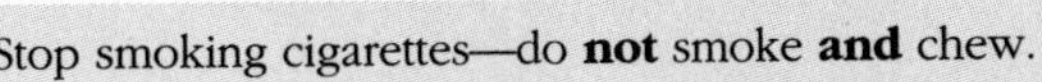

FIGURE 3: The Seven Ss

Stop smoking cigarettes—do **not** smoke **and** chew.

Substitute the chewing piece for a cigarette when you feel the urge to smoke.

Slowly bite the chewing piece, only about 2 or 3 times per minute. The nicotine is released similar to a cigarette, so you should "park" the chewing piece between the cheek and gum just like you pause between puffs of a cigarette.

Several pieces per day—approximately 1 piece for every 1 or 2 cigarettes to a maximum of 20 pieces a day. It is important to take enough daily to build an adequate blood level of nicotine to prevent nicotine withdrawal.

Stay on the therapy for a maximum of 6 months.

Staged reduction—gradually reduce the number of pieces used per day over a period of several weeks.

Stop using the nicotine pieces. To help deal with the urge to smoke, you might want to carry pieces with you at all times, just in case.

Adapted with permission from: Butting out for life. A smoking cessation counselling program for pharmacists. Laval, PQ: Merrell Dow Pharmaceuticals (Canada) Inc., 1993. Wilson DMC. The role of the family physician in cigarette abstention. Mod Med Can 1989;44(8):802–11.

constituents, possible interaction with denture adhesives and denture cleaning compounds.

Nicotine resin products are contraindicated in nonsmokers, children and pregnant or breast-feeding women. It has been suggested, however, that particularly for pregnant women who are heavy smokers, nicotine replacement is a less hazardous option than continuing to smoke if nonpharmacological methods are not successful, since the fetus is exposed to more nicotine from maternal smoking than from nicotine replacement therapy. Patients suffering from angina, high blood pressure and disease or inflammation of the mouth or stomach should consult with their physician prior to initiating therapy and use nicotine replacement products with caution.

The manufacturer suggests that patients be advised to limit use of these products to 6 months. Patients should be told to gradually reduce the number of pieces used over a 6-month period. Long-term use has been reported quite rarely (0 to 3% at 24 months). Some authors suggest that prolonged use of nicotine replacement therapy should not be a concern in view of the demonstrated dangers of smoking.

The risk of poisoning by swallowing the nicotine resin products is small due to the slow and incomplete absorption from the stomach in the absence of chewing as mentioned above. In human studies, ingesting ten 4 mg nicotine polyacrilex pieces produced a blood level of nicotine no greater than that produced by smoking a mild cigarette (5 ng/mL), and pieces of the gum containing 68% of the nicotine were recovered in the feces. An overdose could occur if many pieces were chewed simultaneously or in rapid succession. The lethal dose of nicotine for adults is 40 to 60 mg. Acute nicotine poisoning causes nausea and vomiting; abdominal pain; cold sweat; headache; dizziness; disturbed hearing and vision; mental confusion and weakness. Further effects may be faintness; hypotension; difficulty breathing; rapid weak and irregular pulse; circulatory collapse and convulsions. Death could result from respiratory failure due to paralysis of the respiratory muscles.

When patients select nicotine replacement therapy, review the proper use, precautions and storage with them (Figure 3). It is important that patients realize this product is not an innocuous chewing gum and is not to be chewed continually. The patient should also be advised not to drink acidic beverages (e.g., carbonated beverages, coffee, tea, apple, orange or grape juice) with the chewing piece as it may decrease the absorption of the nicotine.

Herbal Preparations: Some herbal cigarettes are sold in health shops and by mail order in Canada. In Australia, such products have been found to contain levels of tar and particulate matter similar to that of conventional cigarettes. One product, (*Paipo*), is a plastic tube filled with a mixture of natural herb extracts, flavored with either cinnamon or mint. This is not intended to be lighted, just to be held like a cigarette. There is no scientific evidence suggesting these products promote smoking cessation.

Citric Acid or Ascorbic Acid Aerosols: There have been some investigations of the use of either citric acid or ascorbic acid in an aerosol formulation for inhalation, which may produce a tracheobronchial sensation similar to that from inhaling cigarette smoke. This may help alleviate the craving for cigarettes. No products of this type are currently available, although there has been some research into prototypes. The studies involve small groups over a short time and do not provide definitive results.

RECOMMENDED READING

Glynn TJ, Manley MW. How to help your patients stop smoking: A National Cancer Institute manual for physicians. Washington DC. US Dept of Health and Human Services (Public Health Service), National Institutes of Health. 1990. Publication. NIH 90-3064.

Gourlay SG, McNeill JJ: Antismoking products. Med J Aust 1990;153:699-704.

The health benefits of smoking cessation: A report of the Surgeon General. Washington, DC: U.S. Department of Health and Human Services, Public Health Service, Center for Chronic Disease Prevention and Health Promotion, Office on Smoking and Health, 1990. DHHS publication no. (CDC) 90-8416.

The health consequences of involuntary smoking: A report of the Surgeon General. Washington, DC: U.S. Department of Health, Education and Welfare, 1986.

The health consequences of smoking: cardiovascular disease. A report of the Surgeon General. Washington, DC: U.S. Department of Health and Human Services, 1983. DHHS (PHS) 84-50204.

The health consequences of smoking: Nicotine addiction: A Report of the Surgeon General. Washington, DC: U.S. Department of Health and Human Services, Public Health Service, Center for Chronic Disease Prevention and Health Promotion, Office on Smoking and Health, 1988. DHHS publication no. (CDC) 88-8406.

Schwartz JL. Review and Evaluation of Smoking Cessation Methods: The United States and Canada, 1978-1985. Washington, DC: U.S. Department of Health and Human Services, 1987.

Smoking Tobacco and Health: A Fact Book. Washington, DC: Department of Health and Human Services, 1987.

Viswervaran C, Schmidt FL. A meta-analytic comparison of the effectiveness of smoking cessation methods. J Appl Psychol 1992;77(4): 554-61.

Wilson DMC, Lindsay EA, Best JA, et al. A smoking cessation intervention for family physicians. Can Med Assoc J 1987;137(7):613-9.

24

SPORTS MEDICINE PRODUCTS

LILY LUM

CONTENTS

Sports Injuries 613
- Prevention
- Treatment
- Sports Injuries and Their Management
- First Aid Supplies for Sports Injuries

Heat-Related Disorders 617
- Heat Cramps
- Heat Syncope
- Heat Exhaustion
- Heat Stroke

Drug Abuse in Sports 619
- Ergogenic Aids
- Banned Substances

Recommended Reading 622

SPORTS INJURIES

Canadians are becoming more health conscious and participating in more exercise programs and sports activities. Although commonly associated with health benefits, sport and exercise can cause injuries. Physiotherapists and pharmacists are often approached for guidance and help in their prevention and treatment.

Sports injuries can be caused by trauma, overuse or environmental factors. The type of injury varies: trauma or acute injury is more likely due to contact sports; overuse or chronic injuries are more commonly associated with repetitive movements. The acronym of 3 Fs, too **fast**, too **far**, and too **frequent**, is often used to describe the cause of overuse injuries. Musculoskeletal disorders that result include muscle pain and stiffness following exercise, bursitis, capsulitis, tendonitis, tenosynovitis, and tennis elbow. Acute injuries include ligament sprains and muscle strains. Other problems encountered are blisters and friction burns, and environmental injuries, e.g., heat stroke.

PREVENTION

Proper conditioning and training prevent many sports-related injuries. Training should always begin with stretching and low intensity exercise. Warning signs of impending injury are extreme fatigue, lack of enthusiasm for training and pain. Protective equipment and proper footwear are essential for those participating in high-risk sports requiring direct contact with playing equipment or other players.

TREATMENT

The four essentials of early management of soft-tissue injuries can be remembered by the acronym RICE: **R**est, **I**ce, **C**ompression, **E**levation. The RICE regimen may be followed by heat, massage, drug treatment and rehabilitation.

Rest: Immobilization is recommended for at least the first 24 hours to avoid aggravating the injury. If long-term rest is indicated, the unaffected joint(s) should be moved to prevent tissue atrophy and loss of coordination. Prolonged rest for muscle injuries is usually discouraged.

Ice: Cold packs (cryotherapy) applied to an injured area reduce local blood flow by constricting blood vessels, limiting the swelling. Plain ice, wrapped in a towel to prevent skin damage or frostbite, or commercial ice packs should be administered for 15 minutes, then reapplied every 2 waking hours for the first 24 hours. Cold therapy should be applied with caution to patients with poor circulation (e.g., diabetes, Raynaud's disease).

Compression: An elasticized bandage applied to an injured area for at least the first 24 hours can reduce swelling, provide support for a weak joint or a protective layer for wounds.

Elevation: The injured area should be raised above the level of the heart to help drain fluid and reduce swelling.

Heat Versus Cold Therapy

As a general rule, the application of cold is the preferred immediate treatment for most musculoskeletal injuries. Many physicians recommend heat therapy after the first 48 hours, when the swelling has subsided, and during the chronic rehabilitative phases of the injury. Local heat is also a useful therapeutic adjunct in the treatment of minor muscle and tendon injuries. It produces analgesia through its effect on free nerve endings, decreases the incidence of painful muscle spasm by relaxing muscles and reduces joint stiffness by decreasing synovial fluid viscosity. Heat causes vasodilation. Increased blood flow helps provide a greater local supply of nutrients, oxygen, antibodies, leukocytes and enzymes to the injured area; waste products from the inflammatory process are carried away with the increased circulation.

Heat may be applied for 20 to 30 minutes, every 2 to 4 hours as needed.

Contraindications include patients who are unconscious, those with impaired skin sensitivity, poor circulation or open wounds.

Hot water bottles, electric heating pads, heat packs and infrared heat lamps supply local heat, but care should be taken to avoid burns: follow the instructions carefully; hot water bottles and heat packs can be wrapped with a towel or cloth for comfort and safety; heating pads and heat lamps should be kept on low to moderate settings.

Oral and Topical Analgesics

Oral analgesics such as acetaminophen and the nonsteroidal anti-inflammatory drugs (NSAIDs) ASA and ibuprofen can provide effective relief of musculoskeletal pain when used alone or in conjunction with other treatments. They may be useful in acute as well as chronic injuries.

Topical analgesics and counterirritants have been a traditional remedy for the treatment of general aches and pains. The most common ingredients are methyl salicylate and triethanolamine salicylate. Although of limited value, they may be useful in rehabilitation. They should not be used in acute injury where there is risk of bleeding, under dressings or on open wounds.

Refer to the Pain and Fever Products chapter for further discussion of internal and external analgesics.

SPORTS INJURIES AND THEIR MANAGEMENT

Ankle Sprains

A sprain is a ligament injury caused by overstretching or twisting. In the ankle, it is mainly the lateral ligaments of the joint that tear. Symptoms include pain, swelling, tenderness, and later bruising around the injury. Initial treatment should be the RICE regimen and the ankle taped or braced. The doctor may want to x-ray the joint to rule out a fracture. NSAIDs and physiotherapy may be prescribed. Severely damaged ligaments may require surgical repair. For rehabilitation, it is necessary to regain strength, flexibility and balance. Ligaments generally take 12 months to fully heal.

Strains

A strain is an injury to the muscle, usually due to overstretching, characterized by pain and swelling. Muscle strains vary in severity from damage to the fibres with muscle sheath intact to complete rupture of the muscle. Treatment should be the RICE regimen. Complete rupture of the muscle may require surgical repair.

Blisters

A small pocket of fluid under the skin surface may be formed during sports or exercise from repeated friction between the skin and a hard object (e.g., ill-fitting or new shoes). Intact blisters are best left untreated and may be protected with a sterile nonadherent dressing. If the blister is aspirated or punctured, the equipment (e.g., needle) should be sterile and the skin left to prevent infection. Apply a topical antiseptic and cover with a sterile, nonadherent dressing; change as necessary.

Friction Burns

Friction burns commonly occur in falls on a synthetic surface or floor and generally affect only the outer layer of skin. The mildest form causes only superficial redness that requires no treatment. Broken skin should be cleansed and covered with a sterile nonadherent dressing.

Overuse Injuries

Muscle pain and stiffness following exercise, bursitis, capsulitis, tendonitis, stress fractures, tenosynovitis, and tennis elbow are examples of overuse injuries. Generally, initial treatment is the RICE regimen and possibly drug therapy with NSAIDs. Most of the NSAIDs are indicated or used in the treatment of painful nonrheumatic inflammatory conditions such as athletic injuries, bursitis, capsulitis, tendonitis or tenosynovitis. For self-treatment of mild to moderate pain, the usual adult dose for ibuprofen is 200 to 400 mg every 4 to 6 hours, not to exceed 1.2 g daily. Treatment should not extend beyond 10 days without the advice of a physician. A rehabilitative program of gradually increasing exercise should be implemented, except in more serious conditions where complete rest is indicated. Initially, the athlete can cross train for fitness with activities such as cycling, swimming or pool running.

Muscle pain and stiffness commonly occurs 24 to 28 hours after unaccustomed intense physical activity. Warm-up exercises and conditioning with a gradual increase in the intensity and duration of the workouts will help prevent or reduce it. Fluid replacement as well as pre- and postexercise stretching are very important. NSAIDs have been shown to help delay the onset of muscle soreness.

Bursitis is inflammation of the bursa, a fluid-filled sac where friction would otherwise develop such as the shoulder, knee, or elbow. The bursa facilitate the motion of tendons and muscle over bony prominences. With overuse, inflammation causes pain, tenderness and swelling, and is often associated with tendonitis (e.g., subacromial bursitis, rotator cuff tendonitis).

Capsulitis is inflammation of the joint capsule, the fibrous supporting tissue surrounding the shoulder joint.

Tendonitis is inflammation of a tendon (the bundles of collagen fibres that attach muscles to bones), commonly the shoulder and Achilles tendon that connects the heel to calf muscle.

Tenosynovitis is inflammation of the tendon sheaths (their outer covering), commonly occurring in the forearm, often from overuse.

Tennis elbow, lateral epicondylitis, is tendonitis of the lateral (outer) side of the elbow caused by overuse of the forearm muscles. It commonly occurs in racquet sports and activities that require repetitive, one-sided movements. Protective braces prevent and treat the injury.

Stress fractures (e.g., of tibia-fibula) result from repeated impact on hard surfaces or excessive muscle stress leading to fatigue fracture of the bone. Treatment includes cross training, strength and flexibility training. Good shoes and orthotics are recommended if there is excessive foot involvment.

FIRST AID SUPPLIES FOR SPORTS INJURIES

The following chart summarizes suggested medical supplies for a first aid kit or first aid station at sporting events.

TABLE 1: First Aid Supplies for Sports Injuries

Medical Supply	Indication	Examples
Bandages		
compression	Provide pressure to reduce the flow of blood and inflammatory exudate	Elastic adhesive bandage
retention	Hold dressings in place Apply pressure to stop bleeding	
support	Provide support for an injured area during active movement	
laceration	Minor lacerations	*Steri-Strip*
Cooling aids	Reduce blood flow in soft tissue injuries Minimize swelling	Ice, ice packs
Disinfectants and cleansers	Cleanse and disinfect skin and wounds	Cetrimide; chlorhexidine; povidone-iodine; normal saline (sterile solutions may also be used for eye irrigation)
Dressings		
absorbent	Absorb wound exudate Provide protection	An absorbent pad surrounded partly or completely by a piece of extension plaster
adhesive	Cover minor wounds	
hemostatic	Stop bleeding	Calcium alginate dressing (e.g., *Kaltostat, Algoderm*)
standard	Used for severely bleeding wounds	An absorbent pad and retention bandage in one complete sterile dressing
tulle	Apply to abrasions, burns, and other skin injuries Usually beneath an absorbent dressing	*Sofra-tulle* or equivalent
water jel	For blisters and burns	*2nd Skin*
athletic tape	Provide support to prevent initial or further tearing of a ligament	
Forceps, scissors, safety pins	General surgical use Cut up dressings	
Surgical adhesive tape	Secure dressings	
Swabs	Apply disinfectants and cleansers	Cotton gauze
Thermos (wide-necked) or insulated bag	Carry ice or ice packs	
Thermometer	Measure body temperature in heat-related injuries	
Towels	General cleaning purposes	
Massage creams	To prevent muscle cramps and to treat pre-event stiffness	
Miscellaneous		Finger splints, sling

HEAT-RELATED DISORDERS

Exercising, playing, or working in hot weather can lead to a number of disorders such as heat cramps and heat syncope (fainting). Heat exhaustion and heat stroke are life threatening.

HEAT CRAMPS

Excessive loss of electrolytes and fluids through heavy sweating during physical exertion in very hot, humid weather may bring on muscle cramps. They usually begin in the most worked muscles (e.g., arms in tennis players, legs in runners) and often occur after the activity ends. Gently massaging the cramped muscle, cooling the body with tepid water and wet towels, and oral administration of salt and water can provide relief.

HEAT SYNCOPE

Fainting occurs in athletes, workers or travellers unacclimatized to hot, humid weather. Prolonged standing in the heat (e.g., military personnel), standing suddenly from a lying or sitting position and standing at the end of a race can lead to blood pooling in the legs, reducing the amount sent to the head. Symptoms prior to fainting may be dizziness, lightheadedness, and clammy skin. The best treatment is to get away from the heat, lie down with the legs raised and replace fluids.

HEAT EXHAUSTION

Heat exhaustion is more serious, affecting the cardiovascular and other body systems. It often develops slowly over several days or weeks and involves severe dehydration. Symptoms include: profuse perspiration, flu-like malaise, fatigue, rapid pulse, thirst, lightheadedness, pale and clammy skin, and slightly elevated temperature. The recommended treatment is rest in a cool place and oral rehydration with salted fluids. Five mL (1 tsp) of salt to 500 mL of water is adequate, but moderately salty soup is more palatable.

HEAT STROKE

Heat stroke is a more severe and advanced form of heat exhaustion and is considered a medical emergency. Cessation of sweating results in

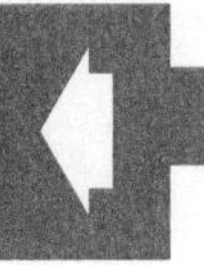

ADVICE FOR THE PATIENT

Preventing Heat-Related Disorders

- Acclimatize the body gradually by increasing heat exposure slowly; training and fitness are important.
- Minimize physical activities and outdoor exposure during the hottest part of the day (e.g., 11:00 a.m. to 3:00 p.m.).
- Use physical protection from the sun's rays (e.g., wide-brimmed hats, umbrellas).
- Wear loose, light-weight, light-colored clothing (preferably cotton).
- Take frequent cool showers or baths.
- Replace fluids before and during vigorous exercise.
- Do not run or exercise during periods of illness.
- Avoid drugs that can predispose to heat-related illnesses. Some of the more common drugs are listed below:

alcohol

antihistamines
(with significant anticholinergic effects)
- brompheniramine
- chlorpheniramine
- dimenhydrinate
- diphenhydramine
- hydroxyzine

anticholinergic drugs
- atropine
- clidinium
- dicyclomine
- glycopyrrolate
- homatropine
- hyoscyamine
- propantheline
- scopolamine

tricyclic antidepressants
- amitriptyline
- imipramine

phenothiazines
- chlorpromazine
- prochlorperazine
- trimeprazine

hyperthermia, a dangerously high body temperature, possibly reaching above 41°C (106°F). Other symptoms include: agitation, restlessness, confusion, bizarre behavior, rapid pulse, hot and dry reddened skin, staggering gait, diarrhea, seizures, and unconsciousness.

Prompt recognition of the symptoms is very important. As much clothing as possible should be removed while awaiting medical assistance, the body cooled by fanning, spraying or sponging with cool water. Hospital medical treatment usually includes spraying tepid water on the skin of the patient. Small ice packs may be placed on the neck, groin, and armpits (areas close to the major blood vessels). Dehydration is treated with intravenous fluids. Total body immersion in a tub of ice water is no longer indicated as it causes vasoconstriction, decreasing rather than accelerating body cooling. The patient's cardiac function is monitored in case of cardiac arrest.

Salt Tablet Versus Fluid Replacement

The use of salt tablets is not generally indicated during exercise. The ingestion of sodium chloride may lead to an increase in gastric emptying and an inhibition of sweating due to hyperosmolarity. The replenishment of fluids is of greater importance than sodium supplementation since fluid losses during exercise are much greater than electrolyte losses.

Whether plain water or some type of carbohydrate-electrolyte solution is superior in terms of preventing dehydration and hyperthermia, and improving performance has been the subject of extensive study and remains a controversial topic among exercise physiologists and practitioners, e.g., coaches, trainers, team physicians. Some researchers favor the use of a hypotonic glucose-balanced electrolyte (isomolar) solution (e.g., *Gatorade*). Other experts feel that plain water is the safest, least expensive drink for athletes, exercisers and marathoners.

Fluids should be replaced at regular intervals during heavy exercise to prevent dehydration.

Alcoholic beverages and caffeinated drinks (e.g., coffee, tea, colas) should be avoided. They are diuretics promoting fluid loss.

DRUG ABUSE IN SPORTS

Olympic athletes in ancient Greece are believed to have used herbs and mushrooms to improve athletic performance. In the late 19th century, French athletes drank a mixture of coca leaves and wine to reduce fatigue and hunger associated with prolonged exercise. In the modern sports era, drug abuse was recognized as a problem when the use of stimulants was reported at the 1952 Winter Olympics in Oslo, Norway. More recently, at the 1988 Summer Olympics in Seoul, South Korea, a Canadian athlete tested positive for anabolic steroids and was denied a gold medal. Drug abuse has most often been associated with weight lifting, track and field, swimming, cycling, and football. It is now a major concern.

Sports organizations have developed policies and drug testing programs as competition has intensified to the point that increasing numbers of athletes are striving to upgrade their performance by any means to obtain success. Some turn to ergogenic (performance-enhancing) drugs. Although the drugs carry potential adverse effects, most athletes that use them view the risk-to-benefit ratio as favorable. The majority of drugs with abuse potential (e.g., anabolic steroids) are obtained as prescription drugs or illegally via the underground black market.

ERGOGENIC AIDS

The International Olympic Committee defines ergogenic drug use or doping as "the administration of or use by a competing athlete of any substance foreign to the body or any physiological substance taken in abnormal quantity or taken by an abnormal route of entry into the body with the sole intention of increasing in an artificial manner his/her performance in competition." In this section, nonprescription drugs used as ergogenic aids are described.

Caffeine: Caffeine is widely consumed as an ingredient in coffee, tea, soft drinks, and many nonprescription drug products (e.g., cold preparations). It has been used by athletes as an ergogenic aid. Studies have shown that caffeine can improve the efficiency of fuel utilization by releasing free fatty acids as an alternative fuel source and by sparing glycogen, the primary source of energy during athletic performance. Caffeine is also a CNS stimulant, increasing alertness and reducing the perception of fatigue.

Adverse effects include nervousness, instability, and insomnia at a variety of doses. Excessive doses (e.g., adult toxic effects may begin at 15 mg/kg; 150-200 mg/kg may be lethal) have been reported to cause delirium, seizures, coma, and death.

In drug testing, a urine sample will be considered positive if the concentration of caffeine exceeds 12 mcg/mL. The normal ingestion of coffee, tea or colas will not cause this limit to be exceeded or even remotely approached. However, the ingestion of excess caffeine tablets (600 to 1,000 mg ingested within 50 to 60 minutes) may result in a positive doping test.

Codeine: Codeine is commonly found in a number of nonprescription combination analgesic products. Although narcotic analgesics are not generally considered ergogenic aids, there is the potential for misuse among athletes. Treatment of serious pain that allows an athlete to participate may lead to further aggravation of the injury. For this reason, the International Olympic Committee has banned the use of narcotic analgesics. The use of ASA, acetaminophen, and nonsteroidal anti-inflammatory agents (e.g., ibuprofen) for the treatment of less serious pain is allowed.

ADVICE FOR THE ATHLETE

Drug Abuse

- No list should be considered complete. Different sport associations may ban different substances. Check with your national or local sport organization.
- If in doubt, do not take the medicine or substance.
- Some vitamin preparations may contain banned substances.
- Some medications have similar brand names; one may contain banned substances, the other not. For example, Robitussin contains guaifenesin and is permitted but Robitussin-PE contains pseudoephedrine, a banned substance.

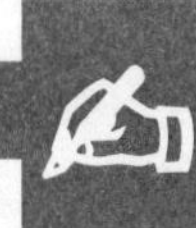

Resource List

Cardinal Health Systems
Sports medicine: injury and treatment (computer program). IBM PC and compatible; Cyberlog, 1990.
4600 West 77th Street, Suite 150
Edina, MN 55435
(612) 835-6941; Fax (612) 835-7141

Canadian Centre for Drug-free Sport
Suite 702, 1600 James Naismith Drive
Gloucester, ON K1B 5N4
(613) 748-5755; Fax (613) 748-5746

The Canadian Centre for Drug-free Sport (CCDS) offers a number of reference materials:

- Drug-free sport doping control handbook—Information for athletes and coaches. (CCDS publication B-001)
- Banned and restricted doping classes and methods booklet. (CCDS publication B-003)
- The drug-free sport video. (CCDS videotape M-005)
- Doping in sport and athletic training: literature review. (CCDS research and report R-003)

Cyproheptadine: Cyproheptadine is a serotonin and histamine antagonist used to promote appetite and weight gain. It is popular among young athletes who wish to gain weight without taking anabolic steroids.

Nutritional supplements: Nutritional supplements promoted as containing individual amino acids or high in protein are often excessively consumed by athletes in the belief that protein builds muscle and increases strength. Some athletes believe that these amino acid supplements are easier to digest and absorb than protein from regular food sources. Research has demonstrated that excessively high protein diets and supplements are not necessary. The body cannot store protein. Excess protein, not balanced by calorie intake, will not be converted into muscle protein. It will be used as a calorie source and excess nitrogen will be excreted by the kidney. Excessive nitrogen excretion may lead to kidney damage. These nutritional supplements, often considered fads, should not replace a well-balanced diet and good nutrition in general.

Sympathomimetic drugs: Sympathomimetic drugs, such as ephedrine, pseudoephedrine, and phenylpropanolamine, are commonly found in cold preparations. Because these drugs are banned, they are thought to possess ergogenic effects. However, there is little data to prove they enhance athletic performance; the potential for abuse is more likely due to their easy availability as nonprescription products. Athletes using pseudoephedrine as a nasal decongestant may unintentionally be at risk for a positive urine drug test.

Minor adverse effects include nervousness, irritability, insomnia, and headaches; the more serious reactions reported include agitation, confusion, paranoia, hypertension, and arrhythmias.

Vitamins and minerals: Vitamins and minerals are widely consumed among athletes in the belief they are ergogenic aids. However, studies have not shown that amounts in excess of recommended daily intake are associated with any performance-enhancing benefits. The fitness literature often praises the virtues of megavitamin supplementation. The vitamins most often taken in megadoses are C, E, and B complex. These excess vitamins are excreted unused by the body. Megavitamin supplementation is not harmless. Adverse effects associated with megadoses of vitamin C include uricosuria, kidney stones and diarrhea. Adverse effects reported with megadoses of vitamin E include coagulation abnormalities, weakness, muscle fatigue, and headache.

BANNED SUBSTANCES

Athletes should only be taking drugs for a justified medical condition that is being treated by a physician. The International Olympic Committee and other sports organizations began drug testing to protect amateur athletes from any potential unfair advantage gained by those who take the drugs to enhance athletic performance and any potential harmful side effects.

The following categories of drugs are considered banned substances in amateur sports:

- stimulants
- narcotic analgesics
- anabolic agents
- beta blockers

- diuretics
- peptide hormones and analogues, e.g., growth hormones, erythropoietin
- substances that alter the integrity of the urine samples, e.g., sodium bicarbonate loading

The majority of banned substances are prescription drugs. However, a few nonprescription drugs are on the list. For example, the category includes caffeine, ephedrine, phenylephrine, phenylpropanolamine, and pseudoephedrine (ingredients commonly found in cold preparations) as banned substances. In the narcotic analgesic category, codeine was recently delisted and is now permitted for medical use, but should still be declared.

A list of banned substances can be obtained from the Canadian Centre for Drug-free Sport (see Resource List).

RECOMMENDED READING

Smith NJ, Stanitski CL. Sports Medicine—A Practical Guide. Philadelphia; Toronto: Saunders, 1987.

Strauss RH, ed. Drugs and Performance in Sports. Philadelphia; Toronto: Saunders, 1987.

Strauss RH, ed. Sports Medicine. 2nd ed. Philadelphia; Toronto: Saunders, 1991.

Thomas JA, ed. Drugs, Athletes and Physical Performance. New York: Plenum Publishing, 1988.

Tver DF, Hunt HF. Encyclopedic Dictionary of Sports Medicine. New York; London: Chapman and Hall, 1986.

25

SUNSCREEN AND TANNING PRODUCTS

Sanna G. Pellatt

CONTENTS

Solar Radiation 623
UV Intensity
UV Index
Effects of UV Radiation 626
Sunburn
Tanning
Photosensitivity
Photoaging
Cancer
Protection 633
Nonpharmacological Protection
Topical Protection
Pharmaceutical Agents 638
Chemical Sunscreens
Physical Sunscreens
Possible Adverse Effects of Sunscreens
Systemic Protection
Pigmenting or Tanning Agents
Depigmenting Agents
Recommended Reading 642

SOLAR RADIATION

Sunlight consists of electromagnetic radiation of various wavelengths ranging from gamma rays to radio waves (Figure 1). Ultraviolet radiation is subdivided into UVC, UVB and UVA.

The shortest wavelength in the UV spectrum is UVC (200 to 290 nm), also referred to as germicidal radiation. Effectively screened by the atmosphere's ozone layer, UVC radiation from sunlight does not reach the earth's surface. It is also emitted by artificial sources such as germicidal lamps, welding arcs, and high and low pressure mercury arc lamps, which can cause sunburn.

The next longest wavelength, UVB (290 to 320 nm), is 5 to 10% of solar ultraviolet light reaching the ground. It is responsible for sunburn, delayed tanning (melanogenesis) and the conversion of 7-dehydrocholesterol in the skin to vitamin D_3. It has also been implicated in damage to DNA, immune suppression, skin cancer and wrinkling.

The remaining 90 to 95%, UVA, extends from 320 to 400 nm. Because of its longer wavelength, UVA penetrates deeper into the dermis causing both immediate pigment darkening and delayed tanning. It can cause a weak sunburn, but requires 1,000 times the dose of UVB to produce erythema. UVA radiation is responsible for photosensitivity reactions to certain chemicals and drugs and can enhance the acute and chronic effects of UVB radiation. It has no known benefit to human health and, since it penetrates deep into the dermis, poses potential short-term and long-term hazards to the eyes and skin. These rays can cause cataracts and retinal damage, premature aging of the skin, suppression of the immune system and an increased risk of skin cancer.

UV INTENSITY

Several factors modify the intensity of UV radiation reaching the skin: UVA radiation is present all day and throughout the year; UVB radiation varies according to the time of day and the season. About 30 to 50% of the total daily sunburning energy is received between 11 a.m. and 1 p.m., when the angle of incoming radiation is perpendicular to the earth's surface. In the early morning and late after-

Solar Radiation

noon more UVB radiation is filtered out as it travels a greater distance through the ozone layer at a lower angle. At latitudes other than the equator, the thickness of the ozone layer varies with the season: thickest in late winter, thinnest in late summer and early fall. Because some chemicals such as chlorofluorocarbons used in refrigerators, halons in fire extinguishers and methylchloroform in cleaners deplete ozone, there is an international agreement to phase out and ultimately eliminate their use.

At higher altitudes, UV intensity is greater. In general, UVB increases by 4% for every 300 m increase in altitude, while UVA remains practically constant. The intensity also increases as one travels toward the equator. Clouds and air pollution can filter out infrared and visible radiation, letting through as much as 80% of UV radiation as scattered light. Therefore sunburn can occur on a relatively cool, sunless day. High humidity and air movement across the skin surface can increase the severity of sunburn. The components of this "windburn" effect are not yet known. Window glass and mylar plastic filter out UVB radiation but allow UVA rays to pass through.

Sunlight can be reflected from a variety of sources. A covered porch or beach umbrella does not protect against reflected radiation and sunburn may occur. Reflected light can be damaging because it often strikes normally shaded parts of the body, such as the eyes. A green lawn scatters about 3% of radiation; dry sand reflects about 25%. Fresh snow may reflect 80% or more of sunlight. White paint, sheets of aluminum and even glossy magazine pages reflect 70 to 90% of UV radiation. Reflection from water is usually minimal (4%) unless the sun is directly overhead. At least 40% of UV radiation is transmitted through 50 cm of clear water. Swimming in either the sea or an outdoor

FIGURE 1

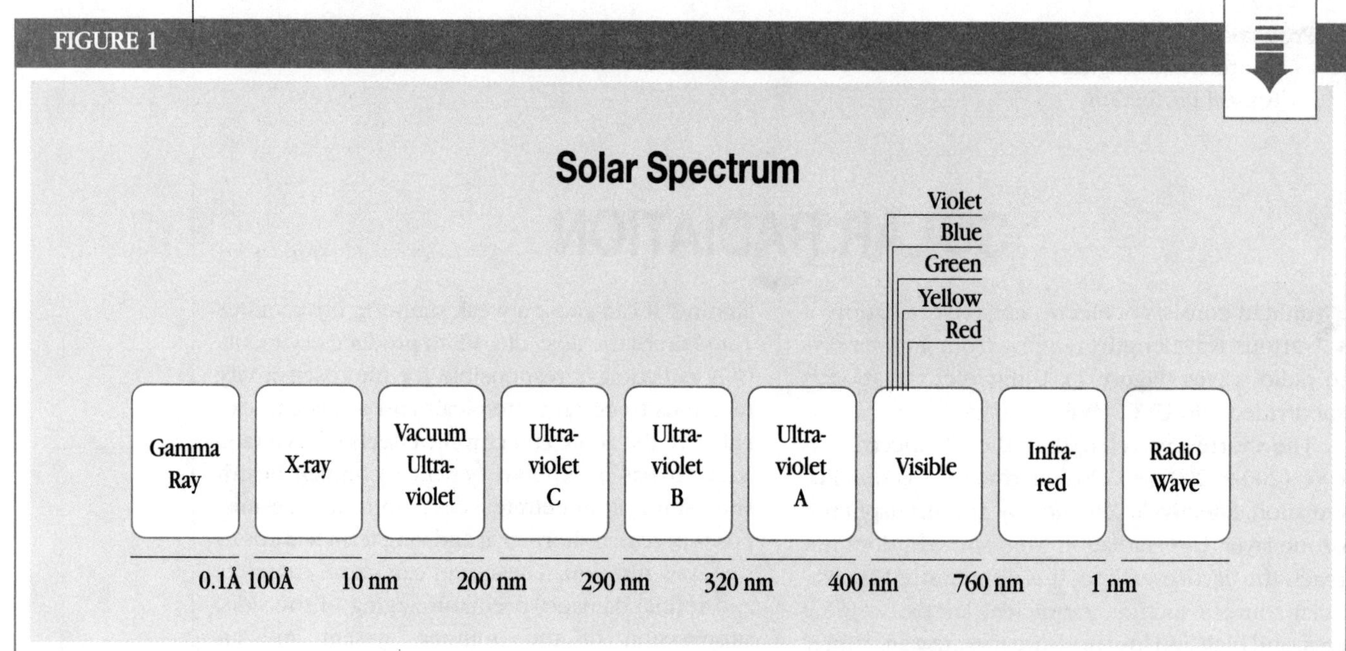

TABLE 1: The UV Index and Estimated Time to Burn For a Fair-Skinned Person

UV Index	Category	Sunburn Time
Over 9	Extreme	Less than 15 minutes
7-9	High	About 20 minutes
4-7	Moderate	About 30 minutes
0-4	Low	More than 1 hour

pool offers little protection against sunburn. Figure 2 illustrates important environmental factors that affect UV radiation.

UV INDEX

In 1992, Environment Canada scientists developed a method to predict the intensity of UV radiation based on daily changes in the ozone layer. The UV Index provides a forecast of the expected local clear-sky intensity of UV rays for the coming day. It is broadcast on radio and television, run in newspapers and available at weather offices across the country. On a scale of 0 to 10, 10 is a typical noon value for a summer day in the tropics. The UV Index, categories and estimated time to burn for a fair-skinned person are given in Table 1.

FIGURE 2: Environmental Factors Affecting Ultraviolet Radiation (UVR)

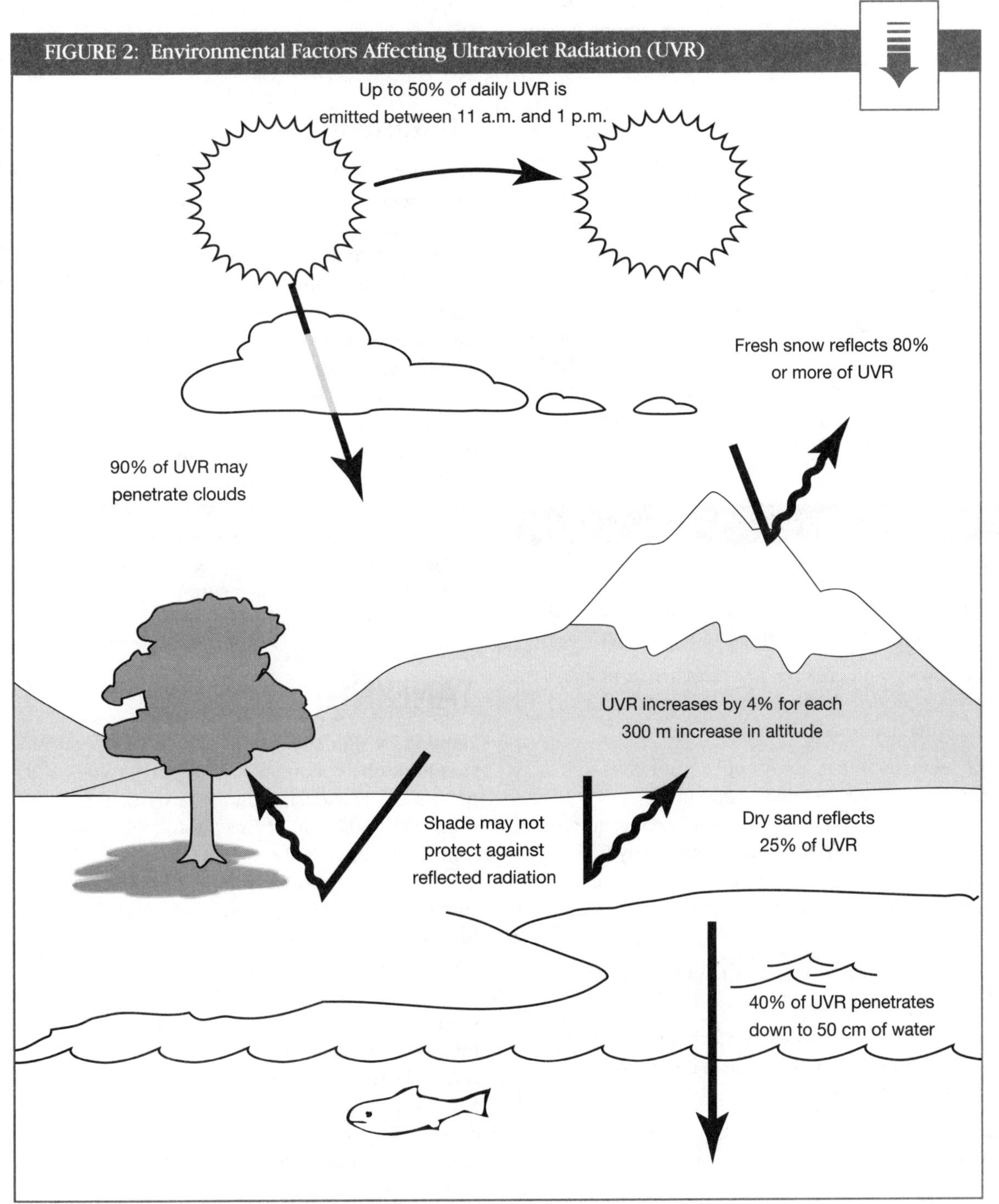

EFFECTS OF UV RADIATION

SUNBURN

Sunlight acts on normal skin to produce a variety of short term effects. The most common is sunburn, which in its mildest form appears as a reddening of the skin (erythema). UVB radiation causes 85% of erythema, UVA the remaining 15%. Sunburn is usually evident 2 to 12 hours after exposure to UV light. It peaks in 20 to 48 hours and gradually subsides over the following 3 to 5 days.

Symptoms

The skin response is complex and not fully understood. It has an early inflammatory phase characterized by redness and tenderness, followed by a delayed repair phase. It has been suggested that several vasoactive substances such as histamine, prostaglandins, arachidonic acid metabolites, kinins and cytokines may be responsible for the inflammatory response. Epidermal changes involve the formation of "sunburn" cells, thought to arise when keratinocytes (cells that synthesize keratin) are in a phase of the cell cycle when the replicating DNA is especially vulnerable and receives a lethal dose of UV radiation.These damaged cells form within 24 hours, followed by elimination by phagocytosis within 72 hours. With longer exposure, the initial erythema may be accompanied by edema, itching, fever and pain. Blistering occurs in more severe reactions. Systemic symptoms such as nausea, chills, abdominal cramping and headache may also accompany the local reactions if large areas of the body are involved.

ADVICE FOR THE PATIENT

Treating Sunburn

Sunburn is dangerous and should be avoided, but if it does occur, follow these steps:

- For sunburns in children less than 1 year of age, severe sunburn, or where headache, fever or shivering occur, contact a physician.
- For minor sunburn, apply cool compresses to the red areas for 20 minutes and take acetylsalicylic acid or acetaminophen if required to relieve pain. A moisturizing lotion may be used to relieve dryness. Avoid acetylsalicylic acid in children because of its association with Reye's syndrome.
- Avoid anesthetic sprays; they could cause a hypersensitivity reaction.
- Rest in a cool, dark room and stay out of the sun while sunburn heals, because damaged skin is more prone to burning again.
- Dryness and peeling following a sunburn can be treated with a moisturizing lotion.

Treatment

Treatment of sunburn depends on its severity. Mild cases can be treated like any other minor burn with cool water soaks or compresses for 20 minutes. Taking ASA or acetaminophen often alleviates the pain. Acetaminophen is the drug of choice for children or teenagers because ASA is associated with the development of Reye's syndrome. Topical anesthetic sprays should be avoided because they pose the risk of sensitization. Resting and staying out of the sun while the sunburn heals is essential since damaged skin is more prone to burning again. Mild sunburn is self-limiting and usually heals without scarring. For sunburn in children under a year, a more severe sunburn, or where headache, shivering or fever result, a physician should be contacted. Peeling following a sunburn can be treated with a moisturizer.

TANNING

Tanning, a sign that skin damage has occurred, should not be encouraged. It involves two distinct processes: immediate pigment darkening (IPD) from UVA radiation, due to photo-oxidation of the skin pigment melanin, usually disappears in 1 to 4 hours; delayed hyperpigmentation, the classic suntan caused by increased melanin formation (melanogenesis) in the lower epidermal layer, takes several days to become noticeable.

Whether a person burns or tans after a single sun exposure depends on the amount of melanin in their skin and their capacity for melanogenesis. The degree of sunburn is inversely proportional to the amount of melanin in the dermal layers of the skin: darker skinned individuals, who have more melanin, are rarely affected by sunburn; those with fairer complexions are highly susceptible. The six types of human skin are based on the tendency to burn and subsequent ability to tan (Table 2).

Repeated exposure to sunlight makes the skin less sensitive due to increased melanin production (tanning) and increased thickening of the stratum corneum that accompanies epidermal hyperplasia. The skin feels rough and dry, an effect that may persist for months.

The photoprotective role of thickened stratum corneum is evident in albinos and individuals with vitiligo who do not produce melanin, yet become resistant to sunburn on repeated exposure to sunlight. Melanin pigmentation is stimulated, and the resistance of unprotected skin to solar radiation is increased by gradually increasing exposure to sunlight.Unfortunately, this natural defence requires dangerous amounts of UV exposure.

Contrary to tanning parlors' claims, there is no safe tan. The skin is damaged by exposure to sunlight or artificial sources of UV radiation. Commercial tanning units are promoted and used to induce a suntan for cosmetic purposes. Pigmentation from tanning parlors can only produce a maximum SPF of 4 and does not occur without cell damage.

Tanning booths are small rooms in which a patron is exposed to several lamps emitting UV radiation. Most of these lamps produce more than 95% UVA and less than 5% UVB. As UV bulbs age they emit less radiation, so burning can occur with the same exposure time when old bulbs are replaced with new ones. Patrons should be aware of the maximum exposure time recommended for a particular unit, and timers used to prevent overexposure. Protective eye wear should be worn while the lamps are in operation. Susceptible individuals risk photosensitivity reactions.

The Canadian Dermatology Association urges consumers to avoid tanning booths and to refrain from using sun-lamps.

PHOTOSENSITIVITY

An adverse reaction to the sun, photosensitivity encompasses both phototoxicity and photoallergy. Drug photosensitivity reactions are adverse skin responses to the combination of UV (usually UVA) radiation and topical or systemic exposure to a

TABLE 2: Skin Types* and Recommended Sun Protection Factor (SPF) to Protect Against Sunburn†

Skin Type	Sunburn/Suntan History	Examples	SPF
I	Poor ability to tan; burns easily and severely, then peels	Very fair skin, freckles Unexposed skin is white Blue, green or grey eyes Blonde, red or brown hair	15+
II	Tans minimally or lightly following exposure; usually burns easily resulting in a painful burn	Fair skin Unexposed skin is white Blue, green, grey or brown eyes Blonde, red or brown hair	15+
III	Tans gradually following exposure; burns moderately	"Average" Unexposed skin is white Eye and hair color usually brown	15+
IV	Tans well with initial exposure; burns minimally	Unexposed skin is white or light brown Dark eye and hair color (Mediterraneans, Orientals, Hispanics)	10 to 15
V	Tans easily and profusely; rarely burns	Unexposed skin is brown (American Indians, East Indians, Latin Americans)	10 to 15
VI	Deeply pigmented; never burns	Unexposed skin is black (African and American blacks, Australian and South Indian Aborigines)	6 to 10

*Determined by the reaction to the first 30 minutes of sun exposure after winter season or no sun exposure.
†Canadian Dermatology Association recommends a sunscreen of at least SPF 15 to protect against chronic effects of UV exposure.
Adapted with permission from: Pathak MA, Fitzpatrick TB. Preventative treatment of sunburn, dermatoheliosis and skin cancer with sun-protective agents. In: Fitzpatrick TB, et al, editors. Dermatology in General Medicine. 4th ed. New York: McGraw Hill, 1993:1689–717.

chemical, often prescription and nonprescription medications. UVA is readily transmitted through window glass and produced by fluorescent lamps commonly found in offices and factories. A susceptible person is not necessarily protected by being indoors.

Phototoxic reactions can occur in almost anyone if the photosensitizing agent absorbs enough of the appropriate radiation to cause cellular damage. They can occur on first exposure to the agent, within a few minutes to several hours after UV exposure and peak within hours to several days later, are dose related and confined to unprotected areas of the skin. They resemble an exaggerated sunburn reaction characterized by erythema, edema and blister formation. Most phototoxic reactions can be treated the same way as an ordinary sunburn.

Photoallergic reactions are less common, occurring in a small proportion of the people exposed to the drug. They are allergic reactions involving the immune system and require prior sensitization to the drug and UV radiation. Photoallergens combine with proteins in the skin to form complete antigens, which then initiate the immune response. Photoallergic reactions may look like urticarial lesions, developing within a few minutes after exposure, or may resemble papular or eczematous lesions and appear 24 hours or later. Itching frequently occurs before the appearance of lesions and often subsides in an hour. These reactions regularly show cross-sensitivity with chemically related compounds. Avoiding further exposure to the agent usually results in complete clearance of the eruption within 1 week. If continued use of the drug is vital, the patient should be instructed to avoid sun exposure between 10 a.m. and 4 p.m. and use a broad-spectrum sunscreen. People taking medications or using topical agents known to cause photosensitivity reactions should follow the same advice.

Various drug products and chemicals cause photosensitivity reactions (Table 3). The same agent can cause both a phototoxic and photoallergic reaction. The oils found in the rinds of citrus fruits as well as several chemicals added to soaps, cosmetics and perfumes for their antibacterial properties have been implicated.

Photodermatoses are disease states caused or exacerbated by exposure to sunlight, ranging from photosensitivity reactions to degenerative and neoplastic changes (Table 4). Patients that exhibit photosensitivity reactions after exposure to UV light not only have increased sensitivity to light, but may also have increased sensitivity to chemicals. In addition to cautioning them to avoid sunlight when possible, these patients should be advised to use a fragrance-free broad-spectrum sunscreen routinely on all exposed areas.

PHOTOAGING

Long-term exposure to sunlight causes considerable cumulative damage to the skin. The major changes in pigment and skin texture, known as photoaging and commonly called actinic damage or skin aging, are manifested as atrophy, wrinkling, dryness, telangiectasia (capillary dilation) and the splotchy hypo-hyperpigmentation often seen on sun-exposed areas of middle-aged or older persons. Despite increased public awareness of the harmful effects of UV radiation, sun-damaged skin is no longer restricted to older people. It is estimated that a person receives about 75% of the total lifetime dose of UV radiation before age 20.

Solar elastosis refers to the loss of normal elastic and connective tissue in the upper dermis. This loss often results in easy bruising and stellate scar formation due to degeneration of the supportive structures. "Turkey skin" is characteristic of this condition. Solar lentigo is a flat, evenly pigmented macule commonly referred to as an age spot or liver spot. Fair-skinned individuals are more susceptible to skin changes caused by chronic exposure to sunlight, although pigmented skin only partly resists photoaging.

Abnormal epidermal hyperplasia, known as actinic or solar keratosis, is premalignant and develops after years of sun exposure. These lesions are reddened patches often covered with a scale that can be pulled off but quickly returns. They are usually asymptomatic. People with these lesions should be referred to a physician. They are most common in older people but may occur in younger individuals who have had prolonged exposure to sunlight (e.g., sailors, farmers, lifeguards).

CANCER

Cancer is the most serious long-term effect of sunlight on the skin. The incidence is higher when UV radiation exposure is greater. The risk of skin cancer is inversely proportional to the amount of natural pigmentation.

The most common skin cancers are basal cell carcinoma, squamous cell carcinoma and malignant melanoma. Most often seen on sun-exposed areas, such as the head, neck, rim of the ears, chin and back of the hands of fair-complexioned

TABLE 3: Agents That May Cause Photosensitivity Reactions

Anticancer Drugs
Dacarbazine*
Fluorouracil
Methotrexate
Pentostatin
Procarbazine
Vinblastine

Antidepressants
Amoxapine
Doxepin
Isocarboxazid
Maprotiline
Tricyclics

Antihistamines
Astemizole
Azatadine
Cyproheptadine
Diphenhydramine

Antimicrobials
Azithromycin
Chlortetracycline
Demeclocycline*
Doxycycline
Griseofulvin
Minocycline
Nalidixic acid*
Norfloxacin
Ofloxacin
Sulfonamides
Tetracycline

Antiparasitics
Pyrvinium pamoate
Quinine

Antipsychotics
Chlorprothixene
Flupenthixol
Fluspirilene
Haloperidol
Loxapine
Nefazodone
Paroxetine
Phenothiazines
Pimozide
Thiothixene
Trazodone

Cardiovascular Agents
ACE inhibitors
Amiodarone
Diltiazem
Disopyramide
Felodipine
Flecainide
Fluvastatin
Metoprolol
Pravastatin
Sotalol
Terazosin

CNS Drugs
Carbamazepine
Diazepam
Estazolam
Selegiline

Diuretics
Acetazolamide
Amiloride
Chlorthalidone
Furosemide
Indapamide
Metolazone
Quinethazone
Thiazides
Triamterene

Nonsteroidal Anti-inflammatory Drugs
Diclofenac
Ketoprofen
Nabumetone
Naproxen
Phenylbutazone
Piroxicam
Sulindac
Tenoxicam

Others
5-Aminosalicylic acid
Auranofin
Aurothioglucose
Benzocaine
Bergamot oil, oils of citron, lavender, lime, sandalwood, cedar (used in many perfumes and cosmetics; also topical exposure to citrus rind oils)*
Chlorhexidine
Coal tar derivatives (acridine, anthracene, phenathrene)*
Gold salts
Hexachlorophene
Interferon 2α
Methazolamide
6-methylcoumarin (used in perfumes, shaving lotions and sunscreens)
Musk ambrette (used in perfumes)
Olsalazine
Omeprazole
Pentosan polysulfate sodium
Porfimer
Sulfonylureas
Terconazole
Tretinoin

*Reactions often occur.
Source: Krogh CME, ed. Compendium of Pharmaceuticals and Specialties. 30th ed. Ottawa: Canadian Pharmaceutical Association, 1995.

individuals; they seem to occur less in black populations living in the same geographic area. Unlike other forms of skin cancer, melanoma may occur on areas of the body not routinely exposed to sunlight.

In recent years the incidence of malignant melanoma has increased markedly: in Canada from 735 in 1980 to an estimated 3,100 in 1994 in both males and females. Melanoma in men is rising faster than any other cancer (4.5% per year); the incidence in women is also increasing rapidly (1% per year). In the United States, the lifetime risk of developing malignant melanoma is 1:1,500 for a person born in 1935 in contrast to 1:105 for someone born in 1991. The projected risk for a person born in the year 2,000 is 1:90. During the 1980s, the rise in incidence of malignant melanoma was approximately 7% per year, the most rapidly increasing rate for any cancer in the United States. Investigators have concluded that this increase is related to increased sun exposure.

Studies show that the risk of developing skin cancer is associated with an individual's tendency to burn easily and tan poorly. A history of repeated blistering sunburns in childhood or adolescence also correlates with a higher risk of melanoma. It has been suggested that the use of sunblocking agents to prevent sunburn may well reduce this risk. An Australian study showed that regular use of sunscreens prevented the development of solar keratoses, precursors of squamous cell carcinomas, and hastened the remission of existing ones.

Melanomas may form in or near a mole; because they spread easily once they reach a certain size, it is important to differentiate them from normal moles. The characteristic features of early malig-

Effects of UV Radiation

nant melanoma can be remembered by the acronym ABCD: A for asymmetry; B for border irregularity; C for color variegation; and D for diameter greater than 6 mm (top of a pencil eraser). Early melanomas have an irregular shape and border, may become inflamed and have a reddish edge and rarely, may bleed, ooze or crust. A melanoma may be itchy, grows in size, is usually greater than 6 mm in diameter and irregularly colored in shades of brown or black. These signs are not characteristic of ordinary moles. A person who displays such lesions should seek medical advice. Monthly self-examination of moles can increase early detection of both melanoma and non-melanoma skin cancers. Any change in a mole or birthmark or the development of a new mole should be reported to a physician immediately. Those at highest risk for malignant melanoma are fair-skinned with red or blonde hair, have several moles and freckle easily in sunlight. A family history of melanoma and blistering sunburns during childhood and adolescence also increase this risk.

Changes in the immune system from habitual sun exposure may contribute to the risk of skin cancer. A lifetime exposure to UV radiation may also cause eye damage resulting in decreased transmission of visible light by the lens and an increase in cataract formation.

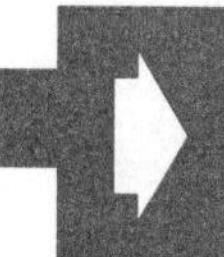

ADVICE FOR THE PATIENT

Preventing Cancer

The risk of skin cancer is related to the skin type and the amount of time spent in the sun. Fair-haired, blue-eyed individuals who burn and freckle easily are at particular risk. A person with a family history of melanoma, or who has several moles, or who had two or more blistering sunburns during childhood is at a higher risk for melanoma.To diminish the risk of developing skin cancer, these steps should be followed:

- Keep sun exposure to a minimum especially between the peak times of 10 a.m. and 3 p.m.
- Wear protective clothing including a broad-brimmed hat and sunglasses, long-sleeved shirt and long pants or skirt.
- Apply a broad-spectrum sunscreen generously to all exposed areas 30 minutes before sun exposure and reapply every 2 to 3 hours and after swimming or exercise. Remember that reapplying the sunscreen does not extend protection, it just ensures the SPF will be maintained.
- Be aware that clouds, fog and haze do not filter out the sun's harmful rays, and that they are reflected off sheets of aluminum, snow, water, sand and glossy magazine pages.
- Avoid tanning booths and sun-lamps since their use is associated with premature aging of the skin, cataract formation and an increased risk of skin cancer.
- Examine your skin and your children's skin regularly for any changes in size, shape or color of any moles.
- Protect children by keeping them out of the sun. Infants over 6 months of age should be protected by an SPF 15 or more sunscreen when exposed to sunlight.
- Teach children and teenagers to practise safe sun, since damage starts with the first exposure and accumulates over a lifetime.

TABLE 4: Action Spectra of Various Normal and Abnormal Responses of Human Skin to Solar Radiation

Condition	Range of Effectiveness Wavelengths (nm)	Maximum Reaction (nm)
I Normal individuals		
Sunburn reaction (solar)	290-320	305-307
Sunburn reaction (artificial light source)	250-320	250-275
Immediate pigment darkening (IPD) or tanning reaction	320-700	340-380
Delayed tanning (melanogenesis)	290-480	290-320
II Photosensitivity		
A. Phototoxic reaction		
Systemic drugs (see Table 2)	300-400	320-380
Topical drugs (see Table 2)	300-400	320-380
Phytophotodermatitis (plants)	320-400	320-360
Phototoxicity in chemically induced porphyria or hematoporphyrins	380-600	380-420
B. Photoallergic reaction		
Drug photoallergy (delayed hypersensitivity, topical or systemic) (see Table 2)	290-450	320-380
Certain solar urticarias (immediate hypersensitivity)	290-380	290-320 320-400
C. Persistent photosensitivity (persistent light reactions or actinic reticuloid)	290-400	290-320
III Degenerative and neoplastic		
Chronic actinic elastosis	290-400	290-320
Actinic keratosis	290-320	290-315
Basal cell epithelioma	290-320	290-315
Squamous cell carcinoma	290-320	290-315
Malignant melanoma	290-320	290-315
IV Genetic and metabolic		
Xeroderma pigmentosum	290-320	290-320
Albinism	290-400	290-320
Ephelides (freckles)	290-400	290-320
Erythropoietic porphyria	390-600	390-420
Erythropoietic protoporphyria	390-600	390-420
Porphyria cutanea tarda	390-600	390-420
Variegate porphyria	390-600	390-420
Vitiligo (macules)	290-320	290-315
Hartnup syndrome	290-320	
Cockayne's syndrome	290-320	
Darier-White disease	290-320	
Bloom's syndrome	290-320	
Rothmund-Thomson syndrome	290-320	
Haily-Haily disease	290-320	
V Nutritional		
Kwashiorkor	290-400	
Pellagra	290-400	
VI Infections *(viral)*		
Lymphogranuloma venereum	290-320	
Herpes simplex	290-320	

TABLE 4: Action Spectra of Various Normal and Abnormal Responses of Human Skin to Solar Radiation *(cont'd)*

Condition	Range of Effectiveness Wavelengths (nm)	Maximum Reaction (nm)
VII Miscellaneous *(light and normal skin or diseases)*		
Hydroa aestivale	290-400 infrared	290-320
Hydroa vacciniforme	290-400 infrared	290-320
Polymorphous photodermatoses, including variants such as papular, plaques, papulovesicular and eczematous eruptions	290-400	290-320
Disseminated superficial actinic porokeratosis	290-320	290-320
Discoid lupus erythematosus	290-320	290-320
Systemic lupus erythematosus	290-320	
Dermatomyositis	290-320	
Photosensitive eczema	290-320	

Adapted with permission from: Pathak MA. Sunscreens: topical and systemic approaches for protection of human skin against harmful effects of solar radiation. J Am Acad Dermatol 1982;7(3):285-312.

PROTECTION

NONPHARMACOLOGICAL PROTECTION

Nonpharmacological measures can ensure protection in addition to, or as an alternative to sunscreens. The easiest strategy is to avoid sun exposure between 10 a.m. and 3 p.m. Dry, dark colored, tightly woven clothing offers physical protection. If light can be seen through clothing held to the sun, then UV rays can penetrate it. Wet clothing loses some of its ability to block out the sun's rays. Some examples of the SPF of dry clothing are given below:

Cotton/polyester T-shirt	SPF 15
Cotton shirt	SPF 7
Cotton denim jacket	SPF 1,700
Polyester/lycra surf shirt	SPF 35

Broad-brimmed and Legionnaire style hats made of tightly woven fabric (not straw or plastic weave) protect the face and neck. Baseball caps should be avoided; they do not protect the cheeks, ears and neck. Shade offers protection from direct UV radiation, but reflected radiation is still a problem. Sunglasses that contain UV filters are recommended. The *SLIP SLAP SLOP* program of the Canadian Cancer Society and the Canadian Dermatology Association advises everyone to seek shade and SLIP on clothing to cover arms and legs, SLAP on a wide-brimmed hat and SLOP on a sunscreen with SPF 15 or higher.

TOPICAL PROTECTION

Sunscreens can be grouped in two broad categories: topical and systemic, and topical sunscreens subdivided further into physical and chemical. Table 5 lists the sun-protection agents considered safe and effective by Health Canada.

Sun Protection Factor

The degree of protection offered by preparations available in Canada is indicated by the sun protection factor (SPF) listed on product labels. This value is the quotient of the dose of UV radiation neces-

TABLE 5: Sunscreen Agents Recognized as Safe and Effective by Health Canada

Sunscreen Agent	Synonyms	Concentration
Chemical Agents		
UVA Absorbers		
Butyl methoxydibenzoylmethane	Parsol 1789, Avobenzone	5%
Benzophenone-3	Oxybenzone	2-6%
Benzophenone-4	Sulisobenzone	5-10%
Benzophenone-8	Dioxybenzone	3%
Menthyl anthranilate	Methyl 2-aminobenzoate	3.5-5%
Terephthalylidene dicamphor sulfonic acid	Mexoryl SX	0.5-10%
UVB Absorbers		
2-ethoxyethyl p-methoxycinnamate	Cinoxate	1-3%
Diethanolamine p-methoxycinnamate		8-10%
Ethyldihydroxypropyl PABA	4-[bis 2-(hydroxypropyl) amino] benzoic acid	1-5%
Octocrylene	2-ethylhexyl 2-cyano-3,3 diphenylacrylate	7-10%
Octyl methoxycinnamate	2-ethylhexyl p-methoxycinnamate	2-7.5%
Octyl salicylate	2-ethylhexyl salicylate	3-5%
Glyceryl PABA	Glyceryl p-aminobenzoate	3%
Homosalate	Homomenthyl salicylate	4-15%
PABA	Aminobenzoic acid	5-15%
Amyl dimethyl PABA	Padimate A	1-5%
Octyl dimethyl PABA	Padimate O	1.4-8%
2-phenylbenzimidazole-5-sulfonic acid		1-4%
Triethanolamine salicylate	Trolamine salicylate	5-12%
Physical Agents		
Titanium dioxide		2-25%
Zinc oxide		20%

Adapted with permission from: Health Protection Branch Standard Proprietary Medicine Monograph Sunburn Protectants. Ottawa: Health Canada, 1995.

sary to produce perceptible redness (minimal erythemal dose or MED) using a sunscreen divided by the amount necessary to produce this erythema without the sunscreen.

$$SPF = \frac{\text{MED of sunscreen-protected skin}}{\text{MED of unprotected skin}}$$

The higher the SPF, the more protection the product offers. In practical terms, the SPF means that if a person can stay in the sun unprotected for 15 minutes before experiencing erythema, a sunscreen with an SPF of 4 extends this period to 1 hour. Reapplying the sunscreen after the first hour does not extend protection for another hour since the skin has already received enough UV radiation to bcgin a sunburn.

Sunscreens with an SPF of 15 block about 93% of UVB radiation. Many sunscreens labelled SPF 30 or higher have recently become available, providing about 97% protection. This high level may not be necessary, since in most regions the maximum dose of UV radiation does not exceed 15 MED during an entire day of exposure. Patients with photodermatoses, who have exquisite photosensitivity and cannot be exposed to sunlight without incurring serious sunburn, may benefit from them. SPF values are determined experimentally under ideal conditions with indoor solar simulators and may be as much as 50% higher than measurements obtained outdoors. In natural sunlight the protective efficacy of a sunscreen product may vary considerably due to differences in individual characteristics, environmental conditions and sunscreen properties. These factors are summarized in Table 6.

Measuring UVA Efficacy

The SPF value of a sunscreen is a measure of its degree of protection primarily from UVB radiation. To date, there is no standard measure for UVA protection, making it difficult to compare products. Testing for UVA efficacy is complicated since erythema (the endpoint for measuring SPF) is not easily obtained with UVA. Several measures for UVA protection have been proposed, but until a standard method has been established, patients should be advised to base their selection on the ingredients listed on the sunscreen product.

Choice of a Sunscreen

Sunscreen products are available in creams (oily or vanishing), lotions (clear or milky), gels, sprays and solids (lip balm). Counselling people on the prevention of sunburn, skin cancer, photoaging and various forms of sun sensitivity, the choice and recommendation of a sunscreen depends on several factors.

Skin Type: To prevent sunburn, people with fair complexions and blue, green or grey eyes, who burn easily and tan poorly (skin types I and II), should use sunscreens with an SPF of at least 15. Those with skin type III, who burn moderately but tan well, may also use a sunscreen with a similar SPF. Darker-skinned people (skin type IV or V), who tan easily and burn minimally or rarely, may use a sunscreen with an SPF rating of 10 to 15. Those with skin type VI may use a sunscreen with SPF 6 to 10 (Table 1). Both UVB and UVA rays are erythrogenic and all individuals, irrespective of skin type, will burn if exposed to a dose of UV radiation that exceeds their individual MED value. To protect against the long-term effects of sun exposure the Canadian Dermatology Association recommends a sunscreen with SPF 15 on all individuals.

Type of Activity: Before recommending a sunscreen product, the type of activity and duration of sun exposure should be considered. Persons engaging in water sports (e.g., swimming, water skiing or windsurfing), profuse sweating from exercise or prolonged sunbathing require a product not easily washed off. Snow-skiers or mountain climbers might need a higher SPF because of the added effects of UV radiation at a higher altitude and reflection off snow.

Site of Application: The lips and nose are particularly sensitive to UV radiation. Normal skin has a thick stratum corneum, melanin, keratin and protein, which protect against moderate exposure to UV light. The stratum corneum on the lips is thin and melanin is absent, so maximum protection is required. Patients should be advised to apply a waterproof sunscreen on the lips before sun exposure and to repeat application to restore protection after eating or drinking. While in the sun, re-application is required immediately after swimming. Women may use an opaque lipstick after applying the sunscreen. Some people with recurrent sunlight-induced herpes labialis may benefit from a high SPF sunscreen.

Condition of Skin: People with dry skin often benefit from a cream or lotion base. Those with oily skin, especially if prone to acne, do better with an alcohol solution or gel. Some alcohol-based vehicles may irritate during energetic activity and should not be used on eczematous or inflamed skin. Some of these products may contain up to 70% alcohol, which renders them highly flammable. Smokers and persons exposed to open flames (e.g., outdoor barbecues) should avoid applying alcohol-based sunscreens near these activities.

Sun Sensitivity: Individuals who have a photosensitivity reaction or a condition exacerbated by sunlight need protection from both UVA and UVB radiation. Products containing para-aminobenzoic acid (PABA) or PABA esters alone are not suitable since they do not absorb the UVA radiation responsible for most photosensitivity reactions. A combination product containing butyl methoxydibenzoylmethane (Parsol 1789), a UVB absorbing agent, and a physical sunscreen with a high SPF should be used. People with skin carcinomas require maximum protection from UV radiation. These patients should also be advised to protect themselves by wearing a hat, long-sleeved shirt and long pants or skirt. The most effective preventive measure is avoiding sun exposure.

Cross-sensitivity: Certain drugs (e.g., sulfonamides and thiazide diuretics) may show cross-

TABLE 6: Factors Affecting Sunscreen Efficacy

Factor	Description
Individual Characteristics	
Test subjects:	Variations in skin type, melanin content, skin thickness, degree of vascularity, amount of hair on test site, age of subject
Sweating:	Skin temperature, rate of production and evaporation of sweat, amount of urocanic acid (a natural sunscreen present in sweat)
Swimming:	Duration of swimming, water (whether chlorinated or salted), state of hydration of the skin
Environmental Conditions	
UV intensity:	Irradiation dose of UVA and UVB, season, latitude, altitude, clouds, air pollution, time of day, reflectivity of the ground
Temperature	
Degree of humidity	
Direct and scattered radiation	
Snow	
Sand	
Wind velocity	
Sunscreen Properties	
Concentration:	Differences in the concentration of the UV-absorbing active ingredients
Vehicle:	Composition, chemical properties (lipophilic or hydrophilic nature), pH, emollient properties
Thickness of applied film:	Uniform application of about 2 mg/cm^2 or 2 mL/cm^2 (equivalent to a film thickness of 0.02 mm on the skin) has been recommended. It takes about nine 2.5 mL measures of sunscreen to achieve that thickness of film on the skin. On average, one measure (2.5 mL) is to be used for the face and neck, one for each arm and shoulder, one for the front of the torso, one for the back and two for each leg and top of the foot. Studies examining the effect of film irregularities on sunscreen efficacy report discrepancies of approximately 50% in SPF values.
Other ingredients:	Some impurities or additives can act as photosensitizers (e.g., ortho and meta esters of PABA, and 6-methylcoumarin, a fragrance).
Substantivity:	It refers to the ability of a sunscreen to maintain efficacy when subjected to moisture (such as swimming and sweating). This property is a function of both the sunscreen agent and the vehicle. Sunscreen substantivity varies with its hydrophilic and lipophilic properties, pH, heat stability, emollient nature, percutaneous absorptivity, ionized state and diffusion capacity, and with ingredient absorption and conjugation to the stratum corneum proteins. Products with cream, oil or gel bases are more resistant to removal by water than those with alcohol bases. In addition, a water-in-oil base has a greater resistance to water removal than gel or oil-in-water emulsion. Development of new vehicles combining an oil-in-water emulsion with an acrylate film polymer that adheres to the skin has led to increased water resistance. Combination products are more substantive than those containing a single ingredient. Emollients in creams or lotions lower the substantivity of the sunscreen agent. The substantivity of a product is optimized by applying it 30 minutes prior to sun exposure to allow enough time for protein binding. **Water resistant** implies that a sunscreen will maintain its photoprotective effect after 40 minutes of active immersion (e.g., swimming), and **waterproof** sunscreens remain effective after 80 minutes of immersion. Reapplying sunscreens after swimming or sweating does not extend the duration of photoprotection but ensures that the said SPF will be maintained.

sensitivity with PABA and its derivatives (Table 7). Individuals sensitive to these agents should not use sunscreens containing PABA or its esters. In rare instances, there is sensitivity to an ingredient other than the active sunscreen in the product. There have been reports of allergic contact dermatitis in response to the vehicle (e.g., triethanolamine stearate), the fragrance (e.g., 6-methylcoumarin), the preservative (e.g., parabens) and the lubricant (e.g., phenyl dimethicone) present in a sunscreen product. New users can test a product by applying a small amount to a small patch of skin at least 24 hours before using it on a larger area.

Other factors that may influence the choice of a sunscreen are past experience with various products, motivation for its use, ease of application, cosmetic acceptability, fragrance and cost. The Canadian Dermatology Association recommends protecting the skin from the sun every day from spring right through to fall, and during the winter if participating in an outdoor sport. Individuals should be reminded that it is never too late to start using sun protection to help prevent further skin damage.

Sunscreens on Children

Chemical sunscreens are not recommended for infants under the age of 6 months, primarily because skin development is immature, absorption through young skin is very high and metabolic and excretory systems are underdeveloped. Sunburn occurs readily in young babies because the amount of melanin present is less than it will ever be in the infant's life. Babies should wear protective clothing or be kept out of the sun for their first 6 months. Sunscreens with SPF 15 or more are recommended for infants over 6 months as well as children and adolescents. Creams or milky lotions are preferred as alcoholic lotions and gel sunscreens can cause stinging, irritation and burning of the eyes. The recommended sunscreen for children is an SPF 15 milky lotion for total body application and a physical block for sun-sensitive areas such as the nose and shoulders.

Since the number of blistering sunburns suffered during childhood and adolescence is associated with an increased risk of malignant melanoma later in life, it is essential to adequately protect youngsters. One study demonstrated that parents who had been educated by their child's physician regarding sun protection were twice as likely to use sunscreen on their child as parents who did not recall receiving any information. Other studies showed that teenagers are more likely to use sunscreens if their parents had insisted on their use early in life and that they are more compliant with nongreasy formulations that do not aggravate acne. Investigators project that regular use of sunscreen with a sun protection factor of 15 during the first 18 years can decrease the lifetime risk of nonmelanoma skin cancers by 78%. Teaching children and parents to practise sun protection early in life can reduce sun-related skin damage since it begins with the first exposure and accumulates over a lifetime. Parents can involve young children by getting them to do the "shadow test." The sun's rays are strongest when the sun is directly overhead and short shadows are cast. If the shadow is shorter than the child, then it is time to go indoors or find some shade. When the shadow is longer than the child, it is safe to play outside.

TABLE 7: Examples of Drugs that Cross-react with PABA and its Esters

Sulfonamide antibiotics Sulfamethoxazole Sulfisoxazole	**Ester-type anesthetics** Benzocaine Procaine Tetracaine
Sulfonamide-based oral hypoglycemics Chlorpropamide Glyburide Tolbutamide	**Artificial sweeteners** Saccharin Sodium cyclamate
Thiazide diuretics Chlorothiazide Hydrochlorothiazide	**Para-amino type azo dyes** Aniline Paraphenylenediamine

Adapted from: Mathias CGT. Commentary and update: cutaneous sensitivity to monoglyceryl para-aminobenzoate. Cleve Clin Q 1983;50(2):85–86.

PATIENT ASSESSMENT QUESTIONS

?

***Q** Are you requesting a sunscreen product for yourself or someone else? Will exposure to the sun be intense or limited?*

It is important to determine the skin type of the person using the sunscreen (Table 2). Depending on the sunburning/suntanning history of the individual and the degree of sun exposure, an appropriate sunscreen product with a high or low sun protection factor (SPF) may be selected.

***Q** Do you require the sunscreen for outdoor work or for recreational activities? Do you plan to swim, ski, climb mountains or participate in strenuous activities while using the product?*

The type of activity helps determine the product to recommend. An individual who swims or sweats requires a product not easily washed off.

***Q** What sunscreens have you used in the past? Have you ever reacted to a sunscreen product?*

A person's past experience (successful or unsuccessful) may help in the selection of an appropriate sunscreen. Individuals who have experienced any allergic reactions to a sunscreen formulation should choose a product with different ingredients.

***Q** Have you had any allergic reactions to oral or topical medications?*

Although sunscreens do not generally produce hypersensitivity reactions, PABA has shown cross-sensitivity with chemically related drugs. A person who reports an allergic reaction to drugs such as sulfonamide antibiotics, hypoglycemics, thiazides or ester-type anesthetics should be cautioned against using products containing PABA and its derivatives (Table 7).

***Q** What medications are you currently taking?*

Certain drugs may cause photosensitivity reactions (Table 3). A person taking a medication that may be photosensitizing requires a broad spectrum sunscreen that protects against both UVB and UVA radiation.

***Q** Do you have any medical conditions that predispose you to skin problems (such as a rash or severe sunburn) on exposure to sunlight or ultraviolet radiation? Has your physician advised you to use a sunscreen when exposed to sunlight?*

Certain medical conditions may be caused or aggravated by exposure to sunlight (Table 4). A person with abnormal responses to sunlight should be referred to a physician. A sunscreen product should offer protection against the radiation responsible for precipitating the skin reactions.

***Q** Is your skin dry or oily?*

The condition of a person's skin should be considered when recommending a sunscreen. Individuals with dry skin often benefit from a cream-based formulation; those with oily skin may benefit from an alcohol-based product.

***Q** Have you ever had cold sores caused by sun exposure?*

Sunlight may be a precipitating factor in recurrent herpes labialis. An adequate lip sunscreen may block the effect of solar radiation and prevent cold sore recurrence in some people.

***Q** Are you prone to acne?*

Patients with acne should use a noncomedogenic and/or nonacnegenic sunscreen.

PHARMACEUTICAL AGENTS

CHEMICAL SUNSCREENS

Chemical sunscreens absorb, reflect or scatter a certain portion of UV light away from the skin to prevent penetration of the dermis. Not containing any visible-light absorbing chemicals, they are usually colorless, therefore cosmetically acceptable to most individuals.

The molar absorptivity of a chemical sunscreen refers to its ability to absorb UV radiation. A large molar absorptivity at a particular wavelength indicates good absorption at that wavelength. To be effective against sunburn, a sunscreen should have a range of maximum absorption that overlaps the range of UV radiation responsible for sunburn. An agent with a low molar absorptivity may be made more effective by increasing its concentration in a formulation.

Para-aminobenzoic acid (PABA) and its esters absorb UVB but not UVA radiation. PABA and glycerol PABA absorb between 260 and 313 nm, and PABA esters, amyl dimethyl PABA (padimate A) and octyl dimethyl PABA (padimate O) protect between 280 and 315 nm. PABA is most effective in a concentration of 5% in a 70% ethanol solution. Its use has declined in recent years because of the incidence of irritation and hypersensitivity reactions. Its main advantage is its ability to penetrate the stratum corneum and bind to proteins.Continued use of PABA leads to an accumulation that gets trapped in the skin and may provide extended UVB protection even after swimming, sweating or showering. Padimate A and padimate O have low water solubility and are poorly removed by water. They can be incorporated into lotion or cream bases, which are less irritating than alcohol bases and more resistant to removal by water. Sunscreens with PABA and PABA ester should be applied 30 minutes before sun exposure to allow for binding to the stratum corneum. To assure maximum protection, it is best to reapply sunscreens every 2 to 3 hours and after swimming or profuse sweating.

PABA can stain clothes and fibreglass yellow, especially after exposure to sunlight. Allergic contact dermatitis may develop from the use of PABA and certain esters, mainly glyceryl PABA. In addition, certain drugs have been reported to cross-react with PABA and its esters (Table 8). People with a history of hypersensitivity to these agents should avoid sunscreens containing PABA and its derivatives.

Cinnamic acid derivatives commonly used are **cinoxate** (2-ethoxyethyl p-methoxycinnamate) and **octyl methoxycinnamate** (2-ethylhexyl p-methoxycinnamate) (Parsol MCX). They absorb primarily in the UVB region (270 to 328 nm). They do not bind to the stratum corneum, so wash off easily and must be reapplied frequently. Cinnamic acid derivatives used in combination with benzophenones appear to effectively protect against UVB and UVA radiation up to 360 nm. Adverse effects with octyl methoxycinnamate are few, although there have been reports of contact dermatitis with cinnamate-containing sunscreens, as well as cross-sensitization among cinnamon derivatives such as cinnamon oil, Balsam of Peru, cinnamic acid and aldehyde.

Salicylic acid derivatives, such as **homosalate** (homomenthyl salicylate) and **octyl salicylate** (2-ethylhexyl salicylate), absorb primarily in the UVB region (260 to 310 nm), but have about one-third the absorbency of PABA. Weak in absorbing UV, they have to be used in relatively high concentrations.They are useful in solubilizing other non-soluble sunscreens such as benzophenones. Homosalate, with an absorbency range between 290 and 315 nm, must be used in a concentration of 4 to 15% to be effective. It does not bind to the skin, is easily removed by sweating or swimming and rarely, may cause contact and photocontact allergy.

Benzophenone derivatives, such as **oxybenzone**, **dioxybenzone** and **sulisobenzone**, absorb UVB and the shorter UVA wavelengths. Oxybenzone absorbs between 270 and 350 nm (max 287 to 290 nm), dioxybenzone absorbs between 260 and 380 nm (max 289 to 327 nm) and sulisobenzone absorbs between 270 and 360 nm (max 286 to 324 nm). Since they absorb radiation within the UVA range, they may be useful for photosensitivity reactions or conditions exacerbated by sunlight. Unfortunately, their absorption falls sharply at wavelengths over 330 nm, and they may not provide complete UV protection. When used in higher concentrations (6 to 10%), they cover the entire UVR spectrum, with the higher concentrations giving increased absorptive properties.

Products containing benzophenones in combination with PABA or PABA esters provide better protection than either agent used alone. Adverse effects are rare, but contact dermatitis and photocontact reactions may occasionally develop.

Menthyl anthranilate, the only anthranilic acid derivative currently available in sunscreen products, has the weakest molar absorptivity of all sunscreen agents. It absorbs UV radiation in the range of 300 to 360 nm; maximum absorption is between 332 and 345 nm. It has about one-twentieth the absorbency of PABA, is used in combination with other sunscreens to provide an effective product, and rarely causes sensitization problems.

Dibenzoylmethane derivatives such as **butyl methoxydibenzoylmethane** (Parsol 1789, avobenzone) and **4-isopropyl dibenzoylmethane** (Eusolex 8020) are a new class of sunscreen. Eusolex is not available in Canada. They absorb radiation in most of the UVA region (310-390 nm) with peak absorption at 358 nm.They are formulated in concentrations of 2 to 3% and are usually combined with UVB filters. They are indicated for photosensitivity reactions or conditions exacerbated by sunlight. Allergic reactions and photocontact dermatitis have been reported with these agents especially with Eusolex 8020. Cross-sensitivity between these two agents has occasionally been observed. Because of the high incidence of contact and photocontact allergy with Eusolex 8020, the manufacturers have withdrawn this compound from the European market.

Terephthalidene dicamphor sulfonic acid (Mexoryl SX) is a new sunscreen that absorbs UV radiation between 290 and 400 nm with a peak at 345 nm. It is highly photostable with a capacity for reversing to its original isomer after excitation of the molecule by UV light. This property prevents degradation of the sunscreen and maintains protective ability. It is formulated in concentrations up to 10% with other UVA and UVB filters to provide a broad-spectrum sunscreen product.

PHYSICAL SUNSCREENS

Physical sunscreens form an occlusive barrier that reflects and scatters light.They include zinc oxide, talc (magnesium trisilicate), titanium dioxide, kaolin, ferric (or ferrous) oxide and red veterinary petrolatum, which must be applied in a thick layer to be effective. They are cosmetically unacceptable, may stain clothing and are often messy to use. However, they help protect particularly sun sensitive areas such as the nose and lips and may be more appealing now that they are available in a variety of bright colors.

Physical blockers, such as zinc oxide and titanium dioxide, have the advantage of not being sensitizers, but their occlusive nature may cause acne, folliculitis and miliaria (heat rash). Recently developed preparations of microfine titanium dioxide and micronized zinc oxide are almost invisible on the skin and more cosmetically elegant. They may prove useful in conditions exacerbated by sunlight where chemical sunscreens are not tolerated. Physical sunscreens do not wash off easily when the skin is immersed in water, but melt with the heat of the sun.

POSSIBLE ADVERSE EFFECTS OF SUNSCREENS

The most common side effects of sunscreens are skin irritation and staining mainly due to PABA or alcohol-containing products. Contact and photocontact dermatitis may sometimes occur with chemical sunscreens, rarely with excipients in the product. Switching to another product with different ingredients usually alleviates the problem.

The role of sunscreens in the rate of increase of malignant melanoma has been questioned. UVB-blocking sunscreens may allow prolonged periods of sun exposure (particularly to UVA) not possible without them. Prevention of sunburn may give users a false sense of security and excessive amounts of UVA radiation might place them at a higher risk for melanoma. Broad-spectrum sunscreens will help diminish this concern. It should be stressed that sunscreens should not be used to prolong sun exposure, just to protect the skin.

Routine use of sunscreens may be associated with a blockage of vitamin D_3 photosynthesis. UVB radiation is necessary for the conversion of 7-dehydrocholesterol in the skin to vitamin D_3. Elderly sunscreen users who depend on UV-induced vitamin D_3 to meet their requirements may risk vitamin D deficiency, which may lead to osteomalacia and bone fractures. If they are unable to tolerate dairy products, oral vitamin D supplements or limited sun exposure without sunscreen should be recommended.

Vitamin D deficiency is not a concern in children and adolescents who have casual sun exposure and an adequate diet. Infants under 6 months do not require vitamin D conversion; this is bypassed by administration of vitamin D supplements.

In 1988, the FDA of the United States reported the discovery of NPABAO (2-ethylhexyl (4-N-methyl-N-nitrosamino) benzoate), a new nitrosamine in some sunscreens. It has not yet been determined if NPABAO is a carcinogen. Because ultraviolet radiation is known to be carcinogenic, the use of sunscreens should continue to be encouraged.

SYSTEMIC PROTECTION

The desire for systemic photoprotectants to reduce skin reaction to solar radiation has inspired much research. Agents such as PABA, antihistamines, vitamins A, C and E, ASA, unsaturated fatty acids and steroids have been investigated but not proven successful. Three systemic agents that have shown limited efficacy are beta-carotene, antimalarials and some of the psoralen derivatives. Beta-carotene is no longer available in Canada as a systemic photoprotective agent.

PIGMENTING OR TANNING AGENTS

Low SPF sunscreens or products containing no sunprotective agent in oil or emollient-rich bases are promoted as "suntan" products. The low SPF (less than 3) provides minimal protection, and the oily base makes the skin more permeable to UV radiation, resulting in inflammation and postinflammatory hyperpigmentation, not tanning.

The use of systemic agents that modify skin color, **beta-carotene** and **canthaxanthin**, has declined in recent years. Canthaxanthin is a carotenoid, but unlike beta-carotene it possesses no vitamin A activity. It is commonly used in low concentrations as a coloring agent in foods such as cheese and ketchup.

Canthaxanthin is dosed by body weight using a 20-day schedule; subsequent maintenance doses are necessary to maintain the color. Its use to produce an artificial suntan has been associated with retinal deposits and in some cases resulted in impaired vision. The development of brick-red stools can mask lower gastrointestinal tract bleeding.

After ingestion, beta-carotene and canthaxanthin accumulate in subcutaneous fat and in the epidermis. In individuals with skin types I, II and III, the skin colors orange-brown. People with erythropoietic protoporphyria or generalized vitiligo may find this color more appealing than the yellowish color produced by beta-carotene alone. Some do not like the unnatural coloring of the palms, soles and skin behind the ear lobes.

Since the photoprotective ability as well as the long-term systemic effects of the canthaxanthin/beta-carotene mixture have not been fully evaluated, recommending its use must await further investigation. Aplastic anemia associated with cathaxanthin use has been reported. Despite a warning by the United States Food and Drug Administration to not use cathaxanthin as an oral tanning agent, the drug is readily available through mail-order advertisements.

Applying **dihydroxyacetone** (DHA) to the skin slowly produces a brown color similar to a tan. The topical formulation containing DHA becomes oxidized and stains the skin, probably by binding to the keratin of the stratum corneum to form a dark pigment. No new melanin is produced, and the color washes off with soap and water or solvents such as acetone or alcohol. These formulations offer no photoprotection against UVA or UVB radiation but protect from the visible spectrum (400 to 500 nm). They may be useful for people with erythropoietic protoporphyria who require protection from visible radiation.

Dihydroxyacetone in concentrations of 4 to 8% has been used in creams and lotions. DHA is incorporated into camouflaging creams for people with vitiligo. A single application of DHA may give a patchy appearance, especially when applied to large areas of vitiliginous skin. Repeated application after the lotion dries results in progressive darkening. Although products are available in only one color, most people find they can adequately camouflage lesions once they know how many applications are required to achieve the desired skin tone. To maintain pigmentation once the desired skin color is achieved, DHA may be applied every 1 to 3 days. When treatment is stopped, the color starts to fade in about 2 days and disappears completely within 8 to 14 days as the epidermal cells of the stratum corneum are sloughed.

DEPIGMENTING AGENTS

Depigmenting agents lighten hyperpigmented areas caused by medical disorders (lentigines, freckles, melasma) or drugs (tetracyclines, antimalarials, hormones and chemotherapeutics such as busulfan, 5-fluorouracil, cyclophosphamide, nitrogen mustard and bleomycin). Melasma, brownish macules on the face, may occur in pregnant women, women on oral contraceptives or in people taking phenytoin or mephenytoin and is aggravated by sun exposure. A sunscreen with UVB and broad-spectrum UVA coverage should be used.

Hydroquinone is an antioxidant that inhibits the conversion of tyrosine to dihydroxyphenylalanine (a precursor of melanin). It does not injure or decrease the number of melanocytes and is available without prescription in concentrations of 2 to 4% in bleaching creams and ointments. To depigment hyperpigmented areas, it should be applied in a thin uniform layer twice a day to intact skin and kept away from the eyes. Since its action is only temporary, repeat applications are needed at frequent intervals, usually twice a day for weeks to months. It may cause irritation and is best stored in airtight containers, protected from light.

Hydroquinone is relatively safe in low concentrations (2%); the incidence of side effects greatly increases at higher concentrations. Adverse reactions include stinging sensations, erythema, and allergic and contact dermatitis. Toxic reactions resulting in complete depigmentation of the treated areas instead of a mere lightening have been reported. Minimal exposure to sunlight may reverse the bleaching effect of hydroquinone. Using sunscreens or protective clothing, and avoiding unnecessary sun exposure during treatment achieves best results and prevents repigmentation. Some preparations contain a combination of hydroquinone and sunscreen agents and should be used during the day.

Monobenzone, the monobenzyl ether of hydroquinone, is available as a 20% cream, gel or emulsion. It, too, inhibits the conversion of tyrosine to dihydroxyphenylalanine, preventing formation of melanin pigment in the skin. Its pigment-decreasing action is irreversible, somewhat erratic and unpredictable. Areas of normal skin distant to the site of treatment have often become permanently depigmented. Monobenzone is only indicated for use in extensive vitiligo when permanent depigmentation is desired. It is contraindicated for use in freckling, melasma or hyperpigmentation where less but not absent pigmentation is desired. It may cause irritation and sensitization of the skin. Although a nonprescription drug, therapy with this medication is generally supervised by a dermatologist.

RECOMMENDED READING

Buescher LS. Sunscreens and photoprotection. Otolaryngol Clin North Am 1993; 26(1):13-22.

Pathak MA, Fitzpatrick TB. Preventative treatment of sunburn, dermatoheliosis and skin cancer with sun-protective agents. In: Fitzpatrick TB, et al , eds. Dermatology in General Medicine. 4th ed. New York: McGraw-Hill, 1993:1689-1717.

Rapaport MJ. Choosing a broad-spectrum sunscreen with UVA protection. Dermatol Nursing 1991; 3(2):83-9, 102.

26

TRAVEL HEALTH PRODUCTS

HELEN NG

CONTENTS

Travellers' Diarrhea 643
- Signs and Symptoms
- Prophylaxis
- Treatment

Water Purification 646
- Methods of Purification

Motion Sickness 648
- Signs and Symptoms
- Treatment

Travel First Aid 650
- First Aid Kit
- Storage of Medication

Pharmaceutical Agents 652

Recommended Reading 654

TRAVELLERS' DIARRHEA

Travellers' diarrhea is characterized by an increase in frequency of loose stool and linked to fecally contaminated food or water. Although often associated with travelling from an industrialized region to a developing country, it has also been reported in the reverse situation. The term traveller includes not only tourists but also those studying or working in foreign countries.

The risk of developing travellers' diarrhea is determined mainly by the destination, the highest risk areas being Latin America, Africa, Asia, and the Middle East. It is also more common during the rainy seasons. Other risk factors include the use of histamine type 2 (H_2) blockers (e.g., ranitidine), proton pump inhibitors (e.g., omeprazole), and patients with insulin-dependent diabetes, gastrectomy, achlorhydria or acquired immune deficiency syndrome (AIDS). Approximately 20 to 50% of all travellers are affected. It is not gender specific and is more prevalent in the young than the old, possibly due to more adventurous lifestyles or a lack of acquired immunity.

The main causes are bacteria, with enterotoxigenic *Escherichia coli* (up to 40%) the most common (Table 1). Viral pathogens such as Rotavirus and Norwalk virus account for 10 to 15% of

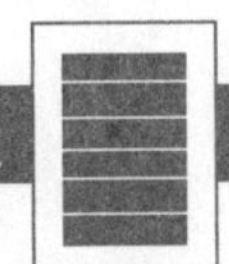

TABLE 1: Organisms Causing Travellers' Diarrhea

(in approximate order of frequency)

Bacteria	Viruses	Parasites
Enterotoxigenic *Escherichia coli*	Rotavirus	*Giardia lamblia*
Shigella species	Norwalk virus	*Cryptosporidium* species
Aeromonas species		*Entamoeba histolytica*
Plesiomonas shigelloides		
Salmonella species		
Campylobacter jejuni		
Noncholera vibrios		

cases, parasitic infections (e.g., *Giardia lamblia, Entamoeba histolytica*) for up to 6%, and mixed infections for about 10 to 20%.

SIGNS AND SYMPTOMS

Defined as a twofold or greater increase in the frequency of loose stools, travellers' diarrhea is often accompanied by abdominal pain, nausea, vomiting, bloating, fecal urgency, and tenesmus (a painful sphincter spasm).

The onset is abrupt, usually within the week of arrival but can also occur 7 to 10 days after returning home, depending on the incubation period of the enteropathogen.

It is often self-limiting with an average duration of 3 to 4 days. About 10% of cases persist for longer than a week and 2% longer than a month. Patients with persistent diarrhea should be tested for parasitic infections.

Travellers' diarrhea can be classified as invasive or noninvasive. Noninvasive diarrhea has localized symptoms such as watery diarrhea due mainly to the enterotoxin produced by the pathogen. Invasive diarrhea (about 10% of cases) has serious systemic symptoms such as dysentery (e.g., bloody diarrhea), chills, fever, cramps and vomiting, believed to occur when the bacteria penetrates the mucosa of the gut. These patients should not self-treat with nonprescription products but be referred to a physician for treatment.

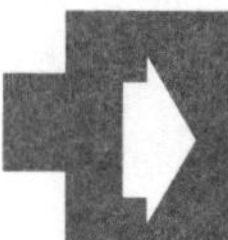

ADVICE FOR THE PATIENT

Travellers' Diarrhea

Individuals visiting areas where travellers' diarrhea is common should follow the dietary restrictions below:

- Eat only freshly prepared foods that are served steaming hot.
- Drink only bottled beverages, treated water (see Water Purification section in this chapter), hot coffee or tea.
- Wet cans or bottles should be wiped dry before opening and the surface that contacts the mouth wiped clean.
- Eat only fruits that can be peeled.
- Bread, jellies, and syrups are considered safe.
- Avoid raw meat, raw seafood, and raw vegetables.
- Avoid unpasteurized milk and dairy products.
- Avoid cold cuts and cream-filled desserts.
- Avoid ice cubes (alcohol will not disinfect ice cubes).

PROPHYLAXIS

Nonpharmacological Prophylaxis

Because contaminated food or water is the main cause of travellers' diarrhea, educating patients to avoid risk factors is the key to prevention. The basic rule is: Boil it, cook it, peel it, or forget it while abroad. See ADVICE FOR THE PATIENT for dietary recommendations for travellers.

Pharmacological Prophylaxis

Prophylactic therapy may give a false sense of security to travellers who otherwise would be more cautious in the selection of food and beverages. The decision to use prophylaxis is based on the importance of the trip, the traveller's underlying health, willingness to follow dietary restrictions and desire to use it. Prophylactic agents are not recommended for children or pregnant women. Pregnant women are encouraged to postpone unnecessary trips to high risk areas.

In general, prophylactic therapy should begin on the first day of travel and continue for 1 to 2 days after returning home, but should be restricted to only 3 weeks. For longer stays, pharmacological prophylaxis is not recommended due to its financial burden, increased risk of side effects and prevention of acquired immunity.

Bismuth subsalicylate, considered the drug of choice, is believed to act through its antimicrobial effects. It can be given in liquid form or as a chewable tablet at an adult dose of 60 mL or 2 tablets four times daily at meals and bedtime. Taken at the recommended dosage, the reported efficacy is about 60%. The best protection is given when the total daily dose is divided into 4; divided into 2, the efficacy rate is reduced to about 40%. Bismuth subsalicylate should be avoided in persons with salicylate allergy, gout, or peptic ulcers. For those taking anticoagulants, ASA, or probenecid, it should be used with caution as there are potential drug interactions. It may inhibit the absorption of doxycycline, so should not be taken within 1 to 3 hours of it. Bismuth-induced encephalopathy is unlikely in reasonably healthy people due to its poor absorption but may develop in patients with AIDS if taken in excessive doses.

Lactobacillus preparations, which contain bacteria that metabolize carbohydrate in the gut to lactic acid, reduce the intraluminal pH and inhibit the growth of enteropathogens. Because the reported efficacy ranges from 0 to 14%, they should not be recommended.

Antidiarrheal agents (e.g., loperamide) and activated charcoal do not have a role in prophylactic therapy. Antimicrobials remain controversial due to the risk of serious adverse reaction, the development of resistance and the lack of effective agents available if treatment is required.

TREATMENT

Nonpharmacological Treatment

Replenishing fluids and electrolytes to prevent dehydration is important. For most patients, taking flavored mineral water with saltine crackers is usually adequate. For the very young and elderly patients, who are more prone to dehydration, an oral rehydration solution is recommended. Homemade solutions are discouraged as any inaccuracy in measurement can result in serious problems. An oral solution of a commercial rehydration product is given as needed. It is important that infants continue breast or bottle feeding.

Medical attention should be sought for a patient with signs of moderate to severe dehydration (e.g., rapid and weak pulse, sunken eyes, absence of tears, reduced, concentrated urine or greater than 6% loss in body weight), bloody diarrhea, fever greater than 39°C (102°F), persistent diarrhea and/or vomiting.

Pharmacological Treatment

Although travellers' diarrhea is rarely life-threatening, its symptoms may be uncomfortable and treatment is often sought. For children under 2 years of age and for pregnant women, therapy should consist mainly of fluid and electrolyte replacement.

Loperamide, the only nonprescription antidiarrheal agent available in Canada, is considered more effective than bismuth subsalicylate. It has a more rapid onset of action and antisecretory activity.

Concern about the use of loperamide stems from the risk of prolonging the presence of the pathogen in the stool. It should not be used if fever or blood in the stool is present since it may exacerbate invasive travellers' diarrhea. It is contraindicated in children under 2 years of age.

Loperamide use should be limited to 48 hours. Patients with persistent, severe diarrhea should seek medical advice as antibiotic therapy may be required. Adverse effects include constipation, drowsiness, and dizziness.

Bismuth subsalicylate decreases the frequency and duration of travellers' diarrhea of both bacterial and viral origin by as much as 50%. This is probably due to the antisecretory action of its salicylate moiety although it also possesses antimicrobial and anti-inflammatory activity.

Treatment should be limited to 48 hours with no more than 8 doses in a 24-hour period. Due to the risk of Reye's syndrome, bismuth subsalicylate should be avoided in children and adolescents with chickenpox or the flu. Travellers should be warned about transient blackening of the tongue and stools by the drug. Other side effects include nausea, constipation, and, rarely, tinnitus. It is not recommended in children under 3 years of age.

Adsorbent agents such as activated charcoal and aluminum hydroxide have been found ineffective in the treatment of diarrhea and should not be recommended. Few studies exist that compare the efficacy of absorbant agents to other antidiarrheals. Among the absorbant agents, only two are found effective in diarrhea: attapulgite and polycarbophil. Attapulgite may be used in pregnant patients as it is not absorbed systemically. Polycarbophil has been shown to increase stool consistency and decrease the frequency of bowel movements, but a large dose is required and its onset of action is slow.

WATER PURIFICATION

Diseases such as cholera, typhoid fever, hepatitis A, and travellers' diarrhea can be contracted through contaminated drinking water. In areas of poor sanitation or where chlorinated tap water is not available, travellers should purify their drinking water.

METHODS OF PURIFICATION

The three current methods of purification are: heat, chemical agents and filtration. The efficacy of the various methods cannot be quantitatively evaluated due to the lack of published studies. At present, boiling for 15 minutes (20 minutes at higher altitudes) is considered the most effective.

Iodination is preferred when boiling is not feasible. Chlorination is no longer recommended by the Centers for Disease Control (CDC) as its activity is dependent on pH, temperature and organic content of the water.

Although filtration is not recognized by the CDC, various portable filters with an iodine exchange resin are recommended by some travel clinics. Only those recommended, which will vary with the clinic and availability, should be used. Filters without an exchange resin do not remove certain microbes and viruses and generally are not recommended. Table 2 summarizes the various water purification methods.

TABLE 2: Summary of Water Purification Methods

Method	Procedure	Advantages	Disadvantages	Comments
HEAT	Maintain water at a vigorous boil for 15 minutes (20 minutes at high altitudes)	Reliable and effective	Not always practical	Most effective method May add a pinch of salt or pour water several times between containers to improve taste Do not add ice to cool water
CHEMICAL **A) Iodination** i) Tincture of Iodine 2%	Use 5 drops/L of clean water or 10 drops if water is cold or cloudy; let stand for at least 30 minutes before use A slight taste of iodine should be apparent in treated water or the above procedure should be repeated	Inexpensive and reliable	Avoid long term use (greater than 3 weeks) Use with caution in persons with thyroid diseases, pregnant women, infants and children Slight iodine taste Stains	In cold water, contact time should be increased up to several hours For very cold water, it is more effective to warm the water before iodination Powdered drink mix may be added to treated water to improve taste
ii) Tetraglycine hydroperiodide (e.g., *Potable Aquaxcell* tablets)	1 tablet/L of water; let stand for 15 minutes prior to use 2 tablets/L of cold or turbid water; let stand for 20 minutes prior to use	As per tincture of iodine	As per tincture of iodine, except does not stain	As per tincture of iodine

TABLE 2: Summary of Water Purification Methods *(cont'd)*

Method	Procedure	Advantages	Disadvantages	Comments
B) Chlorination				
i) Liquid chlorine bleach (4–6% available chlorine)	Add 2 drops (0.1 mL) of household bleach/L of water; let stand for 30 minutes before use; double the bleach and the time if water is cold or cloudy Treated water should have a slight chlorine taste or the above procedure should be repeated	Readily available Inexpensive	Questionable efficacy Chlorine taste	No longer recommended by the CDC
FILTRATION DEVICES[a]	**Filtration is not recognized by CDC as a method of purification**			
A) Passport Purification Devices	Water is passed through an iodinated resin with special filtration membranes A secondary carbon bed is built-in to improve taste	Portable device Water can be used immediately Carbon filter to improve taste Collapsible	User must keep track of usage Should not be used to purify very turbid water	
B) PUR Antimicrobial Water Purifier	Available in hand pump or cup devices Water is passed through a microfilter and a tri-iodine resin matrix	Lightweight and portable Water can be used immediately Replaceable iodine resin matrix Hand pump device is convenient for large groups	Should not be used to purify very turbid water User must keep track of usage	Optional carbon cartridge is available
C) Water Tech Water Purifier	Cup device where water is passed through a pentiodide matrix	Lightweight and portable	User must keep track of usage Should not be used for very turbid water Lack of microfilter and carbon bed	
D) Katadyn Water Filters	With 0.2 micron ceramic filter device where water is passed through with or without a pump, depending on the device	No chemical taste	Expensive Does not have an iodine resin and water is not completely safe Microfilter may be plugged up and periodic replacement may be required	

[a] As the manufacturer frequently changes the filtration devices to improve efficacy, the current issue of *CPS (Compendium of Pharmaceuticals and Specialties)* should be used as a supplement to this chart for specific details with respect to the filtration devices.

MOTION SICKNESS

Historically, motion sickness was thought to be caused by trauma to the gastrointestinal tract. Not until the late 19th century were the symptoms associated with the function of the inner ear.

The term motion sickness is a misnomer. It is not a sickness but a normal physiologic response to an unusual stimulus. Individuals, however, vary in their susceptibility. The cause is thought to be a mismatch of information received by the brain from the inner ear and the eyes. This hypothesis, known as the sensory conflict theory, explains why an individual with vestibular dysfunction is immune.

With continuous exposure to the stimulus, tolerance will develop. This may account for individuals over 50 years of age rarely suffering from motion sickness; it is most common in children between the ages of 2 and 12.

SIGNS AND SYMPTOMS

Generally, the symptoms follow a certain pattern. The first sign, skin pallor, is followed by restlessness, yawning and a cold sweat. Malaise and drowsiness may set in and the individual experience gastric awareness. The symptoms progress to hypersalivation, nausea and vomiting. Symptoms vary with the individual and may occur rapidly.

ADVICE FOR THE PATIENT

Motion Sickness

Helpful hints to minimize motion sickness:

- Stay in a position where there is least motion (e.g., the front seat of a car, the deck of a ship, the seats over the wings of a plane).
- Lie back in a semi-reclined position, keeping the head as still as possible.
- Focus on distant objects as they appear more stationary, or closing eyes; children may be placed in the front seat in raised car seats allowing them to look out the front windshield.
- Distract the child's attention from the moving vehicle; although reading can worsen motion sickness, occupying children with coloring books and games may be helpful.
- Avoid overeating or drinking prior to the trip as it may predispose to nausea and vomiting.
- Avoid tobacco smoke or offending odors from food.

TREATMENT

Nonpharmacological Treatment

The key to controlling motion sickness is prevention. This is done by minimizing conflict between vestibular and visual receptors. See ADVICE FOR THE PATIENT for helpful tips.

Behavior modification or biofeedback, where one learns to control the early symptoms, has been relatively successful for NASA (National Aeronautics and Space Administration) personnel and others in occupations that expose them to motion sickness.

Powdered ginger root (*Zingiber officinale*) in capsules is thought to increase gastric motility and absorb toxins and acids, thus inhibiting nausea feedback by the gastrointestinal tract. The efficacy of ginger is questionable as the few studies evaluating this use have conflicting results. Doses up to 1 g, given 30 minutes to 1 hour prior to exposure to stimulus, were used.

Sea-Band has 2 wristbands with non-corrosive buttons that when worn correctly (3 finger widths from the first wrist crease) maintain a constant pressure at the Nei-Kuan acupressure point. It is intended for both prophylaxis and treatment. Various studies evaluating acupressure wristbands have not found them better than placebo.

Pharmacological Treatment

The nonprescription drugs used to control motion sickness include the anticholinergic agent scopolamine and the antihistamines dimenhydrinate and promethazine.

While scopolamine prevents motion sickness, its effectiveness in treatment is questionable. Clinical trials of transdermal scopolamine have not shown it to be more effective than dimenhydrinate. One study evaluating the effect of ephedrine did not find it improved the efficacy of scopolamine.

Various nonprescription antihistamines are effective. Their mechanism of action is thought to be both antihistaminic and anticholinergic as both types of receptors are found in the afferent vomiting pathways.

Dimenhydrinate is considered the gold standard

for both the prevention and treatment of motion sickness. Neither diphenhydramine nor promethazine appear to offer an advantage.

The most common adverse effect of these drugs is drowsiness, and the use of alcohol, sedatives and tranquillizers can intensify sedation. Because anticholinergic effects such as blurred vision and dry mouth have been reported, caution is recommended in patients with glaucoma and prostate hypertrophy.

Preliminary studies in space motion sickness have shown terfenadine, but not astemizole, moderately efficacious in motion sickness with large individual variability. Until further studies have evaluated these second generation antihistamines, they should not be recommended.

TRAVEL FIRST AID

Travellers may find they are ill more often while abroad than at home. They are often reluctant to seek medical help for minor illnesses because of the language barrier, high cost and questionable quality of service, especially in developing countries. Therefore, all travellers should take a first aid kit, for self-treatment of minor ailments.

FIRST AID KIT

Organize all ingredients in a self-sealing bag using plastic containers, where possible, instead of glass. A first aid kit for travellers can be divided into two sections: medications and first aid supplies (Table 3). For detailed information on the agents listed below, refer to the appropriate chapter.

Medications

Analgesic: ASA, acetaminophen or ibuprofen relieve mild to moderate pain and reduce fever.

Antihistamine: can be used to treat minor allergic conditions. Sedating antihistamines (e.g., diphenhydramine) are effective mild tranquillizers for jet lag. Certain antihistamines (e.g., dimenhydrinate) control motion sickness.

Decongestant: oral decongestants (e.g., pseudoephedrine) or topical nasal sprays (e.g, xylometazoline) relieve congested eustachian tubes during aircraft descent.

Calamine lotion: useful for mild dermatitis and pruritus.

Antiseptic: (e.g., povidone-iodine) to disinfect minor cuts or abrasions to prevent skin infections.

Sunscreen: broad spectrum with SPF 15 or greater needed to prevent sunburn.

Insect repellant: those containing DEET (N,N-diethyl-m-toluamide) protect against a variety of mosquitos, ticks, fleas, chiggers, and flies.

Oil of cloves: for relief of dental pain until care is available.

Antacid: (e.g., aluminum and magnesium hydroxide) relieves indigestion and heartburn. Bismuth subsalicylate prevents and treats travellers' diarrhea.

Antifungal skin cream: A preparation containing clotrimazole or miconazole is effective for fungal skin infections.

Ear drops: an analgesic (e.g., antipyrine/benzocaine) for minor ear pain.

Patient-specific medication: extra amounts of medications used on a regular basis should be taken along with a written prescription (using the generic drug name) in case of an emergency.

First Aid Supplies

The following are recommended:

- adhesive bandages;
- sterile gauze;
- adhesive tape;
- safety pins;
- disposable thermometer;
- scissors; and
- fine tweezers (for the removal of splinters or ticks).

TABLE 3: Travel First Aid Kit

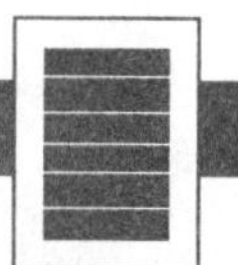

Medications		First Aid Supplies	
Analgesic	Oil of cloves	Adhesive bandages	Safety pins
Antihistamine	Antiseptic agent	Sterile gauze	Fine tweezers
Decongestant	Sunscreen	Adhesive tape	Disposable thermometer
Antacid	Insect repellant	Scissors	
Calamine lotion	Patient-specific medication		

STORAGE OF MEDICATION

Store all medication in the original labelled container to avoid problems at borders and facilitate drug identification in case of emergency.

Keep all medication in the carry-on luggage in case of delays or misplaced luggage.

Diabetics required to bring hypodermic syringes and needles should carry a physician's letter authorizing possession. Insulins can be kept cool in a wide-mouth insulated bottle: fill the bottle with cold or iced water until the internal temperature is lowered, empty and then put in the insulin vials, which should be refrigerated once the destination is reached. Insulin should be carried in the hand luggage and not in the luggage compartment of the aircraft where it may be exposed to extreme temperatures.

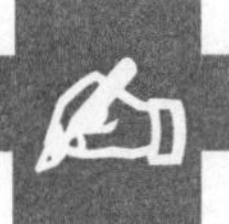

Resource List

The local travel clinic, which has current information on vaccinations and antimalarial therapy, should be contacted at least 4 weeks prior to travel to ensure adequate time for vaccinations.

A list of travel clinics in Canada can be obtained from the Canadian Society for International Health, 170 Laurier Avenue West, Suite 902, Ottawa ON K1P 5V5. Tel: (613) 230-2654; Fax: (613) 230-8401.

Travellers seeking English-speaking physicians can inquire at their hotel reception, tour couriers or Canadian embassies. The International Association for Medical Assistance to Travellers (IAMAT) will supply a directory of English-speaking physicians in 125 countries and territories. IAMAT physicians have agreed to provide services with set fee schedules. Membership in IAMAT is free, although a small donation is requested to help support its work. Detailed information can be obtained from one of their two offices:

40 Regal Road
Guelph ON
N1K 1B5
Tel: (519) 836-0102
Fax: (519) 836-3412

1287 St Clair Ave W
Toronto ON
M6E 1B8
Tel: (416) 652-0137

Airlines will accommodate travellers on special diets if informed at least 24 hours in advance.

Other useful resources include:

Health Canada

Travel Information Office
301 Elgin Street
Ottawa ON
Tel: (613) 954-6594
(for government employees)

Quarantine Health Services
Laboratory Centre for Disease Control
Tel: (613) 957-8739
Fax: (613) 952-8286
(general travel and tropical health information)

PHARMACEUTICAL AGENTS

(For a detailed discussion of antidiarrheal agents, including adsorbents, bismuth subsalicylate and loperamide, see the chapter Gastrointestinal Products.)

Antihistamines

The mechanism of action of antihistamines is thought to be both antihistaminic and anticholinergic as both types of receptors are found in the afferent vomiting pathways.

The most common side effect is drowsiness. Other adverse effects, which do not require medical attention, include headache, dryness of mouth and blurred vision. Side effects requiring medical referral are: incoordination, palpitation or hypotension.

The use of alcohol, sedatives and tranquillizers is not recommended as it can intensify sedation. Antihistamines should be used with caution in patients with glaucoma and prostate hypertrophy.

Dimenhydrinate: Composed of approximately 53% diphenhydramine and 47% 8-chlorotheophylline, it is well absorbed following oral administration, and antiemetic effects occur within 15 to 30 minutes.

Considered one of the most effective nonprescription agents for both the prevention and the treatment of motion sickness, it should be taken 30 minutes to 1 hour before exposure to motion. For dosing information, refer to Table 4.

Dimenhydrinate is available in tablet, chewable tablet, capsule, oral liquid, suppository and injectable forms.

Diphenhydramine: Also an effective agent in the prevention and treatment of nausea and/or vomiting due to motion sickness, it is well absorbed after oral administration, but undergoes first-pass metabolism in the liver with only 40-60% of an oral dose reaching systemic circulation. After a single oral dose of diphenhydramine, the drug appears in the plasma within 15 minutes with peak plasma concentration ranging from 1 to 4 hours. For dosing information, refer to Table 4.

Diphenydramine is available in capsule, caplet, oral liquid or injectable forms.

Promethazine: Structurally similar to the phenothiazines, it exhibits marked antihistamine activity. Although not shown superior to dimenhydrinate, it

TABLE 4: Summary of Agents Used in Motion Sickness

Agent	Dosage
Dimenhydrinate	**Adults** 50–100 mg every 4–6 hours as needed, up to a maximum of 400 mg/day **Children** 12 years of age and over: 50 mg every 4 hours as needed, up to a maximum of 300 mg/day 6–12 years of age: 25–50 mg every 6–8 hours as needed, up to a maximum of 150 mg/day 2–6 years of age: 15–25 mg every 6–8 hours as needed, up to a maximum of 75 mg/day
Diphenhydramine	**Adults** 25–50 mg every 4 hours if needed, up to a maximum of 300 mg/day **Children** 6–12 years of age: 12.5–25 mg every 4–6 hours if needed, up to a maximum of 100 mg/day 2–5 years of age: 6.25 mg every 4–6 hours if needed, up to a maximum of 4 doses/day less than 2 years of age: 3–12 mg every 4 hours if needed, up to a maximum of 4 doses/day
Promethazine	**Adults** 25 mg initially, followed by 10–25 mg every 4–6 hours if needed, up to a maximum of 100 mg/day **Children** 2 years of age and over: 0.25–0.5 mg/kg every 4–6 hours if needed
Scopolamine	**Adults** Apply 1 patch every 72 hours up to a maximum of 2 patches/course

is effective for the prevention and treatment of motion sickness. Promethazine is well absorbed following oral administration with onset of action within 20 minutes.

To prevent motion sickness, promethazine should be taken 30 minutes before exposure to motion. For dosing information, refer to Table 4. Promethazine is contraindicated in children under 2 years of age due to the depression of arousal and respiratory mechanisms with the potential induction of sleep apnea.

Promethazine is available in tablet, oral liquid or injectable forms.

Anticholinergics

Scopolamine: Although the mechanism by which scopolamine controls motion sickness is still not clear, it has been proposed that cholinergic neurotransmitters may be involved in the afferent vomiting pathways.

Scopolamine has been shown as effective as dimenhydrinate in the prevention of motion sickness, but its use in treatment is questionable and should not be recommended.

The oral use of scopolamine has been limited by its short duration of action and high incidence of adverse effects. Transdermal scopolamine was developed to decrease the frequency of adverse effects as well as the need for frequent administration. However, central nervous system side effects have been reported to be similar to the oral form.

The transdermal system consists of a 2.5 cm^2 flexible disc with four layers: 1) a backing layer of polyester film; 2) a drug reservoir containing 1.5 mg of scopolamine; 3) a rate controlling membrane; and 4) an adhesive layer.

The patch is designed to release 1 mg of scopolamine over 3 days. It should be applied over the post-auricular skin approximately 12 hours before exposure to the stimulus. The patch is removed after 72 hours or earlier if the journey is shorter. If therapy is needed after 72 hours, a second disc may be applied behind the other ear. Patients should wash their hands thoroughly after handling the disc to avoid getting scopolamine in their eyes.

Side effects of transdermal scopolamine include dry mouth, blurred vision, and drowsiness. Anisocoria, an unequal dilatation of pupils, has been reported as a transient side effect. Transient tachycardia followed by paradoxical bradycardia has been reported with both transdermal and oral scopolamine. Rare cases of psychosis have also been reported, particularly in children and the elderly. Withdrawal symptoms such as nausea, vomiting, and headache are also possible, especially with prolonged use. Scopolamine is contraindicated in patients with angle-closure glaucoma. It is not recommended in children, the elderly, pregnant or breastfeeding women. It should be used with caution in patients with urinary retention (e.g., prostate hypertrophy), open angle glaucoma, or intestinal obstruction (e.g., pyloric stenosis). The use of alcohol is not recommended as it may potentiate the adverse effects of scopolamine.

Scopolamine is available in transdermal patches.

RECOMMENDED READING

Canadian Immunization Guide. 4th ed. Ottawa, Ontario: Health Protection Branch (updated periodically). Available from the Canadian Medical Association, Membership Services, 1867 Alta Vista Dr., Ottawa, Ontario K1G 3Y6.

1993 Canadian Recommendations for the Prevention and Treatment of Malaria Among International Travellers. Canada Communicable Disease Report 1993 (July); (updated periodically). Available from Health Canada, Quarantine Health Services, Laboratory Centre for Disease Control, Tunney's Pasture, Ottawa, Ontario K1A 0L2.

Health Information for International Travel. Atlanta, GA: Department for Health and Human Services, 1994 (updated annually). Available from the Department of Health and Human Services, Public Health Service, Centers for Disease Control, Atlanta, GA 30333, U.S.A.

Hill DR, Pearson RD. Health advice for international travel. Ann Intern Med 1988;108:839–52.

International Travel and Health: Vaccination Requirements and Health Advice. Geneva: World Health Organization, 1994 (updated annually). Available from the Canadian Public Health Association, 1565 Carling Ave., Suite 400, Ottawa, Ontario K1Z 8R1.

Skjenna OW, Evans JF, Moore M, et al. Helping patients travel by air. Can Med Assoc J 1991; 144(3):287–93.

Repchinsky C. Principles of immunization for the pharmacist. Can Pharm J 1986;119:428.

World Immunization Chart. Available from International Association for Medical Assistance to Travellers (IAMAT), 40 Regal Rd., Guelph, Ontario N1K 1B5.

27

WOMEN'S HEALTH CARE PRODUCTS

LAURA-LYNN POLLOCK

CONTENTS

General Principles of Feminine Hygiene 655
- Anatomy and Physiology
- Genital Hygiene
- Vaginal Dryness
- Hair Removal

Menstrual Care 661
- Menstrual Cycle
- Toxic Shock Syndrome
- Dysmenorrhea
- Premenstrual Syndrome

Vaginal Infections 671
- Physiology
- When to Recommend Self-Treatment
- Vulvovaginal Candidiasis

Contraception 678
- Physiology
- Contraceptive Methods
- Contraception and Sexually Transmitted Diseases

Pharmaceutical Agents 689

Recommended Reading 692

GENERAL PRINCIPLES OF FEMININE HYGIENE

ANATOMY AND PHYSIOLOGY

The visible external genitalia, or the vulva, includes the area of the mons pubis, the labia minora and majora, and the perineum (Figure 1). Protected within this region are the clitoris and the vaginal and urethral openings. The anus is posterior to the perineum.

The vagina, a tube-like structure, is at a 45° angle to the vulva, extending upward to the uterus. Transverse folds in the vaginal wall provide the flexibility of shape and size required for intercourse and childbirth.

Epithelial cells line the vagina. During childbearing years, increased estrogen levels cause proliferation of the basal cells in the epithelium. The glycogen stored by these cells is broken down to lactic acid by vaginal *Lactobacilli* or Döderlein's *bacilli*, making the vaginal environment acidic with a pH of 3.5 to 5.5.

Vaginal discharge from a variety of sources—cervical glands, uterus, fallopian tubes and a transudate from the capillaries in the vaginal walls—is normal and healthy. The quantity and consistency of the secretions vary in response to monthly estrogen and progesterone fluctuations. Sometimes the discharge is pasty, white, and scanty. Other times it is more copious with the consistency of uncooked egg white. No discharge is apparent on other days. Secretions are important for cleansing the vagina and maintaining its pH and normal bacterial environment.

A mild odor is produced when vaginal secretions combine with secretions from glands in the external genitalia. Normally this odor is not unpleasant and should not cause concern.

GENITAL HYGIENE

Proper genital hygiene is simple and easy. The perineal area can be cleansed by washing regularly with water and mild soap throughout the menstrual cycle. The vagina is cleansed by natural secretions and generally does not require further care.

General Principles of Feminine Hygiene

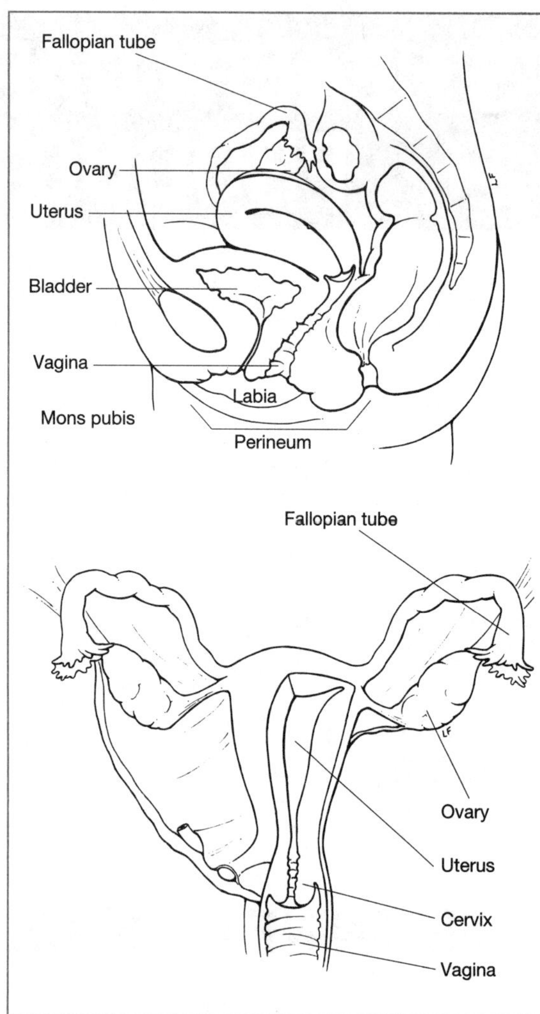

FIGURE 1: Female Reproductive System

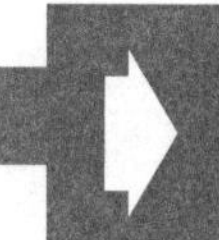

ADVICE FOR THE WOMAN

Genital Hygiene

- The perineum should be washed regularly with water and mild soap.
- The vagina does not generally require washing or rinsing.
- Mild genital odor is normal and common. It can be minimized by following proper genital hygiene.
- Poor hygiene, infection, sensitivity reaction to a product or a forgotten vaginal tampon may be responsible for unpleasant odor or irritation. If proper genital hygiene does not alleviate these symptoms then consult your physician.

Although normal genital hygiene does not need pharmacological products, many women still wish to use the various nonprescription products available: vaginal douches, genital towelettes and feminine deodorant sprays provide a wide range of choices. Their use is rarely necessary and some of them carry significant risks for certain users.

Vaginal douching is a process of instilling fluid into the vagina to flush the cavity. It can be used for cleaning, to decrease vaginal itching or irritation, to alter vaginal pH and occasionally to treat vaginal infections. There is no substantiated benefit to routine douching, and there are concerns that it may disrupt the normal vaginal flora or increase the occurrence of genital irritation. Douching may also play a role in the development of ascending infections of the genital tract (e.g., salpingitis) in susceptible individuals.

Although not recommended, occasional douching (2 or 3 times monthly, or less) is not harmful if appropriate solutions and technique are used, and a vaginal infection is not present.

The simplest and safest douching liquid is warm water. There is no risk of irritation or allergic reactions.

Vinegar and water provide a mildly acidic solution that may be used for general hygiene or to relieve vaginal irritation. Alkaline douches using sodium bicarbonate have also been used. Acidic douches are generally preferred for women of child-bearing age as the normal vaginal pH is acidic. These douches can be prepared from home ingredients (Table 1) or a commercially prepared product used. Vinegar and water douches are usually the best alternative to water alone.

The addition of perfumes, astringents, proteolytic agents and antimicrobial agents to commercial douching solutions increases the risk of adverse reactions to the product. Perfumes alone can be irritating or cause allergic reactions in sensitive individuals. Many of the products contain these and other additives. It is best to recommend an unscented product that contains few ingredients.

Douches are instilled using a syringe. There are two main types: fountain and bulb; neither is preferred over the other. Disposable douching equipment is usually similar to the bulb syringe.

A fountain syringe consists of a rubber bag (similar to a hot water bottle), tubing, and a rounded plastic nozzle with holes for insertion into the vagina. Gravity creates the flow of fluid from the bag to the vagina. A bulb syringe has no tubing. The small bag or bottle is filled with fluid and the vaginal tip attached directly to it. The fluid is forced out of the bulb, either by squeezing the device, or by the inward pressure exerted by the distended walls of the bulb.

Correct technique is important when douching. Excessive fluid pressure on the vagina and cervix may cause reflux of the solution and possibly of bacteria into the uterus or peritoneal cavity via the fallopian tubes.

Genital towelettes are disposable wipes moistened with astringents, emollients, surfactants, counterirritants, antimicrobials and perfumes. They are convenient for genital hygiene but not superior to water and mild soap, and irritation and sensitivity reactions are possible.

Aerosol sprays are marketed for controlling genital odor; however, normal genital odor does not require the use of feminine deodorants, and mask-

TABLE 1: Preparation of Vinegar or Sodium Bicarbonate Douches

Vinegar and Water	Sodium Bicarbonate and Water
Add 15–30 mL of vinegar to 1 L of warm water	Mix 15–30 mL of sodium bicarbonate powder in 1 L of warm water

ADVICE FOR THE WOMAN

Vaginal Douches

General information:

- Thoroughly clean reusable douching apparatus with hot water and soap after each use.
- Do not use douches during pregnancy unless otherwise advised by a physician.
- Douching is not an effective means of birth control.
- If a vaginal spermicide has been used for contraception, do not douche for at least 6 hours after intercourse.
- Vulvovaginal irritation may indicate an infection. Although douching may temporarily relieve the symptoms, it is important to see a physician and receive the correct treatment for the infection if irritation continues or recurs frequently.
- Do not douche for at least 24 hours before examination for a suspected vaginal infection. Douching may hinder the diagnosis and delay treatment.

Technique: The correct technique is important to decrease the risk of problems.

Fountain syringe:

Fill the bag with the douching solution, clamp off the tubing and hang or hold positioned about 60 cm above the hips, then:

Bulb syringe:

Fill the bulb or bottle with the douching solution, then:

- Lie on your back in the tub with your knees bent.
- Insert the vaginal tip into the vagina. With gentle downward pressure, slip it in as far as it will comfortably go.
- Release the clamp of the fountain syringe or gently squeeze the bulb of the syringe to instill the fluid into the vagina.
- A feeling of fullness in the pelvic region will indicate that sufficient fluid has been instilled.
- Gently remove the tip from the vagina.
- Hold the labia together with one hand to contain the fluid in the vagina.
- Release after about 1 minute and the fluid will be expelled.

ing an unusual or unpleasant odor may delay the seeking of necessary medical treatment. There is also a significant incidence of local irritation reactions to the propellants, perfumes and antimicrobials in these products.

If a woman is intent on using a genital deodorant, it is important that she be informed of its limitations and be aware of the proper technique for use.

VAGINAL DRYNESS

All women will have periods of time when their vaginal lubrication is decreased, and they experience vaginal dryness. When estrogen levels are low, such as during and after menopause, after childbirth, or at certain times in the menstrual cycle, vaginal lubrication can be inadequate. Sometimes tampons can decrease lubrication, and occasionally oral contraceptives or other medications alter the normal vaginal environment.

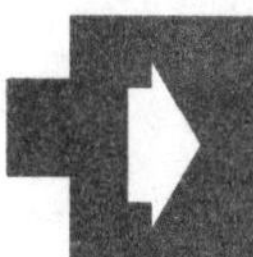

ADVICE FOR THE WOMAN

Feminine Deodorant Sprays

- Genital sprays are for use on the external genitalia only. Do not apply to the vagina.
- The spray should not be applied just before sexual intercourse as it may irritate the vagina or penis.
- To apply, hold the canister at least 20 cm from the body and press down on the nozzle to release the spray. Irritation may occur if the product is applied in excessive amounts or from the chilling effect of the propellants.
- If irritation or redness occurs, wash the affected area with water and mild soap. Discontinue use of the product.
- If the condition does not improve, a physician should be consulted.
- Do not use genital sprays when wearing a menstrual pad. Pads may increase the risk of irritation by increasing the time the spray contacts the body.
- Tampons should not be inserted immediately after using the spray. The vaginal tissue may be irritated.
- Do not apply to broken skin or skin lesions, e.g., herpes.

Symptoms

Vaginal dryness may go unnoticed or cause genital itching, burning or pain during daily activities and/or sexual intercourse.

Treatment

Water soluble vaginal moisturizers are useful for women bothered by vaginal dryness. These products are usually in a gel form and can be applied intravaginally or to the external genitalia.

As there are no pharmacologically active components in these preparations, they can be used frequently and for long periods of time.

Many of thc products require frequent reapplication and can be bothersome due to leakage. Newer products provide longer adherence and remoisturize the vaginal tissue. One long-lasting preparation claims to be effective for up to 3 days after each intravaginal application and gives the best results when used regularly. It provides immediate lubrication when applied but its long-term effect is said to be due to its ability to replenish moisture in vaginal tissue.

Vaginal lubricants and moisturizers have few side effects apart from the potential for local irritation in very sensitive individuals. They offer relief for temporary conditions, and newer ones are progressing towards useful treatment of the long-term vaginal changes seen during or after menopause.

HAIR REMOVAL

Personal care for some women includes the removal of unwanted hair from the underarms, legs, bikini line or the face. This is usually for cosmetic purposes and is not required for personal hygiene. Racial and cultural factors play a strong role in normal hair growth patterns and attitudes to them.

Hypertrichosis is excess hair growth with normal distribution while hirsutism describes hair distribution that is inconsistent with the usual for sex or possibly race. Hirsutism is usually due to endocrine influences, e.g., excessive androgens or progestins.

Hair grows in a cyclical manner, going through two distinct phases: growth (anagen) and resting (telogen). The amount of hair a person has is, in part, determined by the relative lengths of each of these periods. If the rest phase is long and the follicle devoid of hair for a period of time prior to new growth, the person appears to have less hair than someone with a short rest period and very little time when a follicle is hairless.

There are two basic types of hair. Soft, fine hair, known as vellus hair, is found on many parts of the body. Coarse hair, such as found on the head, is terminal hair. Hair may be considered unsightly if coarse growth happens in an area where vellus hair would be expected. Androgens can influence the follicle to produce terminal hair, often the cause of facial hair changes seen in some older women.

There are a number of ways to temporarily remove hair. The method chosen is determined by personal preference, amount of hair to be removed, ease of removal, how often the procedure needs to be repeated and any adverse reactions that have occurred with previous methods.

Shaving is the most common method employed for depilation (removal of the hair by affecting the shaft). To decrease skin irritation, lubrication is recommended prior to hair removal. Shaving creams, soap or other mild lubricant can be used. Hair will begin growing back immediately and be visible within 2 days. The regrowth may feel bristly. Shaving does not cause hair to come back in greater amounts or to become thicker.

Individual hairs are often removed by **plucking**—pulling the hair out of the follicle with tweezers. As the hair is removed from deep within the follicle the regrowth takes several weeks to become noticeable. This is a method of epilation or the detachment of hair from the hair root.

Waxing is an efficient means of removing large quantities of hair from the follicle. Wax is applied to the area in need of epilation, then covered with a fabric strip that sticks to the wax. When the wax is set, the strip is pulled off, taking the wax and hair with it. This is repeated in patches until the desired area has been treated. Technique is important with this method. Some waxes are applied directly from the package at room temperature, and others require warming prior to use.

Devices that mechanically remove hair from the follicle vary in nature but look somewhat like an electric shaver. As the head of the device is moved over an area, it entraps the hair in its mechanism and twists or pulls the hair out.

With **electrolysis**, hair follicles are destroyed by a mild current passed through an inserted needle. This should not be done with home equipment. Trained professionals are recommended for this procedure to increase the effectiveness as well as decrease the risk of scarring, infection or other damage.

Products are available that chemically destroy the hair shaft. Thioglycollates (e.g., calcium thioglycollate) are the common ingredient in these creams and lotions. They are combined with agents that react with them, such as calcium hydroxide. When applied to hair they chemically change the keratin and the hair turns to a soft mass that can be wiped off. This process is fairly fast (usually <15 minutes). These products are more effective on soft, fine hair than on coarse terminal hair. Large areas can be covered and treated with one application. The regrowth is less prickly than with shaving. Technique is important to the effect and safety of the chemical hair removal products. Local irritation can occur, so a patch test on the forearm or other small area of skin is recommended before using. The cream should be applied to the area, left on for about 15 minutes and then removed. If irritation occurs within the following 24 hours, the product should be avoided.

There is an odor to chemical hair removal products that bothers some people, and water increases it. It is removed once the product is wiped off.

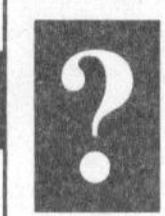

PATIENT ASSESSMENT QUESTIONS

***Q* Why do you wish to use a douche? Are you experiencing vaginal irritation or unusual discharge?**

When a woman asks for advice regarding a douching product, it is important to assess the situation before making a recommendation. Vaginal infections are often characterized by vulvovaginal irritation and itching, or increased vaginal discharge. Douches should not be used when a vaginal infection is suspected unless recommended by a physician. In some instances, povidone-iodine douches are prescribed to assist in controlling the infection.

***Q* Do you know how to use this douching product?**

Some products must be diluted or mixed correctly to avoid irritation. Douching apparatus may be confusing to someone who has never used it before. Use of the apparatus and proper technique must be explained to the consumer. Only gentle pressure is required when instilling the solution.

***Q* Do you have any allergies to soaps, chemicals or perfumes?**

Some ingredients in douching products can cause hypersensitivity reactions. Always check allergy potential with the consumer before recommending a product.

ADVICE FOR THE WOMAN

Hair Removal Products

The correct use of hair removal products is outlined in the package information with each product, but some general guidelines can be followed:

Waxing:

- If using the type of wax that requires warming, check that it is not too hot before applying.
- When pulling the fabric strips, use a firm quick motion.
- After the wax has been removed, it may be helpful to apply a cool moist towel to the treated area. This may help to decrease the redness that sometimes occurs.
- Hair should be allowed to grow for several weeks prior to waxing. Waxing is more effective on longer hair and repeat treatments spaced too close together can be irritating to the skin.

Depilatory lotions and creams:

- It is important to test skin sensitivity to the product before using it.
- Apply cream or lotion to a small patch of skin and leave on for 15 minutes.
- Wipe off, wash with water and soap, then observe the area for 24 hours.
- If redness or a rash occurs, do not use the depilatory.
- Apply the cream or lotion with an applicator stick or wear plastic gloves. Bare hands are not recommended.
- Avoid touching eyes, mouth or genital area with the product.
- Discontinue use of the product if irritation occurs.
- Water can increase the odor of the chemicals. Wipe the excess cream or lotion off prior to washing to keep the odor to a minimum.

MENSTRUAL CARE

MENSTRUAL CYCLE

Menstruation is the cyclical, physiological, desquamation of the endometrium that occurs during a woman's reproductive years. Although the menstrual cycle is usually discussed in the context of 28 days, there is much individual variability. The normal range can be anywhere from 20 to 40 days, often with minor variations from one month to another.

The menstrual cycle is hormonally driven. It is due to an interdependent cycling of estrogen, progesterone, luteinizing hormone and follicle-stimulating hormone (Figure 2). The average woman experiences about 450 menstrual cycles in her lifetime. Menarche commonly occurs around 12 years of age, and menstruation usually ceases around or after the age of 50.

The average length of menses is 5 days with a range of 2 to 8 days. During any one menstrual period the characteristics of the flow may vary. Sometimes it can be heavy with red clots, at other times it may be scant, with a brownish tinge.

Blood, cervical and uterine secretions, endometrial tissue, mucus and vaginal secretions make up the material discharged during menstruation. On average, 30 to 50 mL of blood is lost with each menstrual period. About 1% of women lose more than 200 mL.

Amenorrhea, lack of menstruation, can be due to physiologic causes or secondary causes, such as stress, dramatic weight fluctuation, nutrition, excessive physical activity or discontinuation of oral contraceptives. Failure to menstruate should be assessed by a physician.

Although there may be cultural or personal taboos surrounding physical or sexual activities during menses, there are no physiological reasons why such activities need to be curtailed.

Menstrual Hygiene

Regular genital hygiene practices are important during menses to decrease odor and genital irritation. Sanitary pads or tampons are used to absorb the flow. The decision to use either pads or tampons is a personal choice.

Pads are worn against the perineum and secured to undergarments by adhesive strips or pins, or suspended in place by use of a sanitary belt. Disposable pads are made from absorbent cotton, rayon or cellulose. Reusable, washable cotton fabric pads are also available.

Maxi or superabsorbant pads are suitable for times of heavy flow; mini pads and panty liners are used for light flow or between periods to absorb vaginal discharge. Longer pads and ones with tabs that wrap around the edge of the underwear help prevent soiling of the undergarment.

Tampons are wads of cotton, rayon or cellulose inserted intravaginally using a plunger-style applicator or by pushing the tampon into the vagina with a finger or applicator stick. The application method varies from brand to brand. Various absorbencies are available as is a slimmer version that may provide a more comfortable insertion for some women.

Millions of women have used tampons successfully. There is, however, evidence of three important consequences: vaginal or cervical ulcers, vaginal mucosal changes and toxic shock syndrome. This is particularly apparent when superabsorbent tampons are used during periods of light flow. Repetitive use may increase the risk of transient mucosal changes progressing to clinical ulceration. Frequent insertion and removal of tampons can also cause transient mucosal damage. This is particularly true when a relatively dry tampon is pulled across the vaginal mucosa during removal. It is important that tampons be inserted and removed gently and that the absorbency of the tampon corresponds to the degree of menstrual flow.

Both pads and tampons come in scented and unscented versions. Scented or deodorant products are not recommended, nor required. There is the risk of allergic reactions to perfumes in the products.

TOXIC SHOCK SYNDROME

Toxic shock syndrome (TSS) is an acute illness caused by the toxin-producing *Staphylococcus aureus*. Those at risk for TSS include women who use tampons, postpartum women and anyone with surgical wound infections or staphylococcal infections. Tampons are believed to increase the risk of the condition due to their potential for damaging vaginal and cervical tissue.

Staphylococcus aureus, commonly found on vulvar tissue, may be introduced into the vagina

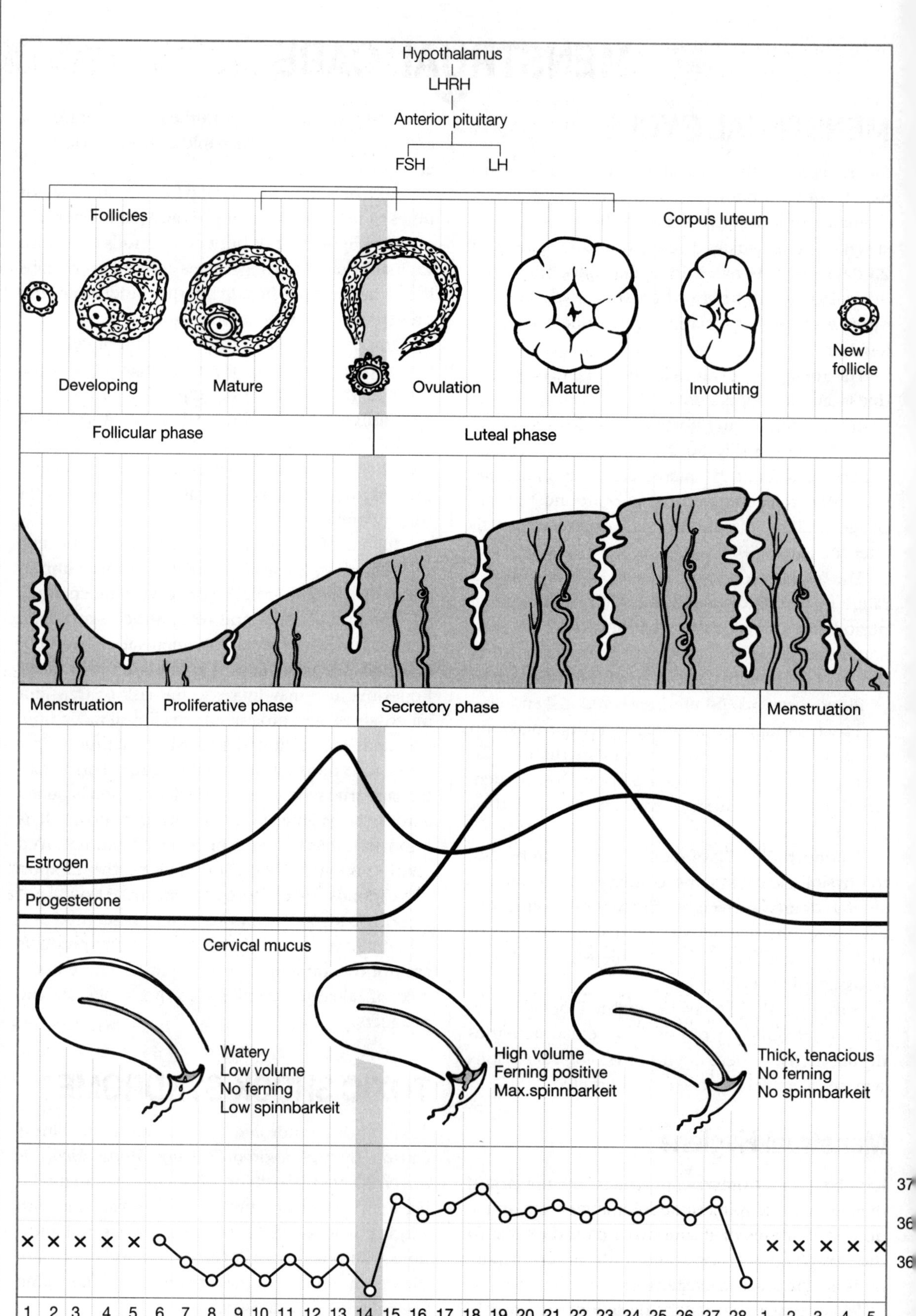

FIGURE 2: The Menstrual Cycle

when the tampon is inserted and can proliferate in the supportive vaginal environment. If a toxin is produced, it can be absorbed into the systemic circulation through a vaginal wall damaged by the use of the tampons.

Symptoms

The complex of symptoms includes: sudden high fever; a diffuse sunburn-like rash and erythema on the palms of hands and soles of feet; desquamation of skin on the palms and soles within 2 weeks of initial symptoms and low blood pressure (systolic <90 mm Hg) leading to severe hypotension and shock.

In addition, people with TSS present with three or more of the following:

- nausea;
- vomiting or diarrhea at the onset of illness;
- sore throat or redness of the conjunctiva of the eye;
- severe myalgias;
- oliguria (decreased urine output) and renal impairment;
- elevated hepatic enzymes and bilirubin indicating hepatic failure;
- low platelet counts, abnormal bruising and bleeding;
- confusion, disorientation and loss of consciousness;
- cardiac arrhythmias.

Treatment

A menstruating woman with symptoms of TSS should seek medical help immediately. If she has a tampon in place, it should be removed. TSS is rare but can be fatal if not recognized early and treated correctly. Treatment is supportive and aimed at eradicating the toxin-producing organism.

DYSMENORRHEA

Over half the women of reproductive age experience some cramping or abdominal discomfort just prior to menses or during the first 2 days. In the vast majority of cases there is no discernible abnormality, and it is therefore labelled primary dysmenorrhea. Secondary dysmenorrhea can be caused by endometriosis, pelvic infections and the use of intrauterine devices, etc.

ADVICE FOR THE WOMAN

Menstrual Care

- Regular washing of the genital area is important for good hygiene. Use water and mild soap.
- Pads and tampons should be changed regularly (about 4 to 6 times daily).
- Avoid the use of superabsorbent tampons during periods of light flow. This may decrease the risk of damage to the vaginal tissue.
- Alternate between pad and tampon use during menses (e.g., use tampons during the day and pads at night). This may decrease risk of tampon damage to vaginal tissue.
- After vaginal surgery, childbirth or any other procedure that may have damaged the vaginal epithelium, do not use tampons until healing is complete (6 to 8 weeks).
- The use of tampons should be avoided for at least 6 months following TSS.
- If TSS symptoms occur during menstruation, (e.g., high fever, nausea, diarrhea, vomiting, a sunburn-like rash or lightheadedness on rising), the tampon should be removed and medical attention sought.

PATIENT ASSESSMENT QUESTIONS

Q *Have you used this brand of tampons before?*

The method of application varies from brand to brand. Some have plunger-type applicators, others have applicator sticks or are inserted with a finger. The consumer may not realize the difference and accidentally purchase an unsuitable product.

Q *Do you know the symptoms of toxic shock syndrome?*

Although toxic shock syndrome is rare, if the following symptoms occur during menstruation the woman should seek medical attention immediately: sudden fever, diarrhea, vomiting and sunburn-like rash.

Primary dysmenorrhea has been associated with uterine ischemia caused by exaggerated uterine contractility. High levels of prostaglandins that can stimulate uterine contractility have been found in women experiencing painful menses. These prostaglandins can cause the release of intracellular substances that in turn can contribute to dysmenorrhea. Bradykinins and histamine can promote pain while heparin, histamine and serotonin may reduce homeostasis and cause longer and heavier periods.

Prostaglandins have a short life span and are synthesized just prior to their release. Estrogen, luteal phase levels of progesterone, and the state of the endometrium all contribute to the ultimate synthesis of prostaglandins in the female genital tract.

Symptoms

Cramping and abdominal discomfort usually begin on the first day of menses, often just prior to the first sign of bleeding. The discomfort peaks shortly thereafter and is usually gone by the second day. The pain is spasmodic and centres in the lower abdomen with some radiation to the back and possibly the upper thighs.

FIGURE 3

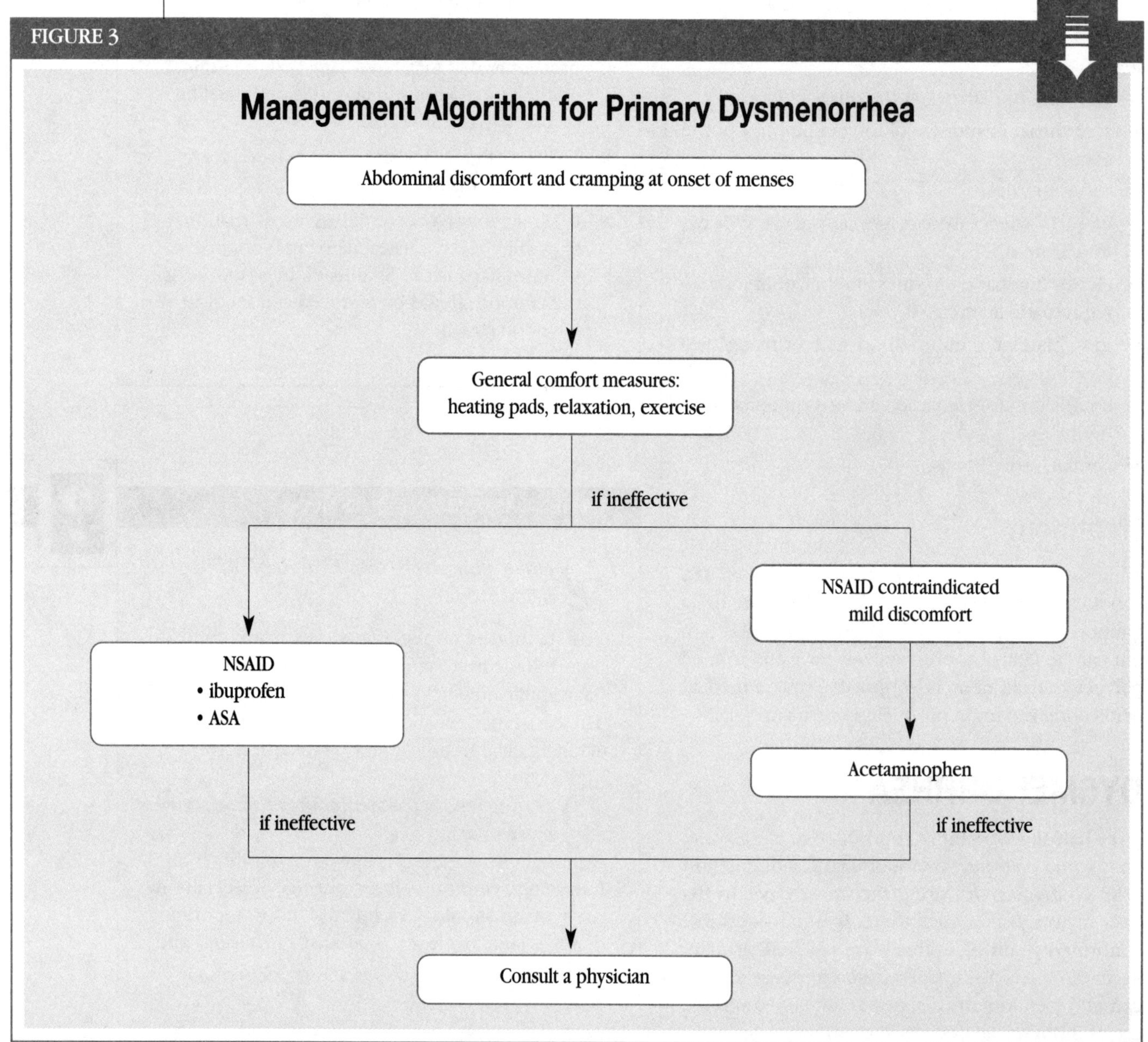

For most women the symptoms are mild to moderate and do not interfere with daily activities. About 10 to 15% of dysmenorrheic women will suffer severe symptoms that are debilitating.

Symptoms seem to abate with advancing age and after childbirth, but this postpartum improvement may only be temporary.

Treatment

There are a number of supportive and pharmacological therapies for treating primary dysmenorrhea. See Figure 3 for the management algorithm.

Nonpharmacological Treatment

Warm baths and heating pads or hot water bottles applied to the abdomen may help to reduce discomfort. Relaxing activities or exercise bring relief for some women.

Pharmacological Treatment

Nonprescription analgesics are the mainstay of treatment for mild to moderate cases of primary dysmenorrhea. In combination with general comfort measures they will relieve the symptoms of the majority of women. Selection of a medication is based on the severity of the symptoms, patient characteristics and patient preference.

Interest in the treatment of dysmenorrhea has increased markedly since prostaglandins have been implicated in the pathogenesis of the condition. Drugs that inhibit prostaglandin synthesis, such as nonsteroidal anti-inflammatory agents (NSAIDs), decrease uterine contractility and provide pain relief. Ibuprofen is available without a prescription and is an excellent choice for treatment of dysmenorrhea provided the woman has no contraindications to its use. Studies show that up to 80% of women with primary dysmenorrhea will record improvement with the use of a NSAID. Regular analgesic doses of ibuprofen can be used: 200 to 400 mg every 4 to 6 hours (after food to decrease stomach irritation).

Gastrointestinal problems are common with ibuprofen, as they are with all NSAIDs. Ibuprofen will have to be discontinued in up to 15% of users due to epigastric pain, abdominal discomfort, nausea and vomiting, abdominal bloating and gas. Gastrointestinal ulceration and hemorrhage can occur, but it is rare when the drug is used for short term, acute treatment, such as in dysmenorrhea. Caution should be exercised when recommending ibuprofen for a woman also taking warfarin. There is a theoretical increased risk of gastric ulcer bleeding with the two drugs in combination.

Cautious use is also recommended in women with a history of gastrointestinal ulceration, in those with known hypersensitivity to ASA or other NSAIDs, and in women who have experienced asthma-like symptoms, urticaria or rhinitis with ASA or NSAIDs.

ASA has mild antiprostaglandin synthesis activity as well as analgesic properties. It has been shown effective in about 30% of users although some studies refute these results and seem to indicate that ASA is not superior to placebo. Studies aside, many women use ASA-containing products for relief of symptoms.

Doses range from 325 to 1,000 mg every 4 to 6 hours to a daily maximum of 4 g. A suitable dose will depend upon the woman's response and

ADVICE FOR THE WOMAN

Cautions for the Use of ASA and Ibuprofen

- Follow the dosing on the package.
- Take the medication with food or milk to decrease the chance of stomach irritation.
- Check with your pharmacist or physician before using ASA or ibuprofen if any of the following situations exist for you:
  - a history of peptic ulcer disease or gastrointestinal bleeding;
  - recent or current use of anticoagulants (blood thinners);
  - asthma (especially if triggered by allergies) or history of hives;
  - allergy or sensitivity to anti-inflammatory medication;
  - history of chronic alcohol consumption;
  - current use of medications that may possibly cause gastrointestinal ulceration; e.g., prednisone and other oral cortisone-like medication, anti-inflammatory drugs.
- ASA is not recommended if you also have flu-like symptoms (e.g., fever, aching joints): there may be an association with the development of further complications.

acceptance of the drug. The following symptoms may be an indication that the dose of ASA is too high: ringing in the ears; changes in vision; headache; confusion; dizziness; stomach upset.

Prior to recommending ASA, the potential for adverse effects must be assessed. Women should also be informed that some users observe an apparent increase in menstrual flow while using ASA. If this is bothersome then ASA should be discontinued and alternate therapy tried.

Acetaminophen provides relief due to its analgesic properties. It is the least likely nonprescription analgesic to cause side effects, and most women are able to tolerate it. It is a reasonable choice for those with mild discomfort and in particular for women who cannot tolerate the

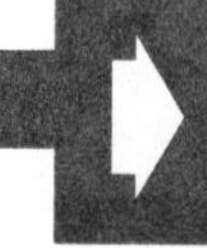

ADVICE FOR THE WOMAN

Dysmenorrhea

- Abdominal cramping and discomfort are common occurrences at the start of menses. In the majority of cases there are no underlying medical conditions causing the symptoms.
- General comfort measures, such as heating pads on the abdomen, warm baths, relaxing activities or exercise, can be helpful.
- Begin your medication at the first sign of symptoms.
- Medication with ASA or ibuprofen should be taken with food to reduce stomach irritation.
- Symptoms usually disappear within the first 3 days of menses.
- Continue with the medication until the discomfort is gone. Depending on your symptoms, this could be after the first dose or you may need to use the medication for several days.
- Follow the dosing recommendations on the package or those given to you by your health care provider.
- If you have used nonprescription treatment for several menstrual cycles and have not had adequate relief, see your physician for further assessment.

?

PATIENT ASSESSMENT QUESTIONS

Q ***Please describe your menstrual pain.***

Dysmenorrhea is a cramping, labor-like pain centred in the abdomen and lower back. It begins just before or at the onset of menses and lasts for 1 to 3 days. If the pain lasts through menses and increases in severity or is felt at other times in the menstrual cycle, there may be an underlying medical disorder that should be assessed by a physician.

Q ***Have you tried any medication in the past for menstrual pain? Did it help?***

If nonprescription analgesics have been used for several cycles with no success, prescription therapy may be indicated. Refer the individual to a physician.

Q ***Do you have a history of stomach or duodenal ulcers?***

Individuals with any of the above should avoid the use of ASA and ibuprofen if possible. ASA, and to a lesser degree, ibuprofen can cause gastrointestinal irritation and ulceration. Acetaminophen is the nonprescription drug of choice for these individuals.

Q ***Are you taking other medication?***

ASA can interact with a number of medications, including phenytoin, warfarin and probenecid. Ibuprofen appears to have fewer interactions, but should be used with caution in combination with oral anticoagulants, lithium, triamterene and other ulcerogenic agents. Acetaminophen is the drug of choice if a drug interaction is possible with ASA.

other options, such as ibuprofen. Its dosage range parallels that of ASA at 325 to 1,000 mg every 4 to 6 hours to a daily maximum of 4 g. Effectiveness varies depending on the severity of the cramping and pain. Overall, the response rate is similar to that seen with ASA (≤30%).

Nonprescription products are available containing acetaminophen or ASA in combination with mild diuretics (e.g., pamabrom, caffeine), antihistamines (e.g., pyrilamine maleate) and/or weak muscle relaxants (e.g., cinnamedrine). Although these products are specifically marketed for the symptomatic treatment of dysmenorrhea, they are of no greater benefit than the analgesic components alone. Some of the side effects from these combination products, such as drowsiness from the antihistamine, may actually be bothersome to the user. Diuretics, antihistamines and muscle relaxants are not recommended for the treatment of primary dysmenorrhea.

Single-entity products of ibuprofen, ASA or acetaminophen are the suitable choices for nonprescription therapy of abdominal discomfort and cramping. Ibuprofen has proven to be the most effective agent, ASA and acetaminophen less so. For mild symptoms, however, any of the three drugs could be tried. The final selection will depend on the severity of the symptoms, patient characteristics and patient preference.

PREMENSTRUAL SYNDROME

Premenstrual syndrome is a complex disorder with a variety of somatic, emotional and behavioral symptoms prior to menses. It was downplayed and made the brunt of jokes for many years but has now been recognized as having a significant impact on women's lives.

Over 90% of women of reproductive age have some symptoms, about 5% are severely affected. Women in their 30s and 40s have a higher incidence and severity of PMS than younger women.

Numerous theories have been presented to explain this condition; however, there is little conclusive evidence to support an etiology or the various treatments.

It is generally believed that normal ovarian function triggers biochemical activity in the central nervous system (CNS) and other target tissues that is transposed into PMS symptoms in susceptible women. When ovarian function is suppressed by drugs or surgery, PMS symptoms disappear. They are also decreased by drugs that block the neuroendocrine response to ovarian function, such as serotonin reuptake inhibitors like fluoxetine.

While estrogen or progesterone may play some role in PMS, it is not simply explained by an excess or deficiency of either. Neurotransmitters in the CNS may be responsible for mediating the response of PMS sufferers to ovarian steroids. β-endorphins seem to be decreased in the luteal phase of women with PMS, and there is research into the possible relationship to decreased serotonin activity seen in some cases.

The role of sodium and water retention is not scientifically supported. Recent information indicates that women who experience feelings of bloatedness and abdominal distention prior to menses do not have an associated gain in weight, total body water, extracellular fluid volume or any other indication of excess fluid.

It is likely that the cause of PMS is complex; until the puzzle is unravelled further, treatments will remain numerous and varied. Each woman should try therapeutic measures that target her specific needs and symptoms.

Symptoms

There are a variety of symptoms and presentations of PMS (Table 2). Each woman will experience her own unique combination, course and severity of symptoms, which can range from very mild to extremely severe. In rare cases they have led to suicide and homicide.

It is the timing of the symptoms that helps with the diagnosis rather than the symptoms themselves. They begin during the luteal phase of the

TABLE 2: Symptoms of PMS

Psychological	Physical
Anxiety, tension, loss of control, depression, crying, mood swings, increased appetite, cravings, binges, lethargy, fatigue, sleep disturbances, confusion, clumsiness, aggression, phobias	Abdominal discomfort and bloating, edema, possible weight gain, breast discomfort and tenderness, headaches, backaches, acne, rhinitis, palpitations

menstrual cycle and may increase in intensity as menses approaches. The onset of menses often brings about a rapid cessation of symptoms, although some women will have symptoms through menses. There is a symptom-free period prior to ovulation.

PMS must be distinguished from other conditions, such as dysmenorrhea or psychiatric disorders. Dysmenorrhea occurs at the start of menses rather than during the luteal phase and has somewhat different symptoms. Psychiatric disorders, such as depression or bipolar affective disorder, may be exacerbated around menses but the symptoms would be present at all stages of the menstrual cycle. There would be no symptom-free period. Failure to accurately diagnose the conditions has led to ineffective and inappropriate treatment.

Treatment

Treatment of PMS is supportive, symptomatic and aimed at reversing the cause of the condition. See Figure 4 for the management algorithm.

Nonpharmacological Treatment

Once other medical conditions have been ruled out and the diagnosis of PMS made, the first step is to reassure the woman that the symptoms are PMS related and that other women experience similar

FIGURE 4

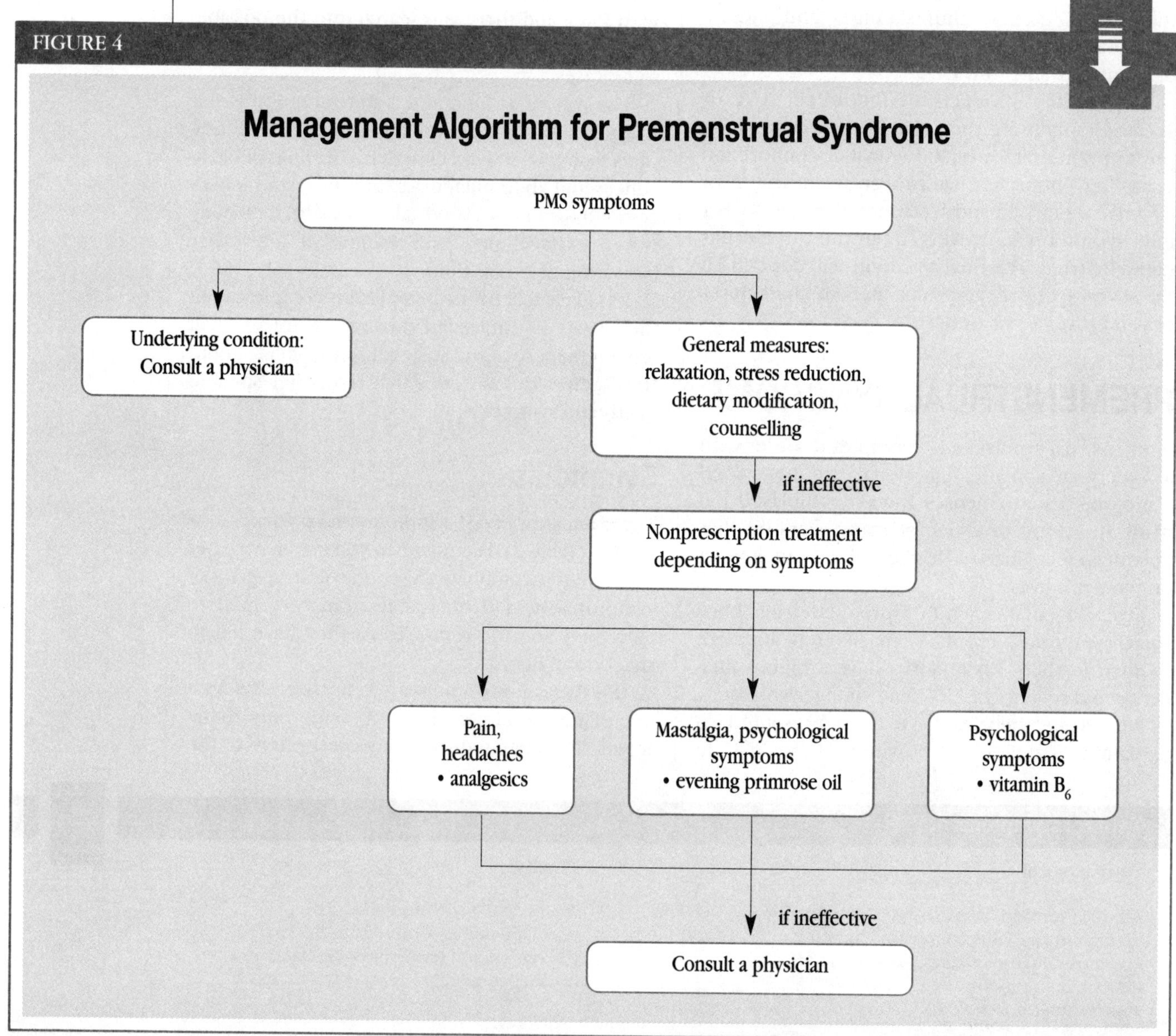

problems. Treatment recommendations depend on the specific symptoms and their severity.

Health care professionals advising women with PMS can recommend several general measures to help alleviate the symptoms. Stress reduction along with regular exercise are considered helpful by some. Reduction of caffeine and alcohol intake may decrease irritability, depression or fatigue, and reduction of salt and carbohydrates may help control feelings of bloatedness and decrease weight gain.

Pharmacological Treatment

Available nonprescription therapy is generally limited in its effectiveness. Little has been found to be supported by scientific scrutiny. Much of the information about various treatments comes from poorly designed studies or anecdotal reports. Any recommendations for pharmacological treatment should be combined with general measures to obtain the maximum relief. A woman whose symptoms are not relieved by nonprescription therapy should be referred to her physician for assessment and prescription medication.

Analgesics such as ASA, acetaminophen and ibuprofen are commonly used to relieve mild pain and headaches associated with PMS. Ibuprofen shows no superiority over the others in the treatment of PMS as prostaglandins have an uncertain role in this condition. The choice of analgesic depends mainly on the woman and whether there are any contraindications to the use of the agent.

Doses of 325 to 1,000 mg every 4 to 6 hours, not to exceed 4 g daily, are recommended for ASA and acetaminophen. Ibuprofen can be taken in doses of 200 to 400 mg every 4 to 6 hours (for more detailed information see section on Dysmenorrhea).

There are products marketed specifically for PMS that contain ASA or acetaminophen plus an antihistamine (e.g., pyrilamine maleate) and a mild diuretic (e.g., pamabrom, caffeine). Although unlikely to cause significant problems for most users, they are not a rational way to approach treatment.

Antihistamines have no proven value in the treatment of PMS. They may have been included to try to decrease symptoms such as irritability and tension through their sedative properties. The amount of antihistamine in the product is well below usual adult doses and is unlikely to be helpful or harmful, but it may increase the fatigue and lethargy felt by some women with PMS.

Diuretics were once widely used for PMS. Fluid and water retention are no longer considered major causes of PMS symptoms, and the role of diuretics is greatly reduced. Mild diuretics found in nonprescription products are of no proven value. Reduction of dietary salt intake would likely be more effective. If a woman has significant water retention, a prescription diuretic would be more suitable.

There is some indication that certain women with PMS have low levels of a fatty acid required for the synthesis of prostaglandins. Commercial preparations of evening primrose oil contain at least 9% gamma-linoleic acid, the fatty acid that is a precursor of prostaglandin E_1 and arachidonic acid. Uncontrolled studies have supported the use of the oil for treatment of depression, mastalgia and anxiety, while other studies show no advantage over placebo. There is considerable anecdotal evidence to support its use, however.

The oil is available in 0.5 g capsules, the usual dose 2 to 4 capsules daily. Even with the use of 12 capsules daily no significant side effects have been reported.

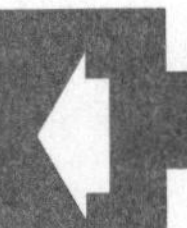

ADVICE FOR THE WOMAN

Premenstrual Syndrome

- Reduce stress factors and practice stress management activities. Pamper yourself.
- Eliminate or reduce caffeine or alcohol intake. Anxiety, irritability, depression and fatigue can be increased by these substances.
- Reduce your salt intake. Avoid very salty foods. This may help to decrease the feeling of bloatedness.
- Exercise regularly.
- Limit intake of sweets and other carbohydrate sources during PMS. Acute increases in carbohydrate intake can cause rapid weight gain in some women.
- There is also a belief that high sugar-containing foods may enhance PMS symptoms.
- Nontraditional therapies such as acupuncture, hypnosis and yoga have been tried. Their benefits are difficult to assess, but some women believe they are very helpful in promoting a feeling of well-being.

Vitamin therapy has also been advocated. Vitamin B_6 (pyridoxine) has been used for PMS and for oral contraceptive induced depression. As a cofactor in the synthesis of several neurotransmitters (e.g., serotonin, dopamine), it was hoped that pyridoxine supplementation might affect mood and behavioral symptoms. The results of studies are contradictory with the nay-sayers predominating. This vitamin is widely used for PMS, however, and a number of anecdotal reports support its benefits.

Pyridoxine toxicity is well documented. Partially reversible neuropathies with sensory loss have occurred with doses as low as 200 mg daily. At low doses these symptoms may take many months to appear while at high doses (greater than 1 g daily) the neurological symptoms were detected more quickly.

Considering the questionable effectiveness of the vitamin and the risk of toxicity, vitamin B_6 doses should not exceed 100 mg daily unless prescribed by a physician. If toxicity is suspected, the vitamin should be discontinued immediately.

Other vitamin and mineral deficiencies have been suggested as contributors to PMS—vitamins A and E, magnesium and calcium. There is no evidence to support supplementation with any of these. There are some prescription vitamin and mineral products designed for PMS therapy. They too carry the risk of toxicity and are used only under careful medical supervision.

Often, more than one medication will be tried concurrently. Possible interactions should always be considered although common PMS treatments have little interactive potential.

There has been more success in PMS treatment with some of the prescription therapies. If a woman does not gain relief from the general measures and nonprescription options, she should see her physician. Possible alternatives at that stage are oral contraceptives, bromocriptine, diuretics, progesterone suppositories, danazol, estrogen patches, antidepressants, gonadotropin-releasing hormone agonists or surgery.

PATIENT ASSESSMENT QUESTIONS

Q *What symptoms lead you to believe you have PMS and when did they begin?*

PMS symptoms are many and varied. They usually peak 2 to 3 days before onset of menstruation and resolve rapidly once menses begins. They can begin on or any time after ovulation. It is important to rule out any underlying medical condition that may cause the symptoms. Once PMS is suspected, nonprescription treatment can be tried. Women with severe incapacitating symptoms should be referred to a physician.

Q *Are you trying any general measures that may help decrease PMS symptoms?*

A number of lifestyle modifications may help decrease PMS symptoms. They include stress reduction, increased exercise and dietary changes, such as reduction of caffeine, alcohol, salt and carbohydrate intake.

Q *What have you used in the past for PMS relief?*

A review of past therapy indicates whether nonprescription options are still available or whether the woman must try prescription therapy next.

VAGINAL INFECTIONS

Women commonly seek health care advice because of bothersome genital symptoms, such as abnormal vaginal discharge or perineal irritation and itching. Examination usually confirms a diagnosis of a vaginitis or vaginosis, the majority attributable to a vaginal infection. About 90% of all vaginal infections are either bacterial vaginosis (formerly nonspecific vaginitis or gardnerella vaginitis), candidiasis or trichomoniasis. Only vulvovaginal candidiasis is recommended for self-treatment.

PHYSIOLOGY

Within the transverse folds of the healthy vaginal wall live numerous indigenous organisms. Common examples are *Lactobacilli, Streptococci* species, *Staphylococci* species, *Gardnerella vaginalis*, anaerobes, *Candida albicans* and *Ureaplasma urealyticum*. There is wide variation in types and numbers of these normal flora from woman to woman. Variations are due to many factors, such as the woman's age, sexual history, pregnancy, contraceptive methods used, menstruation, antibiotic use, vaginal trauma (e.g., surgery) and even tampon use.

In most instances the organisms exist in harmony with the vaginal environment, a balance that produces no adverse effects. Changes to the vaginal epithelium, the normally acidic vaginal pH or the structure of the vagina can allow for overproduction of host organisms or the colonization of externally acquired pathogens.

WHEN TO RECOMMEND SELF-TREATMENT

The decision to recommend self-treatment must be made with care. There are a number of other types of vaginitis that must be ruled out, sexually transmitted diseases to consider and allergic or sensitivity reactions to topical products that may be implicated in the woman's symptoms.

Vaginitis covers a group of conditions that have similar symptoms but a variety of causes. In general, there may be abnormalities of vaginal discharge and odor, itching or burning, spotting, and occasionally dyspareunia. The common ones: trichomonas vaginitis, candida vulvovaginitis and bacterial vaginosis all have distinguishing features (Table 3), but it is often difficult to distinguish one from the other by signs and symptoms alone. Atrophic vaginitis occurs in postmenopausal women due to changes in the vaginal mucosa and pH brought about by the decrease in estrogen. Vaginal discharge, irritation or burning, and spotting can occur.

A brief sexual history may be helpful in determining if a sexually transmitted condition is a possibility. Trichomonas vaginitis is sexually acquired, but vulvovaginal candidiasis and atrophic vaginitis are not. The role of sexual transmission of bacterial vaginosis is unclear. Cervicitis due to chlamydial or gonococcal infection can cause increased vaginal discharge and/or odor and if left untreated can lead to serious medical sequelae such as pelvic inflammatory disease and systemic complications.

TABLE 3: Characteristics of Common Types of Vaginitis/Vaginosis

Cause	Common Symptom(s)	pH
Bacterial vaginosis	"Fishy" odor Creamy discharge (grey/yellow)	5-6
Vulvovaginal candidiasis	Severe pruritus (vulvovaginal) "Cottage cheese" discharge Stinging/burning sensation	<4.5
Trichomoniasis	Genital wetness or frothy discharge May be pruritic	6+
Atrophy	Vaginal discharge Spotting Soreness and burning	7

It is important to remember that vulvovaginal candidiasis is generally not associated with systemic symptoms, such as fever, chills or lower abdominal pain, and that their presence warrants further medical investigation by a physician. Women most at risk for sexually transmitted disease are those who have unprotected intercourse and/or multiple sexual partners.

Feminine deodorant sprays, douches, perfumed soaps and powders, laundry detergent and vaginal spermicides are some of the substances that have caused allergic or sensitivity reactions in susceptible women. They can cause a chemical vulvovaginal irritation that must be distinguished from an infectious etiology. Women who routinely use feminine deodorant sprays and vaginal douches may be wise to discontinue their use until the cause of the vulvovaginal irritation is determined.

The wide variety of etiologies that may be responsible for vulvovaginal symptoms makes it very difficult to determine the cause based solely on those symptoms. Vulvovaginal candidiasis is the only condition that will respond to antifungal agents thus making the correct diagnosis essential. Self-treatment with nonprescription antifungal agents should only be recommended when the woman has had at least one previous episode of identical symptoms diagnosed as candidiasis, and has no apparent risk for a sexually transmitted or hypersensitivity condition. Pregnant women, those with recurrent episodes of vulvovaginal candidiasis (<2 months between episodes), young females (<12 years of age) and those with conditions that predispose them to candidiasis (e.g., diabetes mellitus) should be referred to a physician.

VULVOVAGINAL CANDIDIASIS

Vulvovaginal candidiasis has a number of predisposing factors associated with it (Table 4). They all affect the vaginal epithelium or vaginal environment in ways that upset the normal balance and permit the colonization with or overproduction of *Candida* strains (e.g., *C. albicans*).

Symptoms

A woman is usually alerted to the existence of a problem by the development of bothersome symptoms. The classic symptom is severe vulvovaginal itching. There may also be a "cottage cheese" vaginal discharge, or burning or stinging during urination. The latter is due to the effect of urine on the irritated vulvar tissue. Symptoms such as fever or lower abdominal pain are not associated with vulvovaginal candidiasis. In general, these include all or some of the following: a change in amount, appearance or smell of vaginal secretions; vaginal and perineal irritation or pruritus; and pain or discomfort on intercourse. Each type of vaginitis or vaginosis has characteristic symptoms that help to distinguish it from all the others (Table 3).

Nonpharmacological Treatment

Candida is the second most common cause of vaginal infections. Many women are prone to recurrent or resistant infections. They, in particular, might be interested in trying some preventive measures to enhance their recovery or for prophylaxis. Such measures could include good genital hygiene, wearing of loose fitting undergarments to allow ventilation and dietary changes, such as increasing yogurt in the diet.

Pharmacological Treatment

The intravaginal application of antifungal agents is the mainstay of treatment of vaginal candidiasis. Imidazoles (e.g., clotrimazole, miconazole, etc.) are the agents commonly used in Canada. They are about 90% effective, can be given in short-course regimens, appear to decrease symptoms quickly and are well tolerated. There are a number of drugs available in this class, all of which appear to be

TABLE 4: Predisposing Factors for Vulvovaginal Candidiasis

Physiological Conditions	Medications	Medical Conditions	Other
Pregnancy, menses	Antibiotics, corticosteroids, chemotherapy, oral contraceptives, estrogen supplements	Uncontrolled diabetes mellitus, immunocompromised states e.g., HIV infection, multiple environmental sensitivities	Diet, poorly ventilated underclothing, chemical irritants, stress

equally effective. The recent move to deregulate several of them, e.g., clotrimazole, miconazole and tioconazole, to nonprescription status, has dramatically improved the available nonprescription options. See Figure 5 for the management algorithm.

A number of treatment regimens have proven effective (Table 5). Traditional dosing provides for a 7-day or greater course of treatment. With the newer, more concentrated products, courses of 1 to 3 days are possible. For a woman experiencing the occasional, acute bout of vaginal candidiasis, the shorter courses are often preferred as reflected by good compliance. Women who have recurrent or tenacious infections may need extended courses of treatment. In some cases the usual 6 to 7 day treatments must be continued for up to 3 or 4 weeks. Extended treatment should only be used on the advice of a physician. Combo-paks (topical cream plus vaginal inserts) are recommended when topical therapy is required to treat vulvar irritation accompanying the vaginal irritation. Cream can also be used by the male partner if it has been determined he is contributing to reinfection. It is not common to treat the male partner, but it may be appropriate in specific circumstances, e.g., if the infection seeded from the penis of an uncircumcised male.

Imidazole antifungals have generally replaced other nonprescription therapies. Some references still mention the use of gentian violet 1% solution as a vaginal paint. Although effective, it is messy and stains clothing. It is a rare situation when this would be the recommended treatment.

Vinegar and water douches and yogurt douches have been used to try to stabilize the vaginal environment and return to the ecological balance where *Candida* is kept under control. The vinegar douches were used to help maintain vaginal pH in the optimal acidic range and yogurt douches were supposed to restore *Lactobacilli* activity in the vagina and thereby maintain acidity and balance the normal vaginal flora. They were used for acute treatment of symptoms as well as prophylactically. Neither of these two treatments have proven track records. Some women may still wish to use them, particularly if recurrent infections are a problem. Health care providers can help to ensure that proper douching technique is followed, that reusable equipment is well cleaned after each use to prevent reinfection and that women seek alternative treatment if they remain symptomatic after douching.

Boric acid has shown effectiveness against vaginal candidiasis. Gelatin capsules containing 600 mg of boric acid inserted into the vagina once or twice daily for 14 to 28 days have been found effective in up to 92% of women. Despite the apparent success with the drug, this is not

ADVICE FOR THE WOMAN

Vulvovaginal Candidiasis—Preventive Measures

To help increase the effectiveness of your treatment or to decrease the chance of recurrence:

- Maintain good genital hygiene.
- Wear loose-fitting undergarments and pants.
- Wear cotton underwear and panty hose with cotton crotch pieces to aid ventilation. Avoid synthetic fabrics.
- Modify your diet—increase yogurt intake, avoid high sugar foods.

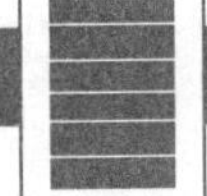

TABLE 5: Nonprescription Treatment Regimens for Vulvovaginal Candidiasis

Clotrimazole	Miconazole
1% vaginal cream —1 applicatorful at bedtime (6 days) 2% vaginal cream —1 applicatorful at bedtime (3 days) 100 mg vaginal insert—1 tablet at bedtime (6 days) 200 mg vaginal insert—1 tablet at bedtime (3 days) 500 mg vaginal insert—1 tablet at bedtime (1 day)	2% vaginal cream—1 applicatorful at bedtime (7 days) 100 mg vaginal suppository—1 vaginal suppository at bedtime (7 days) 400 mg vaginal ovule—1 ovule at bedtime (3 days)
Tioconazole	
6.5% vaginal ointment—1 applicatorful at bedtime (1 day) 300 mg vaginal ovule—1 ovule at bedtime (1 day)	

FIGURE 5

Suggested Approach for Treating Vulvovaginal Candidiasis (VVC)

Question	Answer	Medical Referral
Symptoms consistent with vulvovaginal candidiasis (vaginal itch or irritation, curdy white discharge, external dysuria)	no	A condition other than VVC may exist and accurate diagnosis required.
↓ yes		
Determine presence of other symptoms: • fever • pain (pelvic, abdominal) • rash/sores • odor/colored profuse discharge	yes	Presence of such symptoms is not typical of VVC and accurate diagnosis is required prior to therapy.
↓ no		
First episode	yes	Nonprescription vaginal antifungals are indicated only for the treatment of VVC in females who have prior medical confirmation of the diagnosis and who are currently experiencing the **same symptoms.**
↓ no		
Recurrence <2 months	yes	Recurrence may imply treatment failure or the presence of medical conditions which require further attention by a physician.
↓ no		
Pregnant	yes	Although the imidazole vaginal antifungals appear to be safe for use during pregnancy, **they are not approved for OTC use in pregnancy.**
↓ no		
Age <12 years	yes	VVC is uncommon in young females and other diagnosis must be considered.
↓ no		
Unstable medical conditions: • AIDS • diabetes • immunocompromised	yes	Certain medical conditions may require additional interventions to obtain satisfactory resolution.
↓ no		
High risk sexual behavior	yes	There is a higher risk that symptoms are due to STD or that an STD may exist concomitantly. Medical assessment is advised.
↓ no		
Treat with nonprescription vaginal antifungals		

Adapted with permission from: Travill L. New nonprescription antifungal preparations. Ottawa: Travill Consulting, 1994.

considered a first line therapy. It is generally kept as an alternative for women who are not responsive to the vaginal or systemic antimycotic products or for those who are unable to use them.

The decision to recommend nonprescription treatment for a suspected vaginal candidiasis, without a thorough examination, must be made with care. Classic symptoms (e.g., severe vulvovaginal itching), a past history of vaginal candidiasis plus one or more risk factors are strong indicators that vaginal antimycotics are indicated. Women who have never experienced the problem before, those whose symptoms are less definitive or those who have had an unsuccessful trial with clotrimazole, miconazole or tioconazole should be referred to their physician for further investigation.

When recommending therapy, it may be wise to suggest the short course treatments. Early recognition of nonresponders will ensure that suitable treatment is not delayed. If vaginal candidiasis is confirmed after further investigation an alternate antimycotic or extended course of treatment will be prescribed.

Women with recalcitrant or recurrent infections (more than one episode in a 2-month period) should be referred to their physician.

Hormonal changes in pregnancy increase the occurrence of vaginal infections due to *Candida* species. Although clotrimazole and miconazole have been used safely in pregnant women, self-treatment is not advisable. A pregnant woman should be seen by her physician if vaginitis is suspected.

Sometimes with vaginal infections the vulvovaginal irritation or pruritus is severe. Local anesthetic and antipruritic creams or gels are sometimes used to decrease the discomfort prior to the antimicrobial therapy taking effect. Benzocaine is the most common local anesthetic used. Health care providers should be wary of situations when these topical preparations are used for symptomatic relief. They are not recommended due to the risk of skin sensitization. If a woman insists on using them, it is important that she use them only on the external genitalia and for short periods of time. Application of a topical antimycotic cream to the perineal area would be a more suitable way to help symptoms of pruritus and irritation. Although it is not officially indicated, nystatin topical cream could be used for this purpose.

Acidophilus capsules are widely used to help decrease recurrence of vulvovaginal candidiasis. They can be taken by mouth or in some cases, administered intravaginally. As with increased dietary yogurt intake, the attempt is to reset the vaginal environment to keep *Candida* under control. There is no strong scientific evidence to support the use of acidophilus products, but they are generally safe to use.

PATIENT ASSESSMENT QUESTIONS

Q *What symptoms are you experiencing?*

Assessment of the symptoms will help identify the appropriate treatment. Self-medication is only suitable for the treatment of vaginal candidiasis. Other suspected infections require prescription therapy.

Q Do you have a previous history of vaginal infections? When was your last infection and how did you treat it?

It is important to determine if this is a new infection or a recurrence of one that was not treated adequately. Knowledge of the types of past infections may help in the differential diagnosis and in selecting a treatment that has been useful in the past. Women with chronic vaginal candidiasis can also be counselled on preventive measures.

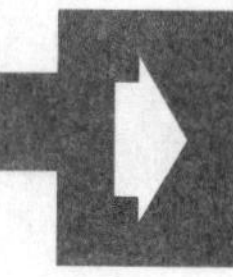

ADVICE FOR THE WOMAN

Vulvovaginal Candidiasis

For the treatment to be effective, it must be used correctly:

- Follow the dosing instructions on the package. Continue using the medication until it is all finished even if your symptoms disappear before that time.
- Bedtime is a good time to use the medication as lying down will stop the medication from leaking out. This will be more comfortable for you.
- If leakage is a problem, a sanitary pad or panty liner can be used for protection of undergarments.
- If your symptoms do not start to improve within 3 days or if the condition exists beyond 7 days despite treatment, you should consult your physician.
- Prevention may be helpful in decreasing recurrent infection.
- Do not stop using this medication if your menstrual period starts during treatment. Use sanitary pads instead of vaginal tampons since tampons may soak up the medicine.

Advice on the insertion of vaginal creams, jellies, foams and suppositories:

Insertion of vaginal creams, jellies:

- Remove the cap from the tube, invert the top and puncture the seal at the tube opening.
- Screw the applicator onto the tube.
- Squeeze the tube gently until the applicator plunger is fully extended. This will give you the correct dose.
- Unscrew the applicator from the tube.
- You can lubricate the applicator by applying a small amount of cream to the outside of the barrel.

Insertion of vaginal foams:

- Shake the canister vigorously before each use.
- With the canister in an upright position and the applicator positioned over the nozzle, press down or sideways on the nozzle with the applicator. This will release the foam.
- When the plunger is fully extended, the applicator is full and can be removed from the nozzle. Do it carefully as the foam has a tendency to continue flowing from the canister.

THEN:

- Lie on your back with your knees drawn up and apart.
- While holding the applicator by the barrel, insert it into the vagina as far as it will comfortably go.
- Hold the barrel and push the plunger all the way in to deposit the cream in the vagina.
- Remove the applicator from the vagina taking care to leave the plunger depressed.

Insertion of vaginal tablets, ovules and suppositories:

- This medication is for use in the vagina. Do not swallow it.
- Unwrap the tablet/ovule/suppository.
- If there is no applicator then the medication will be inserted with your finger.
- Moistening a hard tablet with lukewarm water may make insertion easier.
- Gently push the medication into the vagina as high up as is possible or comfortable.
- If an applicator is supplied, the medication is inserted into the end and the applicator is gently inserted into the vagina as far as it can comfortably go.
- Depress the plunger to release the tablet and then withdraw the applicator from the vagina.
- Insertion is best done while lying on your back, knees drawn up and spread apart.

ADVICE FOR THE WOMAN (*cont'd*)

Points to remember:

- Disposable applicators should be discarded after use. Reusable ones should be well cleaned with warm water and soap and then dried thoroughly after each use.
- Bedtime is a good time to use the medication as lying down will stop the medication from leaking out. This will be more comfortable for you.
- If leakage is a problem a sanitary pad can be used for protection of undergarments.
- If you still have symptoms after finishing all your medication then seek further medical advice.
- Prevention may be helpful in decreasing recurrent infection of this nature.

CONTRACEPTION

Despite the availability of effective contraceptive methods, there are thousands of unplanned pregnancies each year. The reasons are many, including lack of knowledge and method failure. Health care providers can assist by providing unbiased, practical information to women and their partners so suitable contraceptives can be chosen and used correctly.

A sound understanding of the female reproductive cycle is important for health care providers explaining contraceptive issues and helping with the choice of method.

PHYSIOLOGY

The female menstrual cycle, which is controlled by monthly hormonal variations, can be divided into two phases: follicular (preovulatory) and luteal (postovulatory). The follicular phase begins the first day of menses (day one of menstrual cycle). Ovarian follicles start to mature under the control of follicle-stimulating hormone (FSH) secreted by the anterior pituitary gland. Over time the FSH secretion is inhibited in response to rising estrogen levels produced by the developing follicles. About day 7 of the cycle, one follicle predominates and arrests the development of the others. Estrogen continues to rise and just prior to ovulation, causes a dramatic release or surge of luteinizing hormone (LH). This triggers the final maturation of the dominant follicle and subsequent release of the ovum. This occurs at approximately midcycle (day 14).

After release of the ovum (luteal phase) the ruptured follicle becomes the corpus luteum, a body capable of estrogen and progesterone production. These hormones continue to rise until they reach their peak about 18 to 22 days into the cycle. If fertilization of the ovum did not occur, the corpus luteum degenerates and estrogen and progesterone levels drop quickly. Menses then occurs and the cycle begins again.

Although the menstrual cycle is usually discussed in the context of 28 days, there is much individual variation—20 to 40 days, often with changes month to month. Differences occur most commonly in the timing of ovulation at the end of the follicular phase. The luteal phase is more consistent in length (14 days). As an example, in a cycle shorter than 28 days, ovulation occurs before the midpoint of the cycle, sometimes as early as day 7. The converse is true when menstruation occurs at intervals greater than 4 weeks.

The misjudging of the timing of ovulation is sometimes a factor in unplanned pregnancies. It is not accurate to judge the timing of ovulation strictly by determining the midpoint of the cycle or by assuming day 14.

There are other uninformed beliefs that can contribute to a pregnancy. A woman is not somehow protected by the fact that she is having her first sexual experience. Once a woman has passed puberty she can become pregnant. It can happen the first time she has sexual intercourse or any subsequent time. The risk of accidental pregnancy with unprotected intercourse is approximately 90% per year.

Breast-feeding may delay the resumption of ovulation (and menstruation), but it is not a reliable method of contraception. Its effects are not absolute, and hormonal activity can still return to levels where ovulation occurs, often before menses resumes. Lack of menses (amenorrhea) is not always a signal that ovulation is suppressed.

CONTRACEPTIVE METHODS

There are many contraceptive options available. Each has its own factors that may or may not make it suitable for a particular person. The final choice of method is a personal decision reached by weighing the benefits and risks. Health care providers can help with the decision by providing balanced information on all the methods, including factors that help the woman determine the suitability of the method to her lifestyle and health profile.

The main considerations, for those who are choosing a contraceptive method, are effectiveness, acceptability and safety.

Concerns about the risk of pregnancy are uppermost in most people's minds when looking for the right contraceptive. They generally want to know if the method works and the chance of pregnancy if the method is used correctly.

Actual efficacy is difficult to determine. It is often significantly higher than the theoretical estimate. The discrepancies could be due to improper use of the method, motivation of the user to prevent pregnancy, frequency of intercourse, or differences or bias in the study design. There is no 100% reliable method. Table 6 lists the expected and reported failure rates of the various methods. There is quite a range of effectiveness displayed in this table so it is important to keep in mind that most methods do offer good protection against pregnancy when used consistently and correctly. Although much of the information focuses on the effectiveness of hormonal contraceptives, they are not the answer for everyone. As more becomes known about their potential side effects (e.g., thromboembolic disorders, questions about association with cancer), and with the increase in information about sexually transmitted diseases, the barrier methods have shown an increase in popularity.

Some commonly used methods are ineffective. Withdrawal of the penis from the vagina prior to ejaculation (coitus interruptus) is not a reliable method. It is not always possible for the man to withdraw his penis from his partner's vagina and ejaculate far enough away that no sperm is deposited into the vagina. There may also be semen leakage prior to the actual ejaculation.

Douching with water or other solutions is used by some to try to flush semen from the vagina after intercourse. This has no spermicidal action and may actually help the transport of sperm into the uterus.

All contraceptives involve some risk to the user, which must be balanced with the efficacy and acceptability of the method. In general the barrier methods and spermicidal agents carry fewer significant risks than the systemic hormonal contraceptives.

Personal considerations are very important for the selection of a contraceptive. Only the woman and her partner can decide what makes a method an acceptable choice. Health care providers can help with that choice by asking questions that allow the woman to consider various issues.

Fertility Awareness Techniques

Fertility awareness techniques are used to predict the most likely time for ovulation so that a couple can abstain from sexual intercourse or use contraception during that fertile period. These techniques take time, commitment, education and support. Motivated couples in stable relationships are generally the most successful candidates for this type of contraception.

The prediction of the fertile period is achieved by the daily charting of various aspects of a woman's menstrual cycle. These include length of the cycle (calendar, rhythm), basal body temperature, cervical mucus changes, position and texture of the cervix and possibly other miscellaneous

TABLE 6: Failure Rates for Selected Contraceptive Methods*

Method (%)	Expected (Theoretical) Failure (%)	Reported Failure (%)
Chance (no contraceptive)	90	90
Douching		40
Withdrawal (coitus interruptus)	4	20-27
Fertility awareness (calendar, rhythm, mucous method, basal temperature, sympto-thermal method)	2-10	~20
Spermicides	3	21
Contraceptive sponge (nulliparous women have lower failure rates than parous women)	5-9	18-28
Male condom	2	12
Female condom	~3	~18
Diaphragm (+ spermicide)	3	18
Cervical cap	5	18
IUD	1-2	5-6
Oral contraceptive pill: combined	0.1	3
progestogen only	0.5	3
Implants—Norplant rods	<0.1	<0.1
Depo-Provera	0.3	0.3

*Based on results for the first year of use.

physical symptoms experienced during the cycle. Some women will chart only the cycle length or the basal body temperature while others will use a combination of predictors (sympto-thermal) to determine fertility.

The charting of cycle length allows for a general prediction of when ovulation will occur. Basal body temperature (BBT) is the daily body temperature or basal temperature that occurs prior to rising in the morning or prior to any activity. It can be taken orally, rectally or vaginally but must be done the same way each time. It is not the actual temperature that indicates ovulation but rather the pattern that is significant. About 12 to 24 hours prior to ovulation it is sometimes possible to detect a small drop in temperature. In response to progesterone secreted by the corpus luteum, the temperature usually rises sharply immediately following ovulation. This elevation continues for several days (Figure 2). BBT is useful for determining the end of a fertile period but is less reliable as an advance predictor of ovulation. Febrile illness will interfere with BBT readings, and they will not be reliable while fever is present.

Basal thermometers are recommended when taking a BBT. They are similar to a regular thermometer, but the calibrations are set wider apart to allow for easy determination of the small variations in temperature that are expected with BBT.

Cervical mucus changes in the stages of the menstrual cycle. As ovulation approaches, mucus increases in volume and becomes thin, clear and stretchable (like uncooked egg white). Volume and changes in color are easy to detect. Other characteristic changes are less obvious and require detailed observation. Close to or at the time of ovulation, a mucous thread can be formed when mucus is blown onto a glass slide and then is drawn along the slide by a glass cover. The formation of this thread is known as spinnbarkeit. A dried specimen of mucus will also show a fern-like pattern around the time of ovulation. This "ferning" is symbolic of high estrogen levels seen just prior to ovulation.

Vaginal spermicides and lubricant products may interfere with cervical mucus assessments. It would be wise to avoid the use of such products at critical cycle times when using this method to detect ovulation.

The approach of ovulation can also be detected by the softening of the cervix. This can be detected by the woman performing regular digital exploration of the external cervical area.

Self discipline is very important with fertility awareness methods. Charting of symptoms or changes must be done routinely, often daily, for many months (6 to 12) before the fertile periods can be estimated. The information gathered during those months is considered a representative sample of the variations seen in ovulation times for that particular woman. The earliest and latest ovulation times are used to help set the outside parameters of the fertile period. Continued charting of the pertinent information will enhance the effectiveness of the method. Two considerations that also affect the setting of the fertile period are the assumptions that the sperm are viable for up to 3 days and that the ovum will live for 24 hours after release. The final assessment of fertility is based on all the available factors.

When several characteristics are used in the prediction, and the charting is done without fail, natural family planning can be effective. This is particularly so if intercourse is avoided prior to ovulation and confined to the postovulatory period.

Detailed instruction should be provided for couples wishing to use fertility awareness monitoring as a contraceptive. It takes experience with the method and understanding of the female fertility cycle to accurately carry out and assess the results of the monitoring. Women's health clinics, centres for birth control information, and organizations specifically focusing on fertility awareness methods are often available in communities and can be very helpful in providing the couple with information, education and follow-up support.

Vaginal Spermicides

Spermicides are chemicals that can rapidly kill sperm and help to block the passage of sperm into the uterus. The majority are surfactants that disrupt the sperm cell making the sperm unviable.

Nonoxynol-9 and octoxynol are two agents found in spermicidal products. There may be bactericidal components added, such as benzethonium chloride.

Products usually consist of the spermicide in an inert vehicle. The vehicle provides some benefit as a barrier to sperm motility as well as disperses and suspends the spermicide in the upper part of the vagina covering the cervical os. Foams, gels, creams and suppositories are available. As well as contraceptives, these products can also be used as vaginal or condom lubricants during intercourse.

Foams are generally considered the most acceptable type of spermicidal product for intravaginal use. They disperse quickly when applied, providing almost immediate efficacy. There is less leakage of the foams than gels and some creams, making them more aesthetically pleasing and discreet. Foams can be used alone or in combination with condoms.

Jellies and creams can be used alone, in combination with condoms or applied to diaphragms or cervical caps. In general, the higher concentrations are intended for use alone while the lower concentrations are to be used with diaphragms and caps. Jellies are water soluble and readily disperse over the vagina and cervix. Vaginal secretions and sexual activity aid in this process. Leakage is more of a problem when the gels and creams are inserted intravaginally as they become more liquid with addition of vaginal secretions and body temperature. When the spermicide is applied directly onto the diaphragm or cervical cap, leakage is reduced as the cream or gel is held in place by the device.

Creams disperse less readily than foams and jellies. This can be a problem if they are not positioned over the cervix on application. After a few minutes they will spread; however, the coverage is somewhat unpredictable. Leakage is reduced compared with jellies so there are some aesthetic advantages to the use of creams over the gels.

Vaginal suppositories require time to dissolve after insertion into the vagina. It can take 10 to 30 minutes depending on the circumstances and

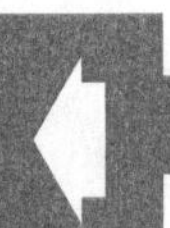

ADVICE FOR THE WOMAN

Vaginal Spermicides (Foams, Jellies, Creams and Suppositories)

Vaginal spermicides give short-term contraceptive coverage. They can be used alone or in combination with diaphragms, cervical caps and condoms. Your health care provider can help you select a product that best suits your needs.

The following general information will help you with the use of vaginal spermicides when used alone.

- The spermicide must be inserted into the vagina prior to sexual intercourse. Generally, this can be up to 30 to 60 minutes before.
- If intercourse has not occurred within 1 hour of application then insert a second dose. Spermicides will begin to lose their effectiveness after a while.
- Suppositories must be inserted into the vagina at least 10 to 15 minutes before intercourse to ensure they dissolve in time to be effective.
- The dosage for each product varies. Foams, creams and jellies usually call for 1 or 2 applicatorsful (this is product specific). One suppository is usually the recommended dose.
- A product will come with its own applicator. Use only this device to ensure the correct dose.
- Applicators for foams, creams, and jellies must be completely filled to equal one dose.
- Follow the recommended insertion technique and ensure that the spermicide is deposited high in the vagina at the cervix.
- One dose of spermicide must be used prior to each ejaculation. This may mean that you need to use several doses of spermicide during intercourse.
- Once ejaculation has occurred, do not douche or bathe for 8 hours afterwards. It is important that the spermicide remain in place for an extended period to be fully effective.
- You may wish to wear a sanitary pad after intercourse if leakage of the spermicide bothers you.
- Clean the applicators after each use. If you are using cream, jellies or foam, place the applicator in a glass of water immediately after using to help with the cleaning.
- It is safe to use this product while menstruating.
- Spermicides will have an expiry date on the container. Do not use the product after the expiry date.

there are occasions when dissolution remains incomplete long after that. It is important that insertion occur in time to allow the suppository to disperse (minimum 10 to 15 minutes before intercourse). If a suppository fails to dissolve, the effectiveness is reduced, and there may be irritation on intercourse. New and more efficient methods of applying vaginal spermicides are always being sought. One product recently released in the United States and yet to come on the Canadian market is a vaginal spermicide film that is inserted to cover the vaginal and cervical areas. More experience will be required before one can fairly compare this new method with ones already on the market.

Vaginal spermicides are free of systemic side effects and are generally safe to use. It is possible for these topical agents to cause local irritation or allergic reactions to either the male or female partner. A change to a different product is sometimes all that is needed to alleviate the problem. Vehicle components, perfumes, active ingredients and the spermicide concentration can all play a role in these local adverse reactions. If a local reaction occurs, the woman should stop using the product and wash off as much as possible. If intercourse has taken place within the last 6 hours, it is inadvisable to remove the spermicide from the vagina by bathing or douching unless the irritation is severe or bothersome. The risk of pregnancy must be weighed against the potential effects of the local reaction to the product.

Spermicide use at the time of conception or during pregnancy was once investigated as a cause of fetal defects. Subsequent studies have not supported this concern; however, it is usually recommended that spermicides not be used if pregnancy is suspected.

Correct application is important to ensure the highest effectiveness of vaginal spermicides. Product information should be reviewed for directions that are product specific as well as following some general recommendations.

Some people find vaginal spermicides unpleasant or inconvenient to use. The insertion of the product in proximity to intercourse is seen as an unwanted disruption, and there are those who object to the smell or the taste. Leakage or mild vulvovaginal irritation from the product may also cause rejection of this method.

There is one major noncontraceptive benefit of spermicides that has become important in the last few years. Several studies have shown that the woman has a reduced risk of acquiring cervical gonorrhea or chlamydia infections if spermicides are used. Protection against some forms of sexually transmitted disease may be very useful for certain women. Their use in those circumstances should be encouraged.

The effectiveness against human immunodeficiency virus (HIV) is not well established. In vitro evidence suggests that spermicides may be useful against HIV, but this has not been established in vivo. Spermicides alone should not be recommended to decrease the risk of HIV infection. Latex condoms should be used in combination, as they have shown a benefit against HIV transmission.

One of the reasons that spermicides may be less effective in preventing HIV transmission in vivo than in vitro is that their effect is usually high in the vagina by the cervix. HIV is thought to possibly enter the body through damaged vaginal mucosa. Spermicides may not cover the vagina completely enough to stop the transmission of HIV. Gonorrhea and chlamydia are stopped at the cervix, their typical point of entry.

Diaphragm

Diaphragms are latex domes with flexible steel rings around the edge (Figure 6). The rings are encased in rubber. It is positioned across the upper portion of the vagina over the cervix and acts as a physical barrier to sperm. Spermicidal jelly or cream is applied to one side of the dome and held against the cervical os by the device. The spermicide substantially increases the diaphragm's effectiveness and should always be used.

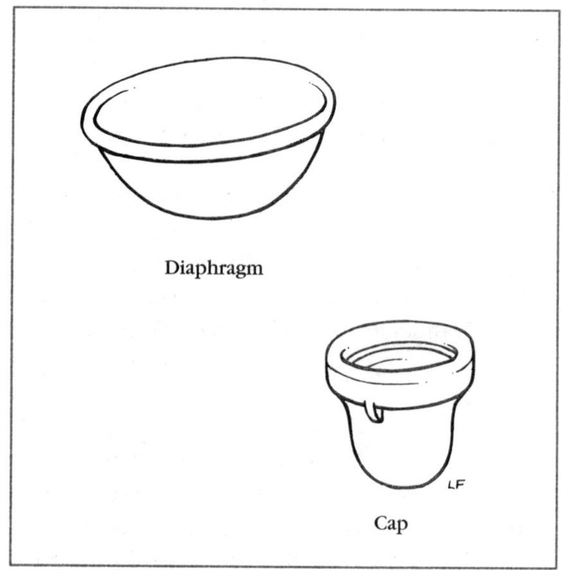

FIGURE 6: Diaphragm and Cervical Cap

The diaphragm can be purchased without a prescription, but it requires precise fitting. The sizes range from 50 to 105 mm. A trained clinician should determine the correct size prior to purchase. It is based on the depth of the vagina and also vaginal muscle tone. A poorly fitted diaphragm may cause wearer discomfort and increase the chance of the device becoming dislodged or disrupted by the penis during intercourse.

As well as the size, there must be assessment of the appropriate rim type. There are several types of springs or steel structures inside the rim of the diaphragm. The coil spring and flat spring are the commonly available models.

The coil steel spring allows for a flexible but firm diaphragm ring that folds easily for insertion. It exerts mild pressure on the vaginal wall and is comfortable for most women with average vaginal muscle tone and pubic arch notch. The arch notch is the indentation behind the pubic bone in which the front of the diaphragm sits. The flat spring may be more comfortable for women with very firm muscle tone or who have a narrow pubic arch notch. It is easily flexed for insertion. The coil spring is the more commonly prescribed type of diaphragm. If a flat spring is required, this is usually indicated on the prescription. If the type is not indicated, the coil spring can be considered suitable.

Many women are fitted for a diaphragm, given cursory instructions and then proceed home with the package insert. This is unsatisfactory as insertion usually requires practice and guidance before a woman feels comfortable using the device. Women's health centres and birth control clinics often offer detailed counselling and follow-up for diaphragm users. Correct procedures as well as becoming comfortable with one's own body are important features of the counselling that can be provided.

The diaphragm fits in the upper half of the vagina, held in place by the pressure of the device against the vaginal wall and by inserting the front rim into the pubic arch notch. It is inserted with the fingers or with an introducer. When in place the cervix must be completely covered by the diaphragm (Figure 7).

The introducer is a plastic handle with notches on it. The diaphragm is stretched between two notches (based on diaphragm size), and the handle with the diaphragm is gently inserted into the vagina. With a twisting motion the diaphragm is displaced from the introducer and fits into place in the vagina. Some women find the introducer easier than inserting the diaphragm by hand. Most women, however, comfortably perform hand insertion without problems.

Removal of the diaphragm is simple. With a finger or the end of the introducer hooked behind the front rim of the diaphragm, it can be untucked from the pubic arch notch and slowly pulled from the vagina.

A diaphragm size does not usually change in a short period of time unless there has been a precipitating event. Refitting should occur if there has been a weight change of >4 kg, birth of a child, pelvic surgery or if the diaphragm is causing discomfort. In some women urinary tract infections increase with the diaphragm. Pressure on the bladder or rectum may be due to a poorly fitted diaphragm. A change in size or rim type may be helpful.

Allergic reactions or irritation are possible due to the latex or the spermicide. If an unpleasant odor occurs while using the diaphragm, it may be due to poor hygiene or a vaginal infection. Regular cleaning of the diaphragm is important. It should not be worn for longer than 24 hours without removing and cleaning it.

Toxic shock syndrome has been associated with diaphragm use, but it is not considered a major contributor to the development of the condition. While it provides virtually no protection against HIV transmission, it does give some protection against other sexually transmitted diseases. Risk of a cervical neoplasia is also reduced with diaphragm use.

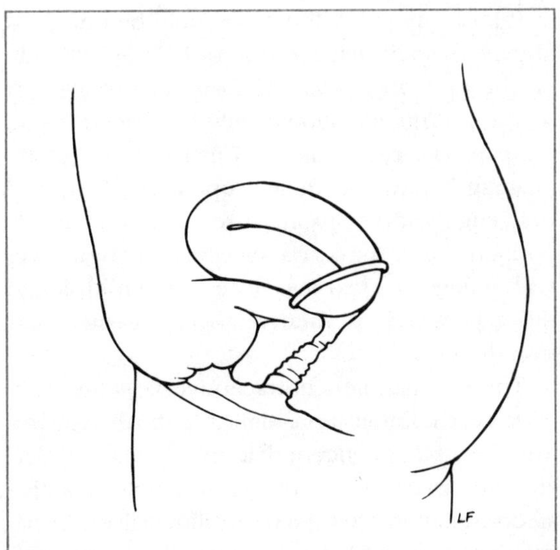

FIGURE 7: Diaphragm Placement

Diaphragms with spermicide offer a reliable method of contraception if they are used consistently and correctly. There are few side effects commonly associated with a properly fitted diaphragm so safety is generally not an issue. They can be used safely during menstruation and provide an aesthetic benefit of catching the menstrual discharge. Someone wishing to use a diaphragm must be comfortable with the idea of inserting the device internally and that it requires motivation to insert it when needed. To be effective it must be used.

Cervical Cap

The cervical cap offers protection similar to that of the diaphragm. It is a small, soft rubber dome held in place over the cervix by suction (Figure 6). Prior to attaching the cap, spermicidal cream or gel is placed in the cup. On insertion of the cap the spermicide is held against the cervix. It must be fitted by trained individuals, and there are relatively few of those in Canada. Though not readily available, women's health centres and birth control clinics may be helpful if a woman wishes to try the cap.

Caps come in several sizes and designs and must be fitted so that the cap fits neatly over the cervix. Suction must be formed between the cap and the base of the cervix. Not all women will be able to wear the cap, a reported 6 to 30% may have difficulty finding one that fits correctly. Structural differences around or of the cervix often make it difficult to get a good seal between the cap and the cervix.

Prior to insertion the cap should be one-third filled with spermicidal cream or jelly. Spermicide on the rim can hinder the formation of suction so the spermicide should only be placed inside the cap. The cap is inserted manually by gently pushing it into the vagina, open end first, and pinching the dome to increase suction once it is positioned over the cervix. A gentle downward pull with a finger tucked inside the rim will dislodge the cap, which is then removed, washed and stored.

The cap has noncontraceptive benefits, side effects and complications similar to the diaphragm. And there is the concern that cap use may accelerate the development of cervical abnormalities associated with the human papillomavirus. Cervical abrasions and lacerations have also occurred with cervical cap use. Regular Pap smears (prior to use, then yearly) are recommended to monitor any other serious cervical tissue changes.

Cervical caps offer an alternative to the common barrier methods. Although not widely available, some women may find the cap the best choice for them.

Female Condom

The newest barrier method is the female condom. Available in Europe for a couple of years, it was expected on the Canadian market in early 1994. There has been a delay in its release, and it is not yet available.

The condom is a disposable, soft, polyurethane sheath with flexible rings at each end. This loose-fitting tube is about 18 cm in length, closed at one end and open at the other. The closed end is inserted high up into the vagina, over the cervix and anchored in place using the upper ring. It fits in place like a diaphragm. The lower ring is at the open end and it is placed outside the vagina against the body. This ring keeps the condom from being pushed inside the vagina during intercourse. The outer side of the condom is lubricated with a spermicide. It comes in one size only.

It should be inserted prior to intercourse and like the male condom is removed after coitus and discarded. A new condom is used each time. The procedure for insertion and removal is similar to that of the diaphragm. Insertion and removal can happen any time in relation to coitus. After ejaculation the condom can remain in place as long as desired provided there is no risk of leakage of the semen.

Effectiveness is about equal to other barrier methods. The main perceived benefit is that the entire vaginal mucosa is covered during intercourse, which decreases the theoretical risk of the transmission of STDs including HIV. Some also find it less disruptive than the male condom as it does not require insertion close to the time of intercourse.

The main drawback to the use of the female condom is that some people find it aesthetically unacceptable. The lubrication makes it slippery while trying to insert it and once in, there is a portion of it visible as it hangs outside the body.

The female condom provides another means for women to protect their sexual health. It may be particularly useful for women with multiple partners or those who have a series of monogamous relationships.

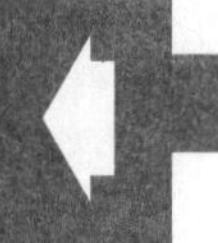

ADVICE FOR THE WOMAN

Diaphragm or Cervical Cap

It is important to be comfortable with the insertion of your diaphragm or cap before you use it. Ask your health care provider to discuss insertion in detail and provide an opportunity to practice using the device. Once you are comfortable with insertion, be sure to remember the following points:

- If using a diaphragm: Always use the diaphragm with vaginal jelly or cream. Place 5 to 15 mL of spermicide on the side of the diaphragm to be next to your cervix. Rub it over the surface to cover. It can also be placed around the rim, however, this may make the diaphragm slippery and difficult to insert. If so, avoid placing it on the rim.
- If using a cap: Fill the cap approximately one-third full with spermicidal cream or jelly. Do not apply it to the rim.
- The diaphragm or cap can be inserted just prior to intercourse or some time before; 30 to 60 minutes prior to intercourse is often recommended for the diaphragm but the cap has no such guidelines. In either case, it is better to put it in when convenient, regardless of the timing, rather than not use it at all.
- Leave your diaphragm or cap in for at least 6 to 8 hours after intercourse.
- Diaphragm users should insert an intravaginal application of spermicide prior to repeating intercourse during the 6 to 8 hour time frame. Do not remove your diaphragm for this application. The applicatorful of spermicide is deposited directly into the vagina not on the diaphragm itself. Cap users may also wish to follow this same precaution, but it is not required.
- The diaphragm or cap should not remain in place for longer than 24 hours without removal and washing. It can then be placed back in the vagina with fresh cream or jelly. Longer use can increase odor or risk of infection.
- In very rare instances toxic shock syndrome has been associated with diaphragm and cap use. All diaphragm and cap users should follow these safety precautions:
  - Wash your hands before inserting the diaphragm or cap.
  - Wear the diaphragm or cap for no longer than 24 hours at a stretch.
  - Do not use cap during menstruation.
  - Seek medical attention if you experience the following symptoms: high fever; diarrhea; vomiting; muscle aches; or sunburn-like rash.
- It is important to wash the diaphragm or cap with warm water and mild soap, dry it well and store it in its case when not in use. With care the diaphragm or cap can last for several years.
- Diaphragms and caps can get small tears and holes. Always check before using by holding it up to the light to help identify any damage. Small tears commonly appear where the rim and dome join.
- The fabric of the diaphragm or cap can be damaged by the use of petroleum jelly products (e.g., *Vaseline*), strong detergents and perfumes. If you require vaginal lubrication do not use petrolatum preparations such as *Vaseline*. A water-soluble gel is recommended.
- The diaphragm or cap should cause you no discomfort nor hinder your activities. If you notice any problems, see your clinician for refitting.

CONTRACEPTION AND SEXUALLY TRANSMITTED DISEASES

Sexually transmitted diseases (STDs) are common and sometimes difficult to cure. The consequences of STDs may be devastating: infertility and ectopic pregnancies if the infections progress to the upper genital tract, cervical neoplasia or, in the case of HIV infection, the ultimate consequence, death.

Reduction of the spread of STDs is a major focus for health care. Women are at more risk of acquiring STDs from one act of coitus with an infected male than a man is from an infected woman. Every sexually active person should have good information on ways to reduce the risks of infection. It is everyone's responsibility to keep sex safe.

Contraceptives can play a role in the transmission of STDs. Some can decrease risks while others may help in the transmission or increase the consequences of the infection. It is important for health care providers to be familiar with the effects of contraception on STDs and pass this information on.

Sexually Transmitted Disease and the Effects of Contraception

Health care providers can provide the following information:

- Abstinence is the most effective way to avoid STDs.
- An uninfected couple in a monogamous relationship is virtually safe from STDs.
- Risk increases as the number of different partners increases.
- Sexual intimacy should be avoided with a partner who has any symptoms that may be related to an STD.
- Discuss previous sexual history with a new partner before becoming sexually involved.
- Sexual activities that have a high risk of STD transmission are: vaginal intercourse without a condom; oral-anal, penile-rectal, oral-vulvar or oral-penile contact.

Effects of contraceptives on STDs:

- Spermicides:
  - reduce risk of cervical gonorrhea and *Chlamydia* infections;
  - uncertain effect on HIV in vivo, should use with a condom to increase protection against HIV;
  - very high concentrations can alter normal vaginal flora and increase risk of vaginal infection such as candidiasis.
- Diaphragms and cervical caps:
  - decrease the risk of cervical involvement with STDs, e.g., cervical gonorrhea, *Chlamydia* infection and trichomoniasis;
  - uncertain effect on HIV transmission because vaginal mucosa is not totally covered.
- Female condoms:
  - decrease the risk of cervical involvement with STDs, e.g., cervical gonorrhea, *Chlamydia* infection and trichomoniasis;
  - HIV protection is predicted as vaginal mucosa protected during intercourse.
- Male condoms:
  - decrease the risk of cervical involvement with STDs, e.g., cervical gonorrhea, *Chlamydia* infection and trichomoniasis;
  - best contraceptive protection against HIV, especially in combination with spermicides.
- Oral contraceptives:
  - increase the risk of chlamydia infections (e.g., 200%) as indicated by epidemiological and biological evidence;
  - have an uncertain role in HIV transmission with conflicting results—do not rely on this method to decrease the risk of transmission of HIV;
  - decrease the risk of severe pelvic inflammatory disease (PID) possibly due to change in cervical mucus and other physiological changes to uterus and cervix.
- Intrauterine devices:
  - increase the risk of PID;
  - no protection against HIV, may increase risk.

Contraception

PATIENT ASSESSMENT QUESTIONS

When helping with the selection of a contraceptive method, it is important to get a medical history to determine if there are contraindications to the use of any of the methods. As well, health care providers should consider assessing some of these issues:

Q *What effect would an unplanned pregnancy have on the woman (couple)?*

It is important to consider the failure rates of each method. If pregnancy is definitely not desired, then a method with a very low failure rate may be desirable.

Q *Which methods interest her? Are there any that she feels are absolutely not suitable? Why?*

Answers to these questions can help rule out certain methods as well as detect misunderstandings or concerns that the woman might have.

Q *Is she in a monogamous relationship or does she have more than one partner?*

This helps to assess the woman's risk for acquiring a sexually transmitted disease.

Spermicides and barrier methods may be the best choices for women who are at risk.

Q *How often does she require contraception (e.g., how often does she have sexual intercourse)? Is the timing fairly predictable?*

Contraceptives that provide constant protection (e.g., hormonal contraceptives) are sometimes preferred if there is frequent sexual activity and/or if intercourse is likely to happen at unpredictable times.

Q *Do her religious or moral beliefs have any impact on her use of contraception?*

Sometimes sexually active women who are contravening their religious or family teachings may be ambivalent about the use of contraceptives, and need some counselling to come to terms with this. There are also methods such as the IUD that are sometimes rejected on moral grounds by those who object to its proposed method of action (i.e., inhibiting implantation).

Q *Is she comfortable with using a method that requires her to insert something into her vagina? Is she physically able to do it?*

Spermicides and barrier methods may not be suitable if the answer to either of the above questions is no.

Q *Is cost a factor?*

It is important to select a contraceptive within the woman's financial means to ensure she can have it when needed. In certain locations there are birth control clinics that will supply contraceptives at a modest cost to those in need.

Q *Does she want to become pregnant at some time in the future?*

There is a recommended waiting period of several months prior to conception after discontinuing oral contraceptives. Intrauterine devices increase the risk of pelvic inflammatory disease. Infertility is a possible consequence of PID. Although the risk is low, it may be a consideration.

PHARMACEUTICAL AGENTS

Acetaminophen and ASA

Both of these internal analgesics are used for relief of pain and discomfort associated with dysmenorrhea or premenstrual syndrome. Doses, side effects, contraindications and precautions are the same as for the relief of any other pain. (See the Pain and Fever Products chapter.)

Benzocaine

Benzocaine is a local anesthetic of the ester type. It is found in topical creams and gels, some of which are marketed for the relief of vulvovaginal irritation and itching. A 5 to 10% preparation is considered helpful for temporary relief of symptoms. Benzocaine-containing preparations can be applied to the affected area up to 4 times daily.

Local sensitivity or allergic reactions are possible with topical anesthetics and increased irritation or redness should be watched for. There is the risk of cross sensitivity to other local anesthetics of the same type (e.g., procaine). Benzocaine can be absorbed through mucous membranes and should be applied in moderate amounts. It is not meant for application into the vagina.

The use of benzocaine preparations should not be recommended; if used it should be short term only. It should not be used in place of appropriate curative therapy, which is available for most causes of vulvovaginal irritation. It provides symptomatic relief only and risks delaying effective therapy by masking the symptoms.

Boric Acid

Boric acid, a mild disinfectant with weak bacteriostatic and fungistatic action, is applied intravaginally for the treatment or prophylaxis of vaginal candidiasis. Gelatin capsules can be prepared containing boric acid powder in a preweighed amount, and a variety of treatment regimens have been used. The intravaginal use of capsules containing 600 mg of boric acid powder once or twice daily for 2 weeks is common. It is sometimes used once daily, during menses only, as a prophylaxis against candidiasis that occurs in menstrual bleeding.

Boric acid has a number of systemic toxicities so it is only used topically. Most toxic events have occurred after the accidental ingestion of boric acid by children. Others have developed when high doses of boric acid preparations have been applied to abraded skin, often when straight boric acid powder was used. Symptoms include erythematous rash with desquamation, nausea and vomiting (blue-green color of vomitus and feces), circulatory collapse, coma, convulsions, shock and possibly death. It is unlikely that toxicity will occur with the intravaginal use described above.

It has been used safely in a large number of women for the treatment of vaginal candidiasis. It is a second line choice of treatment; there are superior treatments available. It has shown benefit in the treatment of women with chronic infection that have not responded to usual antimycotic therapy.

Caffeine

Caffeine is a xanthine derivative that has mild diuretic and stimulant action. It is incorporated into preparations for dysmenorrhea and PMS to help decrease fatigue and fluid retention. Stimulant effects of caffeine are usually noticeable at about 100 to 200 mg doses. The amount of caffeine in the products for dysmenorrhea and PMS are much less than that and unlikely to be sufficient to help with fatigue and lethargy. Diuresis would not be significant at these doses either.

The adverse effects of caffeine can be seen at doses in the therapeutic range (100 to 300 mg every 3 to 4 hours). These include headache, nausea, insomnia and irritability. In some cases they can be similar to symptoms that the user is experiencing already due to her condition (e.g., PMS). Caffeine is generally not a useful agent in the treatment of dysmenorrhea or PMS.

Imidazole Antifungal Agents

Clotrimazole, miconazole and tioconazole are antifungal agents of the imidazole class. Imidazoles are fungistatic and may have some fungicidal action at higher concentrations. Their action is aimed at a variety of dermatophytes, *Candida albicans* and some protozoa. They can damage the cell wall membrane of the organism, cause the buildup of intracellular toxins in the organisms, e.g., high concentration of hydrogen peroxide, and also inhibit the transformation of *Candida albicans* into the invasive mycelial form. Imidazoles are first-line therapy for the treatment of vulvovaginal candidiasis with success rates of >90%. Drugs in this class are considered equal in their effectiveness when compared with one another.

These agents are only effective topically, and various treatment regimens are effective. The shorter courses use higher concentrations per dose than the longer courses. None is superior, although the shorter courses increase the user's compliance and perhaps treatment outcome. The correct application technique is important for treatment to be as effective as possible.

Adverse effects are few. Sometimes there is mild vulvovaginal irritation or burning on application. Rarely there may be abdominal cramping or headache. If severe, the medication should be discontinued and medical attention sought. Clotrimazole and miconazole have been used intravaginally during pregnancy without apparent harm to the fetus. It is recommended that pregnant women use the product only under medical advice.

Evening Primrose Oil

The evening primrose provides a dietary source of gamma-linoleic acid (GLA), a precursor to the production of prostaglandins. It is believed by some that advantageous prostaglandins may be low in women with PMS, due to a deficiency of GLA.

Results are varied with respect to efficacy. Much of the support for its use is anecdotal. There is some evidence to support the trial of evening primrose oil in premenstrual women who experience mastalgia. Other symptoms that some believe will benefit from this medication are depression, vasoactive symptoms of menopause, and irritability. Although its efficacy is largely supported by anecdotal evidence alone, it does appear safe to use, with no significant side effects reported.

The dosage is variable, usually 2 to 4 of the 0.5 g capsules daily. Doses up to 12 capsules daily have been reported with no adverse effects.

Ibuprofen

Ibuprofen is a nonsteroidal anti-inflammatory drug (NSAID) useful in the treatment of various conditions including dysmenorrhea. Its action is similar to that of other NSAIDs—inhibition of cyclooxygenase activity resulting in decreased formation of prostaglandin precursors and thus of prostaglandins. It is believed to be the inhibition of prostaglandin synthesis that makes NSAIDs so effective in the treatment of dysmenorrhea.

A decrease in intrauterine prostaglandins allows a decrease in uterine muscle contractility, an increase in blood flow to the uterine muscle, thus a decrease in uterine ischemic pain. Headache and nausea may also be relieved as a result, possibly due to a decrease in extrauterine prostaglandin production.

NSAIDs are a first line therapy in dysmenorrhea and, as a nonprescription option, ibuprofen is one of the most commonly used for the condition. It and several other NSAIDs (e.g., naproxen, mefenamic acid) have been proven effective in >80% of women with discomfort or pain during menstruation. It is also helpful in some cases of secondary dysmenorrhea, e.g., with IUD use.

Doses vary but are usually recommended in the range of 200 to 400 mg every 4 to 6 hours. The maximum total daily dose should not exceed 1.2 g if used without medical supervision. It has an onset of action of about 30 minutes, a duration of action between 4 to 6 hours. Best results are achieved if the drug is initiated at the first sign of symptoms. There is no apparent benefit to beginning the drug a few days prior to the expected onset of symptoms.

While very effective, there are some side effects and precautions that make it unsuitable for some people. NSAIDs, ibuprofen included, are notable for their effects on the gastrointestinal tract. Gastrointestinal irritation, nausea and vomiting can occur. It may be reduced if the medication is taken with food. Rarely gastritis or, more seriously, gastric ulceration has occurred. Women with a history of gastrointestinal irritation or ulceration should use this medication with caution, short term only.

Skin rashes are possible in <10% of users. This is likely an allergic response to the drug. Anaphylaxis has also been reported and cross sensitivity possible with ASA and other NSAIDs. A review of the user's medical history would be helpful prior to recommending ibuprofen.

It is possible that a woman who does not respond to ibuprofen may respond to another NSAID.

Pamabrom

A theophylline derivative, pamabrom is included in nonprescription products for its mild diuretic effect. The maximum daily recommended dose is 200 mg. It is present in subtherapeutic doses in nonprescription products.

Pyridoxine

Vitamin B_6 or pyridoxine is classed as a nutritional supplement. It is used by some for the treatment of irritability and depression associated with PMS but there is poor scientific support for its use. It acts in the body to indirectly assist in various metabolic functions such as protein, fat and carbohydrate utilization. It is also involved in the conversion of tryptophan to serotonin, the synthesis of heme and the synthesis of gamma-aminobutyric acid (GABA) in the central nervous system.

Dietary sources include whole grain cereals, bananas, eggs and meats. It is not readily degraded during cooking. It is available in a vitamin B complex or as a single entity product. Oral supplements are readily absorbed from the gastrointestinal tract.

The daily adult requirement is small (2 mg) and usually readily available in the diet. Pyridoxine deficiency may be exhibited by the following: irritability, muscle twitching, dermatitis near the eye, oral lesions and glossitis, convulsions and peripheral neuropathy.

The usual supplemental dose for PMS symptoms and for the treatment of depression and other symptoms in women using the oral contraceptive begins at 50 mg daily. When daily doses of 200 mg or more have been used, for periods of >30 days, symptoms mimicking deficiency have occurred when the vitamin was discontinued. High doses (2 to 6 g daily) with prolonged use have also caused cases of pyridoxine toxicity as characterized by partially reversible sensory neuropathies—numbness of feet and hands. It is recommended that doses be kept at or below 100 mg daily unless treatment is for actual deficiency, and a physician is monitoring the response.

There are a number of possible drug interactions with pyridoxine. Among the drugs that can interact are levodopa, isoniazid, immunosuppressants and estrogens or oral contraceptives.

Pyrilamine Maleate

This antihistamine is included in nonprescription products for its side effect rather than its usual therapeutic effect. As with many antihistamines, drowsiness is common. The theory of pyrilamine's inclusion in products for PMS is that a sedative may help decrease the tension and irritability experienced by some women.

The usual adult dose is 100 mg. PMS products contain 12.5 to 25 mg of the drug—doses substantially below those recommended. Although unlikely to cause significant drowsiness, there is still the possibility of additive CNS depression with other drugs and alcohol. Women who require alertness in their daily activities or who are experiencing fatigue with PMS may not be good candidates for the use of this medication.

Thioglycollates

Thioglycollates are chemical depilatories found in hair removal creams. They are recommended for use in concentrations of 2 to 4%. They act by destroying disulfide bonds in the hair keratin, which allows increased osmotic pressure and swelling in the fibres, and hair turns into a soft mass.

The cream is usually applied to the area to be treated using a plastic glove or applicator stick. A liberal layer of cream is needed. The cream is left on for 5 to 15 minutes (product specific), then wiped off. Water can increase the chemical odor from the product so it is recommended that washing with soap and water occur after removal of the bulk of the cream. Treatment can be repeated when necessary, usually in several weeks time.

Skin irritation is the most common adverse effect. If irritation does occur, the affected area should be well washed with mild soap and water. If severe, mild topical corticosteroids may be necessary to reduce the reaction. Medical assessment and treatment may be necessary. Patch testing for sensitivity prior to application is recommended.

RECOMMENDED READING

General

Hatcher RA, Stewart F, Trussell J, et al. Contraceptive Technology 1990-92. 15th revised ed. New York: Irvington, 1992. (or more recent edition as published approximately every 2 years)

Vaginal Douches

Rosenberg MJ, Phillips RS, Holmes MD. Vaginal douching. Who and why? J Reprod Med 1991; 36:753-58.

Dysmenorrhea

Weitzman MD, Malinak LR. Dysmenorrhea: rational medical treatment. Drug Therapy 1988;Oct: 102-10.

Toxic Shock Syndrome

Todd JK. Therapy of toxic shock syndrome. Drugs 1990;39(6):856-61.

Premenstrual Syndrome

Chihal HJ. Premenstrual syndrome: an update for the clinician. Obstet Gynecol Clin North Am 1990; 17:457-77.

O'Brien PMS. Helping women with premenstrual syndrome. BMJ 1993;307:1471-75.

Vaginal Infections

Centers for Disease Control. 1993 Sexually Transmitted Diseases Treatment Guidelines. MMWR 1993;42: 1-25.

Hopkins M. Vaginal infections. Pharmacy Practice 1994;10:39-47.

Foreman A, Smith CB. Vaginitis, systemically solving a bothersome problem. Postgrad Med 1990; 88:123-33.

Contraception

Coccodrilli Coley K. Contraception: what pharmacists should tell their patients. Am Pharm 1993; NS33:55-64.

Hatcher RA, Stewart F, Trussell J, et al. Contraceptive Technology 1990-92. 15th revised ed. New York: Irvington, 1992.

REFERENCES

CHAPTER 1—Nonprescription Drugs in Health Care

Anderson M. The economics of Self-Medication. Queen's Health Policy. Kingston, Ont: Queen's University, 1995:53.

Cohen L. OTC ibuprofen: One year later. Pharm Pract 1990;6:115.

Decima Research. Attitudes, perceptions and behaviour relating to ethical medicine. Ottawa: Supply and Services, 1990:9.

Hanley R. Shoppers confused by OTC offerings. Pharm Post 1994;2:15.

Kogan MD, Pappas G, Yu SM, et al. Over-the-counter medication use among US preschool-age children. JAMA 1994;272:1025-30.

Leibowitz A. Substitution between prescribed and over-the-counter medications. Med Care 1989;27:85-94.

Segall A. Age differences in lay conceptions of health and self-response to illness. Can J Aging 1987;6:47-65.

Stoller E. Prescribed and over-the-counter medicine use by the ambulatory elderly. Med Care 1988;26:1149-57.

CHAPTER 2—Consumer Counselling

The Health Professional and Self-Care

Charupatanapong N. Perceived likelihood of risks in self-medication practices. J Soc Adm Pharm 1994;11(1):18-28.

Chiles VK. Self-medication in perspective. In: Chiles VK, ed. Canadian Self-medication. Ottawa: Canadian Pharmaceutical Association, 1980:x-xix.

Community pharmacists and self-medication. Toronto: ABM Research Ltd., June 1992.

Consumer usage and attitude survey. Toronto: Canadian Facts, October 1991.

Final report of the task force on responding to the self-medicating patient. Presented to the Canadian Pharmaceutical Association Council of Delegates, 1984.

Gore P, Madhaven S. Credibility of the sources of information for nonprescription medicines. J Soc Adm Pharm 1993;10(3):109-22.

Health for all: the role of self-medication. Proceedings of the sixth general assembly. Ottawa: World Federation of Proprietary Medicine Manufacturers, 1981.

Kleoppel JW, Henry DW. Teaching patients, families, and communities about their medications. In: Smith CE, ed. Patient Medication: Nurses in Partnership with Other Health Professionals. Orlando: Grune & Stratton, 1987:271-96.

Lilja J. Consumer behaviour. Int J Pharm Pract 1994;(June):192-93.

Skinner D. Consumer use of nonprescription drugs. Can Pharm J 1985; 118(5):206-13.

Taylor J, Greer M. NPM Consultations: an analysis of pharmacist availability, accessibility, and approachability. J Soc Adm Pharm 1993; 10(3):101-08.

To the year 2000: the changing roles of nonprescription medicines and the practice of pharmacy. Ottawa: Nonprescription Drug Manufacturers Association of Canada, August 1991.

Information-Gathering Communication Skills

Anon. Obtaining additional specific information; direct questioning, system review and physical examination. In: Enelow AJ, Swisher SN. Interviewing and Patient Care. New York: Oxford University Press, 1979:51-65.

Benson MA, Cribb A. In their own words: community pharmacists and their health education role. Int J Pharm Pract 1995;3:74-77.

Enelow AJ, McKinney Adler A. Adler A. Basic interviewing. In: Enelow AJ, Swisher SN. Interviewing and Patient Care. New York: Oxford University Press, 1979:19-50.

Interviewing and assessment. In: Tindall WN, Beardsley RS, Kimberlin CL. Communication in Pharmacy Practice: A Practical Guide for Students and Practitioners. Philadelphia: Lea & Febiger, 1994:110-21.

King M, Novik L, Citrenbaum C. Irresistible Communication: Creative Skills for the Health Professional. Philadelphia: Saunders, 1980.

Kitching JB. Communication and the community pharmacist. Pharm J 1986;237(6401):449-54.

McBean Cochran B. The art of questioning. Pharm Pract 1989;5(1):21-24.

Morrow N, Hargie O, Donnelly H, et al. "Why do you ask?" A study of questioning behaviour in community pharmacist-client consultations. Int J Pharm Pract 1993;2:90-94.

Pillow WF. Communicating with the patient. Concepts and skills for inter-personal communication. Indianapolis: Eli Lilly and Company, 1985:39-41.

Ray MD, ed. Basic Skills in Clinical Pharmacy Practice. Carrboro: American Society of Hospital Pharmacists, 1983.

Reiser DE, Klein Schroder A. The interview process. Patient interviewing—the human dimension. Baltimore: Waverly Press, 1980:111-36.

Russell CG, Wilcox EM, Hicks CI. Interpersonal Communication in Pharmacy: An Interactionist Approach. New York: Appleton-Century-Crofts, 1982.

The Schering report VII. What's right with pharmacy—the pharmacist's growing influence in the expanding otc market. Kenilworth: Schering Laboratories, 1985.

Systematic Approach to Self-Care Counselling

Ackerman SJ. Doing more harm than good with children's medications. FDA Consumer 1989;23(2):28-31.

Balon ADJ. Counselling. Pharm J 1986;236(6401):452-54.

Barber ND, Raynor DK. Understanding medicine labels: the effect of plain English. Pharm J 1989;242(6521)(Suppl):R13-17.

Basara LR, Juergens JP. Patient package insert readability and design. Am Pharm 1994;NS34(8):48-53.

Bates D, McIntosh D, Chambers CR. An evaluation of verbal and written methods in counselling cancer patients. Can J Hosp Pharm 1995;48(2): 98-99.

Becker MH, Rosenstock IM. Compliance with medical advice. In: Streptoe A, Mathews A, eds. Health Care and Human Behavior. London: Academic Press, 1984:75-203.

Bradley B, Singleton M, Li Wan Po A. Readability of patient information leaflets on over-the-counter (OTC) medicines. J Clin Pharm Ther 1994;19:7-15.

Cheung A. Visual acuity in reading nonprescription drug labels. Can Pharm J 1995;127(10):47-51.

Decima Research. Attitudes, perceptions and behaviour relating to ethical medicines. A research report to the Department of National Health and Welfare. Drugs Directorate, Health Protection Branch, Department of National Health and Welfare. Ottawa: Minister of Supply and Services Canada, 1990.

Doak C, Doak L, Root J. Teaching Patients with Low Literacy Skills. Philadelphia: JB Lippincott, 1985.

Edwards C, Stillman P. Minor Illness or Major Disease? Responding to Symptoms in the Pharmacy. 2nd ed. London: Pharmaceutical Press, 1995.

Galloway R, McGuire J. Determinants of compliance with iron supplementation: supplies, side effects, or psychology? Soc Sci Med 1994; 39(3):381-90.

Glynn RJ, Buring JE, Manson JE, et al. Adherence to aspirin in the prevention of myocardial infarction: the physicians' health study. Arch Intern Med 1994;154:2649-59.

Holt GA, Dorcheus L, Hall EL, et al. Patient interpretation of label instructions. Am Pharm 1992;NS32(3):58-62.

Holt GA, Hollon JD, Hughes SE, et al. OTC labels: can consumers read and understand them? Am Pharm 1990;NS30(11):51-54.

Holt GA. How adults learn. Am Pharm 1981;NS21(7):46-47, 70.

Inciardi JA. Over the counter drugs: epidemiology, adverse reactions, over-dose deaths and mass-media promotion. Addict Dis Int J 1977; 3(2):253-72.

Kishi DT, Watanabe AS. A systematic approach to drug therapy for the pharmacist. Am J Hosp Pharm 1974;31:494-97.

Komiya T, Kudo M, Urabe T, et al. Compliance with antiplatelet therapy in patients with ischemic cerebrovascular disease: assessment by platelet aggregation testing. Stroke 1994;25(12):2337-42.

Lamb GC, Green SS, Heron J. Can physicians warn patients of potential side effects ... without fear of causing those side effects? Arch Intern Med 1994;154(Dec):2753-56.

LaPierre G, Mallet L. Readability of materials. Can Pharm J 1987;120(12): 718-28.

Ley P. Communicating with Patients. Improving Communication, Satisfaction and Compliance. New York: Croom Helm, 1988.

Lively BT, Baldwin HJ, Carleton BR, et al. The relationship of knowledge to perceived benefits and risks of oral contraceptives. Drug Information J 1981;15:153-59.

Maiman LA, Becker MH, Katlic AW. How mothers treat their children's physical symptoms. J Community Health 1985;10(3):136-55.

Matte DA, McLean WM. Self medication, abuse or misuse? Drug Intell Clin Pharm 1978;12:603-11.

McBean BJ, Blackburn JL. An evaluation of four methods of pharmacist conducted patient education. Can Pharm J 1982;115(5):167-72.

McBean Cochran B. The elderly patient: "But I couldn't see the directions." Pharm Pract 1988;4(5):25-31.

McBean Cochran B. Discussing side effects. Pharm Pract 1988;4(7): 23-27.

McBean Cochran B. Effective patient information. Pharm Pract 1989;5(8):20-24.

McKenzie MW. How to conduct a patient medication history interview. In: Ray MD, ed. Basic Skills in Clinical Pharmacy Practice. Carrboro: American Society of Hospital Pharmacists, 1983:79-128.

Meyer LE, Reis JC, Reeder W, et al. Impact of perception on side effects. Drug Intell Clin Pharm 1985;19:213.

Morgan P. Illiteracy can have major impact on patients' understanding of health care information. Can Med Assoc J 1993;148(7):1196-203.

Myers ED, Clavert EJ. The effect of forewarning in the occurrence of side effects and discontinuance of medication in patients on dothiepin. J Int Med Res 1976;4:237-40.

Myers ED, Clavert EJ. The effect of forewarning in the occurrence of side effects and discontinuance of medication in patients on amitriptyline. Br J Psychiatry 1973;122:461-64.

Nichol MB, McCombs JS, Johnson KA, et al. The effects of consultation on over-the-counter medication purchasing decisions. Med Care 1992; 30(11):989-1003.

Ranelli PL. Rediscovering the act of interviewing by pharmacists. J Clin Pharm Ther 1990;15(5):377-80.

Rantucci M, Segal HJ. Hazardous non-prescription analgesic use by the elderly. J Soc Adm Pharm 1991;8(3):108-20.

Rantucci M, Segal HJ. Over-the-counter medication. J Soc Adm Pharm 1986;3(3):81-91.

Reading skills of adults in Canada. Statistics Canada. Labour and Household Surveys Division. Ottawa: Minister of Industry, Science and Technology, 1992.

Reiser DE, Klein Schroder A. Components of the medical history. In: Patient Interviewing—the Human Dimension. Baltimore: Waverly Press, 1980:163-82.

Rogers A. Teaching adults. Philadelphia: Open University Press, 1986.

Rudd CC. Teaching and counselling patients about drugs. In: Ray MD, ed. Basic Skills in Clinical Pharmacy Practice. Carrboro: American Society of Hospital Pharmacists, 1983:153-86.

Russell CG, Wilcox EM, Hicks CI. Interpersonal Communication in Pharmacy: An Interactionist Approach. New York: Appleton-Century-Crofts, 1982:107-19.

Rymes-Barley C. A secret inability to comply; the price of illiteracy. Can Pharm J 1989;122(2):86-94.

Schommer JC, Sullivan DL, Haugtvedt CL. Patients' role orientation for pharmacist consultation. J Soc Adm Pharm 1995;12(1):33-41.

Sumner ED. Handbook of Geriatric Drug Therapy for Health Care Professionals. Philadelphia: Lea & Febiger, 1983:11.

Tabor M. Minimizing the menace of otc drugs. Occup Health Saf 1982;51(5):14-19.

Woods D. Drug labelling—plainer English needed. Can Med Assoc J 1987;136(4):321.

Yung DK, Farrell ET. What consumers recalled. Can Pharm J 1995; 125(9):394-98.

Nonverbal Communication

Asbell B. What They Know About You. Toronto: Random House, 1991.

Barnard D, Barr JT, Schumacher GE. Person to Person—"Empathy." Bethesda: American Association of Colleges of Pharmacy, 1982:13.

Barnard D, Barr JT, Schumacher GE. Person to Person—"Nonverbal Communication." Bethesda: American Association of Colleges of Pharmacy, 1985.

Condon JC, Yousef FS. An Introduction to Intercultural Communications. Indianapolis: The Bobbs-Merrill Co Inc., 1975.

Cresswell S. Doctor/patient communications: a review of the literature. Ont Med Rev 1983;Nov:559-66.

DiMatteo MR, Taranta A, Friedman HA, et al. Predicting patient satisfaction from physicians' nonverbal communication skills. Med Care 1980; 18(4):376-87.

Hall ET. The Silent Language. New York: Doubleday, 1959:163-64. (Cited in Barnard D, Barr JT, Schumacher GE. Person to Person—"Nonverbal Communication." Bethesda: American Association of Colleges of Pharmacy, 1985:8.)

King M, Novik L, Citrenbaum C. Nonverbal communication. In: Irresistible Communication. Creative Skills for the Health Professional. Philadelphia: WB Saunders, 1983:63-74.

Knapp ML. Nonverbal Communication in Human Interaction. New York: Holt, Rinehart, Winston, 1978. (Cited in Russell CG, Wilcox EM, Hicks CI. Interpersonal Communication in Pharmacy: An Interactionist Approach. New York: Appleton-Century-Crofts, 1982:75-90.)

Larsen KM, Smith KC. Assessment of nonverbal communication in the patient/physician interview. J Fam Pract 1981;12(3):481-88.

McBean Cochran B. Non-verbal communication: watching what you 'say'. Pharm Pract 1988;4(9):23-26.

Mehrabian A. Silent Messages. Belmont: Wadsworth Publishing, 1971. (Cited in Barnard D, Barr JT, Schumacher GE. Person to Person—"Nonverbal Communication." Bethesda: American Association of Colleges of Pharmacy, 1985:3.)

Nonverbal communication in pharmacy. In: Tindall WN, Beardsley RS, Kimberlin CL. Communication in Pharmacy Practice; A Practical Guide for Students and Practitioners. Philadelphia: Lea & Febiger, 1994: 38-47.

Ranelli PK. The utility of nonverbal communication in the profession of pharmacy. Soc Sci Med 1979;13A:733-36.

Russell CG, Wilcox EM, Hicks CI. Nonverbal variables. In: Interpersonal Communication in Pharmacy: An Interactionist Approach. New York: Appleton-Century-Crofts, 1982:75-90.

Samovar LA. Understanding Intercultural Communication. Belmont: Wadsworth, 1981.

Spencer H. The hidden meaning of body language. Am Pharm 1981; NS21(7):48-49, 56.

Stewart M, Brown JB, Weston WW, et al. Patient Centered Medicine: Transforming the Clinical Method. Thousand Oaks, CA: Sage Publications, 1995.

Stewart, MA. Effective physician-patient communication and health outcomes: a review. Can Med Assoc J 1995;152(9):1423-33.

Special Counselling Situations

Anon. Courtesy to the hard of hearing (Pamphlet). Toronto: The Canadian Hearing Society, no date.

Anon. Emotional and behavioral responses to illness and to the interviewer. In: Enelow AJ, Swisher SN, eds. Interviewing and Patient Care. New York: Oxford University Press, 1978:102-24.

Anon. Focus on aging: communication disorders and aging. Toronto: Programme in Gerontology, 1981:2(2).

Anon. Tips on one-one communication with a deaf person (Pamphlet). Toronto: The Canadian Hearing Society.

Ascione FJ, Shimp LA. Effectiveness of four education strategies in the elderly. Drug Intell Clin Pharm 1984;18:926-31.

Barnard D, Barr JT, Schumacher GE. Person to Person—"Empathy." Bethesda: American Association of Colleges of Pharmacy, 1982.

Burns B, Phillipson C. Drugs, Aging and Society. Social and Pharmacologic Perspectives. London: Croom Helm, 1986:1-9.

Chermak G, Jinks M. Counselling the hearing-impaired older adult. Drug Intell Clin Pharm 1981;15:377-82.

Columbo JR, ed. The Canadian Global Almanac. Toronto: Macmillan Canada, 1994:56.

Darnell JC, Murray MD, Martz BL, et al. Medication use by ambulatory elderly—an in-home survey. J Am Geriatr Soc 1986;34(1):1-4.

Denton FT, Spencer BG. Canada's population and labour force, past, present and future. In: Marshall VW, ed. Aging in Canada. Don Mills: Fitzhenry and Whiteside, 1980:21.

Ellor JR, Kurz DJ. Misuse and abuse of prescription and nonprescription drugs by the elderly. Nurs Clin North Am 1982;17(2):319-30.

Jinks MJ, Fuerst RH. Geriatric therapy. In: Young LY, Koda-Kimble MA, eds. Applied Therapeutics, the Clinical Use of Drugs. Vancouver, WA: Applied Therapeutics, 1992:79/1-79/19.

Klein LE, German PS, Levine DM, et al. Medication problems among outpatients. A study with emphasis on the elderly. Arch Intern Med 1984;114:1185.

Lamy PP. Over the counter medication: the drug interactions we overlook. J Am Geriatr Soc 1982;30(suppl 11):69-75.

Liebgott AR, Reiser DE. Obtaining the medical history. In: Reiser DE, Klein Schroder A., eds. Patient Interviewing—The Human Dimension. Baltimore: Waverly Press, 1980:202-08.

Lojholm P. Self medication by the elderly. In: Kayne RC, ed. Drugs and the Elderly. Los Angeles: Ethel Percy Andrus Gerontology Center, University of Southern California, 1978:8-28.

Mant A, Whicker S, Kwok YS. Over-the-counter self-medication: the issues. Drugs Aging 1992;2(4):257-261.

McBean Cochran B. "I didn't quite catch what you said." Pharm Pract 1988;4(4):15-20.

McBean Cochran B. Discussing personal matters. Pharm Pract 1988; 4(8):29-32.

McBean Cochran B. Responding to patients' emotions: listening styles. Pharm Pract 1989;5(2):19-22, 42.

McBean Cochran B. Responding to patients' emotions: empathy. Pharm Pract 1989;5(3):21-24.

McBean Cochran B. Reaching the over-talkative patient. Pharm Pract 1988;4(3):15-18.

Oliver CH. Communication awareness: Rx for embarrassing situations. Am Pharm 1982;NS22(10):21-23.

Ostrom JR, Hammarlund ER, Christensen DB, et al. Medication usage in an elderly population. Med Care 1985;23:157.

Smith MC, Sharpe TR. A study of pharmacists' involvement in drug use by the elderly. Drug Intell Clin Pharm 1984;18(6):525-29.

Sumner ED. Handbook of Geriatric Drug Therapy for Health Care Professionals. Philadelphia: Lea & Febiger, 1983.

Vestal RE. Drug use in the elderly: a review of problems and special considerations. Drugs 1978;16:358.

Summary

Gore MR, Thomas J. Nonprescription informational services in pharmacies and alternative stores: implications for a third class of drugs. J Soc Adm Pharm 1995;12(2):86-99.

Popcorn F. The Popcorn Report. New York: Doubleday, 1991:64-68.

Rachlis M, Kushner C. Second Opinion—What's Wrong with Canada's Health Care System and How to Fix It. Toronto: Collins Publishers, 1989.

Srnka QM. Implementing a self-care-consulting practice. Am Pharm 1993;NS33(1):61-71.

CHAPTER 3—Special Patient Groups

Older Individuals

Anderson RJ, Miller SW. Geriatric drug therapy. In: Herfindale ET, Gourley DR, Lloyd-Hart L, eds. Clinical Pharmacy and Therapeutics. 5th ed. Baltimore: Williams & Wilkins, 1992:969-1010.

Beard K. Adverse reactions as a cause of hospital admissions in the aged. Drugs Aging 1992;2:356-67.

Bender AD. Effect of aging on intestinal absorption: implications for drug absorption in the elderly. J Am Geriatr Soc 1968;16:1331-39.

Bowles S, Knowles S. Drug disposition—in the elderly. On Cont Pract 1992;19:2-4.

Brownridge E. Nutrition needs of the elderly. Pharmacy Practice 1992;9:33-37.

Campion EW, deLabry LO, Glynn RJ. The effect of age on serum albumin in healthy males: report from the normative aging study. J Gerontol 1988;43:M18-20.

Campbell AJ. Drug treatment as a cause of falls in old age. A review of the offending agents. Drugs Aging 1991;1:289-302.

Canada Health Survey, The Health of Canadians, 1981.

Castleden CM, George CF. The effect of aging on the hepatic clearance of propranolol. Br J Clin Pharmacol 1979;7:49-54.

Crooks J, Stevenson IH. Drug response in the elderly—sensitivity and pharmacokinetic considerations. Age Aging 1981;10:73-80.

Dawling S, Crome P. Clinical pharmacokinetic considerations in the elderly. An update. Clin Pharmacokinet 1989;17:236-63.

Erwin WG. Geriatics. In: DiPiro JT, Talbert RL, Hayes PE, et al, eds. Pharmacotherapy; A Pathophysiologic Approach. 2nd ed. New York: Elsevier, 1992:64-69.

Everitt D, Avorn J. Drug prescribing for the elderly. Arch Intern Med 1986;146:2393-96.

Geokas MC, Haverback BJ. The aging gastrointestinal tract. Am J Surg 1969;117:881-92.

Hansten PD, Horn JR. Drug interactions. Philadelphia: Lea and Febiger, 1992.

Hollenberg NK, Adams DF, Solomon HS, et al. Senescence and the renal vasculature in normal man. Circ Res 1974;34:309-16.

Iber FL, Murphy PA, Connor ES. Age-related changes in the gastrointestinal system. Drugs Aging 1994;5:34-48.

James OFW. Gastrointestinal and liver function in old age. Clin Gastroenterol 1983;132:671-91.

Kelly JG, McGarry K, O'Malley K, et al. Bioavailability of labetalol increases with age. Br J Clin Pharmacol 1982;14:305.

Knowles S. Drug use in the elderly. On Cont Pract 1988;15:37-40.

Mayersohn M. Special pharmacokinetic considerations in the elderly. In: Evans WE, Schentag JJ, Jusko WJ, eds. Applied Pharmacokinetics. Principles of Therapeutic Drug Monitoring. 2nd ed. Spokane: Applied Therapeutics, 1986:229-93.

Miller RR. Drug surveillance utilizing epidemiologic methods: a report from the Boston Collaborative Drug Surveillance Program. Am J Hosp Pharm 1973;30:584-92.

Montgomery RD, Haeny MR, Ross IN, et al. The aging gut: a study of intestinal absorption in relation to nutrition in the elderly. Q J Med 1978;47:197-211.

O'Malley K, Crooks J, Duke E, et al. Effect of age and sex on human drug metabolism. BMJ 1971;3:607-09.

Procacci P, Bozza G, Buzzelli G. The cutaneous pricking pain threshold in old age. Gerontol Clin 1970;12:213.

Pucino F, Beck CL, Seifert RL, et al. Pharmacogeriatrics. Pharmacother 1985;5:314-26.

Ritschel WA. Pharmacokinetics in the aged. In: Pagliaro LA, Pagliaro AM, eds. Pharmacologic Aspects of Aging. St. Louis: Mosby, 1983:219-56.

Robertson D. Physiologic changes and clinical manifestations of aging. In: Pagliaro LA, Pagliaro AM, eds. Pharmacologic Aspects of Aging. St. Louis: Mosby, 1983:111-27.

Svennson CK, Woodruff MN, Lalka D. Influence of protein binding and use of unbound (free) drug concentration. In: Evans WE, Schentag JJ, Jusko WJ, eds. Applied Pharmacokinetics. Principles of Therapeutic Drug Monitoring. 2nd ed. Spokane: Applied Therapeutics, 1986: 187-219.

Tsujimoto G, Hashimoto K, Hoffman BB. Pharmacokinetic and pharmacodynamic principles of drug therapy in old age. Part 1. Int J Clin Pharmacol Ther Toxicol 1989;27:13-26.

Weale RA. The aging eye. New York: HK Lewis, 1963.

Weksler ME. Biologic basis and clinical significance of immune senescence. In: Rossman I, ed. Clinical Geriatrics. 4th ed. Philadelphia: Lippincott, 1986:57-67.

Williamson J, Chopin JM. Adverse reaction to prescribed drugs in the elderly. A multi-centre investigation. Age Aging 1980;9:73-80.

Compliance

Haynes RB. A critical review of the 'determinants' of patient compliance with therapeutic regimens. In: Sackett DL, Haynes RB, eds. Compliance with Therapeutic Regimens. Baltimore: Johns Hopkins University Press, 1976:26.

MacFarlane LL, Tonks RS. Seniors and their medicines. A pilot study in public housing. Can Pharm J 1992;125:167-72.

Rivers PH. Compliance aids—do they work? Drugs Aging 1992;2:103-11.

Stewart RB. Noncompliance in the elderly. Is there a cure? Drugs Aging 1991;1:163-67.

Infants and Children

General

Avery GB, Randolph JG, Weaver T. Gastric acidity in the first day of life. Pediatrics 1966;37:1005-07.

Benitz WA, Tatro DS. The Pediatric Drug Handbook. 2nd ed. Mosby Year Book, 1988.

Boreus LO. Principles of Pediatric Clinical Pharmacology. New York: Churchill Livingstone, 1982.

Evans WE, Schentag JJ, Jusko WJ, eds. Applied Pharmacokinetics: Principles of Therapeutic Drug Monitoring. 3rd ed. Vancouver, WA: Applied Therapeutics, 1992.

Friis-Hansen B. Body water compartments in children: Changes during growth and related changes in body composition. Pediatrics 1961; 28:325-30.

Goodman Gillman A. Goodman and Gillman's The Pharmacological Basis of Therapeutics. 8th ed. New York: Pergamon Press, 1990.

Institutional Care Section, Health Division, Statistics Canada per Ross Laboratories. Acute diarrhea in infants and children (undated).

Loggie JMH, Kleinman LI, Van Maanen EF. Renal function and diuretic therapy in infants and children. Part I. J Pediatr 1975;86:485-96.

Morselli PL, Franco-Morselli R, Bossi L. Clinical pharmacokinetics in newborns and infants: age-related differences and therapeutic implications. Clin Pharmacokinet 1980;5:485-527.

Nahata MC. Pediatrics. In: DiPiro JT, Talbert RL, Hayes PE, et al, eds. Pharmacotherapy; A Pathophysiologic Approach. 2nd ed. New York: Elsevier, 1992:56-63.

Rane A. Basic principles of drug disposition and action in infants and children. In: Yaffe JF, ed. Pediatric Pharmacology: Therapeutic Principles in Practice. New York: Grune and Stratton, 1980:7-28.

Stewart CF, Hampton EM. Effect of maturation on drug disposition in pediatric patients. Clin Pharm 1987;6:548-64.

Yaffe SJ, Juchau MR. Perinatal pharmacology. Ann Rev Pharmacol 1974;14:219-38.

Yoshioka H, Iseki K, Fujita K. Development and differences of intestinal flora in the neonatal period in breast-fed and bottle-fed infants. Pediatrics 1983;72:317-21.

Reye's Syndrome

Drwal-Klein LA, Phelps SJ. Antipyretic therapy in the febrile child. Clin Pharm 1992;11:1005-21.

Fitzgerald JF. Management of acute diarrhea. Pediatr Infect Dis J 1991;8:564-69.

Forsyth BW, Horwitz RI, Acampora D, et al. New epidemiologic evidence confirming that bias does not explain the aspirin/Reye's syndrome association. JAMA 1989;261:2517-24.

Halpin TJ, Holtzhauer FJ, Campbell RJ, et al. Reye's syndrome and medication use. JAMA 1982;248:687-91.

Hurwitz ES, Barrett MJ, Bregman D, et al. Public Health Service study on Reye's syndrome and medications: report of the pilot phase. N Engl J Med 1985;313:849-57.

Hurwitz ES, Barrett MJ, Bregman D, et al. Public Health Service study on Reye's syndrome and medications: report of the main study. JAMA 1987;257:1905-11.

Kluger MJ. Is fever beneficial? Yale J Biol Med 1986;59:89-95.

Kluger MJ. The adaptive value of fever. In: Mackowiak PA, ed. Fever: Basic Mechanisms and Management. New York: Raven, 1991:105-24.

Starko KM, Ray CG, Dominguez LB, et al. Reye's syndrome and salicylate use. Pediatrics 1980;66:859-64.

Waldman RJ, Hall WN, McGee H, et al. Aspirin as a risk factor in Reye's syndrome. JAMA 1982;247:3089-94.

General Administration Instructions

Extemporaneous oral liquid dosage preparations. Ottawa: Canadian

Society of Hospital Pharmacists, 1988.

Nahata MC, Hipple TF, ed. Pediatric Drug Formulations. Cincinnati: Harvey Whitney Books, 1990.

Rappaport PL. Extemporaneous dosage preparations for pediatrics. Can J Hosp Pharm 1983;36:66-70.

Pregnancy and Lactation

Briggs GG, Freeman RK, Yaffe SJ. Drugs in Pregnancy and Lactation: A Reference Guide to Fetal and Neonatal Risk. 4th ed. Baltimore: Williams & Wilkins, 1994.

Busser J, Rudolph S. Drug use in pregnancy. Pharmacy Practice 1994;10:28-36.

Cheung M. Counseling the pregnant patient. On Cont Pract 1988; 15:7-15.

Ito S, Blajchman A, Stephanson M, et al. Prospective follow-up of adverse reactions in breast-fed infants exposed to maternal medication. Am J Obstet Gynecol 1993;168:1393-99.

Piper JM, Baum C, Kennedy DL. Prescription drug use before and during pregnancy in a medicaid population. Am J Obstet Gynecol 1987;157:148-56.

Schardein JL. Chemically Induced Birth Defects. New York: Dekker, 1993.

Nausea and vomiting

Briggs GG, Freeman RK, Yaffe SJ. Drugs in Pregnancy and Lactation: A Reference Guide to Fetal and Neonatal Risk. 4th ed. Baltimore: Williams & Wilkins, 1994.

Cheung M. Counselling the pregnant patient. On Cont Pract 1988;15: 7-15.

Heinonen OP, Slone D, Shapiro S, et al. Birth defects and drugs in pregnancy. Littleton: Publishing Sciences Group, 1977.

Lee A, Schofield S. Drug use in pregnancy. General principles. Pharm J 1994;253:27-30.

MacMahon B. More on Bendectin (editorial). JAMA 1981;246:371-72.

McCombs J. Therapeutic considerations during pregnancy and lactation. In: DiPiro JT, Talbert RL, Hayes PE, et al, eds. Pharmacotherapy; A Pathophysiologic Approach. 2nd ed. New York: Elsevier, 1992: 1195-210.

Nelson MM, Forfar JO. Association between drugs administered during pregnancy and congenital abnormalities of the fetus. BMJ 1971; 1:523-27.

Pharmacy Service of the Clinical Institute. Can I take this if I'm pregnant. Toronto: Addiction Research Foundation, 1990.

Rayburn W, Wible-Kant J, Bledsoe P. Changing trends in drug use during pregnancy. J Reprod Med 1982;27:569-75.

Sahakian V, Rouse D, Sipes S, et al. Vitamin B6 is effective therapy for nausea and vomiting of pregnancy; a randomized, double-blind placebo-controlled study. Obstet Gynecol 1991;78:33-36.

Saxen I. Cleft palate and maternal diphenhydramine intake. Lancet 1974;1:407-08.

Wheatley D. Drugs and the embryo. BMJ 1964;1:630.

Allergic rhinitis

Cheung M. Counseling the pregnant patient. On Cont Pract 1988; 15:7-15.

Heartburn

Baron TD, Ramirez B, Richter JE. Gastrointestinal motility disorders during pregnancy. Ann Intern Med 1993;118:366-75.

Brown GR. Antacids, antiflatulents and antireflux agents. In: Carruthers-Czyzewski P, ed. Self-Medication Reference for Health Professionals. 4th ed. Ottawa: Canadian Pharmaceutical Association, 1988:245-56.

Cheung M. Counselling the pregnant patient. On Cont Pract 1988; 15:7-15.

Collins E. Maternal and fetal effects of acetaminophen and salicylates in pregnancy. Obstet Gynecol 1981;58:575-625.

Lee A, Schofield S. Drug use in pregnancy. General principles. Pharm J 1994;253:27-30.

Pharmacy Service of the Clinical Institute. Can I take this if I'm pregnant. Toronto: Addiction Research Foundation, 1990.

Rayburn W, Wible-Kant J, Bledsoe P. Changing trends in drug use during pregnancy. J Reprod Med 1982;27:569-75.

Van Thiel DH, Wald A. Evidence refuting a role for increasing abdominal pressure in the pathogenesis of heartburn associated with pregnancy. Am J Obstet Gynecol 1981;140:420-22.

Constipation

Baron TH, Ramirez B, Richter JE. Gastrointestinal motility disorders during pregnancy. Ann Intern Med 1993;118:366-75.

Berkowitz RL, Cousten DR, Mochizcki TK, eds. Handbook for Prescribing Medications During Pregnancy. Boston: Little, Brown, 1981.

Cheung M. Counselling the pregnant patient. On Cont Pract 1988; 15:7-15.

Lee A, Schofield S. Drug use in pregnancy. General principles. Pharm J 1994;253:27-30.

Lum L. Constipation and laxatives. In: Carruthers-Czyzewski P, ed. Self-Medication Reference for Health Professionals. 4th ed. Ottawa: Canadian Pharmaceutical Association, 1988:309-18.

McCombs J. Therapeutic considerations during pregnancy and lactation. In: DiPiro JT, Talbert RL, Hayes PE, et al, eds. Pharmacotherapy; A Pathophysiologic Approach. 2nd ed. New York: Elsevier, 1992: 1195-210.

Pharmacy Service of the Clinical Institute. Can I take this if I'm pregnant. Toronto: Addiction Research Foundation, 1990.

Hemorrhoids

Cheung M. Counselling the pregnant patient. On Cont Pract 1988; 15:7-15.

Lee A, Schofield S. Drug use in pregnancy. General principles. Pharm J 1994;253:27-30.

McCombs J. Therapeutic considerations during pregnancy and lactation. In: DiPiro JT, Talbert RL, Hayes PE, et al, eds. Pharmacotherapy; A Pathophysiologic Approach. 2nd ed. New York: Elsevier, 1992: 1195-1210.

Backache, headache

Cheung M. Counselling the pregnant patient. On Cont Pract 1988; 15:7-15

Lee A, Schofield S. Drug use in pregnancy. General principles. Pharm J 1994;253:27-30.

Pharmacy Service of the Clinical Institute. Can I take this if I'm pregnant. Toronto: Addiction Research Foundation, 1990.

Rayburn W, Wible-Kant J, Bledsoe P. Changing trends in drug use during pregnancy. J Reprod Med 1982;27:569-75.

Common cold

Lee A, Schofield S. Drug use in pregnancy. General principles. Pharm J 1994;253:27-30.

Pharmacy Service of the Clinical Institute. Can I take this if I'm pregnant. Toronto: Addiction Research Foundation, 1990.

Rayburn W, Wible-Kant J, Bledsoe P. Changing trends in drug use during pregnancy. J Reprod Med 1982;27:569-75.

Vitamin and mineral supplementation

Cheung M. Counselling the pregnant patient. On Cont Pract 1988; 15:7-15

Pharmacy Service of the Clinical Institute. Can I take this if I'm pregnant. Toronto: Addiction Research Foundation, 1990.

Lactation

American Academy of Pediatrics Committee on Drugs. The transfer of drugs and other chemicals into human milk. Pediatrics 1994; 93: 137-50.

Anderson PO. Drug use during breast-feeding. Clin Pharm 1991; 10:594-624.

Atkinson SA. Drugs in breast milk. In: Raddle IC, MacLeod SM, ed. Pediatric Pharmacology and Therapeutics. 2nd ed. St. Louis: Mosby, 1993:443-56.

Briggs GG, Freeman RK, Yaffe SJ, ed. Drugs in Pregnancy and Lactation: A Reference Guide to Fetal and Neonatal Risk. 4th ed. Baltimore: Williams & Wilkins, 1994.

Jason J. Breast-feeding in 1991. N Engl J Med 1991;325:1036-37.

Kacew S. Adverse effects of drugs and chemicals in breast milk on the nursing infant. J Clin Pharmacol 1993;33:213-21.

Komuvesh M. Infant nutrition. A guide for professionals. Toronto: Ministry of Health, Ontario, April 1984.

Pray WS. Medications and breast-feeding: A pharmacist's guide. US Pharm 1990;15:14-18.

Chronic Diseases

Hypertension

Brooks PM, Day RO. Nonsteroidal antiinflammatory drugs. Differences and similarities. N Engl J Med 1991;324:1717-25.

Cass E, Kadar D, Stein HA, et al. Hazards of phenylephrine topical medication in persons taking propranolol. Can Med Assoc J 1979; 120:1261-62.

Drew CD, Knight GT, Hughes DT, et al. Comparison of the effects of D-(-)-ephedrine and L-(+)-pseudoephedrine on the cardiovascular and respiratory systems in man. Br J Clin Pharmacol 1978;6:221-25.

Empey D, Young G, Letley E, et al. Dose-response study of the nasal decongestant and cardiovascular effects of peudoephedrine. Br J Clin Pharmacol 1980;9:351-58.

Girgis L, Brooks P. Nonsteroidal anti-inflammatory drugs. Differential use in older patients. Drugs Aging 1994;4:101-12.

Horowitz JD, Lang WJ, Howes LG, et al. Hypertensive responses induced by phenylpropanolamine in anorectic and decongestant preparations. Lancet 1980;1:60-61.

Houston MC. Non steroidal anti-inflammatory drugs and antihypertensives. Am J Med 1991;90:42S-47S.

Johnson AG, Nguyen TV, Day RO. Do nonsteroidal anti-inflammatory drugs affect blood pressure. A meta-analysis. Ann Intern Med 1994; 121:289-300.

Marchessault J, Bold J, Crocker J, et al. First report of the Expert Advisory Committee on nonprescription cough and cold remedies to the Health Protection Branch: Antihistamines, nasal decongestants, and anticholinergics. Ottawa: Health and Welfare Canada, 1988.

Marchessault J, Boyd J, Crocker J, et al. Third report of the Expert Advisory Committee on nonprescription cough and cold remedies to the Health Protection Branch: Phenylpropanolamine, lozenges and combination. Ottawa: Health and Welfare Canada, 1989.

Morgan JP, Funderburk FR. Phenylpropanolamine and blood pressure: a review of prospective studies. Am J Clin Nutr 1992;55:206S-10S.

Radack K, Deck C. Do nonsteroidal anti-inflammatory drugs interfere with blood pressure control in hypertensive patients. J Gen Intern Med 1987;2:108-12.

Saltzman MB, Dolan MM, Doyne N. Comparison of effects of two dosage regimens of phenylpropanolamine on blood pressure and plasma levels in normal subjects under steady-state conditions. Drug Intell Clin Pharm 1983;17:746-50.

Taylor JG. The common cold. In: Carruthers-Czyzewski P, ed. Self-Medication Reference for Health Professionals. 4th ed. Ottawa: Canadian Pharmaceutical Association, 1988:191-212.

Unger DL, Unger L, Temple DE. Effect of an antiasthmatic compound on blood pressure of hypertensive asthmatic patients. Ann Allergy 1967;25:260-61.

White WB, Riotte K. Drugs for cough and cold symptoms in hypertensive patients. Am Fam Pract 1985;31:183-87.

Cardiovascular Disease

Friedman PL, Brown EF Jr, Gunther S, et al. Coronary vasoconstrictor effect of indomethacin in patients with coronary artery disease. N Engl J Med 1981;305:1171-75.

Girgis L, Brooks P. Nonsteroidal anti-inflammatory drugs. Differential use in older patients. Drugs Aging 1994;4:101-12.

Hansten PD, Horn JR. Drug Interactions. Philadelphia: Lea and Febiger, 1993.

Knowles S. Astemizole and terfenadine-induced cardiovascular effects. Can J Hosp Pharm 1992;45:33-37.

Taylor JG. The common cold. In: Carruthers-Czyzewski P, ed. Self-Medication Reference for Health Professionals. 4th ed. Ottawa: Canadian Pharmaceutical Association, 1988:191-212.

White WB, Riotte K. Drugs for cough and cold symptoms in hypertensive patients. Am Fam Pract 1985;31:183-87.

Hyperthyroidism

Dong BJ. Thyroid and parathyroid disorders. In: Herfindal ET, et al, ed. Clinical Pharmacy and Therapeutics. 4th ed. Baltimore: Williams & Wilkins, 1988:137-75.

Taylor JG. The common cold. In: Carruthers-Czyzewski P, ed. Self-Medication Reference for Health Professionals. 4th ed. Ottawa: Canadian Pharmaceutical Association, 1988:191-212.

Glaucoma

Abel SR. Drug-induced potentiation of glaucoma. US Pharm 1981; (Dec):76-81.

Soll DB, Saxon AM. Drugs and glaucoma. Am Fam Pract 1986;34:181-85.

Lesar TS. Glaucoma. In: Pharmacotherapy; A Pathophysiologic Approach. 2nd ed. New York: Elsevier, 1992:1374-75.

Rumelt MB. Blindness from misuse of over-the-counter eye medications. Ann Ophthalmol 1988;20:25-30.

Benign Prostatic Hypertrophy and Bladder Neck Obstruction

Lepor H. Alpha adrenergic antagonists for the treatment of symptomatic BPH. Int J Clin Pharmacol Ther Toxicol 1989;27:151-55.

The Diabetic Patient

Caloric content

Krogh CME, ed. Compendium of Pharmaceuticals and Specialties. 30th ed. Ottawa: Canadian Pharmaceutical Association, 1995.

Naylor M. Caloric and carbohydrate contents of oral pharmaceutical products in Canada. Toronto: Canadian Society of Hospital Pharmacists and Connaught-Novo, 1986.

Medications that may affect blood glucose levels

Cornish WR. Diabetes care. In: Carruthers-Czyzewski P, ed. Self-Medication Reference for Health Professionals. 4th ed. Ottawa: Canadian Pharmaceutical Association, 1988:349-82.

Koda-Kimble MA. Diabetes mellitus. In: Applied Therapeutics; The Clinical Use of Drugs. 5th ed. Vancouver, WA: Applied Therapeutics, 1992:72-74.

Taylor JG. The common cold. In: Carruthers-Czyzewski P, ed. Self-Medication Reference for Health Professionals. 4th ed. Ottawa: Canadian Pharmaceutical Association, 1988:191-212.

Nonprescription medications that interfere that blood glucose testing

Rice GK, Galt KA. In vitro drug interference with home blood-glucose-measurement systems. Am J Hosp Pharm 1985;42:2202-07.

Diabetic Foot Care

Cornish WR. Diabetes care. In: Carruthers-Czyzewski P, ed. Self-Medication Reference for Health Professionals. 4th ed. Ottawa: Canadian Pharmaceutical Association, 1988:349-82.

CHAPTER 4—Acne

Pathophysiology and Pathogenesis

Habif TP. Acne, rosacea, and related disorders. In: Klein EA, Menczer BS, eds. Clinical Dermatology. Toronto: Mosby, 1990:756.

Holland KY, Cunliffe WJ, Roberts CD. The role of bacteria in acne vulgaris, a new approach. Clin Exp Dermatol 1978;3:252-57.

Leyden J, Shalita AR. Rational therapy for acne vulgaris: an update on topical treatment. J Am Acad Dermatol 1986;15:907-14.

Marples RR, Leyden JJ, Steward RN, et al. The skin microflora in acne vulgaris. J Invest Dermatol 1974;62:37-41.

Plewig G, Kligman AM. The dynamics of primary comedone formation. In: Plewig G, Kligman AM, eds. Acne: Morphogenesis and Treatment. New York: Springer-Verlag, 1975:58-107.

Pochi PE, Shalita AR, Strauss JS, et al. Report of the consensus conference on acne classification. J Am Acad Dermatol 1991;24(3):495-500.

Puhvel SM, Reisner RM. The production of hyaluronidase by Corynebacterium acnes. J Invest Dermatol 1972;58:66-70.

Puhvel SM, Sakamoto M. The chemoattractant properties of comedonal components. J Invest Dermatol 1978;71:324-29.

Puissegur-Lupo M. Acne vulgaris, treatments and their rationale. Postgrad Med 1985;78(7):76-88.

Rebello T, Hawk JLM. Skin surface glycerol levels in acne vulgaris. J Invest Dermatol 1978;70:352-54.

Shalita AR. Genesis of free fatty acids. J Invest Dermatol 1974;62:332-35.

Tucker SB, Rogers RS, Winkelman RK. Inflammation in acne vulgaris: leukocyte attraction and cytotoxicity by comedonal material. J Invest Dermatol 1985;74:21-25.

Webster GF, Fsai CC, Leyden JJ. Neutrophil lysosomal release in response to P. acnes. J Invest Dermatol 1979;72:209.

Webster GF, Leyden JJ. Characterization of serum independent polymorphonuclear leukocyte chemotactic factors produced by Propionibacterium acnes. Inflammation 1980;4:261-69.

Winston MH, Shalita AR. Acne vulgaris. Pediatr Clin North Am 1991; 38(4):889-903.

Predisposing Factors

Danby FW. Spironolactone. J Am Acad Dermatol 1992;26(1):137.

Feldman W, Hodgson C, Corber S, et al. Health concerns and health-related behaviours of adolescents. Can Med Assoc J 1986;134:489-93.

Forest MG, Cathiard A, Bertrand JA. Evidence of testicular activity in early infancy. J Clin Endocrinol Metab 1973;37:148.

Hitch JM. Acneform eruption induced by drugs and chemicals. JAMA 1969;200:879.

Kelly AP. Acne and related disorders. In: Sams WM, Lynch PJ, eds. Principles and Practice of Dermatology. New York: Churchill Livingstone, 1990:1014.

Koo JYM, Smith LL. Psychologic aspects of acne. Pediatr Dermatol 1991;8(3):185-88.

Krowchuk DP, Stanclin R, Keskinen R, et al. The psychosocial effects of acne on adolescents. Pediatr Dermatol 1991;8(4):332-38.

MacDonald Hull S, Cunliffe WJ. The use of a corticosteroid cream for immediate reduction in the clinical signs of acne vulgaris. Acta Derm Venereol 1989;69(5):452-53.

Mills OH, Kligman AM. Comedogenicity of sunscreens. Experimental observations in rabbits. Arch Dermatol 1982;118(6):417-19.

Plewig G, Kligman AM. Acne cosmetica. In: Plewig G, Kligman AM, eds. Acne: Morphogenesis and Treatment. New York: Springer-Verlag, 1975:226-29.

Rosenberg EW. Acne diet reconsidered. Arch Dermatol 1981;117(4): 193-95.

Shalita AR. Acne vulgaris: pathogenesis and treatment. Cosmet Toiletries 1983;98:57-60.

Taylor JS. Chloracne. A continuing problem. Cutis 1974;13:585.

Zatulove A, Konnerth NA. Comedogenicity testing of cosmetics. Cutis 1987;39(6):521.

Treatment

American Academy Guidelines: Guidelines of care for acne vulgaris. Am Acad Dermatol 1990;22(4):676-80.

Flandermeyer KL. Clear skin: a step by step program to stop pimples, blackheads, acne. Boston: Little, Brown, 1979:211.

Plewig G, Kligman AM. Treatment—general statement. In: Plewig G, Kligman AM, eds. Acne: Morphogenesis and Treatment. New York: Springer-Verlag, 1975:270-325.

Nonpharmacological Treatment

Epinette WW, Greist MC, Osols II. The role of cosmetics in postadolescent acne. Cutis 1982;29(5):500-514.

Walzer RA. Acne: some answers to a complexion problem. In: Walzer RA, ed. Skintelligence: How to be Smart About Your Skin. New York: ACC, 1981:53-69.

Pharmaceutical Agents

Plewig G, Kligman AM. Acne detergicans. In: Plewig G, Kligman AM, eds. Acne: Morphogenesis and Treatments. New York: Springer-Verlag, 1975:270-325.

Ponte CD. Maprotiline-induced acne (Corres). Am J Psychiatry 1982; 139(1):141.

Shalita AR. Treatment of mild and moderate acne vulgaris with salicylic acid in an alcohol-detergent vehicle. Cutis 1981;28(11):556-58.

Stoughton RB. Comparative in vitro bioassay of skin penetration and activity of chlorhexidine preparations and other topical agents against P. acnes; an assessment of their potential use in the treatment of acne vulgaris (HIB 8-286-10-2). ICI Americans Inc, Research Report on File, CLR-120, March 1979.

Stoughton RB, Leyden JJ. Efficacy of 4 percent chlorhexidine gluconate skin cleanser in the treatment of acne vulgaris. Cutis 1987; 39(6):551-53.

Exfoliants

Arndt KA. Acne. In: Arndt KA, ed. Manual of Dermatologic Therapeutics. Toronto: Little, Brown, 1989:3-13.

Arndt KA. Treatment principles and formulary. In: Arndt KA, ed. Manual of Dermatologic Therapeutics. Toronto: Little, Brown, 1989:263.

Belknap BS. Treatment of acne with 5% benzoyl peroxide gel or 0.05% retinoic acid cream. Cutis 1982;29(6):638-40, 644-45.

Brown S. Therapeutic potpourri. Dermatol Clin 1989;7(1):71-74.

Cunliffe WJ. The conventional treatment of acne. Semin Dermatol 1983;2(2):138-44.

Epstein W. Topical deodorized polysulfides. Broadscope acne therapy. Cutis 1981;28(10):468-72.

Fulghum CC, Catalano PM, Childers RC, et al. Abrasive cleansing in the management of acne vulgaris. Arch Dermatol 1982;118(9):658-59.

Kligman A. Topical tretinoin: indications, safety, and effectiveness. Cutis 1987;39(6):486-88.

Thomas JR, Doyle JA. The therapeutic use of topical vitamin A acid. J Am Acad Dermatol 1981;4:505-13.

Benzoyl Peroxide

Borgludn E, Kristensen B, Larsson-Stymne B, et al. Topical meclocycline sulfosalicylate, benzoyl peroxide, and a combination of the two in the treatment of acne vulgaris. Acta Derm Venereol 1991;71:175-78.

Burke B. Benzoyl peroxide versus topical erythromycin in the treatment of acne vulgaris. Br J Dermatol 1983;108:199-204.

Cotterill JA. Benzoyl peroxide. Acta Derm Venereol 1980;89(suppl): 57-63.

Cunliffe WJ, Burke B. Benzoyl peroxide: lack of sensitization. Acta Derm Venereol 1982;62(5):458-59.

Cunliffe WJ, Dodman B, Eady R. Benzoyl peroxide in acne. Practitioner 1978;220(3):479-82.

Cunliffe WJ, Holland KT. The effect of benzoyl peroxide on acne. Acta Derm Venereol 1981;61(3):267-69.

Ferand O, Jakobsen HB. Water-based versus alcohol-based benzoyl peroxide preparations in the treatment of acne vulgaris. Dermatologica 1986;172:263-67.

Fluckiger R, Furrer HJ, Rufli T. Efficacy and tolerance of a miconazole-benzoyl peroxide cream combination versus a benzoyl peroxide gel in the topical treatment of acne vulgaris. Dermatologica 1986; 172:108-12.

Hogan DJ, To T, Royce Wilson E, et al. A study of acne treatment as risk factors for skin cancer of the head and neck. Br J Dermatol 1991;125:343-48.

Lassus A. Local treatment of acne. A clinical study and evaluation of the effect of different concentrations of benzoyl peroxide gel. Curr Med Res Opin 1981;7(6):370-73.

Maddin S. Benzoyl peroxide. Can J Dermatol 1989;1(4):92.

Mills OH, Kligman AM, Pochi P, et al. Comparing 2.5%, 5%, and 10% benzoyl peroxide on inflammatory acne vulgaris. Int J Dermatol 1986;25(12):664-67.

Montes LF. Therapeutics for the clinic: topical treatment of acne rosacea with benzoyl peroxide acetone gel. Cutis 1983;32:185-90.

Nacht S, Yeung D, Beasley JN, et al. Benzoyl peroxide: percutaneous penetration and metabolic disposition. J Am Acad Dermatol 1981;4(1):31-37.

Prince RA, Harris JM, Maroc J. Comparative trial of benzoyl peroxide versus benzoyl peroxide with urea in inflammatory acne. Cutis 1982;8:323-26.

Report of the Expert Advisory Committee on Dermatology. The carcinogenic activity of benzoyl peroxide. Information Letter. Ottawa: Health and Welfare Canada, 1987;722:1-9.

Rietschel RL, Duncan SH. Benzoyl peroxide reactions in an acne study group. Contact Dermatitis 1982;8:323-26.

Shear NH, Maddin S. Benzoyl peroxide-miconazole cream vs. erythromycin lotion in patients with moderate to severe acne vulgaris. Can J Dermatol 1992;4(2):216-19.

Smith EB, Padilla RS, McCabe JM, et al. Benzoyl peroxide lotion (20 percent) in acne. Cutis 1980;25(1):90-92.

Swinyer LJ, Baker MD, Swinyer TA, et al. A comparative study of benzoyl peroxide and clindamycin phosphate for treating acne vulgaris. Br J Dermatol 1988;119:615-22.

Tkach JR. Allergic contact urticaria to benzoyl peroxide. Cutis 1982; 29(2):187-88.

Van Neste D, Tennstedt D, Decroix J. Imidazole and benzoyl peroxide: a comparative trial of two treatment schedules. Dermatologica 1986; 172:108-12.

Other Antibacterials

Degrect H, Van den Borsche G. Double blind evaluation of a miconazole benzoyl peroxide combination for the topical treatment of acne vulgaris. Dermatologica 1982;164:201-08.

Gamborg Nielsen P. Topical metronidazole gel: use in acne vulgaris. Int J Dermatol 1991;30(9):662-66.

Kurokawa I, Akamatsu H, Nishijima S, et al. Clinical and bacteriologic evaluation of OPC-7251 in patients with acne: a double-blind group comparison study versus cream base. J Am Acad Dermatol 1991; 25:674-81.

Antibiotics

Dalzeil K, Dykes PJ, Marks R. The effect of tetracycline and erythromycin in a model of acne-type inflammation. Br J Exp Pathol 1987;68:67-70.

Eady EA, Holland KT, Cunliffe WH. Should topical antibiotics be used for the treatment of acne vulgaris. Br J Dermatol 1982;107:235-46.

Hughes BR, Murphy CE, Barnett J, et al. Strategy of acne therapy with long-term antibiotics. Br J Dermatol 1989;121:623-28.

Leyden JJ, Shalita AR, Saatjian GD, et al. Erythromycin 2% gel in comparison with clindamycin phosphate 1% solution in acne vulgaris. J Am Acad Dermatol 1987;16:822-27.

Parker F. A comparison of clindamycin 1% solution versus clindamycin 1% gel in the treatment of acne vulgaris. Int J Dermatol 1987; 26(2):121-22.

Sheehan-Dare RA, Papworth-Smith A, Cunliffe WJ. A double-blind comparison of topical clindamycin and oral minocycline in the treatment of acne vulgaris. Acta Derm Venereol 1990;70:534-37.

Antisebum Agents

Cunliffe WJ, MacDonald Hull S. Spironolactone in dermatology. J Am Acad Dermatol 1992;26(1):137-38.

Anti-inflammatory Agents

MacDonald Hull S, Cunliffe WJ. The use of a corticosteroid cream for immediate reduction in the clinical signs of acne vulgaris. Acta Derm Venereol 1989;69(5):452-53.

Other Agents

Bladon PT, Burke BM, Cunliffe WJ, et al. Topical azaleic acid and the treatment of acne: a clinical and laboratory comparison with oral tetracycline. Br J Dermatol 1986;114:493-99.

Cunliffe WJ, Holland KT. Clinical and laboratory studies on treatment with 20% azaleic acid cream for acne. Acta Derm Venereol 1989; 143(suppl):31-34.

Dreno B, Amblard P, Agache P, et al. Low doses of zinc gluconate for inflammatory acne. Acta Derm Venereol 1989;69(6):541-43.

Elbaum DJ. Comparison of the stability of topical isotretinoin and topical tretinoin and their efficacy in acne. J Am Acad Dermatol 1988;19:486-91.

Habbema L, Koopman B, Menke HE, et al. A 4% erythromycin and zinc combination versus 2% erythromycin in acne vulgaris: a randomized, double-blind comparative study. Br J Dermatol 1989;121:497-502.

Layton AM, Cunliffe WJ. Guideline for optimal use of isotretinoin in acne. J Am Acad Dermatol 1991;27:S2-7.

Schachner L, Eaglstein W, Kittles C, et al. Topical erythromycin and zinc therapy for acne. J Am Acad Dermatol 1990;22:253-60.

Shalita AR, Chalker DK, Parish LC, et al. The effects of topical nicotinamide on acne vulgaris. J Invest Dermatol 1992;98(4):318.

Verschoore M, Langer A, Wolska H, et al. Efficacy and safety of CD 271

CHAPTER 5—Allergy and Cold Products

Allergic Rhinitis

Epidemiology

Austen KF. Diseases of immediate type hypersensitivity. In: Wilson J, Braunwald E, Isselbacker K, et al, eds. Harrison's Principles of Internal Medicine. New York: McGraw-Hill, 1991:1426–28.

Norman PS. Allergic rhinitis. J Allergy Clin Immunol 1985;75:531–45.

Price JF. Allergy in infancy and childhood. In: Lessof MH, ed. Allergy: Immunology and Clinical Aspects. Chichester: John Wiley and Sons, 1984:127–73.

Viner AS, Jackman N. Retrospective survey of 1271 patients diagnosed as perennial rhinitis. Clin Allergy 1976;6:251–59.

Welch M, Kemp J. Allergy in children. Primary Care 1987;14:575–89.

Anatomy and Physiology

Naclerio R, Proctor D. The anatomy and physiology of the upper airway. In: Middleton E Jr, Reed C, Ellis E, et al, eds. Allergy: Principles and Practice. St. Louis: Mosby, 1988:579–91.

Pathophysiology

Berman B. Allergic rhinitis: mechanisms and management. J Allergy Clin Immunol 1988;81:980–84.

Bousquet J, Chanez P, Michel F. Pathophysiology and treatment of seasonal allergic rhinitis. Resp Med 1990;84(supplA)11–17.

Garrison J, Rall T. Autacoids: drug therapy of inflammation. In: Goodman L, Gilman A, Rall T,et al, eds. The Pharmacological Basis of Therapeutics. New York: Macmillan, 1990:574–99.

Langer H. Allergic rhinitis: a medical insight. J Otolaryngol 1989;18: 158–64.

Marone G, Casolaro V, Cirillo R, et al. Pathophysiology of human basophils and mast cells in allergic disorders. Clin Immunol Immunopathol 1989; 50:S24–S40.

Marquardt DL, Wasserman SI. Mast cells in allergic diseases and mastocytosis. West J Med 1982;137:195–212.

Naclerio R. The pathophysiology of allergic rhinitis: impact of therapeutic intervention. J Allergy Clin Immunol 1988;82:927–34.

Naclerio R. The role of histamine in allergic rhinitis. J Allergy Clin Immunol 1990;86:628–32.

Smith T. Allergy and pseudoallergy: an overview of basic mechanisms. Primary Care 1987;14:421–34.

Widdicombe J. Nasal pathophysiology. Resp Med 1990;84(suppl A):3–10.

Zweiman B. Pathogenesis of IgE-mediated allergic respiratory diseases. J Resp Diseases 1989;Nov(suppl):S4–S9.

Allergens

Bernstein D, Bernstein I. Allergic rhinitis caused by inhalant factors. In: Rakel E, ed. Conn's Current Therapy. Philadelphia: Saunders, 1986: 598–603.

Green AR. An updated assessment of the critical environmental factors involved in the prevention of allergic disease. Ann Allergy 1979;42: 372–83.

Kuo PH, Roth A. Canada. In: Roth A, ed. Allergy in the World. A Guide for Physicians and Travellers. Honolulu: University Press of Hawaii, 1978:25–28.

Pollart S, Chapman M, Platts-Mills T. House dust sensitivity and environmental control. Primary Care 1987;14:591–603.

Schumacher M. Allergic rhinitis due to aeroallergens. In: Rakel R, ed. Conn's Current Therapy. Philadelphia: Saunders, 1991:708–12.

Weber R. Allergens. Primary Care 1987;14:435–45.

Symptoms

Conner BL, Georgitis JW. Practical diagnosis and treatment of allergic and nonallergic rhinitis. Primary Care 1987;14:457–73.

Frazer J. Allergic rhinitis and nasal polyps. Ear Nose Throat J 1984;63: 172–76.

Middleton E. Chronic rhinitis in adults. J Allergy Clin Immunol 1988;81: 971–75.

Price JF. Allergy in infancy and childhood. In: Lessof M, ed. Allergy: Immunology and Clinical Aspects. Chichester: John Wiley and Sons, 1984:127–73.

Vogt H. Rhinitis. Primary Care 1990;17:309–22.

Wodell RA, Burg FD. Pediatric problem-solving: allergic rhinitis. Drug Ther 1984;14:136–55.

Differential Diagnosis of Allergic Rhinitis

Kaslow J, Novey H. When hay fever doesn't quit. Postgrad Med 1989; 85(6):164–72.

Meltzer E, Schatz M, Zeiger R. Allergic and nonallergic rhinitis. In: Middleton E Jr, Reed C, Ellis E, et al, eds. Allergy: Principles and Practice. St. Louis: Mosby, 1988:1253–89.

Simons F. Allergic rhinitis: recent advances. Pediatr Clin North Am 1988; 35:1053–74.

General Treatment

Busse W. New directions and dimensions in the treatment of allergic rhinitis. J Allergy Clin Immunol 1988;82:890–900.

Jones H. Allergic rhinitis: a study on the prescribing preferences in general practice. Br J Clin Pract 1989;43:30–32.

Ophir D, Elad Y, Dolev Z, et al. Effects of inhaled humidified warm air on nasal patency and nasal symptoms in allergic rhinitis. Ann Allergy 1988;60:239–42.

Pollart S, Chapman M, Platts-Mills T. House dust sensitivity and environmental control. Primary Care 1987;14:591–603.

Reisman R, Mauriello P, Davis G, et al. A double-blind study of the effectiveness of a high-efficiency particulate air (HEPA) filter in the treatment of patients with perennial allergic rhinitis and asthma. J Allergy Clin Immunol 1990;85:1050–57.

The Common Cold

Epidemiology

Cohen S, Tyrrell D, Smith A. Psychological stress and susceptibility to the common cold. N Engl J Med 1991;325:606–12.

Hendley J, Gwaltney J. Mechanisms of transmission of rhinovirus infections. Epidemiol Rev 1988;10:242–58.

Stickler G, Smith T, Broughton D. The common cold. Eur J Pediatr 1985;144:4–8.

The Respiratory Tract

Irwin R, Rosen M, Braman S. Cough: a comprehensive review. Arch Intern Med 1977;137:1186–91.

Kucera L, Myrvik Q. Fundamentals of Medical Virology. Philadelphia: Lea & Febiger, 1985:208–34.

Proud D, Naclerio R, Gwaltney J,et al. Kinins are generated in nasal secretions during rhinovirus colds. J Infect Dis 1990;161:120–23.

Richardson P, Phipps R. The anatomy, physiology, pharmacology and pathology of tracheobronchial mucous secretion and the use of expectorant drugs in human disease. Pharmacol Ther 1978;3:441–79.

Pathophysiology

Dolin R. Common viral respiratory infections. In: Wilson J, Braunwald E, Isselbacher K, et al, eds. Harrison's Principles of Internal Medicine. New York: McGraw-Hill, 1991:700–20.

Grave J, Davis G, Meyer A, et al. The major human rhinovirus receptor is ICAM-1. Cell 1989;56:839–47.

Kapikian A. The common cold. In: Wyngaarden J, Smith L Jr, eds. Cecil

Textbook of Medicine. Philadelphia: Saunders, 1988;1753-57.

Levandowski R. Rhinoviruses. In: Belshe R, ed. Textbook of Human Virology. Littleton: Publishing Services Group, 1984:391-405.

Proud D, Reynolds C, Lacapra S, et al. Nasal provocation with bradykinin induces symptoms of rhinitis and a sore throat. Am Rev Respir Dis 1988;137:613-16.

Rabinowitz H. Upper respiratory tract infections. Primary Care 1990; 17:793-809.

Signs and Symptoms

Fed Reg 1983;48(203):48576-95.

Gwaltney J Jr. Rhinoviruses. In: Evans A, ed. Viral Infections of Humans: Epidemiology and Control. New York: Plenum Medical Book, 1982: 491-517.

Phillpotts R, Tyrrell D. Rhinovirus colds. Br Med Bull 1985;41:386-90.

Pharyngitis

Embree J. Pharyngitis. Med North Am 1990;9:1050-53.

Huovinen P, Lahtonen R, Ziegler T, et al. Pharyngitis in adults: the presence and coexistence of viruses and bacterial organisms. Ann Intern Med 1989;110:612-16.

Lang S, Singh K. The sore throat: when to investigate and when to prescribe. Drugs 1990;40:854-62.

Lundberg C, Nord CE. Streptococcal throat infections: still a complex clinical problem. Scand J Infect Dis 1988;57(Suppl):7-11.

Influenza

Anon. National Advisory Committee on Immunization: statement on influenza vaccination for the 1991-1992 season. Canada Disease Weekly Report 1991;17-24(15 June):121-26.

Dolin R. Influenza. In: Wilson J, Braunwald E, Isselbacher K, et al, eds. Harrison's Principles of Internal Medicine. New York: McGraw-Hill, 1991:695-700.

Douglas R Jr. Influenza. In: Wyngaarden J, Smith L Jr, eds. Cecil Textbook of Medicine. Philadelphia: Saunders, 1988:1762-67.

Perlman P, Ginn D. Respiratory infections in ambulatory adults. Postgrad Med 1990;87(1):175-84.

Van Exan R. In case you're asked—influenza in perspective. Pharm Pract 1990;6(7):9-14.

Sinusitis

Panje W. Sinusitis. In: Rakel R, ed. Conn's Current Therapy. Philadelphia: Saunders, 1991:178-80.

Shapiro G. Sinusitis in children. J Allergy Clin Immunol 1988;81:1025-27.

General Treatment

Anon. Disinfectants. In: Reynolds J, ed. Martindale: The Extra Pharmacopoeia. London: Pharmaceutical Press, 1989:949-72.

Bryant BG, Lombardi TP. Selecting OTC products for coughs and colds. Am Pharm 1993;33:19-24.

Eby G, Davis D, Halcomb W. Reduction in duration of common colds by zinc gluconate lozenges in a double-blind study. Antimicrob Agents Chemother 1984;25:20-24.

Farr B, Conner E, Betts R, et al. Two randomized controlled trials of zinc gluconate lozenge therapy of experimentally induced rhinovirus colds. Antimicrob Agents Chemother 1987;31:1183-87.

Fed Reg 1982;47(101):22776-81.

Hilding DA. Literature review: the common cold. Ear Nose Throat J 1994;73:639-47.

Kyriakos T. What's hot in self-medication. Drug Merch 1989;70(1):34-37.

Macknin M, Mathew S, Medendorp S. Effect of inhaling heated vapor on symptoms of the common cold. JAMA 1990;264:989-91.

McBean Cochran B. "What should I take for my cold?" Pharm Pract 1990;6(9):33-38.

Saketkhoo K, Januszkiewicz A, Sackner M. Effects of drinking hot water, cold water, and chicken soup on nasal mucous velocity and nasal airflow resistance. Chest 1978;74:408-10.

Saroea GH. Common colds: causes, potential cures and treatment. Can Fam Physician 1993;39:2215-20.

Turner H, Garner W, Lanese R. A comparative study of a phenol-based mouthwash as a gargle or a spray with a saline gargle. Am Coll Health Assoc J 1980;29:129-32.

Tyrrell D. Some recent work at the Common Cold Unit, Salisbury. Infection 1988;16:261-62.

Tyrrell D. Hot news on the common cold. Annu Rev Microbiol 1988; 42:35-47.

Tyrrell D, Barrow I, Arthur J. Local hyperthermia benefits natural and experimental common colds. BMJ 1989;298:1280-83.

Antihistamines

Anon. Antihistamine drugs. In: McEvoy GK, ed. American Hospital Formulary Service Drug Information. Bethesda: American Society of Hospital Pharmacists, 1991:2-30.

Anon. Antihistamines. In: Reynolds JE, ed. Martindale: The Extra Pharmacopoeia. London: Pharmaceutical Press, 1989:443-65.

Anon. Antihistamines. In: USP DI: Drug Information for the Health Care Provider. Rockville: United States Pharmacopeial Convention, 1991: 382-449.

Anon. Teenagers take OTC drug to induce euphoria. Can Pharm J 1987; 120(1):14.

Berman B. Perennial allergic rhinitis: clinical efficacy of a new antihistamine. J Allergy Clin Immunol 1990;86:1004-08.

Bruttmann G, Charpin D, Germouty J, et al. Evaluation of the efficacy and safety of loratadine in perennial allergic rhinitis. J Allergy Clin Immunol 1989;83:411-16.

Brandon ML. Newer non-sedating antihistamines: will they replace older agents? Drugs 1985;30:377-81.

Burns JF, Conney AH, Koster R. Stimulatory effect of chronic drug administration on drug-metabolizing enzymes in liver microsomes. Ann NY Acad Sci 1963;104:881-93.

Bye CE, Cooper J, Empey DW, et al. Effects of pseudoephedrine and triprolidine, alone and in combination, on symptoms of the common cold. BMJ 1980;281:189-90.

Callier J, Engelen RF, Ianniello I, et al. Astemizole (R 45 512) in the treatment of hay fever: an international double-blind study comparing a weekly treatment (10 mg and 25 mg) with a placebo. Curr Ther Res 1981;29:24-35.

Campoli-Richards D, Buckley M, Fitton A. Cetirizine: a review of its pharmacological properties and clinical potential in allergic rhinitis, pollen-induced asthma, and chronic urticaria. Drugs 1990;40:762-81.

Carruthers SG, Shoeman DW, Hignite CE, et al. Correlation between plasma diphenhydramine level and sedative and antihistamine effects. Clin Pharmacol Ther 1978;23:375-82.

Chan K, Chan G. A study of prescribed H1-antihistamine preparations over a period of 12 months in community pharmacy. J Clin Pharm Ther 1987;12:1-9.

Chiou WL, Athanikar NK, Huang S-M. Long half-life of chlorpheniramine (Letter). N Engl J Med 1979;300:501.

Chu T, Yamate M, Biedermann A, et al. Once versus twice daily dosing of terfenadine in the treatment of seasonal allergic rhinitis: US and European studies. Ann Allergy 1989;63:612-15.

Church M, Gradidge C. Inhibition of histamine release from human lung in vitro by antihistamine and related drugs. Br J Pharmacol 1980;69: 663-67.

Clissold S, Sorkin E, Goa K. Loratadine: a preliminary review of its pharmacodynamic properties and therapeutic efficacy. Drugs 1989;37: 42-57.

Collins-Williams C. Antihistamines in asthma. J Asthma 1987;24:55-58.

Corey JP. Advances in the pharmacotherapy of allergic rhinitis: second-generation H1-receptor antagonists. Otolaryngol Head Neck Surg 1993;109:584-92.

Craft T. Torsades de pointes after astemizole overdose. BMJ 1986; 292:660.

Creticos P. Antihistamines in the treatment of allergic rhinitis. J Resp Diseases 1989;Nov(suppl):S10–S12.

Crutcher JE, Kantner TR. The effectiveness of antihistamines in the common cold. J Clin Pharmacol 1981;21:9–15.

Davies AJ, Harindra V, McEwan A, et al. Cardiotoxic effect with convulsions in terfenadine overdose. BMJ 1989;298:325.

Del Carpio J, Kabbash L, Turenne Y, et al. Efficacy and safety of loratadine (10 mg once daily), terfenadine (60 mg twice daily), and placebo in the treatment of seasonal allergic rhinitis. J Allergy Clin Immunol 1989;84: 741–46.

Delafuente J, Davis T, Davis J. Pharmacotherapy of allergic rhinitis. Clin Pharm 1989;8:474–85.

Drouin MA. H1 antihistamines: perspective on the use of the conventional and new agents. Ann Allergy 1985;55:747–52.

Evans L. Psychological effects caused by drugs in overdose. Drugs 1980;19:220–42.

Falliers C, Brandon M, Buchman E, et al. Double-blind comparison of cetirizine and placebo in the treatment of seasonal rhinitis. Ann Allergy 1991;66:257–62.

Fed Reg 1985;50(10):2200–18.

Fed Reg 1976;41(176):38312–423.

Fed Reg 1987;52(163):31892–914.

Feldman MD, Behar M. A case of massive diphenhydramine abuse and withdrawal from use of the drug (Letter). JAMA 1986;255:3119–20.

Filderman R. Inhibition of skin reactivity by antihistamines. Cutis 1988; 42:19–21.

Flowers FP, Araujo O, Nieves C. Antihistamines. Int J Dermatol 1986;25: 224–31.

Hansten P, Horn J, eds. Drug Interactions and Updates. Malvern: Lea & Febiger, 1990.

Hays DP, Johnson BF, Perry R. Prolonged hallucinations following a modest overdose of tripelennamine. Clin Toxicol 1980;16:331–33.

Gendreau-Reid L, Simons K, Simons E. Comparison of the suppressive effect of astemizole, terfenadine and hydroxyzine on histamine-induced wheals and flares in humans. J Allergy Clin Immunol 1986; 77:335–40.

Girard JP, Sommacal-Schopf D, Bigliardi P, et al. Double-blind comparison of astemizole, terfenadine and placebo in hay fever with special regard to onset of action. J Int Med Res 1985;13:102–08.

Holgate S, Emanuel M, Howarth P, et al. Astemizole and other H1-antihistaminic drug treatment of asthma. J Allergy Clin Immunol 1985;76: 375–80.

Holgate ST, Howarth PH. Treating hay fever. BMJ 1985;291:92.

Howard JC Jr, Kantner TR, Lilienfield LS, et al. Effectiveness of antihistamines in the symptomatic management of the common cold. JAMA 1979;242:2414–17.

Howarth PH, Emanuel MB, Holgate ST. Astemizole, a potent histamine H1-receptor antagonist: effect in allergic rhinoconjunctivitis, on antigen and histamine induced skin wheal responses and relationship to serum levels. Br J Clin Pharmacol 1984;18:1–8.

Howarth PH, Holgate ST. Comparative trial of two non-sedative H1 antihistamines, terfenadine and astemizole, for hay fever. Thorax 1984;39: 668–72.

Kahn A, Hasaerts D, Blum D. Phenothiazine-induced sleep apneas in normal infants. Pediatrics 1985;75:844–47.

Kaiser H. H1-receptor antagonist treatment of seasonal allergic rhinitis. J Allergy Clin Immunol 1990; 86:1000–03.

Kemp J, Falliers C, Fox R, et al. A multicenter, open study of the non-sedating antihistamine, terfenadine (Seldane), in the maintenance therapy of seasonal allergic rhinitis. Ann Allergy 1988;60:349–54.

Krogh CME, ed. Compendium of Pharmaceuticals and Specialties. 30th ed. Ottawa: Canadian Pharmaceutical Association, 1995.

Lucas BD, Purdy CY, Scarim SK, et al. Terfenadine pharmacokinetics in breast milk in lactating women. Clin Pharmacol Ther 1995;57: 398–402.

Maibach H. The relative safety and effectiveness of antihistamines. Cutis 1988;42:2–4.

Mann K, Crowe J, Tietze K. Nonsedating histamine H1-receptor antagonists. Clin Pharm 1989;8:331–44.

McTavish D, Goa K, Ferrill M. Terfenadine: an updated review of its pharmacological properties and therapeutic efficacy. Drugs 1990;39: 552–74.

Meltzer E. Antihistamine- and decongestant-induced performance decrements. J Occup Med 1990;32:327–34.

Meltzer E. The use of antihistamines for the treatment of airway disease. Cutis 1988;42:22–25.

Milavetz G, Smith J. Pharmacotherapy of asthma and allergic rhinitis. Primary Care 1990;17:685–701.

Morris E. Pharmacotherapy of allergic disease. Primary Care 1987;14: 605–21.

Naclerio R, Kagey-Sobotka A, Lichtenstein L, et al. Terfenadine, an H1-anti-histamine inhibits histamine release in vivo in the human. Am Rev Respir Dis 1990;142:167–71.

Naclerio RM. The effect of antihistamines on the immediate allergic response: a comparative review. Otolaryngol Head Neck Surg 1993; 108:723-30.

Nicholson AN. Central effects of H1- and H2-antihistamines. Aviat Space Environ Med 1985;56:293–98.

Norman PS. Newer antihistaminic agents. J Allergy Clin Immunol 1985; 76:366–68.

Paton DM, Webster DR. Clinical pharmacokinetics of H1-receptor antagonists (the antihistamines). Clin Pharmacokinet 1985;10:477–97.

Richards DM, Brogden RN, Heel RC, et al. Astemizole: a review of its pharmacodynamic properties and therapeutic efficacy. Drugs 1984;28: 38–61.

Schuller DE, Turkewitz D. Adverse effects of antihistamines. Postgrad Med 1986;79:75–86.

Scheffer A, Samuels L. Cetirizine: antiallergic therapy beyond traditional H1 antihistamines. J Allergy Clin Immunol 1990;86:1040–46.

Sibbald B, Hilton S, D'Souza M. An open cross-over trial comparing two doses of astemizole and beclomethasone diproprionate in the treatment of perennial rhinitis. Clin Allergy 1986;16:203–11.

Simons FE, Luciuk GH, Simons KJ. Pharmacokinetics and efficacy of chlorpheniramine in children. J Allergy Clin Immunol 1982;69:376–81.

Simons F, Lukowski J, Becker A, et al. Comparison of the effects of single doses of the new H1-receptor antagonists loratadine and terfenadine versus placebo in children. J Pediatrics 1991;118:298–300.

Simons FE, Simons KJ. H1-receptor antagonists: clinical pharmacology and use in allergic disease. Pediatr Clin North Am 1983;30:899–914.

Simons F, Simons K. Optimum pharmacological management of chronic rhinitis. Drugs 1989;38:313–31.

Simons FER. H1-receptor antagonists. Comparative tolerability and safety. Drug Safety 1994;10:350–80.

Skassa-Brociek W, Bousquet J, Montes F, et al. Double-blind placebo-controlled study of loratadine, mequitazine, and placebo in the symptomatic treatment of seasonal allergic rhinitis. J Allergy Clin Immunol 1988;81:725–30.

Tarnasky P, Van Arsdel P. Antihistamine therapy in allergic rhinitis. J Fam Pract 1990;30:71–80.

Trzeciakowski JP, Mendelsohn N, Levi R. Antihistamines. In: Middleton E Jr, Reed C, Ellis E, et al, eds. Allergy: Principles and Practice. St. Louis: Mosby, 1988:715–38.

Uden DL, Huska DR, Kellenberger TA, et al. Antihistamines: a study of pediatric usage and incidence of toxicity. Vet Hum Toxicol 1984;26: 469-72.

Uzan A, Le Fur G, Malgouris C. Are antihistamines sedative via a blockade of brain H1 receptors? J Pharm Pharmacol 1979;31:701–02.

Vanden Bussche G, Emanuel MB, Rombaut N. Clinical profile of astemizole. A survey of 50 double-blind trials. Ann Allergy 1987;58:184–88.

von Maur K. Antihistamine selection in patients with allergic rhinitis. Ann Allergy 1985;55:458–62.

Woodward J. Pharmacology and toxicology of nonclassical antihistamines. Cutis 1988;42:5–9.

Review Articles

Bye C, Cooper J, Empey D, et al. Effects of pseudoephedrine and triprolidine, alone and in combination, on symptoms of the common cold. BMJ 1980;281:189–90.

Crutcher J, Kantner T. The effectiveness of antihistamines in the common cold. J Clin Pharmacol 1981;21:9–15.

Dechant K, Goa K. Levocabastine: a review of its pharmacological properties and therapeutic potential as a topical antihistamine in allergic rhinitis and conjunctivitis. Drugs 1991;41:202–24.

Fed Reg 1985;50(10):2220–41.

Gaffey M, Gwaltney J Jr, Sastre A, et al. Intranasally and orally administered antihistamine treatment of experimental rhinovirus colds. Am Rev Respir Dis 1987;136:556–60.

Grant S, Goa K, Fitton A, et al. Ketotifen: a review of its pharmacodynamic and pharmacokinetic properties, and therapeutic use in asthma and allergic disorders. Drugs 1990;40:412–48.

Holmberg K, Pipkorn U, Bake B, et al. Effects of topical treatment with H1 and H2 antagonists on clinical symptoms and nasal vascular reactions in patients with allergic rhinitis. Allergy 1989;44:281–87.

Howard J Jr, Kantner T, Lillienfield L, et al. Effectiveness of antihistamines in the symptomatic management of the common cold. JAMA 1979; 242:2414–17.

McTavish D, Sorkin E. Azelastine: a review of its pharmacodynamic and pharmacokinetic properties, and therapeutic potential. Drugs 1989;38: 778–800.

Pruitt A. Rational use of cold and cough preparations. Pediatr Ann 1985;14(4):289–91.

Weiler J, Donnelly A, Campbell B, et al. Multicenter, double-blind, multiple-dose, parallel groups efficacy and safety trial of azelastine, chlorpheniramine, and placebo in the treatment of spring allergic rhinitis. J Allergy Clin Immunol 1988;82:801–11.

West S, Brandon B, Stolley P, et al. A review of antihistamines and the common cold. Pediatrics 1975;56(1):100–07.

Decongestants

Paull B. The role of decongestants in allergic rhinitis management. J Resp Diseases 1989;Nov(suppl):S13–S17.

Storms W, Bodman S, Nathan R, et al. SCH 434: a new antihistamine/ decongestant for seasonal allergic rhinitis. J Allergy Clin Immunol 1989;83:1083–90.

Nasal Decongestants

Anon. Decongestants and analgesics. In: USP DI. Drug Information for the Health Care Provider. Rockville: United States Pharmacopeial Convention, 1991:1084–97.

Anon. Sympathomimetic agents. In: McEvoy G, ed. American Hospital Formulary Service Drug Information. Bethesda: American Society of Hospital Pharmacists, 1991:671–719.

Bale J Jr, Fountain M, Shaddy R. Phenylpropanolamine-associated CNS complications in children and adolescents. Am J Dis Child 1984;138: 683–85.

Black M, Remsen K. Rhinitis medicamentosa. Can Med Assoc J 1980; 122:881–84.

Capel L, Swanston A. Beware congesting nasal decongestants. BMJ 1986;293:1258–59.

Chaplin S. Adverse reactions to sympathomimetics in cold remedies. Adverse Drug Reaction Bull 1984;107:396–99.

Dougherty R. Pseudo-speed: look-alikes or pea-shooters. NY State J Med 1982;82:74–75.

Drew C, Knight G, Hughes D, et al. Comparison of the effects of D-ephedrine and L-pseudoephedrine on the cardiovascular and respiratory systems in man. Br J Clin Pharmacol 1978;6:221–25.

Elis J, Laurence D, Mattie H, et al. Modification by monoamine oxidase inhibitors of the effect of some sympathomimetics on blood pressure. BMJ 1967;2:75–78.

Empey D, Medder K. Nasal decongestants. Drugs 1981;21:438–43.

Fed Reg 1976;41(176):38312–423.

Fed Reg 1985;50(10):2200–18.

Empey D, Young G, Letley E, et al. Dose-response study of the nasal decongestant and cardiovascular effects of pseudoephedrine. Br J Clin Pharmacol 1980;9:351–58.

Griffiths R, Brady J, Snell J. Relationship between anorectic and reinforcing properties of appetite suppressant drugs: implications for assessment of abuse liability. Biol Psychiatry 1978;13:283–90.

Herridge C, A'Brook M. Ephedrine psychosis (Letter). BMJ 1968;2:160.

Higgins J, Oppenheimer E, Gershman M. Phenylpropanolamine-associated headaches (Letter). Am J Dis Child 1985;139:331.

Hoffman B, Lefkowitz R. Catocholamines and sympathomimetic drugs. In: Goodman L, Gilman A, Rall T, et al, eds. The Pharmacological Basis of Therapeutics. New York: Macmillan, 1990: 187–220.

Jordan P. CNS stimulants sold as amphetamines (Letter). Am J Hosp Pharm 1981;38:29.

Marchessault J, Boyd J, Crocker J, et al. First report of the Expert Advisory Committee on nonprescription cough and cold remedies to the Health Protection Branch: Antihistamines, nasal decongestants, and anticholinergics. Ottawa: Health and Welfare Canada, 1988.

Marchessault J, Boyd J, Crocker J, et al. Third report of the Expert Advisory Committee on nonprescription cough and cold remedies to the Health Protection Branch: Phenylpropanolamine, lozenges, and combinations. Ottawa: Health and Welfare Canada, 1989.

Mueller S. Phenylpropanolamine (Letter). N Engl J Med 1984;310:395.

Pentel P. Phenylpropanolamine and blood pressure (Letter). JAMA 1985; 253:2491–92.

Pentel P. Toxicity of over-the-counter stimulants. JAMA 1984;252: 1989–903.

Sankey R, Nunn A, Sills J. Visual hallucinations in children receiving decongestants. BMJ 1984;288:1369.

Soederman P, Sahlberg D, Wiholm B-E. CNS reactions to nose drops in small children (Letter). Lancet 1984;1:573.

Waggoner W. Phenylpropanolamine issue (Letter). Neurology 1984; 34:1526.

Waters B, Lapierre Y. Secondary mania associated with sympathomimetic drug use. Am J Psychiatry 1981;138:837–38.

White W, Riotte K. Drugs for cough and cold symptoms in hypertensive patients. Am Fam Physician 1985;31(3):183–87.

Evaluating Coughs

Bamer S. Cough: physiology, evaluation, and treatment. Lung 1986; 164:79–92.

Braman S, Corrao W. Chronic cough: diagnosis and treatment. Primary Care 1985;12:217–25.

Chou D, Wang S. Studies on the localization of central cough mechanism: site of action of antitussive drugs. J Pharmacol Exp Ther 1973;194: 499–505.

Fuller R, Jackson D. Physiology and treatment of cough. Thorax 1990; 45:425–30.

Toop L, Howie J, Paxton F. Night cough and general practice research. J R Coll Gen Pract 1986;36:74–77.

Cough Medicines

Anon. Antitussives, expectorants and mucolytic agents. In: McEvoy G, ed. American Hospital Formulary Service Drug Information. Bethesda: American Society of Hospital Pharmacists, 1991:1593–607.

Anon. Supplementary drugs and other substances. In: Reynolds J, ed. Martindale: The Extra Pharmacopoiea. London: Pharmaceutical Press, 1989:1552, 1586.

Boyd E. A review of studies on the pharmacology of the expectorants and inhalants. Int J Clin Pharmacol Ther Toxicol 1970;3:55–60.

Committee on drugs. Use of codeine- and dextromethorphan-containing cough syrups in pediatrics. Pediatrics 1978;62:118–22.

Croughan-Minibane MS, Petitti DB, Rodnick JE, et al. Clinical trial examining effectiveness of three cough syrups. J Am Board Fam Pract 1993;6:109–15.

Domino E, Krutak-Krol H, Lal J. Evidence for a central site of action for the antitussive effects of caramiphen. J Pharmacol Exp Ther 1985;233: 249–53.

Fed Reg 1982;47(132):30002–10.

Fed Reg 1987;52(155):30042–57.

Fleming P. Dependence on dextromethorphan hydrobromide. BMJ 1986; 293:597.

Krogh CME, ed. Compendium of Pharmaceuticals and Specialties. 26th ed. Ottawa: Canadian Pharmaceutical Association, 1991:265, 539, 1097.

Lilienfield L, Rose J, Princiotto J. Antitussive activity of diphenhydramine in chronic cough. Clin Pharmacol Ther 1976;19:421–25.

Loder R. Safe reduction of the cough reflex with noscapine: a preliminary communication on a new use for an old drug. Anaesthesia 1969;24: 355–58.

Marchessault J, Boyd J, Crocker J, et al. Second report of the Expert Advisory Committee on nonprescription cough and cold remedies to the Health Protection Branch: Antitussives, expectorants, and bronchodilators. Ottawa: Health and Welfare Canada, 1989.

Orrell M, Campbell P. Dependence on dextromethorphan hydrobromide (Letter). BMJ 1986;293:1242–43.

Von Muehlendahl K, Krienke E, Scherf-Rahne B, et al. Codeine intoxication in childhood. Lancet 1976;2:303–05.

Expectorants

Anon. Guaiphenesin and iodide. Drug Ther Bull 1985;23(16):62–64.

Buchanan G, Martin V, Levine P, et al. The effects of "anti-platelet" drugs on bleeding time and platelet aggregation in normal human subjects. Am J Clin Pathol 1977;68:355–59.

Chodosh S, Medici T. Expectorant effect of glyceryl guaiacolate (Letter). Chest 1973;64:543–45.

Cohen B. Antitussive effect of guaifenesin (Letter). Chest 1983;84: 118–19.

Hirsch S, Viernes P, Kory R. The expectorant effect of glyceryl guaiacolate in patients with chronic bronchitis. Chest 1973;63:9–14.

Kuhn J, Hendly J, Adams K, et al. Antitussive effect of guaifenesin in young adults with natural colds: objective and subjective assessment. Chest 1982;82:713–18.

Robinson R, Cumming W, Deffenbaugh E. Effectiveness of guaifenesin as an expectorant: a cooperative double-blind study. Curr Ther Res 1977; 22:284–96.

Thomson M, Pavia D, McNicol M. A preliminary study of the effect of guaiphenesin on mucociliary clearance from the human lung. Thorax 1973;28:742–47.

Anticholinergics

Gaffey M, Gwaltney J Jr, Dressler W, et al. Intranasally administered atropine methonitrate treatment of experimental rhinovirus colds. Am Rev Respir Dis 1987;135:241–44.

Gaffey M, Hayden F, Boyd J, et al. Ipratropium bromide treatment of experimental rhinovirus infection. Antimicrob Agents Chemother 1988;32:1644–47.

Nonsteroidal Anti-inflammatory Drugs

Graham N, Burrell C, Douglas R, et al. Adverse effects of aspirin, acetaminophen and ibuprofen on immune function, viral shedding, and clinical status in rhinovirus-infected volunteers. J Infect Dis 1990;162:1277–82.

Sperber S, Sorrentino J, Riker D, et al. Evaluation of an alpha agonist alone and in combination with a nonsteroidal antiinflammatory agent in the treatment of experimental rhinovirus colds. Bull NY Acad Med 1989;65:145–60.

Sperber S, Hayden F. Chemotherapy of rhinovirus colds. Antimicrob Agents Chemother 1988;32:409–19.

Vitamin C

Anderson T, Suranyi G, Beaton G. The effect on winter illness of large doses of vitamin C. Can Med Assoc J 1974;111:31–36.

Anderson T, Reid D, Beaton G. Vitamin C and the common cold: a double-blind trial. Can Med Assoc J 1972;107:503–08.

Anderson T, Beaton G, Corey P, et al. Winter illness and vitamin C: the effect of relatively low doses. Can Med Assoc J 1975;112:823–26.

Coulehan J. Ascorbic acid and the common cold: reviewing the evidence. Postgrad Med 1979;66(3):153–60.

Dykes M, Meier P. Ascorbic acid and the common cold: evaluations of its efficacy and toxicity. JAMA 1975;231:1073–79.

Elwood P, Hughes S, St. Leger A. A randomized controlled trial of therapeutic effect of vitamin C in the common cold. Practitioner 1977;218: 133–37.

Karlowski T, Chalmers T, Frenkel L, et al. Ascorbic acid for the common cold: a prophylactic and therapeutic trial. JAMA 1975;231:1038–42.

Murray T, Carroll K, Davignon J, et al. Nutrition recommendations: the report of the scientific review committee. Ottawa: Health and Welfare Canada, 1990:99–102.

Pauling L. Vitamin C and the Common Cold. San Francisco: WH Freeman, 1970:39–52.

Pitt H, Costrini A. Vitamin C prophylaxis in marine recruits. JAMA 1979;241:908–11.

Rivers J. Safety of high-level vitamin C ingestion. Ann N Y Acad Sci 1987;198:445–54.

CHAPTER 6—Antiparasitic and Anthelmintic Products

Pediculosis

Arndt KA. Infestations: pediculosis, scabies, and ticks. In: Arndt KA. Manual of Dermatologic Therapies with Essentials of Diagnosis. 4th ed. Boston: Little, Brown, 1989:94–100.

Billstein SA, Mattaliano VJ. The "nuisance" sexually transmitted diseases: molluscum contagiosum, scabies, and crab lice. Med Clin North Am 1990;74:1487–1505.

Blondell RD. Parasites of the skin and hair. Prim Care 1991;18:167–83.

Chunge RN, Scott FE, Underwood JE, et al. A review of the epidemiology, public health importance, treatment and control of head lice. Can J Public Health 1991;82:196–200.

Chunge RN, Scott FE, Underwood JE, et al. A pilot study to investigate transmission of head lice. Can J Public Health 1991;82:207–08.

Elgart ML. Scabies. Dermatol Clin 1990;8:253–63.

Hogan DJ, Schachner L, Tanglertsampan C. Diagnosis and treatment of childhood scabies and pediculosis. Pediatr Clin North Am 1991;38: 941–57.

La Piana Simonsen L. Head lice: what to tell parents. Pharm Times 1994;60(8):36.

Levine GI. Sexually transmitted parasitic diseases. Prim Care 1991;18: 101–28.

Taplin D, Meinking TL. Scabies, lice and fungal infections. Prim Care 1989;16:551–68.

Taplin D, Meinking TL. Pyrethrins and pyrethroids in dermatology. Arch Dermatol 1990;126:213–20.

Pediculosis—Nonpharmacological Treatment

Arndt KA. Infestations: pediculosis, scabies, and ticks. In: Arndt KA. Manual of Dermatologic Therapies with Essentials of Diagnosis. 4th ed. Boston: Little, Brown, 1989:94–100.

Benmur P, Lusthaus S, Weinberg A, et al. Facial chemical burn (Letter). Burns 1994;20:282.

Billstein SA, Mattaliano VJ. The "nuisance" sexually transmitted diseases: molluscum contagiosum, scabies, and crab lice. Med Clin North Am 1990;74:1487–1505.

Blondell RD. Parasites of the skin and hair. Prim Care 1991;18:167–83.

Burns DA. The treatment of human ectoparasite infection. Br J Dermatol 1991;125:89–93.

Chunge RN, Scott FE, Underwood JE, et al. A review of the epidemiology, public health importance, treatment and control of head lice. Can J Public Health 1991;82:196–200.

Gossel TA. Head lice: coping with the yearly infestation. US Pharm 1990;15(9):39–46.

Hogan DJ, Schachner L, Tanglertsampan C. Diagnosis and treatment of childhood scabies and pediculosis. Pediatr Clin North Am 1991;38: 941–57.

La Piana Simonsen L. Head lice: what to tell parents. Pharm Times 1994;60(8):36.

Pediculosis—Pharmacological Treatment

Arndt KA. Infestations: pediculosis, scabies, and ticks. In: Arndt KA. Manual of Dermatologic Therapies with Essentials of Diagnosis. 4th ed. Boston: Little, Brown, 1989:94–100.

Billstein SA, Mattaliano VJ. The "nuisance" sexually transmitted diseases: molluscum contagiosum, scabies, and crab lice. Med Clin North Am 1990;74:1487–1505.

Blondell RD. Parasites of the skin and hair. Prim Care 1991;18:167–83.

Brandenburg K, Deinard AS, DiNapoli J, et al. 1% permethrin cream rinse vs 1% lindane shampoo in treating pediculosis capitis. Am J Dis Child 1986;140:894–96.

Briggs GC, Freeman RK, Yaffe SJ. Drugs in Pregnancy and Lactation. 4th ed. Baltimore: Williams & Wilkins, 1994.

Burns DA. The treatment of human ectoparasite infection. Br J Dermatol 1991;125:89–93.

Carson DS, Tribble PW, Weart WC. Pyrethrins combined with piperonyl butoxide (RID) vs 1% permethrin (NIX) in the treatment of head lice. Am J Dis Child 1988;142:768–69.

Chunge RN, Scott FE, Underwood JE, et al. A review of the epidemiology, public health importance, treatment and control of head lice. Can J Public Health 1991;82:196–200.

Culver CA, Malina JJ, Talbert RL. Probable anaphylactoid reaction to a pyrethrin pediculicide shampoo. Clin Pharm 1988;7:846–49.

DeSimone EM, McCracken G. September lice alert. US Pharm 1994; 19(9):32–40.

DiNapoli JB, Austin RD, Englender SJ, et al. Eradication of head lice with a single treatment. Am J Public Health 1988;78:978–80.

Drugs for parasitic infections. Med Lett Drugs Ther 1995;37(961):99–108.

Gossel TA. Head lice: coping with the yearly infestation. US Pharm 1990;15(9):39–46.

Hogan DJ, Schachner L, Tanglertsampan C. Diagnosis and treatment of childhood scabies and pediculosis. Pediatr Clin North Am 1991;38: 941–57.

Levine GI. Sexually transmitted parasitic diseases. Prim Care 1991; 18:101–28.

Mathias RG, Wallace JF. The hatching of nits as a predictor of treatment failure with lindane and pyrethrin shampoos. Can J Public Health 1990;81:237–39.

Taplin D, Meinking TL. Scabies, lice and fungal infections. Prim Care 1989;16:551–68.

Taplin D, Meinking TL. Pyrethrins and pyrethroids in dermatology. Arch Dermatol 1990;126:213–20.

Voelker Phipps M. Permethrin: treatment of head lice infestations. Am Pharm 1991;NS31(10):53–56.

Scabies

Amer M, El-Gharib I. Permethrin versus crotamiton and lindane in the treatment of scabies. Int J Dermatol 1992;31:357–58.

Arndt KA. Infestations: pediculosis, scabies, and ticks. In: Arndt KA. Manual of Dermatologic Therapies with Essentials of Diagnosis. 4th ed. Boston: Little, Brown, 1989:94–100.

Billstein SA, Mattaliano VJ. The "nuisance" sexually transmitted diseases: molluscum contagiosum, scabies, and crab lice. Med Clin North Am 1990;74:1487–1505.

Blondell RD. Parasites of the skin and hair. Prim Care 1991;18:167–83.

Elgart ML. Scabies. Dermatol Clin 1990;8:253–63.

Fisher TF. Lindane toxicity in a 24-year-old woman. Ann Emerg Med 1994;24:972–74.

Hogan DJ, Schachner L, Tanglertsampan C. Diagnosis and treatment of childhood scabies and pediculosis. Pediatr Clin North Am 1991;38: 941–57.

Lane AT. Scabies and head lice. Pediatr Ann 1987;16:51–54.

Levine GI. Sexually transmitted parasitic diseases. Prim Care 1991; 18:101–28.

Pruksachatkunakorn C, Duarte AN, Schachner L. Scabies. How to find and stop the itch. Postgrad Med 1992;91(6):263–69.

Sterling GB, Janniger CK, Kihiczak G, et al. Scabies. Am Fam Physician 1992;46:1237–41.

Taplin D, Meinking TL. Scabies, lice and fungal infections. Prim Care 1989;16:551–68.

Scabies—Pharmacological Treatment

Amer M, El-Gharib I. Permethrin versus crotamiton and lindane in the treatment of scabies. Int J Dermatol 1992;31:357–58.

Arndt KA. Infestations: pediculosis, scabies, and ticks. In: Arndt KA. Manual of Dermatologic Therapies with Essentials of Diagnosis. 4th ed. Boston: Little, Brown, 1989:94–100.

Billstein SA, Mattaliano VJ. The "nuisance" sexually transmitted diseases: molluscum contagiosum, scabies, and crab lice. Med Clin North Am 1990;74:1487–1505.

Blondell RD. Parasites of the skin and hair. Prim Care 1991;18:167–83.

Briggs GC, Freeman RK, Yaffe SJ. Drugs in Pregnancy and Lactation. 4th ed. Baltimore: Williams & Wilkins, 1994.

Burns DA. The treatment of human ectoparasite infection. Br J Dermatol 1991;125:89–93.

DeSimone EM, McCracken G. September lice alert. US Pharm 1994; 19(9):32–40.

Drugs for parasitic infections. Med Lett Drugs Ther 1995;37(961):99–108.

Elgart ML. Scabies. Dermatol Clin 1990;8:253–63.

Hogan DJ, Schachner L, Tanglertsampan C. Diagnosis and treatment of childhood scabies and pediculosis. Pediatr Clin North Am 1991;38: 941–57.

Lane AT. Scabies and head lice. Pediatr Ann 1987;16:51–54.

Levine GI. Sexually transmitted parasitic diseases. Prim Care 1991; 18:101–28.

Permethrin for scabies. Med Lett Drugs Ther 1990; 32(813):21-22.

Pruksachatkunakorn C, Duarte AN, Schachner L. Scabies. How to find and stop the itch. Postgrad Med 1992;91(6):263-69.

Scabene Product Monograph. Stiefel Canada Inc. 1991, Mar 11.

Scabicides/Pediculicides. In: Drug Facts and Comparisons. St. Louis: Facts and Comparisons, Oct 1991:584a-86.

Schultz MW, Gomez M, Hansen RC, et al. Comparative study of 5% permethrin cream and 1% lindane lotion for the treatment of scabies. Arch Dermatol 1990;126:167-70.

Sterling GB, Janniger CK, Kihiczak G, et al. Scabies. Am Fam Physician 1992;46:1237-41.

Taplin D, Meinking TL. Pyrethrins and pyrethroids in dermatology. Arch Dermatol 1990;126:213-20.

Enterobiasis

Cook GC. Enterobius vermicularis infections. GUT 1994;35:1159-62.

Cook GC. Threadworm infection and its treatment. Pharm J 1990; 244(Jun 23):765-67.

Gossel TA. Pinworms. US Pharm 1984;56(9):32-56.

Intestinal nematode infections. WHO model prescribing information—drugs used in parasitic diseases. Geneva: World Health Organization, 1990:83-93.

Kollias G, Kyriakopoulos M, Tiniakos G. Epididymitis from Enterobius vermicularis: case report. J Urol 1992;147:1114-16.

MacLeod CL, ed. Parasitic Infections in Pregnancy and the Newborn. New York: Oxford University Press, 1988:192-207.

McKay T. Enterobius vermicularis infection causing endometritis and persistent vaginal discharge in three siblings (Letter). N Z Med J 1989;102:56.

Pray WS. Pinworms: a common family nuisance. US Pharm 1993; 18(4):30-35.

Richard A, Zhanel GG. Treatment of vaginal pinworms. Can J Hosp Pharm 1989;42:208-09.

Sheahan SL, Seabolt JP. Management of common parasitic infections encountered in primary care. Nurse Pract 1987;12(8):19-33.

Tellier R, Keystone J. Intestinal parasites—current therapy. On Cont Pract 1992;19(3):13-22.

Williams DR, Stajich GV, Matthews HW. Common intestinal parasitic infections. Pharm Times 1986(Nov);52:120-31.

Enterobiasis—Nonpharmacological Treatment

Cook GC. Enterobius vermicularis infections. GUT 1994;35:1159-62.

Cook GC. Threadworm infection and its treatment. Pharm J 1990;244(Jun 23):765-67.

Katz M. Anthelmintics: current concepts in the treatment of helminthic infections. Drugs 1986;32:358-71.

Pray WS. Pinworms: a common family nuisance. US Pharm 1993; 18(4):30-35.

Sheahan SL, Seabolt JP. Management of common parasitic infections encountered in primary care. Nurse Pract 1987;12(8):19-33.

Enterobiasis—Pharmacological Treatment

Committee on Antimicrobial Agents, Canadian Infectious Disease Society. Treatment of parasitic infections: Canadian versus US recommendations. Can Med Assoc J 1988;139:849-51.

Cook GC. Enterobius vermicularis infections. GUT 1994;35:1159-62.

Cook GC. Threadworm infection and its treatment. Pharm J 1990;244 (Jun 23):765-67.

Drugs for parasitic infections. Med Lett Drugs Ther 1995;37(961):99-108.

Gossel TA. Pinworms. US Pharm 1984;56(9):32-56.

Intestinal nematode infections. WHO model prescribing information—drugs used in parasitic diseases. Geneva: World Health Organization, 1990:83-93.

Leach FN. Management of threadworm infestation during pregnancy. Arch Dis Child 1990;65:399-400.

MacLeod CL, ed. Parasitic Infections in Pregnancy and the Newborn. New York: Oxford University Press, 1988:192-207.

Pray WS. Pinworms: a common family nuisance. US Pharm 1993; 18(4):30-35.

Rosenblatt JE. Antiparasitic agents. Mayo Clin Proc 1992;67(3):276-87.

Safety of antimicrobial drugs in pregnancy. Med Lett Drugs Ther 1987;29(743):61-63.

Sheahan SL, Seabolt JP. Management of common parasitic infections encountered in primary care. Nurse Pract 1987;12(8):19-33.

Tellier R, Keystone J. Intestinal parasites—current therapy. On Cont Pract 1992;19(3):13-22.

Turner JA. Drug therapy of gastrointestinal parasitic infections. Am J Gastroenterol 1986;81:1125-37.

van Riper G. Pyrantel pamoate for pinworm infestation. Am Pharm 1993;NS33(2):43-45.

White NJ. Antiparasitic drugs in children. Clin Pharmacokinet 1989; 17(suppl 1):138-55.

Williams DR, Stajich GV, Matthews HW. Common intestinal parasitic infections. Pharm Times 1986;52(Nov):120-31.

Pharmaceutical Agents

Benzyl Benzoate

Billstein SA, Mattaliano VJ. The "nuisance" sexually transmitted diseases: molluscum contagiosum, scabies, and crab lice. Med Clin North Am 1990;74:1487-1505.

Burns DA. The treatment of human ectoparasite infection. Br J Dermatol 1991;125:89-93.

Haustein U, Hlawa B. Treatment of scabies with permethrin versus lindane and benzyl benzoate. Acta Derm Venereol 1989;69:348-51.

Hogan DJ, Schachner L, Tanglertsampan C. Diagnosis and treatment of childhood scabies and pediculosis. Pediatr Clin North Am 1991;38: 941-57.

Rasmussen JE. The problem of lindane. J Am Acad Dermatol 1981; 5:507-16.

Crotamiton

Blondell RD. Parasites of the skin and hair. Prim Care 1991;18:167-83.

Rasmussen JE. The problem of lindane. J Am Acad Dermatol 1981; 5:507-16.

Sterling GB, Janniger CK, Kihiczak G, et al. Scabies. Am Fam Physician 1992;46:1237-41.

Lindane

Arndt KA. Infestations: pediculosis, scabies, and ticks. In: Arndt KA. Manual of Dermatologic Therapies with Essentials of Diagnosis. 4th ed. Boston: Little, Brown, 1989:94-100.

Billstein SA, Mattaliano VJ. The "nuisance" sexually transmitted diseases: molluscum contagiosum, scabies, and crab lice. Med Clin North Am 1990;74:1487-1505.

Blondell RD. Parasites of the skin and hair. Prim Care 1991;18:167-83.

Burns DA. The treatment of human ectoparasite infection. Br J Dermatol 1991;125:89-93.

Davies JE, Dedhia HV, Morgade C, et al. Lindane poisonings. Arch Dermatol 1983;119:142-44.

Fisher TF. Lindane toxicity in a 24-year-old woman. Ann Emerg Med 1994;24:972-74.

Fraser J. Permethrin: a top end viewpoint and experience (Letter). Med J Aust 1994;160(12):806.

Friedman SJ. Lindane neurotoxic reaction in nonbullous congenital ichthyosiform erythroderma. Arch Dermatol 1987;123:1056-58.

Ginsburg CM, Lowry W, Reisch JS. Absorption of lindane (gamma benzene hexachloride) in infants and children. J Pediatr 1977;91: 998-1000.

Haustein U, Hlawa B. Treatment of scabies with permethrin versus lindane and benzyl benzoate. Acta Derm Venereol 1989;69:348-51.

Hogan DJ, Schachner L, Tanglertsampan C. Diagnosis and treatment of childhood scabies and pediculosis. Pediatr Clin North Am 1991;38: 941-57.

Hosler J, Ischanz C, Hignite CE, et al. Topical application of lindane cream (Kwell) and antipyrine metabolism. J Invest Dermatol 1979;74:51-53.

Lane AT. Scabies and head lice. Pediatr Ann 1987;16:51-54.

Lee B, Groth P. Scabies: transcutaneous poisoning during treatment (Letter). Pediatrics 1977;59:643.

Levine GI. Sexually transmitted parasitic diseases. Prim Care 1991;18: 101-28.

Matsuoka LY. Convulsions following application of gamma benzene hexachloride (Letter). J Am Acad Dermatol 1981;5:98-99.

Permethrin for scabies. Med Lett Drugs Ther 1990;32(813): 21-22.

Pramanik AK, Hansen RC. Transcutaneous gamma benzene hexachloride absorption and toxicity in infants and children. Arch Dermatol 1979;115:1224-25.

Pruksachatkunakorn C, Duarte AN, Schachner L. Scabies. How to find and stop thc itch. Postgrad Med 1992,91(6):263-69.

Rasmussen JE. The problem of lindane. J Am Acad Dermatol 1981;5: 507-16.

Rasmussen JE. Lindane. A prudent approach. Arch Dermatol 1987;123: 1008-10.

Rauch AE, Kowalsky SF, Lesar TS, et al. Lindane (Kwell)-induced aplastic anemia. Arch Intern Med 1990;150: 2393-95.

Schultz MW, Gomez M, Hansen RC, et al. Comparative study of 5% permethrin cream and 1% lindane lotion for the treatment of scabies. Arch Dermatol 1990;126:167-70.

Soloman LM, Fahrner L, West DP. Gamma benzene hexachloride toxicity. Arch Dermatol 1977;113:353-57.

Sterling GB, Janniger CK, Kihiczak G, et al. Scabies. Am Fam Physician 1992;46:1237-41.

Taplin D, Meinking TL. Scabies, lice and fungal infections. Prim Care 1989;16:551-68.

Taplin D, Meinking TL. Pyrethrins and pyrethroids in dermatology. Arch Dermatol 1990;126:213-20.

Telch J, Jarvis DA. Acute intoxications with lindane (gamma benzene hexachloride). Can Med Assoc J 1982;126:662-63.

Piperazine Adipate

Gossel TA. Pinworms. US Pharm 1984;56(9):32-56.

Katz M. Anthelmintics: current concepts in the treatment of helminthic infections. Drugs 1986;32: 358-71.

Keusch GT. Anthelmintic therapy: the worm has turned. Drug Ther 1982;12(Aug):213-17, 220-22.

Rosenblatt JE. Antiparasitic agents. Mayo Clin Proc 1992;67(3):276-87.

Tellier R, Keystone J. Intestinal parasites—current therapy. On Cont Pract 1992;19(3):13-22.

Turner JA. Drug therapy of gastrointestinal parasitic infections. Am J Gastroenterol 1986;81:1125-37.

Williams DR, Stajich GV, Matthews HW. Common intestinal parasitic infections. Pharm Times 1986;52(Nov):120-31.

Pyrantel Pamoate

Gossel TA. Pinworms. US Pharm 1984;56(9):32-56.

Katz M. Anthelmintics: current concepts in the treatment of helminthic infections. Drugs 1986;32:358-71.

Keusch GT. Anthelmintic therapy: the worm has turned. Drug Ther 1982;12(Aug):213-17, 220-22.

Rosenblatt JE. Antiparasitic agents. Mayo Clin Proc 1992;67(3):276-87.

Tellier R, Keystone J. Intestinal parasites—current therapy. On Cont Pract 1992;19(3):13-22.

Turner JA. Drug therapy of gastrointestinal parasitic infections. Am J Gastroenterol 1986;81:1125-37.

Williams DR, Stajich GV, Matthews HW. Common intestinal parasitic infections. Pharm Times 1986;52(Nov):120-31.

Pyrethrins, Synthetic

Amer M, El-Gharib I. Permethrin versus crotamiton and lindane in the treatment of scabies. Int J Dermatol 1992;31:357-58.

Andrews EB, Joseph MC, Magenheim MJ, et al. Postmarketing surveillance study of permethrin creme rinse. Am J Public Health 1992;82: 857-61.

Arndt KA. Infestations: pediculosis, scabies, and ticks. In: Arndt KA. Manual of Dermatologic Therapies with Essentials of Diagnosis. 4th ed. Boston: Little, Brown, 1989:94-100.

Billstein SA, Mattaliano VJ. The "nuisance" sexually transmitted diseases: molluscum contagiosum, scabies, and crab lice. Med Clin North Am 1990;74:1487-1505.

Blondell RD. Parasites of the skin and hair. Prim Care 1991;18:167-83.

Burns DA. The treatment of human ectoparasite infection. Br J Dermatol 1991;125:89-93

Chunge RN, Scott FE, Underwood JE, et al. A review of the epidemiology, public health importance, treatment and control of head lice. Can J Public Health 1991;82:196-200.

DeSimone EM, McCracken G. September lice alert. US Pharm 1994; 19(9):32-40.

Haustein U, Hlawa B. Treatment of scabies with permethrin versus lindane and benzyl benzoate. Acta Derm Venereol 1989;69:348-51.

Hogan DJ, Schachner L, Tanglertsampan C. Diagnosis and treatment of childhood scabies and pediculosis. Pediatr Clin North Am 1991;38: 941-57.

Pruksachatkunakorn C, Duarte AN, Schachner L. Scabies. How to find and stop the itch. Postgrad Med 1992;91(6):263-69.

Sterling GB, Janniger CK, Kihiczak G, et al. Scabies. Am Fam Physician 1992;46:1237-41.

Taplin D, Porcelain SL, Meinking TL, et al. Community control of scabies: a model based on use of permethrin cream. Lancet 1991;337:1016-18.

Taplin D, Meinking TL. Scabies, lice and fungal infections. Prim Care 1989;16:551-68.

Taplin D, Meinking TL. Pyrethrins and pyrethroids in dermatology. Arch Dermatol 1990;126:213-20.

vanderRhee HJ, Farquhar JA, Vermeulen NPE. Efficacy and transdermal absorption of permethrin in scabies patients. Acta Derm Venereol 1989;69:170-82.

Pyrethrins with piperonyl butoxide

Arndt KA. Infestations: pediculosis, scabies, and ticks. In: Arndt KA. Manual of Dermatologic Therapies with Essentials of Diagnosis. 4th ed. Boston: Little, Brown, 1989:94-100.

Billstein SA, Mattaliano VJ. The "nuisance" sexually transmitted diseases: molluscum contagiosum, scabies, and crab lice. Med Clin North Am 1990;74:1487-1505.

Blondell RD. Parasites of the skin and hair. Prim Care 1991;18:167-83.

Burns DA. The treatment of human ectoparasite infection. Br J Dermatol 1991;125:89-93.

Chunge RN, Scott FE, Underwood JE, et al. A review of the epidemiology, public health importance, treatment and control of head lice. Can J Public Health 1991;82:196-200.

Culver CA, Malina JJ, Talbert RL. Probable anaphylactoid reaction to a pyrethrin pediculicide shampoo. Clin Pharm 1988;7:846-49.

DeSimone EM, McCracken G. September lice alert. US Pharm 1994; 19(9):32-40.

Elgart ML. Scabies. Dermatol Clin 1990;8:253-63.

Gossel TA. Head lice: coping with the yearly infestation. US Pharm 1990;15(9):39-46.

Hogan DJ, Schachner L, Tanglertsampan C. Diagnosis and treatment of childhood scabies and pediculosis. Pediatr Clin North Am 1991;38: 941-57.

Lane AT. Scabies and head lice. Pediatr Ann 1987;16:51-54.

La Piana Simonsen L. Head lice: what to tell parents. Pharm Times 1994;60(8):36.

Taplin D, Meinking TL. Pyrethrins and pyrethroids in dermatology. Arch Dermatol 1990;126:213-20.

Pyrvinium Pamoate

Drugs that cause photosensitivity. Med Lett Drugs Ther 1986; 28(713): 51-52.

Tellier R, Keystone J. Intestinal parasites—current therapy. On Cont Pract 1992;19(3):13-22.

Williams DR, Stajich GV, Matthews HW. Common intestinal parasitic infections. Pharm Times 1986;52(Nov):120-31.

Sulfur

Blondell RD. Parasites of the skin and hair. Prim Care 1991;18:167-83.

Elgart ML. Scabies. Dermatol Clin 1990;8:253-63.

Hogan DJ, Schachner L, Tanglertsampan C. Diagnosis and treatment of childhood scabies and pediculosis. Pediatr Clin North Am 1991; 38:941-57.

Lane AT. Scabies and head lice. Pediatr Ann 1987;16:51-54.

Rasmussen JE. The problem of lindane. J Am Acad Dermatol 1981;5: 507-16.

CHAPTER 7—Dermatitis, Seborrhea, Dandruff and Dry Skin Products

Normal Skin

Baadsgaard O, Fisher GJ, Voorhees JS, et al. Interactions of epidermal cells and T-cells in inflammatory skin disease. J Am Acad Dermatol 1990; 23:1312-17.

Ebling JF . The normal skin. In: Rook AR, Wilkinson DS, et al, eds. Textbook of Dermatology. Oxford: Blackwell Scientific Publications, 1986.

Jamoulle J-C, Schafer H. Topical modalities. In: Fitzpatrick TB, Eisen AZ, Wolff K, et al, eds. Dermatology in General Medicine. New York: McGraw-Hill, 1993: 2829-46.

Sams WM. Structure and function of the skin. In: Sams WM, Lynch PJ, eds. Principles and Practices of Dermatology. New York: Churchill Livingstone, 1990:3-14.

Atopic Dermatitis

Clark RAF, Nicol N, Adinoff AD. Atopic dermatitis. In: Sams WM, Lynch PJ, eds. Principles and Practices of Dermatology. New York: Churchill Livingstone, 1990:365-88.

Cooper KD. Atopic dermatitis: recent trends in pathogenesis and therapy. J Invest Dermatol 1994;102(1):128-37.

Ghadially R, Halkier-Sorenson L, Elias PM. Effects of petrolatum on stratum corneum structure and function. J Am Acad Dermatol 1992;26:387-96.

Hanifin JM. Atopic dermatitis: new therapeutic considerations. J Am Acad Dermatol 1991;24(6 Part 2):1097-101.

Linde YW. Dry skin in atopic dermatitis. Acta Derm Venereol 1992;Suppl 177:9-13.

Przybilla B, Eberlein-Konig B, Rueff F. Practical management of atopic eczema. Lancet 1994;343:1342-46.

Leung DM. Role of IgE in atopic dermatitis. Curr Opin Dermatol 1993; 5(6):956-62.

Sampson HA. Atopic dermatitis. Ann Allergy 1992;69(6):469-79.

Yoshida H. Guidelines of care for atopic dermatitis. J Am Acad Dermatol 1992;26(3):485-88.

Contact Dermatitis

Fisher AA. The role of nonsensitizing alternatives in the management of allergic contact dermatitis. Semin Dermatol 1986;5:263-72.

Gossel TA. Therapeutic relief of contact dermatitis. US Pharm 1990; 5:12-16.

Hogan DH. Contact dermatitis. Med North Am 1989;31:5740-46.

Janniger CK, Thomas I. Diaper dermatitis: an approach to prevention employing effective diaper care. Cutis 1993;52:153-55.

Keefner KR, DeSimone EM. Contact dermatitis: skin reactions to irritants. US Pharm 1991;6:36-39.

Lynde CW. Poison ivy dermatitis. Med North Am 1989;31(3):5748-53.

Martini MC, Marks JG. Contact dermatitis and contact urticaria. In: Sams WM, Lynch PJ, eds. Principles and Practices of Dermatology. New York: Churchill Livingstone, 1990:389-402.

Mathias CGT. Prevention of occupational contact dermatitis. J Am Acad Dermatol 1990;23:742-48.

Seborrhea and Dandruff

Binder RL, Jonelis FJ. Seborrheic dermatitis: a newly reported side effect of neuroleptics. J Clin Psychiatry 1984;45:125-26.

Dubois M. Dandruff and seborrheic dermatitis of the scalp. Can Pharm J 1985;118:434-36.

Janniger CK. Infantile seborrheic dermatitis: an approach to cradle cap. Cutis 1993;51:233-35.

Kligman AM, Leyden JJ. Seborrheic dermatitis. Semin Dermatol 1983;2(1):57-59.

White SW. Localized erythematous disease. In: Sams WM, Lynch PJ, eds. Principles and Practices of Dermatology. New York: Churchill Livingstone, 1990:403-16.

Dry Skin

Arndt KA. Manual of Dermatologic Therapeutics. Boston: Little, Brown, 1989:55-57.

Steinbaugh JR. Dry skin. Am Fam Physician 1983;27(3):171-74.

Walther RR, Harber LC. Expected skin complaints of the geriatric patient. Mod Med Can 1985;40(9):874-78.

Antipruritics

Arndt KA, Mendenhall PV, Sloan KB, et al. The pharmacology of topical therapy. In: Fitzpatrick TB, Eisen AZ, Wolff K, et al, eds. Dermatology in General Medicine. New York: McGraw-Hill, 1993:2837-44.

Harvey SC. Topical drugs. In: Gennaro AR, ed. Remington's Pharmaceutical Sciences. Easton: Mack Publishing, 1985:773-91.

Local anesthetics. In: Reynolds JEF, ed. Martindale The Extra Pharmacopoeia. London: Pharmaceutical Press, 1993:995-1018.

Pramagel monograph. In: Krogh CME, ed. Compendium of Pharmaceuticals and Specialties. 30th ed. Ottawa: Canadian Pharmaceutical Association, 1995:1079.

Ritchie JM, Greene NM. Local anesthetics. In: Goodman Gilman A, Rall TW, Nies AS, et al, eds. The Pharmacological Basis of Therapeutics. New York: Pergamon, 1990:311-31.

Tong AKF, Vickers CFH. Topical noncorticosteroid therapy. In: Fitzpatrick TB, Eisen AZ, Wolff K, et al, eds. Dermatology in General Medicine. New York: McGraw-Hill, 1993:2851-57.

Astringents

Bond CA. Skin disorders Part 1. In: Young LY, Koda-Kimble MA, eds. Applied Therapeutics: The Clinical Use of Drugs. Vancouver, WA: Applied Therapeutics, 1988:1397–416.

Edwards L. Medical therapy. In: Sams WM, Lynch PJ, eds. Principles and Practices of Dermatology. New York: Churchill Livingstone, 1990: 47–62.

Harvey SC. Topical drugs. In: Gennaro AR, ed. Remington's Pharmaceutical Sciences. Easton: Mack Publishing, 1985:773–91.

Bath Products

Arndt KA. Manual of Dermatologic Therapeutics. Boston: Little, Brown, 1989:55–57.

Aveeno monograph. In: Krogh CME, ed. Compendium of Pharmaceuticals and Specialties. 30th ed. Ottawa: Canadian Pharmaceutical Association, 1995:132.

Bond CA. Skin disorders Part 1. In: Young LY, Koda-Kimble MA, eds. Applied Therapeutics: The Clinical Use of Drugs. Vancouver, WA: Applied Therapeutics, 1992:64.1–16.

Wehr RF, Krochmal L. Considerations in selecting a moisturizer. Cutis 1987;39(6):512–15.

Cleansing Products

Ricciatti-Sibbald DJ. Dermatitis. In: Carruthers-Czyzewski P, ed. Self-medication Reference for Health Professionals. Ottawa: Canadian Pharmaceutical Association, 1992:63–81.

Strube DD. The irritancy of soaps and syndets. Cutis 1987;39:544–45.

Corticosteroids

Anon. Topical corticosteroids general statement. In: McEvoy G, ed. AHFS Drug Information. Bethesda: American Society of Hospital Pharmacists, 1994:2316–19.

Gossel TA. Hydrocortisone for self-therapy. US Pharm 1992;17(8):18, 20-25, 62–63.

Emollients and Moisturizers

Arndt KA. Manual of Dermatologic Therapeutics. Boston: Little, Brown, 1989:55–57.

Arndt KA, Mendenhall PV, Sloan KB, et al. The pharmacology of topical therapy. In: Fitzpatrick TB, Eisen AZ, Wolff K, et al, eds. Dermatology in General Medicine. New York: McGraw-Hill, 1993:2837–46.

Bond CA. Skin disorders Part 1. In: Young LY, Koda-Kimble MA, eds. Applied Therapeutics: The Clinical Use of Drugs. Vancouver, WA: Applied Therapeutics, 1988:1397–416.

Swinyard EA, Lowenthal W. Pharmaceutical necessities. In: Gennaro AR, ed. Remington's Pharmaceutical Sciences. Easton: Mack Publishing, 1985:1278–320.

Tong AKF, Vickers CFH. Topical noncorticosteroid therapy. In: Fitzpatrick TB, Eisen AZ, Wolff K, et al, eds. Dermatology in General Medicine. New York: McGraw-Hill, 1993:2851–57.

Wehr RF, Krochmal L. Considerations in selecting a moisturizer. Cutis 1987;39(6):512–15.

Soaks

Arndt KA, Mendenhall PV, Sloan KB, et al. The pharmacology of topical therapy. In: Fitzpatrick TB, Eisen AZ, Wolff K, et al, eds. Dermatology in General Medicine. New York: McGraw-Hill, 1993:2837–46.

Edwards L. Medical therapy. In: Sams WM, Lynch PJ, eds. Principles and Practices of Dermatology. New York: Churchill Livingstone, 1990: 47–62.

Harvey SC. Topical drugs. In: Gennaro AR, ed. Remington's Pharmaceutical Sciences. Easton: Mack Publishing, 1985:773–91.

CHAPTER 8—Ear Care Products

Anatomy and Physiology

Anderson JE, ed. Grant's Atlas of Anatomy. 8th ed. Baltimore: Williams & Wilkins, 1983:7-142-7-146.

Basmajian JV, ed. Grant's Method of Anatomy. 10th ed. Baltimore: Williams & Wilkins, 1981:534–54.

Brunner LS, Suddarth DS, Bare BG, et al, eds. Textbook of Medical and Surgical Nursing. 6th ed. New York: Lippincott, 1988:1371.

Guyton AC, ed. Textbook of Medical Physiology. 6th ed. Philadelphia: Saunders, 1991:570–80.

Disorders of the Ear

Ballenger JJ. Diseases of the Nose, Throat, Ear, Head, and Neck. 14th ed. Philadelphia: Lea and Febiger, 1991:1069–1118.

Dukes MNG, ed. Myler's Side Effects of Drugs. 11th ed. Amsterdam: Elsevier Publishers, 1988.

Farb SN. Otorhinolaryngology. 3rd ed. New York: Medical Examination Publishing, 1983:41–94.

Hanger HC, Mulley GP. Cerumen: its fascination and clinical importance: A review. J R Soc Med 1992;85:346–49.

Hendricks WM. Complications of ear piercing. Cutis 1991;48:386–94.

Hirsch BE. Infections of the external ear. Am J Otolaryngol 1992; 13:145–55.

Lucente FE. Fungal infections of the external ear. Otolaryngol Clin North Am 1993;26:995–1006.

Paparella MM, Shumrick DA, Gluckman JL, et al, eds. Otolaryngology. 3rd ed. Philadelphia: Saunders, 1991:1137–60.

Pullen FW. Otitis externa (swimmer's ear). Presentation at the Medicine of Diving Seminar. Grand Cayman: Medical Seminars Inc., 1992:31–32.

Ruddy J, Bickerton RC. Optimum management of the discharging ear. Drugs 1992;43:219–35.

Rybak LP. Drug ototoxicity. Ann Rev Pharmacol Toxicol 1986;26:79–99.

Strome M, Kelly JH, Fried MP, eds. Manual of Otolaryngology: Diagnosis and Therapy. 2nd ed. Boston: Little, Brown, 1992:49–106.

Yelland M. Otitis externa in general practice. Med J Aust 1992; 156: 325–30.

Zivic RC, King S. Cerumen impaction management for clients of all ages. Nurse Pract 1993;18:29, 33–37.

Pharmaceutical Agents

Budavari, S, ed. The Merck Index. 11th ed. Rahway: Merck and Company, 1989.

Fahmy S, Whitefiels M. Multicentre clinical trial of exterol as a cerumenolytic. Br J Clin Prac 1982;36:197–204.

Gennar AR, Chase CD, Marderosian AD, et al, eds. Remington's Pharmaceutical Sciences. 18th ed. Easton: Mack Publishing Company, 1990.

Gossel TA, O'Hara JD. Counseling patients to treat ear afflictions. US Pharmacist 1993;18:26–35.

Mehta AK. An in vitro comparison of the disintegration of human ear wax by five cerumenolytics commonly used in general practice. Br J Clin Pract 1985;39:200–03.

Reynolds JEF, ed. Martindale: The Extra Pharmacopoeia. 30th ed. London: Pharmaceutical Press, 1993.

CHAPTER 9—Eye Care Products

General

Chawla HB. Ophthalmology. Edinburgh: Churchill Livingstone, 1993.

Ellis PP. Handbook of Ocular Therapeutics and Pharmacology. St. Louis: Mosby, 1985.

Frith P, Gray R, MacLennan S, et al. The Eye in Clinical Practice. London: Oxford-Blackwell Scientific, 1994.

Fraunfelder FT, Roy FH, eds. Current Ocular Therapy. Philadelphia: Saunders, 1990.

Freidlaender MH. Ocular allergy—scratching the surface of the red eye. Postgrad Med 1986;79(5):261-71.

Halperin JA, ed. The United States Pharmacopoeia-23. The National Formulary-18. Rockville, MD: United States Pharmacopoeial Convention, 1995.

Jose JF, Polse KA, Holden EK. Optometric Pharmacology. Orlando: Grune and Stratton, 1984.

Kanski JJ. Clinical Ophthalmology—A Systematic Approach. Toronto: Butterworths, 1989.

Krogh CME, ed. Compendium of Pharmaceuticals and Specialties. 29th ed. Ottawa: Canadian Pharmaceutical Association, 1994.

Lund W, ed. The Pharmaceutical Codex. London: Pharmaceutical Press, 1994.

McEvoy Gk, ed. AHFS '94 Drug Information. Bethesda: American Society of Hospital Pharmacists, 1994.

Reynolds J, ed. Martindale: The Extra Pharmacopoeia. London: Pharmaceutical Press, 1993.

Mandell GL, Douglas RG, Bennett JE, eds. Principles and Practice of Infectious Diseases. New York: Churchill Livingstone, 1990.

Mauger TF, Craig EL, eds. Havener's Ocular Pharmacology. St. Louis: Mosby, 1994.

Newell FW. Ophthalmology: Principles and Concepts. St Louis: Mosby, 1991.

Ophthalmic drug products for over-the-counter human use. Establishment of a monograph, proposed rulemaking. Federal Register 1980;45(89):30002-50.

Ostler HB, ed. Diseases of the External Eye and Adnexa—a Text and Atlas. Baltimore: Williams & Wilkins, 1993.

Robin JS, Ellis PP. Ophthalmic ointments. Surv Ophthalmol 1978;2: 335-40.

Stock EL. External eye diseases. Postgrad Med 1985;78(8):102-11.

Van Heuven WA, Zwaan JT, eds. Decision Making in Ophthalmology. St. Louis: Mosby, 1992.

Disorders of the Eyelids

Diegel JT. Eyelid problems—blepharitis, hordeola, and chalazia. Postgrad Med 1986;80(2):271-72.

Jacobs PM, Thaller VT, Wong D. Intralesional corticosteroid therapy of chalazia: a comparison with incision and curettage. Br J Ophthalmol 1984;68:836-37.

Mathers WD, Shields WJ, Sachdev MS, et al. Meibomian gland dysfunction in chronic blepharitis. Cornea 1991;10(4):277-85.

Watson AP, Austin DJ. Treatment of chalazions with injection of a steroid suspension. Br J Ophthalmol 1984;68:833-35.

Wilson LA, Julian AJ, Ahearn MS, et al. The survival and growth of microorganisms in mascara during use. Am J Ophthalmol 1975;79: 596-601.

Disorders of the Conjunctiva

Anon. Lodoxamide for vernal keratoconjunctivitis sicca. Med Lett Drugs Ther 1994;36(318):23-26.

Anon. Ophthalmic levocabastine for allergic conjunctivitis. Med Lett Drugs Ther 1994;36(920):35-36.

Belzer D. Conjunctivitis treatment (Letters). Ped Ann 1993;22(10):594.

Dechant KL, Goa KL. Levocabastine: a review of its pharmacological properties and therapeutic potential as a topical antihistamine in allergic rhinitis and conjunctivitis. Drugs 1991;41(2):202-24.

Ehlers W, Donshik PC. Allergic ocular disorders: a spectrum of diseases. CLAO J 1992;18(2):117-24.

Fisher AA. Allergic reactions to contact lens solutions. Cutis 1985; 36(3):209-11.

Leino M, et al. The effect of sodium cromoglycate eyedrops compared to the effect of terfenadine on acute symptoms of seasonal allergic conjunctivitis. Acta Ophthalmologic 1992;70(3):341-45.

Munson M, Yeykal T. Secrets of sneezin'. Prevention 1994;46(8):26-28.

Parys W, Blockhuys S, Janssens M. New trends in the treatment of allergic conjunctivitis. Doc Ophthalmol 1992;82:353-60.

Sendele DD. Chemical hypersensitivity reactions. Int Ophthalmol Clin 1986;26(1):25-34.

Sohoel P, Freng BA, Kramer J. Topical levocabastine compared with orally administered terfenadine for the prophylaxis and treatment of seasonal rhinoconjunctivitis. J Allergy Clin Immunol 1993;92(1):73-81.

Tovey ER, Woolcock AJ. Direct exposure of carpets to sunlight can kill all mites. J Allergy Clin Immunol 1994;93(6):1072-74.

Troeme SD, Raizman MB, Bartley GB. Medical therapy for ocular allergy. Mayo Clin Proc 1992;67:557-65.

Weiss AH. Chronic conjunctivitis in infants and children. Pediatr Ann 1993;22(6):366-68.

Dry Eye

Holly FJ, Lemp MA. Tear physiology and dry eyes. Surv Ophthalmol 1977;22(2):69-87.

Laibovitz RA, Solch S, Adriano K, et al. Pilot trial of cyclosporine 1% ophthalmic ointment in the treatment of keratoconjunctivitis sicca. Cornea 1993;12(4): 315-23.

Lamberts DW. Dry eye and tear deficiency. Int Ophthalmol Clin 1983; 23(1):123-30.

Mather WD. Ocular evaporation in meibomian gland dysfunction and dry eye. Ophthalmology 1993;100(3):347-51.

Trauma

Born CP. Ocular injuries—treat or refer? Postgrad Med 1983;73(2): 311-17.

Administration of Ophthalmic Solutions and Ointments

Annable WL. Therapy for ocular infections. Pediatr Clin North Am 1983;30(2):389-96.

Anon. Achieving patient compliance. Nurs Times 1993;89(13):50-52.

Anon. Here's how to teach the "depot" method for eye drops. Pharm Pract 1977:(Aug)56.

Anon. How to instil ophthalmic medication in a child's eyes. Pharm Pract 1975;10(12):2.

Fritz M. Eyedrops. Alaska Med 1977;19(3):43-44.

Law S. Development and utilization of the eyedropper adaptation device: an example of interdisciplinary cooperation. Home Healthc Nurse 1987;5(4):50-51.

Letocha CE. Methods for self-administration of eyedrops. Ann Ophthalmol 1985;17(12):768-69.

Schein OD, et al. Microbial contamination of in-use-ocular medications. Arch Ophthalmol 1992;110:82-85.

Sheldon GM. Self-administration of eyedrops. Ophthalmic Surg 1987; 18(5):393-94.

Weisbecker C, Linkewich J. Dealing with ophthalmic needs—common ocular problems. On Cont Pract 1983;10(1):33-36.

Winfield AJ, Jessiman D, Williams A, et al. A study of the causes of non-compliance by patients prescribed eyedrops. Br J Ophthalmol 1990;74(8):477-80.

Contact Lens Care—General

Bailey NJ. Making contact (Editorial). Contact Lens Forum 1978;(Aug):47.

Borska L. Contact lenses in the 21st century. Rev Optom 1991; (Jul):44-48.

Fontana F, Weiner B. A new approach to compliance. Supply'em, drill'em, and grill'em. Rev Optom 1990;127:63-65.

Gordon K. A pharmacist's guide through the complexities of contact lens care. Part I. Drug Merch 1981;62:48-52.

Middleton D. Product Manager—Solutions, Barnes-Hind Inc. (Letter to D. Wing, author) 1987, Oct. 8.

Talamo JH, Larkin DS. Bilateral Acanthamoeba keratitis and gas-permeable contact lenses (Letter). Am J Ophthalmol 1993;116:651-52.

Weissman BA, Donzis PB, Hoft RH. Keratitis and contact lens wear: a review. J Am Optom Assoc 1987;58:799-803.

Hard (PMMA) Lenses

Abel SR, Gourley DR. Eye diseases. In: Katcher BS, Young LY, Koda-Kimble MA, eds. Applied Therapeutics, The Clinical Use of Drugs. San Francisco: Applied Therapeutics, 1983:1201-37.

Appen RE, Hutson CF. Traumatic injuries: office treatment of eye injury. 1. Injury due to foreign materials. Postgrad Med 1976;60:233-35.

Cooper RL, Constable IJ. Infective keratitis in soft contact lens wearers. Br J Ophthalmol 1977;61:250-54.

Karp EJ. A guide to cosmetic contact lenses. Sight Sav Rev 1977;47:3-8.

Koetting RA. Contact lens update. J Am Pharm Assoc 1975;15:575-77, 587.

Mandell RB. Contact Lens Practice. Springfield: CC Thomas, 1981: 296-312, 383-430.

Ruben M. The pros and cons of hard and soft contact lenses. Nurs Times 1976;72:1018-20.

Sweeney DF. Corneal exhaustion syndrome with long term wear of contact lenses. Optom Vis Sci 1992;69:601-08.

Gas Permeable Lenses

Anon. Contact lenses now. Drug Ther Bull 1988;26:39-40.

Garnett B. Gas-permeable hard contact lenses. Can J Optom 1980; 42:45-49.

Kame R, Asno G, Lee J. Hard lens solutions with the Polycon. Contact Lens Forum 1981;(Aug):43-46.

Shovlin J. Protect your RGP wearers. Optom Manage 1992;(Oct):69.

Soft (Hydrogel) Lenses

Lum VJ, Lyle WM. Chemical components of contact lens solutions. Can J Optom 1981;43:136-51.

Mandell RB. Contact Lens Practice. Springfield: CC Thomas, 1981: 495-518.

Sutherland RL, VanLeeuwen WN. Soft contact lenses. Can Med Assoc J 1972;107:49-50.

Silicone Lenses

Birdsall AA. Silicone: material of the future. Contact Lens Forum 1982; (May):89-97.

Herrin S. Reliving Dow Corning's nightmare. Rev Optom 1985;122: 35-44.

Mandell RB. Contact Lens Practice. Springfield: CC Thomas, 1981: 650-51.

Flexible Wear Contact Lenses

Alfonso E, Mandelbaum S, Fox MJ, et al. Ulcerative keratitis associated with contact lens wear. Am J Ophthalmol 1986;101:429-33.

Anon. Disposable extended-wear contact lenses (Editorial). Lancet 1988;1:1437.

Anon. Soft contact lenses. Med Lett Drugs Ther 1990;32:69-70.

Baldone JA, Kaufman HE. Extended wear contact lenses (Editorial). Ann Ophthamol 1983;15:595-96.

Barr J. Extended wear with minimal corneal compromise. Int Contact Lens Clin 1984;11:10-15.

Baum J, Barza M. Pseudomonas keratitis and extended-wear soft contact lenses (Editorial). Arch Ophthalmol 1990;108:663-64.

Bennett ES, Andrasko G. Facing the hard facts. Rev Optom 1985;122: 37-44.

Binder PS. Myopic extended wear with the Hydrocurve II soft contact lens. Ophthalmology 1983;90:623-26.

Bruce AS, Brennan NA. Corneal pathophysiology with contact lens wear. Surv Ophthalmol 1990;35:25-58.

Cavanagh HD. Extended wear—what happened? CLAO J 1987;13:194.

Chalupa E, Swarbrick, HA, Holden BA, et al. Severe corneal infections associated with contact lens wear. Ophthalmology 1987;94:17-22.

Cohen EJ, Laibson PR, Arentsen JJ, et al. Corneal ulcers associated with cosmetic extended wear soft contact lenses. Ophthalmology 1987;94:109-14.

Coster DJ. Medical aspects of contact lens wear. Med J Aust 1984; 140:455-57.

Cuhna MC, Thomassen TS, Cohen EJ, et al. Complications associated with soft contact lens use. CLAO J 1987;13:107-11.

Dart JK, Badenoch PR. Bacterial adherence to contact lenses. CLAO J 1986;12:220-24.

Dart JK. Bacterial keratitis in contact lens users. BMJ 1987;295:959-60.

Dister RE, Harris MG. Legal consequences of the FDA's 7-day extended wear (Letter). J Am Optom Assoc 1990;61:212-14.

Donzis PB, Mondino BJ, Weissman BA, et al. Microbial contamination of contact lens care systems. Am J Ophthalmol 1987;1004:325.

Duran JA, Refojo MF, Gipson IK, et al. Pseudomonas attachment to new hydrogel contact lenses. Arch Ophthalmol 1987;105:106-09.

Erie JC, Nevitt MP, Hodge DO, et al. Incidence of ulcerative keratitis in a defined population from 1950 through 1988. Arch Ophthalmol 1993;11:1665-71.

Farkas P, Kassalow TW, Farkas B. Parts 1 and 2. Clinical overview of the management and fitting of the extended wear patient. J Am Optom Assoc 1981;52:187-92, 397-402.

Fonn D, Holden B. Rigid gas-permeable vs. hydrogel contact lenses for extended wear. Am J Optom Physiol Opt 1988;65:536-44.

Fontana F, Ghormley NR, Kame R, et al. Targeting extended wear trouble spots. Rev Optom 1986;123:33-48.

Franks WA, Adams GGW, Dart JKG, et al. Relative risks of different types of contact lenses. BMJ 1988;297:524-25.

Galentine PG, Cohen EJ, Laibson PR, et al. Cornea ulcers associated with contact lens wear. Arch Ophthalmol 1984;102:891-94.

Graham CM, Dart JKG, Buckley RJ. Extended wear hydrogel and daily wear hard contact lenses for aphakia—success and complications compared in a longitudinal study. Ophthalmology 1986;93:1489-94.

Hart DE, Shih K. Surface interactions on hydrogel extended wear contact lenses: microflora and microfauna. Am J Optom Physiol Opt 1987;64: 739-48.

Hirano J, Hirano M. Extended wear of our gas-permeable hard contact lenses. Contact Lens J 1989;17:213.

Holden BA, Mertz GW, McNally JJ. Corneal swelling response to contact lenses worn under extended wear conditions. Invest Ophthalmol Vis Sci 1983;24:218-26.

Holden BA, Sweeney DF, Vannas A, et al. Effects of long-term extended contact lens wear on the human cornea. Invest Ophthalmol Vis Sci 1985;26:1489-501.

Holden BA, Swarbrick HA, Sweeney DF, et al. Strategies for minimizing the ocular effects of extended contact lens wear—a statistical analysis. Am J Optom Physiol Opt 1987;64:781-89.

Koenig SB, Solomon JM, Hyndiuk RA, et al. Acanthamoeba keratitis associated with gas-permeable contact lens wear. Am J Ophthalmol 1987;103:832.

Lamer L. Extended wear contact lenses for myopes. A follow-up study of 400 cases. Ophthalmology 1983;90:156-61.

Lebow K. The Boston IV lens. Rev Optom 1985;122:65-71.

Levy B. Rigid gas-permeable lenses for extended wear—a 1-year clinical evaluation. Am J Optom Physiol Opt 1985;62:889-94.

Mandell RB, Liberman G. The paraperm lens. Rev Optom 1985; 122:75-76.

Martin NF, Kracher GP, Stark WJ, et al. Extended wear soft contact lenses for aphakic correction. Arch Ophthalmol 1983;101:39-41.

Mayo MS, Schlitzer RL, Ward MA, et al. Association of Pseudomonas and Serratia corneal ulcers with use of contaminated solutions. J Clin Microbiol 1987;25:1398-400.

Millodot M. Clinical evaluation of an extended wear lens. Int Contact Lens Clin 1984;11:16-20.

Nightingale SL. From the Food and Drug Administration. Maximum wearing time shortened for extended-wear lenses. JAMA 1989;262:1916.

Omerod LD, Smith RE. Contact lens-associated microbial keratitis. Arch Ophthalmol 1986;104:79-83.

Parsons MR, Holland EJ, Agapitos PJ. Nocardia asteroides keratitis associated with extended-wear soft contact lenses. Can J Ophthalmol 1989;24:120-22.

Piccolo MG. Soft lens extended wear. Rev Optom 1985;122:80-90.

Polse KA, Rivera RK, Bonanno J. Ocular effects of hard gas-permeable-lens extended wear. Am J Optom Physiol Opt 1988; 65:358-64.

Rosenfeld SI, Mandelbaum S, Corrent GF, et al. Granular epithelial keratopathy as an unusual manifestation of Pseudomonas keratitis associated with extended-wear soft contact lenses. Am J Ophthalmol 1990;109:17-22.

Schein OD, Buehler PO, Stamler JF, et al. Impact of overnight wear on the risk of contact lens-associated ulcerative keratitis. Arch Ophthalmol 1994;112:186-90.

Schein O, Hibberd P, Kenyon KR. Contact lens complications: incidental or epidemic? (Editorial) Am J Ophthalmol 1986;102:116-17.

Schein OD, Glynn RJ, Poggio EC, et al. Microbial Keratitis Study Group. The relative risk of ulcerative keratitis among users of daily-wear and extended-wear soft contact lenses. A case-control study. N Engl J Med 1989;321:773-78, 824-26.

Schwartz CA. Frequent replacement: it works for astigmats. Rev Optom 1994;(May):35-40.

Shovlin J. Why reconsider 7-day extended wear? Optom Manage 1993; (Feb):82.

Stapleton F, Dart JKG, Minassian D. Risk factors with contact lens related suppurative keratitis. CLAO J 1993;19:204-10.

Stenson S. Soft contact lenses and corneal infection (Editorial). Arch Ophthalmol 1986;104:1287-89.

Tomlinson A. The Airlens. Rev Optom 1985;122:57-60.

Vilforth JC. The Food and Drug Administration is requesting manufacturers of cosmetic extended-wear soft contact lenses to indicate a recommended wearing time in the product labeling (News). Arch Ophthalmol 1989;107:969.

Wilhelmus, KR. Review of clinical experience with microbial keratitis associated with contact lenses. CLAO J 1987;13:211-14.

Young G, Port M. Rigid gas-permeable extended wear: a comparative clinical study. Optom Vis Sci 1992;69:214-26.

Disposable Contact Lenses

Auran JD, Starr MB, Jakobiec FA. Acanthamoeba keratitis: a review of the literature. Cornea 1987;6:2-26.

Boshnick E. Why my patients prefer disposables. Contact Lens Spectrum 1993;8(10):31-34.

Boswell GJ, Ehlers WH, Luistro A, et al. A comparison of conventional and disposable extended wear contact lenses. CLAO J 1993;19:158-65.

Buehler PO, Schein OD, Stamler JF, et al. The increased risk of ulcerative keratitis among disposable soft contact lens users. Arch Ophthalmol 1992;110:1555-58.

Cohen EJ, Gonzalez C, Leavitt KG, et al. Corneal ulcers associated with contact lenses including experience with disposable lenses. CLAO J 1991;17:173-76.

Doren GS, Cohen EJ, Higgins SE, et al. Management of contact lens associated Acanthamoeba keratitis. CLAO J 1991;17:120-25.

Dornic DI, Wolf T, Dillon WH, et al. Acanthamoeba keratitis in soft contact lens wearers. J Am Optom Assoc 1987;58:482-86.

Dunn JP Jr, Mondino BJ, Weissman BA, et al. Corneal ulcers associated with disposable hydrogel contact lenses. Am J Ophthalmol 1989; 108:113-17.

Farris RL. Extended wear contact lenses: boon or bane? CLAO J 1994; 20:73-77.

Ficker L, Hunter P, Seal D, et al. Acanthamoeba keratitis occurring with disposable contact lens wear (Letter). Am J Ophthalmol 1989;108:453.

Gellatly KW. Disposable contact lenses: a clinical performance review. Can J Optom 1993;55:166-73.

Heidemann DG, Verdier DD, Dunn SP, et al. Acanthamoeba keratitis associated with disposable contact lenses. Am J Ophthalmol 1990; 110:630-34.

International Committee on Contact Lenses. Contact lens maintenance systems. Int Contact Lens Clin 1992;19:153-56.

John T. How safe are disposable soft contact lenses? Am J Ophthalmol 1991;111:766-68.

John T, Desai D, Sahm D. Adherence of Acanthamoeba castellani cysts and trophozoites to unworn soft contact lenses. Am J Ophthalmol 1989;108:658-64.

Kame RT, Farkas B, Lane I, et al. Patient response to disposable contact lenses worn on a daily disposable regimen. Contact Lens Spectrum 1993;8(6):45-49.

Kaye DB, Hayashi MN, Schenkein JB. A disposable contact lens program: a preliminary report. CLAO J 1988;14:33-37.

Kershner RM. Infectious corneal ulcer with over extended wearing of disposable contact lenses (Letter). JAMA 1989;261:3549-50.

Killingsworth DW, Stern GA. Pseudomonas keratitis associated with the use of disposable soft contact lenses. Arch Ophthalmol 1989; 107:795-96.

Kotow M, Holden BA, Grant T. The value of regular replacement of low water content contact lenses for extended wear. J Am Optom Assoc 1987;58:461-64.

Larkin DFP, Kilvington S, Easty DL. Contamination of contact lens storage cases by Acanthamoeba and bacteria. Br J Ophthalmol 1990; 74:233-35.

Levy B. Complications of rigid gas permeable lenses for extended wear. Optom Vis Sci 1991;68:624-28.

MacRae S, Heerman C, Stulting RD, et al. Corneal ulcer and adverse reaction rates in premarket contact lens studies. Am J Ophthalmol 1991; 111:457-65.

Marshall EC. Disposable vs. non-disposable contact lenses—the relative risk of ocular infection. J Am Optom Assoc 1992;63:28-34.

Marshall EC, Begley CG, Nguyen CHD. Frequency of complications among wearers of disposable and conventional soft contact lenses. Int Contact Lens Clin 1992;19:55-60.

Matthews TD, Fraser DG, Minassian DC, et al. Risks of keratitis and patterns of use with disposable contact lenses. Arch Ophthalmol 1992;110:1559-62.

Mertz PHV, Bouchard CS, Mathers WD, et al. Corneal infiltrates associated with disposable extended wear soft contact lenses: a report of nine cases. CLAO J 1990;16:269-72.

Moore MB. Parasitic infections. In: Kaufman HE, Barron BA, McDonald MB, et al, eds. The Cornea. New York: Churchill Livingstone, 1988: 271-79.

Parker WT, Wong SK. Keratitis associated with disposable soft contact lenses. Am J Ophthalmol 1989;107:195.

Poggio EC, Abelson MB. Complications and symptoms with disposable daily wear contact lenses and conventional soft daily wear contact lenses. CLAO J 1993;19:95-102.

Rabinovitch J, Fook TC, Hunter WS, et al. Acanthamoeba keratitis in a soft-contact-lens wearer. Can J Ophthalmol 1990;25:25-28.

Rabinowitz SM, Pflugfelder SC, Goldberg M. Disposable extended-wear contact lens-related keratitis (Case report). Arch Ophthalmol 1989;107:1121.

Serdahl CL, Mannis MJ, Shapiro DR, et al. Infiltrative keratitis associated with disposable soft contact lenses (Case reports). Arch Ophthalmol 1989;107:322-23.

Shovlin JP. Who needs one-day disposables? Rev Optom 1993;(Nov):89.

White G Jr, Thiese SM, Olafsson HE, et al. Disposable contact lenses. Prac Optom 1991;2:144-46.

Contact Lenses and Drugs—Oral Contraceptives

Caron GA. Contact lenses and oral contraceptives (Letter). BMJ 1966; 1:980.

Chizek DJ, Franceschetti AT. Oral contraceptives: their side effects and ophthalmological manifestations. Surv Ophthalmol 1969;14:90-105.

De Vries Reilingh A, Reiners H, Van Bijsterveld OP. Contact lens tolerance and oral contraceptives. Ann Ophthalmol 1978;10:947-52.

Dixon JM. Twenty years and twenty thousand contact lens patients. Trans Am Ophthalmol Soc 1981;79:64-73.

Goldberg JB. A commentary on oral contraceptive therapy and contact lens wear. J Am Optom Assoc 1970;41:237-41.

Guyton AC. Basic Human Physiology: Normal Function and Mechanisms of Disease. Toronto: Saunders, 1977:242, 343-51, 856-66.

Kaufman A. The effects of contraceptives on contact lens performance. Contact Lens J 1980;6:15-18.

Koetting RA. The influence of oral contraceptives on contact lens wear. Am J Optom 1966;43:268-74.

Manchester PJ Jr. Hydration of the cornea. Trans Am Ophthalmol Soc 1970;68:427-61.

Petursson GJ, Fraunfelder FT, Meyer SM. Pharmacology of ocular drugs. Oral contraceptives. Ophthalmology 1981;88:368-71.

Reid IS. Prenatal sex-hormone exposure and congenital limb-reduction defects (Letter). Lancet 1976;2:373.

Ruben M. Contact lenses and oral contraceptives (Letter). BMJ 1966; 1:1110.

Sabell AG. Oral contraceptives and the contact lens wearer. Br J Physiol Opt 1970;25:127-37.

Sarwar M. Contact lenses and oral contraceptives (Letter). BMJ 1966; 1:1235.

Contact Lenses and Drugs—Ophthalmics

Anon. Contact lens questions and answers. Fading away. Rev Optom 1985;122:89.

Fraunfelder FT. Drug-induced Ocular Side Effects and Drug Interactions. Philadelphia: Lea & Febiger, 1982:251.

Garber JM. "Film" solution (Letter). Contact Lens Forum 1980;(Sept):15.

Krezanoski JZ. Topical medications. Int Ophthalmol Clin 1981; 21:173-76.

Lea SJH, Loades J, Rubinstein MP. The interaction between hydrogel lenses and sodium fluorescein. Theoretical and practical considerations. Acta Ophthalmol (Copenh) 1989;67:441-46.

Miller D, Brooks SM, Mobilia E. Adenochrome staining of soft contact lenses. Ann Ophthalmol 1976;8:65-67.

Miranda MN, Garcia-Castineiras S. Effects of pH and some common topical ophthalmic medications on the contact lens Permalens. CLAO J 1983;9:43-48.

Sugar J. Adenochrome pigmentation of hydrophilic lenses. Arch Ophthalmol 1974;91:11-12.

Contact Lenses and Drugs—Systemic Medications

Aucamp A. Drug excretion in human tears and its meaning for contact lens wearers. South Afr Optom 1980;39:128-36.

Barber JC. Management of the patient with dry eyes. Contact Intraoc Lens Med J 1977;3:10-15.

Bergmanson JPG, Rios R. Adverse reaction to painkiller in hydrogel lens wear. J Am Optom Assoc 1981;52:257-58.

Chang FW. The possible adverse effects of over-the-counter medications on the contact lens wearer. J Am Optom Assoc 1977;48:319-23.

Farber AS. Ocular side effects of antihistamine-decongestant combinations. Am J Ophthalmol 1982;94:565.

Fraunfelder FT. Drug-induced Ocular Side Effects and Drug Interactions. Philadelphia: Lea & Febiger, 1982:88-97, 112-31, 165-70, 186-87, 190-94, 206-07, 297-305, 306-08, 311-15.

Garston M. When meds disrupt contact lens wear. Rev Optom 1993;(Apr):49-50.

Harris J, Jenkins P. Discoloration of soft contact lenses by rifampicin (Letter). Lancet 1985;2:1133.

Koffler BH, Lemp MA. The effect of an antihistamine (chlorpheniramine maleate) on tear production in humans. Ann Ophthalmol 1980; 12:217-19.

Lemp MA, Hamill JR Jr. Factors affecting tear film breakup in normal eyes. Arch Ophthalmol 1973;89:103-05.

Litovitz GL. Amitriptyline and contact lenses (Letter). J Clin Psychiatry 1984;45:188.

Lyons RW. Orange contact lenses from rifampin (Letter). N Engl J Med 1979;300:372-73.

Miller D. Systemic medications. Int Ophthalmol Clin 1981;21:177-83.

Onofrey B. The odd case of the blurry-eyed cruise passenger. Rev Optom 1991;(Oct):93.

Riley SA, Flegg PJ, Mandal BK. Contact lens staining due to sulphasalazine (Letter). Lancet 1986;1:972.

Simmerman JS. Contact lens fitting after Accutane treatment. Rev Optom 1985;122:102.

Troiano G. Amitriptyline and contact lenses (Letter). J Clin Psychiatry 1985;46:199.

Valentic JP, Leopold IH, Dea FJ. Excretion of salicylic acid into tears following oral administration of aspirin. Ophthalmology 1980; 87:815-20.

Contact Lenses and Drugs—Smoking

Stewart BV. Soft contact lens discoloration and the use of tobacco. Int Contact Lens Clin 1978;6:269-75.

Contact Lenses and Compliance

Adams CP Jr, Cohen EJ, Laibson PR, et al. Corneal ulcers in patients with cosmetic extended-wear contact lenses. Am J Ophthalmol 1983; 96:705-09.

Asbell PA, Dunn MJ, Schechter CB, et al. Compliance in the care of disposable contact lenses: the effect of patients' health beliefs. CLAO J 1993;19:150-52.

Bowden FW, Cohen E, Arentsen J, et al. Patterns of lens care practices and lens product contamination in contact lens associated microbial keratitis. CLAO J 1989;15:49-54.

Chun MW, Weissman BA. Compliance in contact lens care. Am J Optom Physiol Opt 1987;64:274-76.

Collins MJ, Carney LG. Patient compliance and its influence on contact lens wearing problems. Am J Optom Physiol Opt 1986;63:952-56.

Collins M, Coulson J, Shuley V, et al. Contamination of disinfection solution bottles used by contact lens wearers. CLAO J 1994;20:32-36.

Jones DB. Acanthamoeba—the ultimate opportunist? Am J Ophthalmol 1988;102:527-30.

Kleinstein R, Stone G. Helping patients to follow their treatment plans. J Am Optom Assoc 1978;49:1144-46.

Kanpolat A, Kalayci D, Arman D, et al. Contamination in contact lens care systems. CLAO J 1992;18:105-07.

Mayo MS, Cook WL, Schlitzer RL, et al. Antibiograms, serotypes, and plasmid profiles of Pseudomonas aeruginosa associated with corneal ulcers and contact lens wear. J Clin Microbiol 1986;24:372-76.

Sager DP, Lunsfor MJ, Stein JM, et al. ReNu system: a compliance study. Spectrum 1992;(Dec):39-44.

Sokol JL, Mier MG, Bloom S, et al. A study of patient compliance in a contact lens-wearing population. CLAO J 1990;16:209-13.

Stehr-Green JK, Barley TM, Visvesvara GS. The epidemiology of Acanthamoeba keratitis in the United States. Am J Ophthalmol 1989; 197:331-36.

Stehr-Green JK, Bailey TM, Brandt FH, et al. Acanthamoeba keratitis in soft contact lens wearers. A case-control study. JAMA 1987;258:57-60.

Trick LR. Patient compliance—don't count on it! J Am Optom Assoc 1993;64:264-70.

Turner FD, Gower LA, Stein JM, et al. Compliance and contact lens care: a new assessment method. Optom Vis Sci 1993;70:998-1004.

Anesthetics-Local

Brancaccio RR, Milburn PB, Silvi E. Iatrogenic contact dermatitis to proparacaine: an ophthalmic topical anesthetic. Cutis 1993;52(5): 296-98.

Duffin RM, Olson RJ. Tetracaine toxicity. Ann Ophthalmol 1984;16(9): 836-38.

Henkes HE, Waubke TN. Keratitis from abuse of corneal anaesthetics. Br J Ophthalmol 1978;62:62-65.

Kintner JC, Grossniklaus HE, Lass JH, et al. Infectious crystalline keratopathy associated with topical anesthetic abuse. Cornea 1990; 9(1):77-80.

Norden LC. Adverse reactions to topical ocular anesthetics. J Am Optom Assoc 1976;47(6):730-33.

Rosenwasser GO. Complications of topical ocular anesthetics. Int Ophthalmology Clin 1989;29(3):153-58.

Rosenwasser GO, Holland S, Pflugfelder SC, et al. Topical anesthetic abuse. Ophthalmol 1990; 97(8):967-72.

Zagelbaum BM, Tostanoski JR, Hochman MA, et al. Topical lidocaine and proparacaine abuse. Am J Emerg Med 1994;12(1):96-97.

Antihistamines

Abelson MB, Allansmith MR, Friedlaender MH. Effects of topically applied ocular decongestant and antihistamine. Am J Ophthalmol 1980; 90:254-57.

Abelson MB, Paradis A, George MA, et al. Effects of Vasocon-A in the allergen challenge model of acute allergic conjunctivitis. Arch Ophthalmol 1990;108(4):520-24.

Anon. Safety of terfenadine and astemizole. Med Lett Drugs Ther 1992; 34(863):9.

Estelle F, Simons R, Simons KJ. Pharmacokinetic optimisation of histamine H1-receptor antagonist therapy. Clin Pharmacokinet 1991; 21(5):372-93.

Miller J, Wolf EH. Antazoline phosphate and naphazoline hydrochloride, singly and in combination for the treatment of allergic conjunctivitis; a controlled, double-blind clinical trial. Ann Allergy 1975;35(1):81-86.

Artificial Tears

Doughty M. What is really new and where do we go from here for dry and irritated eyes? Optom Vis Sc 1990;67(7):567-71.

Gilbard JP, Rossi SR, Heyda KG, et al. Stimulation of tear secretion and treatment of dry-eye disease with 3-isobutyl-1-methylxanthine. Arch Ophthalmol 1991; 109(5):672-76.

Gilbard JP, Farris RL. New concepts in the therapy of keratoconjunctivitis sicca. In: Srinivasan D, ed. Ocular Therapeutics. New York: Masson Publishers, 1980:213-17.

Gilbard JP, Kenyon KR. Tear diluents in the treatment of keratoconjunctivitis sicca. Ophthalmology 1985;92(5):646-50.

Gobbels M, Spitznas M. Influence of artificial tears on corneal epithelium in dry-eye syndrome. Graefes Arch Clin Exp Ophthalmol 1989; 227(2):139-41.

Holly FJ. Artificial tear formulations. Int Ophthalmol Clin 1980;20(3): 171-184.

Holly FJ. Diagnostic methods and treatment modalities of dry eye conditions. Int Ophthalmol 1993;17:113-25.

Lamberts DW, Potter DE. Clinical Ophthalmic Pharmacology. Boston: Little, Brown, 1987.

Lemp MA, Goldberg M, Robby MR. The effect of tear substitutes on tear film break-up time. Invest Ophthalmol 1975;14(3):255-58.

Lemp MA. Design and development of an artificial tear. Paper presented at 80th annual meeting American Academy of Ophthalmology and Otolaryngology. Dallas, 1975;21:5.

Limberg MB. Topical application of hyaluronic acid and chondroitin sulfate in the treatment of dry eyes. Am J Ophthalmol 1987;103(2): 194-97.

Liotet S, Van Bijsterveld OP, Kogbe O, et al. A new hypothesis on tear film stability. Ophthalmologica 1987;195(3):119-24.

Mauger TF, Craig EL, eds. Haveners Ocular Pharmacology. St. Louis: Mosby, 1994.

Motolko M, Breslin CW. The effect of pH and osmolarity on the ability to tolerate artificial tears. Am J Ophthalmol 1981;1:781-84.

Moudgil SS, Khurana AK, Singh M, et al. Effect of methylcellulose on tear film break-up-time in health and disease. Acta Ophthalmologica 1987; 65(4):397-99.

Nelson JD, Farris RL. Sodium hyaluronate and polyvinyl alcohol artificial tear preparations. Arch Ophthalmol 1988;106(4):484-87.

Prakash UBS, Rosenow EC. Pulmonary complications from ophthalmic preparations. Mayo Clin Proc 1990;65(4):521-29.

Rieger G. Contrast sensitivity in patients with keratoconjunctivitis sicca before and after artificial tear application. Graefes Arch Clin Exp Ophthalmol 1993;231:577-79.

Rieger G. Lipid-containing eyedrops: a step closer to natural tears. Ophthalmologica 1990;201(4):206-12.

Versura P. Dry eye before and after therapy with hydroxypropyl methylcellulose. Ophthalmologica 1989;198(3):152-62.

Wright P, Cooper M, Gilvarry AM. Effect of osmolarity of artificial tear drops on relief of dry eye symptoms: BJ6 and beyond. Br J Ophthalmol 1987;71(2):161-64.

Wright P. Other forms of treatment of dry eyes. Trans Ophthalmol Soc U K 1985;104:497-98.

Decongestants

Anon. Babies' blood pressure raised by eye drops. BMJ 1974;1:2-3.

Fraunfelder FT. Drug-induced Ocular Side Effects and Drug Interactions. Philadelphia: Lea & Febiger, 1989.

Hugues FC, Le Jeunne C. Systemic and local tolerability of ophthalmic drug formulations—an update (rev). Drug Safety 1993;8(5):365-80.

Mindlin RL. Accidental poisoning from tetrahydrozoline eyedrops (Letter). N Engl J Med 1966;275:112.

Patton TF, Robinson JR. Pediatric dosing considerations in ophthalmology. J Pediatr Ophthalmol 1976;13(3):171-78.

Rumelt MB. Blindness from misuse of over-the-counter eye medications. Ann Ophthalmol 1988;20(1):26-30.

Semla TP, Beizer JL, Higbee MD. Geriatric Dosage Handbook. Ohio: Lexi-Comp, 1993.

Preservatives

Burstein NL. The effects of topical drug and preservatives on the tears and corneal epithelium of dry eye. Trans Ophthalmol Soc U K 1985; 104:402-09.

Lemp MA, Zimmerman LE. Toxic endothelial degeneration in ocular surface disease treated with topical medications containing benzalkonium chloride. Am J Ophthalmol 1988;105(6):670-73.

Mullen W, Shepherd W, Labovitz J. Ophthalmic preservatives and vehicles. Surv Ophthalmol 1973;17(6):469-93.

Stern GA, Killingsworth DW. Complications of topical antimicrobial agents. Int Ophthalmol Clin 1989;29(3):137-42.

Tan B. Hypersensitivity and allergic reactions to ophthalmic drugs. Aust J Optom 1974;57:114-21.

Tosti A, Tosti G. Thimerosal: a hidden allergen in ophthalmology. Contact Dermatitis 1988;18(5):268-73.

Formulations

Feldman EG, ed. Handbook of Nonprescription Drugs. Washington: American Pharmaceutical Association, 1991.

Routine Care of Contact Lenses

Anon. Contact lens care: no easy solutions. Rev Optom 1980;117:24-25.

Anon. Drugstores take their cue from doctors. Rev Optom 1994;(Feb):9.

Gordon K. A pharmacist's guide through the complexities of contact lens care. Part II. Drug Merch 1981;62:36-40.

Smith RE, MacRae SM. Contact lenses—convenience and complications (Editorial). N Engl J Med 1989;321:824-26.

Cleaning Solutions

Anon. Contact lens questions and answers. All in good order. Rev Optom 1986;123:77.

Arons IJ. Your guide to contact lens care products. Contact Lens Forum 1978;(Aug):49-55.

Bailey NJ. Contact lens coating: the effect on service life. J Am Optom Assoc 1975;46:214-18.

Bergenske P. Enzymatic cleaning of silicone co-polymer rigid lenses. Am J Optom Physiol Opt 1983;60:540-41.

Butrus SI, Klotz SA. Contact lens surface deposits increase the adhesion of Pseudomonas aeruginosa. Curr Eye Res 1990;9:717-24.

Clements L. Soft lens spoilage. Contact Lens J 1980;6:5-14.

Eriksen S. Cleaning hydrophilic contact lenses: an overview. Ann Ophthalmol 1975;7:1223-32.

Farkas P, Kassalow TW, Farkas B. The use of enzyme tablets to control grade III GPC with PMMA lenses. J Am Optom Assoc 1984;55:836-37.

Feldman GL, Bailey WR. Clinical experiences with chemical vs. thermal disinfection of hydrophilic lenses. Contact Lens J 1974;8:17-20.

Fontana FD, Meier GD, Becherer D. Opti-Clean for hydrophilic lenses. Contact Lens Forum 1982;(Nov):57-65.

Fowler SA, Korb DR, Finnemore VM, et al. Surface deposits on worn hard contact lenses. Arch Ophthalmol 1984;102:757-59.

Fowler SA, Allansmith MR. The surface of the continuously worn contact lens. Arch Ophthalmol 1980;98:1233-36.

Grosvenor TP. Contact Lens Theory and Practice. Chicago: Professional Press, 1963:236-46.

Hathaway RA, Lowther GE. Soft lens cleaners: their effectiveness in removing deposits. J Am Optom Assoc 1978;48:259-66.

Houlsby RD, Ghajar M, Chavez G. Microbiological evaluation of soft contact lens disinfecting solutions. J Am Optom Assoc 1984;55:205-11.

Jones RA. Assistant product manager, Personal Products Division, Bausch and Lomb. (Personal communication to D. Wing, author) 1991, Sept 10.

Jose JG, Polse KA. Optometric Pharmacology. Orlando: Grune & Stratton, 1984:69-87.

Josephson JE, Haber R, Pope CA, et al. Clinical evaluation of a new cleaner for hard and soft lenses. Can J Optom 1981;43(suppl):179-85.

Kilvington S, Larkin DFP. Acanthamoeba adherence to contact lenses and removal by cleaning agents. Eye 1990;4(Pt 4):589-93.

Kleist F, Thorson JC. How effective are soft lens cleaners? Rev Optom 1978;115:43-49.

Koetting RA. What improved cleaning techniques can do. Contact Lens Forum 1978;(Mar):33-37.

Korb DR, Greiner JV, Finnemore VM, et al. Treatment of contact lenses with papain. Increase in wearing time in keratoconic patients with papillary conjunctivitis. Arch Ophthalmol 1983;101:48-50.

Missotten L, Maudgal PC, Houttequiet I. Surface deterioration of soft contact lenses. Contact Intraocul Lens Med J 1981;7:27-38.

Myers RI, Larsen DW, Tsao M, et al. Quantity of protein deposited on hydrogel contact lenses and its relation to visible protein deposits. Optom Vis Sci 1991;68:776-82.

Poggio EC, Glynn RJ, Schein OD, et al. The incidence of ulcerative keratitis among users of daily-wear and extended-wear soft contact lenses. N Engl J Med 1989;321:779-83.

Reynolds JEF, ed. Martindale: The Extra Pharmacopoeia. London: Pharmaceutical Press, 1982:370. (A newer edition is available)***

Sibley MJ, Shih KL, Hu JC. The microbiological benefit of cleaning and rinsing contact lenses. Int Contact Lens Clin 1985;12:235-42.

Sibley MJ. Cleaning solutions for contact lenses. Int Contact Lens Clin 1982;9:291-94.

Stein H, Harrison K. The safety and effectiveness of Polyclens—an all purpose cleaner for hydrophilic soft contact lenses. CLAO J 1983;9:39-42.

Tsuda S, Ando N, Anan N. Fitting and analysis of the Menicon soft lens—part 1. Int Contact Lens Clin 1977;4:55-66.

Isopropyl Alcohol

Ghajar M, Houlsby RD, Chavez G. Microbiological evaluation of Mira-Flow. J Am Optom Assoc 1989;60:592-95.

Inns HDE. Soft contact lenses and solutions in Canada. Can J Optom 1980;42:27-37.

Lowther GE, Hilbert JA. Deposits on hydrophilic lenses: differential appearance and clinical causes. Am J Optom Physiol Opt 1975;52: 687-92.

Ruben M. Ocular pathogens and contact lens hygiene. In: Ruben M, ed. Soft Contact Lenses: Clinical and Applied Technology. Toronto: J Wiley & Sons, 1978:335-47.

Unorthodox Cleaners

Diefenbach CB, Seibert CK, Davis LJ. Analysis of two "home remedy" contact lens cleaners. J Am Optom Assoc 1988;59:518-21.

Hess RJ, Kneisser G, Fukushima A, et al. Soft contact lens cleaning: a scanning electron microscopic study. Contact Intraocul Lens Med J 1982;8:23-28.

Lutzi D. Contact lens solution compatibility. Contact Lens J 1980;6:2-4.

To K. Artificial tears or lens cleaner. Am J Ophthalmol 1989;108:610.

Enzymes

Allansmith MR, Korb DR, Greiner JV, et al. Giant papillary conjunctivitis in contact lens wearers. Am J Ophthalmol 1977;83:697-708.

Allen K, Bui C, Grosvenor T. Is it necessary to enzyme-clean programmed replacement soft lenses for daily wear? Int Contact Lens Clin 1992; 19:205-09.

Aswad MI, John T, Barza M, et al. Bacterial adherence to extended wear soft contact lenses. Ophthalmology 1990;97:296-302.

Baines MG, Cai F, Backman HA. Adsorption and removal of protein bound to hydrogel contact lenses. Optom Vis Sci 1990;67:807-10.

Begley CG, Paragina S, Sporn A. An analysis of contact lens enzyme cleaners. J Am Optom Assoc 1990;61:190-94.

Bellemare F. Compatibility of enzymatic cleaning with cold contact lens disinfection. Int Contact Lens Clin 1979;6:219-22.

Bernstein DI, Gallagher JS, Grad M, et al. Local ocular anaphylaxis to papain enzyme contained in a contact lens cleansing solution. J Allergy Clin Immunol 1984;74:258-60.

Bosmann HB, Gutheil RL, Anderson JA. Residual enzyme activity on soft contact lenses and its inhibition by tears. Int Contact Lens Clin 1980;7:156-61.

Breen W, Fontana F, Hansen D, et al. Clinical comparison of pancreatin-based and subtilisin-based enzymatic cleaners. Contact Lens Forum 1990;15:32-38.

Davis RL. Animal versus plant enzyme. Int Contact Lens Clin 1983;10: 277-84.

Fowler SA, Allansmith MR. The effect of cleaning soft contact lenses: a scanning electron microscopic study. Arch Ophthalmol 1981;99: 1382-86.

Gold RM, Kaplan AI, Orenstein J. Reducing failure in cold disinfection systems. Contact Lens Forum 1979;(Dec):57-65.

Gold RM, Orenstein J. Surfactant cleaners vs the enzyme cleaner. Contact Lens Forum 1980;(Jan):39-40.

Hill RM, Goings J. Enhancing the enzyme action. Contact Lens Forum 1980;(Sept):53-55.

Kleist FD. Soft lens cleaners compared. Contact Lens Forum 1980; (Aug):47-53.

Krezanoski JZ. Contact lens products. J Am Pharm Assoc 1970;10:13-18.

Lieblein JS. How important is enzymatic cleaning? An in-office evaluation. Int Contact Lens Clin 1979;6:151-53.

Morgan JF. Maintenance and care of soft lenses. In: Ruben M, ed. Soft Contact Lenses: Clinical and Applied Technology. Toronto: J Wiley & Sons, 1978:285-90.

Sibley MJ. Cleaning solutions for contact lenses. Contact Lens Clin 1982;9:291-94.

Stern GA, Zam ZS. The pathogenesis of contact lens-associated Pseudomonas aeruginosa corneal ulceration: I. The effect of contact lens coatings on adherence of Pseudomonas aeruginosa to soft contact lenses. Cornea 1986;5:41-45.

Disinfection

Ernst RR. Sterilization by heat. In: Block SS, ed. Disinfection, Sterilization and Preservation. Philadelphia: Lea & Febiger, 1977:481-521.

McLaughlin WR, Hallberg KB, Tuovinen OH. Chemical inactivation of microorganisms on rigid gas permeable contact lenses. Optom Vis Sci 1991;68:721-27.

Sibley MJ. Disinfection solutions. Int Ophthalmol Clin 1981;21:237-47.

Organomercurials

Cioletti KR. Determination of thimerosal content in contact lens polymers. Int Contact Lens Clin 1980;7:3-7.

Connor CG, Hopkins SL, Salisbury RD. Effectivity of contact lens disinfection systems against Acanthamoeba culbertsoni. Optom Vis Sci 1991;68:138-41.

Harrison DP. Thimerosal and anterior crystalline lens vacuoles. Rev Optom 1985;122:55-56.

Harvey SC. Antiseptics and disinfectants; fungicides; ectoparasiticides. In: Gilman AG, Goodman LS, Gilman A, eds. Goodman and Gilman's The Pharmacological Basis of Therapeutics. New York: Macmillan, 1980: 964-87.

Johnsson J, Nygren B, Sjogren E. Disinfection of soft contact lenses in liquid. Contact Lens J 1978;6:3-10.

Kleist F. Appearance and nature of hydrophilic contact lens deposits—part 1: protein and other organic deposits. Int Contact Lens Clin 1979;6:120-30.

Kleist F. Appearance and nature of hydrophilic contact lens deposits—part 2: inorganic deposits. Int Contact Lens Clin 1979;6:177-86.

Lieblein JS. Overview of soft contact lens hygiene. Rev Optom 1978;15:29-32.

Ludwig IH, Meisler DM, Rutherford I, et al. Susceptibility of Acanthamoeba to soft contact lens disinfection systems. Invest Ophthalmol Vis Sci 1986;27:626-28.

McBride RJ, Mackie MAL. Evaluation of the antibacterial activity of contact lens solutions. J Pharm Pharmacol 1974;26:899-900.

Morgan JF. Evaluation of a cleaning agent for hydrophilic contact lenses. Can J Ophthalmol 1975;10:214-17.

Norton DA, Davies DJG, Richards NE, et al. The antimicrobial efficiencies of contact lens solutions. J Pharm Pharmacol 1974;26:841-46.

Refojo MF. Reversible binding of chlorhexidine gluconate to hydrogel contact lenses. Contact Intraocul Lens Med J 1976;2:47-56.

Sibley MJ, Yung G. A technique for the determination of chemical binding to soft contact lenses. Am J Optom 1973;50:710-14.

Stewart-Jones JH, Hopkins GA, Phillips AJ. Drugs and solutions in contact lens practice and related microbiology. In: Stone J, Phillips AJ, eds. Contact Lenses: A Textbook for Practitioners and Students. London: Butterworths, 1980:59-90, 365-75.

Wechsler S, George NC. Disinfection of hydrophilic lenses. J Am Optom Assoc 1981;52:179-86.

Zand LM. Review: the effect of nontherapeutic ophthalmic preparations on the cornea and tear film. Aust J Optom 1981;64:44-70.

EDTA

Anon. Contact lens questions and answers. Read the label. Rev Optom 1986;123:61.

Anon. AMA Drug Evaluations. New York: J Wiley & Sons, 1980:402-03.

Dabezies OH. Contact lens hygiene: past, present and future. Contact Lens Med Bull 1979;3:2-15.

Kleist FD. Prevention of inorganic deposits on hydrophilic contact lenses. Int Contact Lens Clin 1981;8:44-47.

Lemp MA. Bandage lenses and the use of topical solutions containing preservatives. Ann Ophthalmol 1978;10:1319-21.

Phillips AJ. Contact lens solutions. Contact Lens J 1977;6:3-23.

Snyder AC, Hill RM, Bailey NJ. Home sterilization: fact or fiction. Contact Lens Forum 1977;(Feb):41-43.

Lens Storage

Benjamin WJ, Hill RM. Ultra-thins: the case for continuous care. J Am Optom Assoc 1980;51:277-79.

Simmons PA, Edrington TB, Hsieh L, et al. Bacterial contamination rate of soft contact lens cases. Int Contact Lens Clin 1991;18:188-91.

Chemical Disinfection Products

Anger CB, Ambrus KJ, Stoecker J, et al. Antimicrobial efficacy of hydrogen peroxide for contact lens disinfection. Contact Lens Spectrum 1990;5(11):46-51.

Anon. Contact lens questions and answers. Generic peroxide. Rev Optom 1986;123:77.

Anon. Doctors go "cold." Rev Optom 1984;121:28.

Bass SJ. When parasites take up residence in the eye. Rev Optom 1993;(Oct):61-69.

Beattie AM, Slomovic AR, Rootman DS, et al. Acanthamoeba keratitis with two species of Acanthamoeba. Can J Opthalmol 1990;25:260-62.

Billig H, Bailey N, Fleischman W, et al. A new, rapid hydrogen peroxide system for contact lens disinfection. CLAO J 1984;10:341-45.

Conn H, Langer R. Iodine disinfection of hydrophilic contact lenses. Ann Ophthalmol 1981;13:361-64.

Courtney RC, Jarantino N, Brown P. Clinical safety and acceptability of a catalase tablet for hydrogen peroxide neutralization. Int Contact Lens Clin 1990;17:67-73.

Epstein AB, Freedman JM. Keratitis associated with hydrogen peroxide disinfection in soft lens wearers. Int Contact Lens Clin 1990;17:74-81.

Fonn D, Anderson R, Sorbara L, et al. A survey of optom contact lens use in Canada. Can J Optom 1990;52:90.

Garnett B. A clinical comparison of two soft lens chemical disinfection regimens. Optom Monthly 1982;73:260-63.

Gasset AR, Ramer RM, Katzin D. Hydrogen peroxide sterilization of hydrophilic contact lenses. Arch Ophthalmol 1975;93:412-15.

Gordon KD. The effect of oxidative disinfecting systems on tinted hydrogel lenses. Can J Optom 1989;51:175-76.

Gottardi W. Iodine and iodine compounds. In: Block SS, ed. Disinfection, Sterilization and Preservation. Philadelphia: Lea & Febiger, 1983: 183-96.

Gregoire J. A retrospective study using Barnes-Hind Soft Mate II system. Contact Lens Forum 1989;14:51.

Harris MG, Hernandez GN, Nuno DM. The pH of hydrogen peroxide disinfection systems over time. J Am Optom Assoc 1990;61:171-74.

Harris MG, Kirby JE, Tornatore CW, et al. Microwave disinfection of soft contact lenses. Optom Vis Sci 1989;66:82-86.

Harris MG. Practical considerations in the use of hydrogen peroxide disinfection systems. CLAO J 1990;16(1 suppl):S53-60.

Hart DE, Reindel W, Proskin HM, et al. Microbial contamination of hydrophilic contact lenses: quantitation and identification of microorganisms associated with contact lenses while on the eye. Optom Vis Sci 1993;70:185-91.

Holden B. A report card on hydrogen peroxide for contact lens disinfection. CLAO J 1990;16(1 suppl):S61-64.

Inns HDE. The Septicon system. Can J Optom 1979;41:144-46.

Inns HDE. The Griffin lens. Am J Optom 1973;50:977-83.

Janoff LE. The Septicon system: a review of pertinent scientific data. Int Contact Lens Clin 1984;11:274-82.

Josephson JE, Caffery BE. Exploring the sting. J Am Optom Assoc 1987;58:288-89.

Kaplan EN, Gundel RE, Sosale A, et al. Residual hydrogen peroxide as a function of platinum disc age. CLAO J 1992;18:149-54.

Knopf HLS. Reaction to hydrogen peroxide in a contact-lens wearer. Am J Ophthalmol 1984;97:796.

Koetting RA. Cosmetics. Int Ophthalmol Clin 1981;21:185-93.

Krezanoski JZ, Houlsby RD. A comparison of new hydrogen peroxide disinfection systems. J Am Optom Assoc 1988;59:193-97.

Krezanoski JZ. Where are we in the development of pharmaceutical products for soft (hydrophilic) lenses? Contacto 1976;20:12-16.

Lavery KT, Cowden JW, McDermott HML. Corneal toxicity secondary to hydrogen peroxide saturated contact lens (Letter). Arch Ophthalmol 1991;109:1352.

Levy B, Gross ML. Clinical evaluation of a chlorine based disinfection system for contact lenses. Can J Optom 1988;50:16.

Littlefield S, Bao N, Kreutzer P. Comparative antimicrobial capacity of soft contact lens storage solutions. Int Contact Lens Clin 1990;17:272-75.

Lowe R, Valias V, Brennan NA. Comparative efficacy of contact lens disinfection solutions. CLAO J 1992;18:34-40.

Lowther GE. Disinfection of extended wear lenses. Int Contact Lens Clin 1984;11:14.

Lutzi D, Callender M. Safety and efficacy of a new hydrogen peroxide disinfection system for soft lenses—In-a-Wink. Can J Optom 1985; 47:30-33.

Marques MS, Lluch S, Merindano MD, et al. Effect of different disinfecting contact lens solutions against ocular bacterial strain growth. Contact Lens J 1991;19(1):9-12.

McNally J. Clinical aspects of topical application of dilute hydrogen peroxide solutions. CLAO J 1990;16(suppl 1):S46-52.

Morgan JF. Complications associated with contact lens solutions. Ophthalmology 1979;86:1107-19.

Penley CA, Ahearn DG, Schlitzer RL, et al. Laboratory evaluation of chemical disinfection of soft contact lenses. II. Fungi as challenge organisms. Contact Intraocul Lens Med J 1981;7:196-204.

Penley CA, Schlitzer RL, Ahearn DG, et al. Laboratory evaluation of chemical disinfection of soft contact lenses. Contact Intraocul Lens Med J 1981;7:101-10.

Penley CA, Liabres C, Wilson LA, et al. Efficacy of hydrogen peroxide disinfection for soft contact lenses contaminated with fungi. CLAO J 1985;11:65-68.

Persico J. Keep the bugs out. Optom Manage 1993;(Feb):59-64.

Petricciani R, Krezanoski J. Preservative interaction with contact lenses. Contacto 1977;21:6-10.

Piccolo MG, Leach NE, Boltz RL. Rigid lens base curve stability upon hydrogen peroxide disinfection. Optom Vis Sci 1990;67:19-21.

Preschel N. A simple, effective method for sterilization of contact lens cases. Invest Ophthalmol Vis Sci 1992;33(suppl):938.

Reynolds JEF, ed. Martindale: The Extra Pharmacopoeia. London: Pharmaceutical Press, 1982:1232, 1292-93. (A newer edition is available)***

Sagan W, Schwaderer KN. A new cleaning technique for hydrophilic contact lenses. J Am Optom Assoc 1974;45:266-69.

Shih KL, Raad MK, Hu JC, et al. Disinfecting activities of non-peroxide soft contact lens cold disinfection solutions. CLAO J 1991;17:165-68.

Sibley MJ, Shih KL, Hu J. Evaluation of a new thimerosal-free 5-minute hydrogen peroxide disinfection lens care regimen. Can J Optom 1982;44(suppl):5-7.

Sibley MJ, Chu V. Understanding sorbic acid-preserved contact lens solutions. Int Contact Lens Clin 1984;11:531-42.

Sickler SG, Bao N, Littlefield SA. Comparative antimicrobial activity of three leading soft contact lens disinfection solutions. Int Contact Lens Clin 1992;19:19-24.

Silvany RE, Dougherty JM, McCulley JP. Effect of contact lens preservatives on Acanthamoeba. Ophthalmology 1991;98:854-57.

Silvany RE, Wood TS, Bowman RW, et al. The effect of contact lens solutions on two species of Acanthamoeba (Abstract). Invest Ophthalmol Vis Sci 1988;29(suppl):253.

Steel SA. Patient preference study compares top lens care systems. Contact Lens Spectrum 1990;5:56-59.

Tarantino N, Courtney RC, Lasswell LA. Simultaneous enzymatic cleaning and hydrogen peroxide disinfection of hydrogel lenses. CLAO J 1988;15:189-96.

Tse LSY, Callender MG, Charles AM. Antimicrobial effectiveness of some soft contact lens care systems. Am J Optom Physiol Opt 1987;64: 824-28.

Wardlaw JC, Sarver MD. Discoloration of hydrogel contact lenses under standard care regimens. Am J Optom Physiol Opt 1986;63:403-08.

Wickliffe B, Entrekin DN. Relation of pH to preservative effectiveness. II. Neutral and basic media. J Pharm Sci 1964;53:769-73.

Wilson LA, McNatt J, Reitschel R. Delayed hypersensitivity to thimerosal in soft contact lens wearers. Ophthalmology 1981;88:804-09.

Wilson LA, Sawant AD, Simmons RB, et al. Microbial contamination of contact lens storage cases and solutions. Am J Ophthalmol 1990;110: 193-98.

Allergic Reactions

Allansmith MR. Treatment of external diseases with immunological properties. Int Ophthalmol Clin 1973;13:193-210.

Anon. A three-eyed look at cold disinfection. Contact Lens Forum 1978;(Jul):21-35.

Anon. Symposium: how to solve flexible lens care problems. Contact Intraocul Lens Med J 1981;7:89-100.

Binder PS. Myopic extended wear with the Hydrocurve II soft contact lens. Ophthalmology 1983;90:623-26.

Binder PS, Rasmussen DM, Gordon M. Keratoconjunctivitis and soft contact lens solutions. Arch Ophthalmol 1981;99:87-90.

Callender M, Lutzi D. The incidence of adverse ocular reactions among soft contact lens wearers using chemical disinfection procedures. Can J Optom 1979;41:138-40.

Courtney RC, Lee JM. Predicting ocular intolerance of a contact lens solution by use of a filter system enhancing fluorescein staining detection. Int Contact Lens Clin 1982;9:302-10.

Coward B, Neumann R, Callendar M. Solution intolerance among users of 4 chemical soft lens regimens. Am J Physiol Opt 1984;61:523-27.

Crook TG, Freeman JJ. Reactions induced by the concurrent use of thimerosal and tetracycline. Am J Optom Physiol Opt 1983;60:759-61.

Dabezies OH, ed. Soft contact lens care—the state of the art. Minutes of a symposium held at the 1980 Contact Lens Association of Ophthalmologists meetings; 1980 January 10; Las Vegas, NV. Princeton: Communications Media for Education, 1980.

Fagedes H. The problem with thimerosal. Contact Lens Forum 1980;(Sept):45-49.

Fichman S, Baker VV, Horton HR. Iatrogenic red eyes in soft contact lens wearers. Int Contact Lens Clin 1978;5:20-24.

Greenberger MH. A chlorhexidine-free chemical regimen for hydrophilic contact lenses. Int Contact Lens Clin 1981;8:13-15.

Harrison DP. Contact lens wear problems: implications of penicillin allergy, diabetic relatives, and use of birth control pills. Am J Optom Physiol Opt 1984;61:674-78.

Josephson JE. The "multi-purge" procedure and its application for hydrophilic lens wearers utilizing preserved solutions. J Am Optom Assoc 1978;49:280-81.

Josephson JE. Hydrogel lens statistics drawn from private practice. Int Contact Lens Clin 1978;5:99-103.

Josephson JE, Caffery BE. Hydrogel lens solutions. Int Ophthalmol Clin 1981;21:163-71.

Kline LN, DeLuca TJ. Thermal vs chemical disinfection. Contact Lens Forum 1979;(Feb):28-31.

McMonnies CW. Allergic complications in contact lens wear. Int Contact Lens Clin 1978;5:182-89.

Molinari JF, Nash R, Badham D. Severe thimerosal hypersensitivity in soft contact lens wearers. Int Contact Lens Clin 1982;9:323-29.

Rahi AHS, Garner A. Immunopathology of the eye. London: Blackwell Scientific, 1976:4-5.

Rietschel RL, Wilson LA. Ocular inflammation in patients using soft contact lenses. Arch Dermatol 1982;118:147-49.

Robertson IF. Continuous-wear hydrophilic contact lenses versus intraocular lenses. Adv Ophthalmol 1978;37:150-55.

Roth HW. The etiology of ocular irritation in soft lens wearers: distribution in a large clinical sample. Contact Intraocul Lens Med J 1978;4:38-47.

Shank RA. Chemical disinfection. Contact Lens Forum 1979;(Oct):57-59.

van Ketel WG, Melzer-van Riemsdijk FA. Conjunctivitis due to soft lens solutions. Contact Dermatitis 1980;6:321-24.

Yamane SJ. Complex questions surround increased allergic reactions in wearers of soft contact lenses. Int Contact Lens Clin 1980;7:152-55.

Zadnik K. Severe allergic reaction to saline preserved with thimerosal. J Am Optom Assoc 1984;55:507-09.

Thermal Disinfection

Anon. FDA mail alert to 50,000 eye care providers on hazards of Acanthamoeba. AOA News 1989;28:4.

Bailey NJ. Cleaning of coated soft lenses. J Am Optom Assoc 1974;45:1049-52.

Bailey NJ. Making contact (Editorial). Contact Lens Forum 1979;(Nov):15.

Bailey NJ. Making contact (Editorial). Contact Lens Forum 1979;(Jun):21.

Bailey NJ. Where the salt has gone. Contact Lens Forum 1980;(Jan):19-23.

Bilbaut T, Gachon AM, Dastugue B. Deposits on soft contact lenses. Electrophoresis and scanning electron microscopic examinations. Exp Eye Res 1986;43(2):153-65.

Callender M, Lutzi D. Comparing the clinical findings of Soflens wearers using thermal and cold disinfection procedures. Int Contact Lens Clin 1978;5:119-23.

Carmichael CA. Heat or chemical disinfection: does it really matter? Rev Optom 1983;121(Aug):71-74.

Chandler JW. Biocompatibility of hydrogen peroxide in soft contact lens disinfection: antimicrobial activity vs. biocompatibility—the balance. CLAO J 1990;16(1 suppl):S43-45.

Dolman PJ, Dobrogowski MJ. Contact lens disinfection by ultraviolet light. Am J Ophthalmol 1989;108:665-69.

Donzis PB, Mondino BJ, Weissman BA. Bacillus keratitis associated with contaminated contact lens care systems. Am J Ophthalmol 1988;105:195-97.

Gold RM, Melman E. Salt tablets: what price economy? Contact Lens Forum 1981;(Aug):35-39.

Gordon KD. Disinfection efficacy of soft lens care systems. Prac Optom 1991;2:149-150.

Gottschalk-Katsev N, Weissman BA. Disinfection: choose your weapons wisely. Here's a simple guide to today's infection fighters. Rev Optom 1990;127:46-50.

Gritz DC, Lee TY, McDonnell PJ, et al. Ultraviolet radiation for the sterilization of contact lenses. CLAO J 1990;16:294-98.

Harris MG, Higa CK, Lacey LL, et al. The pH of aerosol saline solution. Optom Vis Sci 1990;67:84-88.

Harris MG, Rechberger J, Grant T, et al. In-office microwave disinfection of soft contact lenses. Optom Vis Sci 1990;67:129-32.

Hathaway R, Lowther CE. Appearance of hydrophilic lens deposits as related to chemical etiology. Int Contact Lens Clin 1976;3:27-35.

Hill RM. Escaping the sting. Int Contact Lens Clin 1979;6:43-45.

Hill RM. How "pure" are the waters? Int Contact Lens Clin 1981;8:33-34.

Hind HW. Contact lens solutions: yesterday, today, and tomorrow. Contact Lens Forum 1979;(Nov):17-27.

Houlsby RD, Ghajar M, Chavez G. Microbiological quality of water used by pharmaceutical manufacturers and soft lens wearers. Int Contact Lens Clin 1981;8:9-14.

Josephson JE, Caffery BE. The dangers of distilled water in contact lens maintenance. J Am Optom Assoc 1988;59:219-20.

Krezanoski JZ. Water and the care of soft contact lenses. Int Contact Lens Clin 1975;2:48-55.

Lowther GE, Hilbert JA. Deposits on hydrophilic lenses: differential appearance and clinical causes. Am J Optom Physiol Opt 1975;52:687-92.

Lowther GE. Hydrogel lens solutions (Editorial). Int Contact Lens Clin 1982;9:272-73.

Lowther G. Lens material—an overview. J Am Optom Assoc 1984;55:186-87.

Lubert GP, Caplan L. Comparing thermal and chemical disinfection systems for the etafilcon A 58% water content contact lens. Am J Optom Physiol Opt 1984;61:683-88.

MacRae SM, Cohen EJ, Andre M. Guidelines for safe contact lens wear. Am J Ophthalmol 1987;103:832-33.

Merindano MD, Marques MS, Lluch S, et al. Domestic microwave oven in contact lens disinfection. Contact Lens J 1990;18:241-46.

Phillips AJ. Selection of contact lens solutions. Ophthalmic Optician 1969;9:394-95.

Pitts RE, Krachmer JH. Evaluation of soft contact lens disinfection in the home environment. Arch Ophthalmol 1979;97:470-72.

Riedhammer TM, Falcetta JJ. Effects of long-term heat disinfection on Soflens (polymacon) contact lenses. J Am Optom Assoc 1980; 51:287-89.

Riordan-Eva P, Eykyn SJ, Muir MGK. Pseudomonas aeruginosa corneal ulcer associated with an aerosol can of preservative-free saline. Case report. Arch Ophthalmol 1988;106:1506.

Rohrer MD, Terry MA, Bulard RA, et al. Microwave sterilization of hydrophilic contact lenses. Am J Ophthalmol 1986;101:49-57.

Ruben M, Tripathi RC, Winder AF. Calcium disposition as a cause of spoilation of hydrophilic soft lenses. Br J Ophthalmol 1975;59:141-48.

Spizziri LJ. Stromal corneal changes due to preserved saline solution used in soft contact lens wear: report of a case. Ann Ophthalmol 1981;13:1277-78.

Sposato P. A "bouquet" of new solutions: take your pick. Contact Lens Forum 1981;(Aug):15-23.

Wilson LA, Sawant AD, Ahearn DG. Comparative efficacies of soft contact lens disinfectant solutions against microbial films in lens cases. Arch Ophthalmol 1991;109:1155-57.

Wilson LA, Schlitzer RL, Ahearn DG. Pseudomonas corneal ulcers associated with soft contact-lens wear. Am J Ophthalmol 1981;92:546-54.

Yamane SJ. Studies with a unit dose saline solution. Contact Lens Forum 1979;(Aug):91-95.

Wetting and Viscosity Agents

Anon. Contact lens questions and answers. Tracks of my tears. Rev Optom 1985;122:53.

Brennan NA, Efron N. Symptomatology of HEMA contact lens wear. Optom Vis Sci 1989;86:834-38.

Caffery BE, Josephson JE. Is there a better "comfort drop"? J Am Optom Assoc 1990;61:178-82.

Carney LG, Hill RM, Habenicht BL. Ageing lubricant solutions—a clinical comment. Contact Lens J 1990;18:157-58.

Efron N, Golding TR, Brennan NA. The effect of soft lens lubricants on symptoms and lens dehydration. CLAO J 1991;17:114-19.

Ghormley NR. Rewetting solutions for soft contact lenses (Editorial). Int Contact Lens Clin 1984;11:588.

Hill RM, Mauger TF. The solution label's phantom features. Contact Lens Forum 1981;(Apr):115-17.

Lemp MA, Holly FJ. Recent advances in ocular surface chemistry. Am J Optom 1970;47:669-72.

Maeda AY. Discomfort from drying with hydrogel contact lenses. Int Contact Lens Clin 1982;9:143-45.

Mauger TF, Hill RM. A key to solution effects? Contact Lens Forum 1982;(Apr):23-25.

Mauger TF, Hill RM. Solutions that soothe. Contact Lens Forum 1982;(Feb):75-77.

Poster MG. Optical efficacy of rewetting and lubricating solutions. Contact Lens Forum 1981;(Dec):25-31.

Zografi G. Interfacial phenomena. In: Osol A, ed. Remington's Pharmaceutical Sciences. Easton: Mack Publishing, 1980:253-65.

Multifunction Solutions

House HO, Leach NE, Edrington TB, et al. Contact lens cleaner efficacy: multipurpose versus single-purpose products. Int Contact Lens Clin 1991;18:238-45.

Lapierre M, Duplessis L, Zanga P. Single versus multi-product care systems: a comparison of cleaning efficacy. Can J Optom 1993;55:209-19.

Leisring J, Gill L. The clinical safety of a new generation chemical disinfecting agent. Spectrum 1990;(Oct):63-67.

Marquardt R, Roth HW, Laux U. Experiences with a new large diameter soft contact lens. Contact Lens J 1975;8:9-19.

Mulford MB, Houlsby RD, Langston JB, et al. Rigid lens care revisited. Contact Lens Forum 1980;(Sept):33-43.

Roth HW. Soft hydrophilic contact lenses: results of a long-term study. J Japan Contact Lens Soc 1979;21:18-21.

Roth HW, Roth-Wittig M. Multipurpose solutions for soft lens maintenance. Int Contact Lens Clin 1980;7:92-95.

Accessory Solutions

Shively CD. Accessory solutions in contact lens care and practice. In: Ruben M, ed. Soft Contact Lenses: Clinical and Applied Technology. Toronto: J Wiley & Sons, 1978:383-424.

Shovlin JP. Acanthamoeba keratitis in rigid lens wearers: the issue of tap water rinse. Int Contact Lens Clin 1990;19:47-49.

Weissman BA, Tari LA. A solution for the dry eye. Contact Lens Forum 1982;(Feb):5-7.

Buffers

Committee of revision. The United States Pharmacopeia. Rockville: United States Pharmacopeial Convention, 1980:1100-01.

Demas GN. pH consistency and stability of contact lens solutions. J Am Optom Assoc 1989;60:732-34.

Lamy PP, Shangraw RF. Physico-chemical aspects of ophthalmic and contact lens solutions. Am J Optom 1971;48:37-51.

MacKeen DG, Bulle K. Buffers and preservatives in contact lens solutions. Contacto 1977;21:31-36.

Troy G. Contact lens solutions: your first aid to a successful fit. Optom Manage 1975;11:49-75.

Preservatives

Burstein NL. Corneal cytotoxicity of topically applied drugs, vehicles and preservatives. Surv Ophthalmol 1980;25:15-30.

Dabezies OH. Soft contact lens hygiene. Contact Intraocul Lens Med J 1975;1:103-08.

Havener WH. Ocular Pharmacology. St Louis: Mosby, 1978:425-37.

MacKeen DL, Green K. Chlorhexidine kinetics of hydrophilic contact lenses. J Pharm Pharmacol 1978;30:678-82.

Mandell RB. Contact Lens Practice. Springfield: CC Thomas, 1981: 313-41.

Mondino BJ, Salamon SM, Zaidman GW. Allergic and toxic reactions of soft contact lens wearers. Surv Ophthalmol 1982;26:337-44.

Mondino BJ, Weissman BA, Farb MD, et al. Corneal ulcers associated with daily-wear and extended-wear contact lenses. Am J Ophthalmol 1986;102:58-65.

Rosenthal P, Chou MH, Salamore JC, et al. Quantitative analysis of chlorhexidine gluconate and benzalkonium chloride adsorption on silicone/acrylate polymers. CLAO J 1986;12:43-50.

Mixing Solutions

Shovlin J. Don't let patients "mix and match" solutions. Optom Manage 1994;(May):61.

Shovlin JP. Hard luck with enzymes and wetting solution. Rev Optom 1994;(Jan):115.

Sibley MJ, Shovlin JP. Are you having mixed reactions? Switching solutions can make for bad chemistry. Rev Optom 1990;127:52-56.

CHAPTER 10—First Aid Products

General

The Canadian Red Cross Society. First Aid: The Vital Link. 1st ed. St. Louis, MO: Mosby-Year Book, 1994.

Cooper DM. Wound assessment and evaluation of healing. In: Bryant RA, ed. Acute and Chronic Wounds: Nursing Management. 1st ed. St. Louis, MO: Mosby, 1992:69-90.

Doughty DB. Principles of wound healing and wound management. In: Bryant RA, ed. Acute and Chronic Wounds: Nursing Management. 1st ed. St. Louis, MO: Mosby, 1992:31-68.

McEvoy GK, Litvak K, Welsh OH, eds. AHFS 95. Drug Information. 37th ed. Bethesda, MD: American Society of Health-System Pharmacists, 1995.

Montgomery RL. Basic Anatomy for the Allied Health Professions. 1st ed. Baltimore, MD: Urban and Schwarzenberg, 1980:23-26.

Wilson JD, Braunwald E, Isselbacher KJ, eds. Harrison's Principles of Internal Medicine. 12th ed. New York: McGraw-Hill, 1991: 310-11, 339.

Minor Cuts and Wounds

Leaper D. Antiseptics and their effect on healthy tissue. Nurs Times 1986; May 28:45-47.

Lee D, Mavinil S. Home nursing care skin care program. Victoria, BC: Capital Regional District Health, Aug 1993.

McCreadie D. Penetrating wounds. Practitioner 1993;237:867-69.

Modic BM. Myths and facts...about chronic wound care. Nursing90 1990; Dec:68.

Rodeheaver G. Controversies in topical wound management. Wounds 1989;1(1):19-34.

Shur-Clens and SAF-Clens product monographs. Calgon-Vestal Laboratories, St. Louis, MO. July 1993.

Infection

Kahn RM, Goldstein EJ. Common bacterial skin infections. Postgrad Med 1993;93(6):175-82.

Mandell GL, Douglas GR, Bennett JE, eds. Principles and Practice of Infectious Diseases. 3rd ed. New York: Churchill Livingstone, 1990.

McCreadie D. Penetrating wounds. Practitioner 1993;237:867-69.

Ross EV, Baxter DL Jr. Widespread Candida folliculitis in a nontoxic patient. Cutis 1992;49(4):241-43.

Sanford JP, Gilbert DN, Gerberding JL. The Sanford Guide to Antimicrobial Therapy. 23rd ed. Dallas, Tex: Antimicrobial Therapy Inc., 1994.

Smith DJ, Thomas PD, Garner WL, et al. Burn wounds: infection and healing. Am J Surg 1994;167(1A) Suppl:46S-48S.

Williams RE, MacKie RM. The staphylococci. Importance of their control in the management of skin disease. Dermatologic Clinics 1993;11(1): 201-06.

Fungal Skin Infections

Bergus GR, Johnson JS. Superficial tinea infections. Am Fam Physician 1993;48(2):259-68.

Frieden IJ, Howard R. Tinea capitas: epidemiology, diagnosis, treatment, and control. J Am Acad Dermatol 1994;31(3):S42-S46.

Habif TP. Clinical Dermatology. A Color Guide to Diagnosis and Therapy. 2nd ed. St Louis, MO: Mosby, 1990: 301-39.

Hall JH, Lesher JL Jr. Superficial fungal infections. Pediatrician 1991; 18:224-32.

Hay RJ. Dermatophytosis and other superficial mycoses. In: Mandell GL, Douglas RG, Bennett JE, eds. Principles and Practice of Infectious Diseases. 3rd ed. New York: Churchill Livingstone, 1990:2017-34.

Howard R, Frieden IJ. Tinea capitis: new perspectives on an old disease. Semin Dermatol 1995;14(1):2-8.

Schwartz RA, Janniger CK. Pediatric dermatology: tinea capitis. Cutis 1995;55:29-33.

Travill L. New Nonprescription Antifungal Preparations. Pharmacy Home Study Program. 1st ed. Nepean, Ont: Travill Consulting, 1994:51-56.

Viral Skin Infections

Chan CY, Wallander KA. Diphenhydramine toxicity in three children with varicella-zoster infection. DICP 1991;25(2):130-32.

Habif TP. Clinical Dermatology. A Color Guide to Diagnosis and Therapy. 2nd ed. St Louis, MO: Mosby, 1990:285-90.

McGrath NE. Pediatric update. Children with chickenpox: emergency department care and teaching. J Emerg Nursing 1992;18(4):353-54.

Thompson DF. Diphenhydramine, topical—use in varicella infections. In: Drugdex Drug Consults. Oklahoma City, Okla: Micromedex, Sept 1990.

Burns

Baxter CR. Management of burn wounds. Dermatol Clin 1993; 11(4): 709-14.

Drueck C. Emergency department treatment of hand burns. Emerg Med Clin North Am 1993;11(3):797-809.

Peate WF. Outpatient management of burns. Am Fam Physician 1992;45(3):1321-30.

Punch JD, Smith DJ Jr, Robson MC. Hospital care of major burns. Postgrad Med 1989;85(1):205-15.

Smith DJ, Thomson PD, Garner WL, et al. Burn wounds: infection and healing. Am J Surg 1994;167(1A) Suppl:46S-48S.

Waitzman AA, Neligan PC. How to manage burns in primary care. Can Fam Physician 1993;39:2394-400.

Frostbite

The Canadian Red Cross Society. First Aid: The Vital Link. 1st ed. St. Louis, MO: Mosby-Year Book, 1994.

Drueck C. Emergency department treatment of hand burns. Emerg Med Clin North Am 1993;11(3):797-809.

Poisoning

Jawary D, Cameron PA, Dziukas L, et al. Drug overdose—reducing the load. Med J Aust 1992;156:343-46.

Krenzelok EP, Dunmire SM. Acute poisoning emergencies: resolving the gastric decontamination controversy. Postgrad Med 1992; 91(2): 179-86.

Kulig K. Current concepts: initial management of ingestions of toxic substances. N Engl J Med 1992;326(25):1677-81.

Phillips S, Gomez H, Brent J. Pediatric gastrointestinal decontamination in acute toxin ingestion. J Clin Pharmacol 1993;33:497-507.

Insect Bites And Stings

Couch P, Johnson CE. Prevention of Lyme disease. Am J Hosp Pharm 1992;49:1164-73.

Elgart GW. Insect bites and stings. Dermatol Clin 1990;8(2):230-36.

Freeman Kent DA, Willis GA, eds. The British Columbia Drug and Poison Information Centre Poison Management Manual. 3rd ed. Ottawa, Ont: Canadian Pharmaceutical Association, 1989:223-25.

Johnstone T, Deputy Medical Health Officer, Capital Regional District, Victoria, BC (personal communication). Lyme disease in Canada. March 1995.

Karch FE, Weintraub M. Drug therapy of itching. In: Drugdex Drug Consults. Denver, CO: Micromedex, May 1989.

Moffitt JE, Yakes AB, Stafford CT. Allergy to insect stings. Postgrad Med 1993;93(8):197-208.

Murdoch L, Duncan C, Edwards S, eds. Insect repellent use in children. Ontario College of Pharmacists Drug Information Centre Newsletter: New Drugs Drug News 1990(May-June);8(3).

Reisman RE. Stinging insect allergy. Med Clin North Am 1992; 76(4): 883-94.

Tortorice KL, Heim-Duthoy KL. Clinical features and treatment of Lyme disease. Pharmacotherapy 1989;9(6):363-71.

Anesthetics (Topical)

Anon. New OTC products. Am Pharm 1994;N834(2):37.

Anon. New OTC products. Am Pharm 1992;N832(2):32.

Continuing Education Highlights: Sulfonamide cross-allergenicity: answers to common questions. Vancouver, BC: College of Pharmacists of British Columbia, 1989(March, April, May);14(2):1-3.

Karch FE, Weintraub M. Drug therapy of itching. In: Drugdex Drug Consults. Denver, CO: Micromedex, May 1989.

McEvoy GK, Litvak K, eds. AHFS: Drug Information '94. 36th ed. Bethesda, MD: American Society of Hospital Pharmacists, 1994: 2331-35.

Reynold JEF, ed. Martindale: The Extra Pharmacopoeia. 29th ed. London: Pharmaceutical Press, 1989:1062-63.

Rocky Mountain Drug Consultation Centre. Topical medications—cross sensitization with systemic medications. In: Drugdex Drug Consults. Denver, CO: Micromedex, Mar 1987.

Schatz M. Adverse reactions to local anesthetics. Immunol Allergy Clin North Am 1992;12(3):585-609.

Thompson DF, Collier T. Emla cream use for topical anesthesia. In: Drugdex Drug Consults. Denver, CO: Micromedex, May 1993.

USP DI. Volume I. 13th ed. Rockville, MD: The United States Pharmacopeial Convention, 1993:144-49.

Antibiotics

Kucers A, Bennett N, Kemp R. The Use of Antibiotics: a Comprehensive Review with Clinical Emphasis. 4th ed. Philadelphia: Lipincott, 1987: 751-55.

Sanford JP, Gilbert DN, Gerberding JL. The Sanford Guide to Antimicrobial Therapy. 23rd ed. Dallas: Antimicrobial Therapy, 1994.

Suleman P, Manager Medical Information, Warner-Lambert (personal communication), 1995. Polysporin.

Antihistamines (Topical)

McGann KP, Pribanich S, Graham JH, et al. Diphenhydramine toxicity in a child with Varicella. A case report. J Fam Pract 1992;35(2):213-14.

Rocky Mountain Drug Consultation Centre. Topical medications—cross sensitization with systemic medications. In: Drugdex Drug Consults. Denver, CO: Micromedex, Mar 1987.

Sisca TS, Callahan AK. Topical antihistamines efficacy. In: Drugdex Drug Consults. Easton, MD: Micromedex, Aug 1987.

Thompson DF. Diphenhydramine, topical—use in Varicella infections. In: Drugdex Drug Consults. Oklahoma City, Okla: Micromedex, Sept 1990.

Other Antipruritics

AfterBite product information. Tender Corporation, Littleton, NH. Jan 1995.

Karch FE, Weintraub M. Drug therapy of itching. In: Drugdex Drug Consults. Denver, CO: Micromedex, May 1989.

Keats C, Director International Sales, Tender Corporation (personal communication), 1995. AfterBite.

McGrath NE. Pediatric update. Children with chickenpox: emergency department care and teaching. J Emerg Nursing 1992;18(4):353-54.

McLean WH, Ariano R. Evening primrose oil therapy of polyunsaturated fat deficiency. In: Drugdex Drug Consults. Ottawa, Ont: Micromedex, Mar 1984.

Antiseptics

Anon. Wound-care update 91: culturing wounds, dressing choices, packing trends and more. Nursing91 1991;April:47-50.

Baxter CR. Management of burn wounds. Dermatol Clin 1993; 11(4):709-14.

Kjolseth D, Frank MJ, Barker JH, et al. Comparison of the effects of commonly used wound agents on epithelialization and neovascularization. J Am Cell Surg 1994;179:305-12.

Krogh CME, ed. Compendium of Pharmaceuticals and Specialties. 29th ed. Ottawa: Canadian Pharmaceutical Association, 1994:553-54.

Larson E. Guideline for use of topical antimicrobial agents. Am J Infection Control 1988;16(6):253-65.

Leaper D. Antiseptics and their effect on healing tissue. Nurs Times 1986;May 28:45-47.

Modic BM. Myths and facts...about chronic wound care. Nursing90 1990;Dec:68.

Rodeheaver G. Controversies in topical wound management. Wounds 1989;1(1):19-34.

Russell L. Healing alternatives. Nurs Times 1993;89(42):88-90.

Thompson DF. Dakin's solution—cellular toxicity. In: Drugdex Drug Consults. Oklahoma City, Okla: Micromedex, Oct 1989.

Astringents

Anon. New OTC products. Am Pharm 1994;N834(2):37.

Anon. New OTC products. Am Pharm 1992;N832(2):32.

Bond CA. Skin disorders I. In: Koda-Kimble MA, Young LY, eds. Applied Therapeutics: The Clinical Use of Drugs. 5th ed. Vancouver WA: Applied Therapeutics, 1992:64-2-64-3.

Federal Register (US) 1989 Apr 3;54(62):13490-99.

Federal Register (US) 1994 Jun 3;59(106):29767-68.

Freeman Kent DA, Willis GA, eds. The British Columbia Drug and Poison Information Centre Poison Management Manual. 3rd ed. Ottawa, Ont: Canadian Pharmaceutical Association, 1989:223-25.

Harvey SC. Topical drugs. In: Osol A, Hoover JE, eds. Remington's Pharmaceutical Sciences. Easton, PA: Mack Publishing, 1976:712-19.

Korting HC, Schafer-Korting M, Hart H, et al. Anti-inflammatory activity of hamamelis distillate applied topically to the skin: influence of vehicle and dose. Eur J Clin Pharmacol 1993;44:315-18.

Cleansers

Paye M, Simion FA, Pierara GE. Dansyl chloride labelling of stratum corneum: its rapid extraction from skin can predict skin irritation due to surfactants and cleansing products. Contact Dermatitis 1994; 30(2):91-96.

Rodeheaver G. Controversies in topical wound management. Wounds 1989;1(1):19-34.

Shur-Clens and SAF-Clens product monographs. Calgon-Vestal Laboratories, St. Louis, MO. July 1993.

Simion FA, Rhein LD, Grove GL, et al. Sequential order of skin responses to surfactants during a soap chamber test. Contact Dermatitis 1991; 25(4):242-9.

Ultra-Klenz product monograph. Carrington Laboratories, Dallas, Tex. July 1991.

Dressings

Anon. Wound care update 91: culturing wounds, dressing choices, packing trends, and more. Nursing91 1991;Apr:47-50.

Baxter CR. Management of burn wounds. Dermatol Clin 1993; 11(4):709-14.

Lee D, Mavinil S. Home nursing care skin care program. Victoria, BC: Capital Regional District Health, Aug 1993.

Modic BM. Myths and facts...about chronic wound care. Nursing90 1990;Dec:68.

Peate WF. Outpatient management of burns. Am Fam Physician 1992; 45(3):1321-30.

Waitzman AA, Neligan PC. How to manage burns in primary care. Can Fam Physician 1993;39:2394-400.

Wood L, enterostomal therapy nurse, Greater Victoria Hospital Society, Victoria, BC (personal communication). Wound Dressing. July 1994.

Insect Repellents

Anon. Advice for travellers. Med Lett Drugs Ther 1992;34(869):41-44.

Anon. Insect repellents. Med Lett Drugs Ther 1989;31(792):45-47.

Claxton M, Marketing Assistant, Shering-Plough (personal communication). Muskol.

Magnon GJ, Robert LL, Kline DL, et al. Repellency of two DEET formulations and Avon Skin-So-Soft against biting midges in Honduras. J Am Mosquito Control Assoc 1991;7(1):80-82.

MMWR 1989. Deet-induced seizures - 1989 CDC Report. In: Drugdex Drug Consults. Denver, CO: Micromedex, Aug 1991.

Registered pest control products (sorted by register's code). Ottawa, Ont: Agriculture and Agri- food Canada, Sept 20 1994:2-10.

Reynold JEF, ed. Martindale: The Extra Pharmacopoeia. 29th ed. London: Pharmaceutical Press, 1989:1062-63.

Ipecac

Jawary D, Cameron PA, Dziukas L, et al. Drug overdose—reducing the load. Med J Aust 1992;156:343-46.

Krenzelok EP, Dunmire SM. Acute poisoning emergencies: resolving the gastric decontamination controversy. Postgrad Med 1992;91(2): 179-86.

Kulig K. Current concepts: initial management of ingestions of toxic substances. N Engl J Med 1992;326(25):1677-81.

Phillips S, Gomez H, Brent J. Pediatric gastrointestinal decontamination in acute toxin ingestion. J Clin Pharmacol 1993;33:497-507.

Corticosteroids

Anon. Topical corticosteroids. Med Lett Drugs Ther 1991;33(857): 108-10.

Giannotti B, Pimpinelli N. Topical corticosteroids: which drug and when? Drugs 1992; 44(1):65-71.

CHAPTER 11—Foot Care Products

Popovich NG. Foot Care Products. In: Feldmann EG, Blockstein WL, et al, eds. Handbook of Nonprescription Drugs. Washington: American Pharmaceutical Association, 1990.

Athlete's Foot

Abramson C. A new look at dermatophytosis and atopy. In: McCarthy DJ, Montgomery RA. Podiatric Dermatology. Baltimore: Williams and Wilkins, 1986.

DeSimone EM, McCracken G. Common fungal infections of the skin. US Pharmacist 1994;(August):30-35.

Leyden JJ, Aly R. Tinea pedis. Semin Dermatol 1993;12(4):280-84.

Page JC, Abramson C, Lee WL, et al. Diagnosis and treatment of tinea pedis. A review and update. J Am Podiatr Med Assoc 1991;81 (6):304-16.

Pariser DM. Superficial fungal infections. A practical guide for primary care physicians. Postgrad Med 1990;87(5):205-14.

Smith EB. Topical antifungal drugs in the treatment of tinea pedis, tinea cruris and tinea corporis. J Am Acad Dermatol 1993;28(5Pt1):S24-28.

Calluses and Corns

Richards RN. Calluses, corns and shoes. Semin Dermatol 1991; 10(2): 112-14.

George DH. Management of hyperkeratotic lesions in the elderly patient. Clin Podiatr Med Surg 1993;10(1):69-77.

Silfverskiold JP. Common foot problems. Relieving the pain of bunions, keratoses, corns and calluses. Postgrad Med 1991;89(5):183-88.

Plantar Warts

Anderson FE. Warts—fact or fiction. Drugs 1985;30:368-75.

Campbell BJ. The treatment of warts. Prim Care 1986;13(3):465-76.

Glover MG. Plantar warts. Foot and Ankle 1990;11(3):172-78.

Steele K, Irwin WG. Treatment options for cutaneous warts in family practice. Fam Pract 1988;5:314-19.

Steele K. Management of cutaneous warts. Aust Fam Physician 1988; 17(11):950-52.

Ingrown Toenails

Iseli A. The management of ingrown toenails. Aust Fam Physician 1990;19(9):1414-19.

Murtagh J. Ingrowing toenails. Aust Fam Physician 1993;22(2):206.

Taylor MB. Successful treatment of warts. Choosing the best method for each situation. Postgrad Med 1988;84(8):126-36.

Bunions

Holmes GB. Surgical management of foot disorders: bunions and bunionettes. Curr Opin Rheumatol 1991;3:98-101.

Silfverskiold JP. Common foot problems. Relieving the pain of bunions, keratoses, corns and calluses. Postgrad Med 1991;89(5):183-88.

CHAPTER 12—Gastrointestinal Products

Dyspepsia

Barbara L, Camilleri M, Corinaldesi R, et al. Definition and investigation of dyspepsia: consensus of an international ad hoc working party. Dig Dis Sci 1989;34:1272-76.

Berstad A. Non-ulcer dyspepsia and gastritis—clinical aspects. J Physiol Pharmacol 1993;44(3 suppl 1):41-59.

Berstad A, Weberg R. Antacids in the treatment of gastroduodenal ulcer. Scand J Gastroenterol 1986;21:385-91.

Bond CM. Guidelines for dyspepsia treatment. Pharm J 1994;252(6776): 228-29.

Chamberlain CE. Acute hemorrhagic gastritis. Gastroenterol Clin North Am 1993;22:843-73.

Ching CK, Lam SK. Antacids: indications and limitations. Drugs 1994;47: 305-17.

Crean GP, Holden RJ, Knill-Jones RP, et al. A database on dyspepsia. Gut 1994;35(2):191-202.

Crotty B, Smallwood RA. What's new? Med J Aust 1993;159:627-29.

Davis WM. Is aluminum an etiologic contributor to alcoholic amnesia and dementia? Med Hypotheses 1993;41:341-43.

Dunn BE. Pathogenic mechanisms of Helicobacter pylori. Gastroenterol Clin North Am 1993;22:43-57.

Eckstein RP, Hoschl R, Lam SK, et al. Intragastric distribution and gastric emptying of solids and liquids in functional dyspepsia. Lack of influence of symptom subgroups and H. pylori-associated gastritis. Dig Dis Sci 1993;38:2247-54.

Goggin PM, Collins DA, Jazrawi RP, et al. Prevalence of Helicobacter pylori infection and its effect on symptoms and non-steroidal anti-inflammatory drug induced gastrointestinal damage in patients with rheumatoid arthritis. Gut 1993;34(12):1677-80.

Gudjonsson H, Oddsson E, Bjornsson S, et al. Efficacy of sucralfate in treatment of non-ulcer dyspepsia. A double-blind placebo-controlled study. Scand J Gastroenterol 1993;28(11):969-72.

Halter F. Clinical use of antacids. J Physiol Pharmacol 1993;44(3 suppl 1):61-74.

Heading RC. Definitions of dyspepsia. Scand J Gastroenterol 1991;26(suppl 182):1-6.

Isenberg JI, Peterson WL, Elashoff JD, et al. Healing of benign gastric ulcer with low-dose antacid or cimetidine. N Engl J Med 1983;308: 1319-24.

Laine L. Helicobacter pylori, gastric ulcer, and agents noxious to the gastric mucosa. Gastroenterol Clin North Am 1993;22:117-25.

Lambert JR. The role of Helicobacter pylori in nonulcer dyspepsia: a debate—for. Gastroenterol Clin North Am 1993;22:141-51.

MacCara ME, Nugent FJ, Garner JB. Acid neutralization capacity of Canadian antacid formulations. Can Med Assoc J 1985;132:523-27.

Muris JW, Starmans R, Pop P, et al. Discriminant value of symptoms in patients with dyspepsia. J Fam Pract 1994;38(2):139-43.

Nyren O. Therapeutic trial in dyspepsia: its role in the primary care setting. Scand J Gastroenterol 1991;26(suppl 182):61-69.

Richter JE. Dyspepsia: organic causes and differential characteristics from functional dyspepsia. Scand J Gastroenterol 1991;26(suppl 182): 11-16.

Scott AM, Kellow JE, Shuter B, et al. Intragastric distribution and gastric emptying of solids and liquids in functional dyspepsia. Lack of influence of symptom subgroups and H. pylori-associated gastritis. Dig Dis Sci 1993;38:2247-54.

Talley NJ. Spectrum of chronic dyspepsia in the presence of the irritable bowel syndrome. Scand J Gastroenterol 1991;26(suppl 182):7-10.

Talley NJ. Drug treatment of functional dyspepsia. Scand J Gastroenterol 1991;26(suppl 182):47-60.

Talley NJ. The role of Helicobacter pylori in nonulcer dyspepsia: a debate—against. Gastroenterol Clin North Am 1993;22:153-67.

Talley NJ. Nonulcer dyspepsia: current approaches to diagnosis and management. Am Fam Physician 1993;47:1407-16.

Talley NJ, Weaver AL, Tesmer DL, et al. Lack of discriminant value of dyspepsia subgroups in patients referred for upper endoscopy. Gastroenterology 1993;105(5):1378-86.

Talley NJ, Weaver AL, Tesmer DL, et al. Smoking, alcohol and nonsteroidal anti-inflammatory drugs in outpatients with functional dyspepsia and among dyspepsia subgroups. Am J Gastroenterol 1994; 89:524-28.

Tarnawski A, Hollander D, Gergely H. Antacids: new perspectives in cytoprotection. Scand J Gastroenterol 1990;25(suppl 174):9-14.

Veldhuyzen van Zanten SJO, Sherman PM. Helicobacter pylori infection as a cause of gastritis, duodenal ulcer, gastric cancer and nonulcer dyspepsia: a systematic overview. Can Med Assoc J 1994;150:177-85.

Witteman EM, Hopman WP, Becx MC, et al. Short report: smoking habits and the acquisition of metronidazole resistance in patients with Helicobacter pylori-related gastritis. Aliment Pharmacol Ther 1993; 7:683-87.

Gastroesophageal Reflux

Ahmed AM, al-Karawi MA, Shariq S, et al. Frequency of gastroesophageal reflux in patients with liver cirrhosis. Hepatogastroenterology 1993;40:478-80.

Anon. Cisapride for nocturnal heartburn. Med Lett Drugs Ther 1994; 36(915):11-13.

Collen MJ, Johnson DA, Sheridan MJ. Basal acid output and gastric acid hypersecretion in gastroesophageal reflux disease. Correlation with ranitidine therapy. Dig Dis Sci 1994;39(2):410-17.

Goldstein JL, Schlesinger PK, Mozwecz HL, et al. Esophageal mucosal resistance: a factor in esophagitis. Gastroenterol Clin North Am 1990;19:565-86.

Irwin RS, French CL, Curley FJ, et al. Chronic cough due to gastroesophageal reflux. Clinical, diagnostic, and pathogenetic aspects. Chest 1993;104:1511-17.

Kahrilas PJ. Esophageal motor activity and acid clearance. Gastroenterol Clin North Am 1990;19:537-50.

Kerr P, Shoenut JP, Steens RD, et al. Nasal continuous positive airway pressure. A new treatment for nocturnal gastroesophageal reflux? J Clin Gastroenterol 1993;17(4):276-80.

Kuster E, Ros E, Toledo-Pimentel V, et al. Predictive factors of the long term outcome in gastro-oesophageal reflux disease: six year follow up of 107 patients. Gut 1994;35(1):8-14.

Peters JH, DeMeester TR. Gastroesophageal reflux. Surg Clin North Am 1993;73:1119-44.

Raiha I, Impivaara O, Seppala M, et al. Determinants of symptoms suggestive of gastroesophageal reflux disease in the elderly. Scand J Gastroenterol 1993;28:1011-14.

Richter JE. Gastroesophageal reflux disease: a review of medical therapy. In: Castell DO, Wu WC, Ott DJ, eds. Gastroesophageal Reflux Disease: Pathogenesis, Diagnosis, Therapy. Mount Kisco, NY: Futura, 1985: 221-41.

Robinson M. Gastroesophageal reflux disease. Selecting optimal therapy. Postgrad Med 1994;95(2):88-90, 93-94, 99-102.

Soffer EE, Wilson J, Duethman G, et al. Effect of graded exercise on esophageal motility and gastroesophageal reflux in nontrained subjects. Dig Dis Sci 1994;39(1):193-98.

Sontag SJ. The medical management of reflux esophagitis: role of antacids and acid inhibition. Gastroenterol Clin North Am 1990;19:683-712.

Tucci F, Resti M, Fontana R, et al. Gastroesophageal reflux and bronchial asthma: prevalence and effect of cisapride therapy. J Pediatr Gastroenterol Nutr 1993;17(3):265-70.

Gastrointestinal Gas

Levitt MD. Excessive gas: patient perception vs. reality. Hosp Pract 1985;20(11):163.

Levitt MD. How to handle complaints of "too much gas". Drug Therapy 1987;17(10):76-79, 83-86.

Sutalf LO, Levitt MD. Follow-up of a flatulent patient. Dig Dis Sci 1979;24:652-56.

Tomlin J, Lowis C, Read NW. Investigation of normal flatus production in healthy volunteers. Gut 1991;32:665-69.

Infantile Colic

Becker N, Lombardi P, Sidoti E, et al. Mylicon drops in the treatment of infant colic. Clin Ther 1988;10:401-05.

Sethi KS, Sethi JK. Simethicone in the management of infant colic. The Practitioner 1988;232:508.

Vesterfelt KL, Steinberg SK. The pharmacist's role in counselling new parents. Infant Care 1989;(May):14-18.

Constipation

Alabaster O, Tang ZC, Frost A, et al. Potential synergism between wheat bran and psyllium: enhanced inhibition of colon cancer. Cancer Lett 1993;75:53-58.

Almond P. Constipation: a family-centred approach. Health Visit 1993; 66:404-05.

Barrish JO, Gilger MA. Colon cleanout preparations in children and adolescents. Gastroenterol Nurs 1993;16:106-09.

Bingham SA, Cummings JH. Effect of exercise and physical fitness on large intestinal function. Gastroenterology 1989;97:1389–99.

Brown SR, Cann PA, Read NW. Effect of coffee on distal colon function. Gut 1990;31:450–53.

Coenen C, Wegener M, Wedmann B, et al. Does physical activity influence bowel transit time in healthy young men? Am J Gastroenterol 1992;87:292–95.

Elliot DL, Watts WJ, Girard DE. Constipation: mechanisms and management of a common clinical problem. Postgrad Med 1983;74:143–49.

Gattuso JM, Kamm MA. The management of constipation in adults. Aliment Pharmacol Ther 1993;7:487–500.

Hogue VW. Diarrhea and constipation. In: Herfindal ET, Gourley DR, Hart LL, eds. Clinical Pharmacy and Therapeutics. 5th ed. Baltimore: Williams & Wilkins, 1992:436–49.

Kinnunen O, Winblad I, Koistinen P, et al. Safety and efficacy of a bulk laxative containing senna versus lactulose in the treatment of chronic constipation in geriatric patients. Pharmacology 1993;47(suppl 1):253–55.

Klauser AG, Peyerl C, Schindlbeck NE, et al. Nutrition and physical activity in chronic constipation. Eur J Gastroenterol Hepatol 1992; 4:227–33.

Klauser AG, Muller-Lissner SA. How effective is nonlaxative treatment of constipation? Pharmacology 1993;47(suppl 1):256–60.

Lennard-Jones JE. Clinical management of constipation. Pharmacology 1993;47(suppl 1):216–23.

Lindsay A. Smart Cooking. Toronto: Macmillan of Canada, 1986:235–37.

Loening-Baucke V. Constipation in early childhood: patient characteristics, treatment, and longterm follow up. Gut 1993;34:1400–04.

Loening-Baucke V. Chronic constipation in children. Gastroenterology 1993;105:1557–64.

Loening-Baucke V. Management of chronic constipation in infants and toddlers. Am Fam Physician 1994;49:397–400, 403–06, 411–13.

Muller-Lissner SA. Adverse effects of laxatives: fact and fiction. Pharmacology 1993;47(suppl 1):138–45.

Murray FE, Bliss CM. Geriatric constipation: brief update on a common problem. Geriatrics 1991;46(3):64–68.

Oettle GJ. Effect of moderate exercise on bowel habit. Gut 1991; 32:941–44.

Passmore AP, Wilson Davies K, Flanagan PG, et al. A comparison of Agiolax and lactulose in elderly patients with chronic constipation. Pharmacology 1993;47(suppl 1):249–52.

Passmore AP, Wilson Davies K, Stoker C, et al. Chronic constipation in long stay elderly patients: a comparison of lactulose and a senna-fiber combination. BMJ 1993;307:769–71.

Sonnenberg A, Koch TR. Epidemiology of constipation in the United States. Dis Colon Rectum 1989;34:606–11.

Sprague-McRae JM, Lamb W, Homer D. Encopresis: a study of treatment alternatives and historical and behavioral characteristics. Nurse Pract 1993;18(10):52–53, 56–63.

Tolia V, Lin CH, Elitsur Y. A prospective randomized study with mineral oil and oral lavage solution for treatment of faecal impaction in children. Aliment Pharmacol Ther 1993;7:523–29.

van der Horst ML, Sykula JA, Lingley K. The constipation quandary. Can Nurse 1994;90(1):25–30.

Ziegenhagen DJ, Tewinkle G, Kruis W, et al. Adding more fluid to wheat bran has no significant effects on intestinal functions of healthy subjects. J Clin Gastroenterol 1991;13(5):525–30.

Diarrhea

Avendano P, Matson DO, Long J, et al. Costs associated with office visits for diarrhea in infants and toddlers. Pediatr Infect Dis J 1993; 12: 897–902.

Banwell JG. Pathophysiology of diarrheal disorders. Rev Infect Dis 1990;12(suppl 1):S30–S35.

Barrett MJ. Association of Reye's syndrome with use of Pepto-Bismol (bismuth subsalicylate). Pediatr Infect Dis J 1986;5:611.

Bennett RG, Greenough WB. Approach to acute diarrhea in the elderly. Gastroenterol Clin North Am 1993;22:517–33.

Bierer DW. Bismuth subsalicylate: history, chemistry, and safety. Rev Infect Dis 1990;12(suppl 1):S3–S8.

Brown KH, Peerson JM, Fontaine O. Use of nonhuman milks in the dietary management of young children with acute diarrhea: a meta-analysis of clinical trials. Pediatrics 1994;93:17–27.

Brown KR, Phillips SM. Tropical diseases of importance to the traveler. Adv Int Med 1984;29:59–84.

Centers for Disease Control. Health information for international travel 1992. Atlanta: National Center for Prevention Services, June 1992. HHS publication no. (CDC) 92-8280.

Chak A, Banwell JG. Traveller's diarrhea. Gastroenterol Clin North Am 1993;22:549–61.

DuPont HL, Sullivan P, Pickering LK, et al. Symptomatic treatment of diarrhea with bismuth subsalicylate among students attending a Mexican university. Gastroenterology 1977;73:715–18.

DuPont HL, Ericsson CD, Johnson PC, et al. Use of bismuth subsalicylate for the prevention of travelers' diarrhea. Rev Infect Dis 1990;12(suppl 1):S64–S67.

Figueroa Quintanilla D, Salazar Lindo E, Sack RB, et al. A controlled trial of bismuth subsalicylate in infants with acute watery diarrheal disease. N Engl J Med 1993;328:1653–58.

Gryboski JD, Kocoshis S. Effect of bismuth subsalicylate on chronic diarrhea in childhood: a preliminary report. Rev Infect Dis 1990;12 (suppl 1):S36–S40.

Harvey SC. Antimicrobial drugs. In: Remington's Pharmaceutical Sciences. Easton: Mack Publishing, 1990:1166.

Laney DW, Cohen MB. Approach to the pediatric patient with acute diarrhea. Gastroenterol Clin North Am 1993;22:499–516.

Lange WR, Kreider DS. Food and water acquisition abroad: guidelines for finding safe sustenance. Postgrad Med 1983;73(5):325–32.

Mitchell DK, Van R, Morrow AL, et al. Outbreaks of astrovirus gastroenteritis in day care centers. J Pediatr 1993;123:725–32.

Park S, Giannella RA. Approach to the adult patient with acute diarrhea. Gastroenterol Clin North Am 1993;22:483–97.

Pothoulakis C, LaMont JT. Clostridium difficile colitis and diarrhea. Gastroenterol Clin North Am 1993;22:623–37.

Powell DW, Szauter KE. Nonantibiotic therapy and pharmacotherapy of acute infectious diarrhea. Gastroenterol Clin North Am 1993;22: 683–707.

Reves RR, Morrow AL, Bartlett AV, et al. Child day care increases the risk of clinic visits for acute diarrhea and diarrhea due to rotavirus. Am J Epidemiol 1993;137:97–107.

Sack RB. Travelers' diarrhea: microbiologic bases for prevention and treatment. Rev Infect Dis 1990;12(suppl 1):S59–S67.

Soriano-Brucher H, Avendano P, O'Ryan M, et al. Bismuth subsalicylate in the treatment of acute diarrhea in children: a clinical study. Pediatrics 1991;87:18–27.

Steffen R. Worldwide efficacy of bismuth subsalicylate in the treatment of travelers' diarrhea. Rev Infect Dis 1990;12(suppl 1):S80–S86.

Steinhoff MC, Douglas RG, Greenberg HB, et al. Bismuth subsalicylate therapy of viral gastroenteritis. Gastroenterology 1980;78:1495–99.

Irritable Bowel Syndrome

Aggarwal A, Cutts TF, Abell TL, et al. Predominant symptoms in irritable bowel syndrome correlate with specific autonomic nervous system abnormalities. Gastroenterology 1994;106:945–50.

Almy TP. Wrestling with the irritable colon. Med Clin North Am 1978;62:203–10.

Brostoff J. Irritable bowel syndrome. N Engl J Med 1994;330:1390.

Dancey CP, Backhouse S. Towards a better understanding of patients with irritable bowel syndrome. J Adv Nurs 1993;18:1443-50.

Friedman G. Diet and the irritable bowel syndrome. Gastroenterol Clin North Am 1991;20:313-24.

Friedman G. Treatment of the irritable bowel syndrome. Gastroenterol Clin North Am 1991;20:325-33.

Hall MJ, Barry RE. Current views on the aetiology and management of the irritable bowel syndrome. Postgrad Med J 1991;67:785-89.

Harvey RF, Pomare EW, Heaton KW. Effects of increased dietary fibre on intestinal transit. Lancet 1973;1:1278-80.

Ivey KJ. Are anticholinergics of use in the irritable colon syndrome? Gastroenterology 1975;68:1300-07.

Jones R. Irritable bowel syndrome. Practitioner 1991;235:811-14.

Jones R, Lydeard S. Irritable bowel syndrome in the general population. BMJ 1992;304:87-90.

Lambert JP, Brunt PW, Mowat NA, et al. The value of prescribed 'high-fibre' diets for the treatment of the irritable bowel syndrome. Eur J Clin Nutr 1991;45:601-09.

Lind CD. Motility disorders in the irritable bowel syndrome. Gastroenterol Clin North Am 1991;20:279-95.

Lynn RB, Friedman LS. Irritable bowel syndrome. N Engl J Med 1993;329:1940-45.

Mendeloff AI. Dietary fiber and human health. N Engl J Med 1977; 297:811-14.

Mullin GE. Food allergy and irritable bowel syndrome. JAMA 1991; 265:1736.

O'Keefe E, Talley NJ. Irritable bowel syndrome in the elderly. Clin Geriatr Med 1991;7:265-86.

Pattee PL, Thompson WG. Drug treatment of the irritable bowel syndrome. Drugs 1992;44:200-06.

Rhodes JB, Abrams JH, Manning RT. Controlled clinical trial of sedative-anticholinergic drugs in patients with irritable bowel syndrome. J Clin Pharmacol 1978;18:340-45.

Ritchie JA, Truelove SC. Comparison of various treatments for irritable bowel syndrome. BMJ 1980;281:1317-19.

Schuster MM. Diagnostic evaluation of the irritable bowel syndrome. Gastroenterol Clin North Am 1991;20:269-78.

Soltoft J, Gudmand-Hoyer E, Krag B, et al. A double-blind trial of the effect of wheat bran on symptoms of irritable bowel syndrome. Lancet 1976;1:270-72.

Sullivan MA, Cohen S, Snape WJ. Colonic myoelectrical activity in irritable-bowel syndrome: effect of eating and anticholinergics. N Engl J Med 1978;298:878-83.

Talley NJ. Why do functional gastrointestinal disorders come and go? Dig Dis Sci 1994;39:673-77.

Talley NJ, Zinsmeister AR, Van-Dyke C, et al. Epidemiology of colonic symptoms and the irritable bowel syndrome. Gastroenterology 1991; 101:927-34.

Talley NJ, O'Keefe EA, Zinsmeister AR, et al. Prevalence of gastrointestinal symptoms in the elderly: a population-based study. Gastroenterology 1992;102:895-901.

Talley NJ, Weaver AL, Zinsmeister AR. Smoking, alcohol, and nonsteroidal anti-inflammatory drugs in outpatients with functional dyspepsia and among dyspepsia subgroups. Am J Gastroenterol 1994;89:524-28.

Thompson WG. Symptomatic presentations of the irritable bowel syndrome. Gastroenterol Clin North Am 1991;20:235-47.

Thompson WG. Irritable bowel syndrome. Strategy for the family physician. Can Fam Physician 1994;40:307-10, 313-16.

Toskes PP, Connery KL, Ritchey TW. Calcium polycarbophil compared with placebo in irritable bowel syndrome. Aliment Pharmacol Ther 1993;7:87-92.

Van Outryve M, Milo R, Toussaint J, et al. "Prokinetic" treatment of constipation-predominant irritable bowel syndrome: a placebo-controlled study of cisapride. J Clin Gastroenterol 1991;13:49-57.

Weber FH, McCallum RW. Clinical approaches to irritable bowel syndrome. Lancet 1992;340:1447-52.

West L, Warren J, Cutts T. Diagnosis and management of irritable bowel syndrome, constipation, and diarrhea in pregnancy. Gastroenterol Clin North Am 1992;21:793-802.

Whitehead WE, Crowell MD. Psychologic considerations in the irritable bowel syndrome. Gastroenterol Clin North Am 1991;20:249-67.

Nausea and Vomiting

Kousen M. Treatment of nausea and vomiting in pregnancy. Am Fam Physician 1993;48:1279-84.

Mitchelson F. Pharmacological agents affecting emesis. A review (part I). Drugs 1992;43:295-315.

Simons K. Emetics and antiemetics. In: Carruthers-Czyzewski P, ed. Self-Medication Reference for Health Professionals. 4th ed. Ottawa: Canadian Pharmaceutical Association, 1992:257-65.

Stainton MC; Neff EJ. The efficacy of SeaBands for the control of nausea and vomiting in pregnancy. Health Care Women Int 1994;15:563-75.

Takeda N, Morita M, Hasegawa S, et al. Neuropharmacology of motion sickness and emesis. Acta Otolaryngol Suppl 1993;501:10-15.

Thomas RE, Wyer M. Nausea, vomiting, diarrhea, and constipation. In: Herfindal ET, Gourley DR, Hart LL, eds. Clinical Pharmacy and Therapeutics. 4th ed. Baltimore: Williams & Wilkins, 1988:290-99.

Pharmaceutical Agents

Awouters F, Megens A, Verlinden M, et al. Loperamide. Survey of studies on mechanism of its antidiarrheal activity. Dig Dis Sci 1993;38:977-95.

Balasa RW, Murray RL, Kondelis NP, et al. Phosphate-binding properties and electrolyte content of aluminum hydroxide antacids. Nephron 1987;45:16-21.

Bhutta TI, Tahir KI. Loperamide poisoning in children. Lancet 1990; 335:63.

Charritat JL, Corbineau D, Guth S, et al. Évaluation thérapeutique de l'attapulgite de Mormoiron dans les diarrhées aïgues du nourrisson et de l'enfant. Étude multicentrique en pratique libérale controlée versus placebo chez 113 patients. Ann Pediatr Paris 1992;39:326-32.

Contardi I. Batterioterapia orale quale prevenzione della diarrea da antibiotici in eta pediatrica. Clin Ter 1991;136:409-13.

De Luca A, Coupar IM. Difenoxin and loperamide: studies on possible mechanisms of intestinal antisecretory action. Naunyn Schmiedebergs Arch Pharmacol 1993;347:231-37.

Eherer AJ, Santa Ana CA, Porter J, et al. Effect of psyllium, calcium polycarbophil, and wheat bran on secretory diarrhea induced by phenolphthalein. Gastroenterology 1993;104:1007-12.

Gaginella TS, Mascolo N, Izzo AA, et al. Nitric oxide as a mediator of bisacodyl and phenolphthalein laxative action: induction of nitric oxide synthase. J Pharmacol Exp Ther 1994;270:1239-45.

Gorbach SL. Bismuth therapy in gastrointestinal diseases. Gastroenterology 1990;99:863-75.

Gordon MF, Abrams RI, Rubin DB, et al. Bismuth toxicity. Neurology 1994;44:2418.

Gump DW, Nadeau OW, Hendricks GM, et al. Evidence that bismuth salts reduce invasion of epithelial cells by enteroinvasive bacteria. Med Microbiol Immunol Berl 1992;181:131-43.

Hill MA, Greason FC. Loperamide dependence. J Clin Psychiatry 1992;53:450.

Isolauri E, Kaila M, Mykkanen H, et al. Oral bacteriotherapy for viral gastroenteritis. Dig Dis Sci 1994;39:2595-2600.

Jungreis AC, Schaumburg HH. Encephalopathy from abuse of bismuth subsalicylate (Pepto-Bismol). Neurology 1993;43:1265.

Kaila M, Isolauri E, Soppi E, et al. Enhancement of the circulating antibody secreting cell response in human diarrhea by a human Lactobacillus strain. Pediatr Res 1992;32:141-44.

Kline MD, Koppes S. Acidophilus for sertraline-induced diarrhea. Am J Psychiatry 1994;151:1521-22.

Kune GA. Laxative use not a risk for colorectal cancer: data from the Melbourne Colorectal Cancer Study. Z Gastroenterol 1993;31:140-43.

Leng-Peschlow E. Sennoside-induced secretion and its relevance for the laxative effect. Pharmacology 1993;47(suppl 1):14-21.

McKeigue PM, Lamm SH, Linn S, et al. Bendectin and birth defects: I. A meta-analysis of the epidemiologic studies. Teratology 1994;50:27-37.

Motola C, Mann MD, Bowie MD. Effect of loperamide on stool output and duration of acute infectious diarrhea in infants. J Pediatr 1990; 117:467-71.

Musial F, Enck P, Kalveram KT, et al. The effect of loperamide on anorectal function in normal healthy men. J Clin Gastroenterol 1992; 15:321-24.

Nusko G, Schneider B, Muller G, et al. Retrospective study on laxative use and melanosis coli as risk factors for colorectal neoplasms. Pharmacology 1993;47(suppl 1):234-41.

Oggero R, Garbo G, Savino F, et al. Dietary modifications versus dicyclomine hydrochloride in the treatment of severe infantile colics. Acta Paediatr 1994;83:222-25.

Rambout L, Sahai J, Gallicano K, et al. Effect of bismuth subsalicylate on ciprofloxacin bioavailability. Antimicrob Agents Chemother 1994; 38:2187-90.

CHAPTER 13—Hemorrhoidal Products

Alexander-Williams J. The nature of piles. BMJ 1982;285:1064.

Altman DF. Diseases of the rectum and anus. In: Wyngaarden J, Smith L, eds. Textbook of Medicine. 18th ed. Philadelphia: Saunders, 1988:789.

Anon. Getting to the seat of the problem. FDA Consumer 1980;14(7): 19-23.

Bassford T. Treatment of common anorectal disorders. Am Fam Physician 1992;45:1787-94.

Birkett DH. Hemorrhoids: diagnostic and treatment options. Hosp Pract 1988;23:99-108.

Carden ABG. Management of hemorrhoids and associated anorectal conditions. Drugs 1972;4:75-80.

Cocchiara JL. Hemorrhoids: a practical approach to an aggravating problem. Postgrad Med 1991;89:149-52.

Dennison AR, Wherry DC, Morris DL. Hemorrhoids: nonoperative management. Surg Clin North Am 1988;68:1401-09.

Dennison AR, Whiston RJ, Rooney S, et al. The management of hemorrhoids. Am J Gastroenterol 1989;84:475-81.

Dicaire P, Boucher PC. The treatment of hemorrhoids. Can Pharm J 1985;118(3):121-22.

Driscoll DF, DeFelice MD, Baptista RJ. Hemorrhoids: etiology and treatment. US Pharmacist 1981;6(5):43-58.

Gibbons CP, Bannister JJ, Read NW. Role of constipation and anal hypertonia in the pathogenesis of haemorrhoids. Br J Surg 1988;75:656-60.

Gossel TA. Anorectal disorders. US Pharmacist 1985;10(8):23-24.

Gossel TA. Hemorrhoidal products. US Pharmacist 1989;14(7):37-42.

Griffith CDM, Morris DL, Ellis I, et al. Out-patient treatment of haemorrhoids with bipolar diathermy coagulation. Br J Surg 1987;74:827.

Hancock BD. Haemorrhoids. BMJ 1992;304:1042-44.

Hodes B. Hemorrhoidal products. In: Handbook of Nonprescription Drugs. Washington: American Pharmaceutical Association, 1992: 469-78.

Holt RL. Hemorrhoids: Cure and Prevention. Turnbridge Wells: Abascus Press, 1990:3-119.

Leff E. Hemorrhoids; current approaches to an ancient problem. Postgrad Med 1987;82:95-101.

Loder PB, Kamm MA, Nicholls RJ, et al. Hemorrhoids: pathology, pathophysiology and aetiology. Br J Surg 1994;81:946-54.

Mazier WP. Hemorrhoids, fissures and pruritus ani. Surg Clin North Am 1994;74:1277-92.

Miller B. Hemorrhoids. In: Carruthers-Czyzewski P, ed. Self-Medication Reference for Health Professionals. 4th ed. Ottawa: Canadian Pharmaceutical Association, 1992:329-35.

Sause RB. Self-treatment of hemorrhoids. US Pharmacist 1995;20:32-36, 39-40.

Schussman LC, Lutz LJ. Outpatient management of hemorrhoids. Prim Care 1986;13:527-41.

Smith LE. Hemorrhoids: a review of current techniques and management. Gastroenterol Clin North Am 1987;16:79-91.

Sun WM, Read NW, Shorthouse AJ. Hypertensive anal cushions as a cause of the high anal canal pressures in patients with haemorrhoids. Br J Surg 1990;77:458-62.

Van Ketel WG. Contact allergy to different anti-hemorrhoidal anesthetics. Contact Dermatitis 1983;9(6):512.

CHAPTER 14—Herbal Products

General

Chandler RF. Herbal medicine. In: Clarke C, ed. Self-Medication A Reference for Health Professionals. 3rd ed. Ottawa: Canadian Pharmaceutical Association, 1988:517-32.

Chandler RF. Herbal medicine. In: Carruthers-Czyzewski P, ed. Self-Medication Reference for Health Professionals. 4th ed. Ottawa: Canadian Pharmaceutical Association, 1992:493-511.

Foster S. Herbal Renaissance. Salt Lake City: Gibbs Smith, 1993:6-14.

Ullman D. The mainstreaming of alternative medicine. Healthcare Forum J 1993;36:24-30.

Introduction

Anon. Alternative medicine: the facts. Consumer Reports 1994;59:51-59.

Anon. Canadian adverse drug reaction newsletter. Ottawa: Health Canada, 1994;4(2):1-3.

Anon. Canadians make use of alternative therapies, Canada health monitor survey finds. Pharm Pract 1991;7:8.

Anon. Jin Bu Huan toxicity in children—Colorado, 1993. MMWR Morb Mortal Wkly Rep 1993;42:633-35.

Anon. Lead poisoning associated with use of traditional ethnic remedies—California, 1991-1992 (Editorial). JAMA 1993;270:808.

Aslam M, Shaw J. Problems of identity with traditional Asian remedies. Pharm J 1992;248:20-21, 23.

Atherton DJ. Towards the safer use of traditional remedies. BMJ 1994; 308:673-74.

But PP-H, Tal Y-T, Young K. Three fatal cases of herbal aconite poisoning. Vet Hum Toxicol 1994;36:212.

Chan TYK, Tse LKK, Chan JCN, et al. Aconitine poisoning due to Chinese herbal medicines: a review. Vet Hum Toxicol 1994;36: 453-55.

Cronan TA, Kaplan RM, Posner L, et al. Prevalence of the use of unconventional remedies for arthritis in a metropolitan community. Arthritis Rheum 1989;32:1604-07.

D'Arcy PF. Adverse reactions and interactions with herbal medicines. Part 1. Adverse reactions. Adverse Drug React Toxicol Rev 1991;10: 189-208.

D'Arcy PF. Adverse reactions and interactions with herbal medicines. Part 2. Drug interactions. Adverse Drug React Toxicol Rev 1993;12: 147-62.

Der Marderosian AH. Natural medicine. Am Drug 1994;210:61-68.

De Smet PAGM. Drugs used in nonorthodox medicine. In: Dukes MNG, Beeley L, eds. Side Effects of Drugs Annual 14. Amsterdam: Elsevier, 1990:429-51.

De Smet PAGM, Keller K, Hansel R, et al. Adverse Effects of Herbal Drugs. Vol. 1. Berlin: Springer-Verlag, 1992.

De Smet PAGM, Keller K, Hansel R, et al. Adverse Effects of Herbal Drugs. Vol. 2. Berlin: Springer-Verlag, 1993.

Eisenberg DM, Kessler RC, Foster C, et al. Unconventional medicine in the United States. N Engl J Med 1993;328:246-52.

Graham-Brown RAC, Bourke JF, Bumphrey G. Chinese herbal remedies may contain steroids. BMJ 1994;308:473.

Harper J. Traditional Chinese medicine for eczema. BMJ 1994;308: 489-90.

Hofferberth B. The efficacy of EGb 761 in patients with senile dementia of the Alzheimer type, a double-blind, placebo-controlled study on different levels of investigation. Hum Pharmacol Clin Exp 1994;9: 215-22. In: Inpharma 1994;949:12.

Houghton P. Echinacea. Pharm J 1994;253:342-43.

Houghton P. Ginkgo. Pharm J 1994;253:122-23.

Kleijnen J, Knipschild P. Ginkgo biloba. Lancet 1992;340:1136-39.

Maher EJ, Young T, Feigel I. Complementary therapies used by patients with cancer. BMJ 1994; 309:671-72.

Markowitz SB, Nunez CM, Klitzman S, et al. Lead poisoning due to Hai Ge Fen. JAMA 1994;271:932-34.

Mitchell S. Healing without doctors. Am Demographics 1993;15:46-49.

Murray RH, Rubel AJ. Physicians and healers—unwitting partners in health care. N Engl J Med 1992;326:61-64.

Solecki RS. Shanidar IV: a Neanderthal flower burial in northern Iraq. Science 1975;190:880-81.

Tyler VE. Phytomedicines in Western Europe: their potential impact on herbal medicine in the United States. Herbalgram 1994;30:24-31, 67-68, 77.

Umstead GS. Unapproved drug therapies; geriatrics, arthritis and cancer. J Pharm Technol 1988;4:97-106.

Walker AF. What is ginseng? Lancet 1994;344:619.

Allopathic Medicines

Canadian Drug Identification Code. Ottawa: Health and Welfare Canada, 1993.

Chandler RF. Licorice, more than just a flavor. Can Pharm J 1985;118(9): 421-24.

Der Marderosian A, Liberti L. Natural Product Medicine. Philadelphia: GF Stickley, 1988.

Farnsworth NR. The role of medicinal plants in drug development. In: Krogsgaard-Larsen P, Christensen SB, Kofod H, eds. Natural Products Drug Development. Copenhagen: Munksgaard, 1983:17-30.

Farnsworth NR. The role of ethnopharmacology in drug development. Ciba Foundation Symposium 154. Bioactive compounds from plants. Toronto: John Wiley and Sons, 1990:2-21.

Farnsworth NR, Bingel AS. Problems and prospects of discovering new drugs from higher plants by pharmacological screening. In: Wagner H, Wolff P, eds. New Natural Products and Plant Drugs with Pharmacological, Biological or Therapeutical Activity. New York: Springer-Verlag, 1977:1-22.

Gibson MR. Glycyrrhiza in old and new perspectives. Lloydia 1978;41: 348-54.

Grieve M. A Modern Herbal. New York: Hafner Publishing, 1967:487-93, 520-21.

Krogh CME, ed. Compendium of Pharmaceuticals and Specialties. 29th ed. Ottawa: Canadian Pharmaceutical Association, 1994.

Leung AY. Encyclopedia of Common Natural Ingredients Used in Food, Drugs, and Cosmetics. New York: John Wiley and Sons, 1980.

Tyler VE, Brady LR, Robbers JE. Pharmacognosy. Philadelphia: Lea & Febiger, 1988:176, 203-25, 482-85.

Youngken HW. Textbook of Pharmacognosy. Toronto: Blakiston, 1948: 520-21, 785-96, 812-22.

Alternative Medicine

Anon. Interest in alternative medicine growing. Am Pharm 1994;34: 12-13.

D'Arcy PF. Adverse reactions and interactions with herbal medicines. Part 2. Drug interactions. Adverse Drug React Toxicol Rev 1993;12:147-62.

Der Marderosian AH. Natural medicine. Am Drug 1994;210:61-68.

Eisenberg DM, Kessler RC, Foster C, et al. Unconventional medicine in the United States. N Engl J Med 1993;328:246-52.

Mitchell S. Healing without doctors. Am Demographics 1993;15:46-49.

Reynolds W, Executive Director, Canadian Health Food Association (personal communication). Jan 26 1995.

Rowe PM. Pharmaceutical populism at issue in USA. Lancet 1994;344: 1764.

Schwartz JD. Selling middle America on nature's way of curing illness. Brandweek 1992;33:30-32.

Weisz P. A healthier choice? Herbal, homeopathic gain acceptance. Brandweek 1994;35:26-29.

Plants Generally Regarded as Foods

Chandler RF, Anderson LA, Phillipson JD. Laetrile in perspective. Can Pharm J 1984;117(10):517-20.

Departmental consolidation of the Food and Drugs Act and of the Food and Drugs Regulations. Ottawa: Health and Welfare Canada, 1985.

Dreisbach RH. Handbook of Poisoning: Prevention, Diagnosis and Treatment. Los Altos: Lange Medical Publications, 1980:246-50.

Duke JA. Handbook of Medical Herbs. Boca Raton: CRC Press, 1985.

Frohne D, Pfander HJ. A Colour Atlas of Poisonous Plants. London: Wolfe Publishing, 1984:13-29, 63-64.

Hardin JW, Arena JM. Human Poisoning from Native and Cultivated Plants. Durham: Duke University Press, 1974:69-73, 118-19.

Lewis WH, Elvin-Lewis MPF. Medical Botany: Plants Affecting Man's Health. New York: John Wiley and Sons, 1977:5, 32, 90-91, 97-100, 213-19.

Liberti LE, ed. The Lawrence Review of Natural Products. Collegeville: Pharmaceutical Information Associates, Sept 1986.

Trease GE, Evans WC. Pharmacognosy. Philadelphia: Lea & Febiger, 1988:176, 203-25, 482-85.

Tyler VE, Brady LR, Robbers JE. Pharmacognosy. Philadelphia: Lea & Febiger, 1988:176, 203-25, 482-85.

Tyler VE. The New Honest Herbal. Philadelphia: GF Stickley, 1987.

Youngken HW. Textbook of Pharmacognosy. Toronto: Blakiston, 1948: 520-21, 785-96, 812-22.

Flavors and Spices

Anon. Report of the Expert Advisory Committee on herbs and botanical preparations. Ottawa: Health Protection Branch, Health and Welfare Canada, 1986.

Anon. Review of 171 herbs used in brewing teas. FDA Special Publication, 1975:1-32.

Canadian Drug Identification Code. Ottawa: Health and Welfare Canada, 1993.

Chandler RF. Juniper, an inconspicuous but insidious drug. Can Pharm J 1986;119(10):562-66.

Departmental consolidation of the Food and Drugs Act and of the Food and Drugs Regulations. Ottawa: Health and Welfare Canada, 1985.

Duke JA. Handbook of Medical Herbs. Boca Raton: CRC Press, 1985.

Grieve M. A Modern Herbal. New York: Hafner Publishing, 1967:487-93, 520-21.

Hawkes D, Chandler RF. Aniseed—a spice, a flavor, a drug. Can Pharm J 1984;117(1):28-29.

Leung AY. Encyclopedia of Common Natural Ingredients Used in Food, Drugs, and Cosmetics. New York: John Wiley and Sons, 1980.

Liberti LE, ed. The Lawrence Review of Natural Products. Collegeville: Pharmaceutical Information Associates, Sept 1986.

Marcus C, Lichtenstein EP. Interactions of naturally occurring food plant components with insecticides and pentobarbital in rats and mice. J Agric Food Chem 1982;30:563-68.

Miller EC, Swanson AB, Phillips DH, et al. Structure-activity studies of the carcinogenicities in the mouse and rat of some naturally occurring and synthetic alkenylbenzenes related to safrole and estragole. Cancer Res 1983;43:1124-34.

Morton JF. Atlas of Medicinal Plants of Middle America. Springfield: CC Thomas, 1981.

Osol A, Hoover JE, eds. Remington's Pharmaceutical Sciences. Easton: Mack Publishing,1975:1228.

Spoerke DG Jr. Herbal medication: use and misuse. Hosp Formul 1980;15:941-42, 945, 949-51.

Tierra M. The Way of Herbs. Santa Cruz: Unity Press, 1980:29-30, 69, 89-90.

Tyler VE, Brady LR, Robbers JE. Pharmacognosy. Philadelphia: Lea & Febiger, 1988:176, 203-25, 482-85.

Tyler VE. The New Honest Herbal. Philadelphia: GF Stickley, 1987.

Windholz M, ed. The Merck Index. Rahway, NJ: Merck Sharpe and Dohme, 1983.

Medicinal Teas

Chandler RF, Hopper SN, Harvey MJ. Ethnobotany and phytochemistry of yarrow, Achillea millefolium compositae. Econ Bot 1982;36:203-23.

Der Marderosian A. Medicinal teas—boon or bane? Drug Ther 1977;7(2): 178-81, 184-85, 188.

Duke JA. Handbook of Medical Herbs. Boca Raton: CRC Press, 1985.

Leung AY. Encyclopedia of Common Natural Ingredients Used in Food, Drugs, and Cosmetics. New York: John Wiley and Sons, 1980.

Mitchell J, Rook A. Botanical Dermatology. Vancouver: Greengrass, 1979:186-87, 212.

Montgomery B. First US report connecting death to popular Chicano, Indian herbal tea. JAMA 1977;238:1233-34.

Rodriguez E, Towers GHN, Mitchell JC. Biological activities of sesquiterpene lactones. Phytochemistry 1976;15:1573-80.

Roland AE, Smith EC. The Flora of Nova Scotia. Halifax: The Nova Scotia Museum, 1969:697-701.

Tierra M. The Way of Herbs. Santa Cruz: Unity Press, 1980:29-30, 69, 89-90.

Tyler VE. The New Honest Herbal. Philadelphia: GF Stickley, 1987.

Common Herbal Medicines

Anon. The British Pharmaceutical Codex. London: Pharmaceutical Press, 1934:569-70, 689-90, 695, 712-13, 738, 914-15.

Awang DVC. Comfrey. Can Pharm J 1987;120(2):100-04.

Awang DVC. Feverfew. Can Pharm J 1989;122(5):266-70.

Beliveau J. Valeriana officianalis. Can Pharm J 1986;119(1):24-27.

Bounthanh C, Bergmann C, Beck JP, et al. Valepotraites, a new class of cytotoxic and antitumor agents. Planta Med 1981;41:21-28.

Bradley PR. British Herbal Pharmacopeia. Bournemouth, UK: Megaron Press, 1983.

Canada Gazette Part II:1652. Schedule No. 670, 1988.

Chandler RF. Herbs as foods and medicines. Drugs Ther Maritime Pract 1987; 10(5).

Chandler RF. Juniper, an inconspicuous but insidious drug. Can Pharm J 1986;119(10):562-66.

Cooper CR, ed. Herbal remedies. Hosp Formul 1982;17:1387, 1391-92.

Der Marderosian A, Liberti L. Natural Product Medicine. Philadelphia: GF Stickley, 1988.

Duke JA. Handbook of Medical Herbs. Boca Raton: CRC Press, 1985.

Frohne D, Pfander HJ. A Colour Atlas of Poisonous Plants. London: Wolfe Publishing, 1984:13-29, 63-64.

Hamon NW. Garlic and the genus Allium. Can Pharm J 1987;120(8): 492-97.

Johnson ES, Kadam NP, Hylands DM, et al. Efficacy of feverfew as prophylactic treatment of migraine. BMJ 1985;291:569-73.

Leung AY. Encyclopedia of Common Natural Ingredients Used in Food, Drugs, and Cosmetics. New York: John Wiley and Sons, 1980.

Locock RA. Acorus calamus. Can Pharm J 1987;120(5):340-42, 344.

Locock RA. Mistletoe. Can Pharm J 1986;119(3):124-27.

Montgomery B. First US report connecting death to popular Chicano, Indian herbal tea. JAMA 1977;238:1233-34.

Olin BR, ed. Comfrey. The Lawrence Review of Natural Products. St Louis: Facts and Comparisons, Oct 1990.

Olin BR, ed. Valerian. The Lawrence Review of Natural Products. St Louis: Facts and Comparisons, Oct 1991.

Roulet M, Laurini R, Rivier L, et al. Hepatic venoocclusive disease in newborn infant of a woman drinking herbal tea. J Pediatr 1988;112: 433-36.

Spoerke DG Jr. Herbal Medications. Santa Barbara: Woodbridge Press, 1990.

Tyler VE. The New Honest Herbal. Philadelphia: GF Stickley, 1987.

Warren RG. The anti-migraine activity of feverfew (Tanacetum parthenium). Aust J Pharm 1986;67:475-77.

Safety Concerns

Anon. Canadian adverse drug reaction newsletter. Ottawa: Health Canada 1994;4(2):1-3.

Anon. Report of the Expert Advisory Committee on herbs and botanical preparations. Ottawa: Health and Welfare Canada, 1986.

Anon. Second report of the Expert Advisory Committee on herbs and botanical preparations. Ottawa: Health and Welfare Canada, 1993.

Reynier PJP, De Cremiers F. Plant-based medicinal products in France. Drug Inf J 1994;28:571-73.

Westendorf J. Pyrrolizidine alkaloids—general discussion. In: De Smet PAGM, Keller K, Hansel R, et al, eds. Adverse effects of herbal drugs. Vol. 1. Berlin: Springer-Verlag, 1992:193-206.

Westendorf J. Pyrrolizidine alkaloids—Cynoglossum officinale. In: De Smet PAGM, Keller K, Hansel R, et al, eds. Adverse Effects of Herbal Drugs. Vol. 1. Berlin: Springer-Verlag, 1992:207-10.

Westendorf J. Pyrrolizidine alkaloids—Petasites species. In: De Smet PAGM, Keller K, Hansel R, et al, eds. Adverse Effects of Herbal Drugs. Vol. 1. Berlin: Springer-Verlag, 1992:211-14.

Westendorf J. Pyrrolizidine alkaloids—Senecio species. In: De Smet PAGM, Keller K, Hansel R, et al, eds. Adverse Effects of Herbal Drugs. Vol. 1. Berlin: Springer-Verlag, 1992:215-18.

Westendorf J. Pyrrolizidine alkaloids—Symphytum species. In: De Smet PAGM, Keller K, Hansel R, et al, eds. Adverse Effects of Herbal Drugs. Vol. 1. Berlin: Springer-Verlag, 1992:219-22.

Westendorf J. Pyrrolizidine alkaloids—Tussilago farfara. In: De Smet PAGM, Keller K, Hansel R, et al, eds. Adverse Effects of Herbal Drugs. Vol. 1. Berlin: Springer-Verlag, 1992:223-26.

Poisonous Plants

Anon. Dorland's Pocket Medical Dictionary. London: Saunders, 1959.

Frohne D, Pfander HJ. A Colour Atlas of Poisonous Plants. London: Wolfe Publishing, 1984:13-29, 63-64.

Pre- and Perinatal Issues

Anon. Jin Bu Huan toxicity in children—Colorado, 1993. MMWR Morb Mortal Wkly Rep 1993;42:633-35.

Bunce KL. The use of herbs in midwifery. J Nurse Midwifery 1987;32: 255-59.

Chan TYK. The prevalence of use and harmful potential of some Chinese herbal medicines in babies and children. Vet Human Toxicol 1994; 36:238.

Der Marderosian A, Liberti L. Natural Product Medicine. Philadelphia: GF Stickley, 1988:68-69.

Hutchings DE. Issues of risk assessment: lessons from the use and abuse of drugs during pregnancy. Neurotoxicol Teratol 1990;12:183-89.

Keeler RF, Stuart LD. The nature of congenital limb defects induced in lambs by maternal ingestion of Veratrum californicum. Clin Toxicol 1987;25:273-86.

Keeler RF. Early embryonic death in lambs induced by Veratrum californicum. Cornell Vet 1990;80:203-07.

Ehudin-Pagano E, Paluzzi PA, Ivory LC, et al. The use of herbs in nurse-midwifery practice. J Nurse Midwifery 1987;32:260-62.

Kline J, Stein A, Hutzler M. Cigarettes, alcohol and marijuana: varying associations with birthweight. Int J Epidemiol 1987;16:44-51.

Lewis WH, Elvin-Lewis MPF. Medical botany. New York: John Wiley & Sons, 1977.

Pruitt AW, Jacobs EA, Schydlower M, et al. Drug-exposed infants. Pediatrics 1990;86:639-42.

Roulet M, Laurini R, Rivier L, et al. Hepatic venoocclusive disease in newborn infant of a woman drinking herbal tea. J Pediatr 1988;1(12): 433-36.

Smith CG, Asch RH. Drug abuse and reproduction. Fertil Steril 1987;48: 355-73.

Srisuphan W, Bracken MB. Caffeine consumption during pregnancy and association with late spontaneous abortion. Am J Obstet Gynecol 1986;154:14-20.

Talalaj S, Czechowicz A. Are herbal remedies safe? Med J Aust 1988;148: 102-03.

Talalaj S, Czechowicz A. Cautions in the use of herbal remedies during pregnancy and for small children. Med J Aust 1990;152:52.

Talalaj S, Czechowicz A. Hazardous herbal remedies are still on the market. Med J Aust 1990;153:302.

Westendorf J. Pyrrolizidine alkaloids—general discussion. In: De Smet PAGM, Keller K, Hansel R, et al, eds. Adverse Effects of Herbal Drugs. Vol. 1. Berlin: Springer-Verlag, 1992:193-206.

Westendorf J. Pyrrolizidine alkaloids—Cynoglossum officinale. In: De Smet PAGM, Keller K, Hansel R, et al, eds. Adverse Effects of Herbal Drugs. Vol. 1. Berlin: Springer-Verlag, 1992:207-10.

Westendorf J. Pyrrolizidine alkaloids—Petasites species. In: De Smet PAGM, Keller K, Hansel R, et al, eds. Adverse Effects of Herbal Drugs. Vol. 1. Berlin: Springer-Verlag, 1992:211-14.

Westendorf J. Pyrrolizidine alkaloids—Senecio species. In: De Smet PAGM, Keller K, Hansel R, et al, eds. Adverse Effects of Herbal Drugs. Vol. 1. Berlin: Springer-Verlag, 1992:215-18.

Westendorf J. Pyrrolizidine alkaloids—Symphytum species. In: De Smet PAGM, Keller K, Hansel R, et al, eds. Adverse Effects of Herbal Drugs. Vol. 1. Berlin: Springer-Verlag, 1992:219-22.

Westendorf J. Pyrrolizidine alkaloids—Tussilago farfara. In: De Smet PAGM, Keller K, Hansel R, et al, eds. Adverse Effects of Herbal Drugs. Vol. 1. Berlin: Springer-Verlag, 1992:223-26.

Drug Interactions

Akhtar MS, Athar MA, Yaqub M. Effect of Momordica charantia on blood glucose levels of normal and alloxan diabetic rabbits. Planta Med 1981;42:205-12.

Anon. Kelp diets can produce myxedema. JAMA 1975;233:9-19.

Anon. Herbal medicines containing germander withdrawn. Geneva: World Health Organization. PHA Information Exchange Service. Alert no. 27. 19 May 1992.

Aslam M, Stockley IH. Interaction between curry ingredient (karela) and drug (chlorpropamide). Lancet 1979;1:607.

Blumenthal M. Debunking the ginseng abuse syndrome. Whole Foods 1991;(Mar). Via Classical Botanical Reprint No. 223.

Bo-Linn GW, Morawski SG, Fordtran JS. Starch blockers their effect on calorie absorption from a high-starch meal. N Engl J Med 1982;307: 1413-16.

Bradley PR, ed. British Herbal Pharmacopeia. Bournemouth, UK: Megaron Press, 1983.

But PP-H, Tal Y-T, Young K. Three fatal cases of herbal aconite poisoning. Vet Hum Toxicol 1994;36:212.

Caley MJ, Clarke RA. Cardiac arrhythmia after mushroom ingestion. BMJ 1977;2:1633.

Chandler RF. Licorice, more than just a flavor. Can Pharm J 1985;118(9): 421-24.

Cosyns J-P, Jadoul M, Squifflet J-P, et al. Chinese herbs nephropathy: a clue to Balkan endemic nephropathy? Kidney Int 1994;45:1680-88. Via Inpharma 1994;947:21.

D'Arcy PF. Adverse reactions and interactions with herbal medicines. Part 1. Adverse reactions. Adverse Drug React Toxicol Rev 1991;10: 189-208.

D'Arcy PF. Adverse reactions and interactions with herbal medicines. Part 2. Drug interactions. Adverse Drug React Toxicol Rev 1993;12: 147-162.

Der Marderosian A, Liberti L. Natural Product Medicine. Philadelphia: GF Stickley, 1988:68-69.

De Smet PAGM, Stricker BHC, Wilderink F, et al. Hyperthyreoidie tijdens her gebruik van kelptabletten. Ned Tijdschr Geneeskd 1990;134: 1058-59.

De Smet PAGM. Toxicological outlook on the quality assurance of herbal remedies. In: De Smet PAGM, Keller H, Hansel R, et al, eds. Adverse Effects of Herbal Drugs. Berlin: Springer-Verlag, 1992:1-72.

De Smet PAGM. Drugs used in nonorthodox medicine. In: Dukes MNG, ed. Meyler's Side Effects of Drugs. 12th ed. Amsterdam: Elsevier, 1992:1209-32.

De Smet PAGM, Keller K, Hansel R, et al. Adverse Effects of Herbal Drugs. Vol. 2. Berlin: Springer-Verlag, 1993.

De Smet PAGM, Smeets OSNM. Potential risks of health food products containing yohimbe extracts. BMJ 1994;309:958.

Dukes MNG. Remedies used in nonorthodox medicine. In: Dukes MNG, ed. Side Effects of Drugs, annual 1. Amsterdam: Excerpta Medica, 1977:371-78.

Farnsworth NR, Kinghorn AD, Soejarto DD, et al. Siberian ginseng (Eleutherococcus scuticosus): current status as an adaptogen. Econ Bot Plant Res 1987;1:156.

Fleminger R.Visual hallucinations and illusions with propranolol. BMJ 1978;1:1182.

Fushimi R, Tachi J, Amino N, et al. Chinese medicine interfering with digoxin immunoassays. Lancet 1989;1:339.

Griffin JP. Drug-induced disorders of mineral metabolism. In: D'Arcy P, Griffin JP, eds. Iatrogenic Diseases. 2nd ed. Oxford: Oxford University Press, 1979:226-38.

Heald GE, Poller L. Anticoagulants and treatment for children. BMJ 1974;1:455.

Hogan RP. Hemorrhagic diathesis caused by drinking a herbal tea. JAMA 1983;249:2679-80.

Huupponen R, Seppala P, Lisalo E. Effect of guar gum, a fibre preparation, on digoxin and penicillin absorption in man. Eur J Clin Pharmacol 1984;26:279-81.

Jones BD, Runikis AM. Interaction of ginseng with phenelzine. J Clin Psychopharmacol 1987;7:201-02.

Jori A, Bianchetti A, Prestini PE. Effect of essential oils on drug metabolism. Biochem Pharmacol 1969;18:2081-85.

Karunanithy R, Sumita KP. Undeclared drugs in Chinese antirheumatoid medicine. Int J Pharm Pract 1991;1:117-19.

Kempin SJ. Warfarin resistance caused by broccoli. N Engl J Med 1983; 308:1229-30.

Koreich OM. Ginseng and mastalgia. BMJ 1978;1:1566.

Koren G, Randor S, Martin S, et al. Maternal ginseng use associated with neonatal androgenization. JAMA 1990;264:2866.

Koren G, Gladstone D, Martin S, et al. Periploca in disguise—the need for regulation of herbal products. Can J Clin Pharmacol 1994;1:13-16.

Leatherdale BA, Panesar RK, Singh G, et al. Improvement in glucose tolerance due to Momordica charantia (karela). BMJ 1981;282: 1823-24.

Lewis WH, Elvin-Lewis MPF. Medical Botany. New York: John Wiley & Sons, 1977.

Miyazaki S, Inoue H, Nadai T. Effect of antacids on the distribution behaviour of tetracycline and methacycline. Chem Pharm Bull 1977; 27:2523-27.

Nemirovskii ON. Toxicological characteristics of some essential oils according to the results of single and repeated exposures. Trening Sanit-gig-Med Inst 1975;111:61-65. Via Chem Abst 89:85417.

Palmer BV, Montgomery AC, Monteiro JC. Ginseng and mastalgia. BMJ 1978;1:1284.

Perlmann BB. Interaction between lithium salts and ispaghula husk. Lancet 1990;335:416.

Punnonen R, Lukola A. Oestrogen-like effect of ginseng. BMJ 1980; 281:1110.

Radford AP. Ink caps and mushrooms. BMJ 1978;1:112.

Seawright AA, Steele DP, Menrath RE. Seasonal variation in hepatic microsomal oxidation metabolism in vitro and susceptibility to carbon tetrachloride in a flock of sheep. Aust Vet J 1972;48:488-94.

Shader RI, Greenblatt DJ. Phenelzine and the dream machine-ramblings and reflections (editorial). J Clin Psychopharmacol 1985;5:65.

Shima K, Tanaka A, Ikegami H, et al. Effect of dietary fiber, glucomannan, on absorption of sulfonylurea in man. Horm Metab Res 1983;15:1-3.

Talalaj S, Czechowicz A. Are herbal remedies safe? Med J Aust 1988;148: 102-03.

Tanner LA, Bosco LA. Gynecomastia associated with calcium channel blocker therapy. Arch Intern Med 1988;148:379-80.

Udall JA, Krock LB. A modified method of anticoagulant therapy. Curr Ther Res 1968;10:207-1.

Walker FB. Myocardial infarction after diet-induced warfarin resistance. Arch Intern Med 1984;144:3089-90.

Watson AJ, Pegg M, Green JRB. Enteral feeds may antagonise warfarin. BMJ 1984;288:557.

Welihinda J, Karunanayke EH, Sherrif MHR, et al. Effect of Momordica charantia on the glucose tolerance in maturity onset diabetes. J Ethnopharmacol 1986;17:277-82.

White RD, Swick RA, Cheeke PR. Effects of microsomal enzymes induction the toxicity ofpyrrolizidine (Senecio) alkaloids. J Toxicol Environ Health 1983;12:633-40.

Wilkins RW. Clinical usage of Rauwolfia alkaloids including reserpine (Serpasil). Ann N Y Acad Sci 1954;59:36-44.

Young RE, Milroy R, Hutchison S, et al. The rising price of mushrooms. Lancet 1982;1:213-15.

CHAPTER 15—Homeopathic Products

History

Bradford L. The Life and Letters of Dr. Samuel Hahnemann. Philadelphia: Boericke and Tafel, 1895.

Brown PS. Nineteenth-century American health reformers and the early nature cure movement in Britain. Medical History 1988:32:174-94.

Coutler HL. Divided Legacy: The Conflict Between Homeopathy and the American Medical Association (volume III). Berkeley: North Atlantic Books, 1981.

Cummings S, Ullman D. Everybody's Guide to Homeopathic Medicines. Los Angeles: Jeremy P. Tarcher, 1984.

Danziger E. The Emergence of Homeopathy: Alchemy into Medicine. London: Century, 1987.

Grossinger R. Planet Medicine: From Stone-Age Shamanism to Post-Industrial Medicine. Berkeley: North Atlantic Books, 1987.

Kaufman M. Homeopathy in America. Baltimore: Johns Hopkins University Press, 1971.

Robinson K. Homeopathy: Questions and Answers (pamphlet), 1980.

Starr P. Social Transformation of American Medicine. New York: Basic, 1982.

Ullman D. Homeopathy: Medicine for the 21st Century Man. Berkeley, CA: North Atlantic Books, 1991.

Current Use of Homeopathy

Anon. Magic or Medicine. Which? 1986:443-447.

Anon. Taking the Alternative Path to Health. Times (London) 1985 March 13.

Chase A. Options: Homeopathy. Washington Post 1983 April 28;D5.

Eizayaga FX. Homeopathy. World Homeopathic Directory. New Delhi: Harjeet, 1982:36-7.

Eizayaga FX. Homeopathy in American Spanish-Speaking Countries. A Presentation at the Annual Conference of the National Center for Homeopathy; 1985 October 4-5.

Furnam A, Smith C. Choosing alternative medicine: A comparison of the beliefs of patients visiting a general practitioner and a homeopath. Soc Sci Med 1988;26(7):685-9.

Kishore J. Homeopathy: The Indian experience. World Health Forum 1983;3:107.

Knipschild P, Kleijnen J, ter Riet G. Belief in the efficacy of alternative medicine among general practitioners in the Netherlands. Soc Sci Med 1990;31(5):625-6.

McKee J. Holistic health and the critique of Western medicine. Soc Sci Med 1991;26(8):775-84.

Poll IFOP. Médecines douces: la revanche de l'Homéopathie. Le Nouvel Observateur 1985; avril 12:36-41.

Swayne J. Survey of the use of homeopathic medicine in the U.K. health system. J R Coll Gen Pract 1989;Dec:503-6.

Thomas K, Carr J, Westlake L, et al. Use of non-orthodox and conventional care in Great Britain. BMJ 1991;302(6770):207-10.

Wharton R, Lewith G. Complementary medicine and the general practitioner. BMJ 1986;292(June 7):1498-5000.

What is homeopathy?

Grossinger R. Planet Medicine: From Stone-Age Shamanism to Post-Industrial Medicine. Berkeley, CA: North Atlantic Books, 1987.

Ullman D. Homeopathy: Medicine for the 21st Century Man. Berkeley, CA: North Atlantic Books, 1991.

Law of Similars

Cummings S, Ullman D. Everybody's Guide to Homeopathic Medicines. Los Angeles: Jeremy P. Tarcher, 1984.

Danziger E. The Emergence of Homeopathy: Alchemy into Medicine. London: Century, 1987.

Ford JM. Principles of homeopathy. Midwives Chronicle and Nursing Notes 1988;May:148-9.

Moore E. Homeopathy. On Cont Pract 1989;16(1):21-4.

Ullman D. Homeopathy: Medicine for the 21st Century Man. Berkeley, CA: North Atlantic Books, 1991.

Vithoulkas G. Homeopathy: Medicine for the New Man. New York: Arco, 1979.

Infinitesimal Doses

Cummings S, Ullman D. Everybody's Guide to Homeopathic Medicines. Los Angeles: Jeremy P. Tarcher, 1984.

Ford JM. Principles of homeopathy. Midwives Chronicle and Nursing Notes 1988;May:148-9.

Picard P, et al. The Canadian Guide to Homeopathic Self-medication. Montreal: Chenelière, 1995.

Ullman D. Homeopathy: Medicine for the 21st Century Man. Berkeley, CA: North Atlantic Books, 1991.

Choosing a Remedy

Grossinger R. Planet Medicine: From Stone-age Shamanism to Post-industrial Medicine. Berkeley, CA: North Atlantic Books, 1987.

Lockie A. Family Guide to Homeopathy. Toronto: Penguin Books, 1989.

Ullman D. Homeopathy: Medicine for the 21st Century Man. Berkeley, CA: North Atlantic Books, 1991.

Basic Science

Cazin JC, et al. A Study of the effect of decimal and centesimal dilution of arsenic on rentention and mobilization of arsenic in the rat. Human Toxicol 1987;July. Vol 6.

Davenas E, Beauvais F, Amara J, et al. Human basophil degranulation triggered by very dilute antiserum against IgE. Nature 1988;333:816-8.

Davenas E, Poitevin B, Benveniste J. Effect on mouse peritoneal macrophages of orally administered very high dilutions of silica. Eur J Pharmacol 1987;135(April):313-319.

Maddox J, et al. 'High-dilution' experiments a delusion. Nature 1988; 334(July 28):443-7.

Now you see it (Editorial). Scientific American 1988;September:19-20.

Silvio M, Paparelli A. Ultrasonic study of homeopathic solutions. Br Homeopath J 1990;79:212-6.

When to believe the unbelievable (Editorial). Nature 1988;333(June 30): 816-8.

Clinical Trials

Ferley JP, et al. A controlled evaluation of a homeopathic preparation in the treatment of influenza-like syndromes. Br J Clin Pharmacol 1989;299(March):365-6.

Fisher P. Research into homeopathic treatment of rheumatological disease: Why and how? Complementary Medical Res 1990;4(3):34-40.

Fisher P. Effect of homeopathic treatment on fibrositis (primary fibromyalgia). BMJ 1989;229(Aug. 5):365-6.

Gibson RG, Gibson SLM, MacNeil AD, et al. Homeopathic therapy in rheumatoid arthritis: evaluation by double-blind clinical therapeutic trial. Br J Clin Pharmacol 1980;9:453-9.

Gibson RG, Gibson SLM, MacNeil AD, et al. Salicylates and homeopathy in rheumatoid arthritis: preliminary observations. Br J Clin Pharmacol 1978;6:391-5.

Kleijnen J, Knipschild P, ter Riet G. Clinical trials of homeopathy. BMJ 1991;302(772):316-22.

Leaman AM, Gorman D. Cantharis in the early treatment of minor burns. Arch Emerg Med 1989;6:259-61.

Reilly DT, Taylor MA, McSharry C, et al. Is homeopathy a placebo response? Controlled trial of homeopathic potency with pollen in hayfever as model. Lancet 1986;Oct 18:881-5.

Shipley M, Berry H, Broster G, et al. Controlled trial of homeopathic treatment of osteoarthritis. Lancet 1983;Jan 15:97-8.

Voziznov AF, Simeonova NK. Homeopathic treatment of patients with adenomas of the prostate. Br Homeopath J 1990;79:148-151.

Alternatives to Classical Homeopathy

Yasgus JA. Dictionary of Homeopathic Medical Terminology. 2nd ed. Vau Hoy Publishers, 1992.

Homeopathic Standards

Krogh CME, ed. Compendium of Pharmaceuticals and Specialties. 29th ed. Ottawa: Canadian Pharmaceutical Association, 1994:B118.

Moore E. Homeopathy. On Cont Pract 1989:16(1):21-4.

Counselling Tips/Advice for the Patient

Cummings S, Ullman D. Everybody's Guide to Homeopathic Medicines. Los Angeles: Jeremy P. Tarcher, 1984.

Lockie A. Family Guide to Homeopathy. Toronto: Penguin Books, 1989.

Picard P, et al. The Canadian Guide to Homeopathic Self-medication. Montreal: Chenelière, 1995.

Homeopathic Medicines in Pharmacies

Cummings S, Ullman D. Everybody's Guide to Homeopathic Medicines. Los Angeles: Jeremy P. Tarcher, 1984.

Picard P, et al. The Canadian Guide to Homeopathic Self-medication. Montreal: Chenelière, 1995.

CHAPTER 16—Medical Devices

Anon. Five therapies account for 60% of home infusion. US Pharmacist 1993; 18(4):16.

Anon. New trial using home infusion therapy for breast cancer patients. Pharm J 1993;251:797.

Beasley R, Cushley M, Holgate ST. A self management plan in the treatment of adult asthma. Thorax 1989;44:200-04.

Bernstein LH. An update on home intravenous antibiotic therapy. Geriatrics 1991;46(6):47-52.

Bettess S. Home diagnostic agents and testing devices. Winnipeg: Canadian Council on Continuing Education in Pharmacy, 1989: XI (3).

Brandt LJ, Steiner-Grossman P, eds. Treating IBD. New York: Raven Press, 1989.

Broadwell DC, Jackson BS. Principles of Ostomy Care. St. Louis: Mosby, 1982.

Caiola SM. The pharmacist and home use pregnancy tests. Am Pharm 1992;NS32(1):57-60.

Charlton I, Charlton G, Broomfield J, et al. Evaluation of peak flow and symptoms, self-management plans for control of asthma in general practice. BMJ 1990;301:1355-59.

Cherniak RM. Chronic and acute asthma: keep to successful management. Postgrad Med 1984;75(2):87-98.

Chrisman CR, Self TH, Rumback MJ. Use of peak flow meters in asthmatics. Am Pharm 1991;NS31(5):24-28.

Clark NM. Asthma self-management education. Chest 1989;95(5): 1110-13.

Cote D, Oruck J, Thickson ND. A Review of the Manitoba home IV antibiotic program. Can J Hosp Pharm 1989;42(4):137-41.

de Champlain J. The clinical evaluation of hypertension. Can Fam Physician 1985;31:307-12.

Eron LJ. Parenteral antibiotic therapy in outpatients: quality assurance and other issues in a protohospital. Chemotherapy 1991;37 (suppl):1-40.

Evans CE, Logan AG. The Canadian consensus on hypertension management. Montreal: Canadian Hypertension Society, 1990:1-12.

Evans CE, Haynes RB, Goldsmith CH, et al. Home blood pressure monitoring: a comparative study of accuracy. J Hypertension 1989;7:133-42.

Finlayson M, Havixbeck K. A post-discharge study on the use of assistive devices. Can J Occup Ther 1992;59(4):201-07.

Fletcher M. Electronic blood pressure monitors. Can Consumer 1987; 17(2):21-24.

Gossell TA. Diagnostic products. US Pharmacist 1986;11(2):68-72.

Graham DR, Keldermans MM, Klem LW, et al. Infectious complications among patients receiving home intravenous therapy with peripheral, central, or peripherally placed central venous catheters. Am J Med 1991;91(suppl 3B):95S-100S.

Gringuaz A. Monoclonal antibodies. US Pharmacist 1985;10(10):38-48.

Horner ES. Urinary incontinence. US Pharmacist 1993;18(4):65-80.

Howard L, Heaphey MS, Fleming CR, et al. Four years of North American registry home parenteral nutrition outcome data and their implications for patient management. JPEN 1991;15:384-93.

Hunter KA, Bryant BG. Educating parents and children about asthma. US Pharmacist 1993;18(11):84-96.

Jaybose S, Escobedo V, Tugal O, et al. Home chemotherapy for children with cancer. Cancer 1992;69(2):574-79.

Lum L. Ovulation predictor tests. Pharm Pract 1990;6(8):31-34.

Mandelstam D. Incontinence and its Management. Dover: Croom Helm, 1986.

McAbee RR, Grupp K, Horn B. Home intravenous therapy: Part I—issues. Home Health Care Services Quarterly 1991;12(3):59-121.

Miyahara RK, Nykamp D. On the shelf and in the future. US Pharmacist 1990;15(3):50-62.

Norman RJ. When a positive pregnancy test isn't. Med J Aust 1991; 154:718-19.

Oed ML. Measuring blood pressure and blood cholesterol: the need for accuracy and precision. US Pharmacist 1990; Cardiovascular Disease Supplemental: 52-56.

Patt RB. PCA: prescribing analgesia for home management of severe pain. Geriatrics 1992;47(3):69-84.

Pedretti MS, Zoltan B. Occupational Therapy Practice Skills for Physical Dysfunction. 3rd ed. Toronto: Mosby, 1990.

Phillips RH. Coping with an Ostomy. Wayne: Avery Publishing Group, 1986.

Rappaport MB, Dibble SL, Ryder MA. Venous access device utilization in home care settings. Home Health Care Services Quarterly 1994;14(4): 141-62.

Schmidt GR, Hoettels Wenig J. An evaluation of home blood pressure monitoring devices. Am Pharm 1989;NS29(91):25-30.

Schoepp G. Winds of change. Drug Merchandising 1991;72(11):9-13.

Thickson ND. Economic of home intravenous services. PharmacoEconomics 1993;3(3):220-27.

Trombly CA, ed. Occupational Therapy for Physical Dysfunction. 3rd ed. Baltimore: Williams & Wilkins, 1987.

Fecal Occult Blood Testing

Anon. Home diagnostic kits for early colorectal cancer detection. Current Trends in Drug Therapy. Rocky Mountain Poison and Drug Foundation 1985;VI(6).

Canadian Task Force on Periodic Health Examination. The periodic health examination. Can Med Assoc J 1979;121:1193-254.

Gilbertsen VA, McHugh RB, Schuman L, et al. The earlier detection of colorectal cancers. A preliminary report of the result of the occult blood study. Cancer 1980;45:2899-901.

Gossel TA. Fecal occult blood testing products. US Pharmacist 1986; 11(4):40-51.

Greegor DH. Diagnosis of large-bowel cancer in the asymptomatic patient. JAMA 1967;201(12):123.

Hoogewerf PE, et al. Patient compliance with screening for fecal occult blood in family practice. Can Med Assoc J 1987;137:195-98.

Pye G, Jackson J, Thomas WM, et al. Comparison of Coloscreen Self-Test and Haemoccult fecal occult blood tests in the detection of colorectal cancer in symptomatic patients. Br J Surg 1990;77:630-31.

Simon JB. Occult blood screening for colorectal carcinoma: a critical review. Gastroenterology 1985;88:820-37.

Simon JB. Occult blood screening of Canadians: wise or unwise? Can Med Assoc J 1985;133:647-49.

Uchida K, Matsuse R, et al. Immunochemical detection of human blood in feces. Clin Chim Acta 1990;189:267.

CHAPTER 17—Men's Health Care Products

Jock Itch

Arndt KA. Manual of Dermatologic Therapeutics. Toronto: Little, Brown and Company, 1986.

Battistini F, Cordero C, Urcuyo FG, et al. The treatment of dermatophytoses of the glabrous skin: a comparison of undecylenic acid and its salt versus tolnaftate. Int J Dermatol 1983;22:388-9.

Bennett JE. Antimicrobial agents: antifungal agents. In: Gilman AG, et al, eds. The Pharmacological Basis of Therapeutics. New York: Pergamon Press, 1990:1165-85.

Clayton YM, Gange RW, MacDonald DM, et al. A clinical double-blind trial of topical haloprogin and miconazole against superficial fungal infections. Clin Exp Dermatol 1979;4:65-73.

Cohn MS. Superficial fungal infections. Postgrad Med 1992;91(2):239.

Federal Register 1992;57:38568.

Fuerst JF, Cox GF, Weaver SM, et al. Comparison between undecylenic acid and tolnaftate in the treatment of tinea pedis. Cutis 1980; 25:544-7, 549.

Male O. A double-blind comparison of clotrimazole and tolnaftate therapy of superficial dermatophytoses. Postgrad Med J 1974;50 (Suppl 1): 75-6.

Mandell, Douglas, Bennett. Principles and Practice of Infectious Diseases. 3rd ed. New York, NY: Churchill Livingstone, 1990.

Lookingbill DP, Marks JG. Principles of Dermatology. Toronto: WB Saunders Company, 1986.

Popovich NG. Foot care products. In: Handbook of Nonprescription Drugs. 9th ed. Washington, DC: American Pharmaceutical Association, 1990:963-1003.

Spiekermann PH, Young MD. Clinical evaluation of clotrimazole. A broad-spectrum antifungal agent. Arch Dermatol 1976;112:350.

Tschen EH, Becker LE, Ulrich JA, et al. Comparison of over-the-counter agents for tinea pedis. Cutis 1979;23:696-8.

VanDersarl JV, Sheppard RH. Clotrimazole vs haloprogin treatment of tinea cruris. Arch Dermatol 1977;113:1233-5.

Contraception

AHFS Drug Information 92. Bethesda, MD: American Society of Hospital Pharmacists, Inc., 1994.

Anon. New condom for men to be made of plastic. Medical Post 1994; 30(17):64.

Anon. Male contraceptive has electric charge to zap sperm dead. Toronto Star 1993 Sept. 15.

Anon. Proper use of condoms. US Pharmacist 1992;17(11):42.

Carrier RS. Contraceptive methods and products. In: Handbook of Nonprescription Drugs. Washington, DC: American Pharmaceutical Association, 1990:715.

Condoms for prevention of sexually transmitted diseases. MMWR 1988; 37(9):133-7.

Gebhart F. Itching for safe sex? Relief may be on the way. Drug Topics 1992; May:46.

Kastrup EK, Olin BR, eds. Facts and Comparisons. St. Louis: JB Lippincott, 1994:107b.

Pray WS. Condoms and preventing HIV transmission. US Pharmacist 1992; 17(1):37.

Verbal communication: Stephan Michael, Okamoto, Stamford CT, USA 06497;(203)375-0003.

Premature Ejaculation

Aycock L. The medical management of premature ejaculation. J Urol 1949;63:432.

Bennet D. Treatment of ejaculation praecox with monoamine oxidase inhibitors. Lancet 1961;2:1309.

Beretta G, et al. Effect of alpha-blocking agent in the management of premature ejaculation. Acta Europa Fertilatis 1986;17:43.

Blachly PM. Management of the opiate abstinence syndrome. Am J Psychiatry 1966;122:742.

Buffum J. Pharmacosexology: The effects of drugs on sexual function: A review. J Psychoact Drugs1982;14:5.

Cooper AG, et al. A clinical trial of the beta blocker propranolol in premature ejaculation. J Psychosom Res 1984;28:331.

Damrau F. Premature ejaculation: Use of ethyl amino benzoate to prolong coitus. J Urol 1963;89:936.

Diagnostic and Statistical Manual of Mental Disorders. 3rd ed. Washington, DC: American Psychiatric Association, 1987.

Fein RL. Intracavernous medication for treatment of premature ejaculation. Urology 1980;35:301.

Frank E, et al. Frequency of sexual dysfunction in "normal" couples. N Engl J Med 1978;299:111.

Girgis SM, et al. A double blind trial of clomipramine in premature ejaculation. Andrologia 1982;14:364.

Goodman RE. An assessement of clomipramine in the treatment of premature ejaculation. J Int Med Res 1980;8 (Suppl 3):53.

Homonnal ZT, et al. Phenoxybenzamine—An effective male contraceptive pill. Contraception 1984;29:479.

Hughes JM. Failure to ejaculate with chlordiazepoxide. Am J Psychiatry 1964;121:610.

Kaplan HS. The New Sex Therapy. New York:Brunner/Mazel, 1974.

Keitner GI, et al. Spontaneous ejaculation and neuroleptics. J Clin Psychopharmacol 1983;3:34.

Masters WH, Johnson VE. Human Sexual Inadequacy. Boston: Little, Brown and Company, 1970.

Mellgren A. Treatment of ejaculation praecox with thioridazine. Psychosomatique 1987;15:454.

Nettelbladt P, et al. Sexual dysfunction and sexual satisfaction in 58 unmarried swedish males. J Urol 1979;23:141.

Nininger JE. Inhibition of ejaculation by amitriptylline. Am J Psychiatry 1978;135:750.

Rapp MS. Two cases of ejaculatory impairment related to phenelzine. Am J Psychiatry 1979;136:1200.

Segraves RT. Treatment of premature ejaculation with lorazepam. Am J Psychiatry 1987;144:1240.

Shapiro B. Premature ejaculation: A review of 1130 cases. J Urol 1943; 50:374.

Stanley E. Premature ejaculation. BMJ 1981;282:1521.

Williams W. Secondary premature ejaculation. Austral N Z J Psychiatry 1984;18:333.

Pharmaceutical Agents

American Hospital Formulary Services—Drug Information. Bethesda: American Society of Hospital Pharmacists, 1994.

Beam TR. Antifungal agents. In: Smith CM, Reynard AM, eds. Textbook of Pharmacology. Philadelphia: WB Saunders Company, 1992:888.

F.D.C. Reports—"The Pink Sheet" March 11, 1985: T&G7.

Popovich NG. Foot care products. In: Handbook of Nonprescription Drugs. 9th ed. Washington DC: American Pharmaceutical Association, 1990:963.

Reynolds JEF. Martindale: The Extra Pharmacopoeia (electronic version). Denver, CO: Micromedex Inc., 1994.

USP-DI Volume II. Advice for the Patient. Rockville MD: United States Pharmacopeial Convention, 1994.

CHAPTER 18—Nutrition Products

General Principles of Nutrition

Normal Nutrition and Canada's Food Guide to Healthy Eating

Bowman A, Stern ML. Parameters in nutritional assessment. In: Bell L, ed. Manual of Nutritional Care. 4th ed. Vancouver: British Columbia Dietitians' & Nutritionists' Association, 1992:71-88.

Garrow JS, Livingstone WPT, eds. Human Nutrition and Dietetics. 9th ed. Edinburgh: Churchill Livingstone, 1993.

Health and Welfare Canada. Canada's food guide to healthy eating. Ottawa: Supply and Services Canada, 1992.

Health and Welfare Canada. Nutrition recommendations: The report of the Scientific Review Committee. Ottawa: Supply and Services Canada, 1990.

Health and Welfare Canada. Canadian guidelines for healthy weights. Reports of Expert Committee. Ottawa: Supply and Services Canada, 1988.

Health and Welfare Canada. Nutrition recommendations update on dietary fat and children. Ottawa: Supply and Services Canada, 1993.

Health and Welfare Canada. Promoting healthy weights: a discussion paper. Ottawa: Supply and Services Canada, 1988.

Holbrook JM, McCarter DN. General nutrition. In: Herfindal ET, Gourley DR, Hart LL, eds. Clinical Pharmacy and Therapeutics. 5th ed. Baltimore: Williams & Wilkins, 1992:122-32.

McCarter DN, Holbrook JM. Vitamins and minerals. In: Herfindal ET, Gourley DR, Hart LL, eds. Clinical Pharmacy and Therapeutics. 5th ed. Baltimore: Williams & Wilkins, 1992:133-49.

Pard J, ed. Nutritional Care Manual. Don Mills: Ontario Hospital Association, 1989:69-96.

Basic Nutrients: A Review

Brownridge E. Foods that fight back. Pharmacy Practice 1993;9(5):40-50.

Choy G, Kali-Rai R, Ferrill M. A review of vitamins and their therapeutic uses. Calif Pharm 1993;(Mar):42-52.

Holbrook JM, McCarter DN. General nutrition. In: Herfindal ET, Gourley DR, Hart LL, eds. Clinical Pharmacy and Therapeutics. 5th ed. Baltimore: Williams & Wilkins, 1992:122-32.

McCarter DN, Holbrook J. Vitamins and minerals. In: Herfindal ET, Gourley DR, Hart LL, eds. Clinical Pharmacy and Therapeutics. 5th ed. Baltimore: Williams & Wilkins, 1992:133-49.

O'Connor D. Folic acid and neural tube defects prevention. Natl Inst Nutr Rev 1993;8(21):1-3.

Pard J. Nutritional Care Manual. Don Mills: Ontario Hospital Association, 1989.

Nutritional Assessment

Bowman A, Stern ML. Parameters in nutritional assessment. In: Bell L, ed. Manual of Nutritional Care. 4th ed. Vancouver: British Columbia Dietitians' & Nutritionists' Association, 1992:71-88.

Teasley-Strausburg KM. Nutritional status assessment. In: Teasley-Strausburg KM, Cerra FB, Lehmann S, et al, eds. Nutritional Support Handbook, A Compendium of Products and Guidelines for Usage. Cincinnati: Harvey-Whitney Books, 1992:1-18.

Infant Formulas

American Academy of Pediatrics. The transfer of drugs and other chemicals into human milk. Pediatrics 1994;93(1):137-50.

Anderson PO. Drug use during breast-feeding. Clin Pharm 1991;10: 594-621.

Barness LA. Pediatric Nutrition Handbook. 3rd ed. Elk Grove Village, Ill: Am Acad Ped, 1993.

Bell L, ed. Manual of Nutritional Care. 4th ed. Vancouver: British Columbia Dietitians' & Nutritionists' Association, 1992.

Bradley CL. Common infant feeding problems. Pharm Prac 1993;10:58-78.

Briggs GG, Freeman RK, Yaffee SJ. Drugs in Pregnancy and Lactation, a Reference Guide to Fetal and Neonatal Risks. 4th ed. Baltimore: Williams & Wilkins, 1994.

Briggs GG. Drugs in pregnancy and lactation. In: Koda Kimble MA, Young LY, eds. Applied Therapeutics: the Clinical Use of Drugs. Vancouver, WA: Applied Therapeutics, 1992.

Buttar HS. Neonatal risks of drugs excreted in breast milk. Can Pharm J 1994;127(8):14-19.

Canadian Pediatric Society, Nutrition Committee. Fluoride supplementation. Contemp Pediatr 1987;3:50-56.

Canadian Pediatric Society, Nutrition Committee. Meeting iron needs in infants and young children: an update. Can Med Assoc J 1991; 144:1451.

Health and Welfare Canada. Feeding babies: a counselling guide on practical solutions to common infant feeding questions. Ottawa: Supply and Services Canada, 1986.

Health and Welfare Canada. Nutrition recommendations: the report of the Scientific Review Committee. Ottawa: Supply and Services Canada, 1990.

Kacew S. Adverse effects of drugs and chemicals in breast milk on the nursing infant. J Clin Pharmacol 1993;33:213-21.

Marshall LL. Infant formula products. Am Pharm 1993;NS33(10):55-60.

Murry L, Seger D. Drug therapy during pregnancy and lactation (Review). Emerg Med Clin North Am 1994;12(1):129-49.

Ontario Dietetic Association, Ontario Hospital Association. Nutritional Care Manual. 6th ed. Don Mills: The Ontario Hospital Assoc, 1989.

Principles of Weight Control

Symptoms of Obesity and Treatment

Appelt GD. Weight control products. In: Covington TR, ed. Handbook of Nonprescription Drugs. Washington: American Pharmaceutical Association, 1993:339-48.

Bjortorp P, VanItalhie TB, eds. The cost of obesity. Pharmacoeconomics 1994;5(1):1-79.

Davis J, Sherer K. Applied Nutrition and Diet Therapy for Nurses. 2nd ed. Philadelphia: Saunders, 1994:584-613.

Energy balance and weight control. In: Whitney EN, Hamilton EMN, Rolfes SR. Understanding Nutrition. 5th ed. St. Paul: West Publishing, 1990:349-90.

Gray DS. Diagnosis and prevalence of obesity. Med Clin North Am 1989; 73:1-13.

Health and Welfare Canada. Canadian guidelines for healthy weight: report of Expert Committee. Ottawa: Supply and Services, 1988.

Health and Welfare Canada. Promoting healthy weights: a discussion paper. 14th ed. Ottawa: Supply and Services Canada, 1988.

Jinks M, Garrison MW. Obesity and eating disorders. In: Herfindal ET, Gourley DR, Hart LL, eds. Clinical Pharmacy and Therapeutics.- Baltimore: Williams & Wilkins, 1992:984-95.

Kendall A, Levitsky DA, Strupp BJ et al. Weight-loss on a low fat diet: consequences of the imprecision of the control of food intake in human. Am J Clin Nutr 1991; 53(5)1124-9.

Lissner L. Causes, diagnosis and risks of obesity. Pharmacoeconomics 1994;2(suppl 1):8-17.

Miller WJ, Stephens T. The prevalence of overweight and obesity in Britain, Canada and United States. Am J Public Health 1987;77:38-41.

Nutrition recommendations update on dietary fat and children. Ottawa: Supply and Services Canada, 1993.

Pi-Sunyer FX. Medical hazards of obesity. Ann Intern Med 1993;119(7 pt 2):655-60.

Prewitt TE, Schmeisser D, Bowen PE, et al. Changes in body weight composition, and energy intake in women fed high- and low-fat diets. Am J Clin Nutr 1991;54 (2):304-10.

Sheppard L, Kristal AR, Kushi L, et al. Weight loss in women participants in a randomized trial of low-fat diets. Am J Clin Nutr 1991;54(2): 821-28.

Smigerowsky N. Eating disorders I: Anorexia nervosa and bulimia nervosa (lecture presentation for MED 413: Nutrition course) April, 1995. Faculty of Medicine, University of Alberta, Edmonton.

VanItallie TB. Worldwide epidemiology of obesity. Pharmacoeconomics 1994;5(suppl 1):1-7.

Special Nutrition Requirements

Nutrition Requirements for Specific Health and Disease States

Abrams B, Duncan D, Hertz-Picciotto I. A prospective study of dietary intake and acquired immune deficiency syndrome in HIV-seropositive homosexual men. J Acquir Immune Defic Syndr 1993;6:949-58.

Armstrong AL, Wallace WA. The epidemiology of hip fractures and methods of prevention (Review). Acta Orthop Belg 1994;1(60 suppl): 85-101.

Bell L, ed. Manual of Nutritional Care. 4th ed. Vancouver: British Columbia Dietitians' & Nutritionists' Association, 1992.

Dwyer J. Overview: dietary approaches for reducing cardiovascular disease risks (Review). J Nutr 1995;125(3 suppl):656S-665S.

Health and Welfare Canada. Nutrition recommendations: the report of the Scientific Review Committee. Ottawa: Supply and Services Canada, 1990.

Joffe I, Epstein S. Osteoporosis associated with rheumatoid arthritis: pathogenesis and management (Review). Semin Arthritis Rheum 1991;20(4):256-72.

Joseph JC. Corticosteroid-induced osteoporosis (Review). Am J Hosp Pharm 1994;51(2):188-97.

Pard J. Nutritional Care Manual. Don Mills: Ontario Hospital Association, 1989.

Whiting SJ. Safety of some calcium supplements questioned (Review). Nutr Rev 1994;52(3):95-97.

Tang AM, Graham NMH, Kirby AJ, et al. Dietary micronutrient intake and risk of progression to AIDS in HIV-I-infected homosexual men. Am J Epidemiol 1993;138:937-51.

Nutrition for Older Individuals

Ahmed FE. Effect of nutrition on the health of the elderly (Review). J Am Diet Assoc 1992;9:1102-08.

Allred JB, Gallagher-Allred CR, Bowers DF. Elevated blood cholesterol: a risk factor for heart disease that decreases with advanced age (brief comm). J Am Diet Assoc 1990;90(4):574-76.

Boyd JA, Hospodka RJ, Bustamate P, et al. Nutritional considerations in the elderly. Am Pharm 1991;NS31(4):293-98.

Brownridge E. Nutrition needs of the elderly. Pharm Prac 1992; 8(7):33-38.

Clintex: product labels for: Nutren products, 1995.

Jarvis L, Swalling J. Enteral nutritional support. In: Bell L, ed. Manual of Nutritional Care. 4th ed. Vancouver: British Columbia Dietitians' & Nutritionists' Association, 1992:123-26.

Keith T, Lyons L. A pharmacist's guide to enteral nutrition. NARD Journal 1992;114(3):33-37.

Koehler KM, Garry PJ. Nutrition and aging (Review). Clin Lab Med 1993;13(2):433-53.

Krause MV, Mahan LK. Nutrition in adulthood and the later years. In: Food, Nutrition and Diet Therapy. 7th ed. Toronto: Saunders, 1984:328-33.

Louie V. Nutrition for the elderly. In: Bell L, ed. Manual of Nutritional Care. 4th ed. Vancouver: British Columbia Dietitians' and Nutritionists' Association, 1992:7-9.

Mead-Johnson: product labels for: Boost, Isocal, Sustacal, 1995.

Ross Laboratories: product monographs for: Ensure products; Tube Feedings (Jevity, Osmolite); Disease-specific products (Glucerna, Nepro, Pulmocare, Suplena); Meal Replacement (Essentials), March 1995.

Rosenberg IH, Miller JW. Nutritional factors in physical and cognitive functions of elderly people (Review). Am J Clin Nutr 1992;55 (6 suppl):1237s-1243s.

Nutrition for the Athlete

Barron RL, Vanscoy GJ. Natural products and the athlete: facts and folklore. Ann Pharmacother 1993;27:607-15.

Beltz SD, Doering PL. Efficacy of nutritional supplements used by athletes. Clin Pharm 1993;12:900-08.

Economos CD, Bortz SS, Nelson ME. Nutritional practices of elite athletes. Practical recommendations. Sports Med 1993;16(6):381-99.

Grunewald KK, Bailey RS. Commercially marketed supplements for body building athletes (Review). Sports Med 1993;15(2):90-103.

Marriage B, Schnurr H. Sports Nutrition Resource Manual. Edmonton: Sports Medicine Council of Alberta, 1993:41.

Pennington J, ed. Bowe and Church's Food Values of Portions Commonly Used. 15th ed. Philadelphia: Lippincott, 1989:160.

Probart CK, Bird PJ, Parker KA, et al. Diet and athletic performance. Med Clin North Am 1993;77(4):757-72.

Smith NJ, Worthington-Roberts B. Food for sport. Palo Alto, CA: Bull Publishing, 1989.

Sobal J, Harquart LF. Vitamin/mineral supplement use among athletes: a review of the literature. Int J Sport Nutr 1994;4(4):320-34.

Williams MH. Ergogenic and ergolytic substances. Med Sci Sports Exerc 1992;24(9 suppl):S344-48.

Alternative Sweeteners

Appelt GD. Weight control products. In: Covington TR, Lawson LC, Young LL, et al, eds. Handbook of Nonprescription Drugs. 10th ed. Washington: American Pharmaceutical Association, 1993:346.

Pray WS. Artificial sweeteners. US Pharmacist 1994;(Jan):41-48.

Sanyude S. Alternative sweeteners. Can Pharm J 1990;123(10):455-60.

Sucralose Information from McNeil Consumer Products, Guelph, Ontario.

White JR Jr, Campbell RK. Diabetes care products and monitoring devices. In: Covington TR, Lawson LC, Young LL, et al, eds. Handbook of Nonprescription Drugs. 10th ed. Washington: American Pharmaceutical Association, 1993:256-57.

Salt Substitutes

Bell L, ed. Manual of Nutritional Care. 4th ed. Vancouver: British Columbia Dietitians' & Nutritionists' Association, 1992.

Desimone JA. Transduction in taste receptors. Nutrition 1991;7(2): 146-49.

Fox GN. Use of salt substitutes (letter; comment). J Fam Pract 1990; 30(6):632, 717.

Swales JD. Salt substitutes and potassium intake (Editorial). BMJ 1991; 303(6810):1084-85.

CHAPTER 19—Oral Health Care Products

Oral Anatomy and Physiology

Anon. Dental caries and community water fluoridation trends—United States. JAMA 1985;253:1377, 1383.

Bailit HL, Braun R. Is periodontal disease the primary cause of tooth extraction in adults? J Am Dent Assoc 1987;114:40-45.

Caplan DJ, Weintraub JA. The oral health burden in the United States: a summary of recent epidemiologic studies. J Dent Educ 1993;57:853-62.

Douglass CW, Gillings D, Sollecito W, et al. National trends in the prevalence and severity of the periodontal diseases. J Am Dent Assoc 1983;107:403-12.

Evans RG. Implications of dental disease: an economist's perspective. J Can Dent Assoc 1980;46:56-59.

Legler DW, Menaker L. Etiology, epidemiology and clinical implications of caries. In: Menaker L, ed. The Biologic Basis of Dental Caries: An Oral Biology Textbook. Hagerstown: Harper-Row, 1980:211-25.

Lizaire AL, Hargreaves JA, Finnigan PD, et al. Oral health status of 13-year-old school children in Alberta, Canada. J Can Dent Assoc 1987; 53:845-48.

Locker D, Slade GD, Leake JL. Prevalence of and factors associated with root decay in older adults in Canada. J Dent Res 1989;68:768-72.

Miller MA. Odontologic diseases. In: Lynch MA, ed. Burket's Oral Medicine. Toronto: Lippincott, 1977:283-301.

Olds GE, Yanchik VA. Preventive dentistry: an educational module for pharmacists. Clin Prev Dent 1979;1:27-30.

Scott JH, Symons NBB. Introduction to Dental Anatomy. Edinburgh: Churchill Livingstone, 1977.

Ship JA, Ship IJ. Trends in oral health in the aging population. Dent Clin North Am 1989;33(1):33-42.

Stamm JW. Some indicators of the oral health status of the North American child population. J Can Dent Assoc 1980;46:21-30.

Dental Caries

American Dental Association Council on Dental Therapeutics. Accepted dental therapeutics. Chicago: Am Dent Assoc, 1984.

Bibby BG. Diet and nutrition and dental caries. J Can Dent Assoc 1980;46:47-55.

Bibby BG, Mundorff SA, Zero DT, et al. Oral food clearance and the pH of plaque and saliva. J Am Dent Assoc 1986;112:333-37.

Caplan DJ, Weintraub JA. The oral health burden in the United States: a summary of recent epidemiologic studies. J Dent Educ 1993;57:853-62.

Catalanotto FA, Wrobel WR, Epstein DW. Sucrose taste thresholds and dental caries: implications for dietary counselling. Clin Prev Dent 1979;1:14-18.

Cooper SA. Oral analgesics used to treat dental pain. Clin Prev Dent 1981;3:28-32.

Derkson GD, Ponti P. Nursing bottle syndrome: prevalence and etiology in a non-fluoridated city. J Can Dent Assoc 1982;48:389-93.

Feigal RJ, Jensen ME, Mensing CA. Dental caries potential of liquid medications. Pediatrics 1981;68:416-19.

Finn SB. The epidemiology of dental caries. In: Stallard RE, ed. A Textbook of Preventive Dentistry. Philadelphia: Saunders, 1982:20-31.

Fleming WJ. Dental and oral hygiene. In: Chiles VK, ed. Canadian Self-Medication. Ottawa: Canadian Pharmaceutical Association, 1980: 85-95.

Grenby TH, Bashaarat AH, Gey KF. A clinical trial to compare the effects of xylitol and sucrose chewing-gums on dental plaque growth. Br Dent J 1982;152:339-43.

Hargreaves JA, Thompson GW. Ultraviolet light and dental caries in children. Caries Res 1989;23:389-92.

Honkala E, Tala H. Total sugar consumption and dental caries in Europe—an overview. Int Dent J 1987;37:185-91.

Horowitz HS. The prevention of oral disease. Established methods of prevention. Br Dent J 1980;149:311-18.

Hunter PB. Risk factors in dental caries. Int Dent J 1988;38:211-17.

Imfled T. Efficacy of sweeteners and sugar substitutes in caries prevention. Caries Res 1993;27(suppl 1):50-55.

Jensen ME. Responses of interproximal plaque pH to snack foods and effect of chewing sorbitol-containing gum. J Am Dent Assoc 1986;113:262-66.

Jones RR, Cleaton-Jones P. Depth and area of dental erosions and dental caries in bulimic women. J Dent Res 1989;68:1275-78.

Kandelman D, Gagnon G. A 24-month clinical study of the incidence and progression of dental caries in relation to consumption of chewing gum containing xylitol in school preventive programs. J Dent Res 1990; 69:1771-75.

Kennon S, Tasch EG, Arm RN, et al. The relationship between plaque scores and the development of caries in adult dentition. Clin Prev Dent 1979;1:26-31.

Kingman A, Little W, Gomez I, et al. Salivary levels of Streptococcus mutans and lactobacilli and dental caries experiences in a US adolescent population. Community Dent Oral Epidemiol 1988;16:98-103.

Klausen B, Helbo M, Dabelsteen E. A differential diagnostic approach to the symptomatology of acute dental pain. Oral Surg Oral Med Oral Pathol 1985;59:297-301.

Kleinberg I. Etiology of dental caries. J Can Dent Assoc 1979;45:661-68.

Korberly BH, Schreiber GF, Kilkuts A, et al. Evaluation of acetaminophen and aspirin in the relief of preoperative dental pain. J Am Dent Assoc 1980;100:39-42.

Legler DW, Menaker L. Etiology, epidemiology and clinical implications of caries. In: Menaker L, ed. The Biologic Basis of Dental Caries: An Oral Biology Textbook. Hagerstown: Harper-Row, 1980:211-25.

Lizaire AL, Hargreaves JA, Finnigan PD, et al. Oral health status of 13-year-old school children in Alberta, Canada. J Can Dent Assoc 1987; 53:845-48.

Locker D, Slade GD, Leake JL. Prevalence of and factors associated with root decay in older adults in Canada. J Dent Res 1989;68:768-72.

Loe H, Kleinman DV, eds. Dental plaque control measures and oral hygiene practices: proceedings from a state-of-the-science workshop. Oxford: IRL Press, 1986:39-116.

Loesche WJ, Grossman NS, Earnest R, et al. The effect of chewing xylitol gum on the plaque and saliva levels of Streptococcus mutans. J Am Dent Assoc 1984;108:587-92.

Makinen KK, Soderling E, Hurttia H, et al. Biochemical, microbiologic and clinical comparisons between two dentifrices that contain different mixtures of sugar alcohols. J Am Dent Assoc 1985;111:745-51.

Morrissey RB, Burkholder BD, Tarka SM Jr. The cariogenic potential of several snack foods. J Am Dent Assoc 1984;109:589-91.

Murray JJ. Efficacy of preventive agents for dental caries: systemic fluorides: water fluoridation. Caries Res 1993;27(suppl 1):2-8.

Newbrun E. Sugar and dental caries: a review of human studies. Science 1982;217:418-23.

Newbrun E. Sugar and dental caries. Clin Prev Dent 1982;4:11-13.

Olds GE, Yanchik VA. Preventive dentistry: an educational module for pharmacists. Clin Prev Dent 1979;1:27-30.

Shaw L, Glenwright HD. The role of medications in dental caries formation: need for sugar-free medication for children. Pediatrician 1989;16(3-4):153-55.

Stamm JW. Some indicators of the oral health status of the North American child population. J Can Dent Assoc 1980;46:21-30.

Vratsanos SM, Mandel ID. The effect of sucrose and hexitol-containing chewing gums on plaque acidogenesis in vivo. Pharmacol Ther Dent 1981;6:87-91.

Walker AR, Cleaton-Jones PE. Sugar intake and dental caries: where do we stand? ASDC J Dent Child 1989;56:30-35.

Periodontal Diseases

Amigoni NA, Johnson GK, Kalkwarf KL. The use of sodium bicarbonate and hydrogen peroxide in periodontal therapy: a review. J Am Dent Assoc 1987;114:217-21.

Anderson DL. Etiology of periodontal disease. J Can Dent Assoc 1979;45:669-72.

Bailit HL, Braun R. Is periodontal disease the primary cause of tooth extraction in adults? J Am Dent Assoc 1987;114:40-45.

Baumert MK, Johnson GK, Kaldahl WB, et al. The effect of smoking on the response to periodontal therapy. J Clin Periodontol 1994;21: 91-97.

Butler RT, Kalkwarf KL, Kaldahl WB. Drug-induced gingival hyperplasia: phenytoin, cyclosporine, and nifedipine. J Am Dent Assoc 1987;114: 56-60.

Capilouto ML, Douglass CW. Trends in the prevalence and severity of periodontal diseases in the US: a public health problem? J Public Health Dent 1988;48:245-51.

Douglass CW, Gillings D, Sollecito W, et al. National trends in the prevalence and severity of the periodontal diseases. J Am Dent Assoc 1983;107:403-12.

Evans RG. Implications of dental disease: an economist's perspective. J Can Dent Assoc 1980;46:56-59.

Dickey RP. Managing contraceptive pill patients. Durant: Creative Infomatics, 1983:68.

Fourel J, Falabregues R, Bonfil JJ. A clinical approach to gingival stimulation. J Periodontol 1981;52:130-34.

Goldhaber P. Oral manifestations of disease. In: Isselbacher KJ, Adams RD, Braunwald E, et al. Harrison's Principles of Internal Medicine. New York: McGraw-Hill, 1980:187-92.

Heasman PA, Offenbacher S, Collins JG, et al. Flurbiprofen in the prevention and treatment of experimental gingivitis. J Clin Periodontol 1993;20:732-38.

Heasman PA, Seymour RA, Kelly PJ. The effect of systemically-administered flurbiprofen as an adjunct to toothbrushing on the resolution of experimental gingivitis. J Clin Peridontol 1994;21:166-70.

Ismail AI, Lewis DW. Periodic health examination, 1993 update: 3. Periodontal disease: classification, diagnosis, risk factors and prevention. Can Med Assoc J 1993;149:1409-22.

Kornman KS. The role of supragingival plaque in the prevention and treatment of periodontal diseases. A review of current concepts. J Periodontol Res 1986;21(suppl 16):5-22.

Mandel ID, Gaffar A. Calculus revisited: a review. J Clin Periodontol 1986;13:249-57.

Prayitno SW, Addy M, Wade WG. Does gingivitis lead to periodontitis in young adults? Lancet 1993;342:471-72.

Robertson PB, Walsh M, Greene J, et al. Periodontal effects associated with the use of smokeless tobacco. J Periodontol 1990;61:438-43.

Serio FG, Siegel MA. Periodontal diseases: a review. Cutis 1991;47:55-62.

Shapiro L, Stallard RE. Etiology of periodontal disease. In: Stallard RE, ed. A Textbook of Preventive Dentistry. Philadelphia: Saunders, 1982: 61-70.

Ship JA, Ship IJ. Trends in oral health in the aging population. Dent Clin North Am 1989;33(1):33-42.

Stallard RE. Epidemiology of periodontal disease. In: Stallard RE, ed. A Textbook of Preventive Dentistry. Philadelphia: Saunders, 1982:50-60.

Taiyeb Ali TB, Waite IM. The effect of systemic ibuprofen on gingival inflammation in humans. J Clin Periodontol 1993;20:723-28.

Thomason JM, Seymour RA, Rice N. The prevalence and severity of cyclosporin and nifedipine-induced gingival overgrowth. J Clin Periodontol 1993;20:37-40.

Weintraub JA, Burt BA. Periodontal effects and dental caries associated with smokeless tobacco use. Public Health Rep 1987;102:30-35.

Wunderlich RC, Caffesse RG, Morrison EC, et al. The therapeutic effect of toothbrushing on naturally occurring gingivitis. J Am Dent Assoc 1985;110:929-31.

Dental Erosion

Giunta JL. Dental erosion resulting from chewable vitamin C tablets. J Am Dent Assoc 1983;107:253-56.

Broken Teeth or Misfitting Restorations

Burket LW. Oral medicine in the edentulous patient. In: Lynch MA, ed. Burket's Oral Medicine. Toronto: Lippincott, 1977:568-81.

Teething Pain

Flynn AA. Counseling special populations on oral health care needs. Am Pharm 1993;33(9):33-39.

Flynn AA. Oral health products. In: Covington TR, ed. Handbook of Nonprescription Drugs. 10th ed. Washington: American Pharmaceutical Association, 1993:428.

Grad H, Grushka M. Dental pain - treatment with nonprescription drugs. On Cont Pract 1986;13(2):16-21.

Cold Sores

Anon. Herpes simplex: an overview of the disease and its treatment. Pharm Advis 1982;4(3)1-2.

Anon. Lipactin gel, Nitrol TSAR kit, MS Contin among Rx/OTC launches. Drug Merch 1986;(Feb):38.

Anon. Probax, Tabinil, Calsan launched. Drug Merch 1985;(Dec):56.

Arndt KA. Herpes simplex. In: Arndt KA, ed. Manual of Dermatologic Therapeutics. Boston: Little, Brown, 1989:75-81.

Danziger S. Ice-packs for cold sores (Letter). Lancet 1978;1:103.

Davis LE, Redman JC, Skipper BJ, et al. Natural history of frequent recurrences of herpes simplex labialis. Oral Surg Oral Med Oral Pathol 1988;66:558-61.

DiGiovanna JJ, Blank H. Failure of lysine in frequently recurrent herpes simplex infection. Arch Dermatol 1984;120:48-51.

Glezerman M, Lunenfeld E, Cohen V, et al. Placebo-controlled trial of topical interferon in labial and genital herpes. Lancet 1988;1:150-52.

Greenberg MS. Ulcerative, vesicular and bullous lesions. In: Lynch MA, ed. Burket's Oral Medicine. Toronto: Lippincott, 1984:163-208.

Guinan ME, MacCalman J, Kern ER, et al. Topical ether and herpes simplex labialis. JAMA 1980;243:1059-61.

Jensen JL, Kanas RJ, DeBoom GW. Multiple oral and labial ulcers in an immunocompromised patient. J Am Dent Assoc 1987;114:235-36.

Mills J, Hauer L, Gottlieb A, et al. Recurrent herpes labialis in skiers. Clinical observations and effect of sunscreen. Am J Sports Med 1987; 15:76-78.

Popovich NG, Popovich JG. What you should know about fever blisters and canker sores. US Pharmacist 1978;3:35-48.

Sketris I. Cold sore/canker sore. In: Chiles VK, ed. Canadian Self-Medication. Ottawa: Canadian Pharmaceutical Association, 1980:51-54.

Taieb A, Body S, Astar L, et al. Clinical epidemiology of symptomatic primary herpetic infection in children. A study of 50 cases. Acta Paediatr Scand 1987;76:128-32.

Wilson IJ. Self treatment of cold cores with ice (Letter). Lancet 1979;1:613.

Young TB, Rimm EB, D'Alessio DJ. Cross-sectional study of recurrent herpes labialis. Prevalence and risk factors. Am J Epidemiol 1988;127: 612-25.

Zimmerman DR. Self treatment of cold sores with ice (Letter). Lancet 1978;2:1260.

Canker Sores

Antoon JW, Miller RL. Aphthous ulcers: a review of the literature on etiology, pathogenesis, diagnosis, and treatment. J Am Dent Assoc 1980;101:803–08.

Arndt KA. Aphthous stomatitis (canker sores). In: Arndt KA, ed. Manual of Dermatologic Therapeutics. Boston: Little, Brown, 1983:19–21.

Axell T, Henricsson V. Association between recurrent aphthous ulcers and tobacco habits. Scand J Dent Res 1985;93:239–42.

Bittoun R. Recurrent aphthous ulcers and nicotine. Med J Aust 1991; 154:471–72.

Burns RA, Davis WJ. Recurrent aphthous stomatitis. Am Fam Physician 1985;32:99–104.

Eversole LR, Shopper TP, Chambers DW. Effects of suspected foodstuff challenging agents in the etiology of recurrent aphthous stomatitis. Oral Surg Oral Med Oral Pathol 1982;54:33–37.

Gallina G, Cumbo V, Messina P, et al. HLA-A, B, C, DR, MT, and MB antigens in recurrent aphthous stomatitis. Oral Surg Oral Med Oral Pathol 1985;59:364–70.

Greenberg MS. Ulcerative, vesicular and bullous lesions. In: Lynch MA, ed. Burket's Oral Medicine. Toronto: Lippincott, 1984:163–208.

Hay KD, Reade PC. The use of an elimination diet in the treatment of aphthous ulceration of the oral cavity. Oral Surg Oral Med Oral Pathol 1984;57:504–07.

Hoover CI, Olson JA, Greenspan JS. Humoral response and cross-reactivity to viridans streptococci in recurrent aphthous ulceration. J Dent Res 1986;65:1101–04.

Hunter L, Addy M. Chlorhexidine gluconate mouthwash in the management of minor aphthous ulceration. A double-blind, placebo-controlled cross-over trial. Br Dent J 1987;162:106–10.

Lindemann RA, Riviere GR, Sapp JP. Oral mucosal antigen reactivity during exacerbation and remission phases of recurrent aphthous ulceration. Oral Surg Oral Med Oral Pathol 1985;60:281–84.

Miller MF, Chilton NW. The effect of an oxygenating agent upon recurrent aphthous stomatitis—a double-blind clinical trial. Pharmacol Ther Dent 1980;5:55–58.

Miller MF. Use of levamisole in recurrent aphthous stomatitis. Drugs 1980;19:131–36.

Miller MF, Garfunkel AA, Ram CA, et al. The inheritance of recurrent aphthous stomatitis. Observations on susceptibility. Oral Surg Oral Med Oral Pathol 1980;49:409–12.

Olson JA, Feinberg I, Silverman S Jr, et al. Serum vitamin B12, folate, and iron levels in recurrent aphthous ulceration. Oral Surg Oral Med Oral Pathol 1982;54:517–20.

Pedersen A, Hougen HP, Klausen B, et al. LongoVital in the prevention of recurrent aphthous ulceration. J Oral Pathol Med 1991;19:371–75.

Pimlott SJ, Walker DM. A controlled trial of the efficacy of topically applied fluocinonide in the treatment of recurrent aphthous ulceration. Br Dent J 1983;154:174–77.

Potoky JR. Recurrent aphthous stomatitis; a proposed therapeutic regimen. J Oral Med 1981;36:44–46.

Scully C, Porter SR. Recurrent aphthous stomatitis: current concepts of etiology, pathogenesis and management. J Oral Pathol Med 1989;18: 21–27.

Thompson AC, Nolan A, Lamey PJ. Minor aphthous oral ulceration: a double-blind cross-over study of beclomethasone dipropionate aerosol spray. Scott Med J 1989;34:531–32.

Wray D, Graykowski EA, Notkins AL. Role of mucosal injury in initiating recurrent aphthous stomatitis. BMJ 1981;283:1569–70.

Wray D, Vlagopoulos TP, Siraganian RP. Food allergens and basophil histamine release in recurrent aphthous stomatitis. Oral Surg Oral Med Oral Pathol 1982;54:388–95.

Wray D. A double-blind trial of systemic zinc sulfate in recurrent aphthous stomatitis. Oral Surg Oral Med Oral Pathol 1982;53:469–72.

Wright A, Ryan FP, Willingham SE, et al. Food allergy or intolerance in severe recurrent aphthous ulceration of the mouth. BMJ 1986;292: 1237–38.

Zissis NP, Hatzioti AJ, Antoniadis D, et al. Therapeutic evaluation of levamisole in recurrent aphthous stomatitis. J Oral Med 1983;38:161–63.

Candidiasis

Arendorf TM, Walker DM. The prevalence and intraoral distribution of Candida albicans in man. Arch Oral Biol 1980;25:1–10.

Arndt KA. Fungal infections—candidiasis. In: Arndt KA, ed. Manual of Dermatologic Therapeutics. Boston: Little, Brown, 1989:63–66.

Cohen L. Oral candidiasis—its diagnosis and treatment. J Oral Med 1972;27:7–11.

DePaola LG, Peterson DE, Overholser CD Jr, et al. Dental care for patients receiving chemotherapy. J Am Dent Assoc 1986;112:198–203.

Hay KD. Candidosis of the oral cavity: recognition and management. Drugs 1988;36:633–42.

Holbrook WP, Rodgers GD. Candidal infections: experience in a British dental hospital. Oral Surg Oral Med Oral Pathol 1980;49:122–25.

Jones HE. Therapy of superficial fungal infection. Med Clin North Am 1982;66:873–93.

Lucas VS. Association of psychotropic drugs, prevalence of denture-related stomatitis and oral candidosis. Community Dent Oral Epidemiol 1993;21:313–16.

Scrafani JT. Superficial fungal infections and their treatment. US Pharmacist 1978;3:26–38.

Other Causes of Oral Lesions

Wright WE, Haller JM, Harlow SA, et al. An oral disease prevention program for patients receiving radiation and chemotherapy. J Am Dent Assoc 1985;110:43–47.

Halitosis

Attia EL, Marshall KG. Halitosis. Can Med Assoc J 1982;126: 1281–85.

Durham TM, Malloy T, Hodges ED. Halitosis: knowing when 'bad breath' signals systemic disease. Geriatrics 1993;48(Aug):55–59.

Tessier JF, Kulkarni GV. Bad breath: etiology, diagnosis and treatment. Oral Health 1991(Oct):19–24.

Dry Mouth

Ettinger RL. Xerostomia—a complication of aging. Aust Dent J 1981;26: 365–71.

Ferguson MM. Pilocarpine and other cholinergic drugs in the management of salivary gland dysfunction. Oral Surg Oral Med Oral Pathol 1993;75:186–91.

Fox PC, van der Ven PF, Sonies BC, et al. Xerostomia: evaluation of a symptom with increasing significance. J Am Dent Assoc 1985; 110:519–25.

Gilbert GH, Heft MW, Duncan RP. Mouth dryness as reported by older Floridians. Community Dent Oral Epidemiol 1993;21:390–97.

Glass BJ, Van Dis ML, Langlais RP, et al. Xerostomia: diagnosis and treatment planning considerations. Oral Surg Oral Med Oral Pathol 1984; 58:248–52.

Gossel TA. Dry mouth and use of saliva substitutes. US Pharmacist 1986;11:22–28, 58.

Grad H, Grushka M, Yanover L. Drug-induced xerostomia: the effects and treatment. J Can Dent Assoc 1985;51:296–300.

Locker D. Subjective reports of oral dryness in an older adult population. Community Dent Oral Epidemiol 1993;21:165–68.

Närhi TO. Prevalence of subjective feelings of dry mouth in the elderly. J Dent Res 1994;73(1):20–25.

Navazesh M. Xerostomia in the aged. Dent Clin North Am 1989;33:75–80.

Nederfors T, Henricsson V, Dahlöf C, et al. Oral mucosal friction and subjective perception of dry mouth in relation to salivary secretion. Scand J Dent Res 1993;101:44–48.

Schubert MM, Izutsu KT. Iatrogenic causes of salivary gland dysfunction. J Dent Res 1987;66:680–88.

Spielman A, Ben-Aryeh H, Gutman D, et al. Xerostomia—diagnosis and treatment. Oral Surg Oral Med Oral Pathol 1981;51:144–47.

Sreebny LM, Valdini A. Xerostomia: a neglected symptom. Arch Intern Med 1987;147:1333–37.

Wu AJ, Ship JA. A characterization of major salivary gland flow rates in the presence of medications and systemic disease. Oral Surg Oral Med Oral Pathol 1993;76:301–06.

Product Information

Dentifrices

Addy M, Mostafa P. Dentine hypersensitivity. II. Effects produced by the uptake in vitro of toothpastes onto dentine. J Oral Rehabil 1989;16: 35–48.

Anon. New rules for tooth whiteners, labels. NDMAC Nonprescription Drug Digest 1991;(Aug):7.

Council on Dental Therapeutics. Acceptance of Sensodyne toothpaste for sensitive teeth. J Am Dent Assoc 1985;110:394–95.

Council on Dental Therapeutics. Evaluation of Denquel sensitive teeth toothpaste. J Am Dent Assoc 1982;105:80.

Council on Dental Therapeutics. Acceptance of Promise with Fluoride and Sensodyne-F toothpastes for sensitive teeth. J Am Dent Assoc 1986;113:673–75.

Deasy MJ, Singh MS, Rustogi KN, et al. Effect of a dentifrice containing triclosan and a copolymer on plaque formation and gingivitis. Clin Prev Dent 1991;13(6):12–19.

Dowell TB. The use of toothpaste in infancy. Br Dent J 1981;150:247–49.

Fed Reg 1980;45:20666.

Goldberg HJ, Enslein K. Effect of an experimental sodium bicarbonate dentifrice on gingivitis and plaque formation: I. in adults. Clin Prev Dent 1979;1:12–16.

Hannah JJ, Johnson JD, Kuftinec MM. Long-term clinical evaluation of toothpaste and oral rinse containing sanguinaria extract in controlling plaque, gingival inflammation, and sulcular bleeding during orthodontic treatment. Am J Orthod Dentofacial Orthop 1989;96:199–207.

Harper DS, Mueller LJ, Fine JB, et al. Clinical efficacy of a dentifrice and oral rinse containing sanguinaria extract and zinc chloride during 6 months of use. J Periodontol 1990;61:352–58.

Harper DS, Mueller LJ, Fine JB, et al. Effect of 6 months use of a dentifrice and oral rinse containing sanguinaria extract and zinc chloride upon the microflora of the dental plaque and oral soft tissues. J Periodontol 1990;61:359–63.

Johannsen G, Redman G, Ryden H. Cleaning effect of toothbrushing with three different toothpastes and water. Swed Dent J 1993;17:111–16.

Jenkins S, Addy M, Newcombe R. The effects of a chlorhexidine toothpaste on the development of plaque, gingivitis and tooth staining. J Clin Periodontol 1993;20:59–62.

Jensen ME, Kohout R. The effect of a fluoridated dentifrice on root and coronal caries in an older adult population. J Am Dent Assoc 1988; 117:829–32.

Johnson MF. Comparative efficacy of NaF and SMFP dentifrices in caries prevention: a meta-analytic overview. Caries Res 1993;27:328–36.

Kanapka JA. Over-the-counter dentifrices in the treatment of tooth hypersensitivity. Dent Clin North Am 1990;34:545–60.

Kazmierczak M, Mather M, Ciancio S, et al. Clinical evaluation of anticalculus dentifrices. Clin Prev Dent 1990;12:13–17.

Kohut BE, Rubin H, Baron HJ. The relative clinical effectiveness of three anticalculus dentifrices. Clin Prev Dent 1989;11:13–16.

Lamb DJ, Howell RA, Constable G. Removal of plaque and stain from natural teeth by a low abrasivity toothpaste. Br Dent J 1984;157:125–27.

Lobene RR. A study to compare the effects of two dentifrices on adult dental calculus formation. J Clin Dent 1989;1:67–69.

Mallatt ME, Beiswanger BB, Drook CA, et al. Clinical effect of a sanguinaria dentifrice on plaque and gingivitis in adults. J Periodontol 1989;60:91–95.

Nagata T, Ishida H, Shinohara H, et al. Clinical evaluation of a potassium nitrate dentifrice for the treatment of dentinal hypersensitivity. J Clin Periodontol 1994;21:217–21.

Petrone M, Lobene RR, Harrison LB, et al. Clinical comparison of the anticalculus efficacy of three commercially available dentifrices. Clin Prev Dent 1991;13(4):18–21.

Rugg-Gunn AJ. A double-blind clinical trial of an anticalculus toothpaste containing pyrophosphate and sodium monofluorophosphate. Br Dent J 1988;165:133–36.

Saxton CA, Huntington E, Cummins D. The effect of dentifrices containing triclosan on the development of gingivitis in a 21-day experimental gingivitis study. Int Dent J 1993;43:423–29.

Schiff TG. The effect of a dentifrice containing soluble pyrophosphate and sodium fluoride on calculus deposits. A 6-month clinical study. Clin Prev Dent 1987;9:13–16.

Stookey GK, DePaola LG, Featherston B, et al. A critical review of the relative anticaries efficacy of sodium fluoride and sodium monofluorophosphate dentifrices. Caries Res 1993;27:337–60.

Svatun B, Saxton CA, Rolla G, et al. One-year study of the efficacy of a dentifrice containing zinc citrate and triclosan to maintain gingival health. Scand J Dent Res 1989;97:242–46.

Svatun B, Saxton CA, Huntington E, et al. The effects of three silica dentifrices containing triclosan on supragingival plaque and calculus formation and on gingivitis. Int Dent J 1993;43:441–52.

Svatun B, Saxton CA. The effects of a silica dentifrice containing triclosan and zinc citrate on supragingival plaque and calculus formation and the control of gingivitis. Int Dent J 1993;43:431–39.

Tarbet WJ, Silverman G, Fratarcangelo PA, et al. Home treatment for dentinal hypersensitivity: a comparative study. J Am Dent Assoc 1982;105: 227–30.

Volpe AR. Dentifrices and mouthrinses. In: Stallard RE, ed. A Textbook of Preventive Dentistry. Philadelphia: Saunders, 1982:170–216.

Volpe AR, Petrone ME, DeVizio W, et al. A review of plaque, gingivitis, calculus and caries clinical efficacy studies with a dentifrice containing triclosan and PVM/MA copolymer. J Clin Dent 1993. IV, special issue:31–41.

Winer RA, Tsamtsouris A. Effects of an experimental sodium bicarbonate dentifrice on gingivitis and plaque formation: II. in teenaged students. Clin Prev Dent 1979;1:17–18.

Zacherl WA, Pfieffer HJ, Swancar JR. The effect of soluble pyrophosphates on dental calculus in adults. J Am Dent Assoc 1985;110:737–38.

Denture Products

Abelson DC. Denture plaque and denture cleansers. J Prosthet Dent 1981;45:376–79.

Augsburger RHH, Elahi JM. Evaluation of seven proprietary denture cleansers. J Prosthet Dent 1982;47:356–59.

Budtz-Jorgensen E. Materials and methods for cleaning dentures. J Prosthet Dent 1979;42:619–23.

Budtz-Jorgensen E. Prevention of denture plaque formation by an enzyme denture cleanser. J Biol Buccale 1977;5:239–44.

Council on Dental Materials, Instruments, and Equipment. Denture cleansers. J Am Dent Assoc 1983;106:77–78.

Dills SS, Olshan AM, Goldner S, et al. Comparison of the antimicrobial capability of an abrasive paste and chemical-soak denture cleaner. J Prosthet Dent 1988;60:467–70.

Ghalichebaf M, Graser GN, Zander HA. The efficacy of denture-cleansing agents. J Prosthet Dent 1982;48:515–20.

Lambert JP, Kolstad R. Effect of a benzoic acid-detergent germicide on denture-borne Candida albicans. J Prosthet Dent 1986;55:699–700.

Moore TC, Smith DE, Kenny GE. Sanitization of dentures by several denture hygiene methods. J Prosthet Dent 1984;52:158–63.

Murray ID, McCabe JF, Storer R. Abrasivity of denture cleaning pastes in vitro and in situ. Br Dent J 1986;161:137–41.

Tarbet WJ, Axelrod S, Minkoff S, et al. Denture cleansing: a comparison of two methods. J Prosthet Dent 1984;51:322–25.

Fluoride

Anon. NDMAC Nonprescription Drug Digest 1991;(Aug):7.

Bagramian RA, Narendran S, Ward M. Relationship of dental caries and fluorosis to fluoride supplement history in a non-fluoridated sample of schoolchildren. Adv Dent Res 1989;3:161–67.

Bayless JM, Tinanoff N. Diagnosis and treatment of acute fluoride toxicity. J Am Dent Assoc 1985;110:209–11.

Beiswanger BB, Gish CW, Mallatt ME. A three-year study of the effect of a sodium fluoride-silica abrasive dentifrice on dental caries. Pharmacol Ther Dent 1981;6:9–16.

Blahut P. Fluoride supplements. Drugs Ther Maritime Pract 1984;7(6)25-30.

Bohannan BM, Stamm JW, Graves RC, et al. Fluoride mouthrinse programs in fluoridated communities. J Am Dent Assoc 1985;111:783–89.

Carlos JP. The prevention of dental caries: ten years later. J Am Dent Assoc 1982;104:193–97.

Clark DC, Robert G, Tessier C, et al. The results after 20 months of a study testing the efficacy of a weekly fluoride mouthrinsing program. J Public Health Dent 1985;45:252–56.

Clovis J, Hargreaves JA, Thompson GW. Caries prevalence and length of residency in fluoridated and non-fluoridated communities. Caries Res 1988;22:311–15.

Driscoll WS, Swango PA, Horowitz AM, et al. Caries-preventive effects of daily and weekly fluoride mouthrinsing in a fluoridated community: final results after 30 months. J Am Dent Assoc 1982;105:1010–13.

Glass RL. Caries reduction by a dentifrice containing sodium monofluorophosphate in a calcium carbonate base. Partial explanation for diminishing caries prevalence. Clin Prev Dent 1981;3:6–8.

Glenn FB, Glenn WD, Duncan RC. Fluoride tablet supplementation during pregnancy for caries immunity: a study of the offspring produced. Am J Obstet Gynecol 1982;143:560–64.

Gossel TA. The role of fluorides in preventing cavities. US Pharmacist 1986;11:28–34.

Horowitz AM. Oral hygiene measures. J Can Dent Assoc 1980;46:43–46.

Horowitz HS. Review of topical applications: fluorides and fissure sealants. J Can Dent Assoc 1980;46:38–42.

Keeping B, Canadian Dental Association. Personal Communication.

Leverett DH. Fluorides and the changing prevalence of dental caries. Science 1982;217:26–30.

Leverett DH, Sveen OB, Jensen OE. Weekly rinsing with a fluoride mouthrinse in an unfluoridated community: results after seven years. J Public Health Dent 1985;45:95–100.

Levy SM. Expansion of the proper use of systemic fluoride supplements. J Am Dent Assoc 1986;112:30–34.

Lu KH, Hanna JD, Peterson JK. Effect on dental caries of a stannous fluoride-calcium pyrophosphate dentifrice in an adult population: one-year results. Pharmacol Ther Dent 1980;5:11–16.

Newbrun E. Systemic fluorides: an overview. J Can Dent Assoc 1980;46: 31–37.

Newbrun E. Effectiveness of water fluoridation. J Public Health Dent 1989;49:279–89.

Nourjah P, Horowitz AM, Wagener DK. Factors associated with the use of fluoride supplements and fluoride dentifrices by infants and toddlers. J Public Health Dent 1994;54(1):47–54.

Popovich NG, Popovich JG. Fluoride dental therapy. US Pharmacist 1981;6:37–61.

Ripa LW. Fluoride rinsing: what dentists should know. J Am Dent Assoc 1981;102:477–81.

Ripa LW. Rinses for the control of dental caries. Int Dent J 1992;42: 263–69.

Rolla G, gaard B, De Almeida Cruz B. Topical application of fluorides on teeth: new concepts of mechanisms of action. J Clin Periodontol 1993;20:105–08.

Smith GE. Fluoride and fluoridation. Soc Sci Med 1988;26:451–62.

Swango PA. The use of topical fluorides to prevent dental caries in adults: a review of the literature. J Am Dent Assoc 1983;107:447–50.

Szpunar SM, Burt BA. Dental caries, fluorosis, and fluoride exposure in Michigan schoolchildren. J Dent Res 1988;67:802–06.

Szpunar SM, Burt BA. Fluoride exposure in Michigan schoolchildren. J Public Health Dent 1990(Winter);50:18–23.

Wei SHY, Yiu CKY. Mouthrinses: recent clinical findings and implications for use. Int Dent J 1993;43:541–47.

Yanover L. Fluoride varnishes as cariostatic agents: a review. J Can Dent Assoc 1982;48:401–04.

Zacherl WA. A three-year clinical caries evaluation of the effect of a sodium fluoride-silica abrasive dentifrice. Pharmacol Ther Dent 1981;6:1–7.

Mouthwashes

Addy M. Pre-brushing mouthrinse PLAX (Letter). Br Dent J 1989;167: 10–11.

Axelsson P, Lindhe J. Efficacy of mouthrinses in inhibiting dental plaque and gingivitis in man. J Clin Periodontol 1987;14:205–12.

Beiswanger BB, Mallatt ME, Mau MS, et al. The relative plaque removal effect of a prebrushing mouthrinse. J Am Dent Assoc 1990;120: 190–92.

Blot WJ, Winn DM, Fraumeni JF Jr. Oral cancer and mouthwash. JNCI 1983;70:251–53.

Brecz M, Netuschil L, Reichert B, et al. Efficacy of Listerine, Meridol, and chlorhexidine mouthrinses on plaque, gingivitis, and plaque bacteria vitality. J Clin Periodontol 1990;17:292–97.

Etemadzadeh H, Ainamo J. Lacking anti-plaque efficacy of 2 sanguinarine mouth rinses. J Clin Periodontol 1987;14:176–80.

Federal Register 1982; 47:22760–930.

Grossman E, Meckel AH, Isaacs RL, et al. A clinical comp of antibacterial mouthrinses: effects of chlorhexidine, phenolics, and sanguinarine on dental plaque and gingivitis. J Periodontol 1989;60:435–40.

Grossman E. Effectiveness of a prebrushing mouthrinse under single-trial and home-use conditions. Clin Prev Dent 1988;10:3–6.

Hornfeldt CS. A report of acute ethanol poisoning in a child: mouthwash versus cologne, perfume and aftershave. Clin Toxicol 1992;30:115–21.

Lamster IB, et al. The effect of Listerine antiseptic on reduction of existing plaque and gingivitis. Clin Prev Dent 1983;5:6.

Leung AKC. Ethanol-induced hypoglycemia from mouthwash (Letter). Drug Intell Clin Pharm 1985;19:480–81.

Mankodi S, Ross NM, Mostler K. Clinical efficacy of Listerine in inhibiting and reducing plaque and experimental gingivitis. J Clin Periodontol 1987;14:285–88.

Mashberg A, Barsa P, Grossman ML. A study of the relationship between mouthwash use and oral and pharyngeal cancer. J Am Dent Assoc 1985;110:731–34.

Minah GE, DePaola LG, Overholser CD, et al. Effects of 6 months use of an antiseptic mouthrinse on supragingival dental plaque microflora. J Clin Periodontol 1989;16:347–52.

Moran J, Addy M, Newcombe R. A clinical trial to assess the efficacy of sanguinarine-zinc mouthrinse (Viadent) compared with chlorhexidine mouthrinse (Corosodyl). J Clin Periodontol 1988;15:612–16.

Overholser CD, Meiller TF, DePaola LG, et al. Comparative effects of 2 chemotherapeutic mouthrinses on the development of supragingival dental plaque and gingivitis. J Clin Periodontol 1990;17:575–79.

Overholser D, et al. Comparative effects of chemotherapeutic agents in reduction of plaque and gingivitis. J Dent Res 1988;67:329.

Parsons LG, Thomas LG, Southard GL, et al. Effect of sanguinaria extract on established plaque and gingivitis when supra-gingivally delivered as a manual rinse or under pressure in an oral irrigator. J Clin Periodontol 1987;14:381-85.

Quirynen M, Marechal M, van Steenberghe D. Comparative antiplaque activity of sanguinarine and chlorhexidine in man. J Clin Periodontol 1990;17:223-27.

Ross NM, Charles CH, Dills SS. Long-term effects of Listerine antiseptic on dental plaque and gingivitis. J Clin Dent 1989;1:92-95.

Singh SM. Efficacy of a prebrushing rinse in reducing dental plaque. Am J Dent 1990;3:15-16.

Weller-Fahy ER, Berger LR, Troutman WG. Mouthwash: a source of acute ethanol intoxication. Pediatrics 1980;66:302-05.

Wynder EL, Kabat G, Rosenberg S, et al. Oral cancer and mouthwash use. JNCI 1983;70:255-60.

Plaque Control Products

Abelson DC, Barton JE, Maietti GM, et al. Evaluation of interproximal cleaning by two types of dental floss. Clin Prev Dent 1981;3:19-21.

Adams RA, Mann WV. Oral hygiene techniques and home care. In: Stallard RE, ed. A Textbook of Preventive Dentistry. Philadelphia: Saunders, 1982:217-40.

Ashley FP, Skinner A, Jackson P, et al. The effect of a 0.1% cetylpyridinium chloride mouthrinse on plaque and gingivitis in adult subjects. Br Dent J 1984;157:191-96.

Axelsson P. Current role of pharmaceuticals in prevention of caries and periodontal disease. Int Dent J 1993;43:473-82.

Balanyk TE, Galustians HJ. Antiplaque efficacy of a prebrushing rinse. Am J Dent 1992;5:46-48.

Beaumont RH. Patient preference for waxed or unwaxed dental floss. J Periodontol 1990;61:123-25.

Bergenholtz A, Olsson A. Efficacy of plaque-removal using interdental brushes and waxed dental floss. Scand J Dent Res 1984;92:198-203.

Bergenholtz A, Brithon J. Plaque removal by dental floss or toothpicks. An intra-individual comparative study. J Clin Periodontol 1980;7:516-24.

Bergenholtz A, Gustafsson LB, Segerlund N, et al. Role of brushing technique and toothbrush design in plaque removal. Scand J Dent Res 1984;92:344-51.

Binney A, Addy M, Newcombe RG. The effect of a number of commercial mouthrinses compared with toothpaste on plaque regrowth. J Periodontol 1992;63:839-42.

Boyd RL, Rose CM. Effect of a rotary toothbrush versus manual toothbrush on decalcification during orthodontic treatment. Am J Orthod Dentofacial Orthop 1994;105:450-56.

Boyd RL, Murray P, Robertson PB. Effect on periodontal status of rotary electric toothbrushes vs manual toothbrushes during periodontal maintenance. I Clinical results. J Periodontol 1989;60:390-95.

Boyd RL, Murray P, Robertson PB. Effect of rotary electric toothbrush versus manual toothbrush on periodontal status during orthodontic treatment. Am J Orthod Dentofacial Orthop 1989;96:342-47.

Brecx M, Theilade J. Effect of chlorhexidine rinses on the morphology of early dental plaque formed on plastic film. J Clin Periodontol 1984;11: 553-64.

Breitenmoser J, Mormann W, Muhlemann HR. Damaging effects of toothbrush bristle end form on gingiva. J Periodontol 1979;50:212-16.

Briner WW, Grossman E, Buckner RY, et al. Effect of chlorhexidine gluconate mouthrinse on plaque bacteria. J Periodontol Res 1986;21(suppl 16):44-52.

Briner WW, Grossman E, Buckner RY, et al. Assessment of susceptibility of plaque bacteria to chlorhexidine after six months oral use. J Periodontol Res 1986;21(suppl 16):53-59.

Ciancio SG. Chemotherapeutics in periodontics. Dent Clin North Am 1980;24:813-26.

Dahlen G. Effect of antimicrobial mouthrinses on salivary microflora in healthy subjects. Scand J Dent Res 1984;92:38-42.

Davies RM. Rinses to control plaque and gingivitis. Int Dent J 1993;42: 276-80.

Deasy MJ, Battista G, Rustogi KN. Antiplaque efficacy of a triclosan/copolymer pre-brush rinse: a plaque prevention clinical study. Am J Dent 1992;5:91-94.

De la Rosa M, Guerra JZ, Johnston DA, et al. Plaque growth and removal with daily toothbrushing. J Periodontol 1979;50:661-64.

Emling RC, Flickinger KC, Cohen DW, et al. A comparison of estimated versus actual brushing time. Pharmacol Ther Dent 1981;6:93-98.

Fardal O, Turnbull RS. A review of the literature on use of chlorhexidine in dentistry. J Am Dent Assoc 1986;112:863-69.

Fine DH, Letizia J, Mandel ID. The effect of rinsing with Listerine antiseptic on the properties of developing dental plaque. J Clin Periodontol 1985;12:660-66.

Gianco SG, Othman S, Mather ML, et al. Clinical effects of a stannous fluoride mouthrinse on plaque. Clin Prev Dent 1992;14(5):27-30.

Glavind L, Zeuner E. The effectiveness of a rotary electric toothbrush on oral cleanliness in adults. J Clin Periodontol 1986;13:135-38.

Glaze PM, Wade AB. Toothbrush age and wear as it relates to plaque control. J Clin Periodontol 1986;13:52-56.

Gordon JM, Lamster IB, Seiger MC. Efficacy of Listerine antiseptic in inhibiting the development of plaque and gingivitis. J Clin Periodontol 1985;12:697-704.

Gossel TA. Mouthwashes: how effective are they against plaque? US Pharmacist 1985;10:23-29, 32.

Gossel TA. Toothbrushes. US Pharmacist 1985;10:22-28.

Graves RC, Disney JA, Stamm JW. Comparative effectiveness of floss and brushing in reducing interproximal bleeding. J Periodontol 1989;60: 243-47.

Grossman E, Reiter G, Sturzenberger OP, et al. Six-month study of the effects of a chlorhexidine mouthrinse on gingivitis in adults. J Periodontol Res 1986;21(suppl 16):33-43.

Honkala E, Nyyssonen V, Knuuttila M, et al. Effectiveness of children's habitual toothbrushing. J Clin Periodontol 1986;13:81-85.

Hull PS. Chemical inhibition of plaque. J Clin Periodontol 1980;7:431-42.

Hellstadius K, sman B, Gustafsson A. Improved maintenance of plaque control by electrical toothbrushing in periodontitis patients with low compliance. J Clin Periodontol 1993;20:235-37.

Jackson CL. Comparison between electric toothbrushing and manual toothbrushing, with and without oral irrigation, for oral hygiene of orthodontic appliances. Am J Orthod Dentofacial Orthop 1991;99: 15-20.

Joyston-Bechal S, Hernanen N. The effect of a mouthrinse containing chlorhexidine and fluoride on plaque and gingival bleeding. J Clin Periodontol 1993;20:49-53.

Kleber CJ, Putt MS, Muhler JC. Duration and pattern of toothbrushing in children using a gel or a paste dentifrice. J Am Dent Assoc 1981;103: 723-26.

Kortsch WE. Challenging the soft brush (Letter). J Am Dent Assoc 1983;106:594.

Kreifeldt JG, Hill PH, Calisti LJP. A systematic study of the plaque removal efficiency of worn toothbrushes. J Dent Res 1980;59:2047-55.

Lamberts DM, Wunderlich RC, Caffesse RG. The effect of waxed and unwaxed dental floss on gingival health. Part I. Plaque removal and gingival response. J Periodontol 1982;53:393-96.

Lang NP, Brecx MC. Chlorhexidine digluconate an agent for chemical plaque control and prevention of gingival inflammation. J Periodontol Res 1986; 21(suppl 16):74-89.

Llewelyn J. A double-blind crossover trial on the effect of cetylpyridinium chloride 0.05% (Merocet) on plaque accumulation. Br Dent J 1980;148:103-04.

Lobene RR, Soparker PM, Newman MB. Use of dental floss: effect on plaque and gingivitis. Clin Prev Dent 1982;4:5-8.

Macgregor IDM. Toothbrushing efficiency in smokers and non-smokers. J Clin Periodontol 1984;11:313-20.

Nelson RF, Rodasti PC, Tichnor A, et al. Comparative study of four over-the-counter mouthrinses claiming antiplaque and/or antigingivitis benefits. Clin Prev Dent 1991;13(6):30-33.

Niemi ML, Sandholm L, Ainamo J. Frequency of gingival lesions after standardized brushing as related to stiffness of toothbrush and abrasiveness of dentifrice. J Clin Periodontol 1984;11:254-61.

Okada K. A study on the preventive effect of dental caries by chlorhexidine mouthwash. J Nihon Univ Sch Dent 1980;22:65-69.

Ong G. The effectiveness of 3 types of dental floss for interdental plaque removal. J Clin Periodontol 1990;17:463-66.

Reitman WR, Whiteley RT, Robertson PB. Proximal surface cleaning by dental floss. Clin Prev Dent 1980;2:7-10.

Ross NM, Mankodi SM, Mostler KL, et al. Effect of rinsing time on antiplaque-antigingivitis efficacy of Listerine. Clin Periodontol 1993;20: 279-81.

Schifter CC, Emling RC, Seibert JS, et al. A comparison of plaque removal effectiveness of an electric versus a manual toothbrush. Clin Prev Dent 1983;5:15-19.

Schonfield SE, Farnoush A, Wilson SG. In vivo antiplaque activity of a sanguinarine-containing dentifrice: comparison with conventional toothpastes. J Periodontol Res 1986;21:298-303.

Segreto VA, Collins EM, Beiswanger BB, et al. A comparison of mouthrinses containing two concentrations of chlorhexidine. J Periodontol Res 1986;21(suppl 16):23-32.

Siegrist BE, Gusberti FA, Brecx MC, et al. Efficacy of supervised rinsing with chlorhexidine digluconate in comparison to phenolic and plant alkaloid compounds. J Periodontol Res 1986;21(suppl 16):60-73.

Smith BA, Collier CM, Caffesse RG. In vitro effectiveness of dental floss in plaque removal. J Clin Periodontol 1986;13:211.

Southard GL, Boulware RT, Walborn DR, et al. Sanguinarine, a new antiplaque agent: retention and plaque specificity. J Am Dent Assoc 1984;108:338-41.

Spolsky VW, Perry DA, Meng Z, et al. Evaluating the efficacy of a new flossing aid. J Clin Periodontol 1993;20:490-97.

Stoltze K, Bay L. Comparison of a manual and a new electric toothbrush for controlling plaque and gingivitis. J Clin Periodontol 1994;21:86-90.

van der Weijden GA, Danser MM, Nijboer A, et al. The plaque-removing efficacy of an oscillating/rotating toothbrush. J Clin Periodontol 1993; 20:273-78.

van der Weijden, GA, Timmerman MF, Reijerse E, et al. The long-term effect of an oscillating/rotating electric toothbrush on gingivitis. J Clin Periodontol 1994;21:139-45.

van der Weijden, GA, Timmerman MF, Nijboer A, et al. A comparative study of electric toothbrushes for the effectiveness of plaque removal in relation to toothbrushing duration. J Clin Periodontol 1993;20: 476-81.

Wade AB. A clinical assessment of the relative properties of nylon and bristle brushes. Br Dent J 1953;94:260-64.

Weitz M, Brownstein C, Deasy M. Effect of a twice daily 0.12% chlorhexidine rinse on the oral health of a geriatric population. Clin Prev Dent 1992;14(3):9-13.

Wennstrom J, Lindhe J. The effect of mouthrinses on parameters characterizing human periodontal disease. J Clin Periodontol 1986;13:86-93.

Wieder SG, Newman HN, Strahan JD. Stannous fluoride and subgingival chlorhexidine irrigation in the control of plaque and chronic periodontitis. J Clin Periodontol 1983;10:172-81.

Worthington HV, Davies RM, Blinkhorn AS, et al. A six-month clinical study of the effect of a pre-brush rinse on plaque removal and gingivitis. Br Dent J 1993;175:322-26.

Wright GZ, Banting DW, Feasby WH. The Dorchester dental flossing study: a final report. Clin Prev Dent 1979;1:23-26.

Wunderlich RC, Lamberts DM, Caffesse RG. The effect of waxed and unwaxed dental floss on gingival health. Part II. Crevicular fluid flow and gingival bleeding. J Periodontol 1982;53:397-400.

Yukna RA, Shaklee RL. Evaluation of a counter-rotational powered brush in patients in supportive periodontal therapy. J Periodontol 1993;64: 859-64.

Zickert I, Emilson CG, Krasse B. Effect of caries preventive measures in children highly infected with Streptococcus mutans. Arch Oral Biol 1982;27:861-68.

Toothache Relievers/Teething Pain

Federal Register 1982; 47:22172-59.

Hume WR. The pharmacologic and toxicologic properties of zinc oxide eugenol. J Am Dent Assoc 1986;113:789-91.

Sveen OB, Yaekel M, Adair SM. Efficacy of using benzocaine for temporary relief of toothache. Oral Surg Oral Med Oral Pathol 1982;53:574-76.

Products for Dry Mouth

Anon. Fights mouth dryness: Biotene. Drug Merch 1986;(Aug):47.

Fischer JM, Schwinghammer T. Are saliva substitute products available, and why would they be used? US Pharmacist 1983;8:9.

Hatton MN, Levine MJ, Margarone JE, et al. Lubrication and viscosity features of human saliva and commercially available saliva substitutes. J Oral Maxillofac Surg 1987;45:496-99.

Klestov AC, Webb J, Latt D, et al. Treatment of xerostomia: a double-blind trial in 108 patients with Sjogren's syndrome. Oral Surg Oral Med Oral Pathol 1981;51:594-99.

Levine MJ, Aguirre A, Hatton MN, et al. Artificial salivas: present and future. J Dent Res 1987;66:693-98.

Wiesenfeld D, Stewart AM, Mason DK. Critical assessment of oral lubricants in patients with xerostomia. Br Dent J 1983;155:155-57.

CHAPTER 20—Pain and Fever Products

Pain

Almekinders LC. The efficacy of nonsteroidal anti-inflammatory drugs in the treatment of ligament injuries. Sports Med 1990;9:137-42.

Almekinders LC. Anti-inflammatory treatment of muscular injuries in sports. Sports Med 1993;15:139-45.

Edmeads J. Headache in the emergency room. Med North Am 1991;22: 2969-73.

Fields HL, Martin JB. Pain: pathophysiology and management. In: Isselbacher KJ, Braunwald E, Wilson JD, et al, eds. Harrison's Principles of Internal Medicine. 13th ed. New York: McGraw Hill, 1994:49-54.

Fine PG, Hare BD. The pathways and mechanism of pain and analgesia: a review and clinical perspective. Hosp Formul 1985;20:972-85.

Goodman CE. Pathophysiology of pain. Arch Intern Med 1983;143: 527-30.

Kubacka RT. Practical approaches to the management of migraine. Am Pharm 1994; NS34:34-73.

McBean Cochran B. Medication-induced headache: strategies for pharmacist identification and management. Halifax: BMC Health Associates, 1994.

Melzack R, Wall PD. Pain mechanisms. Science 1965;150:971-79.

Paget S, Pelicci P, Beary JF, eds. Manual of Rheumatology and Outpatient Orthopedic Disorders. 3rd ed. Boston: Little, Brown, 1993.

Pray WS. Dental pain: refer your patient. US Pharmacist 1994;(Dec):22.

Pryse-Phillips W, Findlay H, Tugwell P, et al. A Canadian population survey on the clinical, epidemiologic and societal impact of migraine and tension type headache. Can J Neurol Sci 1992;19:333-39.

Raj PP, ed. Practical Management of Pain. 2nd ed. St. Louis: Mosby, 1992.

Sjaastad O. Cluster headache syndrome. In: Lord Walton of Detchant, Warlow CP, eds. Major Problems in Neurology Series. Vol 23. London: Saunders, 1992.

Sinatra RS, Hord AH, Ginsberg B, et al, eds. Acute Pain: Mechanism and Management. St. Louis: Mosby, 1992.

Taddeini L, Rotschafer JC. Pain syndromes associated with cancer. Postgrad Med 1984;75:101-08.

Twycross RG, Lack SA. Symptom Control in Far Advanced Cancer: Pain Relief. London: Pitman Books, 1983.

Zambito RF, Sciubba JJ, eds. Manual of Dental Therapeutics. St. Louis: Mosby, 1991.

Fever

Anon. Fever thermometers. Consumer Reports 1988;(Jan): 56-58.

Berg AT. Are febrile seizures provoked by a rapid rise in temperature? Am J Dis Child 1993;147:1101-03.

Bonadio WA. Defining fever and other aspects of body temperature in infants and children. Pediatr Ann 1993;22:467-73.

Camfield PR, Camfield CS, Shapiro SH, et al. The first febrile seizure—antipyretic instruction plus either phenobarbital or placebo to prevent recurrence. J Pediatr 1980;97:16-21.

David CB. Liquid crystal forehead temperature strips. Am J Dis Child 1983;137:87.

Eskerud JR, Brodwall A. General practitioners and fever: a study on perception, self-care and advice to patients. Pharm World Sci 1993;15: 161-64.

Eskerud JR, Andrew M, Stromnes B, et al. Pharmacy personnel and fever: a study on perception, self-care and information to customers. Pharm World Sci 1993;15:156-60.

Garrison RF. Acute poisoning from use of isopropyl alcohol in tepid sponging. JAMA 1953;52:317-318.

Gelfand JA, Dinarello CA, Wolff SM. Fever, including fever of unknown origin. In: Isselbacher KJ, Braunwald E, Wilson JD, et al, eds. Harrison's Principles of Internal Medicine. 13th ed. New York: McGraw Hill, 1994:81-90.

Herzog LW, Coyne LJ. What is fever? Normal temperature in infants less than 3 months old. Clin Pediatr 1993;32:142-46.

Hooker EA. Use of tympanic thermometers to screen for fever in patients in a pediatric emergency department. South Med J 1993;86:855-58.

Ipp M, Jaffe D. Physicians' attitudes towards the diagnosis and management of fever in children 3 months to 2 years of age. Clin Pediatr 1993; 32:66-70.

Lewit EM, Marshall CL, Salzer JE. An evaluation of a plastic strip thermometer. JAMA 1982;247:321-25.

Lorin MI, ed. The Febrile Child: Clinical Management of Fever and Other Types of Pyrexia. New York: John Wiley and Sons, 1982.

Mackowiak PA. Fever: blessing or curse? A unifying hypothesis. Ann Intern Med 1994;120:1037-40.

Mackowiak PA, ed. Fever: Basic Mechanisms and Management. New York: Raven Press, 1991.

Mackowiak PA, Wasserman SS, Levine MM. A critical appraisal of 98.6°F, the upper limit of the normal body temperature, and other legacies of Carl Reinhold August Wunderlich. JAMA 1992;268:1578-80.

May A, Bauchner H. Fever phobia: the pediatrician's contribution. Pediatrics 1992;90:851-54.

Milunsky A, Ulcickas M, Rothman KJ, et al. Maternal heat exposure and neural tube defects. JAMA 1992;268:882-85.

Moltz H. Fever: causes and consequences. Neurosci Behav Rev 1993;17: 237-69.

Moss MH. Alcohol-induced hypoglycemia and coma caused by alcohol sponging. Pediatrics 1970;46:445-47.

Reisinger KS, Koo J, Grant DM. Inaccuracy of the clinitemp skin thermometer. Pediatrics 1979;64:4-6.

Romano MJ, Fortenberry JD, Autrey E, et al. Infrared tympanic thermometry in the pediatric intensive care unit. Crit Care Med 1993;21: 1181-85.

Schmidt BD. Fever phobia. Misconceptions of parents about fevers. Am J Dis Child 1980;134:176-81.

Schmitt BD. Fever in childhood. Pediatrics 1984;74(suppl):929-36.

Scholefield JH, Gerber MA, Dwyer P. Liquid crystal forehead temperature strips. Am J Dis Child 1982;136:198-201.

Selfridge J, Shea SS. The accuracy of the tympanic membrane thermometer in detecting fever in infants aged 3 months and younger in the emergency department setting. J Emerg Nurs 1993;19:127-30.

Styrt B, Sugarman B. Antipyresis and fever. Arch Intern Med 1990;150: 1589-97.

Terndrup TE. An appraisal of temperature assessment of infrared emission detection tympanic thermometry. Ann Emerg Med 1992;21: 1483-92.

Pharmaceutical Agents

Pain and Fever

Anon. Drug Evaluations. 6th ed. Chicago: American Medical Association, 1986.

Bhatt-Mehta V, Rosen D. Management of acute pain in children. Clin Pharm 1991;10:667-85.

Committee on Infectious Diseases. Aspirin and Reye syndrome. Pediatrics 1982;69:810-12.

Doran TF, DeAngelis C, Baumgardner RA, et al. Acetaminophen: more harm than good for chickenpox. J Pediatr 1989;114:1045-48.

Drwal-Klein LA, Phelps S. Antipyretic therapy in the febrile child. Clin Pharm 1992;11:1005-21.

Elliott DP. Preventing upper gastrointestinal bleeding in patients receiving nonsteroidal anti-inflammatory drugs. DICP Ann Pharmacother 1990;24:954-58.

Friedman AD, Barton LL. Sponging Study Group. Efficacy of sponging vs. acetaminophen for reduction of fever. Pediatr Emerg Care 1990;6:6-7.

Fye KH. Recent controversies in the treatment of rheumatoid disease. Hosp Formul 1990;25:1220-32.

Greene JW, Craft L, Ghishan F. Acetaminophen poisoning in infancy. Am J Dis Child 1983;137:386-87.

Insel PA. Analgesics, antipyretics and antiinflammatory agents: drugs employed in the treatment of rheumatoid arthritis and gout. In: Goodman Gilman A, Rall TW, Nies AS, et al, eds. The Pharmacological Basis of Therapeutics. 8th ed. Toronto: Pergamon Press, 1990:638-59.

Kantor TG. Ibuprofen. Ann Intern Med 1979;91:877-82.

Kramer MS, Naimark LE, Roberts-Brauer R, et al. Risks and benefits of paracetamol antipyresis in young children with fever of presumed viral origin. Lancet 1991;337:591-94.

Levy G, Tsuchiya T. Salicylate accumulation kinetics in man. N Engl J Med 1972;287:430-32.

Lovejoy FH. Aspirin and acetaminophen: a comparative view of their antipyretic and analgesic activity. Pediatrics 1978;62(suppl):904-09.

McCormack K. The spinal actions of nonsteroidal anti-inflammatory drugs and the dissociation between their anti-inflammatory and analgesic effects. Drugs 1994;47(suppl 5):28-45.

McEvoy GK, ed. AHFS Drug Information. Bethesda: American Society of Hospital Pharmacists, 1994:1195-1218, 1327-30.

Perneger T, Whelton PK, Klag MJ. Risk of kidney failure associated with the use of acetaminophen, aspirin and nonsteroidal anti-inflammatory drugs. N Engl J Med 1994;331:1675-79.

Newman J. Evaluation of sponging to reduce body temperature in febrile children. Can Med Assoc J 1985;132:641-42.

Rudolf AM. Effects of aspirin and acetaminophen in pregnancy and in the newborn. Arch Intern Med 1981;141:358-63.

Sawynok J, Yakish TL. Caffeine as an analgesic adjuvant: a review of pharmacology and mechanisms of action. Pharm Rev 1993;45:43-85.

Schachtel BP, Fillingim JM, Lance AC, et al. Caffeine as an analgesic. Arch Intern Med 1991;151: 733-37.

Spencer-Green G. Drug treatment of arthritis: update on conventional and less conventional methods. Postgrad Med 1993;93:129-40.

Steele RW, Tanaka PT, Lara RP, et al. Evaluation of sponging and of oral antipyretic therapy to reduce fever. J Pediatr 1970;77:824-29.

Supernaw RB. Therapy of recurrent headache syndromes. US Pharmacist 1991;16:33-54.

USPDI. Drug Information for the Health Care Professional. 14th ed. Rockville: The United States Pharmacopeial Convention, 1994.

Walson PD, Galletta G, Braden NJ, et al. Ibuprofen, acetaminophen and placebo treatment of febrile children. Clin Pharmacol Ther 1989; 46:9-17.

Welch KMA. Drug therapy of migraine. N Engl J Med 1993;329:1476-83.

Whitcomb DC, Block GD. Association of acetaminophen hepatoxicity with fasting and ethanol use. JAMA 1994;272:1845-50.

Wyant GM. Chronic pain: principles and treatment. Drugs 1983;26: 262-67.

External Analgesics

Crossland J, ed. Lewis's Pharmacology. New York: Churchill Livingstone, 1970:560-64.

Food Drug Cosmetic Reporter. Vol. 1 Drugs/Cosmetics. Drug monograph. Washington: Commerce Clearinghouse Inc, 1986:Sec:a)72,068; b)72,091.3; c)72,291.2; d)72,295.

Gammon GD, Starr I. Studies on the relief of pain by counterirritation. J Clin Invest 1941;20:13-20.

Grollman A, ed. Pharmacology and Therapeutics. Philadelphia: Lea & Febiger, 1965:825-32.

Lewis JJ, ed. Introduction to Pharmacology. Edinburgh: E and S Livingstone, 1965:581-88.

Uses

Anon. Sprains, strains and bruises. Drug Ther Bull 1976;14:66-68.

Appenzeller O, Atkinson R, eds. Sports Medicine. Baltimore: Urban and Schwarzenberg, 1983:284-347.

Barker LR, Burton JR, Zieve PD, eds. Principles of Ambulatory Medicine. Baltimore: Williams & Wilkins, 1986:835.

Hoffman GS. Tendinitis and bursitis. Am Fam Physician 1981;23(6): 103-10.

Hurst JW, ed. Medicine for the Practicing Physician. Toronto: Butterworths, 1983:227, 242, 367-80.

Jacknowitz AI. External analgesic products. In: Feldmann EG, ed. Handbook of Nonprescription Drugs. Washington: American Pharmaceutical Association, 1990:871-87.

General Treatment

Sherman M. Hot or cold: which treatment to recommend? Am Pharm 1980; NS20(8):46-49.

Mechanism of Action

Anon. The pain paradox (Editorial). Lancet 1976;1:945-46.

Behbehani M. Physiology of pain. In: Prithvi Raj P, ed. Practical Management of Pain. Chicago: Yearbook Medical Publishers, 1986:61-77.

Collins AJ, Notarianni AJ, Ring EFJ, et al. Some observations on the pharmacology of "deep-heat", a topical rubefacient. Ann Rheum Dis 1984;43:411-15.

Crockford GW, Hellon RF, Heyman A. Local vasomotor responses to rubefacients and ultraviolet radiation. J Physiol 1962;161:21-29.

Dowd PM, Whitefield M, Greaves MW. Hexyl-Nicotinate-induced vasodilation in normal human skin. Dermatologica 1987;174:239-43.

Guy RH, Wester RC, Tur E, et al. Noninvasive assessments of the percutaneous absorption of methyl nicotinate in humans. J Pharm Sci 1983;72:1077-79.

Hannington-Kiff JG. Counterpains. Nurs Times 1977;73(9):312-13.

Hoskins-Michel T, ed. International Perspectives in Physical Therapy I: Pain. New York: Churchill Livingstone, 1971:560-64.

Lange K, Weiner D. The effect of certain hyperkinemics on the blood flow through the skin. J Invest Dermatol 1949;12:263-69.

Maciewicz R, Martin JB. Pain: pathophysiology and management. In: Braunwald E, Isselbacher KJ, Petersdorf RG, et al, eds. Harrison's Principles of Internal Medicine. Montreal: McGraw-Hill, 1987:13-17.

Melzack R, Wall PD. Pain mechanisms: a new theory. Science 1965; 150(3699):973-79.

Morison RAH, Woodmansey A, Young AJ. Placebo responses in an arthritis trial. Ann Rheum Dis 1961;20:179-84.

Peterson JB, Jarber EM, Fulton GP. Responses of the skin to rubefacients. J Invest Dermatol 1959; 35(2):57-64.

Post BS. Effect of percutaneous medication on muscle tissue: an electromyographic study. Arch Phys Med Rehabil 1961;42:791-98.

Post BS, Forster S, Benton JG. The effect of percutaneous medication on motor nerve conduction velocity. Arch Phys Med Rehabil 1964;45: 460-65.

Roskos KV, Bircher AJ, Maiback HI, et al. Pharmacodynamic measurements of methyl nicotinate percutaneous absorption: the effect of aging on microcirculation. Br J Dermatol 1990;122:165-71.

Traut EF, Carstens HP, Thrift CB, et al. Topical treatment in rheumatic disease. IMJ 1962;121:257-60.

Traut EF, Passarelli EW. Placebos in the treatment of rheumatoid arthritis and other rheumatic conditions. Ann Rheum Dis 1957;16:18-21.

Traut EF, Passarelli EW. Study in the controlled therapy of degenerative arthritis. Arch Intern Med 1956;98:181-86.

Vuopala U, Vesterinen E, Kaipainen WJ. The analgesic action of dimethylsulfoxide (DMSO) ointment in arthrosis. Acta Rheum Scand 1971;17: 57-60.

Vuopala U, Isomaki H, Kaipainen WJ. Dimethylsulfoxide (DMSO) ointment in the treatment of rheumatoid arthritis. Acta Rheum Scand 1969;15:139-44.

Wang JK. Stimulation-induced analgesia. Mayo Clin Proc 1976;51:28-30.

White JR, Sage JN. Topical analgesic on induced muscular pain. Phys Ther 1970;50:166-72.

White JR, Sage JN. Effects of a counterirritant on muscular distress in patients with arthritis. Phys Ther 1971;51:36-42.

White JR. Effects of a counterirritant on perceived pain and hand movement in patients with arthritis. Phys Ther 1973;53:956-60.

Allyl Isothiocyanate

Gennaro AR, ed. Remington's Pharmaceutical Sciences. Easton: Mack Publishing, 1985:780-81, 1286, 1291, 1301, 1506, 1512-13.

Macarthur JG, Alstead S. Counter-irritants. A method of assessing their effects. Lancet 1953;2:1060-62.

Reynolds JEF, ed. Martindale: The Extra Pharmacopoeia. London: Pharmaceutical Press, 1989:1064.

Strong Ammonia Solution

Reynolds JEF, ed. Martindale: The Extra Pharmacopoeia. London: Pharmaceutical Press, 1989:1064.

Methyl Salicylate

Brown EW, Scott WO. The absorption of methyl salicylate by the human skin. J Pharmacol Exp Ther 1934;50:32-50.

Chow WH, Cheung KL, Ling HM, et al. Potentiation of warfarin anticoagulation by topical methyl salicylate ointment. J R Soc Med 1989;82: 501-02.

Gordon RR. Poisoning by oil of wintergreen (Letter). BMJ 1968;1:769.

Gosselin RE, Smith RP, Hodge HC, eds. Clinical Toxicology of Commercial Products. Baltimore: Williams & Wilkins, 1984:III-368.

Heng MCY. Local necrosis and interstitial nephritis due to topical methyl salicylate and menthol. Cutis 1987;39:442-44.

Hindson C. Contact eczema from methyl salicylate reproduced by oral aspirin. Contact Dermatitis 1977;3:348-49.

Littleton F. Warfarin and topical salicylates (Letter). JAMA 1990;263:2888.

Morgan JK. Iatrogenic epidermal sensitivity. Br J Clin Pract 1968;22(6): 261-64.

Roberts MS, Favretto WA, Meyer A, et al. Topical bioavailability of methyl salicylate. Aust N Z J Med 1982;12:303-05.

Trapnell K. Salicylate intoxication. J Am Pharm Assoc 1976;16(3):147-49.

Yip ASB, Chow WH, Tai YT, et al. Adverse effect of topical methyl salicylate ointment on warfarin anticoagulation: an unrecognized potential hazard. Postgrad Med J 1990;66:367-69.

Triethanolamine Salicylate

Algozzine GJ, Stein GH, Doering PL, et al. Trolamine salicylate cream in osteoarthritis of the knee. JAMA 1982;247: 1311-13.

Golden EL. A double-blind comparison of orally ingested aspirin and a topically applied salicylate cream in the relief of rheumatic pain. Curr Ther Res 1978;24:524-29.

O'Brien WM. Trolamine salicylate cream in osteoarthritis (Letter). JAMA 1982;248:1577-78.

Rabinowitz JL, Feldman ES, Weinberger A, et al. Comparative tissue absorption of oral 14C aspirin and topical triethanolamine 14C salicylate in human and canine knee joints. J Clin Pharmacol 1982;22:42-48.

Rose FA, Weimer DR. Platelet coagulopathy secondary to topical salicylate use. Ann Plast Surg 1983;11:340-43.

Turpentine Oil

Morgan JK. Iatrogenic epidermal sensitivity. Br J Clin Pract 1968;22(6): 261-64.

Reynolds JEF, ed. Martindale: The Extra Pharmacopoeia. London: Pharmaceutical Press, 1989:1067.

Willis GA, Freeman DA, eds. Poison Management Manual. Ottawa: Canadian Pharmaceutical Association, 1989:439-40.

Capsicum Preparations

Crismon JM, Fox RH, Goldsmith R, et al. Forearm blood flow after inunction of rubefacient substances. J Physiol 1959;145:47P-48P.

Deal CL, Schnitzer TJ, Lipstein E, et al. Treatment of arthritis with topical capsaicin: a double-blind trial. Clin Ther 1991;13:383-93.

Lynn B. Capsaicin: actions on nociceptive C-fibres and therapeutic potential. Pain 1990;41:61-69.

McCarthy GM, McCarthy DJ. Effects of topical capsaicin in the therapy of painful osteoarthritis of the hands. J Rheumatol 1992;19:604-07.

Nolte MJ. Topical capsaicin for postherpetic neuralgia. Drug Intell Clin Pharm 1988;22:488-89.

Rumsfield JA, West DP. Topical capsaicin in dermatologic and peripheral pain disorders. DICP Ann Pharmacother 1991;25:381-87.

Camphor

Aronow R. Camphor poisoning. JAMA 1976;235:1260.

Gosselin RE, Smith RP, Hodge HC, eds. Clinical Toxicology of Commercial Products. Baltimore: Williams & Wilkins, 1984:III-384.

PhelanWJ. Camphor poisoning: over-the-counter dangers. Pediatrics 1976;57:428-31.

Trestrail JH, Spartz ME. Camphorated and castor oil confusion and its toxic results. Clin Toxicol 1977;11:151-58.

Menthol

Papa CM, Shelley WB. Menthol hypersensitivity. JAMA 1964;189:546-48.

Esters of Nicotinic Acid

Nassim JR, Banner H. Skin response to local application of a nicotinic acid ester in rheumatoid arthritis. Lancet 1952;1:699.

Clinical Considerations and Dosage Forms

Idson B. Percutaneous absorption. J Pharm Sci 1975;64: 901-24.

Eucalyptus Oil

Hindle BC. Eucalyptus oil ingestion. N Z Med J 1994;107:185-86.

Webb NJA, Pitt WR. Eucalyptus oil poisoning in childhood: 41 cases in south-east Queensland. J Pediatr Child 1993;29:368-71.

CHAPTER 21—Personal Hygiene Products

Skin and Soaps

Frosch PJ. Irritancy of soaps and detergent bars. In: Frost P, Horowitz SN. Principles of Cosmetics for the Dermatologist. St. Louis: CV Mosby, 1982.

Gennaro A, et al. Remington Pharmaceutical Sciences. 17th ed. Philadelphia: Philadelphia College of Pharmacy and Science, 1985:786.

Grayson M, Eckroth D. Kirk Othmer Encyclopedia of Chemical Technology. 3rd ed, Vol. 21. Toronto: Wiley Interscience, 1993:162-3,176-7.

Jellinek JS. Formulation and function of cosmetics. Toronto: Wiley Interscience, 1970:205-7.

Jungermann E. Specialty soaps: Formulations and processing. In: Spitz L. Soap Technology of the Nineties. Illinois: American Oil Chemist's Society, 1990:230-43.

Morelli JG, Weston WL. Soaps and shampoos in pediatric practice. Pediatrics 1987;80(5):634-7.

Oestreicher M. Detergents, bath preparations, and other skin cleansers. Clinics in Dermatology 1988;6(3):29-36.

Schoen LA, Lazar P. The Look You Like: Medical Answers to 400 Questions on Skin and Hair Care. New York: Marcel Dekker, 1990:153,156.

Simion AF, Rau AH. Sensitive skin: What it is and how to formulate for it. Cosmetics and Toiletries 1994;109:43-9.

Strube DD, Nicoll G. The irritancy of soaps and syndets. Cutis 1987;39: 544-5.

Swern D, ed. Bailey's Industrial Oil and Fat Products. 4th edition. New York: J. Wiley and Sons, 1979.

Umbach W. Cosmetics and Toiletries Development, Production and Use. Toronto: Ellis Horwood, 1991:49-53.

Wilcox MJ, Crichton WP. The soap market: A review of current trends. Cosmetics and Toiletries 1989;104:61-3.

Hyperhidrosis and Antiperspirants

Berkow R, ed. The Merck Manual of Diagnosis and Therapy. 16th ed. New Jersey: Merck Research Laboratories, 1992:2451.

Cosmetics and Toiletries Development, Production and Use. Toronto: Ellis Horwood, 1991:115-21.

Drug Consult: Hyperhidrosis Drug Therapy 1974-1994. Micromedex Inc.

Vol. 81.

Generali JA. What are the differences between antiperspirants and deodorants? US Pharmacist 1988;(Nov):24.

Iklin EK. Antiperspirants and deodorants. Cutis 1987;39:531-2.

Jellinek JS. Formulation and Function of Cosmetics. Toronto: Wiley Interscience, 1970:288-93.

Juhlin L, Hansson H. Topical glutaraldehyde for plantar hyperhydrosis. Arch Derm 1968;97:327-30.

Lione A. The reduction of aluminum intake in patients with Alzheimer's Disease. J Environmental Pathology, Toxicology and Oncology 1985; 6(1):21-32.

Schoen LA, Lazar P. The Look You Like: Medical Answers to 400 Questions on Skin and Hair Care. New York: Marcel Dekker, 1990:182-3.

Walder D, Penneys NS. Antiperspirants and deodorants. Clinics in Dermatology 1988;6(3):37-9.

White JW. Treatment of primary hyperhidrosis. Mayo Clin Proc 1986; 61:951-6.

Wyngaarden JB, Smith LH, Bennett JC. Cecil Textbook of Medicine. 19th ed. Toronto: WB Saunders, 1992:2095.

Hair Care

Anon. Hair care formulary. Cosmetics & Toiletries 1993;108:119.

Bouillon C. Shampoos and hair conditioners. Clinics in Dermatology 1988;6(3):83-92.

Chase D. The New Medically Based No-nonsense Beauty Book. New York: Henry Holt and Company, 1989.

DeVillez RL. The growth and loss of hair. Current Concepts, 1986 (an Upjohn Company publication).

Edwards C, Stillman P. Childhood ailments. Pharm J 1991;252:324-5.

Encyclopedia of Chemical Technology. 3rd ed, Vol. 12. New York: John Wiley & Sons, 1980.

Frangie C. Milady's Standard Textbook of Cosmetology. New York: Milady Publishing Company, 1991.

Harusawa F, Nakama Y, Tanaka M. Anionic-cationic ion-pairs. Cosmetics & Toiletries 1991;106:135-9.

Hunting AL. The use of detoxifying agents in shampoo formulations. Cosmetics & Toiletries 1985;100:49-55.

Krafchik B. Childhood Dermatitis. Infant Care 1990;2(1):10-3.

Morelli JG, Weston WL. Soaps and shampoos in pediatric practice. Pediatrics 1987;80(5):634-7.

Schoen LA, Lazar P. The Look You Like: Medical Answers to 400 Questions on Skin and Hair Care. New York: Marcel Dekker, 1990.

Thomson B, Vincent J, Halloran D. Silicone-in-silicone delivery systems. Soap/Cosmetics/Chemical Specialties 1992; (Oct):25-8.

Tyree DJ, Paloucek F. Personal shampoos and safety considerations. Am J Hosp Pharm 1991;48(5):937-8.

Woodruff J. Staying in condition. Manufacturing Chemist 1994; (Mar):18-20.

Zviak C, ed. The Science of Hair Care. New York: Marcel Dekker, 1986.

CHAPTER 22—Sleep Aids and Stimulants

Introduction

Coleman RM, Dement WC. Falling asleep at work: a problem for continuous operations. Sleep Res 1986;15:265.

Sleep Architecture

Bloom FE. Neurohumoral transmission and the central nervous system. In: Gilman AG, Rall TW, Nies AS, Taylor P, eds. Goodman and Gilman's The Pharmacological Basis of Therapeutics. New York: Maxwell MacMillan, 1990:244.

Rakel RE. Insomnia: concerns of the family physician. J Fam Pract 1993;36(5):551-8.

Rall TW. Hypnotics and sedatives; ethanol. In: Gilman AG, Rall TW, Nies AS, Taylor P, eds. Goodman and Gilman's The Pharmacological Basis of Therapeutics. New York: Maxwell MacMillan, 1990:345.

Insomnia

Berlin RM. Insomnia in hospitalized patients: approaches in management. Psychiatr Med 1987;4:197-208.

Berlin RM, Litovitz GL, Diaz MA, et al. Sleep disorders on a psychiatric consultation. Am J Psychiatry 1984;141:582-84.

Gottlieb GL. Sleep disorders and their management: special considerations in the elderly. Am J Med 1990:88(suppl 3A):29-33S.

Kales A, Kales JD. Sleep lab studies of hypnotic drugs: efficacy and withdrawal effects. J Clin Psychopharmacol 1983;3(2):140-50.

Nofzinger EA, Buysse DJ. Sleep disorders related to another mental disorder. J Clin Psychiatry 1993;54(7):244-55.

Rosekind MR. The epidemiology and occurrence of insomnia. J Clin Psychiatry 1992;53(6 suppl):4-6.

Drug-induced Insomnia

Hill LA. Drug-induced sleep changes. Hosp Pharm 1990;25:1119-20.

Stores G. Sleep disorders in clinical practice. Br J Clin Pract 1992;46(2): 82-84.

Soldatos CR, Kales JD, Scharf MB, et al. Cigarette smoking associated with sleep difficulty. Science 1980;207:551-53.

Walsh JK, Filingim JM. The role of hypnotic drugs in general practice. Am J Med 1990;88(suppl 3A):34-38.

Caffeine-induced Insomnia

Bootzin RR, Perlis ML. Nonpharmacological treatment of insomnia. J Clin Psychiatry 1992;53(6 Suppl):37-41.

Canadian Drug Identification Code. Ottawa: Health and Welfare Canada, 1993.

Narcolepsy

Aldridge MS. Sleep disorders. Curr Opin Neurol Neurosurgery 1992;5: 240-46.

Aldridge MS. Review: narcolepsy. N Engl J Med 1990;323:389-93.

Guilleminault C, Mignol E, Grumet FC. Familial patterns of narcolepsy. Lancet 1989;2:1376-79.

Guilleminault C. Narcolepsy syndrome. In: Kryger MH, Roth T, Dement WC, editors. Principles and Practice of Sleep Medicine. Philadelphia: Saunders, 1994:549-61.

Nonpharmacological Management of Insomnia

Bootzin RR, Perlis ML. Nonpharmacological treatment of insomnia. J Clin Psychiatry 1992;53(6 suppl):37-41.

Coates TJ, Thorsen CE. What to use instead of sleeping pills. JAMA 1978;240:2311-12.

Rakel RE. Insomnia: concerns of the family physician. J Fam Pract 1993; 36(5):555-58.

Wincor MZ. The pharmacist's role in the recognition and management of insomnia. J Clin Psychiatry 1992;53(12 suppl):80-83.

Antihistamines

Rickels K, Morris RJ, Newman H, et al. Diphenhydramine in insomniac family practice patients: a double-blind study. J Clin Pharmacol 1983; 23:235-42.

Briggs G, Freeman K, Yaffe S. Drugs in Pregnancy and Lactation. Baltimore: Williams & Wilkins, 1990.

Parkin DE. Probable Benadryl withdrawal manifestations in a newborn infant. J Pediatr 1974;85:580-82.

L-tryptophan

Nickel A. Triptan: No association with eosinophilia myalgia syndrome. Can Med Assoc J 1990;143(11):1155-56.

Sleep in the Elderly

Monane M. Insomnia in the elderly. J Clin Psychiatry 1992;53 (6 suppl):23-28.

Zorzitto ML. Sleep in the elderly. Mod Med Can 1983;38(1):77-82.

Sleep Apnea

Culebras A. Update on disorders of sleep and sleep-wake cycle. Psychiatr Clin North Am 1992;15(2):467-83.

Kryger MH. Management of obstructive sleep apnea: overview. In: Kryger MH, Roth T, Dement WC, eds. Principles and Practice of Sleep Medicine. Philadelphia: Saunders, 1994:736-47.

Waddhorn RE. Obstructive sleep apnea syndrome: drug and nondrug treatments. Drug Ther 1994;4:48-53.

CHAPTER 23—Smoking Cessation Products

Epidemiology

Decima Research. Attitudes, perceptions, and behaviour relating to ethical medicine. Ottawa: Minister of Supply and Services Canada, 1990:49.

General Social Survey 1985 and 1991, Labour Force Survey Supplements on Smoking Habits, and other selected surveys. Ottawa: Statistics Canada.

Smoking Behavior of Canadians. A National Alcohol and Other Drugs Survey Report (1989), plus update (1991). National Clearinghouse on Tobacco and Health. Ottawa: Health and Welfare Canada.

Pathophysiology

Christen AG. The impact of tobacco use and cessation on oral and dental diseases and conditions. Am J Med 1992; 93(suppl 1A):25S-31S.

Collishaw N, Leahy K. Mortality attributable to tobacco use in Canada, 1989. Chronic Diseases in Canada 1991;12(4):46-9.

Doll R, Hill AB. Mortality in relation to smoking: ten years observations of British doctors. BMJ 1964;1:1399-1410.

Facchini FS, Hollenbeck CB, Jeppesen J. Insulin resistance and cigarette smoking. Lancet 1992; 339:1128-30.

Goodman L, Gilman A, eds. The Pharmacological Basis of Therapeutics. 4th ed. New York: The Macmillan Company, 1971:588-9.

Gossel TA. The physiological and pharmacological effects of nicotine. U.S. Health Professional Supplement; Feb 1992.

The health benefits of smoking cessation: A report of the Surgeon General. Washington, DC: U.S. Department of Health and Human Services, Public Health Service, Center for Chronic Disease Prevention and Health Promotion, Office on Smoking and Health, 1990. DHHS publication no. (CDC) 90-8416.

The health consequences of involuntary smoking: a report of the Surgeon General. Washington, DC: U.S. Department of Health, Education and Welfare, 1986.

The health consequences of smoking: cardiovascular disease. A report of the Surgeon General. Washington, DC: U.S. Department of Health and Human Services, 1983. DHHS(PHS) 84-50204.

Krupski WC. The peripheral vascular consequences of smoking. Ann Vasc Surg 1991;5:291-304.

Lasmes GR, Donofrio KH. Passive smoking: the medical and economic issues. Am J Med 1992; 93(suppl 1A):38S-42S.

Lassila R, Seyberth HW, Hoapanen A, et al. Vasoactive and atherogenic effects of smoking: a study of monozygotic twins discordant for smoking. BMJ 1988;297:955-7.

McCusker K. Mechanisms of respiratory tissue injury from cigarette smoking. Am J Med 1992; 93(suppl 1A):18S-21S.

McGill HC. The cardiovascular pathology of smoking. Am Heart J 1988;115:250-7.

Miller LG. Recent developments in the study of the effects of cigarette smoking on clinical pharmacokinetics and clinical pharmacodynamics. Clin Pharmacokinet 1989;17(2):90-108.

Monograph on the Evaluation of the Carcinogenic Risk of Chemicals to Humans. Tobacco Smoking, Vol. 38. Switzerland: WHO International Agency for Research on Cancer, 1985.

Reducing the health consequences of smoking: 25 years of progress. A report of the Surgeon General's office. Rockville, MD: U.S. Department of Health and Human Services, 1989.

Silverstein P. Smoking and wound healing. Am J Med 1992;93(suppl 1A):22S-24S.

Sherwin MA, Gastwirth CM. Detrimental effects of cigarette smoking on lower extremity wound healing. J Foot Surg 1990;29:84-8.

Smoking Tobacco and Health: A Fact Book. Washington, DC: Department of Health and Human Services, 1987.

Szabo P. Kids' ear infections again tied to passive smoking. The Journal 1992;Aug-Sept:4.

Weiss ST, Tager IB, Schenker M, et al. The health effects of involuntary smoking. Am Rev Respir Dis 1983;128:933-42.

Symptoms: The Smoking Habit

Anon. Scads of smokers trying to quit. Toronto Sun 1992 Aug 13.

Anon. Teen smokers worry more about weight. The Journal 1994; 23(1):6.

Coambs RB, Li S, Kozlowski L. Age interacts with heaviness of smoking in predicting success in cessation of smoking. Am J Epidemiol 1992; 135(3):240-6.

Environics Research Group Ltd. Poll conducted by the Canadian Council on Smoking and Health as reported in Smoking or Health Update, Spring 1991.

Fiore M, Jorenby D, Baker T, et al. Tobacco dependence and the nicotine patch—Clinical guidelines for effective use. JAMA 1992; 268(19): 2687-94.

Freund K, D'Agostino R, Belanger A, et al. Predictors of smoking cessation: The Framingham Study. Am J Epidemiol 1992;135(9):957-964.

Gossel TA. The physiological and pharmacological effects of nicotine. U.S. Health Professional Supplement; Feb 1992.

Gourlay SG, McNeill JJ. Antismoking products. Med J Australia 1990; 153:699-704.

The health consequences of smoking: nicotine addiction: A report of the Surgeon General. Washington, DC: U.S. Department of Health and Human Services, Public Health Service, Centers for Disease Control, Center for Chronic Disease Prevention and Health Promotion, Office on Smoking and Health, 1988. DHHS publication no. (CDC) 88-8406.

Hunt WA, Barnett LW, Branch LG. Relapse rates in addiction programs. J Clin Psychol 1971;27:455-56.

Killen J, Fortmann S, Newman B. Weight change among participants in a large sample minimal contact smoking relapse prevention trial. Addict Behav 1990;15:323-32.

Nunn-Thompson CL, Simon PA. Pharmacotherapy for smoking cessation. Clin Pharm 1989;8:710-20.

Pollin W. The role of the addictive process as a key step in causation of all tobacco related diseases (editorial). JAMA 1984;252:287.

Schwartz JL. Review and evaluation of Smoking Cessation Methods: The United States and Canada, 1978-1985. U.S. Department of Health and Human Services, Public Health Service, National Institute of Health; 1987. NIH Publication no. 87-2940.

Tobacco, Nicotine and Addiction: A committee report prepared at the request of The Royal Society of Canada for the Health Protection Branch. Ottawa: Health and Welfare Canada, 1989.

William M. Effectiveness of clonidine in smoking cessation. Can J Hosp Pharm 1992;45(2):77-8.

Treatment

Anon. Med Lett Drugs Ther 1984; 26(661):47-8.

Bliss RE, Garvey AJ, Heinold JW. The influence of situation and coping on relapse crisis outcomes after smoking cessation. J Consult Clin Psychol 1989;47(3):443-9.

Fagerström KO. Reducing the weight gain after stopping smoking. Addict Behav 1987;12:91-3.

Fagerström KO. A comparison of psychological and pharmacological treatment in smoking cessation. J Behav Med 1982;5:343-51.

Fagerström KO, Melin B. Nicotine chewing gum in smoking cessation: Efficiency, nicotine dependence, therapy duration, and clinical recommendations. In: Grabowski J, Hall SM, eds. Pharmacological adjuncts in the treatment of tobacco dependence. National Institute of Drug Abuse Research Monograph 1985; 53:102-9.

Ferguson T. The Smoker's Book of Health. New York: Putnam, 1987.

Fiore M, Jorenby D, Baker T, et al. Tobacco dependence and the nicotine patch—clinical guidelines for effective use. JAMA 1992;268(19): 2687-94.

General Social Survey 1985 and 1991, Labour Force Survey Supplements on Smoking Habits, and other selected surveys. Ottawa: Statistics Canada.

Glynn TJ, Manley MW. How to help your patients stop smoking—A National Cancer Institute manual for physicians. Washington, DC: US Department of Health and Human Services, Public Health Service, National Institutes of Health; 1990. Publication no. NIH 90-3064.

Goldstein MG, Niaura R, Follick MJ, et al. Effects of behavioural skills training and schedule of nicotine gum administration on smoking cessation. Am J Psychiatry 1989;146(1):56-60.

Gourlay SG, McNeill JJ. Antismoking products. Med J Australia 1990; 153:699-704.

Gross J, Sitzer ML, Maldonado J. Nicotine replacement: Effects on postcessation weight gain. J Consult Clin Psychol 1989;57(1):87-92.

The health benefits of smoking cessation: A report of the Surgeon General. Washington, DC: U.S. Department of Health and Human Services, Public Health Service, Centers for Disease Control, Center for Chronic Disease Prevention and Health Promotion, Office on Smoking and Health, 1990. DHHS publication no. (CDC) 90-8416.

How to help your patients stop smoking—A reference guide for health professionals. Fifth draft. Merrell Dow Pharmaceuticals, 1992.

Jamrozik K, Vessey M, Fowler G, et al. Controlled trial of three different antismoking interventions in general practice. BMJ 1984;288: 1499-1503.

Monograph on the Evaluation of the Carcinogenic Risk of Chemicals to Humans. Tobacco Smoking, Vol. 38. Switzerland: WHO International Agency for Research on Cancer, 1985.

Nicorette® Product Monograph. 1994, Marion Merrell Dow.

Nunn-Thompson CL, Simon PA. Pharmacotherapy for smoking cessation. Clin Pharm 1989;8:710-20.

Pederson LL, Scrimgeour WG, Defcoe NM. Comparison of hypnosis plus counselling, counselling alone and hypnosis alone in a community service smoking withdrawal program. J Consult Clinical Psychol 1975;43(6):920.

Rosenbaum P, O'Shea R. Large-scale study of Freedom from Smoking Clinics—factors in quitting. Public Health Reports 1992;107(2):150-5.

Russell MAH, Merriman R, Stapelton J, Taylor W. Effect of nicotine chewing gum as an adjunct to general practitioner's advice against smoking. BMJ 1983;287:1782-85.

Russell MAH, Wilson C, Taylor CD. Effect of general practitioner's advice against smoking. BMJ 1979;2:231-35.

Schwartz JC. Methods of smoking cessation. Clin Chest Med 1991;12(4): 737-53.

Schwartz JC. Review and evaluation of smoking cessation methods: The United States and Canada, 1978-1985. Washington, DC: U.S. Department of Health and Human Services, Public Health Service, National Institute of Health, 1987. NIH publication no. 87-2940.

Spiegel D, Frischolz EJ, Fleiss JL, Spiegel H. Predictors of smoking abstinence following a single-session restructuring intervention with self-hypnosis. Am J Psychiatry 1993;150(7):1090-7.

Stephens VJ, Hollis JF. Preventing smoking relapse, using an individually tailored skills-training technique. J Consult Clin Psychology 1989; 57(3):420-4.

Tang JL, Law M, Wald N. How effective is nicotine replacement therapy in helping people to stop smoking? BMJ 1994;308(6920):21-6.

Tonnesen P, Fryd V, Hansen M, et al. Effect of nicotine chewing gum in combination with group counselling on the cessation of smoking. N Engl J Med 1988;318:15-8.

Wilson DMC, Lindsay EA, Best JA, et al. A smoking cessation intervention for family physicians. Can Med Assoc J 1987;137(7):613-9.

Viswervaran C, Schmidt FL. A meta-analytic comparison of the effectiveness of smoking cessation methods. J Appl Psychol 1992;77(4): 554-61.

Your guide to a smoke free future. Ottawa: The Canadian Council on Smoking and Health, 1992.

Pharmaceutical Agents

Anon. Med Lett Drugs Ther 1984;26(661):47-8.

Behm FM, Schur C, Levin ED, et al. Clinical evaluation of a citric acid inhaler for smoking cessation. Drug and Alcohol Depend 1993;31(2): 131-8.

Benowitz N. Nicotine replacement therapy during pregnancy. JAMA 1991;266:3174-7.

Fiore M, Jorenby D, Baker T, et al. Tobacco dependence and the nicotine patch—Clinical guidelines for effective use. JAMA 1992;268(19): 2687-94.

Gossel TA. The physiological and pharmacological effects of nicotine. U.S. Health Professional Supplement; Feb 1992.

Gossel TA. Smoking deterrents. U.S. Health Professional 1984;May:10, 12,15-7,72.

Gourlay SG, McNeill JJ. Antismoking products. Med J Australia 1990;153:699-704.

How to help your patients stop smoking—A reference guide for health professionals. Fifth draft. Merrell Dow Pharmaceuticals, 1992.

Hughes JR. Risk-benefit assessment of nicotine preparations in smoking cessation. Drug Safety 1993;8(1):49-56.

Jensen EJ, Schmidt E, Pedersen B, et al. Effect of nicotine, silver and ordinary chewing gum in combination with group counselling on smoking cessation. Thorax 1990;45:831-4.

Levin ED, Behm F, Carnahan E, et al. Clinical trials using ascorbic acid aerosol to aid smoking cessation. Drug and Alcohol Depend 1993; 33(3);211-23.

McNabb ME, Ebert RV, McCusker K. Plasma levels produced by chewing nicotine gum. JAMA 1982;248:865-8.

Nicorette® Product Monograph. 1994, Marion Merrell Dow.

Paipo Product Monograph. 1990, Herdt & Charton.

Wilson DMC. The role of the family physician in cigarette abstention. Mod Med Can 1989;44(8):802-11.

CHAPTER 24—Sports Medicine Products

Anon. Treatment of heat injury. Med Lett Drugs Ther 1990;32(822): 66-68.

Canadian Centre for Drug-free Sport. Banned and restricted doping classes and methods booklet. Gloucester, Ont: Canadian Centre for Drug-free Sport, 1993.

Edwards C, Stillman P. Musculoskeletal disorders. Pharm J 1993; 251(6766):733-38.

Friedman RM, ed. When to ice/when to heat. U C Berkeley Wellness Letter 1994;10(8):6.

Hough DO. Anabolic steroids and ergogenic aids. Am Fam Physician 1990; 41(4):1162-63.

James DW. Improving athletic performance. Am Drug 1987;196(7):1-6.

Johnson SC. Should athletes take salt tablets to replace sodium lost during exercise? US Pharm 1989;8:59-60.

Keeping your cool (how to avoid heat illness). Health News. Toronto: Faculty of Medicine, University of Toronto, 1989;7(8):10-12.

Kyriakos T. Cash in on fitness. Drug Merch 1986;67(3):26.

Merchant WF. Medications and athlete—increasing your sports medicine knowledge. Am Drug 1992;206(5):6-13.

Millard-Stafford M. Fluid replacement during exercise in the heat—review and recommendations. Sports Med 1992;13(4):223-33.

Nykamp D. Sports injuries. US Pharm 1992;17(4):34-55.

Perry PJ. Sport medicine. Canadian Council on Continuing Education in Pharmacy 1991;13(3):1-8.

Peterson L, Renström P. Sports injuries—their prevention and treatment. St. Louis, MO: Mosby Year Book, 1986:60-61, 150-55, 207-11, 466-77.

Pharmacist's checklist—exercise injuries (insert). Can Pharm J 1992; 125(11).

Pray WS. Use of local heat for minor injuries. US Pharm 1993; 18(10):39-45.

Reid DC. Sports injury assessment and rehabilitation. New York: Churchill Livingstone, 1992:1176-77.

Sherman M. A primer on use of hot or cold therapy. US Pharm 1987; 12(1):72-81.

Smith DA, Perry PJ. The efficacy of ergogenic agents in athletic competition. Part II: other performance-enhancing agents. Ann Pharmacother 1992;26(5):653-59.

Sport and exercise. In: Martin J, ed. Handbook of Pharmacy Health Education. London: Pharmaceutical Press, 1991:161-88.

Sport for all—is it cost effective? (Editorial). Drug and Therapy Perspectives 1994;3(9):14-16.

Strauss RH, ed. Sports Medicine. 2nd ed. Philadelphia; Toronto: WB Saunders, 1991:350-57.

Tver DF, Hunt HF. Encyclopedic Dictionary of Sports Medicine. New York: Chapman and Hall, 1986:86-90.

Wagner JC. Abuse of drugs used to enhance athletic performance. Am J Hosp Pharm 1989;46:2059-67.

Wagner JC. Enhancement of athletic performance with drugs—an overview. Sports Med 1991;12(4):250-65.

Walker E, Williams G. First aid while abroad. BMJ 1983;286(6370): 1039-42.

Woolley BH. The latest fads to increase muscle mass and energy. Postgrad Med 1991;89(2):197-205.

CHAPTER 25—Sunscreen and Tanning Products

Solar Radiation

Anon. Sunscreens. Med Lett Drugs Ther 1984;26(663):56-58.

Cavello J, DeLeo VA. Sunburn. Dermatol Clin 1986;4(2):181-87.

Council Report. Harmful effects of ultraviolet radiation. JAMA 1989; 262(3):380-84.

Diffey BL, Larkoe O. Clinical climatology. Photodermatol 1984;1(1): 30-37.

Environment Canada. Canada's ozone layer protection program—a summary. Ottawa: Environment Canada, 1994:1-16.

Environment Canada. UV and you. Living with ultraviolet. Ottawa: Environment Canada, March 1993:1-3.

FDA Formulating Guidelines. Which sunscreens offer the best protection against UVA radiation? Primary Care and Cancer 1991;(Jul-Aug):30-32.

Lowe NJ. Photoprotection. Semin Dermatol 1990;9(1):78-83.

Matsuoka LY, Wortsman J, Hollis BW. Use of topical sunscreen for the evaluation of regional synthesis of vitamin D3. J Am Acad Dermatol 1990;22(5):772-75.

Menter JM. Recent developments in UVA protection. Int J Dermatol 1990;29(6):389-94.

Pathak MA. Sunscreens: topical and systemic approaches for protection of human skin against harmful effects of solar radiation. J Am Acad Dermatol 1982;7(3):285-312.

Pathak MA. Sunscreens: topical and systemic approaches for the prevention of acute and chronic sun-induced skin reactions. Dermatol Clin 1986;4(2):321-34.

Shear NH. Year-round safe sun. Pharmacy Practice 1990;(Jul-Aug):10-14.

Taylor CR, Stern RS, Leyden JJ, et al. Photoaging/photodamage and photoprotection. J Am Acad Dermatol 1990;22(1):1-15.

Sunburn

Anders JE, Leach EE. Sun versus skin. Am J Nurs 1983;83(7):1015-20.

Bickers DR. Sun-induced disorders. Emerg Med Clin North Am 1985;3(4): 659-77.

Cole C, Vanfossen R. Measurement of sunscreen UVA protection: an unsensitized human model. J Am Acad Dermatol 1992;26(1 Pt 1): 178-84.

Drolet BA, Connor MJ. Sunscreens and the prevention of ultraviolet radiation-induced skin cancer. J Dermatol Surg Oncol 1992;18:571-76.

Bickers DR. Photosensitivity and other reactions to light. In: Isselbacher KJ, Braunwald E, Wilson JD, et al, eds. Harrison's Principles of Internal Medicine. New York: McGraw-Hill, 1994:307-12.

Pathak MA, Fanselow DL. Photobiology of melanin pigmentation: dose/response of skin to sunlight and its contents. J Am Acad Dermatol 1983;9(5):724-33.

Warshauer DM, Steinbaugh JR. Sunlight and protection of the skin. Am Fam Physician 1983;27(6):109-15.

Tanning

Boger J, Araujo OE, Flowers F. Sunscreens: efficacy, use and misuse. South Med J 1984;77(11):1421-27.

Kligman LH. Photoaging: manifestations, prevention and treatment. Dermatol Clin 1986;4(3):517-28.

Photobiology Task Force of the American Academy of Dermatology. Risks and benefits from high-intensity ultraviolet A sources used for cosmetic purposes. J Am Acad Dermatol 1985;12(2 Pt 1):380-81.

Photosensitivity

Anon. Drugs that cause photosensitivity. Med Lett Drugs Ther 1986; 28(713):51-52.

Bilsland D, Ferguson J. Contact allergy to sunscreen chemicals in photosensitivity dermatitis/actinic reticuloid syndrome (PD/AR) and polymorphic light eruption. Contact Dermatitis 1993;29:70-73.

Diffey BL, Farr PM. An evaluation of sunscreens in patients with broad action spectrum photosensitivity. Br J Dermatol 1985;112(1):83-86.

Elmets CA. Drug-induced photoallergy. Dermatol Clin 1986;4(2):231-41.

Epstein JH. Phototoxicity and photoallergy in man. J Am Acad Dermatol 1983;8(2):141-47.

McGuffey E. Ask the pharmacist. Are chemical sunscreens beneficial for lupus patients who experience photosensitivity? Am Pharm 1993; NS33(7):20.

Photobiology Task Force of the American Academy of Dermatology. Risks and benefits from high-intensity ultraviolet A sources used for cosmetic purposes. J Am Acad Dermatol 1985;12(2 Pt 1):380-81.

Photoaging

Green HA, Drake L. Aging, sun damage and sunscreens. Clin Plast Surg 1993;20(1):1-8.

Cancer

Canadian Cancer Statistics 1994. Toronto: National Cancer Institute of Canada, 1994:14.

Cancer Statistics Review 1973-1989. Bethesda: National Cancer Institute, 1992:XVI.1.

Cancer in Canada 1980. Ottawa: Statistics Canada, 1983:12-13.

Elwood JM, Gallagher RP, Davison J, et al. Sunburn, suntan and the risk of cutaneous malignant melanoma: the Western Canada melanoma study. Br J Cancer 1985;51(4):543-49.

Epstein JH. Photocarcinogenesis, skin cancer and aging. J Am Acad Dermatol 1983;9(4):487-502.

Friedman RJ, Rigel DS, Silverman MK, et al. Malignant melanoma in the 1990's: the continued importance of early detection and the role of physician examination and self-examination of the skin. CA-A Cancer Journal for Clinicians 1991;41(4):201-26.

Green A, Sisking V, Bain C, et al. Sunburn and malignant melanoma. Br J Cancer 1985;51(3):393-97.

Kopf AW, Friedman RJ, Rigel DS. The many faces of malignant melanoma. New York: The Skin Cancer Foundation, 1987.

Kopf AW, Kripke ML, Stern RS. Sun and malignant melanoma. J Am Acad Dermatol 1984;11(4 Pt 1):674-84.

Pownall M. Suntanning: skin scare. Nurs Times 1985;81(32):19.

Skolnick AA. Medical news and perspectives. Melanoma epidemic yields grim statistics. JAMA 1991;265(24):3217.

Sun awareness program. Ottawa: Canadian Dermatology Association, 1995:1-9.

Sun Sense. Toronto: Canadian Cancer Society, 1993.

Thompson SC, Jolley D, Marks D. Reduction of solar keratoses by regular sunscreen use. N Engl J Med 1993;329(16):1145-51.

Nonpharmacological Protection

Jevtic AP. The sun-protective effect of clothing including beachwear. Aust J Dermatol 1990;31:5-7.

Sun Protection Factor

Azizi E, Kushelevsky AP, Schewach-Millet M. Efficacy of topical sunscreen preparations on the human skin: combined indoor-outdoor study. Isr J Med Sci 1984;20(7):569-77.

Garmyn MA, Murphy GM, Gibbs NK, et al. Are the protection factors assigned to proprietary sunscreen products misleading? Photodermatol 1986;3(2):104-06.

Greaves K, Cripps AJ, Cripps DJ. Actinic reticuloid: action spectra and UVA protection factor sunscreens. Clin Exper Dermatol 1992;17: 94-98.

Kaidbey KH. The photoprotective effect of the new superpotent sunscreens. J Am Acad Dermatol 1990;22(3):449-52.

Luftman DB, Lowe NJ, Moy RL. Sunscreens—update and review. J Dermatol Surg Oncol 1991;17:744-46.

Watson A. Sunscreen effectiveness: theoretical and practical considerations. Aust J Dermatol 1983;24(1):17-22.

Young AR. The use of sunscreens in preventing skin cancer (Reply). Br J Dermatol 1991;124(3):302.

Measuring UVA Efficacy

Anon. Measuring sunscreen protection against UVA. Lancet 1990;(Aug 25):472.

Rapaport MJ. Choosing a broad-spectrum sunscreen with UVA protection. Dermatol Nursing 1991;3(2):83-89,102.

Roelandts R. Which components in broad-spectrum sunscreens are most necessary for adequate UVA protection? J Am Acad Dermatol 1991; 25(6):999-1004.

Stiller MJ, Davis IC, Shupack JL. A concise guide to topical sunscreens: state of the art. Int J Dermatol 1992;31(8):540-43.

Choice of Sunscreen

Basler RSW. Sunscreens. Nebr Med J 1983;68(6):162-65.

Brasier S, Baker K, Mattson K. Screening summer sun. Canadian Consumer 1982;12(6):25-27.

Edwards EK Jr, Edwards EK. Allergic reaction to triethanolamine stearate in a sunscreen. Cutis 1983;31(2):195-96.

Edwards EK Jr, Edwards EK. Allergic reaction to phenyl dimethicone in a sunscreen (Letter). Arch Dermatol 1984;120(5):575-76.

Farr PM, Diffey BL. How reliable are sunscreen protection factors? Br J Dermatol 1985;112(1):113-18.

Gilmore GD. Sunscreens: a review of the skin cancer protection value and education opportunities. J School Health 1989;59(5):211-13.

Hogan D. Potential changes of alcohol-based sunscreens (Letter). JAMA 1992;268(16):2169.

Leroy D, Deschamps P. Influence of formulation on sunscreen water resistance. Photodermatol 1986;3(1):52-53.

Lundeen RC, Langlais RP, Terezhalmy GT. Sunscreen protection for lip mucosa: a review and update. J Am Dent Assoc 1985;111(4):617-21.

O'Neill JJ. Effect of film irregularities on sunscreen efficacy. J Pharm Sci 1984;73(7):888-91.

Pathak MA, Fitzpatrick TB. Preventative treatment of sunburn, dermatoheliosis and skin cancer with sun-protective agents. In: Fitzpatrick TB, et al, eds. Dermatology in General Medicine. 4th ed. New York: McGraw-Hill, 1993:1689-1717.

Proby CM, Baker CS, Morton O, et al. New broad-spectrum sunscreen for polymorphic light eruption (Reply). Lancet 1993:341:1347-48.

Rooney JF, Mannix ML, Wohlenberg CR, et al. Prevention of ultraviolet-light-induced herpes labialis by sunscreen. Lancet 1991;338:1419-22.

Stenberg C, Larkoe O. Sunscreen application and its importance for the sun protection factor. Arch Dermatol 1985;121(11):1400-02.

Sunscreens on Children

Banks BA, Silverman RA, Schwartz RH. Attitudes of teenagers toward sun exposure and sunscreen use. Pediatrics 1992;89(1):40-42.

Maducdoc LR, Wagner RF, Wagner KD. Parents' use of sunscreens on beach-going children. Arch Dermatol 1992;128:628-29.

McGuffey E. Ask the pharmacist. Are sunscreens safe for infants and children? Am Pharm 1992;NS32(8):16.

Morelli JG, Weston WL. What sunscreen should I use for my 3-month-old baby? (Letter) Pediatrics 1993;9(6):882.

Relling MV, Dorr RT. Choosing a sunscreen. Ariz Med 1983;40(8):550-54.

Stern RS, Weinstein MC, Baker SG. Risk reduction for non-melanoma skin cancer with childhood sunscreen use. Arch Dermatol 1986;122(5): 537-45.

Your kids and the sun. Montreal: Canadian Dermatology Association, 1994.

Chemical Sunscreens

Anon. Photoplex—a broad spectrum sunscreen. Med Lett Drugs Ther 1989;31(794):59-60.

Dromgoole SH, Maibach HI. Sunscreening agent intolerance: contact and photocontact sensitization and contact urticaria. J Am Acad Dermatol 1990;22(6):1068-78.

English JSC, White RI, Cronin E. Sensitivity to sunscreens. Contact Dermatitis 1987;17:159-62.

Fisher AA. Sunscreen dermatitis: part II—the cinnamates. Cutis 1992; 50:253-54.

Fisher AA. Sunscreen dermatitis: part III—the benzophenones. Cutis 1992; 50:331-32.

Fisher AA. Sunscreen dermatitis: part IV—the salicylates, the anthranilates, and physical agents. Cutis 1992;50:397-98.

Foley P, Nixon R, Marks R, et al. The frequency of reactions to sunscreens: results of a longitudinal population-based study on the regular use of sunscreens in Australia. Br J Dermatol 1993;128:512-18.

Forestier S. Photostability: a major advance in the field of sun protection. Med Staff Dermatologie 1995;27:13-15.

Fourtanier A, Labat-Robert J, Kern P, et al. In vivo evaluation of photoprotection against chronic ultraviolet-A irradiation by a new sunscreen Mexoryl SX. Photochem Photobiol 1992;55(4):549-60.

Harvey SC. Topical drugs. In: Gennaro AR, ed. Remington's Pharmaceutical Sciences. Easton: Mack Publishing, 1985:790-91.

Lowe NJ. Sunscreens and the prevention of skin aging. J Dermatol Surg Oncol 1990;16(10):936-38.

Mathias CGT. Commentary and update: cutaneous sensitivity to monoglyceryl para-aminobenzoate. Cleve Clin Q 1983;50(2):85-86.

Motley RJ, Reynolds AJ. Photocontact dermatitis due to isopropyl and butylmethoxy dibenzoylmethanes (Eusolex 8020 and Parsol 1789). Contact Dermatitis 1989;21:109-11.

O'Donoghue MN. Sunscreen: one weapon against melanoma. Dermatol Clin 1991;9(4):789-93.

O'Donoghue MN. Sunscreen—the ultimate cosmetic. Dermatol Clin 1991;9(1):99-104.

Patel NP, Highton A, Moy RL. Properties of topical sunscreen formulations. J Dermatol Surg Oncol 1992;18:316-20.

Pathak MA. Sunscreens and their use in the preventative treatment of sunlight-induced skin damage. J Dermatol Surg Oncol 1987;13(7):739-50.

Thune P. Contact and photocontact allergy to sunscreens. Photodermatol 1984;1(1):5-9.

White IR. Risk of contact dermatitis to UVA sunscreens (Reply). Contact Dermatitis 1993;29:229.

Physical Sunscreens

Fed Reg 1978;43(Pt2):38213.

Green C, Catterall M, Hawk JLM. Chronic actinic dermatitis and sunscreen allergy. Clin Exp Dermatol 1991;16:70-71.

Possible Adverse Effects of Sunscreens

Buescher LS. Sunscreens and photoprotection. Otolaryngol Clin North Am 1993;26(1):13-22.

Dobak J, Liu FT. Sunscreens, UVA and cutaneous malignancy: adding fuel to the fire. Int J Dermatol 1992;31(8):544-48.

Garland CF, Garland FC, Gorham ED. Could sunscreens increase melanoma risk? Am J Public Health 1992;82(4):614-15.

Garland CF, Garland FC, Gorham ED. Rising trends in melanoma—an hypothesis concerning sunscreen effectiveness. Ann Epidemiol 1993;3(1):103-10.

Koh HK, Lew RA. Sunscreens and melanoma: implications for prevention. J Natl Cancer Inst 1994;86(2):78-79.

Skolnick AA. Medical news and perspectives. Sunscreen protection controversy heats up. JAMA 1991;265(24):3218-20.

Weinstock MA, Stampfer MJ, Lew RA, et al. Case-control study of melanoma and dietary Vitamin D: implications for advocacy of sun protection and sunscreen use. J Invest Dermatol 1992;98(5):809-11.

Young AR. Senescence and sunscreens. Br J Dermatol 1990;122(35): 111-14.

Systemic Protection

Anon. Pigmenting agents. In: McEvoy GK, Litvak K, Welsh OH, eds. American Hospital Formulary Service—Drug Information 1994. Bethesda: American Society of Hospital Pharmacists, 1994:2367-72.

Anon. Dermatological agents. In: Reynolds JEF, ed. Martindale: The Extra Pharmacopoeia. London: Pharmaceutical Press, 1993:763-64, 771, 1036-37.

Pigmenting or Tanning Agents

Anon. Coloring agents. In: Reynolds JEF, ed. Martindale: The Extra Pharmacopoeia. London: Pharmaceutical Press, 1993:698.

Anon. Dermatological agents. In: Reynolds JEF, ed. Martindale: The Extra Pharmacopoeia. London: Pharmaceutical Press, 1993:757.

Anon. Pigmenting agents. In: McEvoy GK, Litvak K, Welsh OH, eds. American Hospital Formulary Service—Drug Information 1994. Bethesda: American Society of Hospital Pharmacists, 1994:2366-67.

Bluhm R, Branch R, Johnston P, et al. Aplastic anemia associated with canthaxanthine ingested for "tanning" purposes. JAMA 1990;264(9): 1141-42.

Natow AJ. Corrective cosmetics. Cutis 1985;36(2):123-24.

Depigmenting Agents

Anon. Depigmenting agents. In: McEvoy GK, Litvak K, Welsh OH, eds. American Hospital Formulary Service—Drug Information 1994. Bethesda: American Society of Hospital Pharmacists, 1994:2364-65.

Anon. Dermatological agents. In: Reynolds JEF, ed. Martindale: The Extra Pharmacopoeia. London: Pharmaceutical Press, 1993:759, 765.

Anon. Hyperpigmentation and hypopigmentation. In: Arndt KA, ed. Manual of Dermatologic Therapeutics. Boston: Little, Brown, 1983:107-13.

Boyle J, Kennedy CTC. Hydroquinone concentrations in skin lightening creams. Br J Dermatol 1986;114(4):501-04.

Fisher AA. Hydroquinone uses and abnormal reactions. Cutis 1983;31(3): 240-44, 250.

Wintroub BU, Stern RS. Cutaneous drug reactions. In: Isselbacher KJ, Braunwald E, Wilson JD, et al, eds. Harrison's Principles of Internal Medicine. New York: McGraw-Hill, 1994:279-85.

Gossel TA. Skin lighteners. US Pharmacist 1985;10(3):16, 18-20, 22.

Lerner EA, Sober AJ. Chemical and pharmacological agents that cause hyperpigmentation or hypopigmentation of the skin. Dermatol Clin 1988;6(2):327-37.

Tezuka T, Saheki M, Kusuda S, et al. Treatment of non-hairy melanocytic macules by dermabrasion and topical application of 5% hydroquinone monobenzyl ether cream. J Am Acad Dermatol 1993;28:771-72.

Vasquez M, Sanchez JL. The efficacy of broad spectrum sunscreen in the treatment of melasma. Cutis 1983;32(1):92, 95-96.

CHAPTER 26—Travel Health Products

Abramowicz M, ed. Advice for travellers. Med Lett Drugs Ther 1994; 36(922):41-4.

Antibacterials may lessen the misery of travellers' diarrhea (editorial). Drugs and Therapy Perspectives 1994;3(6):12-4.

Becker H. Field water disinfection (letter). JAMA 1988;259(21):3185.

Briggs GG, Freeman RK, Yaffe SJ. Drugs in pregnancy and lactation—a reference guide to fetal and neonatal risk. 3rd ed. Baltimore, MD: Williams and Wilkins, 1990.

Bruce DG, Golding JF, Hockenhull H, et al. Acupressure and motion sickness. Aviat Space Environ Med 1990;61(4):361-5.

Buck ML, Blumer JL. Phenothiazine-associated apnea in two siblings. Ann Pharmacother 1991;3(25):244-6.

Centres for Disease Control. Health Information for International Travel. Atlanta, GA:Department for Health and Human Services, 1994.

Dardick KR. General advice and medical kit. Med Clin North Am 1992; 76(6):1261-74.

Drug consult: nonprescription antiemetics efficacy—FDA report, 1987. Micromedex, Inc. Denver, CO 1987; May:1.

Drug evaluation: ephedrine. Micromedex, Inc. Denver, CO 1993; May:41.

Drug information for the health care provider. Rockville: United States Pharmacopoeial Convention, 1994.

Dukes GE. Over-the-counter antidiarrheal medications used for the self-treatment of acute diarrhea. Am J Med 1990;88(Suppl 6A):245-65.

Dupont HL, Ericsson CD. Prevention and treatment of travellers' diarrhea. N Engl J Med 1993;328(25):1821-6.

Dupont HL. Bismuth subsalicylate in the treatment and prevention of diarrheal disease. DICP Ann Pharmacother 1987;21:687-92.

Dupont HL. Travellers' diarrhea—which antimicrobial? Drugs 1993; 45(6):910-7.

Dyment SZ. The pharmacist and the traveller. Pharmacy Practice 1990; 6(4):31-4.

Ericsson CD, Dupont HL. Travellers' diarrhea: approaches to prevention and treatment. CID 1993;16:616-26.

Ericsson CD. Bismuth subsalicylate in the treatment of travellers' diarrhea. Drug Therapy 1990;Jan:36-40.

First aid kits for travellers (editorial). Pharmacy Today 1993(Oct).

Fung C. Travellers' diarrhea. OCP J 1991;18(2):17-21.

Health and Welfare Canada. Wilderness water—a guide to wilderness drinking water. Ottawa, Ontario: Communications Branch Health and Welfare Canada, 1991.

International Association for Medical Assistance to Travellers. Medical services and the international traveller. Guelph, Ontario: Foundation for the Support of International Medical Training, Inc., 1982.

Jacknowitz AI. Practical advice to help consumers avoid motion sickness. US Pharmacist 1986;11(6):10-20.

Kohl RL, MacDonald S. New pharmacologic approaches to the prevention of space/motion sickness. J Clin Pharmacol 1991;31(10):934-46.

Krogh CME, ed. Compendium of Pharmaceuticals and Specialties. 29th ed. Ottawa:Canadian Pharmaceutical Association, 1994.

Lloyd-Still JD. Treatment of gastroenteritis in children: possible risk of Reye's syndrome? (letter). JAMA 1988;259(12):1875.

McEvoy GK, ed. American Hospital Formulary Services—Drug Information. Bethesda, MD: American Society of Hospital Pharmacists, 1994.

Meyers A. Prevention and treatment of travellers' diarrhea (letter). N Engl J Med 1993(Nov);329(21):1585.

Mitchelson F. Pharmacological agents affecting emesis—a review (part II). Drugs 1992;43(4):443-63.

Murdoch L. Storage and mixing of insulins—part I. New Drugs—Drug News 1987;5(5)1-2.

Murdoch L, ed. Drinking water purification for travellers. New Drugs—Drug News 1986;4(1)1-2.

Okhuysen PC, Ericsson CD. Travellers' diarrhea—prevention and treatment. Med Clin North Am 1992;76(6):1357-73.

Parrot AC. Transdermal scopolamine: a review of its effects upon motion sickness, psychological performance, and physiological functioning. Aviat Space Environ Med 1989;60(1):1-9.

Pray WS. Motion sickness. US Pharmacist 1991; June:20-8.

Rados B. When motion sickness goes along for the ride. FDA Consumer 1985;19(2):6-9.

Ruckenstein MJ, Harrison RV. Motion sickness—helping patients tolerate the ups and downs. Postgrad Med 1991;89(6):139-44.

Sea Bands—anti-sickness wristbands (editorial). Leisure Way 1989; Aug:3.

Seiden H, Cantarutti P, Thayer S. A customized first aid kit for home and vacation. Can Fam Physician 1985;31:2316-8.

Skjenna OW, Evans JF, Moore M, et al. Helping patients travel by air. Can Med Assoc J 1991;144(3):287-93.

Stewart JJ, Wood MJ, Wood CD, et al. Effects of ginger on motion sickness susceptibility and gastric function. Pharmacology 1991;42:111-20.

Tugwood B. Oral rehydration—treatment of acute diarrhea in infants and children. OCP J 1992 (Jul);19(3):11-2.

Walker E, Williams G. ABC of health travel—first aid while abroad. BMJ 1983;286:1039-42.

Wanke LA. Drug consult: ginger prophylaxis for motion sickness. Micromedex, Inc. Denver, CO 1987; April:1.

Wanke L. Drug consult: Transdermal scopolamine—therapy of motion sickness. Micromedex, Inc. Denver, CO 1993; Jan:1-3.

Warwick-Evans LA, Redstone SB. A double-blind placebo controlled evaluation of acupressure in the treatment of motion sickness. Aviat Space Environ Med 1991;62(8):776-8.

CHAPTER 27—Women's Health Care Products

Reproductive Anatomy and Physiology

Fritz MA, Speroff L. Current concepts of the endocrine characteristics of normal menstrual function: the key to diagnosis and management of menstrual disorders. Clin Obstet Gynecol 1983;26:647-87.

Huggins GR, Preti G. Vaginal odors and secretions. Clin Obstet Gynecol 1981;24:335-75.

Sloane E. Biology of Women. New York: J Wiley & Sons, 1985.

Spellacy WN. Abnormal bleeding. Clin Obstet Gynecol 1983;26:702-10.

Ysarkauskas E. Primary female syndromes—an update. N Y State J Med 1990:295-302.

Hygiene and Menstrual Care

Byers JF. To douche or not to douche. Am Fam Physician 1974; 10(3):135-39.

Consumer Reports. Menstrual tampons and pads. The medicine show. New York: Patheon, 1980:214-23.

Freidrich EG. Tampon effects on vaginal health. Clin Obstet Gynecol 1981;24:395-405.

McGowan L. Peritonitis following the vaginal douche and a proposed alternative method of vaginal and vulvar care. Am J Obstet Gynecol 1965;93:506-09.

Rosenberg MJ, Phillips RS, Holmes MD. Vaginal douching. Who and why? J Reprod Med 1991;36:753-58.

Todd JK. Therapy of toxic shock syndrome. Drugs 1990;39(6):856-61.

Zbella EA, Nemec LA, Vermesh M. Vaginal douching: pros, cons and proper technique. Postgrad Med 1984;74(8):93-95.

Dysmenorrhea

Dawood MY. Dysmenorrhea. J Reprod Med 1985;30:154-65.

Dawood MY. Nonsteroidal antiinflammatory drugs and reproduction. Am J Obstet Gynecol 1993;169:1255-65.

Milsom I, Hendner N, Mannheimer C. A comparative study of the effect of high intensity transcutaneous nerve stimulation and oral naproxen on intrauterine pressure and menstrual pain in patients with primary dysmenorrhea. Am J Obstet Gynecol 1994;170:123-29.

Muse KN. Cyclic pelvic pain. Obstet Gynecol Clin North Am 1990;17: 429-40.

Weitzman GA, Malinak LR. Dysmenorrhea: Rational medical treatment. Drug Therapy 1988;(Oct):102-10.

Wenzloff NJ, Shimp L. Therapeutic management of primary dysmenorrhea. Drug Intell Clin Pharm 1984;18:22-26.

Premenstrual Syndrome

Backstrom T. Neuroendocrinology of premenstrual syndrome. Clin Obstet Gynecol 1992;35:612-28.

Briggs CJ. Evening primrose: la belle de nuit, the king's cureall. Can Pharm J 1986;199:249-54.

Chilal HJ. Premenstrual syndrome; an update for the clinician. Obstet Gynecol Clin North Am 1990;17:457-77.

Collins A, Cernin A, Colemand G, et al. Essential fatty acids in the treatment of premenstrual syndrome. Obstet Gynecol 1993;81:93-98.

Donald A. The powerful healing magic of the evening primrose. Bestways 1981;(Sept).

Johnson S. Clinician's approach to diagnosis and management of premenstrual syndrome. Clin Obstet Gynecol 1992;35:637-57.

Kleijnen J, Ter Piet G, Knipschild P. Vitamin B6 in the treatment of premenstrual syndrome—a review. Br J Obstet Gynaecol 1990;97:847-52.

Nader S. Premenstrual syndrome. Tailoring treatment to symptoms. Postgrad Med 1991;90:173-78.

O'Brien PMS. Helping women with premenstrual syndrome. BMJ 1993; 307:1471-75.

O'Brien PMS. The premenstrual syndrome. J Reprod Med 1985;30:11-23.

Rossignol AM, Borlander H. Prevalence and severity of premenstrual syndrome-effects of foods and beverages that are sweet or high in sugar content. J Reprod Med 1991;36:131-36.

True BL, Goodner SM, Burns EA. Review of the etiology and treatment of premenstrual syndrome. Drug Intell Clin Pharm 1985;19:714-21.

Vaginal Infections (including sexually transmitted diseases)

Centers for Disease Control. 1993 Sexually transmitted diseases treatment guidelines. MMWR 1993;42(RR-14):1-25.

Doering PL, Santiago TM. Drugs for the treatment of vulvovaginal candidiasis—the comparative efficacy of agents and regimens. Drug Intell Clin Pharm 1990;24:1078-83.

Drugs for sexually transmitted diseases. Med Lett Drugs Ther 1994; 36(913):1-5.

Esenbach DA. Vaginal infection. Clin Obstet Gynecol 1993;26(1): 186-206.

Foreman E, Smith CB. Vaginitis. Systematically solving the bothersome problem. Postgrad Med 1990;88:123-33.

Hanna NF, Taylor-Robinson D, Kalodiki-Karamanoli M. et al. The relationship between vaginal pH and the microbiological status in vaginitis. Br J Obstet Gynaecol 1985;92:1267-71.

Hopkins M. Vaginal infections. Diagnosis and treatment of bacterial vaginosis, candida vulvovaginitis and trichomonas vaginitis. Pharm Pract 1994;10:39-47.

Jovanovic R, Congema E, Nguyen HT. Antifungal agents vs. borric acid for treating chronic mycotic vulvovaginitis. J Reprod Med 1991;36(8): 593-97.

Krogh CME, ed. Compendium of Pharmaceuticals and Specialties. 29th ed. Ottawa: Canadian Pharmaceutical Association, 1994.

Sobel JD. Candidal vulvovaginitis. Clin Obstet Gynecol 1993;36(1): 153-65.

Sparks JM. Vaginitis. J Reprod Med 1991;36:745-52.

Travill L. New nonprescription antifungal preparations. Pharmacy home study program. Nepean, Ont.: Travill Consulting, 1994.

Contraception

Choice of contraceptives. Med Lett Drugs Ther 1992;34(885):111-14.

Coccodrilli Coley K. Contraception: What pharmacists should tell their patients. Am Pharm 1993;NS33:55-64.

Femidon. Manufacturer's Information. Chartex Int'l, 1993.

Hatcher RA, Stewart F, Trussell J, et al. Contraceptive Technology 1990-91. 15th revised ed. New York: Irvington, 1990.

Women, contraception and HIV. Drug Ther Bull 1993;31(25):97-98.

INDEX

abrasions, 224
abrasives
  in dentifrices, 516
  in soaps, 570
  to treat acne, 67
absorptive dressings, 257
ACE inhibitors
  drug interactions, 41**t**
  photosensitivity reactions, 629**t**
  use in hypertension, 52
acesulfame-K, 484
acetaminophen
  advice for the patient, 542
  breast-feeding, 50**t**
  children, 45, 552**t**
  contraindications, 52, 54-55, 550
  dosages, 553**t**
  effectiveness, 550
  effects of smoking cessation, 606**t**
  indications, 550
  pharmacokinetics, 550
  pharmacology, 550
  pregnancy, 49**t**
  safety, 550
  side effects, 551**t**
  to treat arthritis, 539
  to treat chickenpox, 234
  to treat cold sore pain, 502
  to treat colds, 89
  to treat dental pain, 493, 499, 540
  to treat dysmenorrhea and PMS, 666-67, 669, 689
  to treat ear pain, 151
  to treat fever, 547, 548-49
  to treat headache, 535, 536
  to treat hemorrhoidal pain, 327
  to treat sunburn pain, 626
  to treat teething pain, 500
  to treat wounds and injuries, 543
acetazolamide, 629**t**
acetic acid
  for vaginal douching, 656
  to cleanse wounds, 251
  to prevent otitis externa, 157, 159
  to treat otitis externa, 156, 159
  to treat pediculosis, 104-05
acetylsalicylic acid *see* ASA
achlorhydria, 643
acidulated phosphate fluoride, 495**t**, 517**t**
acne
  advice for the patient, 70
  and seborrheic dermatitis, 134
  defined, 57
  differential diagnosis, 61, 63**t**, 72
  pathogenesis, 57-59, 62**f**
  patient assessment, 63, 64**t**, 71-72
  pharmaceutical agents, 73-75
  predisposing factors, 59-61, 71
  recommended reading, 77
  severity, 61**t**
  signs and symptoms, 61
  skin hygiene, 568
  treatment, 61, 63-69
acne conglobata, 63**t**
acne excoriée, 60, 63**t**
acne fulminans, 63**t**
acne mechanica, 60, 63**t**
acne vulgaris, 61, 63**t**
aconite
  drug and alcohol interactions, 356
  in homeopathic remedies, 369**t**
aconitum napellus
acquired immune deficiency syndrome *see* AIDS
acridine, 629**t**
acrivastine, 93
ACTH *see* corticotropin (ACTH)
activated charcoal
  ineffective for travellers' diarrhea, 645
  to treat poisoning, 240
acupressure, 309, 648
acupuncture
  for smoking cessation, 607
  to treat nausea and vomiting, 309
acute allergic conjunctivitis, 173-74, 199
acute necrotizing ulcerative gingivitis, 497
addiction, nicotine, 600-01, 604
adenine arabinoside, 503**t**
adhesive dressings, 256
adhesives
  dentures, 518
  ostomy, 393
adolescents
  acne, 57
  bismuth subsalicylate, 645
  dimenhydrinate, 313
  smokers, 600
adonis, 356
aerosol formulations, 333
aesculus *see* horse chestnut
age factors
  acne, 57, 71
  arthritis, 538, 539
  constipation, 291
  nutrition, 425
  osteoarthritis, 539
  sleep patterns, 586
agrimony, 356
AIDS, *see also* HIV
  athlete's foot, 261
  nutritional requirements, 472**t**
  seborrheic dermatitis, 134
  travellers' diarrhea, 643
aids for daily living
  bathroom safety, 377-78
  canes and walkers, 379-81
  compression stockings, 381
  crutches, 381
  examples, 377**t**
  patient assessment, 381
  recommended reading, 409
  wheelchairs, 378-80
akee, 357
AKTAC *see* alkyltriethanolammonium chloride

alcloxa
FDA classification, 263t
ineffective for jock itch, 413t
alcohol *see also* ethanol, ethyl alcohol
adverse effects, 434
affecting sleep, 587, 588t, 589, 589t
calories, 434
causing dyspepsia, 276t, 277, 279
causing GER, 283t
causing halitosis, 508
causing incontinence, 384t
comedogenicity, 568t
contributing to heat-related illness, 617-18
diabetes, 53, 434
in homeopathic remedies, 363, 364-65, 366t, 370
in lotions, 141
ineffective for cold sores, 503t
metabolism of, 434
ostomy patients, 396t
PMS, 669
pregnancy, 434
recommended intake, 430t
alcohol-drug interactions
general, 2-3, 434
acetaminophen, 550
ASA, 554t
consumer counselling, 7, 26
dimenhydrinate, 649, 652
diphenhydramine, 652
herbal medicines, 356-57, 358, 359
promethazine, 649, 652
pyrilamine maleate, 691
ranitidine, 316
scopolamine, 649, 653
alcoholism, 473t
alder, 355
aletris *see* unicorn root
alginic acid
pregnancy, 48t
to treat GER, 284, 310
alkanet, 354
alkylamines, 83t
alkyltriethanolammonium chloride, 213
allantoin
in ophthalmic solutions, 202
to treat cankers and cold sores, 515t
to treat hemorrhoids, 328t, 332
allergens
causing dermatitis, 124t, 129t, 133f
causing eye problems, 167t, 173-75, 199, 215-16
causing rhinitis, 79, 81
allergic rhinitis *see* rhinitis
allergies, *see also* atopic dermatitis
confused with acne, 72
frequency in Canada, 3t
self-treatment, 4t
to insect bites and stings, 244-45
allethrin, 103, 118
allium cepa, 369t
allopathic medicines, 336, 355
allopurinol, 540
allyl isothiocyanate, 557
aloe, 320, 344t, 354
alpha agonists, 384t, 385
alpha-blockers
causing incontinence, 384t
risks with hypertension, 52
to treat premature ejaculation, 420
alpha-galactosidase, 304, 310
alpha-hydroxy acids, 145-46
alprazolam, 384t
alternative health care, 337, *see also* homeopathic medicine
alternative sweeteners, 484
althaea, 344t
alum
FDA classification, 263t
ineffective for jock itch, 413t
to treat insect bites, 252
aluminum
breast-feeding, 50t
causing constipation, 292t
contributing to Alzheimer's disease, 310
drug interactions, 41t
pregnancy, 48t
aluminum acetate, *see also* Burow's solution
to prevent otitis externa, 157, 159
to treat athlete's foot, 264, 272
to treat dermatitis, 233, 239, 252
to treat ear disorders, 156, 159
aluminum chlorhydroxide, 572
aluminum chlorhydroxyallantoinate *see* allantoin
aluminum chloride
to decrease perspiration, 572, 583
to treat athlete's foot, 264, 272
to treat insect bites, 246
aluminum chlorohydrate
to decrease perspiration, 572
to treat insect bites, 246
aluminum hydroxide
ineffective for travellers' diarrhea, 645
to treat dermatitis, 129
to treat dyspepsia, 279
to treat dyspepsia and GER, 310-11
to treat hemorrhoids, 332
aluminum potassium sulfate, 515t
aluminum salts
to decrease perspiration, 572, 583
to treat dermatitis, 141
aluminum sulfate
FDA classification, 263t
ineffective for jock itch, 413t
to stop minor bleeding, 252
aluminum zirconium, 572
aluminum zirconylhydroxychloride, 246
Alzheimer's disease
and aluminum, 310
sleep disturbances, 590
amenorrhea, 661
American Dental Association, 514
American Institute of Homeopathy, 361
American Medical Association, 362
amikacin, 152t
amiloride, 629t
amino dietary nutrient acids
for athletes, 486
aminobenzoic acid *see* PABA
aminoglycosides, 152t
5-aminosalicylic acid, 629t
amiodarone, 629t
amitriptyline
causing incontinence, 384t
contributing to heat-related illness, 617
to prevent migraine, 536
weight gain/loss, 453t
ammi, 344t
ammonia, 560
ammonium hydroxide, 245
ammonium lauryl sulfate, 580t
amobarbital, 606t
amoxapine

photosensitivity reactions, 629**t**
weight gain/loss, 453**t**
amphetamine, 453**t**
amphoteric surfactants, 580-81, 582
amphotericin B, 52
ampicillin
causing diarrhea, 297
causing dyspepsia, 276**t**, 277
amyl dimethyl PABA, 633**t**, 638
amylocaine
ophthalmic use, 199
to relieve hemorrhoids, 328**t**, 331
amyltricresols
FDA classification, 263**t**
ineffective for jock itch, 413**t**
anabolic agents, 620
anal exercises, 385
anal fissures, 330
analgesic infusion pumps, 407
analgesics
breast-feeding, 50**t**
causing constipation, 292**t**
effects of smoking, 598
external *see* counterirritants
in first aid kit, 650
to treat dysmenorrhea, 665
to treat hemorrhoidal pain, 327
to treat musculoskeletal pain, 542, 614
to treat PMS, 669
to treat wound pain, 225
use in athletes, 619-20
use in diabetes, 54
use in elderly persons, 41**t**
anaphylaxis
caused by insect bites and stings, 244-45
treatment, 245
androgens, 59, 60**t**
anemia, 473**t**
anesthetics
cause of dermatitis, 133**t**
inappropriate use for burns, 237
ophthalmic use, 199
precautions, 204**t**, 248, 604**t**
side effects, 248
to treat cankers, 504, 514
to treat hemorrhoidal pain, 327, 328**t**, 331
to treat insect bites, 243, 248
to treat minor skin irritations, 248
to treat premature ejaculation, 420, 421
to treat pruritus, 141
to treat sore throat, 98
use in children, 248
anethole, 339
anetholtrithione, 509, 519
angelica, 344**t**
angina
and smoking, 604**t**
nicotine replacement therapy, 610
angular cheilitis, 506
aniline, 636**t**
animal dander, 81, 82
anionic surfactants, 580, 582
anise, 344**t**
anise oil, 339
aniseed, 339
anorexia nervosa
defined, 467
organ system changes, 467**t**
prevalence, 467
treatment, 468, 468**t**
ant stings, 241, 244, 245
antacids
breast-feeding, 50**t**
causing constipation, 292**t**
causing diarrhea, 298
drug interactions, 23, 41**t**, 311, 311**t**
effects of smoking, 599
in first aid kit, 650
ostomy patients, 396**t**
pregnancy, 48**t**
to treat dyspepsia and GER, 278-79, 284, 310-11
to treat insect bites, 246
use in elderly persons, 41**t**, 42
antazoline, 200
anthracene, 629**t**
anthraquinones
to treat constipation, 320
toxicity, 316-17
anti-inflammatories, 243
antianxiety agents, 535
antiarrhythmics, 52
antibiotic sore mouth, 506
antibiotics
association with athlete's foot, 261
causing candidiasis, 506
causing diarrhea, 297
causing ototoxicity, 152**t**
drug interactions, 41**t**
in first aid kits, 246
ostomy patients, 396**t**
topical products, 248-49
to treat ear infection, 154
to treat skin infection, 229
anticancer drugs, 629**t**
anticholinergics
causing constipation, 292**t**
causing dry eye, 177**t**, 193
causing GER, 282, 283**t**
causing incontinence, 383, 384**t**
contributing to heat-related illness, 617
drug interactions, 557
to treat gastrointestinal disorders, 311-12
to treat hemorrhoids, 327, 328**t**, 331
to treat motion sickness, 648-49, 653
to treat rhinitis, 82
anticoagulants
drug interactions, 312, 644
vitamin K antagonism, 357
anticonvulsants, 292**t**, *see also* antiepileptics
antidepressants, *see also* tricyclic antidepressants
affecting sleep, 588**t**
causing incontinence, 383, 384**t**
drug interactions, 52
effects of smoking, 606**t**
photosensitivity reactions, 629**t**
to treat PMS, 670
to treat premature ejaculation, 420
to treat tension-type headache, 535
antidiarrheals
breast-feeding, 50**t**
ostomy patients, 396**t**
to treat diarrhea, 312-13, 645
antiemetics, 313-15
antiepileptics, *see also* anticonvulsants
affecting sleep, 588**t**
causing acne, 59, 60**t**
antifungals
dosage forms for tinea cruris, 414**t**
FDA classification, 263**t**
in first aid kit, 650

to treat athlete's foot, 263-64
to treat candidiasis, 233, 506
to treat jock itch, 412-13, 414**t**, 421-22
to treat ringworm, 231
to treat tinea capitis, 232
to treat tinea versicolor, 232
to treat vaginal infection, 672-73, 689-90
antigens *see* allergens
antihistamines
adverse effects, 94
breast-feeding, 50**t**
causing dry eye, 177**t**, 193
causing incontinence, 383, 384**t**
characteristics, 83**t**-84**t**
classification, 83**t**-84**t**
contraindications, 237
contributing to heat-related illness, 617
dosage, 83**t**-84**t**, 93-94
drug interactions, 52
first-generation, 83**t**, 93
glaucoma, use in, 53
inappropriate use for dysmenorrhea, 667
in first aid kits, 246, 650, 650**t**
in poison treatment, 239
interaction with herbal products, 356-57
photosensitivity reactions, 629**t**
pregnancy, 48**t**, 49**t**
second-generation, 84**t**, 93
to treat anaphylaxis, 245
to treat chickenpox, 234, 247
to treat conjunctivitis, 175, 199-200
to treat dermatitis and dry skin, 126, 129, 137
to treat insect bites, 243
to treat insomnia, 595
to treat motion sickness, 648-49, 652**t**, 652-53
to treat pruritus, 249-50
to treat rhinitis, 82, 89, 93-95
use in children, 45**t**, 95
use in elderly persons, 41**t**, 95, 595
antihypertensives, 292**t**
antimalarials
as sunscreen, 640
causing ototoxicity, 152**t**
cross-sensitivity with clioquinol, 421
antimetabolites, 298
antimicrobials
photosensitivity reactions, 629**t**
to treat diarrhea, 645
to treat sore throat, 98
antimotility drugs, 313, 396**t**
antineoplastics
causing ototoxicity, 152**t**
weight gain/loss, 453**t**
antioxidants, 479
antiparasitics, 629**t**
antiparkinsonian drugs, 588**t**
antiperspirants
effectiveness of dosage forms, 573**t**
pharmaceutical agents, 583
to decrease perspiration, 572
antiplatelet drugs, 554**t**
antipruritics
to treat chickenpox, 234
to treat dermatitis and dry skin, 141
to treat pruritus, 249-50
antipsychotics
causing incontinence, 383, 384**t**
photosensitivity reactions, 629**t**
antipyretics
to treat fever, 548-49
use in diabetes, 54
antipyrine
inappropriate in ear preparations, 159
in ophthalmic solutions, 205
antiseptics
compared to disinfectants, 250
in first aid kits, 650
to cleanse skin, 250-51
to treat blisters, 614
to treat cankers, 515
to treat cold sores, 515
to treat hemorrhoids, 328, 328**t**, 333
antispasmodics
causing constipation, 292**t**
causing incontinence, 383, 384**t**
antitussives, 89, 95**t**, 95-96
use in children, 95**t**, 95-96
anxiolytics, *see also* antianxiety agents
causing constipation, 292**t**
causing incontinence, 384**t**
to treat premature ejaculation, 420
apiol oil, 338
apis mellifica, 369**t**
appetite suppressants
herbal products, 357-58
use, 465-66
arch supports, 266
arnica, 344**t**, 369**t**
arsenicum album, 369**t**
arthritis
gouty, 539-40
osteoarthritis, 539
prevalence, 537
resource group, 408
rheumatoid, 538-39
artificial sweeteners, 636**t**
artificial tears
dosage, 202
indications, 201**t**, 219
polymers in, 201**t**
product solution, 201-02
side effects, 202
to treat conjunctivitis, 173, 175, 176
to treat dry eye, 178
ASA
advice for the patient, 542
affecting contact lenses, 193
breast-feeding, 50**t**
causing dyspepsia, 279
causing ototoxicity, 152**t**
causing peptic ulcer disease, 276
contraindications, 234, 553-54
dosages, 553**t**
drug interactions, 554**t**, 644
indications, 552
pharmacology, 552
precautions, 51, 52, 54, 553-54, 665
pregnancy, 48**t**
Reye's syndrome, 45, 549
side effects, 551**t**
to treat arthritis, 539
to treat bursitis, 540
to treat colds, 89
to treat cold sore pain, 502
to treat dental pain, 493, 499, 540
to treat dysmenorrhea and PMS, 665-67, 669, 689
to treat ear pain, 151
to treat fever, 89, 548-49
to treat headache, 535, 536
to treat musculoskeletal pain, 543, 614

to treat sunburn pain, 626
toxicity, 553
use in children, 45, 549, 552-53
ascorbic acid *see* vitamin C
aspartame, 484, 492
aspidium, 344**t**
assessment *see* patient assessment
asteatotic eczema *see* dry skin
astemizole
adverse effects, 52, 94
characteristics and doses, 84**t**
drug interactions, 52
photosensitivity reactions, 629**t**
to treat colds and rhinitis, 93
weight gain/loss, 453**t**
asthma, 604**t**
astringents
to treat dermatitis, 141-42, 146
to treat hemorrhoids, 327-28, 328**t**, 331
to treat insect bites, 243, 252-53
to treat oily skin, 568
athletes, *see also* sports
drug abuse, 619-21
nutrition, 474-78
nutrition products, 486
athlete's foot
advice for the patient, 263
and jock itch, 411
causative organisms, 230, 261
symptoms, 261-62
treatment, 262-64
types, 262**t**
atopic dermatitis (eczema)
advice for the patient, 125
defined, 123
differential diagnosis, 72, 124**t**
symptoms, 123
treatment, 123-26, 127**t**
atopic keratoconjunctivitis, 174
atrophic candidiasis, 506
atropine
causing dry eye, 177**t**
contributing to heat-related illness, 617
attapulgite, 301, 312, 645
attentive silence (communication skills), 18
auranofin, 629**t**
aurothioglucose, 629**t**
autumn crocus, 344**t**
avobenzone *see* butyl methoxydibenzoylmethane
avulsions, 224
azaleic acid, 75
azatadine
characteristics and doses, 84**t**
photosensitivity reactions, 629**t**
azathioprine, 539
azelastine, 93
azithromycin, 629**t**

BAC *see* benzalkonium chloride
bacitracin
in ophthalmic solutions, 200
to treat blepharitis, 167
to treat conjunctivitis, 173
to treat hordeolum, 169
to treat impetigo, 229
to treat skin infection, 249
backache (pregnancy), 49**t**
baclofen, 384**t**
balsam Peru, 328**t**, 333
bandages
in first aid kits, 246, 650
types for sports injuries, 616**t**
barberry, 345**t**
bath boards, 377
bath mats, 377
bath oil, 142
bath salts, 142
bath seats, 377
bath-tub transfer benches, 377-78
bathing
ostomy patients, 394
to treat varicella zoster, 234
bathroom safety products, 377-78
bearberry *see* uva ursi
beclomethasone
to treat cankers, 505
to treat rhinitis, 82
bed wetting *see* enuresis
bedstraw (sweet-scented), 357
bee stings, 241-42, 244, 245
behavior modification
for weight loss, 465, 466
to treat headache, 535
belching, 286-87
belladonna
as antispasmodic, 311
in homeopathic remedies, 369**t**
to treat hemorrhoids, 328**t**, 331
benign prostatic hypertrophy, 53
benzalkonium chloride
in ophthalmic solutions, 202, 205, 207, 210**t**, 212, 220
to treat cold sores, 502, 515
to treat sore throat, 98
benzethonium chloride
FDA classification, 263**t**
in deodorants, 573, 583
ineffective for jock itch, 413**t**
in otic preparations, 159
to prevent plaque, 521, 522
to treat hemorrhoids, 328**t**, 333
benzocaine
causing dermatitis, 133**t**
cross-sensitivity, 636**t**
for weight loss, 465, 485**t**
in otic preparations, 159
photosensitivity reactions, 629**t**
to treat cankers and cold sores, 502, 514, 515**t**
to treat dental pain, 493
to treat hemorrhoids, 328**t**, 331
to treat minor skin irritations, 248
to treat premature ejaculation, 420, 421
to treat pruritus, 141
to treat sore throat, 98
to treat toothache, 526
to treat vulvovaginal irritation, 689
use in children, 159
benzodiazepines
affecting sleep, 587, 588**t**
causing constipation, 292**t**
causing GER, 282, 283**t**
effects of smoking cessation, 606**t**
benzoic acid
FDA classification, 263**t**
ineffective for jock itch, 413**t**
benzoin, 514, 515**t**
benzophenone-3 *see* oxybenzone
benzophenone-4 *see* sulisobenzone
benzophenone-8 *see* dioxybenzone
benzoxiquine
FDA classification, 263**t**

ineffective for jock itch, 413t
benzoyl peroxide
affecting contact lenses, 192
to treat acne, 67, 68f, 69, 73-75
benzphetamine, 453t
benztropine, 292t
benzyl benzoate, 112, 117
benzyl nicotinate, 559
berberine, 205
bergamot oil, 629t
beta-agonists
causing GER disease, 282, 283t
causing incontinence, 384t
drug interactions, 52
beta-blockers
affecting sleep, 588t
banned in sports, 620
causing dry eye, 177t, 193
causing incontinence, 384t
drug interactions, 41t, 204t
to treat premature ejaculation, 420
to prevent migraine, 536
use in hypertension, 52
weight gain/loss, 453t
beta-adrenergic agonists *see* beta-agonists
beta-adrenergic blockers *see* beta-blockers
beta-butoxyethyl nicotinate, 559
beta-carotene
as antioxidant, 479
as sunscreen, 640
as tanning agent, 640
betanaphthol, 521
betel nut, 345t
bethanechol, 519
betony, 345t
betula, 355, 356
bilberry, 335
bioallethrin, 103, 118
biofeedback
to treat headache, 535, 537
to treat enuresis, 385
to treat motion sickness, 648
biotin
food sources, 443t
function, 443t
recommended nutrient intake, 443t
signs of deficiency, 443t
signs of toxicity, 443t
birch *see* betula
birth control pill *see* oral contraceptives
4-[bis 2-(hydroxypropyl) amino] benzoic acid *see* ethyldihydroxypropyl PABA
bisacodyl, 294, 317t, 320-21
bismuth salts
breast-feeding, 50t
in hemorrhoidal preparations, 332
ostomy patients, 396t
bismuth subsalicylate
drug interactions, 312, 644
to treat diarrhea, 301, 312, 644-45
to prevent diarrhea, 300
use in children, 645
bites (insects)
allergic reactions to, 244-45
patient assessment, 247
prevention, 242-43
treatment, 243-46
types, 241-42
bitter gourd, 357
bittersweet, 354
black cohosh, 345t, 355, 356
blackflies, 241, 245
blackhead (open comedone), 58
bladder neck obstruction, 53
blepharitis
advice for the patient, 172
etiology, 167, 167t
symptoms, 167-68
treatment, 168, 179f-80f, 201t
blessed thistle, 355
blisters, 614-15
bloating (abdominal), 286-88
blood glucose tests, 403-04, 405
blood pressure, high *see* hypertension
blood pressure monitors, 397-98, 405
bloodroot, 345t
blue cohosh, 345t, 355, 356
BMI *see* body mass index
body lice
described, 102
symptoms, 103
treatment, 103
body mass index
correlation with obesity, 433, 452t, 463
determination of, 432-33, 452t
body odor
physiology, 571
prevention, 571-73
body worn urinals, 387
boils *see* furuncles
boldo, 345t, 355, 356
bone fractures, 541
boneset, 345t
borage, 345t
boric acid
FDA classification, 263t
ineffective for jock itch, 413t
incompatibility, 200, 220
in contact lens solutions, 220
in ophthalmic solutions, 200, 205, 220
to treat hemorrhoids, 328t, 333
to treat vaginal candidiasis, 673, 675, 689
bothrops, 371
bran, 317t, 318
breast-feeding, *see also* nursing women
advice for the patient, 456
benefits, 455
composition of breast milk, 455, 456t
contraindications, 455
during infantile diarrhea, 299
establishing, 455
storage of breast milk, 455
vitamin/mineral supplementation, 456, 457t
weaning, 460
briefs fitted, 386
bromhidrosis *see* body odor
bromides, 60t
bromocriptine, 670
brompheniramine
characteristics and doses, 83t
contributing to heat-related illness, 617
pregnancy, 48t
to treat colds and rhinitis, 93, 94
bronchitis, 87
bronchodilators, 588t
broom, 345t, 355, 356
bruises, 224
bryony, 354
buchu, 346t, 355, 356
budesonide, 82

bufexamac, 126, 129, 135, 142
buffers (ophthalmic), 220
bulimia nervosa
    defined, 467
    organ system changes, 467**t**
    prevalence, 467
    treatment, 468, 468**t**
bullous myringitis, 154, 155**t**
bumetanide, 152**t**
bunions, 271
burdock, 346**t**
burns
    classification, 235
    etiology, 235
    friction, 615
    infections, 228, 236
    medical referral, 236
    pathology, 235
    sunburn, 235, 624**t**, 626
    to eye, 181
    treatment, 235-37
Burow's solution, *see also* aluminum acetate
    to treat cold sores, 502
    to treat dermatitis, 126, 129, 146
bursitis, 540, 613, 615
butacaine, 199
butorphanol, 536
butterbur, 354
butyl methoxydibenzoylmethane, 633**t**, 639

cabbage palm, 350**t**
cactus, 371
caffeine
    abuse by athletes, 619, 621
    affecting sleep, 588**t**, 589**t**, 590
    children, 591
    content in foods and beverages, 591**t**
    content in nonprescription drugs, 590**t**
    during homeopathic treatment, 371
    effects of smoking cessation, 606**t**
    recommended intake, 430**t**
    role in PMS, 669
    to treat dysmenorrhea and PMS, 669, 689
    to treat pain, 555-56
    to treat sleep disorders, 595
caffeinism, 590-91
calamine
    in first aid kit, 650
    to treat chickenpox, 234
    to treat dermatitis and pruritus, 129, 141, 239, 252
    to treat hemorrhoids, 328**t**
calamus, 346**t**, 355, 356
calcarea fluorica, 368
calcarea phosphorica, 368
calcarea sulfurica, 368
calcium
    causing constipation, 292**t**
    drug interactions, 41**t**
    food sources, 445**t**
    function, 445**t**
    recommended nutrient intake, 427**t**, 445**t**
    salts, 481**t**
    signs of deficiency, 445**t**
    supplementation, 480-81
    use in athletes, 475
    use in elderly persons, 41**t**, 474
calcium carbonate
    drug interactions, 312
    elemental calcium in, 481**t**
    to treat dyspepsia, 279, 310
calcium channel blockers
    causing constipation, 292**t**
    causing GER, 282, 283**t**
    causing incontinence, 384**t**
    drug interactions, 41**t**
    to prevent migraine, 536
    to treat cluster headache, 537
    use with herbal products
calcium gluconate, 481**t**
calcium hydroxide, 659
calcium lactate, 481**t**
calcium polycarbophil, 304
calcium thioglycolate, 659
calendula, 346**t**
calluses *see* corns and calluses
calories *see* energy (calories)
camphor
    antitussive effect, 96
    during homeopathic treatment, 371
    FDA classification, 263**t**
    ineffective for jock itch, 413**t**
    poisoning, 240
    to treat cankers and cold sores, 515, 515**t**
    to treat ear disorders, 159
    to treat musculoskeletal pain, 557-58
    to treat pediculosis, 104-05
    to treat pruritus, 141
Canada's Food Guide to Healthy Eating, 426, 427, 428**f**-29**f**, 432, 464
Canadian Cancer Society, 604
Canadian Dental Association, 514
Canadian Drug Advisory Committee, 5
Canadian Lung Association, 604, 607
Canadian Pharmaceutical Association, 14
cancer
    advice for the patient to prevent skin cancer, 630
    and dyspepsia, 276**t**, 278
    and smoking, 598, 601
    causing constipation, 292
    causing rectal bleeding, 401-02, 402**t**
    leading to ostomy, 388
    nutritional requirements, 472**t**
    skin cancer caused by sunlight, 628-30
candicidin
    FDA classification, 263**t**
    ineffective for jock itch, 413**t**
candidiasis
    cutaneous, 230, 232-33, 412**t**
    oral, 506
    vulvovaginal, 672-77
canes, 379-81
cankers
    etiology, 504
    foods to avoid, 505**t**
    pharmaceutical agents, 514-15
    predisposing factors, 501**t**
    symptoms, 501**t**, 504
    treatment, 504-05
cannabis, 358
cantharidin, 269
canthaxanthin, 640
capsaicin, 558
capsicum
    medicinal uses and side effects, 346**t**
    to treat musculoskeletal pain, 558
capsulitis, 613, 615
carbamazepine
    causing folliculitis, 60**t**
    photosensitivity reactions, 629**t**
carbamide peroxide
    to soften impacted cerumen, 155, 159

to treat cankers and cold sores, 514, 515t
to treat periodontal disease, 497
to whiten teeth, 527
carbanilides, 67
carbenoxolone, 336
carbinoxamine, 83t
carbohydrates
causing dental caries, 491
dietary nutrient, 430-31
for athletes, 476
recommendations for intake, 430t
requirements in the elderly, 471
carbon monoxide
in tobacco smoke, 597-98
poisoning, 239
carboplatin, 152t
carboxymethylcellulose
for denture adhesion, 518
for weight loss, 485t
in artificial tears, 201t
to treat cankers and cold sores, 514, 515t
carbuncles, 230
carcinoma, ear, 153t
cardiac glycosides, 204t
cardiovascular drugs, 599, 629t
cardiovascular disease, 52
caries *see* dental caries
carnitine, 486
casanthranol *see* cascara
cascara
to treat constipation, 294, 317t, 320
use in pregnancy, 354-55
casein hydrolysate infant formulas, 483
cassava, 338
cassia bark, 358
castor oil
to treat constipation, 321
use in pregnancy, 294, 355
cataplexy, 593
cataracts, 630
catheters
intravenous for home intravenous programs, 407, 408
urinary, 387
cationic surfactants, 581, 582
catnip, 346t
caustic pencils, 252
cavities *see* dental caries
cayenne *see* capsicum
cedar oil, 255, 629t
cefazolin, 60t
celandine, 356
cellulitis, 229
central nervous system depressants, 588t
central nervous system stimulants *see* stimulants
cephalexin
causing folliculitis, 60t
to treat cankers, 514
cephalosporins, 297
cerebral thrombosis, 598
cerumen
ear discharge, 151
impacted, 154-55, 155t
cervical cap
advice for the woman, 685
and STDs, 687
effectiveness, 416, 679t
sizing, 684
cetirizine
characteristics and doses, 84t
to treat dermatitis, 126
to treat rhinitis, 93
cetrimide, 135
cetyl alcohol, 568
cetylpyridinium chloride
in mouthwashes, 521
to prevent plaque, 521, 522, 526
to treat sore throat, 98
chalazion (eyelid cyst), 169
chamomile (chamomilla)
in homeopathic remedies, 369t
medicinal uses and side effects, 341, 346t
to treat itching, 250
chaparral, 346t
charcoal, 50t
chaste tree berry
medicinal uses and side effects, 346t
to treat PMS, 335
cheilitis, 506
chemical disinfection (contact lenses), 211-16, 217t
chemicals
absorption causing poisoning, 239
burns, 181, 235
chickenpox *see* varicella zoster
chicory, 355, 356
chiggers, 241, 245
child-proof containers, 43
chloracne, 60, 63t
chloramphenicol
causing diarrhea, 297
causing folliculitis, 60t
chlorhexidine
in ophthalmic solutions, 212
photosensitivity reactions, 629t
to cleanse wounds, 236, 250-51
to control dental plaque, 517, 521, 526
to treat acne, 67
to treat cankers, 504
to treat skin infection, 230, 250-51
chloride
food sources, 445t
function, 445t
signs of deficiency, 445t
chlorides, 60t
chlorination of water, 646, 647t
chlorine gas poisoning, 239
chlorobutanol
in ophthalmic solutions, 205, 207, 212, 220
not recommended for impacted cerumen, 155, 159
chloroform, 503t
chloroquine, 152t
chlorothiazide, 636t
chlorothymol
FDA classification, 263t
ineffective for jock itch, 413t
chlorpheniramine
characteristics and doses, 83t
contributing to heat-related illness, 617
pregnancy, 48t
to treat chickenpox, 234
to treat colds and rhinitis, 93, 94
to treat dermatitis, 126
treatment of poisoning, 239
use in children, 45t
chlorpromazine
causing incontinence, 384t
contributing to heat-related illness, 617
drug interactions, 115, 118
weight gain/loss, 453t
chlorpropamide, 636t
chlorprothixene, 453t, 629t

chlortetracycline, 629**t**
chlorthalidone, 629**t**
cholecystokinin, 283**t**
cholelithiasis, 276**t**
cholesterol
  in nutrition, 431
  to treat dry skin, 145
cholesterol test kits, 401
chromium
  food sources, 445**t**
  function, 445**t**
  signs of deficiency, 445**t**
chronic disease, nonprescription drug use, 51-55
chronic obstructive pulmonary disease
  and smoking, 598, 604**t**
  peak flow meters, 403
cimetidine
  affecting sleep, 588**t**
  to treat anaphylaxis, 245
  to treat GER, 284, 315-16
  effects of smoking cessation, 606**t**
cinchocaine *see* dibucaine
cinnamedrine, 667
cinnamon *see* cassia bark
cinoxate, 633**t**, 638
circadian rhythm, 587, 589**t**, 589
cisapride, 283**t**, 284, 288
cisplatin
  causing ototoxicity, 152**t**
  drug interactions, 52
citric acid
  effect on skin, 146
  in ophthalmic solutions, 205
  to treat dry mouth, 509, 519
citric acid aerosols, 610
citron oil, 629**t**
citronella oil, 255
citrus fruits, 628
clavus *see* corns and calluses
clay, 568
cleansers
  contact lenses, 207, 210-11
  sports injuries, 616
  stomas, 392
  types, 253
cleansing
  after contact with poison, 239
  burns, 236-37
  chickenpox lesions, 234
  wounds, 226, 253
cleansing creams, 568
cleansing pads for hemorrhoids, 333
cleansing sticks for hemorrhoids, 333
cleavers, 356
clemastine, 83**t**
clidinium, 617
clindamycin, 297
clinical trials (homeopathy), 367
clioquinol
  FDA classification, 263**t**
  to treat athlete's foot, 264, 272
  to treat jock itch, 413, 421
clomipramine, 453**t**
clonidine, 292**t**
clothing as sun protection, 633
clotrimazole
  FDA classification, 263**t**
  to treat athlete's foot, 263-64, 272
  to treat diaper rash, 130
  to treat fungal skin infection, 231, 232, 233
  to treat jock itch, 413, 421
  to treat oral candidiasis, 506
  to treat vaginal infection, 672-73, 673**t**, 689-90
clove oil (eugenol)
  as deodorant, 573
  as insect repellents, 255
  in first aid kit, 650
  to treat toothache, 526
clover (sweet), 357
clozapine, 453**t**
CNS *see* central nervous system
coal tar
  causing acne, 60, 67
  comedogenicity, 568**t**
  FDA classification, 263**t**
  ineffective for jock itch, 413**t**
  photosensitivity reactions, 629**t**
  to treat dandruff and seborrhea, 134
  to treat dermatitis, 126, 143
cobalamin *see* vitamin B_{12}
cobalt
  causing acne, 59
  function, 445**t**
  signs of deficiency, 445**t**
cocoa butter, 60, 332, 568
codeine
  abuse by athletes, 619, 621
  advice for the patient, 542
  breast-feeding, 50**t**
  causing constipation, 292**t**
  causing incontinence, 384**t**
  contraindications, 557
  dosages, 553**t**
  drug interactions, 557
  effectiveness, 557
  indications, 557
  pharmacology, 556-57
  side effects, 551**t**, 557
  to treat colds and rhinitis, 95**t**, 95
  to treat cold sore pain, 502
cohosh, 345**t**, 355, 356
colchicine
  as herbal product, 355
  to treat gouty arthritis, 540
cold (to treat teething pain), 500
cold sores
  etiology and pathophysiology, 501, 501**t**
  ineffective treatments, 503**t**
  pharmaceutical agents, 514-15
  symptoms, 501**t**, 501-02
  treatment, 502
colds
  defined, 86
  differential diagnosis, 80**t**, 87-88, 91**t**
  etiology, 86
  frequency in Canada, 3**t**
  pathophysiology, 86
  patient assessment, 90
  pharmaceutical agents, 93-99
  pregnancy, 49**t**
  recommended reading, 100
  signs and symptoms, 87
  travel tips, 151
  treatment, 4**t**, 88-89, 92**f**
colic
  etiology, 289
  patient assessment, 290
  pharmaceutical agents, 315
  recommended reading, 324
  symptoms, 289-90

treatment, 290
colitis (pseudomembranous), 297-98
collagen, 145
collagen disease, 276t
collagenase, 226
colloidal oatmeal
to treat chickenpox, 234
to treat pruritus and dry skin, 126, 129, 137, 142, 250
colocynth, 354
colorectal cancer
causing rectal bleeding, 401-03
risk factors, 402t
colostomy
irrigation, 391-92
problems, 393-96
reasons for, 388
types, 389f
coltsfoot, 342, 346t
colubrina, 370t
comedogenesis, 568
comedone, 58, 58f
comedone extraction, 66
comfrey, 342-43, 346t, 354, 359
commodes, 386
common cold *see* colds
communication skills
facilitation techniques, 17-18
questioning techniques, 16-17
compliance
contact lens regimen, 193
older consumers, 43
compresses
to treat blepharitis, 168
to treat bursitis, 540
to treat conjunctivitis, 173, 175, 176
to treat dermatitis and dry skin, 146
to treat dry eye, 177
to treat eyelid cyst, 169
to treat insect bites, 243
to treat skin infection, 229-30
compression (bandaging) of injuries, 541, 614
compression stockings, 381
computer-assisted smoking cessation, 608
conditioners
for dry hair, 576
for oily hair, 575
for treated hair, 576
ingredients, 581-82
types, 582
condoms
advantages and disadvantages, 417t
advice for the patient, 418
allergic reactions, 416-18
and STDs, 687
effectiveness, 416, 679t
female, 418, 684
for incontinent men, 387
patient assessment, 417t
types, 416
cone flower, 347t
congestive heart failure, 473t
conjunctiva
anatomy, 164
disorders, 170-76
conjunctivitis
advice for the patient, 172
allergic, 173-75
bacterial, 172-73
chemical/irritative, 175-76
differential diagnosis, 171t
etiology, 170t, 171t, 175t
pharmaceutical agents, 199-200, 201t
symptoms, 170, 172-76
treatment, 172-76, 179f-80f
viral, 173
constipation
advice for the patient, 295
association with hemorrhoids, 326, 329
consumer counselling, 294
defined, 291
etiology, 291-92
ostomy patients, 394
patient assessment, 296
pharmaceutical agents, 316-22
pregnancy, 48t
recommended reading, 324
symptoms, 292
treatment, 292-94
consumer counselling
assessment, 20-22
breast-feeding, 46, 47t, 50t
children, 45
chronic diseases, 51-55
cultural factors, 30
embarrassing subjects, 31-32
follow-up, 26-27
health professional's role, 8, 13, 14, 15f, 36
health education, 2, 7, 8t
hearing-impaired consumers, 33-35
information-gathering skills, 16-18
nondrug treatments, 26
nonverbal communication, 28-30
older consumers, 33-35, 39-43
pregnancy, 46, 47t, 48-49t
product information, 23-26
product selection, 22-23
recommended reading, 37
systematic approach, 19f, 19-27
talkative consumers, 32-33
contact dermatitis
advice for the patient, 130
and skin care products, 568
caused by sunscreens, 636
differential diagnosis, 124t
signs and symptoms, 128
treatment, 128-29, 131f
types, 128, 129f, 129-30
contact lenses
accessory solutions, 219-20
advice for the patient, 194-95
care, 194-95, 207, 208f-09f
causing eye problems, 177t, 181
cleaning solutions, 207, 210-11
compliance issues, 193
composition of debris, 210t
disinfection, 211-17, 217t
disposable, 189-92
extended wear (flexible), 189
gas permeable, 188-89, 191t, 208f
hard (PMMA), 188, 191t, 194-95, 208f
indications, 188
medications affecting, 192-93
multifunction solutions, 218-19
patient assessment, 196f-97f, 198
recommended reading, 222
silicone, 189
smokers, 193
soft (hydrogel), 189, 191t, 194-95, 209f
solution buffers and preservatives, 220
solution combinations, 220-21

storage, 213
types comparison, 190t
viscosity agents, 218
wetting and rewetting agents, 217-18
contraception, *see also* oral contraceptives
advice for the man, 418
advice for the woman, 681
and STDs, 686-87
cervical cap, 684, 685
client assessment, 417, 688
combination, 416
condom, 416-18
diaphragm, 682-84, 685
douching (ineffective), 679
failure rates, 679t
female condom, 684
male implant, 418
physiology, 678
selecting method, 678-79
spermicide, 680-82
sponge, 416, 679t
withdrawal, 679
contusion, eye, 181
COPD *see* chronic obstructive pulmonary disease
copper
food sources, 446t
function, 446t
signs of deficiency, 446t
corns and calluses
advice for the patient, 265
etiology, 265
symptoms, 265
treatment, 266-67
coronary artery disease, 598, 601, 604t
corrosives (poisoning), 240
corticosteroids
affecting sleep, 588t
association with athlete's foot, 261
causing acne, 59, 60t
drug interactions, 52, 554t
ostomy patients, 396t
pregnancy, 48t
to treat arthritis, 539
to treat cankers, 505
to treat dermatitis and dry skin, 126, 137, 143-44
to treat pruritus and inflammation, 243, 254
to treat rhinitis, 82
corticotropin (ACTH), 60t
cosmetics
and contact lenses, 194-95
and eye or eyelid infections, 172
causing acne, 59-60, 63t, 66, 71
causing dermatitis, 128, 129t
photosensitivity reactions, 628
to cover acne, 66
cotrimoxazole
causing diarrhea, 297
causing folliculitis, 60t
couch grass, 356
cough suppressants *see also* antitussives
causing constipation, 292t
pregnancy, 49t
coughs, 87, 89, 98
counselling (by pharmacist) *see* consumer counselling
counselling, smoking cessation, 602-07
Countdown (smoking cessation), 607
counterirritants
advice for the patient, 541
children, 564
dosage forms, 564
effects, 563t
list of, 563t
patient assessment, 544
pharmaceutical agents, 557-61
precautions, 564
recommended reading, 565
selection, 564
to treat hemorrhoids, 327, 328t, 332
to treat musculoskeletal pain, 542, 614
cow's milk protein formulas, 457, 458, 483
cradle cap
differential diagnosis, 124t
in adults, 577
in infants, 134, 135
creams
defined, 144
to treat dermatitis and dry skin, 126, 137, 144-45, 145t
to treat hemorrhoids, 333
cromolyn, 82
crotamiton
to treat dermatitis, 126
to treat scabies, 111, 117
croton oil, 354
crusted scabies, 109
crutches, 381
cryotherapy, 613-14 *see also* ice
cucurbita pumpkin, 346t
culture
and consumer counselling, 30
and pain threshold, 534
curare, 356
cushions for dentures, 518
cyanocobalamin *see* vitamin B_{12}
cyclamate *see* sodium cyclamate
cyclobenzaprine, 384t
cyclophosphamide, 539
cyclosporine
causing acne, 60t
causing gingival hyperplasia, 497
cyproheptadine
abuse by athletes, 620
characteristics and doses, 84t
photosensitivity reactions, 629t
weight gain/loss, 453t
cysts
acne, 59, 63t
eyelid, 169
cytotoxic drugs
affecting sleep, 588t
association with athlete's foot, 261

dacarbazine, 629t
dactinomycin, 60t
daffodil, 354
Dakin's solution *see* sodium hypochlorite
Damsissa, 357
danazol, 670
dandelion, 347t, 356
dandruff
advice for the patient, 135
defined, 134
differential diagnosis, 124t
pharmaceutical agents, 144
signs and symptoms, 134
treatment, 134-35, 136f
danthron
combination with docusate, 321
to treat constipation, 320
toxicity, 317
dantrolene

causing acne, 60**t**
causing incontinence, 384**t**
deadly nightshade, 354, 356
deaf consumers, 34-35
deafness *see* hearing loss
debridement, 226, 229
decongestants, *see also* ophthalmic decongestants
adverse effects, 96-98
children, 96, 204**t**
classes, 96
drug interactions, 98
in first aid kit, 650
pregnancy, 49**t**
to treat colds and rhinitis, 89, 97**t**
decubitus ulcers, 228
DEET *see* diethyltoluamide
deferoxamine, 152**t**
dehydration
from diarrhea, 298, 299, 645
heat-related, 617-18
demeclocycline, 629**t**
dementia, 590
demulcents
to treat canker sores, 514
to treat sore throat, 98
dental caries
advice for the patient, 494
etiology, 491-92, 507
figures, 492**f**, 493**f**
prevention, 493-94, 516-17
symptoms, 492-93
treatment, 493
dental erosion, 499
dental floss, 525-26
dental pain
caused by broken tooth, 499
caused by caries, 492-93
caused by dental procedures, 499
caused by infection, 499
caused by periodontal disease, 497
caused by tooth fracture, 499
caused by tooth grinding, 499
pharmaceutical agents, 526-27
related pain, 540-41
treatment, 540-41
dental staining
caused by smoking, 598
caused by tetracycline, 490
dentifrices
desensitizing, 517
fluoride, 495**t**, 516-17
gingivitis and plaque, 517
tartar control, 517
types and ingredients, 515-16
dentin, 490
dentures
adhesives and cushioning products, 518
cleansing products, 518
ill-fitting, 499
repair kits, 518
stomatitis, 506
deodorants
for body odor, 572-73, 583
for genital odor, 657-58
for ostomy products, 393, 394
2-deoxy-D-glucose, 503**t**
depigmenting agents, 640-41
depilatories, 659, 660
depression, 590
dequalinium chloride, 515, 515**t**
dermatitis
and condom use, 417
atopic, 123-27
contact, 124**t**, 128-32, 636
defined, 121
diaper, 128, 129-30
ear, 153**t**, 155**t**
hand, 128, 129**t**, 132**f**
patient assessment, 140
pharmaceutical agents, 141-46
recommended reading, 147
seborrheic, 134-36
desipramine, 453**t**
detergents *see* soaps
detrusor instability, 383-84
devil's claw, 347**t**
dexbrompheniramine, 83**t**
dextran polymers, 201**t**
dextrin, 431
dextroamphetamine, 453**t**
dextromethorphan, 95**t**, 95-96
di-N-propyl isocinchomeronate, 243
diabetes mellitus
advice for the patient, 54
alcohol, 53, 433
and jock itch, 413
association with athlete's foot, 261, 263
calories in drugs, 53-54
cold products, 89
constipation, 292
drugs affecting blood glucose, 54-55
dyspepsia, 276**t**
foot care, 54-55, 266
glucose monitoring, 403-04
herbal medicines affecting blood glucose, 357
homeopathic remedies, 370
incontinence, 384-85
nutritional requirements, 472**t**
otitis externa, 156
smoking, 604**t**
travelling, 651
diagnostic products
blood pressure monitors, 397-98
cholesterol tests, 401
ear and throat examination kits, 403
fecal occult blood tests, 401-02
glucose tests, 403-04
ovulation predictors, 398, 400-01
patient assessment, 405
peak flow meters, 402-03
pregnancy tests, 398-400
recommended reading, 409
diapers
adult, 386
causing dermatitis, 128, 129-30, 233
diaphragms
advice for the woman, 685
and STDs, 687
effectiveness, 416, 679**t**, 684
figure, 682**f**
placement, 683**f**
sizing, 683
types, 683
diarrhea
advice for the patient, 301
causing fecal incontinence, 386
causing hemorrhoids, 326
defined, 297
drug-induced, 297-98
elderly persons, 299-300

etiology, 297-98, 299**t**
home treatment, 322**t**
infants, 298-99, 322-23
inflammatory vs. noninflammatory, 297**t**
patient assessment, 302
pharmaceutical agents, 312-13, 322-23
pregnancy, 300
recommended reading, 324
travellers', 300-01, 643-45
diazepam
causing constipation, 292**t**
causing incontinence, 384**t**
photosensitivity reactions, 629**t**
dibucaine
to treat hemorrhoids, 328**t**, 331
to treat premature ejaculation, 420
to treat pruritus, 141
dichlorophen
FDA classification, 263**t**
ineffective for jock itch, 413**t**
dichromate, 133**t**
diclofenac, 629**t**
dicyclomine
as antispasmodic, 312
contributing to heat-related illness, 617
to treat colic in infants, 290
diet, *see also* foods; nutrition
acne, 60, 71
arthritis, 539
canker sores, 504, 505**t**
constipation, 291
flatulence potential of foods, 287**t**
gastrointestinal gas, 286, 287-88
GER, 282, 283, 283**t**
halitosis, 508
hemorrhoids, 326, 327
IBS, 303
of athletes, 474-78
of elderly persons, 471, 474
of infants, 455-60, 461**f**, 462
of ostomy patients, 393-94, 395**t**
to manage constipation, 295, 317-18
to manage dry mouth, 509
to manage dyspepsia, 277-78, 279
to manage nausea and vomiting, 307, 309, 648
to manage PMS, 669
to manage vaginal infection, 672
travellers' diarrhea, 301**t**, 644
weight loss, 463-67
diet aids
appetite suppressants, 465-66
herbal products, 357-58
meal replacement products, 466-67
dietary fibre *see* fibre
diethanolamine p-methoxycinnamate, 633**t**
diethylpropion, 453**t**
diethyltoluamide, 243, 254-55
digitalis
causing dyspepsia, 276**t**
herbal products, 356, 358
digoxin, 311**t**, 357
dihydroxyacetone, 640
diltiazem
causing folliculitis, 60**t**
photosensitivity reactions, 629**t**
with herbal products, 358
dimenhydrinate
contributing to heat-related illness, 617
drug interactions, 649, 652
to treat motion sickness, 648-49, 652
to treat nausea, 313, 314**t**
use in children, 45**t**, 313
dimethyl phthalate, 243, 255
dimethylsulfoxide, 508
DIN (Drug Identification Number), 5
dioscorea, 347**t**
dioxybenzone, 633**t**, 638
diphenhydramine
causing incontinence, 384**t**
characteristics and doses, 83**t**
children, 234
contributing to heat-related illness, 617
photosensitivity reactions, 629**t**
pregnancy, 48**t**
to treat anaphylaxis, 245
to treat chickenpox, 234
to treat colds and rhinitis, 94, 95**t**, 96
to treat dermatitis, 126, 129, 141
to treat insomnia, 595
to treat motion sickness, 313-14, 652
to treat pruritus, 249-50
treatment of poisoning, 239
diphenylmethane, 316
diphenylpyraline, 83**t**
disaccharides, 430
diseases
associated with dyspepsia, 276**t**
associated with insomnia, 589**t**, 589-90
associated with obesity, 463**t**
chronic, 51-55
most common (Canada), 3**t**
disinfectants
compared to antiseptics, 250
for contact lenses, 211-16
in deodorants, 583
to treat wounds and injuries, 616**t**
disclosing agents (plaque), 523
dislocation (of joints), 541
disodium edetate, 205, 212-13
disodium phosphate, 220
disopyramide, 629**t**
disposable bed pads, 386
disposable contact lenses
planned replacement programs, 191-92
use, 189-91
disposable pants, 386
diuretics
affecting sleep, 588**t**
banned in sports, 621
causing constipation, 292**t**
causing dry eye, 177**t**, 193
causing incontinence, 383, 384**t**
cross-sensitivity, 635, 636**t**
drug interactions, 41**t**, 52
herbal, 355, 356
ostomy patients, 396**t**
photosensitivity reactions, 629**t**
to treat dysmenorrhea and PMS, 667, 669, 670
diverticulitis, 292
DMP *see* dimethyl phthalate
dock, 355
docusate calcium, 317**t**, 321
docusate sodium
to treat constipation, 317**t**, 321
to treat hemorrhoids, 327
dodecyl trimethyl ammonium bromide, 580**t**
dogbane, 355, 356
domiphen bromide
in mouthwashes, 521
to prevent plaque, 521-22

to treat hemorrhoids, 328**t**, 333
to treat sore throat, 98
domperidone, 283**t**, 284
douches
administration, 656-57
advice for the woman, 657
ineffective as contraceptive, 679
patient assessment, 660
preparation, 657**t**
reason for use, 656
to treat vulvovaginal candidiasis, 673
doxepin
photosensitivity reactions, 629**t**
weight gain/loss, 453**t**
doxycycline
causing GER, 282
drug interactions, 644
photosensitivity reactions, 629**t**
doxylamine
characteristics and doses, 83**t**
pregnancy, 48**t**
dressings
for burns, 237
for sports injuries, 616**t**
selection, 225, 254
types, 254, 256-58
drug abuse
nutritional requirements, 473**t**
resources, 620
sports, 619-21
drug-alcohol interactions
general, 2-3, 434
acetaminophen, 550
ASA, 554**t**
consumer counselling, 7, 26
dimenhydrinate, 649, 652
herbal medicines, 356-57, 358, 359
promethazine, 649, 652
pyrilamine maleate, 691
ranitidine, 316
scopolamine, 649, 653
drug-contact lens interactions, 192-93
drug-drug interactions, 2-3, 22-23, 26 *see also specific drug*
Drug Identification Number (DIN), 5
drug schedules, 5-6, 10
drugs and smoking, 598, 599, 606**t**
drug-vitamin interactions
anticoagulants in herbal products, 357
herbal medicines, 357
vitamin B_6, 691
vitamin K in herbal products, 357
drugs causing
acne, 59, 60**t**, 63**t**, 71
allergic rhinitis, 81
constipation, 292, 292**t**
diarrhea, 297, 299**t**
dry eye, 177**t**
dyspepsia, 276**t**, 276-77
gastric ulcers, 276
GER, 282, 283**t**
halitosis, 508
headache, 537
insomnia, 588**t**, 589**t**
nausea and vomiting, 308
ototoxicity, 152**t**
rhinitis medicamentosa, 81-82
sleep pattern changes, 587, 588**t**
weight gain/loss, 453**t**, 463
dry eye
etiology, 177**t**
symptoms, 177
treatment, 177-78, 179**f**-80**f**, 201**t**
dry mouth
etiology and treatment, 509
pharmaceutical agents, 518-19
dry skin
advice for the patient, 138
defined, 137
differential diagnosis, 124**t**
patient assessment, 140
pharmaceutical agents, 144-46
signs and symptoms, 137
treatment, 137, 139**f**
duodenal ulcer, 275-76, 277**f**
duodenitis, 276**t**
dye-light, 503**t**
dysmenorrhea
advice for the woman, 666
client assessment, 666
etiology, 663-64
symptoms, 664-65
treatment, 664**f**, 665-67
dyspepsia
advice for the patient, 279
defined, 275
etiology, 275-77, 276**t**
patient assessment, 281
pharmaceutical agents, 310-11, 315-16
recommended reading, 323
symptoms, 277
treatment, 277-79, 280**f**

ear, *see also* hearing
anatomy and physiology, 149-50
syringing techniques, 156
ear drops in first aid kit, 650
ear disorders
assessment, 153**t**, 155**t**
boils, 154, 155**t**
bullous myringitis, 154, 155**t**
dermatitis, 128, 129**t**, 153**t**, 155**t**
discharge, 151, 153**t**, 155**t**, 158
drug-induced, 152**t**
foreign body obstruction, 154, 155**t**
hearing loss, 151, 152**t**
impacted cerumen, 154-55, 155**t**
infections, 153-54, 289**t**
otitis externa, 155**t**, 155-57, 158
otitis media, 81, 154, 155**t**, 598
pain, 151, 153**t**, 155**t**, 158, 406
patient assessment, 158
pharmaceutical agents, 159-60
recommended reading, 161
ear piercing
advice for the patient, 154, 156
causing infection, 153
ear wax *see* cerumen
eating disorders
definitions and prevalence, 467-68
organ system changes, 467**t**
patient assessment, 469-70
treatment, 468
echinacea, 335, 347**t**
ecthyma, 229
eczema *see* atopic dermatitis (eczema)
EDTA *see* disodium edetate
ejaculation, premature, 419-20
elastin, 145
elder, 355, 356
electrolysis, 659

electrolytes
content in fluid replacement solutions, 476t
to treat heat-related disorders, 617-18
electromyography, 534
elevation (for injury), 541, 614
EMLA, 248
emmenagogues, 355, 359
emollient dressings, 258
emollients
to treat canker pain, 504
to treat cold sores, 502
to treat cradle cap, 135
to treat dermatitis and dry skin, 125, 129, 137, 144-46
encephalitis, 234
endocrine acne, 63t
enemas, 317t, 321-22
energy (calories)
athletes, 475
older persons, 471
recommended intake, 426t, 427t
restricting, 464
enteral products, 482-83
enteric-coated drugs, 396
enterobiasis
advice for the patient, 114
children, 113
etiology, 113
patient assessment, 116
pharmaceutical agents, 117-19
recommended reading, 120
signs and symptoms, 113-14
treatment, 114-15
enterostomal therapy nurses, 388
enuresis, 385-86, 593
environmental factors and skin disorders, 61, 123, 124t
environmental tobacco smoke, 82, 598, 602
enzyme cleaners, 211
eosinophilic rhinitis, 79
ephedra, 347t, 353, 358
ephedrine
abuse by athletes, 620, 621
as decongestant, 96, 97t, 98
in herbal products, 358
to treat hemorrhoids, 328t, 331, 332-33
use in hypertension, 51
epinephrine
in first aid kits, 246
in ophthalmic medications, 192
to treat anaphylaxis, 245
epoxy resin, 133t
epsom salts, 229-30
ergogenic aids, 478, 619-20
ergotamine, 536, 537
erysipelas, 229
erythrasma, 412t
erythromycin
causing diarrhea, 297
causing dyspepsia, 276t, 277
causing ototoxicity, 152t
drug interactions, 52, 94
erythropoietin, 621
esdepallethrin, 109, 111, 118
esophageal sphincter pressure, 282, 283t
esophagitis, 276t, 282
essential oils
as insect repellents, 255
in deodorants, 573
estazolam, 629t
estrogens
effects of smoking, 598, 606t
to treat PMS, 670
ethacrynic acid
causing ototoxicity, 152t
weight gain/loss, 453t
ethambutol, 60t
ethanol
in mouthwashes, 521
to treat cankers and cold sores, 515, 515t
ethanolamines, 83t
ethionamide
causing acne, 60t
with herbal products, 358
2-ethoxyethyl p-methoxycinnamate *see* cinoxate
ethyl alcohol, 573 *see also* alcohol; ethanol
ethyl ether, 503t, 515
ethyl nicotinate, 559
ethylcellulose, 218t
ethyldihydroxypropyl PABA, 633t
ethylenediamines
causing dermatitis, 133t
classification, 83t
2-ethylhexyl 2-cyano-3,3 diphenylacrylate *see* octocrylene
2-ethylhexyl p-methoxycinnamate *see* octyl methoxycinnamate
2-ethylhexyl salicylate *see* octyl salicylate
ETS *see* environmental tobacco smoke
eucalyptus oil
as insect repellent, 255
during homeopathic treatment, 371
in herbal products, 359
to prevent plaque, 521-22
to treat colds, 96
to treat musculoskeletal pain, 559
to treat sore throat, 98
eugenol *see* clove oil
euphorbia, 355
euphrasia, 370t
Eusol solution *see* sodium hypochlorite
evaporated milk infant formulas, 458
evening primrose oil
to treat PMS, 669, 690
to treat pruritus, 250
exercise
for weight loss, 464-65
to treat arthritis, 538
to treat cluster headache, 537
to treat constipation, 291, 293
to treat PMS, 669
exfoliants, 69, 73
expectorants
pregnancy, 49t
to treat colds, 89, 98
extended wear contact lenses, 189
eye
allergic dermatitis, 128, 129t
anatomy, 163-65, 164f
eye disorders
advice for the patient, 182-83, 184, 185
blepharitis, 167-68, 172, 179f-80f
conjunctivitis, 170-76, 179f-80f
dry eye, 177-78, 179f-80f
frequency and management in Canada, 3t, 4t
patient assessment, 186-87
pharmaceutical agents, 199-206
recommended reading, 222
red eye, 165t
self-treatment, 166
trauma, 181
eye drops, 182-83
eye ointment
comparison with eye solutions, 206t

formulations, 206
instillation techniques, 184
eye whiteners *see* ophthalmic decongestants
eyelid cyst, 169
eyelids
anatomy, 163
disorders, 167-69
glands, 164**t**
eyewash
boric acid in, 200
to treat chemical burn, 181
to treat conjunctivitis, 176, 180**f**

facial contact dermatitis, 129**t**
facilitation techniques (communication), 17-18
Fagerström nicotine tolerance scale, 604, 605**t**, 608
false hellebore, 356
false unicorn root, 355, 356
familial polyposis, 391
family planning *see* fertility awareness techniques
famotidine, 284, 316
fat
daily requirements, 465**t**, 471
dietary nutrient, 431
recommendations for intake, 430**t**
fatty acids
as emollient, 145
comedogenicity, 568**t**
in conditioners, 582
nutrition, 431
fatty alcohols, 582
fatty esters, 582
fecal impaction, 386
fecal incontinence, 386
fecal occult blood testing, 401-03, 405
felodipine
photosensitivity reactions, 629**t**
weight gain/loss, 453**t**
feminine deodorant sprays, 657-58
fenfluramine, 453**t**
fennel, 347**t**
fenugreek, 339, 347**t**
ferric oxide, 639
ferrous fumarate *see* iron
ferrous gluconate *see* iron
ferrous succinate *see* iron
ferrous sulfate *see* iron
ferrum phosphoricum, 368
fertility awareness techniques, 679-80
fever
advice for the patient, 548
children, 547
defined, 545
differential diagnosis, 545
elderly persons, 547
measuring, 545-46
pathophysiology, 545
patient assessment, 549
pregnancy, 547
recommended reading, 565
treatment, 89, 547-49
with colds, 87
feverfew
medicinal uses and side effects, 342, 347**t**
to prevent migraine, 536
to treat migraine headache, 335
fibre
benefits, 432**t**
dyspepsia, 278
food sources, 293**t**, 327
for weight loss, 485**t**
link with hemorrhoids, 326, 327, 329
recommended intake, 432
to treat constipation, 293, 295, 317-18
to treat IBS, 303-04
fibre-containing infant formulas, 458, 483
fibrinolysin-desoxyribonuclease, 226
filtration (water), 646, 647**t**
first aid
anaphylaxis, 245
burns, 235-37
dressings, 254, 256-58
frostbite, 238
insect bites and stings, 243-44, 245-46
pharmaceutical agents, 248-56
poisoning, 239-40
recommended reading, 259
travellers, 650-51
wounds and injuries, 225-27
first aid kits
general, 246
sports, 615, 616**t**
travel, 650
first aid manuals, 246
fissures, anal, 330
flanges (ostomy appliance), 392-93
flatulence, 286-88, 393
flavonoids, 515
flavors and spices, medicinal, 339-40
fleabane, 355
flecainide, 629**t**
flexible wear contact lenses, 189
floctafenine, 298
flu *see* influenza
fluconazole, 506
fluids
comparison of replacement solutions, 476**t**
daily requirements for older individuals, 471
restoring, 299-300, 322-23, 645
flumethasone pivalate, 413
flunarizine, 536
flunisolide, 82
fluorescein, 192
fluoride
children, 516-17, 520**t**, 520
food sources, 446**t**
function, 446**t**, 519
in community water, 495**t**, 519-20
in dentifrices, 516-17
in dry mouth products, 519
in mouthwashes, 495**t**, 523
infant supplements, 457**t**, 459
professionally applied, 495**t**
school programs, 495**t**
signs of deficiency, 446**t**
supplementation, 495**t**, 520**t**, 520-21
to prevent caries, 493-94, 495**t**
toxicity, 520, 521
fluorouracil, 629**t**
fluoxetine
to prevent migraine, 536
weight gain/loss, 453**t**
flupenthixol, 629**t**
flurbiprofen, 498
fluspirilene, 629**t**
fluvastatin, 629**t**
foams, spermicidal, 681
folacin *see* folic acid
folate *see* folic acid
folic acid

food sources, 443**t**
function, 443**t**
neural tube deficiency, 479
pregnancy, 49**t**, 479
recommended nutrient intake, 426**t**, 443**t**
signs of deficiency, 443**t**
signs of toxicity, 443**t**
folliculitis
caused by coal tar products, 59, 126, 143
differential diagnosis, 63**t**
treatment, 229
Food and Drugs Act and Regulations
homeopathic remedies, 368
regulatory process, 5
foods, *see also* diet; nutrition
caffeine content, 591**t**
causing atopic dermatitis, 124, 124**t**
fibre content, 293**t**, 327
flatulence potential, 287**t**
medicinal plants, 338-39
photosensitivity reactions, 628
toxicity of medicinal plants, 338-39
foot care
and diabetes, 54-55, 261, 263, 266
athlete's foot, 261-64
bunions, 271
corns and calluses, 265-67
dermatitis, 129**t**
ingrown toenails, 270
pharmaceutical agents, 272-73
plantar warts, 268-69
recommended reading, 274
foot odor, 3**t**, 4**t**
foot powders, 572
footwear
advice for the patient, 266
and athlete's foot, 262, 263
and bunions, 271
and corns and calluses, 265-66
and warts, 268
testing for size, 267
foreign object
in ear, 154, 155**t**
in eye, 181
formaldehyde
causing dermatitis, 133**t**
as antiperspirant, 572, 583
formulas
elderly persons, 474
infants, 456-59, 483-84
weight loss, 466-67, 482
formulated liquid diet, 482
foxglove
drug interactions, 356
to treat heart disease, 336
frostbite, 238
fructose, 491
fuchsin
FDA classification, 263**t**
ineffective for jock itch, 413**t**
fumitory, 355, 356
fungal foot infections, 3**t**, 4**t**
furosemide
causing folliculitis, 60**t**
causing incontinence, 384**t**
causing ototoxicity, 152**t**
drug interactions, 555
effects of smoking cessation, 606**t**
photosensitivity reactions, 629**t**
weight gain/loss, 453**t**
furuncles
in ear, 154, 155**t**
treatment, 230

galactorrhea, 358
gamboge gum resin, 354
gargles, 88, 89
garlic, 347**t**
gas *see* gastrointestinal gas
gas permeable contact lenses
care, 207, 208**f**
complications, 191**t**
types and uses, 188-89
gasoline poisoning, 240
gastric lavage, 240
gastric ulcer, 276, 277**f**
gastritis, 276**t**
gastroesophageal reflux
advice for the patient, 284
etiology, 282, 283**t**
pathophysiology, 282
patient assessment, 285
pharmaceutical agents, 310-11, 315-16
recommended reading, 324
symptoms, 282-83
treatment, 283-84
gastrointestinal gas
advice for the patient, 286
etiology, 286
infants, 289
patient assessment, 287
recommended reading, 324
symptoms, 286-87
treatment, 287-88, 323
gaultheria procumbens *see* methyl salicylate
gauze dressings, 246, 257
gel dressings, 257-58
gelatin, 518
gels, 137, 143, 145
gelsemium sempervirens, 370**t**
gemmotherapy, 368
gender factors
acne, 57
arthritis, 538, 539
headache, 535
nutrition, 425
seborrheic dermatitis, 134
General Public (GP) number, 5
genital hygiene
men, 412
to prevent infection, 672
women, 655-58, 661, 663
genital towelettes, 657
gentamicin, 152**t**
gentian, 347**t**
gentian violet
to treat enterobiasis, 114
to treat oral candidiasis, 506
GER *see* gastroesophageal reflux
germander, 358-59
giant papillary conjunctivitis, 174
ginger
medicinal uses, 347**t**
to treat motion sickness, 648
ginger (wild), 355
gingival hyperplasia, 497
gingivitis, 496-98, 598
gingivostomatitis, 502
ginkgo, 335, 348**t**

ginseng, 348t, 357, 358
glands of Moll, 164t, 168
glands of Zeis, 164t, 168
glaucoma, 53
glucagon, 283t
glucose tests, 403-04, 405
glues, 239
glutaraldehyde, 572, 583
glutethimide, 606t
glyburide, 636t
glycerin
in conditioners, 582
to treat constipation, 317t, 322
to treat dermatitis and dry skin, 145
to treat ear disorders, 159
to treat hemorrhoids, 328t, 332
glycerin macerate, 368
glyceryl guaiacolate *see* guaifenesin
glyceryl p-aminobenzoate *see* glyceryl PABA
glyceryl PABA, 633t
glycolic acid, 146
glycopyrrolate
contributing to heat-related illness, 617
to treat irritable bowel, 312
goat's milk, 459
gold salts
causing acne, 60t
causing allergic dermatitis, 153, 154
photosensitivity reactions, 629t
to treat arthritis, 539
goldenseal, 348t
gonadotrophin releasing hormone agonists, 670
goosegrass, 356
Gordolobos tea, 341
Gotu Kola, 348t
gout, 539-40
GP (General Public) number, 5
grab bars (bathrooms), 377
gramicidin
in ophthalmic solutions, 200
to treat conjunctivitis, 173
to treat ear disorders, 159-60
to treat eyelid disorders, 168, 169
to treat impetigo, 229
to treat skin infection, 249
green hair, 576-77
green hellebore, 357
gripe water, 315
griseofulvin
causing halitosis, 508
photosensitivity reactions, 629t
with herbal products, 358
groundsel, 354, 355, 356
group support programs (smoking cessation), 607-08
guaifenesin, 98
guanethidine, 204t
guar gum, 357
guarana, 348t
Guillain-Barré syndrome, 234
Gymnema, 348t, 357
gynecomastia, 358

H_1 antagonists, *see* antihistamines
H_2 antagonists
association with travellers' diarrhea, 643
effect of smoking, 599
to treat GER, 284, 315-16
hair
anatomy, 574
care, 577-78
conditioners, 581-82
cradle cap, 577
dry, 575-76
excessive, 658
fine, 576
green, 576-77
growth, 574-75
oily, 575
permed or colored, 576
shampoos, 578-81
split ends, 576
swimmer's, 576
types, 575-76
hair removal (women)
advice for the woman, 660
methods, 658-60
pharmaceutical agents, 691
halitosis, 508, 598
halogenated aromatic hydrocarbons, 60
halogens, 59, 60t
haloperidol
photosensitivity reactions, 629t
weight gain/loss, 453t
haloprogin, 263t
halothane, 60t, 204t
hamamelis *see* witch hazel
hand dermatitis, 128, 129t, 132f
hard (PMMA) contact lenses
care, 194-95, 207, 208f
complications, 191t
types, 188
hawthorn, 335, 348t, 357
head lice
advice for the patient, 104
described, 101-02
symptoms, 102
treatment, 103-05
headache
assessment, 534, 535
cluster, 536-37
management, 4t
medication-induced, 537
migraine, 535-36
pregnancy, 49t
prevalence, 3t, 534-35
tension-type, 535
healing process (skin wounds), 224-25
Health Protection Branch, Health Canada, 1, 5, 9, 368, 514
hearing loss, 151, 152t, 154, 158
hearing-impaired consumers, 33-35
Heart and Stroke Foundation of Canada, 604
heart disease
dyspepsia, 276t
nicotine replacement therapy, 610
nutritional requirements, 473t
risks with herbal medicines, 358
smoking, 598, 601, 604t
heartburn *see also* dyspepsia
and GER, 282
pregnancy, 48t
heartsease, 356
heat-related disorders
cramps, 617
exhaustion, 617
salt replacement, 618
stroke, 617-18
syncope, 617
hellebore, 356, 357
hematoma (ear), 153t
hemlock, 354, 356

hemorrhage, subconjunctival, 176
hemorrhoidectomy, 328
hemorrhoids
- advice for the patient, 329
- anatomy and physiology, 325-26
- causes, 326-27
- causing constipation, 291
- frequency in Canada, 3**t**
- patient assessment, 329
- pharmaceutical agents, 328**t**, 331-33
- pregnancy, 49**t**
- recommended reading, 334
- symptoms, 327
- treatment, 4**t**, 327-28

henbane, 357
hepar sulfur, 371
heparin
- effects of smoking cessation, 606**t**
- to treat cold sores, 515, 515**t**

Herb Trade Association, 339
herbal medicines
- adulteration, 355-58, 359
- alcohol interactions, 356-57, 358, 359
- allopathic, 336
- breast-feeding, 336
- children, 339, 340, 354
- common, 341-43, 344**t**-52**t**
- distinguished from homeopathic medicines, 371
- drug interactions, 355-59
- flavors and spices, 339-40
- foods, 338-39
- for smoking cessation, 610
- guidelines, 336**t**
- history, 335
- labelling, 353**t**
- patient assessment, 359
- pregnancy, 336, 354-55
- recommended reading, 360
- safety concerns, 353
- sales figures, 337
- teas, 340-41

Herpes simplex virus, 501
herpes zoster (ear), 153**t**
hexachlorophene
- causing acne, 67
- photosensitivity reactions, 629**t**

hexylresorcinol
- in mouthwashes, 521
- to treat sore throat, 98

hibiscus, 340-41, 348**t**
hirsutism, 658
HIV, *see also* AIDS
- and condom use, 416, 418
- and spermicides, 682

holly (ground), 356
homatropine, 617
home health care
- aids for daily living, 377-81
- diagnostic devices, 397-404
- incontinence products, 382-87
- intravenous programs, 407-08
- ostomy products, 388-96
- recommended reading, 409
- resource groups, 408
- respiratory aids, 406

home intravenous programs *see* intravenous programs
homeopathic medicine
- availability, 368-69
- children, 370
- choosing, 365-66, 370-71
- clinical trials, 367
- combination products, 363
- counselling tips, 371
- defined, 362-63
- dilutions, 364-65, 365**t**
- dosage forms, 366**t**, 371
- dosages, 363, 370
- drug interactions, 371
- history, 361-62
- homotoxicology, 368
- popularity, 361, 362
- potencies, 365**t**
- principles, 362-63
- recommended reading, 373
- resource list, 372
- side effects, 371
- standards, 368
- tissue salts, 368

homomenthyl salicylate *see* homosalate
homosalate, 633**t**, 638
homotoxicology, 368
hops, 340, 348**t**, 356, 358
hordeolum (stye), 168-69
hormones
- affecting calcium absorption, 480
- causing acne, 60**t**
- causing GER, 282, 283**t**
- to treat PMS, 670

hornets, 241-42, 244, 245
horse chestnut
- medicinal uses and side effects, 348**t**
- to treat hemorrhoids, 328**t**, 333
- drug interactions, 357

horsetail *see* shavegrass
hound's tongue, 354
house dust, 81
human immunodeficiency virus *see* HIV
humectants
- in dentifrices, 516
- in emollients, 145

humidifiers, 88, 406
hyaluronic acid, 201**t**
hydantoin derivatives *see* antiepileptics
hydrangea, 349**t**, 356, 358
hydrastine, 205
hydrochlorothiazide
- causing incontinence, 384**t**
- cross-sensitivity, 636**t**

hydrocolloid dressings, 256-57
hydrocortisone
- children, 143
- to treat dermatitis and dry skin, 129, 135, 137, 143-44
- to treat hemorrhoids, 333
- to treat insect bites, 244

hydrogel dressings, 257-58
hydrogel lenses *see* soft (hydrogel) contact lenses
hydrogen peroxide
- in contact lens solutions, 214-15
- to clean dentures, 518
- to cleanse wounds, 251
- to treat cankers and cold sores, 502, 514, 515**t**
- to treat periodontal disease, 497
- to whiten teeth, 527

hydrolysed protein infant formulas, 457-58, 483
hydroquinone, 69, 75, 641
hydroxychloroquine, 539
hydroxyethylcellulose, 218**t**
hydroxymagnesium aluminate *see* magaldrate
hydroxypropyl methylcellulose
- in artificial tears, 201**t**

in ophthalmic solutions, 218**t**
hydroxyquinolone, 421
hydroxyzine
contributing to heat-related illness, 617
to treat dermatitis, 126, 129, 141
hyoscyamine, 617
hypercholesterolemia, 604**t**
hyperhidrosis, 571, 572
hyperlipidemia, 472**t**
hyperopia, 188**f**
hyperplastic candidiasis, 506
hypertension
and alcohol, 434
and nicotine replacement therapy, 610
and sleep apnea, 593
and smoking, 604**t**
monitors, 397-98, 405
nutritional requirements, 473**t**
risks with herbal medicines, 356-58
cautions with nonprescription drugs, 51
hyperthermia, 545, 618
hyperthyroidism
and dyspepsia, 276**t**
risks with herbal medicines, 358
cautions with nonprescription drugs, 53
hypertrichosis, 658
hypnagogic hallucinations, 593
hypnosis
for smoking cessation, 607
to treat pain, 534
hypnotics
affecting contact lens wear, 193
affecting sleep, 588**t**, 589**t**
causing incontinence, 383, 384**t**
with herbal preparations, 356-57
to treat insomnia, 592, 595
hypoallergenic soaps, 570**f**
hypochlorite solutions, 251
hypothermia, 238
hypothyroidism
and dyspepsia, 276**t**
causing constipation, 292

IBS *see* irritable bowel syndrome
ibuprofen
advice for the patient, 542
breast-feeding, 50**t**
causing dyspepsia, 279
children, 555
contraindications, 555
dosage, 553**t**
drug interactions, 555, 665
indications, 554-55
pharmacology, 554
precautions, 51, 54-55, 555, 665
side effects, 551**t**, 555
to treat arthritis, 539-40
to treat bursitis, 540
to treat cold sore pain, 502
to treat dental pain, 493, 499, 540-41
to treat dysmenorrhea and PMS, 665, 667, 669, 690
to treat ear pain, 151
to treat fever, 548-49
to treat musculoskeletal pain, 614
to treat periodontal disease, 498
ice
in first aid kits, 246
to abort cold sores, 502
to treat headache, 537
to treat wounds and injuries, 225, 541, 613-14, 616**t**
icthyosis vulgaris, 123
ileostomy
potential problems, 394
reasons for, 388
types, 390**f**
imidazoles
drug interactions, 94
to treat athlete's foot, 272
to treat fungal skin infection, 231, 232, 233
to treat vaginal infection, 672-73, 689-90
imidazolines
to treat colds and rhinitis, 96
use in hypertension, 51
imipramine
causing incontinence, 384**t**
contributing to heat-related illness, 617
effects of smoking, 598
weight gain/loss, 453**t**
immunotherapy, 82
impetigo, 229
implants (contraceptive), 679**t**
incontinence
defined, 382
fecal, 386
patient assessment, 387
products, 376**t**, 386-87
recommended reading, 409
resource list, 408
urinary, 382-86
indapamide, 629**t**
indigestion *see* dyspepsia
indomethacin, 152**t**
infant formulas
indications, 456
supplementation, 459
types, 457-59, 483-84
infant soaps, 570**f**
infection
causing diarrhea, 297, 298-99
causing nausea and vomiting, 308
ear, 153**t**, 153-54
skin, 228-34
vaginal, 671-77
Vincent's, 497
wounds, 227, 228-29
inflammation, 534
inflammatory bowel disease, 388
influenza, 88, 91**t**
infrared coagulation (hemorrhoids), 328
infusion pumps, 407
ingrown toenails, 270
injuries
frostbite, 238
heat-related disorders, 617-18
sports-related, 613-16
treatment, 543
types, 541
ink cap, 359
insect repellents, 243, 246, 254-55, 650
insecticides, 239
insects *see* bites (insects); stings (insects)
insomnia
caffeine-induced, 590
causes, 589**t**
infants, 289**t**
treatment, 591-92
types, 589
insulin
and smoking, 598-99
and travelling, 651

interdental cleaning devices, 526
interferon 2, 629**t**
intertrigo, 412**t**
intrauterine devices
- and STDs, 687
- effectiveness, 416, 679**t**

intravenous programs
- criteria, 407**t**
- market, 407
- patient assessment, 407**t**, 408
- problems, 408
- products, 376**t**
- recommended reading, 409
- techniques, 407-08

inulin, 319, 431
iodides
- causing acne, 59, 60**t**
- cross-sensitivity, 421

iodine
- food sources, 446**t**
- function, 446**t**
- purification water, 646**t**
- recommended nutrient intake, 427**t**, 446**t**
- signs of deficiency, 446**t**

iodochlorhydroxyquin *see* clioquinol
iontophoresis, 572
ipecac, 240, 246, 255-56
ipratropium bromide, 82
iron
- adverse effects, 481-82
- causing constipation, 292**t**
- causing dyspepsia, 276**t**, 277
- causing GER, 282
- drug interactions, 41**t**, 311**t**
- food sources, 446**t**
- function, 446**t**
- ostomy patients, 396**t**
- poisoning, 240
- recommended nutrient intake, 427**t**, 446**t**
- salts, 482**t**
- signs of deficiency, 446**t**
- supplementation, 481
- toxicity, 482
- use in athletes, 475
- use in elderly persons, 41**t**, 474
- use in infants, 457**t**, 459

irregularity, 3**t**, 4**t**
irritable bowel syndrome
- advice for the patient, 304
- causing constipation, 292
- defined, 303
- etiology, 303
- patient assessment, 305
- pharmaceutical agents, 311-12
- recommended reading, 324
- support group, 305
- symptoms, 303, 304**t**
- treatment, 303-05

isocarboxazid, 629**t**
isoniazid
- causing acne, 60**t**
- causing folliculitis, 60**t**
- overdose, 240

isopathy, 368
isopropyl alcohol
- contraindicated with open wounds, 251
- to clean contact lenses, 210
- to treat ear disorders, 156, 160

4-isopropyl dibenzoylmethane, 639
isotherapy, 368
isotretinoin, 193
ispaghula, 358
itraconazole
- drug interactions, 94
- to treat oral candidiasis, 506

jalap, 354
jequirity bean, 355
Jesuit's tea, 349**t**
jet lag, 589, 592
jewelry, 128, 129**t**, 133**t**
jimsonweed, 356
jock itch
- advice for the patient, 414
- etiology, 230, 411
- differential diagnosis, 412**t**
- dosage forms, 414**t**
- patient assessment, 415
- signs and symptoms, 411-12
- treatment, 412-14, 421-22

juniper, 349**t**, 355, 356

kaladanna, 354
kalium muriaticum, 368
kalium phosphoricum, 368
kalium sulfuricum, 368
kaolin
- as sunscreen, 639
- to treat diarrhea, 312
- to treat hemorrhoids, 332

karaya gum, 318, 518
karela, 357
kava, 358
Kegel exercises, 385
keloid (ear), 153**t**
kelp, 358
keratin, 145
keratitis, 189-91, 191**t**, 193, 207
keratoconjunctivitis, 174
keratolytics
- to treat corns, calluses and warts, 266-67, 269, 272-73
- to treat dandruff and seborrhea, 134, 146
- to treat hemorrhoids, 328, 328**t**, 332

keratoma, 268
kerosene poisoning, 240
ketoconazole
- drug interactions, 41**t**, 52, 94
- to treat dandruff and seborrhea, 134, 144

ketoprofen, 629**t**
ketotifen, 453**t**
kidney (anatomy), 382**f**
kyushin, 356

L-tryptophan, 595
labelling
- herbal medicines, 353**t**
- usefulness, 7

laceration
- eye, 181
- skin, 224

lachesis, 371
lacrimal apparatus (anatomy), 164-65, 164**f**
lactase, 316, 430
lactating women *see* breast-feeding; nursing women
lactic acid
- to treat dry skin, 137, 145-46
- to treat plantar warts, 269

lactobacillus products
- ineffective for cold sores, 503**t**
- ineffective for travellers' diarrhea, 645

to treat diarrhea, 312-13
lactose
causing dental caries, 491
in homeopathic remedies, 364-65, 366t
intolerance, 430
lactose-free modified cow's milk-based infant formulas, 458, 483
lactulose, 317t, 319
lady's mantle, 356
lamb cecum condoms, 416
lanolin
comedogenicity, 568t
in conditioners, 582
in eye ointments, 202
to treat dry skin, 142, 145
to treat hemorrhoids, 332
lansoprazole, 284
larch, 356
laser therapy, 607
latex condoms, 416
lavender oil
as emmenagogue, 355
as insect repellent, 255
photosensitivity reactions, 629t
law of similars (homeopathy), 362-63
laxatives
breast-feeding, 50t
bulk-forming, 317t, 317-18
causing constipation, 292t
causing diarrhea, 298
classification, 316
combination products, 321
enemas 321-22
herbal, 354-55
lubricant, 317t, 321
osmotic, 317t, 318-19
ostomy patients, 396t
pregnancy, 48t
side effects, 316
stimulant, 317t, 320-21
stool softeners, 317t, 321
suppositories, 322
to treat constipation, 294
toxicity, 316-17
use in children, 45
use in elderly persons, 41t
ledum palustre, 370t
lemon oil
to treat dry mouth, 509, 519
to treat pediculosis, 104-05
lemongrass oil, 255
leukoplakia, 598
levamisole, 505
levocabastine, 93
levodopa, 588t
liberty cap, 358
lice *see* pediculosis
licorice
in herbal products 335, 336, 349t, 355, 356, 357
use in pregnancy, 355
lidocaine
to relieve pruritus, 141
to treat bursitis, 540
to treat cankers and cold sores, 502, 514, 515t
to treat cluster headache, 537
to treat ear disorders, 160
life root, 349t
Lifesign (smoking cessation), 608
lily-of-the-valley, 354, 356
lime oil, 629t
lindane
children, 117
to treat pediculosis, 103-05, 117
to treat scabies, 110, 117
linden flowers, 349t
liniments, 564
lionsear, 355
liquor carbonis detergens *see* coal tar
lithium
causing acne, 59, 60t
causing halitosis, 508
drug interactions, 555
poisoning, 240
to treat headache, 537
weight gain/loss, 453t
with herbal preparations, 358
lithotherapy, 368
lobelia, 349t, 358
loop diuretics, 152t
loperamide
breast-feeding, 50t
to treat diarrhea, 301, 313, 645
to treat IBS, 304-05
use in children, 313
loratadine
characteristics and doses, 84t
to treat rhinitis, 93
to treat pruritus, 126
lotions
defined, 141, 564
to treat dermatitis and dry skin, 126, 129, 137, 141-42, 143
loxapine
photosensitivity reactions, 629t
weight gain/loss, 453t
lozenges, 89, 98
lycopodium, 371
Lyme disease, 242
lysine, 503t

magaldrate
pregnancy, 48t
to treat dyspepsia and GER, 311
magic mushrooms, 358
magnesia phosphorica, 368
magnesium
breast-feeding, 50t
drug interactions, 41t
food sources, 447t
function, 447t
pregnancy, 48t
recommended nutrient intake, 427t, 447t
signs of deficiency, 447t
magnesium citrate, 317t, 319
magnesium hydroxide
side effects, 316
to treat constipation, 317t, 319
to treat dyspepsia, 279, 310-11
magnesium salicylate, 554
magnesium sulfate
contraindications, 316
to treat constipation, 317t, 319
magnesium trisilicate *see* talc
Ma Huang, 347t, 353, 358
maidenhair tree, 335, 348t
malabsorption syndromes, 276t
male fern, 344t
malnutrition
elderly persons, 474, 474t
etiology, 427
mandrake, 357, 358
manganese

food sources, 447t
function, 447t
mannitol
as alternative sweetener, 484
lower risk of caries, 492
to treat constipation, 319
MAO inhibitors *see* monoamine oxidase inhibitors
maprotiline
causing acne, 60t
photosensitivity reactions, 629t
weight gain/loss, 453t
marigold, 346t
marijuana, 358
marjoram, 340
marshmallow, 344t
massage
scalp, 577
to treat musculoskeletal injuries, 562
mate, 349t
mayapple, 354, 355
mazindol, 453t
meal replacement products
brand names, 483
for elderly persons, 474
for weight loss, 466-67, 482-83, 485t
mebendazole, 114
medical devices
daily living, 377-81
diagnostic, 397-404
examples, 376t
incontinence, 382-87
intravenous programs, 407-08
market, 375
ostomy, 388-96
patient assessment, 405
recommended reading, 409
resource list, 408
respiratory, 405
medicated soaps, 67, 568, 570
medicated washes, 67
medicinal teas, 340-41, 359
mefenamic acid, 298
meibomian cyst, 169
meibomian glands, 164t, 167, 168, 169
melilot, 357
meningitis, 234
men's health care products
contraceptives, 416-18
pharmaceutical agents, 421-22
recommended reading, 423
menstrual pads, 661, 663
menstruation
and acne, 57, 71
cycle, 661, 662f, 678
hygiene, 661, 663
toxic shock syndrome, 661, 662
menthol
during homeopathic treatment, 371
FDA classification, 263t
in deodorants, 573
ineffective for jock itch, 413t
to prevent plaque, 521-22
to treat cankers and cold sores, 515, 515t
to treat colds, 96
to treat hemorrhoids, 328t, 332
to treat musculoskeletal pain, 559
to treat pruritus, 141
to treat sore throat, 98
mercurius corrosivus, 371
mercurius cyanatus, 371
mesoridazine, 453t
methacycline, 358
methanol, 240
methazolamide, 629t
methenamine, 573, 583
methotrexate
drug interactions, 554t, 555
photosensitivity reactions, 629t
to treat rheumatoid arthritis, 539
methyl 2-aminobenzoate *see* methyl anthranilate
methyl anthranilate, 633t, 639
methyl nicotinate, 559
methyl salicylate
anti-plaque activity, 521-22
as insect repellent, 255
in herbal medicines, 340, 351t
to treat musculoskeletal pain, 559-60, 614
methylcellulose
for denture adhesion, 518
for weight loss, 465, 485t
in artificial tears, 201t
in ophthalmic solutions, 218t
to treat constipation, 317t, 318
to treat IBS, 304
6-methylcoumarin, 629t
methyldopa
affecting sleep, 588t
causing incontinence, 384t
drug interactions, 204t
interactions with herbal products, 358
methylene blue, 205
methylparaben *see also* parabens
FDA classification, 263t
in ophthalmic solutions, 205
ineffective for jock itch, 413t
methylprednisolone, 540
methysergide
to prevent migraine, 536
to treat cluster headache, 537
metoclopramide
to treat colonic gas, 288
to treat GER, 283t, 284
metolazone, 629t
metoprolol, 629t
MFP *see* sodium monofluorophosphate; monofluorophosphate
miconazole
FDA classification, 263t
to treat athlete's foot, 263-64, 272
to treat diaper rash, 130
to treat fungal skin infection, 231, 232, 233
to treat jock itch, 413, 421
to treat oral candidiasis, 506
to treat vaginal infection, 672-73, 673t, 689-90
micturition, 382-83
migraine, 535-36
milia, 63t
milk
for infants, 459
inappropriate for dyspepsia, 278
milk of magnesia, 294
milk thistle, 335
mineral oil
as emollient, 142, 145
breast-feeding, 50t
causing acne, 60
in conditioners, 582
in eye ointments, 202, 205
to soften impacted cerumen, 154
to treat constipation, 317t, 321

to treat hemorrhoids, 332
use in elderly persons, 41t
minerals
athletes, 475, 620
children, 460
counselling tips, 433
elderly persons, 471, 474
infants, 456, 457t, 459, 460
pregnancy, 49t
supplementation, 480-82
minocycline
causing ototoxicity, 152t
photosensitivity reactions, 629t
mint, 371
miranol, 210t
mistletoe, 349t, 354, 357
mites
causing allergic rhinitis, 81, 82
causing dermatitis, 124, 241
scabies, 108
modified cow's milk-based infant formulas, 458, 483
moisturizers
to treat dermatitis, 125, 129, 137, 144-46
to treat sunburn, 626
mold
causing dermatitis, 124t
causing rhinitis, 81
moleskin
to relieve bunions, 271
to relieve corns and calluses, 266
molybdenum
food sources, 447t
function, 447t
moniliasis *see* candidiasis
monkshood, 356
monoamine oxidase inhibitors
affecting sleep, 587, 588t
drug interactions, 98, 204t
monobenzone, 641
monofluorophosphate, 495t
monosaccharides, 430
Mormon tea, 349t
morning sickness
etiology, 307-08
treatment, 309
mosquitoes, 241, 245
motilin, 283t
motion sickness
advice for the patient, 648
etiology, 307
signs and symptoms, 648
treatment, 308, 648-49
mouth
anatomy and physiology, 489-90
dermatitis, 129t
mouth disorders
and smoking, 598
candidiasis, 506
cankers, 504-05
causing halitosis, 508
cold sores, 501-03
dry mouth, 509
halitosis, 508
patient assessment, 510f, 511f, 512-13
periodontal diseases, 496-98
pharmaceutical agents, 514-15, 518-19, 521-23
mouthwash
children, 521
efficacy for halitosis, 508, 521
fluoridated, 517
ingredients, 521-23
to prevent plaque, 521
to treat cankers, 504, 514
to treat cold sores, 502
to treat dry mouth, 518-19
to treat periodontal disease, 498
mucin, 519
multivitamins
for specific populations, 480
supplementation, 479-80
mupirocin
to treat impetigo, 229
to treat skin infection, 249
musculoskeletal pain
frequency in Canada, 3t
sports injuries, 614-15
treatment, 4t, 543
types, 541, 614
muscle relaxants
to treat dysmenorrhea, 667
to treat premature ejaculation, 420
mushrooms, 358
musk ambrette, 629t
mustard oil, 557
myelitis, 234
myocardial infarction, 604t
myocarditis, 234
myopia, 188f
myringitis, bullous, 154, 155t
myrrh, 515t

n-hexylester nicotinic acid, 559
n-octyl bicycloheptene dicarboximide, 243
nabumetone, 629t
naftifine, 264, 272
naja, 371
nalidixic acid, 629t
naloxone, 313
naphazoline
as decongestant, 96, 97t
to treat hemorrhoids, 328t, 331, 332-33
to treat conjunctivitis, 203t, 204-05
use in hypertension, 51
naproxen
causing folliculitis, 60t
causing ototoxicity, 152t
photosensitivity reactions, 629t
narcolepsy, 587-88, 593
narcotics
causing incontinence, 384t
use in athletes, 619, 620
use in elderly persons, 41t
nasal decongestants
breast-feeding, 50t
use in hypertension, 51
National Drug Scheduling Advisory Committee, 5, 9
natrum muriaticum
natrum phosphoricum, 368
natrum sulfuricum, 368
naturopathy *see* homeopathic medicine
nausea and vomiting
advice for the patient, 307
defined, 306
disease-induced, 308
drug-induced, 308
infectious, 308
motion sickness, 307
patient assessment, 308
pharmaceutical agents, 313-15
physiology, 306-07

pregnancy, 48t, 307-09
treatment, 308-09
NDMAC *see* Nonprescription Drug Manufacturers Association of Canada
nedocromil, 82
neem, 349t
nefazodone, 629t
neomycin
causing dermatitis, 133t
causing ototoxicity, 152t
neonatal acne, 59, 63t
neonatal scabies, 109
nephropathy, 357-58
nettle, 350t, 355, 356
neuralgia, 543
neuroleptics, 420
niacin
food sources, 440t
function, 440t
recommended nutrient intake, 426t, 440t
signs of deficiency, 440t
signs of toxicity, 440t
nickel, 129t, 133t, 153, 154
nicotinamide *see* niacin
nicotine
addiction, 600-01, 604
affecting sleep, 587, 588t, 589t
pharmacological effects, 598
nicotine replacement therapy, 604, 608, 609f, 609-10
nicotine resin complex, 609-10
nicotinic acid *see* niacin
nifedipine
causing gingival hyperplasia, 497
causing incontinence, 384t
weight gain/loss, 453t
with herbal products, 358
nightshade, 354, 356
nit removal, 103
nitrates, 282
nitrofurantoin
discoloring contact lenses, 193
drug interactions, 311t
nitrogen mustard, 152t
nitrous oxide poisoning, 239
nits *see* pediculosis
nodular scabies, 109
nodule (acne), 59
noncompliance *see* compliance
noninflammatory acne, 58
nonionic surfactants
in conditioners, 582
in shampoos, 580
to cleanse wounds, 253
nonoxynol-9, 416, 680
Nonprescription Drug Manufacturers Association of Canada, 2
nonprescription drugs
breast-feeding, 46-47, 47t, 50t
children, 44-45
defined, 1
drug interactions, 2-3
economic issues, 3, 8
industry issues, 8-9
infants, 44-45
market, 1, 10
older consumers, 39-43
patient education, 7, 8t, 10
pregnancy, 46, 47t
professional issues, 8
recommended reading, 11
regulating, 1, 5-6, 10
safety, 2
terminology, 2
use in individuals with chronic disease, 51-55
nonsteroidal anti-inflammatory drugs (NSAIDs)
causing diarrhea, 298
causing dyspepsia, 276t
causing gastric ulcers, 276
causing ototoxicity, 152t
drug interactions, 41t, 554t
photosensitivity reactions, 629t
to treat arthritis, 538-40
to treat bursitis, 540
to treat dental pain, 541
to treat dysmenorrhea and PMS, 665, 669, 690
to treat headache, 535, 536
to treat musculoskeletal pain, 543, 614-15
to treat periodontal disease, 498
use in elderly persons, 41t
use in hypertension, 51-52
nonverbal communication, 28-30
norfloxacin
causing folliculitis, 60t
photosensitivity reactions, 629t
nortriptyline, 453t
Norwegian scabies, 109
noscapine, 96
nosode, 368
NSAIDs *see* nonsteroidal anti-inflammatory drugs (NSAIDs)
nursing women, *see also* breast-feeding
antihistamines, 94-95
codeine, 557
contraception, 678
decongestants, 98
drug use, 46-47, 47t, 50t
enterobiasis, 115, 117
herbal medicines, 336
homeopathic remedies, 370
infantile colic, 289
nicotine products, 610
nutrition, 458
ophthalmic solutions, 200, 204t
pediculicides, 104, 107, 117
resource list, 47
scabicides, 110-11, 117
scopolamine, 653
sleep aids, 595
nutmeg
as insect repellent, 255
as hallucinogenic herb, 358
nutrition, *see also* diet
and weight control, 463-70
assessment, 432-33, 450t-53t, 453-54
athletes, 474-78, 486, 620
basic nutrients, 430-32, 435t-49t
deficiency risk factors, 452t
deficiency symptoms, 450t-52t
elderly persons, 471, 474
for specific diseases, 472t-73t
general recommendations, 430t
infants, 455-62, 483-84
pregnancy, 473t
recommended nutrient intakes, 425-30
recommended reading, 487
nystatin
ineffective for jock itch, 413t
to treat skin infection, 233

oat flour, for oily skin, 568
oatmeal *see* colloidal oatmeal
obesity
associated with seborrhea, 134, 463t

body mass index, 452t
patient assessment, 469-70
symptoms, 463, 464t
treatment, 463-67
occult blood test kits, 401-03, 405
occupation
and acne, 60, 63t
and hand dermatitis, 128
occupational therapists, 377
octocrylene, 633t
octoxynol, 680
octyl bicycloheptene dicarboximide, 243
octyl dimethyl PABA, 633t, 638
octyl methoxycinnamate, 633t, 638
octyl salicylate, 633t, 638
ofloxacin, 629t
oils
comedogenicity, 568t
dietary, 431
volatile, 339, 521-22, 526
ointments
defined, 144, 564
eye, 184, 202, 206t, 206
to treat dermatitis and dry skin, 126, 129, 137, 143, 144
to treat hemorrhoids, 333
older consumers
compliance, 43
counselling, 33-34
pharmacodynamics, 42
pharmacokinetics, 40-42
physiological changes, 40, 42t
population size, 39
special concerns, 39
oligotherapy, 368
olive oil, 154
olsalazine, 629t
omeprazole
association with traveller's diarrhea, 643
photosensitivity reactions, 629t
to treat GER, 284
Ontario Homeopathic Association, 368
ophthalmic anti-infectives, 200-01
ophthalmic decongestants
pharmacokinetics, 203t
potential problems, 204t
precautions, 51, 204t
to treat conjunctivitis, 175, 203-05
ophthalmic solutions
advice for the patient, 185
comparison to ointments, 206t
contact lenses, 207, 210-21
formulations, 206
instillation techniques, 182-83
pharmaceutical agents, 199-206
opiates
causing constipation, 292t
GER, association with, 282, 283t
ostomy patients, 396t
oral contraceptives
affecting contact lens wear, 192
and STDs, 687
and smoking, 599, 604t
causing acne, 60t, 71
effectiveness, 416, 679t
to treat PMS, 670
weight gain/loss, 453t
oral hygiene
pharmaceutical agents, 515-28
recommended reading, 529
to prevent dental caries, 494
to prevent periodontal disease, 497-98
oral rehydration therapy
elderly persons, 299-300
infants and children, 299
solutions, 322-23, 645
oregano, 339-40
Oregon grape, 345t
organomercurials, 205, 212
orthopedic products, 376t
osteoarthritis, 539
osteoporosis, 473t
ostomy
advice for the patient, 388, 392, 393
children, 388
defined, 388
food issues, 393, 394
medication concerns, 396t
problems, 393-96, 395t
products, 391-93
recommended reading, 409
resources, 408
skin care, 392
support groups, 388
types, 388-90
ostomy belts, 393
ostomy products
characteristics, 392-93
irrigation, 391-92
patient assessment, 394
problems, 393-95
OTC (over-the-counter) products *see* nonprescription drugs
otitis externa
differential diagnosis, 155t
etiology, 155
symptoms, 156
treatment, 156-57
otitis media
and environmental tobacco smoke, 598
defined, 154
differential diagnosis, 155t
in association with rhinitis, 81
over-the-counter products *see* nonprescription drugs
overflow incontinence, 383-85
ovulation, 398
ovulation prediction kits
consumer counselling, 400
factors in selecting, 398
mechanism, 400-01
oxidizing agents, 214-15
oxybenzone, 633t, 638
oxygen, 537
oxymetazoline
as decongestant, 96, 97t
to treat conjunctivitis, 203t, 204-05
use in hypertension, 51
oxyquinoline
FDA classification, 263t
ineffective for jock itch, 413t
to treat hemorrhoids, 328t, 333
oxyquinoline sulfate, 263t

PABA
as sunscreen, 633t, 638, 640
causing dermatitis, 133t
cross-sensitivity, 635-36, 636t
to treat cankers and cold sores, 515t
padimate A *see* amyl dimethyl PABA
padimate O *see* octyl dimethyl PABA
pain
acute vs chronic, 531

advice for the patient, 542
caused by inflammation, 534
defined, 531
gate control theory, 533f, 533-34
muscular, 613
pathways, 532f
patient assessment, 543
psychology of, 534
recommended reading, 565
transmission and perception, 531-34
visceral, 540
pain paradox, 562
pain threshold, 534
paints, 239
pamabrom, 667, 669, 690
pancreatin, 211
pancreatitis, 276t
pansy, 356
pantothenic acid
food sources, 441t
function, 441t
recommended nutrient intake, 441t
signs of deficiency, 441t
signs of toxicity, 441t
papain
to clean contact lenses, 211
to treat insect bites, 245
papule (acne), 59
para-aminobenzoic acid *see* PABA
parabens, *see also* methylparaben; propylparaben
as preservatives, 205
causing dermatitis, 133t
ineffective for jock itch, 413t
paradichlorobenzene, 160
Paraguay tea, 349t
paralinguistics, 29
paraphenylenediamine
causing dermatitis, 133t
cross-sensitivity, 636t
pareira brava root, 356
Parkinson's disease
and constipation, 292
and seborrheic dermatitis, 134
paroxetine, 629t
parsley, 338, 350t, 355, 356
parsol 1789 *see* butyl methoxydibenzoylmethane
passion flower, 350t, 356, 358
patches
nicotine, 608
scopolamine, 314-15
to protect eye, 181
to treat corns and calluses, 267
patent medicines, 2
patient assessment, 15t, 16-18, 20-23, 432-33, 453-54
patient comfort aids, 376t
patient counselling *see* consumer counselling
Pau d'Arco, 350t
peak flow meters, 402-03
pectin
as antidiarrheal, 312
breast-feeding, 50t
pediatric scabies, 109
pediculosis
advice for the patient, 104, 106
differential diagnosis, 102
patient assessment, 107
pharmaceutical agents, 117, 118
recommended reading, 120
symptoms, 102-03
treatment, 103-06
types, 101-02
peeling agents *see* exfoliants
PEG-electrolyte lavage, 319
pellitory, 356
pelvic pouch procedure, 391f
penicillamine
causing halitosis, 508
drug interactions, 311t
to treat rheumatoid arthritis, 539
penicillin, 297
pennyroyal, 350t, 355
pentazocine, 606t
pentosan polysulfate sodium, 629t
pentostatin, 629t
peppermint oil, 255
peptic ulcer
and smoking, 277, 604t
associated with dyspepsia, 276, 278f
peptide hormones, 621
perichondritis, 153t, 154
periodontal diseases
defined, 496
etiology, 496, 598
prevention, 498
symptoms, 496-97
treatment, 497-98
peripheral vascular disease
and corns and calluses, 266
and smoking, 604t
periwinkle, 358
permethrin
to treat pediculosis, 103-06, 118
to treat scabies, 110, 111, 118
perphenazine, 453t
personal hygiene products
general, 567
hair care, 574-82
perspiration and body odor, 571-73
pharmaceutical agents, 583
recommended reading, 584
skin care, 568-70
perspiration
anatomy and physiology, 571
contributing to athlete's foot, 263
pharmaceutical agents, 583
prevention, 571-73
pesticide poisoning, 240
petrolatum
as physical sunscreen, 639
in ophthalmic ointments, 202
to treat atopic dermatitis, 125, 145
to treat cradle cap, 135
to treat diaper dermatitis, 130
to treat hemorrhoids, 328t, 332
petroleum oil, 60
petroleum poisoning, 240
pharmacokinetics
children, 44
infants, 44
older individuals, 40-41, 41t
pharyngitis, 87-88
pheasant's eye, 356
phenathrene, 629t
phenazone *see* antipyrine
phenazopyridine, 193
phenelzine
drug interactions, 357
weight gain/loss, 453t
phenindamine, 84t
pheniramine maleate, 200

phenmetrazine, 453t
phenobarbital, 60t
phenol
as antipruritic, 141
FDA classification, 263t
in mouthwashes, 521
ineffective for jock itch, 413t
to treat cankers and cold sores, 515
to treat sore throat, 98
phenolate sodium
FDA classification, 263t
ineffective for jock itch, 413t
phenolphthalein
as stimulant laxative, 294, 317t, 321
discoloring contact lenses, 193
phenothiazines
and herbal products, 358
causing constipation, 292t
classification, 84t
contributing to heat-related illness, 617
drug interactions, 52, 115, 117
effects of smoking cessation, 606t
overdose, 240
photosensitivity reactions, 629t
phenoxymethylpenicillin, 357
phenteramine, 453t
phenyl salicylate
FDA classification, 263t
ineffective for jock itch, 413t
phenylamines
as decongestants, 96
use in hypertension, 51
2-phenylbenzimidazole-5-sulfonic acid, 633t
phenylbutazone
effects of smoking cessation, 606t
photosensitivity reactions, 629t
phenylephrine
as decongestant, 96, 97t
as ophthalmic decongestant, 203t, 204
banned in sports, 621
discoloring contact lenses, 192
use in hypertension, 51
phenylmercuric acetate, 205
phenylmercuric nitrate, 205, 212
phenylpropanolamine
abuse by athletes, 620, 621
and incontinence, 384t, 385
as decongestant, 82, 96-98, 97t
use in hypertension, 51
weight gain/loss, 453t, 465-66, 485t
phenytoin
affecting sleep, 588t
causing constipation, 292t
causing gingival hyperplasia, 497
phosphates
as osmotic laxative, 317t, 319
in ophthalmic solutions, 205
phosphorated carbohydrate solution, 315
phosphorus
food sources, 447t
function, 447t
in homeopathic remedies, 371
recommended nutrient intake, 427t, 447t
signs of deficiency, 447t
photoaging, 628
photoallergy, 628
photodermatoses, 628
photodynamic inactivation, 503t
photosensitivity, 627-28, 629t
phototoxicity, 628
phthiriasis *see* pubic lice
pigmenting agents, 640
piles *see* hemorrhoids
pimozide
photosensitivity reactions, 629t
weight gain/loss, 453t
pine oil, 255
pinworms *see* enterobiasis
piperadines, 84t
piperazine
causing folliculitis, 60t
drug interactions, 115, 117-18
to treat enterobiasis, 114, 115, 115t, 117-18
piperonyl butoxide
to treat pediculosis, 103-05, 118
to treat scabies, 109, 111, 118
pipsessewa, 356
piroxicam, 629t
pitressin, 283t
pityriasis versicolor, 230, 232
pizotyline, 536
plantago, 358
plantain, 356
plantar warts
advice for the patient, 268
mosaic, 268, 269
symptoms, 268
treatment, 268-69, 272-73
plaque
causing periodontal disease, 496
disclosing agents, 523
formation, 491
prevention, 521-23
removing, 494, 497, 523-26
plasters, 267, 273
plucking (hair removal), 659
PMMA lenses *see* hard contact lenses
PMS *see* premenstrual syndrome
pneumonia, 234
podophyllum
to treat plantar warts, 269
use in pregnancy, 354, 355
poison hemlock, 354
poison ivy
causing dermatitis, 124t, 128, 133t
treatment, 239
poison oak
causing dermatitis, 133t
treatment, 239
poison sumac
causing dermatitis, 133t
treatment, 239
poisoning, emergency guidelines, 239
poisons
absorbed (dermal), 124t, 128, 133t, 239
ingested, 239-40, 338-39
inhaled, 239
plants, 354
pokeroot, 338-39, 350t
pollens
causing allergic rhinitis, 81, 82
causing atopic dermatitis, 124, 124t
poloxamer (poloxamer 188), 253
poloxamer (poloxamer 407), 201t, 210t, 218
polyaminopropylbiguanide, 214
polycarbophil
to manage constipation, 317t, 318
to manage diarrhea, 301, 645
polychlorobiphenyls, 60
polyethylene glycol, 201t

polymyxin B
- in ophthalmic products, 200-01
- to treat cankers and cold sores, **515t**
- to treat conjunctivitis, 173
- to treat ear disorders, 160
- to treat eyelid disorders, 168, 169
- to treat impetigo, 229
- to treat skin infection, 249

polyquaternium-1, 214
polysorbate 80, 201**t**, 218
polyvinyl alcohol
- in artificial tears, 201, 201**t**
- in contact lens solutions, 218, 219**t**
- incompatibility, 200, 220

polyvinylmethyl ether maleic acid, 517
polyvinylpyrrolidone *see* povidone
pomade acne, 59, 63**t**
poppy, 356, 358
porfimer, 629**t**
postherpetic neuralgia, 543
potassium
- associated with GER, 282
- drug-induced dyspepsia, 276**t**, 277
- food sources, 448**t**
- function, 448**t**
- signs of deficiency, 448**t**

potassium chlorate, 515**t**
potassium nitrate, 517
potassium sorbate *see* sorbic acid
pouches (ostomy), 392-93
povidone
- in artificial tears, 201**t**
- in contact lens solutions, 219**t**

povidone-iodine
- as antiseptic, 251
- FDA classification, 263**t**
- ineffective for cold sores, 503**t**
- to treat dandruff and seborrhea, 135
- to treat jock itch, 422

powders
- to prevent candidiasis, 233
- to treat diaper dermatitis, 130

pramoxine
- as antipruritic, 141
- to treat hemorrhoids, 328**t**, 331

pravastatin, 629**t**
prazosin, 384**t**
precipitated sulfur, 134
prednisone
- to treat cluster headache, 537
- to treat rheumatoid arthritis, 539

pregnancy
- acne, 71
- alcohol use, 434
- and smoking, 598, 604**t**, 610
- antihistamines, 94-95
- ASA, 553-54
- associated with GER, 283**t**
- associated with hemorrhoids, 326, 329
- caffeine, 590-91
- chickenpox, 234
- codeine, 557
- common medical problems and treatment, **48t-49t**
- constipation, 292, 294, 321
- decongestants, 98
- diarrhea, 300, 644, 645
- diphenhydramine, 595
- drug therapy, 46, 47**t**
- enterobiasis, 114-15, 117-18, 119
- fever, 547
- fluoride, 519
- herbal medicines, 336**t**, 338, 344**t**-52**t**, 354-55
- homeopathic remedies, 370
- ipecac, 240
- minerals (RNI), 427**t**
- nausea and vomiting, 48**t**, 307-09
- nutritional requirements, 473**t**
- ophthalmic preparations, 200
- pediculicides, 104, 107, 117
- scabicides, 110-11, 117
- scopolamine, 653
- sleep aids, 595
- travellers' diarrhea, 644, 645
- vaginal infections, 672**t**, 674**f**, 675
- vitamins (RNI), 426**t**

pregnancy tests
- general, 398
- consumer counselling, 399
- procedure, 398-400
- patient assessment, 405

premature ejaculation, 419-20
premenstrual syndrome
- advice for the woman, 669
- causes, 667
- patient assessment, 670
- symptoms, 667**t**, 667-68
- treatment, 668**f**, 668-70

preservatives (contact lens), 220
prilocaine, 248
primrose oil *see* evening primrose oil
prince's pine, 356
probenecid
- drug interactions, 554**t**, 644
- use in gout, 540

procaine, 636**t**
procarbazine, 629**t**
prochlorperazine
- contributing to heat-related illness, 617
- weight gain/loss, 453**t**

progesterone
- GER, association with, 282, 283**t**
- to treat PMS, 670

promethazine
- characteristics and doses, 84**t**
- drug interactions, 649
- pregnancy, 48**t**
- to treat motion sickness, 648-49, 652**t**, 652-53
- to treat nausea, 314, 314**t**
- to treat pruritus, 129
- use in children, 45**t**, 653
- weight gain/loss, 453**t**

propantheline
- as anticholinergic agent, 312
- causing incontinence, 384**t**
- contributing to heat-related illness, 617

proparacaine
- drug interactions, 199
- ophthalmic use, 199

propionic acid
- FDA classification, 263**t**
- ineffective for jock itch, 413**t**

propolis, 515, 515**t**
propoxyphene, 606**t**
propranolol
- and herbal products, 358
- causing incontinence, 384**t**
- effects of smoking cessation, 606**t**

proprietary medicines, 2
propylene glycol
- in antiperspirants, 573

- to treat ear disorders, 160
- to treat rhinitis, 82

propylparaben, *see also* parabens
- FDA classification, 263**t**
- in ophthalmic solutions, 205
- ineffective for jock itch, 413**t**

prostatic hypertrophy, 53, 358
protectants
- ostomy, 392
- to treat hemorrhoids, 327-28, 328**t**, 332

protein
- athletes, 477-78, 486
- daily requirements, 426**t**-27**t**, 471
- dietary nutrient, 431
- energy equivalency, 430
- in conditioners, 582

protriptyline, 453**t**
proxemics, 29-30
pruritus ani, 330
pseudoephedrine
- abuse by athletes, 620, 621
- and incontinence, 384**t**, 385
- as decongestant, 82, 93, 94, 96-98, 97**t**
- breast-feeding, 50**t**
- use in hypertension, 51

psoralens
- as photoprotectants, 640
- causing acne, 60**t**

psoriasis, 102, 412**t**
psorinum, 371
psyllium
- drug interactions, 358
- as bulk-forming laxative, 317**t**, 318, 321

pubic lice
- advice for the patient, 106
- described, 102
- symptoms, 102
- treatment, 105-06

pulsatilla, 370**t**
puncture wounds, 224
pustule (acne), 59
pyoderma, 102
pyrantel pamoate
- drug interactions, 115, 118
- to treat enterobiasis, 114, 115**t**, 118

pyrethrins, *see also* permethrin
- to treat pediculosis, 103-05, 118
- to treat scabies, 118

pyridoxine *see* vitamin B_6
pyrilamine maleate
- characteristics and doses, 83**t**
- to treat conjunctivitis, 200
- to treat dysmenorrhea and PMS, 667, 669, 691

pyrimethanine, 60**t**
pyrophosphates, 517
pyrvinium pamoate
- photosensitivity reactions, 629**t**
- to treat enterobiasis, 114, 115, 115**t**, 119

quack grass, 355, 356
quaternary ammonium compounds
- to prevent plaque, 522
- to treat dandruff and seborrhea, 135
- to treat sore throat, 98

Quaternium 16 *see* alkyltriethanolammonium chloride
questioning techniques, 16-17
quinethazone, 629**t**
quinidine, 60**t**
quinidine-related agents, 588**t**
quinine
- causing acne, 60**t**
- causing ototoxicity, 152**t**
- photosensitivity reactions, 629**t**
- to treat cankers and cold sores, 515**t**
- to treat malaria, 336

quinolones, 41**t**, 311**t**, 312

race factors
- and lactose intolerance, 430
- and lice, 102
- and pain threshold, 534
- and scabies, 108

radiotherapy
- risk of athlete's foot, 261
- risk of oral problems, 507

ragwort, 354, 355, 356
ranitidine
- alcohol interaction, 316
- associated with travellers' diarrhea, 643
- to treat anaphylaxis, 245
- to treat GER, 284, 316

rash *see* dermatitis; dry skin; skin infections
rauwolfia, 357, 358
rebound hyperemia, 203
recommended nutrient intake
- basic principles, 425-26
- minerals, 427**t**
- vitamins, 426**t**

recurrent aphthous ulcers *see* cankers
recurrent herpes labialis *see* cold sores
red clover, 350**t**
red eye, *see also* conjunctivitis; hemorrhage, subconjunctival, 165**t**
red raspberry leaf, 355
red veterinary petrolatum, 639
regulations
- herbal medicines, 353
- nonprescription drugs, 5-6, 10

regurgitation (infant feeding), 460
rehydration therapy
- elderly persons, 299-300
- infants and children, 299
- solutions, 322-23

reserpine
- causing constipation, 292**t**
- causing incontinence, 384**t**
- drug interactions, 204**t**

resorcinol
- FDA classification, 263**t**
- ineffective for jock itch, 413**t**
- to treat acne, 73
- to treat dandruff and seborrhea, 146

respiratory aids, 376**t**, 406
respiratory system, 86**f**
rest (for injury), 541, 613
retinoic acid, 73
- photosensitivity reactions, 629**t**

rewetting agents, 218
Reye's syndrome
- ASA, 45, 549
- bismuth subsalicylate, 645
- secondary to chickenpox, 234

rheumatoid arthritis
- symptoms, 538
- treatment, 538-39

rhinitis
- causing halitosis, 508
- defined, 79
- differential diagnosis, 80**t**
- etiology, 79, 81
- patient assessment, 90

pharmaceutical agents, 93-98
pregnancy, 48**t**
recommended reading, 100
symptoms, 81-82
treatment, 82, 85**f**
rhinitis medicamentosa, 81-82, 96
rhubarb, 320, 355
rhythm method of contraception, 416
riboflavin *see* vitamin B_2
RICE (injury treatment acronym), 541, 613-14
rifampin, 193
ringworm, 230, 231
ringworm of the groin *see* jock itch
risperidone, 453**t**
RNI *see* recommended nutrient intake
rosacea, 63**t**
rosary pea, 354, 355
rose bengal
discoloring contact lenses, 192
incompatibilities, 212
rubber, 129**t**, 133**t**
rubber band ligation, 328
rubbing alcohol, 156, 157
rue, 355
rupture wort, 356

sabal, 350**t**
saccharin
cross-sensitivity, 636**t**
sweetener, 484
saccharose, 365, 366**t**
safety issues
herbal medicines, 353-59
nonprescription drugs, 2-3, 5
safety products *see* aids for daily living
saffron crocus, 355
salbutamol, 384**t**
salicylanilides, 67
salicylate salts, 554
salicylates
drug interactions, 311**t**
ostomy patients, 396**t**
salicylic acid
affecting contact lens wear, 193
FDA classification, 263**t**
in ophthalmic solutions, 200
ineffective for jock itch, 413**t**
to treat acne, 67, 68**f**, 73
to treat athlete's foot, 264
to treat corns, calluses and warts, 266-67, 269, 272-73
to treat dandruff and seborrhea, 134, 146
to treat fungal skin infection, 232
saline
in first aid kits, 246
to cleanse wounds, 250, 253
to rinse contact lenses, 213, 216
to treat cankers and cold sores, 502, 504
saliva substitutes, to treat dry mouth, 509, 519
salt (dietary)
athletes, 618
recommended daily intake, 430**t**
substitutes, 396, 484-86
sambucus, 371
sandalwood oil, 629**t**
sanguinaria, 517, 521, 522
saponins, 581
sarcode, 368
sarsaparilla, 350**t**
sassafras, 350**t**
savory (summer), 340
saw palmetto, 335, 350**t**, 355, 356
scab formation, 224-25
scabies
advice for the patient, 111
etiology, 108
patient assessment, 112
pharmaceutical agents, 117, 118, 119
recommended reading, 120
symptoms, 108-09
transmission, 108
treatment, 109-12
types, 109
scalp massage, 577
scammony, 354
scarring (acne), 59
scissors (first aid kit), 246, 616
scopolamine
contributing to heat-related illness, 617
drug interactions, 649, 653
risks with benign prostatic hypertrophy, 53
to treat nausea, 314**t**, 314-15, 648, 652**t**, 653
use in elderly persons, 41**t**
scopolia, 356
seborrheic dermatitis
advice for the patient, 135
cradle cap, 135, 577
etiology, 134
differential diagnosis, 102, 124**t**
ear, 153**t**
eye, 167
pharmaceutical agents, 144, 146,
signs and symptoms, 134
treatment, 134-35, 136**f**
secondhand smoke *see* environmental tobacco smoke
secretin, 283**t**
sedatives
affecting contact lens wear, 177**t**, 193
causing incontinence, 383, 384**t**
drug interactions, 649, 652
to treat insomnia, 592, 595
selective serotonin reuptake inhibitors, 536
selegiline
affecting sleep, 588**t**
photosensitivity reactions, 629**t**
selenium
food sources, 448**t**
function, 448**t**
signs of deficiency, 448**t**
selenium sulfide
to treat dandruff and seborrhea, 134, 144
to treat fungal skin infection, 232
to treat seborrheic blepharitis, 168
self-care
defined, 14
equipment, 376**t**
self-treatment
Canadian survey, 2, 3**t**, 4**t**
defined, 14
senega, 351**t**
senna
medicinal uses and side effects, 351**t**, 354
ostomy patients, 396**t**
to treat constipation, 294, 317, 317**t**, 320, 321
sennosides *see* senna
sexually transmitted diseases
and contraception, 416, 682, 684, 686-87
and vaginitis, 671-72
pediculosis, 102
scabies, 108, 112
shampoo trays, 377

shampoos
- factors in selection, 578
- for dry hair, 576
- for fine hair, 576
- for green hair, 576
- for oily hair, 575
- for swimmer's hair, 576
- for treated hair, 576
- ingredients, 578-80
- to treat cradle cap, 135, 577
- to treat dandruff and seborrhea, 134, 143, 144
- types, 581

shark liver oil, 328**t**, 333
shavegrass, 348**t**, 351**t**, 355, 356
shaving (women), 659
shepherd's purse, 356
shoes *see* footwear
shower seats, 377
sialogogues, 509, 518-19
side effects, *see also specific drug*
- consumer counselling, 25-26

silicean, 368
silicone contact lenses, 189
silicone creams, 128
silver nitrate
- in caustic pencils, 252
- ineffective for cankers, 515

silver sulfadiazine
- ineffective for cold sores, 503**t**

simethicone
- to treat colic, 290
- to treat IBS, 304, 323

sinusitis
- causing dental pain, 499
- causing halitosis, 508
- diagnosis, 88, 91**t**

Sjögren's syndrome, 177**t**
skeletal muscle relaxants, 384**t**
skin
- anatomy, 57-58, 121-22, 223
- dry, 568
- effects of smoking, 598
- effects of UV light, 623, 626-30, 631**t**-32**t**
- oily, 568
- sensitive, 568
- wounds to, 224-27

skin barriers (ostomy), 392, 393
skin cancer, 628-30
skin care, *see also* sunscreens
- and acne, 64, 66
- children, 568-69
- depigmenting agents, 640-41
- elderly persons, 568-69
- ostomy patients, 392, 393-94
- pigmenting agents, 640
- tanning agents, 640

skin infections
- bacterial, 228-30
- fungal, 230-33
- pathophysiology of, 223, 228
- patient assessment, 247
- viral, 233-34

skin irritation
- frequency in Canada, 3**t**
- management, 4**t**

skin sealants, 258
skullcap, 351**t**, 355, 356
sleep
- elderly persons, 589-90
- factors affecting, 586-88
- good hygiene, 590, 591, 592
- physiology, 586
- recommended reading, 596
- stages, 586**t**, 587**f**

sleep disorders
- advice for the patient, 595
- apnea, 588, 593
- cost to society, 585
- insomnia, 589-92
- narcolepsy, 593
- patient assessment, 594
- pharmaceutical agents, 595
- recommended reading, 596
- resources, 594

sleep paralysis, 593
slippery elm, 351**t**
smoker's palate, 598
smoking
- and caffeine, 590
- and contact lenses, 193
- and motion sickness, 648
- causing GER, 282, 283**t**
- causing peptic ulcer disease, 277
- drug interactions, 598-99
- epidemiology, 597
- health risks, 598, 604, 604**t**
- physical addiction, 600
- psychological addiction, 600-01

smoking cessation
- general, 597
- advice for the patient, 607
- counselling, 602, 603**f**, 604, 606
- health benefits, 599**t**, 604, 606
- management of dyspepsia, 277, 279
- management of GER, 283
- pharmaceutical agents, 609-10
- recommended reading, 611
- Seven Ss, 609**f**
- treatment, 607-08
- Why Test, 605**f**

snakeroot *see* senega
soaps
- causing dermatitis, 124**t**, 128, 129**t**
- characteristics (common brands), 569**t**
- fragrance-free, 568
- impairs skin's defences, 253
- in first aid kits, 246
- mechanism of action, 569-70
- medicated, 67, 568, 570
- photosensitivity reactions, 628
- surfactant in ophthalmic solutions, 210**t**
- to treat acne, 64
- to treat dermatitis and dry skin, 142-43
- to soften ear wax, 160
- types, 570

sodium
- affecting calcium excretion, 480
- athletes, 476, 618
- deficiency symptoms, 448**t**
- content of medications, 52
- food sources, 448**t**
- function, 448**t**

sodium bicarbonate
- banned in sports, 621
- in contact lens solutions, 220
- to treat dermatitis and dry skin, 137, 142
- to treat insect bites, 246
- pregnancy, 48**t**

sodium bisulfite, 205
sodium borate

FDA classification, 263t
in contact lens solutions, 220
in ophthalmic solutions, 200, 205
incompatibility, 220
ineffective for jock itch, 413t
to prevent plaque, 522
sodium caprylate
FDA classification, 263t
ineffective for jock itch, 413t
sodium carbonate, 220
sodium chloride, 205
sodium citrate, 517
sodium cocoyl isethionate, 580t
sodium cyclamate
cross-sensitivity, 636t
sweetener, 484
sodium fluoride
effectiveness of methods of administration, 495f
in dentifrices, 516, 517t
sodium hypochlorite
in contact lens solutions, 214
to cleanse wounds, 251
sodium laureth sulfate, 580t
sodium lauryl ether sulfate, 104-05
sodium lauryl sulfate
in contact lens solutions, 210t
in shampoos, 580t
to prevent plaque, 522
sodium monofluorophosphate, 516, 517t
sodium perborate
in contact lens solutions, 214
to treat periodontal disease, 497
sodium percarbonate, 515t
sodium peroxide, 214
sodium phosphate, 220
sodium propionate
FDA classification, 263t
ineffective for jock itch, 413t
sodium salicylate
to prevent plaque, 522
to treat pain and fever, 554
sodium sulfide, 270
soft (hydrogel) contact lenses
care, 194-95, 207, 209f
risk of complications, 191t
uses, 189
solvents
causing dermatitis, 128
dermal poisoning, 239
inhalation poisoning, 239
sorbic acid
discoloring contact lenses, 214
in contact lens solutions, 213-14
sorbitol
as alternative sweetener, 484
as emollient, 145
in dry mouth products, 519
lower risk of caries, 492
sore throat
common cold symptom, 87
examination kit, 403, 405
treatment, 89, 98
sotalol, 629t
soy protein infant formulas, 457, 483
spermaceti, 568
spermicides
advice for the man, 418
advice for the woman, 681
allergic reactions, 418
and STDs, 687
defined, 680
effectiveness, 416
formulations, 681-82
on condoms, 416
SPF *see* sun protection factor
sphygmomanometer, 397-98
spironolactone, 358
spitting (infant feeding), 460
sports drinks, 486
sports injuries
advice for the patient, 617
causes, 613
first aid kits, 615, 616t
heat-related, 617-18
prevention, 613
products, 376t
recommended reading, 622
treatment, 541, 543, 613-15
types, 541
sprains, 541, 613, 614
squalene, 145
squash, 346t
squaw vine, 355, 356
squill (white), 356
stannous fluoride
dosages, 517t
effectiveness of methods of administration, 495f
in dentifrices, 516
to prevent plaque, 521
star anise, 344t
starch, 431, 491
starch-blocker, 358
sterculia, 318
steroids
causing acne, 59
to treat cluster headache, 537
Stevens-Johnson syndrome, 177t
stimulants
affecting sleep, 588t
banned in sports, 620
photosensitivity reactions, 629t
to treat sleep disorders, 595
stings (insects)
allergic reactions to, 244-45
ants, 241
bees, 241
hornets and wasps, 241
patient assessment, 247
preventing, 242-43
treatment, 243-46
St. John's Wort, 350t, 356
stone root, 356
stool softeners, ostomy patients, 396
storage (drugs), 26, 651
strains, 541, 613, 614
strep throat, 91t
streptomycin
causing folliculitis, 60t
causing ototoxicity, 152t
stress
affecting sleep, 588, 589t
aggravating PMS, 669
associated with dyspepsia, 277
causing acne, 61
causing dermatitis, 123, 124t
vitamins, 480
stress fractures, 615
stress incontinence, 383, 385
stroke, 292
strontium chloride, 517

strophanthin, 356
strychnine, 240
stye, 168-69
styptic pencils, 252
subconjunctival hemorrhage, 176
subcutaneous infusion pumps, 407
subtilisin, 211
sucralfate, 284
sucralose, 484
sucrose, 430, 491-92
sulfa drugs, 396t
sulfamethoxazole, 636t
sulfasalazine
- discoloring contact lenses, 193
- to treat arthritis, 539

sulfinpyrazone, 554t
sulfisoxazole, 636t
sulfonamides
- causing diarrhea, 297
- cross-sensitivity, 133t, 248, 635, 636t
- drug interactions, 199
- photosensitivity reactions, 629t

sulfonylureas
- drug interactions, 554t
- photosensitivity reactions, 629t

sulfur
- FDA classification, 263t
- food sources, 448t
- function, 448t
- in homeopathic remedies, 371
- ineffective for jock itch, 413t
- to treat acne, 67, 68f, 73
- to treat dandruff and seborrhea, 134, 146
- to treat fungal skin infection, 232
- to treat scabies, 111-12, 119

sulindac, 629t
sulisobenzone, 633t, 638
sumatriptan, 536, 537
sun protection factor (SPF)
- and skin type, 627t
- defined, 633-34

sun-lamps, 627
sunburn
- advice for the patient, 626
- children, 626
- symptoms, 626
- to eye, 181
- treatment, 626
- UV index, 624t

sunscreens
- adverse effects, 639-40
- causing acne, 60
- chemical, 638-39
- children, 636
- efficacy, 634, 635t
- in first aid kits, 246, 650
- patient assessment, 637
- photoprotectants, 640
- physical, 639
- recognized by Health Canada, 633t
- recommended reading, 642
- selection, 634-36
- sun protection factor, 627t, 633-34
- to prevent cold sores, 502

suppositories
- spermicidal (vaginal), 681-82
- to treat constipation, 317t, 322
- to treat hemorrhoids, 333

surfactants
- classification, 210t
- in shampoos, 579, 580-81, 582
- irritation potential, 580t
- to clean contact lenses, 207, 210-11
- to cleanse wounds, 253

sutilains, 226
swabs, 616
sweating *see* perspiration
sweet vernal grass, 357
sweet-scented bedstraw, 357
sweeteners, alternative, 484, 492
swimmer's ear *see* otitis externa
swimmer's hair, 576
sympatholytics, 384t
sympathomimetics
- abuse by athletes, 620
- as ophthalmic decongestants, 203, 203t
- precautions and contraindications, 51, 53, 358
- to treat rhinitis, 82

syncope, 617

taheebo *see* Pau d'Arco
talc, 639
tamarack, 356
tampons, 661, 663
tang, 358
tannic acid
- FDA classification, 263t
- ineffective for jock itch, 413t
- to control perspiration, 572
- to treat cankers and cold sores, 515, 515t
- to treat ingrown toenails, 270

tanning, 626-27
tanning agents, 640
tanning lamps, 627
tansy, 351t
tar *see* coal tar
taxol, 335
TEA *see* triethanolamine salicylate
tea tree, 351t
tear film, 164-65, 165t
teeth *see* tooth
teething, 289t, 500, 547
temazepam, 384t
temperature
- affecting sleep, 587
- and contraception, 679-80
- causing seborrheic dermatitis, 124t
- circadian rhythms, 545, 587
- fever, 545
- frostbite, 238
- heat-related disorders, 617-18
- measuring body temperature, 545-46
- normal body temperature, 545

tendonitis, 613, 615
tennis elbow, 613, 615
tenosynovitis, 613, 615
tenoxicam, 629t
terazosin, 384t, 629t
terconazole, 629t
terephthalidene dicamphor sulfonic acid, 633t, 639
terfenadine
- adverse effects, 94
- characteristics and doses, 84t
- drug interactions, 94
- to treat dermatitis, 126
- to treat motion sickness, 649
- to treat rhinitis, 93-94
- use in cardiovascular disease, 52

tetanus, 228, 236
tetracaine

drug interactions, 199, 636t
ophthalmic use, 199
tetracycline
causing diarrhea, 297
causing folliculitis, 60t
discoloring contact lenses, 193
discoloring teeth, 490
drug interactions, 311t, 312
photosensitivity reactions, 629t
to treat canker sores, 505, 514
with herbal products, 358
tetraglycine hydroperiodide, 646t
tetrahydrozoline
as ophthalmic decongestants, 203t, 204-05
discoloring contact lenses, 192
use in hypertension, 51
theophylline
affecting sleep, 588t
drug-induced dyspepsia, 276t, 277
effects of smoking, 598, 606t
GER, association with, 282, 283t
thermal disinfection (contact lenses), 216-17, 217t
thermometers
basal body temperature, 680
in first aid kits, 616, 650
types, 545-46
thiamine *see* vitamin B_1
thiazides, 629t, 636t
thimerosal
causing dermatitis, 133t
in contact lens solutions, 212
in ophthalmic solutions, 202, 205
thiocarbamide, 508
thioglycollates, 659, 691
thiopropazoate, 453t
thioridazine, 453t
thiothixene
photosensitivity reactions, 629t
weight gain/loss, 453t
thorn apple, 356, 358
thrush, 506
thuya, 371
thyme, 340, 573
thymol
FDA classification, 263t
in mouthwashes, 521
ineffective for jock itch, 413t
to prevent plaque, 521-22
thyroid preparations, 311t, 588t
tick bites, 242, 244
tincture of iodine *see* iodine
tinea capitis, 230, 231-32
tinea corporis, 230, 231
tinea cruris *see* jock itch
tinea pedis *see* athlete's foot
tinea versicolor, 230, 232
tinnitus, 151, 152t, 158
tioconazole, 673t, 689-90
tissue salts, 368
titanium dioxide, 633t, 639
tobacco, 597-98
tobramycin, 152t
toenails
ingrown, 270
involvement in athlete's foot, 262
toilets
raised, 378
splash guards, 378
tissue dispensers, 378
tolbutamide, 636t
tolindate
FDA classification, 263t
ineffective for jock itch, 413t
tolnaftate
FDA classification, 263t
to treat athlete's foot, 264, 273
to treat fungal skin infection, 231
to treat jock itch, 413, 422
tonka bean, 357
tooth
anatomy and physiology, 489-90, 490f
broken, 499
dental caries, 491-95
dental erosion, 499
dental pain, 499
lost fillings, 499
misfitting dentures, 499
patient assessment, 510f, 511f, 512-13
periodontal diseases, 496-98
products, 515-18, 519-21, 523-28
tooth whiteners, 527
toothache *see* dental pain
toothbrushes
children, 524
electric, 525
selection, 523-24
toothbrushing
method, 524-25
to prevent caries, 494, 517
to prevent halitosis, 508
toothpastes, *see also* dentifrices, 515-17
toothpicks, 526
toxic shock syndrome
advice for the woman, 663
etiology, 661, 663, 683
defined, 661
patient assessment, 663
symptoms, 663
treatment, 663
tranquilizers
affecting sleep, 588t, 589t
drug interactions, 649, 652
transient incontinence, 383
trauma (eye), 181
travel health
affecting sleep, 588-89
constipation, 291
diarrhea, 643-45
ear pain, 151, 650
first aid, 650-51
motion sickness, 307, 648-49
ostomy patients, 395
pharmaceutical agents, 652-53
recommended reading, 654
resource list, 651
water purification, 646-47
travellers' diarrhea
advice for the patient, 301, 644
and foods, 301t
etiology, 300, 643-44
organisms involved, 300, 643t
prophylaxis, 300, 644-45
symptoms, 300, 644
treatment, 300-01, 645
trazodone, 629t
trenchmouth, 497
tretinoin *see* retinoic acid
triacetin
FDA classification, 263t
ineffective for jock itch, 413t

triamcinalone, 82
triamterene
drug interactions, 555
photosensitivity reactions, 629t
triazolam, 384t
triclosan
in dentifrices, 517
in deodorants, 573, 583
to prevent plaque, 522
to treat dandruff and seborrhea, 135
tricyclic antidepressants, *see also* antidepressants
affecting contact lens wear, 193
affecting sleep, 587, 588t
causing constipation, 292t
causing dry eye, 177t
contributing to heat-related illness, 617
drug interactions, 204t, 357
effects of smoking cessation, 606t
overdose, 240
photosensitivity reactions, 629t
to treat stress incontinence, 385
triethanolamine lauryl sulfate, 580t
triethanolamine polypeptide oleate, 155, 160
triethanolamine salicylate
as sunscreen, 633t
to treat musculoskeletal pain, 560-61, 614
trifluoperazine, 453t
triglycerides, 431
trihexyphenidyl
causing constipation, 292t
causing incontinence, 384t
trimeprazine, 617
trimethadione, 60t
trimipramine, 453t
tripelennamine
characteristics and doses, 83t
to treat itching, 249-50
triphenylmethane derivatives, 320-21
triprolidine
characteristics and doses, 83t
to treat rhinitis, 93
trolamine salicylate *see* triethanolamine salicylate
tuberculinum, 371
tuberculostatic drugs, 59, 60t
tubocurarine
as skeletal muscle relaxant, 336
medicinal uses and side effects, 351t
turpentine oil, 561
tweezers (first aid), 246
2-deoxy-D-glucose, 503t
tyrothricin, 515t

ulcerative colitis, 388, 391
ulcers
figures, 277f, 278f
link with dyspepsia, 275-76, 276t
vaginal/cervical, 661
ultraviolet light
cancer, 628-30
dermatitis, 124
effects, 631t-32t
environmental factors affecting, 625f
inappropriate to treat acne, 67
index, 624t, 625
intensity, 623-25
photoaging, 628
photosensitivity, 627-28, 629t
protection against, 633-40
sunburn, 626
tanning, 626-27
wavelengths, 623, 624f
undecylenic acid (and its salts)
FDA classification, 263t
to treat athlete's foot, 264, 273
to treat jock itch, 413, 422
undergarments (incontinence), 386-87
unicorn root, 344t, 355, 356
upset stomach, 3t, 4t
urea, 137, 145-46
urea hydrogen peroxide *see* carbamide peroxide
urecholine, 519
ureterostomy, 388, 390f
urge incontinence, 383
urinals (body-worn), 387
urinary alkalinizers, 554t
urinary incontinence
chronic, 383-85
drug-induced, 383, 384t
enuresis, 385-86
micturition, 382-83
predisposing factors, 383t
transient, 383
types, 382t
urinary tract infection, 383, 385
urine glucose tests, 403-04, 406
urostomy
potential problems, 393
reasons for, 388
types, 390f
urticaria, 568
UV *see* ultraviolet light
uva ursi, 351t, 355, 356

vaginal douches *see* douches
vaginal dryness, 658
vaginal infection
characteristics, 671t
physiology, 671
self-treatment, 671-72
vulvovaginal candidiasis, 672-77
vaginitis *see* vaginal infection
vaginosis *see* vaginal infection
valerian, 335, 341-42, 351t, 356
valproic acid, 554t
vancomycin, 152t
vaporizers, 88-89, 406
varicella zoster, 233-34, 249-50
vasoconstrictors
as ophthalmic decongestants, 203-05
to treat hemorrhoids, 327-28, 328t, 332-33
use in hypertension, 51
vasomotor rhinitis, 79
verapamil
causing constipation, 292t
causing incontinence, 384t
interactions with herbal products, 358
vernal keratoconjunctivitis, 174
vertigo
defined, 151
drug-induced, 152t
patient assessment, 158
vinblastine
causing ototoxicity, 152t
photosensitivity reactions, 629t
Vincent's infection, 497
vincristine, 152t
vinegar *see* acetic acid
vipera, 371
visceral pain, 540
viscosity agents, 218

vitamin A
food sources, 435t
function, 435t
recommended nutrient intake, 426t, 435t
signs of deficiency, 435t
signs of toxicity, 435t
use in elderly persons, 471
vitamin B_1
as insect repellent, 255
food sources, 439t
function, 439t
recommended nutrient intake, 426t, 439t
signs of deficiency, 439t
signs of toxicity, 439t
supplementation of breast-fed infants, 457t
vitamin B_2
food sources, 439t
function, 439t
recommended nutrient intake, 426t, 439t
signs of deficiency, 439t
signs of toxicity, 439t
vitamin B_5 *see* pantothenic acid
vitamin B_6
drug interactions, 691
food sources, 441t
function, 441t
pregnancy, 48t
recommended nutrient intake, 441t
signs of deficiency, 441t
signs of toxicity, 441t
to treat morning sickness, 315
to treat PMS, 670, 691
vitamin B_{12}
causing acne, 60t
food sources, 444t
function, 444t
ineffective for cold sores, 503t
recommended nutrient intake, 426t, 444t
signs of deficiency, 444t
signs of toxicity, 444t
supplementation of breast-fed infants, 457t
use in elderly persons, 474
vitamin C
and blood glucose testing, 54-55
and smoking, 598, 606t, 610
as antioxidant, 479
causing dental erosion, 499
food sources, 442t
function, 442t
ineffective for cold sores, 503t
recommended nutrient intake, 426t, 442t
signs of deficiency, 442t
signs of toxicity, 442t
to treat colds, 98-99
vitamin D
and sunscreens, 639
food sources, 436t
function, 436t
improves calcium balance, 480
recommended nutrient intake, 426t, 436t
signs of deficiency, 436t
signs of toxicity, 436t
supplementation of breast-fed infants, 457t
use in elderly persons, 471, 474
vitamin E
as antioxidant, 479
food sources, 437t
function, 437t
ineffective for cold sores, 503t
natural vs. synthetic, 480
recommended nutrient intake, 426t, 437t
signs of deficiency, 437t
signs of toxicity, 437t
topical use, 145
vitamin K
food sources, 438t
function, 438t
in herbal products, 357
recommended nutrient intake, 438t
signs of deficiency, 438t
signs of toxicity, 438t
supplementation of breast-fed infants, 457t
vitamins
breast-feeding, 50t
counselling tips, 433
natural vs. synthetic, 480
ostomy patients, 396
pregnancy, 49t
to treat PMS, 670
use in athletes, 475-76, 620
use in children, 460
use in elderly persons, 471, 474
use in infants, 456, 457t, 459
volatile aromatics, 98
volatile oils
medicinal uses, 339, 557
to prevent plaque, 521-22, 526
vomiting, *see also* nausea and vomiting
causing dental erosion, 499
management of poisoning, 240
vomiting centre, 306f, 306-07
vulvovaginal candidiasis
advice for the woman, 673, 676-77
patient assessment, 675
predisposing factors, 672t
prevention, 673
symptoms, 672
treatment, 672-73, 674f, 675

waist-to-hip ratio, 463
walkers, 379-81
wallflower, 355
warfarin
drug interactions, 23, 554t, 560, 665
effects of smoking, 598
vitamin K antagonism, 357
warts, 63t
warts, plantar, *see* plantar warts
washes, medicated, 67
wasps, 241-42, 244, 245
water
athletes, 476
infants, 460
in shampoos, 579
management of diarrhea, 301
management of hemorrhoids, 327, 329
management of IBS, 304
purification, 300, 646t-47t, 646
recommended intake, 430t, 431-32
to soften impacted cerumen, 154
to treat burns, 235-36
to treat canker sores, 504
to treat cold sores, 502
to treat dermatitis and dry skin, 124-25, 129, 137, 146
to treat fever, 548
to treat heat-related disorders, 617-18
to treat sunburn, 626
water hemlock, 354
water irrigating devices, 525
water plantain, 356

waxing (hair removal), 659, 660
weaning, 460
weight gain
  athletes, 477
  drugs associated with, 453t
  factors associated with, 463
  smoking cessation, 600, 607, 608
weight loss
  advice for the patient, 466
  athletes, 477
  drugs associated with, 453t
  treatment, 463-67
wetting agents, 217-18, 219t
wheelchairs
  accessories, 380t
  advice for the patient, 379
  characteristics, 380t
  common features, 379t
  parts, 378f
  selection, 378-79, 380t
whey hydrolysate infant formulas, 483
white petrolatum, 328t, 332
white squill, 356
whitehead (closed comedone), 58, 61
The Why Test (smoking assessment), 605f
wild carrot, 356
wild ginger, 355
wild lettuce, 356
wintergreen oil *see* methyl salicylate
witch hazel
  in ophthalmic solutions, 205
  to treat hemorrhoids, 328t, 331
  to treat skin irritation, 239, 253
withdrawal (contraception), 679
withdrawal (nicotine), 600
wolfsbane, 356
women's health care products
  contraception, 678-88
  pharmaceutical agents, 689-91
  recommended reading, 692
woodruff (sweet), 352t, 357
wood sorrel, 356
wormwood, 352t
wound-healing agents, 327, 328t, 333
wounds
  and smoking, 598
  burns, 235-37
  classification, 224
  counselling tips, 226-27
  dressings, 225, 254, 256-58
  healing process, 224-25
  medical referral, 236
  patient assessment, 247
  pharmaceutical agents, 248-54
  post-operative, 228
  products, 376t
  recommended reading, 259
  treatment, 225, 226-27, 541
xerostomia
  etiology, symptoms and treatment, 509
  product information, 518-19
xylene, 568t
xylitol, 484, 492
xylometazoline
  as decongestant, 96, 97t
  use in hypertension, 51

yeast, 328t, 333
yeast infections, 230, 232-33
yellow dock, 352t
Yerba mate, 349t
Yerba Santa, 352t
yohimbine, 357, 358
yucca, 352t

zinc
  food sources, 449t
  function, 449t
  ineffective for cold sores, 503t
  recommended nutrient intake, 427t, 449t
  seborrhea, association with, 134
  signs of deficiency, 449t
zinc caprylate
  FDA classification, 263t
  ineffective for jock itch, 413t
zinc chloride, 517
zinc citrate, 517
zinc oxide
  as sunscreen, 633t, 639
  to treat chickenpox, 234, 252
  to treat dermatitis, 129, 141, 239, 252
  to treat diaper rash, 130
  to treat hemorrhoids, 328t, 331
  to treat insect bites, 252
zinc peroxide, 497
zinc phenolsulfonate, 573, 583
zinc propionate
  FDA classification, 263t
  ineffective for jock itch, 413t
zinc pyrithione
  to treat dandruff and seborrhea, 134, 143
  to treat tinea versicolor, 232
zinc salicylate, 515t
zinc sulfate
  in ophthalmic solutions, 202
  to treat cankers and cold sores, 515, 515t
  to treat hemorrhoids, 328t, 331
zinc undecylenate
  to treat athlete's foot, 264, 273
  to treat jock itch, 422
zirconium salts, 572, 583
Zoom, 348t